CDC YELLOW BOOK 2024

Health Information for International Travel

CDC YELLOW BOOK 2024

Health Information for International Travel

Editor in Chief: Jeffrey Nemhauser, MD

SENIOR MEDICAL EDITOR
Regina LaRocque, MD, MPH

MEDICAL EDITORS
Francisco Alvarado-Ramy, MD
Kristina Angelo, DO, MPH&TM
Charles Ericsson, MD
Alida Gertz, MD, MPH, DTM&H
Phyllis Kozarsky, MD
Stephen Ostroff, MD
Edward Ryan, MD, DTM&H
David Shlim, MD
William Stauffer, MD, MPH
Michelle Weinberg, MD, MPH
Mary Elizabeth Wilson, MD

MANAGING EDITORS
Suraj Arshanapally, MPH
Jane Keir, MPH
Laura Leidel, RN, FNP-C, MSN, MPH

ASSISTANT MANAGING EDITOR
Samantha Crowe, MPH

TECHNICAL EDITOR
Amy Guinn, MA

CARTOGRAPHER
Marielle (Ellie) Glynn, MS, MAS

US DEPARTMENT OF HEALTH AND HUMAN SERVICES

CENTERS FOR DISEASE CONTROL AND PREVENTION

NATIONAL CENTER FOR EMERGING AND ZOONOTIC INFECTIOUS DISEASES

DIVISION OF GLOBAL MIGRATION AND QUARANTINE
ATLANTA, GEORGIA

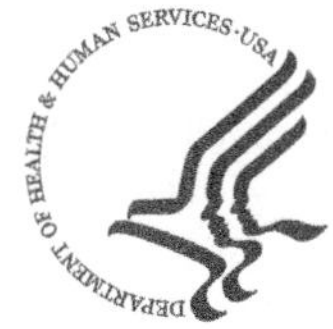

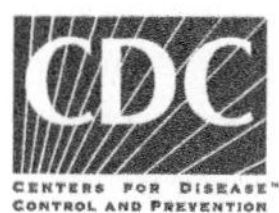

OXFORD
UNIVERSITY PRESS

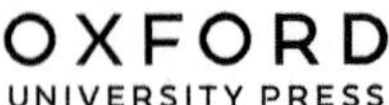

Oxford University Press is a department of the University of Oxford. It furthers the University's objective of excellence in research, scholarship, and education by publishing worldwide. Oxford is a registered trade mark of Oxford University Press in the UK and certain other countries.

Published in the United States of America by Oxford University Press
198 Madison Avenue, New York, NY 10016, United States of America.

CIP data is on file at the Library of Congress
ISBN 978–0–19–757094–4
ISSN 0095–3539 (Print)
ISSN 1939–5574 (Online)

DOI: 10.1093/oso/9780197570944.001.0001

Printed in Canada by Marquis Book Printing

Oxford University Press is proud to pay a portion of its sales from this book to the CDC Foundation. Chartered by Congress, the CDC Foundation began operations in 1995 as an independent, non-profit organization fostering support for the CDC through public-private partnerships.

Further information about the Foundation can be found at www.cdcfoundation.org.

Suggested Citation
Centers for Disease Control and Prevention. CDC Yellow Book 2024: Health Information for International Travel. New York: Oxford University Press, 2023.

Readers are invited to send comments and suggestions regarding this publication in care of Cindy Friedman, MD, Branch Chief, Centers for Disease Control and Prevention, Division of Global Migration and Quarantine, Travelers' Health Branch (proposed), 1600 Clifton Road, NE, Mail Stop H16-4, Atlanta, GA, 30333, USA.

Authorship
CDC Yellow Book authors are identified by their respective CDC Centers as having subject-matter expertise in their field. Contributing authors external to CDC are identified by the editorial staff as experts in their fields. Prior to publication, all content is reviewed by a medical editor, a technical editor, the senior medical editor, and the editor in chief before undergoing final CDC review and clearance.

Newly invited authors are not asked to rewrite chapters previously written by others. All authors (both new and continuing) are, however, expected to conduct a thorough literature search and to update their topic based on currently available science and clinical practice guidelines and recommendations. All authors have provided a signed statement declaring they have no conflict of interest with the content they have written or reviewed for this text and that all content is objective and free from bias.

Disclaimers

COVID-19: All CDC Yellow Book 2024 coronavirus disease 2019 (COVID-19)–related content was reviewed by the CDC COVID-19 Task Force and determined to be accurate as of the date of submission of this manuscript for publication. The information that appears in this print edition, however, may not represent the most current science or public health recommendations available. For the most current information on this rapidly evolving topic, please refer to the CDC website (www.cdc.gov).

Maps: Boundaries and labels shown on maps are not necessarily authoritative.

Names of drugs, biologics, and medical products: Both generic and trade names (without trademark symbols) are used throughout this text. The use of trade names and commercial sources is for identification only and does not imply endorsement by the US Department of Health and Human Services (HHS), the United States Public Health Service (USPHS), or the CDC.

Non-CDC references: References to non-CDC internet sites are provided as a service to readers and do not constitute or imply endorsement of these organizations or their programs by HHS, USPHS, or CDC. CDC is not responsible for the content of these sites. Uniform Resource Locator (URL) addresses provided in the text are current as of the date of publication.

Off-label use descriptions: Descriptions of drugs, biologics, or medical products used for an indication not in the approved labeling or packaging ("off-label" use) do not constitute official HHS approval or endorsement of those products or uses. Off-label uses described in this publication have been identified by subject-matter experts based on published evidence and clinical experience. Clinicians who use a product off-label should be well informed about the product, base its use on firm scientific rationale and sound medical evidence, and maintain records of the product's efficacy and effects.

Notice

This material is not intended to be, and should not be considered, a substitute for medical, legal, or other professional advice. Treatment of the conditions described in this text is highly dependent on individual circumstances. While this text is designed to offer accurate information with respect to the subject matter covered and to be current as of the time it was written, research and knowledge about medical, legal, and health issues are constantly evolving, and dose schedules for medications and vaccines are revised continually, with new side effects recognized and accounted for regularly. Therefore, readers of this text must always confirm the accuracy of any listed product information and clinical procedures with the most up-to-date published product information and data sheets provided by manufacturers and the most recent codes of conduct and safety regulations. Oxford University Press (the Publisher) and the authors and editors make no representations or warranties to readers, express or implied, as to the accuracy or completeness of this material, including without limitation that they make no representations or warranties as to the accuracy or efficacy of the drug dosages provided. The Publisher, the authors, and editors do not accept, and expressly disclaim, any responsibility for any liability, loss, or risk that may be claimed or incurred as a consequence of the use and/or application of any of the contents of this text.

The Publisher, the authors, and editors make all editorial decisions, including content decisions. Neither the Publisher, the authors, nor the editors are responsible for any product information added to this publication by companies purchasing copies for distribution to clinicians.

For additional copies, please contact Oxford University Press. Order online at www.oup.com/us.

cont

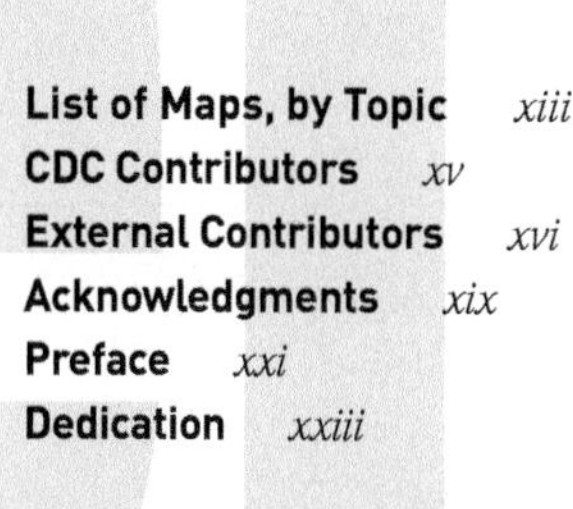

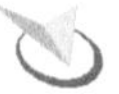

ENVIRONMENTAL HAZARDS & RISKS 181

5 TRAVEL-ASSOCIATED INFECTIONS & DISEASES 243

6 HEALTH CARE ABROAD *549*

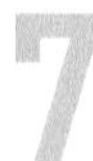

FAMILY TRAVEL *567*

8 TRAVEL BY AIR, LAND & SEA *605*

9 TRAVEL FOR WORK & OTHER REASONS *635*

10 POPULAR ITINERARIES *691*

11 POSTTRAVEL EVALUATION *777*

List of Maps, by Topic

Yellow Fever

POPULAR ITINERARIES

Africa & the Middle East

The Americas & the Caribbean

Asia

CDC Contributors

Abanyie, Francisca
Abe, Karon
Acosta, Anna
Adams, Laura
Ali, Ibne
Allen Tchoukalov, Jessica
Alvarado-Ramy, Francisco
Alvarez, Bianca
Angelo, Kristina
Ansari, Armin
Anstey, Erica
Appiah, Grace
Arshanapally, Suraj
Aubert, Rachael
Azziz-Baumgartner, Eduardo
Ballesteros, Michael
Barton
Behravesh, Casey
Beeler, Jennifer (Jenna)
Benedict, Kaitlin
Benedict, Katharine
Bennett, Sarah
Biggs, Holly
Blain, Amy
Blaney, David
Blanton, Jesse
Bonilla, Luis
Brown, Ashley
Brown, Clive
Bruce, Beau
Buchacz, Katarzyna (Kate)
Caceres, Diego
Cahill, Eric
Cantey, Paul
Chancey, Rebecca
Charles, Macarthur
Chen, Chung (Ken)
Chen, Tai-Ho
Chiller, Tom
Choi, Mary Joung
Collins, Jennifer
Cope, Jennifer
Cossaboom, Caitlin
Crist, Matthew
Desai, Meghna
Dubray, Christine
Edens, William (Chris)
Eidex, Rachel
Estívariz, Concepción
Farrar, Jennifer Loo
Fields, Patricia (Patti)
Fischer, Marc
Francois
Watkins, Louise
Freedman, Mark
Freeland, Amy
Friedman, Cindy
Gaines, Joanna
Galang, Romeo
Galland, G. Gale
Galloway, Renee
García, Macarena
Garcia-
Williams, Amanda
Gastañaduy, Paul
Gee, Jay
Geissler, Aimee
Gershman, Mark
Gertz, Alida
Ghai, Ria
Gimnig, John
Gleason, Brigette
Glynn, Marielle (Ellie)
Gold, Jeremy
Goodson, James
Gould, Carolyn
Green, Michael
Griffin, Patricia
Guagliardo, Sarah Anne
Gutelius, Bruce
Hall, Aron
Ham, D. Cal
Harris, Aaron
Havers, Fiona
Heffelfinger, James
Hendricks, Kate
Herman-Roloff, Amy
Hill, Vincent
Hills, Susan
Hlavsa, Michele
Hughes, Michael
Jackson, Brendan
Jentes, Emily
Jereb, John
Juin, Stanley
Kamb, Mary
Kasule, Juliet
Kersh, Gilbert
Kharod, Grishma
Koama, Timbila
Kroger, Andrew
Lanzieri, Tatiana
Lash, R. Ryan
Laughlin, Mark
Leidel, Laura
Leung, Jessica
Lindsey, Nicole
Liu, Lindy
Logan, Naeemah
Lutgring, Joseph
Macedo de Oliveira, Alexandre
Maloney, Susan
Marano, Nina
Marin, Mona
Marlow, Mariel
Marston, Chung
Martin, Diana
Martin, Stacey
McCollum, Andrea
McCormick, David
McNamara, Lucy
Mead, Paul
Midgley, Claire
Minta, Anna
Mintz, Eric
Mirza, Sara
Mitchell, Tarissa
Mmbuji, Peter
Montgomery, Susan
Montiel, Sonia
Morales, Michelle
Moser, Kathleen
Mott, Joshua
Mutebi, John-Paul
Neblett Fanfair, Robyn
Negrón, María
Nelson, Christina
Nelson, Noele
Nicholson, William
Oduyebo, Titilope
Ojwang, Joseph
Owens, Jasmine
Paddock, Christopher
Park, Ina
Parker, Erin
Payne, Daniel
Paz-Bailey, Gabriela
Pennington, Audrey
Perelygina, Ludmila
Peters, Philip
Petersen, Brett
Phippard, Alba
Pieracci, Emily
Pindyck, Talia
Plumb, Ian
Powers, Ann
Quilter, Laura
Rabold, Elizabeth
Rao, Agam
Reef, Susan
Regan, Joanna
Reno, Hilary
Rey, Araceli
Reyes, Nimia
Rizwan, Aisha
Roellig, Dawn
Routh, Janell

Roy, Sharon
Sánchez-González, Liliana
Sauber-Schatz, Erin
Schafer, Ilana
Secor, W. Evan
Shealy, Katherine
Shoemaker, Trevor
Skoff, Tami
Spradling, Philip
Staples, J. Erin
Stoddard, Robyn
Stoney, Rhett
Straily, Anne
Surie, Diya
Szablewski, Christine
Tack, Danielle
Tan, Kathrine
Tardivel, Kara
Taylor, Melanie
Teshale, Eyasu
Tiller, Rebekah
Tobolowsky, Farrell
Toda, Mitsuru
Tohme, Rania
Traxler, Rita
Treffiletti, Aimee
Vanden Esschert, Kayla
VanderEnde, Kristin
Varela, Kate
Velazquez-Kronen, Raquel
Vieira, Antonio
Walker, Allison
Wallace, Ryan
Wassilak, Steven
Weinberg, Michelle
Weng, Mark
White, Stefanie
Yee, Eileen

External Contributors

Ansdell, Vernon	John A. Burns School of Medicine, University of Hawaii (Honolulu, HI)
Atkinson, Greg	Liverpool John Moores University (Liverpool, United Kingdom)
Aung, Wai Yan	Peace Corps (Yangon, Myanmar)
Backer, Howard	University of California, Berkeley (Berkeley, CA)
Barkati, Sapha	J.D. MacLean Centre for Tropical Diseases, McGill University Health Centre (Montreal, Canada)
Barnett, Elizabeth	Boston Medical Center; Boston University School of Medicine (Boston, MA)
Batterham, Alan	MedConnect North (United Kingdom)
Bégué, Rodolfo	Kapi'olani Medical Center for Women and Children; John A. Burns School of Medicine, University of Hawaii (Honolulu, HI)
Blumberg, Lucille	National Institute for Communicable Diseases (Johannesburg, South Africa)
Borwein, Sarah	Hong Kong SAR, China
Bozkurt, Taylan	MEDARVA Healthcare (Richmond, VA)
Cabada, Miguel	University of Texas Medical Branch (Galveston, TX); Universidad Peruana Cayetano Heredia (Cusco, Peru)
Carroll, I. Dale	The Pregnant Traveler (Spring Lake, MI)
Chen, Lin Hwei	Mount Auburn Hospital (Cambridge, MA); Harvard Medical School (Boston, MA)
Chimiak, James	Diver's Alert Network (Durham, NC)
Connor, Bradley	The New York Center for Travel and Tropical Medicine; Weill Cornell Medical College (New York, NY)
Coyle, Christina	Albert Einstein College of Medicine, Yeshiva University (Bronx, NY)
Dalinkus, Christopher	Piedmont Medical Care Corporation (Atlanta, GA)
Daugherty, Michael	Emory University School of Medicine (Atlanta, GA)
Esposito, Douglas	Administration for Children & Families, US Department of Health & Human Services (Atlanta, GA)

Fairley, Jessica — Emory University School of Medicine (Atlanta, GA)

Fivenson, David — St. Joseph Mercy Health System; Fivenson Dermatology (Ann Arbor, MI)

Flórez-Arango, José — City University of New York Graduate School of Public Health and Health Policy (New York, NY)

Franco-Paredes, Carlos — University of Colorado School of Medicine Anschutz Medical Campus (Aurora, CO); Hospital Infantil de México, Federico Gómez (Mexico City, Mexico)

Freedman, David — Emeritus, University of Alabama at Birmingham (Birmingham, AL)

Gaynor, Kate — Guangzhou United Family Healthcare (Guangzhou, China)

Gracey, Sherry — United States Public Health Service; United States Coast Guard (Honolulu, HI)

Hackett, Peter — University of Colorado School of Medicine Anschutz Medical Campus (Aurora, CO); Institute for Altitude Medicine (Telluride, CO)

Hagmann, Stefan — Baystate Children's Hospital; UMass Chan Medical School–Baystate (Springfield, MA)

Hamer, Davidson — Boston University School of Public Health; Boston University School of Medicine (Boston, MA)

Henao-Martínez, Andrés — University of Colorado Hospital; University of Colorado School of Medicine Anschutz Medical Campus (Aurora, CO)

Hochberg, Natasha — Boston Medical Center; Boston University School of Public Health; Boston University School of Medicine (Boston, MA)

Hynes, Noreen — The Johns Hopkins Hospital; Bloomberg School of Public Health; Johns Hopkins University School of Medicine (Baltimore, MD)

Iamsirithaworn, Sopon — Department of Disease Control, Ministry of Public Health (Nonthaburi, Thailand)

Kayden, Stephanie — Harvard T.H. Chan School of Public Health; Harvard Medical School (Boston, MA)

Keller, Alexander — Special Warfare Operational Medicine Squadron; Uniformed Services University of the Health Sciences (Bethesda, MD)

Killerby, Marie — Vanderbilt University School of Medicine (Nashville, TN)

Kivlehan, Sean — Brigham & Women's Hospital; Harvard Medical School (Boston, MA)

Kohl, Sarah — University of Pittsburgh School of Medicine (Pittsburgh, PA)

Kotton, Camille — Massachusetts General Hospital; Harvard Medical School (Boston, MA)

Kozarsky, Alan — Federal Aviation Administration–Designated Human Intervention Motivation Study (HIMS) Senior Aviation Medical Examiner (AME); Eye Consultants of Atlanta (Atlanta, GA)

Kozarsky, Phyllis — Emerita, Emory University School of Medicine (Atlanta, GA)

Lange, W. Robert — Retired, National Institute on Drug Abuse, US Department of Health & Human Services (Bethesda, MD); Retired, Johns Hopkins University School of Medicine (Baltimore, MD); Retired, University of Maryland (Baltimore, MD)

LaRocque, Regina — Massachusetts General Hospital; Harvard Medical School (Boston, MA)

Lehner, Virginia — Bureau of Consular Affairs, US Department of State (Washington, DC)

Levi, Matt — Virtual Health at CHI Franciscan; CommonSpirit Health (Fox Island, WA)

Libman, Michael — J.D. MacLean Centre for Tropical Diseases, McGill University Health Centre (Montreal, Canada)

McDevitt, Sue Ann — New York University Langone Health (New York, NY)

McLellan, Susan — University of Texas Medical Branch (Galveston, TX)

Meister, Kathleen — ICF (Rockville, MD)

Montgomery, Gary	United States Public Health Service; US Department of Commerce, National Oceanic and Atmospheric Administration (Seattle, WA)
Neumann, Karl	Deceased
Nilles, Eric	Brigham & Women's Hospital; Harvard Medical School (Boston, MA)
Nord, Daniel	Duke University School of Medicine (Durham, NC)
Norton, Scott	Uniformed Services University of the Health Sciences (Bethesda, MD)
Parker, Salim	University of Cape Town Department of Medicine (Cape Town, South Africa)
Raczniak, Gregory	United States Public Health Service; United States Coast Guard (Honolulu, HI)
Riddle, Mark	University of Nevada, Reno School of Medicine (Reno, NV)
Rosselot, Gail	Travel Well of Westchester (Briarcliff Manor, NY)
Ryan, Edward	Massachusetts General Hospital; Harvard T.H. Chan School of Public Health; Harvard Medical School (Boston, MA)
Schumacher, Bryan	United States Navy; Department of Defense Liaison to the Centers for Disease Control and Prevention (Atlanta, GA)
Shlim, David	Jackson Hole Travel & Tropical Medicine (Wilson, WY)
Shurtleff, David	National Center for Complementary & Integrative Health, National Institutes of Health, US Department of Health & Human Services (Bethesda, MD)
Staat, Mary Allen	Cincinnati Children's Hospital Medical Center; University of Cincinnati College of Medicine (Cincinnati, OH)
Stauffer, Kendra	Animal & Plant Health Inspection Service, US Department of Agriculture (Gainesville, FL)
Stauffer, William	University of Minnesota Medical School (Minneapolis, MN)
Stout, Shawn	National Center for Complementary & Integrative Health, National Institutes of Health, US Department of Health & Human Services (Bethesda, MD)
Studer, Nicholas	United States Army Institute of Surgical Research (Fort Sam Houston, TX); Uniformed Services University of the Health Sciences (Bethesda, MD)
Thompson, Andrew	Lane Clark & Peacock LLP (London, United Kingdom)
Valk, Thomas	Jupiter, FL
Van Tilburg, Christopher	Providence Hood River Memorial Hospital (Hood River, OR)
Waggoner, Jesse	Emory University School of Medicine (Atlanta, GA)
Walker, Patricia	HealthPartners Institute; HealthPartners Travel & Tropical Medicine Center (St. Paul, MN); University of Minnesota Medical School (Minneapolis, MN)
Wanat, Karolyn	Medical College of Wisconsin (Milwaukee, WI)
Wanduragala, Danushka	Minnesota Department of Health (St. Paul, MN)
Wangu, Zoon	University of Massachusetts Memorial Children's Medical Center (Worcester, MA); Massachusetts Department of Public Health (Boston, MA)
Weinberg, Nicholas	Dartmouth Geisel School of Medicine (Hanover, NH)
Wilson, Mary Elizabeth	University of California, San Francisco School of Medicine (San Francisco, CA); Harvard T.H. Chan School of Public Health (Boston, MA)
Wu, Henry	Emory University School of Medicine (Atlanta, GA)
Youngster, Ilan	Shamir Medical Center (Zerfin, Israel)

Acknowledgments

To produce a book subtitled "Health Information for International Travel" during an ongoing pandemic takes the right mix of folly, optimism, pluck, and prescience. And who could have predicted that just 2 weeks after delivering our draft to the publisher, the first cases of monkeypox heralding an international outbreak would be diagnosed? Using a travel analogy, putting together CDC Yellow Book 2024 has been a bit like running along the platform and jumping to catch a moving train. After scrapping our plans for CDC Yellow Book 2022 (the release of which had been slated to coincide with the May 2021 Conference of the International Society of Travel Medicine meeting) we rededicated ourselves to publishing this current edition. Written, reviewed, and edited by clinicians and public health professionals over 12 months (roughly April 2021–April 2022), this book reflects not only their generosity but also their steadfast commitment to the philosophy behind this ongoing project.

To all who participated, the editorial team would like to express its sincerest thanks. We would also like to extend our gratitude to Drs. Elise Beltrami and Nicole Cohen for their meticulous reading of the entire volume. They, too, completed their thorough reviews while juggling multiple pandemic-related responsibilities. Their combined breadth and depth of knowledge, keen eye for detail, and artful knack for inserting well-placed, insightful comments significantly improved the manuscript.

The CDC Yellow Book 2024 editorial team would also like to recognize the following authors for their past contributions to the listed chapters in CDC Yellow Book 2020:

Kristina Angelo (Chikungunya, Lung Flukes)
Nelson Arboleda (Dominican Republic)
Paul Arguin (Malaria; Yellow Fever Vaccine & Malaria Prophylaxis Information, by Country)
Henry Baggett (Burma [Myanmar])
Deborah Nicolls Barbeau (Travelers with Chronic Illnesses)
Suzanne Beavers (Air Quality & Ionizing Radiation)
Michele Beckman (Deep Vein Thrombosis & Pulmonary Embolism)
Isaac Benowitz (Medical Tourism)
Holly Biggs (Hand, Foot & Mouth Disease)
Andrea Boggild (Cuba)
John Brooks (HIV Infection)
Clive Brown (Airplanes & Cruise Ships: Illness & Death Reporting & Public Health Interventions; Haiti)
Gary Brunette (Mass Gatherings; South Africa)
William Bunn (The Business Traveler)
Cristina Cardemil (Norovirus)
Roohollah Changizi (China)
Kevin Chatham-Stephens (Campylobacteriosis; Typhoid & Paratyphoid Fever)
Tom Chiller (Histoplasmosis)
Nakia Clemmons (Mumps)
Laura Cooley (Legionnaire's Disease & Pontiac Fever)
Alan Czarkowski (Health Care Workers, Including Public Health Researchers & Medical Laboratorians)
Inés DeRomaña (Study Abroad & Other International Student Travel)
Jodie Dionne-Odom (Sexually Transmitted Infections)
Christine Dubray (Lymphatic Filariasis; Soil-Transmitted Helminths; Cutaneous Leishmaniasis; Onchocerciasis [River Blindness]; Pinworm [Enterobiasis, Oxyuriasis, Threadworm]; African Trypanosomiasis)
Krista Kornylo Duong (Cruise Ship Travel)
Paul Edelson (Air Travel)
John Eichwald (Travelers with Disabilities)
Lacreisha Ejike-King (Haiti)
Stefanie Erskine (Motion Sickness)
Ana Carolina Faria e Silva Santelli (Brazil)
Marc Fischer (Tick-Borne Encephalitis; Zika)
Michael Forgione (US Military Deployments)
Alicia Fry (Influenza)
Joanna Gaines (Brazil; Medical Tourism)
Aimee Geissler (Campylobacteriosis)
Susan Gerber (Middle East Respiratory Syndrome [MERS])
Neela Goswami (Tuberculosis; *Perspectives*: Screening Travelers for Tuberculosis Infection)
J. Nadine Gracia (Haiti)
Brian Gushulak (Humanitarian Aid Workers)

Rebecca Hall (Airplanes & Cruise Ships: Illness & Death Reporting & Public Health Interventions)
Pauline Harvey (India)
Jessica Healy (Salmonellosis)
John Henderson (Burma [Myanmar])
Ronnie Henry (Jet Lag)
Barbara Herwaldt (Neurologic Angiostrongyliasis; Cyclosporiasis; Cysticercosis; Echinococcosis; Cutaneous Leishmaniasis; Visceral Leishmaniasis; Strongyloidiasis; African Trypanosomiasis)
Cynthia Hinton (Travelers with Disabilities)
Michelle Russell Hollberg (Newly Arrived Immigrants & Refugees)
Jennifer Hunter (Diarrheagenic *Escherichia coli*)
Uzma Javed (Safety & Security Overseas)
Emily Jentes (Yellow Fever Vaccine & Malaria Prophylaxis Information, by Country)
Robynne Jungerman (Airplanes & Cruise Ships: Illness & Death Reporting & Public Health Interventions)
Kevin Kain (Tanzania: Kilimanjaro)
Jay Keystone (Sex & Travel; Visiting Friends & Relatives: VFR Travel)
Phyllis Kozarsky (Air Travel; India)
Catherine Law (Complementary & Integrative Health Approaches)
Keun Lee (Promoting Quality in the Practice of Travel Medicine)
Fernanda Lessa (Pneumococcal Disease)
Philip LoBue (Tuberculosis; *Perspectives*: Screening Travelers for Tuberculosis Infection)
Adriana Lopez (Varicella [Chickenpox])
John MacArthur (Thailand)
Sarah Mbaeyi (Meningococcal Disease)
Orion McCotter (Coccidioidomycosis [Valley Fever])
Sue Ann McDevitt (Travelers with Chronic Illnesses)
Elissa Meites (Sex & Travel)
Susan Montgomery (Cysticercosis; Echinococcosis)
Diane Morof (Pregnant Travelers)
Robert Mullan (Taking Animals & Animal Products Across International Borders)
Hammad N'cho (Cholera)
Eric Nilles (Humanitarian Aid Workers)
Stephen Ostroff (Promoting Quality in the Practice of Travel Medicine)
Erin Parker (Injury & Trauma)
Manisha Patel (Poliomyelitis)
Calvin Patimeteeporn (Travel Health Kits)
Hope Pogemiller (Newly Arrived Immigrants & Refugees)
Gary Rhodes (Study Abroad & Other International Student Travel)
Mark Riddle (US Military Deployments)
Candice Robinson (Vaccination & Immunoprophylaxis: General Recommendations)
Katherine Roguski (Influenza)
Pierre Rollin (Tick-Borne Encephalitis)
Gail Rosselot (Travelers with Chronic Illnesses)
Dana Sampson (Haiti)
D. Scott Schmid (B Virus)
Aditya Sharma (Antimicrobial Resistance)
Tyler Sharp (Dengue)
David Sleet (Injury & Trauma; Road & Traffic Safety)
Mark Sotir (Peru; Travel Epidemiology)
Anne Straily (Strongyloidiasis)
Linda Taggart (Cuba)
Kara Tardivel (Airplanes & Cruise Ships: Illness & Death Reporting & Public Health Interventions)
Tejpratap Tiwari (Diphtheria; Tetanus)
Carolina Uribe (Obtaining Health Care Abroad)
Margarita Villarino (Mexico)
Stephen Waterman (Dengue)
Louise Francois Watkins (Shigellosis)
John Watson (Middle East Respiratory Syndrome [MERS])
Simone Wien (International Adoption)
Alison Winstead (Diarrheagenic *Escherichia coli*)
Karen Wong (Cholera)
Kimberly Workowski (Sex & Travel; Sexually Transmitted Infections)

Preface

This edition of the CDC Yellow Book continues a longstanding tradition of providing guidance for the practice of travel medicine. It also serves as a source of US government recommendations for immunizations and prophylaxis for international travel. The goal for this edition, as for previous editions, is to serve as a comprehensive resource for clinicians looking for answers to travel health–related questions. We believe you will find CDC Yellow Book 2024 lives up to the high standards set by its predecessors.

The COVID-19 pandemic interrupted the writing, editing, and publishing of the CDC Yellow Book, delaying the normal biennial production cycle by 2 years. COVID-19 has also created authorship and editorial challenges due to the frequently changing guidance around management, prevention, and treatment of this disease. With the understanding that the science and epidemiology of this disease will continue to evolve, we have endeavored to provide the most "evergreen" COVID-19 information available; for the most up-to-date details on COVID-19, we encourage you to visit the CDC website.

Centers for Disease Control and Prevention
Rochelle Walensky, MD, MPH, Director
National Center for Emerging and Zoonotic Infectious Diseases
Daniel Jernigan, MD, MPH, Acting Director
Division of Global Migration and Quarantine
Lisa Rotz, MD, Acting Director
Travelers' Health Branch
Cindy Friedman, MD, Chief

Dedication

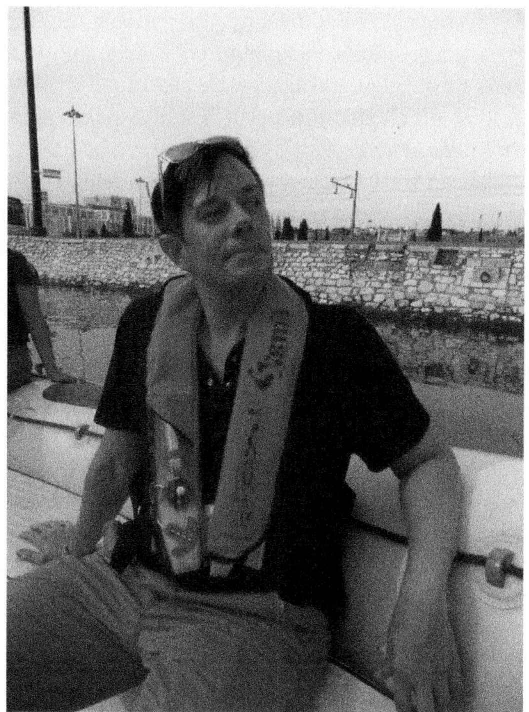

Ronnie Henry (1973–2020)

With this edition of the CDC Yellow Book, we say goodbye to several friends. Martin "Marty" Cetron, who directed the Division of Global Migration and Quarantine (DGMQ) in the National Center for Emerging and Zoonotic Infectious Diseases at CDC since 1996, will retire from the Agency in spring 2023. Over the course of his distinguished career, Marty advanced the practice of global health, mentoring numerous leaders in the field of travel medicine along the way. A list of his accomplishments could easily fill their own volume and his ongoing support of the CDC Yellow Book over the years has helped ensure that this reference remains the respected resource it is. Thank you, Marty, for all you have done. With deep appreciation, we wish you fair winds and Godspeed.

We also are saying goodbye to three physician colleagues and longtime CDC Yellow Book contributors who passed away since we last published: Jay Keystone (September 2019), William Bunn (January 2021), and Karl Neumann (February 2021). We will miss them and their teaching. Their legacy endures, however, and the clinicians and public health professionals who contributed to this edition in their stead, stand on their shoulders.

And last, we remember Ronnie Henry, a dearly loved son, brother, and friend. Ronnie, who began working in medical writing, editing, and publishing in 1996, had experience in a wide range of subjects, including infectious and chronic disease, epidemiology, microbiology, pharmacology, and clinical research. He came to CDC in 2003 as an editor for *Emerging Infectious Diseases*, spent a year in Beijing teaching medical writing and publishing to Chinese researchers, and then worked as an editor for *Preventing Chronic Disease*. Ronnie joined the Travelers' Health Branch in June 2010, as a health communication specialist. He quickly became an encyclopedia of travel health information and served as technical editor for five editions of CDC Yellow Book.

Ronnie helped shape CDC's messaging around healthy international travel for over 10 years, and supported multiple emergency response efforts including Ebola, Zika, and COVID-19. An extraordinary teacher, he influenced authors throughout the agency. He continued writing "Etymologia" features for *Emerging Infections Diseases* long after he left the journal's staff, expanding readers' knowledge with his explanations of the origins of medical and scientific terms. Ronnie had the rare ability to write equally well for scientific and lay audiences. He was also the driving force behind the development of the "Can I Eat This?" app, which delivered accurate and actionable food and water recommendations for international travelers with a dose of Ronnie's trademark humor. The app appeared as an answer to a question on *Jeopardy*, which he claimed as a crowning achievement in his career.

Ronnie traveled the world with his closest friends, exploring the continents of North and South America, Europe, and Asia. He regaled colleagues with tales of his adventures abroad, including the time he ate the entire head of a large fish thinking it was customary to do so in Japan. The shocked expression of the chef and other diners told him otherwise, just a moment too late. Outwardly, Ronnie was a colorful character with many striking qualities that all who met him knew and loved: his ever-changing hair color; his passion for trivia games; his amazing cooking, fermenting, baking, and ice cream–making skills; improv comedy; his fondness for cats and cat memes; his wry wit, astonishing intellect, and eloquence; and the pleasure he took in sharing a well-made meal with good friends. Ronnie was a mainstay in DGMQ and a light to everyone who knew him. At the time of his death (May 2020), Ronnie left behind many friends across CDC, and it is to his memory that this edition of the CDC Yellow Book is dedicated.

Introduction

DISEASE PATTERNS IN TRAVELERS

Allison Walker, Regina LaRocque

Travelers are an important population because of their mobility, their potential for exposure to infectious diseases outside their home country, and the possibility that they could bring those diseases from one country to another. The coronavirus disease 2019 (COVID-19) pandemic is the most recent example of the role travelers can play in the global spread of infectious diseases. Ebola virus, Zika virus, and antimicrobial-resistant pathogens are other examples of health threats whose geographic distribution has been facilitated by international travelers over the past several years. Travelers consequently should be included in general and targeted epidemiologic surveillance—including the use of molecular genomic approaches—to better understand both the exposure risk and impact of current and novel prevention recommendations.

The ability to provide appropriate pretravel guidance—and, when necessary, optimal post-travel evaluation and treatment—is predicated on understanding the epidemiologic features (disease patterns) among different traveling populations. Accounting for behaviors that can influence and potentially increase risk for travel-associated infections and diseases (e.g., attendance at a mass gathering, long-term or adventure travel, visiting friends and family) helps the astute clinician make directed travel health recommendations and focus their attention on the more likely diagnoses from among the lengthy list of travel-associated infections and diseases. An understanding of the epidemiology of the diseases themselves, including modes of transmission, incubation periods, signs and symptoms, duration of infectiousness, and accuracy of diagnostic testing, is also crucial. Including international travelers in epidemiologic surveillance provides additional information about the presence, frequency, seasonality, and geographic distribution of diseases, which might shift over time due to outbreaks, changes in climate and vector habitat, emergence or reemergence in new areas or populations, successful public health interventions, or other factors.

CDC Yellow Book 2024. Jeffrey Nemhauser, Oxford University Press.
DOI: 10.1093/oso/9780197570944.003.0001

1

The risk for travel-related infection can, however, be difficult to ascertain precisely for several reasons. Existing information regarding disease risk for travelers is limited because of the difficulty in obtaining accurate numerators (i.e., number of cases of infection among travelers) and denominators (i.e., number of overall travelers or number of travelers to a specific destination who are susceptible to infection). In cases of mild illness, travelers might never seek health care, or clinicians might not perform diagnostic tests to identify the cause. Travelers often visit multiple destinations, complicating identification of the location of exposure. Data on disease incidence in local populations might be available, but the relevance of such data to travelers—who have different risk behaviors, eating habits, accommodations, knowledge of and access to preventive measures, and activities—might be limited. In addition, epidemiologic investigations involving travelers use various methodologic designs, each with their own strengths and weaknesses, making findings difficult to compare or combine. Many single-clinic or single-destination investigations draw conclusions that might not be generalizable to travelers from different local, national, or cultural backgrounds.

Two existing networks provide epidemiologic data on international travelers from the United States and acquisition of travel-related illness. The GeoSentinel Global Surveillance Network is a worldwide data collection and communication network composed of International Society of Travel Medicine–associated travel and tropical medicine clinics that collect posttravel illness surveillance data. GeoSentinel scientists analyze these data to describe travel-related illness in specific populations of travelers.

Global TravEpiNet (GTEN) is a consortium of health clinics across the United States that deliver pretravel health consultations. Data from GTEN provide a snapshot of travelers seeking pretravel health care, and longitudinal cohort data on risk for and acquisition of travel-associated conditions, including for a subset of travelers who self-collect biological samples for microbiologic and genomic testing.

These travel medicine networks, and travel medicine researchers, increasingly are implementing next-generation sequencing tools to delineate the epidemiology of travel-associated infections and the role of travelers in the global spread of infectious diseases. Advances in the field of genomic sequencing enable high-resolution surveillance that can identify previously unrecognized geographic and epidemiologic associations. These molecular tools are becoming essential to understanding the spread of disease, the emergence of new pathogens or variants of existing ones, and the evolution of antimicrobial resistance. Combining these molecular techniques with traditional surveillance, epidemiologic approaches, and community-based participatory research represents a promising approach to expanding the evidence base underpinning the guidance and recommendations in the field of travel medicine. A broader evidence base will enable better-informed pretravel preparation for the individual traveler, and development of new approaches to mitigating the impact of travel on the global spread of disease.

RESOURCES

HealthMap (https://healthmap.org/en) uses online informal sources and real-time surveillance to provide information on emerging public health threats for diverse audiences.

BIBLIOGRAPHY

Gardy JL, Loman NJ. Towards a genomics-informed, real-time, global pathogen surveillance system. Nat Rev Genet. 2018;19(1):9–20.

LaRocque RC, Rao SR, Lee J, Ansdell V, Yates JA, Schwartz BS, et al. Global TravEpiNet: a national consortium of clinics providing care to international travelers—analysis of demographic characteristics, travel destinations, and pretravel healthcare of high-risk US international travelers, 2009–2011. Clin Infect Dis. 2012;54(4):455–62.

Sotir M, Freedman D. Basic epidemiology of infectious diseases, including surveillance and reporting. In: Zuckerman J, Brunette G, Leggat P, editors. Essential

Travel Medicine. Chichester (UK): John Wiley & Sons; 2015:1–7.

Walz EJ, Wanduragala D, Adedimeji AA, Volkman HR, Gaines J, Angelo KM, Boumi AE, et al. Community-based participatory research in travel medicine to identify barriers to preventing malaria in VFR travellers. J Trav Med. 2019;26(1):tay148.

Wilder-Smith A, Boggild AK. Sentinel surveillance in travel medicine: 20 years of GeoSentinel publications (1999–2018). J Trav Med. 2018;25(1):tay139.

WHY GUIDELINES DIFFER

David Shlim

Numerous international, national, and professional organizations publish guidelines and recommendations for travelers; CDC's Yellow Book is but one example. Travel health providers should be aware of these recommendations, even though they might not follow them in every instance. Through awareness, travel health providers can explain to their patients how their recommendations, and their patients' choices, might be discrepant with what others recommend. It can be unsettling for patients to receive travel medicine advice, vaccines, or an antimalarial drug prescription from a provider, only to find that the advice and prescriptions are contradicted by what other professionals, friends, or destination-country nationals have to say. The skillful travel health provider will be able to help the traveler reconcile seemingly conflicting advice, and travelers will be reassured when providers explain why these differences exist.

HOW GUIDELINES ARE CREATED

In the United States, the Food and Drug Administration (FDA) approves standards for how to use a vaccine or medication, including dosages, ages for which the product is approved, and booster recommendations. Guidance about when to use a product can come from a separate body (e.g., the Advisory Committee on Immunization Practices [ACIP]). To give ACIP the best possible information on which to base their recommendations, working groups of experts hold meetings to review the literature and new studies.

International bodies (e.g., the World Health Organization [WHO]), national committees of other countries, and medical organizations (e.g., the International Society of Travel Medicine and the Infectious Diseases Society of America), also promote their own guidance. Other professional organizations might create consensus clinical practice guidelines based on published medical literature and expert opinion. Travel medicine–specific paid subscription services employ travel medicine experts to organize and present guidelines for health care providers who see international travelers in their practice but who might lack expertise in the subject. Guidance about vaccinations and malaria prophylaxis developed by these organizations and subscription services can differ from CDC advice. Reasons for this are varied and include differences in product availability, licensure standards, cultural perceptions of risk, and opinions among experts, as well as lack of definitive evidence.

Availability of Products

Travel health providers can only use the products available to them. Availability is determined by the regulatory approval status of the product and, to a lesser extent, the marketing and distribution plan of the manufacturer. Regulatory approval processes vary greatly by country. For example, registering a new vaccine or antimalarial drug in the United States is a costly and rigorous process. If the market in a particular country is insufficient to justify the expense of registration, a commercial company might not seek it.

Licensure Standards

Licensure standards also vary. What might be sufficient for one regulatory authority might not suffice for another. For example, primaquine, an option for malaria prophylaxis in the United States, is not registered or commercially available in Switzerland. Atovaquone-proguanil also was available for malaria prophylaxis in the United States before many other countries. In another example, 4 Japanese encephalitis vaccines are available in the world, but only 1 is licensed in the United States.

Differences in Data Interpretation

Even when the same products are available, recommendations for use might not be the same in all countries. The injectable Ty21a typhoid vaccine and the oral typhoid vaccine are examples. In the United States, a booster of the injectable Ty21a vaccine is recommended after 2 years, but in most European countries, a booster is recommended after 3 years. In the United States, health providers dispense a packet of 4 oral typhoid vaccine capsules, whereas in Europe, 3 doses are considered adequate. The regulatory agencies might have reviewed the same data and drawn different conclusions, or they might have reviewed different data at separate times. Regulatory submissions to various agencies rarely occur at the same time. Therefore, for legitimate reasons, the data available for review by each agency might not be the same.

Perception of Risk

People from varying backgrounds can view the same risk data and come to very different conclusions regarding the costs and benefits of minimizing risk to what they consider to be an acceptable level. For example, recommendations to prevent malaria during travel to India vary widely. Germany does not recommend using malaria prophylaxis for any travel to an Indian destination; standby emergency treatment or self-treatment are the only recommendations for identified risk destinations. Guidelines from the United Kingdom recommend only awareness and mosquito bite prevention for more than half the Indian subcontinent, including large cities and popular tourist destinations in the north and south, but suggest prophylaxis consideration for some travelers or for those visiting higher-risk areas. By contrast, CDC recommends malaria prophylaxis for all travelers to any Indian destination, except for some mountainous areas of northern states.

THE IMPACT OF ADVICE

The real question is not just which recommendations each country should adopt, but the possible impact of that advice. Because we do not usually have detailed data on the exact risk to travelers for different vaccine-preventable diseases at a given destination, immunization guidance and recommendations often are based on serologic studies or on the original studies, most often performed in local people, that led to licensing. For example, as noted above, most European countries recommend a booster for the injectable Ty21a typhoid vaccine after 3 years, whereas the United States recommends a booster at 2 years. This difference is based on the perception of falling antibody levels over time, and a decision about where the line of protection against disease falls. Both standards have been in effect for many years, but no current available evidence would lead someone to conclude that one regimen has had a different impact than the other.

An extensive literature review, conducted by the Canadian Committee to Advise on Travel Medicine and Travel, led the committee to limit the recommendation of typhoid vaccine for travelers to South Asia only. This recommendation has not been adopted by CDC or many other international advisory

(continued)

WHY GUIDELINES DIFFER (CONTINUED)

1

boards. Despite this, we have little evidence that Canadian travelers are experiencing more typhoid fever than their counterparts from other countries.

Similar conclusions can be drawn for malaria prophylaxis recommendations. If the guidance provided by one group or organization consistently resulted in more cases of malaria than another, the guidance likely would change. In the absence of that data, however, health professionals continue to use their best judgment, without much knowledge of the true impact of their advice.

CAN WE HARMONIZE GUIDELINES?

The complex nature of how health organizations obtain, evaluate, and verify data, combined with fundamental differences in risk perception, makes it likely that multiple, overlapping, and at times conflicting guidelines will continue to exist. However, conflicting guidelines have decreased in the past decade due to the efforts of several organizations. A recent example has been the collaboration among the WHO, US CDC, and the European Centre for Disease Prevention and Control to develop consistency and clarity in defining travel-associated risk for Zika infection so that providers can more clearly relay that information, particularly to those who are pregnant or planning pregnancy. In addition, more rapid and frequent communication via the internet and regularly held international conferences have narrowed the gaps between conflicting advice.

In summary, the role of the travel health provider is to understand the differences in guidelines, interpret this information, and convey tailored and informed advice in an assured and comforting manner to travelers. There are no absolute right or wrong answers for many existing travel health guidelines. Even with all the data available, recommendations often are based on expert opinion, which can vary.

BIBLIOGRAPHY

Centers for Disease Control and Prevention. Advisory Committee on Immunization Practices (ACIP). Atlanta: The Centers; 2021. Available from: www.cdc.gov/vaccines/acip.

Chiodini P, Patel D, Goodyer L, Ranson H. on behalf of the PHE ACMP. Guidelines for malaria prevention in travellers from the UK 2021. London (UK): Public Health England. Available from: https://assets.publishing.service.gov.uk/government/uploads/system/uploads/attachment_data/file/1002275/Guidelines_for_malaria_prevention_in_travellers_from_the_UK_2021-1.pdf.

Committee to Advise on Tropical Medicine and Travel (CATMAT). Canadian recommendations for the prevention and treatment of malaria. Ottawa (CA): Public Health Agency of Canada; 2021. Available from: http://Canada.ca/en/public-health/services/catmat.html.

German Society for Tropical Medicine and International Health Association (DTG). [Recommendations for the prophylaxis and treatment of malaria of DTG 2018]; 2018. Available from: www.dtg.org.

Hill DR, Ericsson CD, Pearson RD, Keystone JS, Freedman DO, Kozarsky PE, et al. The practice of travel medicine: guidelines by the Infectious Diseases Society of America. Clin Infect Dis. 2006;43(12):1499–539.

Mace KE, Lucchi NW, Tan KR. Malaria surveillance—United States, 2017. MMWR Surveill Summ. 2021;70(2);1–35.

World Health Organization. International health regulations (2005). Geneva: The Organization; 2005. Available from: www.who.int/health-topics/international-health-regulations#tab=tab_1.

World Health Organization. International travel and health. Geneva: The Organization; 2012. Available from: www.who.int/publications/i/item/9789241580472.

. . . perspectives chapters supplement the clinical guidance in this book with additional content, context, and expert opinion. The views expressed do not necessarily represent the official position of the Centers for Disease Control and Prevention (CDC).

MAPS & TRAVEL MEDICINE

Marielle (Ellie) Glynn, Jesse Blanton, R. Ryan Lash

For well over 50 years, the Centers for Disease Control and Prevention (CDC) has used maps to help communicate geographically nuanced information about travel-related disease risks and associated health and safety recommendations. The earliest editions of CDC Yellow Book, a slim pamphlet entitled ***Immunization Information for International Travel***, included reprints of maps produced by the World Health Organization showing areas of risk for malaria (Figure 1-01) and yellow fever (Figure 1-02). Although the number and variety of maps in the CDC Yellow Book have grown over the past 11 editions, from 7 in 2000 to 58 in 2020 (Figure 1-03), most still focus on identifying areas of risk for these same 2 diseases. Over time, as malaria prophylaxis and yellow fever vaccine recommendations for many destinations have become increasingly geographically specific, we have included additional country-specific reference maps in CDC Yellow Book (see Sec. 2, Ch. 5, Yellow Fever Vaccine & Malaria Prevention Information, by Country).

A well-designed map speaks for itself, even when depicting complex features of a disease. Public health maps must accurately reflect the subject matter expert's judgment on best available evidence and clinical practices. CDC Yellow Book maps are subject to multiple constraints, including the spatial and temporal precision of reported disease surveillance data, variation in how data are reported, and the availability of corresponding environmental and demographic data. Decisions also must be made about whether including a map provides additional clarity. For some health risks, a

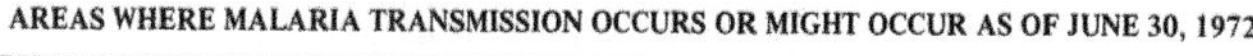

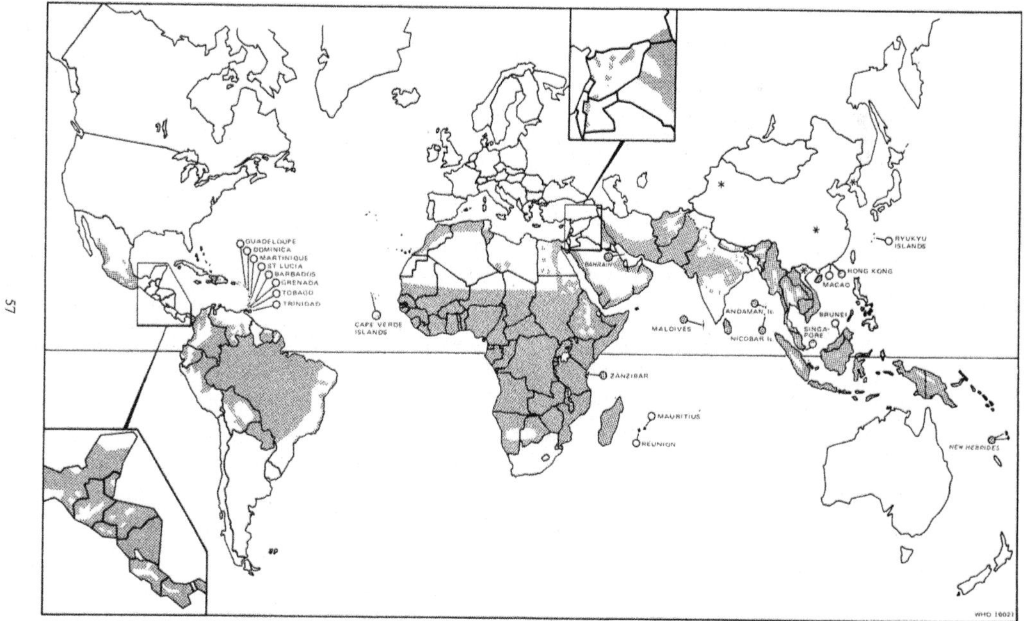

*Status unknown

Adapted from map published in *Weekly Epidemiological Record*, No. 3, 1973

FIGURE 1-01. Reprint of malaria map from Health Information for International Travel 1974 (CDC 1974)

For many years, CDC Yellow Book included World Health Organization global malaria maps, which generally followed the above design style. Small size and lack of labels made these maps difficult to interpret for specific travel itineraries.

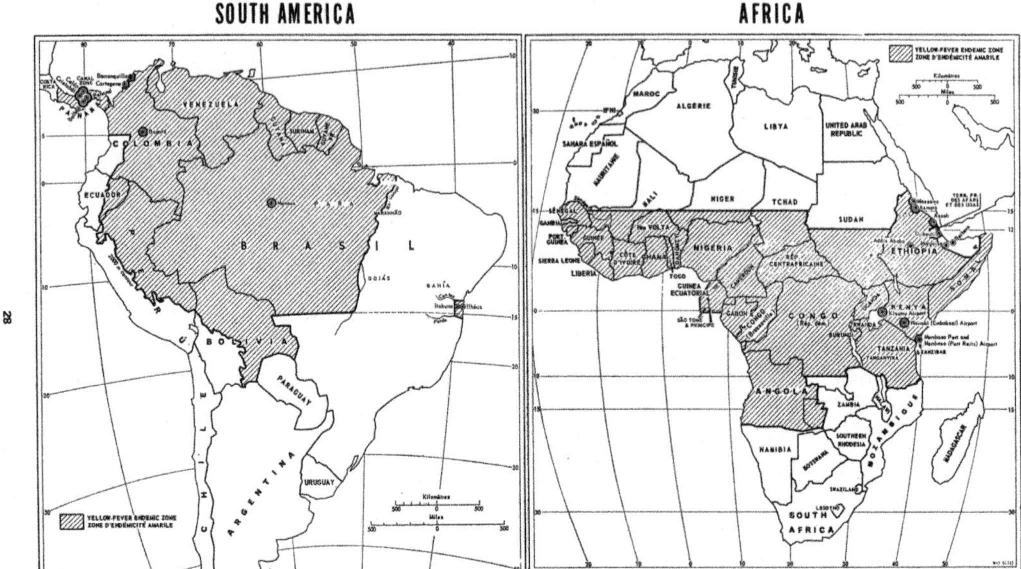

FIGURE 1-02. Reprint of yellow fever endemic zones map from Health Information for International Travel 1977 (CDC 1977)

These World Health Organization maps highlight various ways that boundaries of vectorborne diseases (e.g., yellow fever) can be demarcated. Compare these maps to the most current yellow fever vaccine recommendations in this edition of CDC Yellow Book (see Section 5.2.26, Yellow Fever).

table or textual description is adequate. When vaccination or prophylaxis recommendations apply to an entire country, for example, a map might be unnecessary. Conversely, when risk or recommendations vary based on geographic boundaries that are difficult to describe in words, maps can enhance risk communication, orienting the viewer more quickly and efficiently than a table or text.

In addition to providing vaccination and prophylaxis recommendations, other categories of CDC Yellow Book maps include destination maps, disease distribution maps, and risk maps. The destination maps in Section 10, Popular Itineraries, are included to provide information about the locations of national parks, game preserves, cities, and culturally significant gathering places. These maps serve as visual references to help clinicians understand their patients' travel plans. Disease distribution maps found throughout Section 5, Travel-Associated Infections & Diseases, show the global or regional presence or burden of the diseases described. Disease mapping varies, however. In some cases, a disease prevalence map could be most useful to a clinician; in other instances, risk maps, depicting both disease distribution and other relevant factors (e.g., elevation or access to preventative measures) can help health care providers make specific recommendations. Diseases with complex geographic variation in both prevalence and preventative measures also might have corresponding prophylaxis recommendation maps.

All the static maps from the print edition of CDC Yellow Book are available on the Travelers' Health website (https://wwwnc.cdc.gov/travel/) but advances in online mapping technology have created opportunities to deliver travel health information in novel ways. In March 2017, for example, CDC's Travelers' Health Branch launched a mapping application to aid in the communication of international Zika travel recommendations. This application allows users to search an interactive map; clicking on a destination opens a text box that provides travel health information for the specific location. CDC created a similar map for the coronavirus disease 2019 (COVID-19) pandemic. Efforts are under way to create interactive

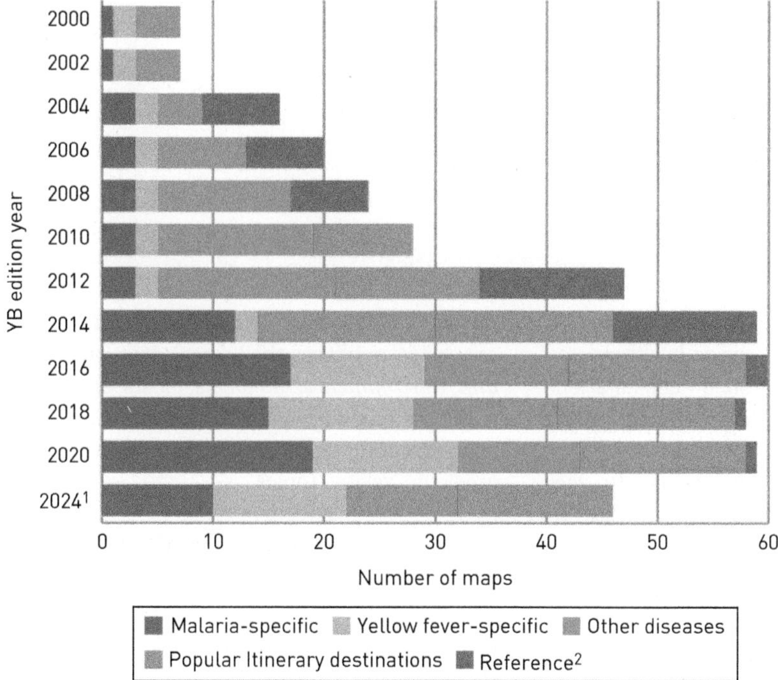

FIGURE 1-03. Number of maps included in CDC Yellow Book (YB) print editions, 2000–2024[1,2]

Over the past 11 editions, the number of CDC YB maps has increased by approximately 10-fold. Many new country-specific malaria and yellow fever risk maps aid in the interpretation of prophylaxis and vaccination recommendations.

[1] YB2022 not published due to the coronavirus disease 2019 pandemic.

[2] Created to supplement written information that appeared in the YB chapter, Yellow Fever Vaccine & Malaria Prevention Information, by Country, reference maps showed cities and provinces of selected countries. It was left to the reader to review these maps along with the written information in the chapter to determine where travelers could be at risk for yellow fever virus and/or malaria transmission. Starting in 2014, YB began replacing reference maps with disease-specific maps depicting risk areas for yellow fever virus and malaria transmission. The last reference map (China) appeared in YB2020.

maps for the online version of CDC Yellow Book that will elucidate the geographic health risks associated with international travel, beyond malaria and yellow fever.

BIBLIOGRAPHY

Center for Disease Control. Health information for international travel 1974: Supplement to the Morbidity and Mortality Weekly Report. MMWR Morb Mortal Wkly Rep. 1974;23(54):1–80.

Center for Disease Control. Health information for international travel 1977: Supplement to the Morbidity and Mortality Weekly Report. MMWR Morb Mortal Wkly Rep. 1977;26(55).

Centers for Disease Control and Prevention. CDC health information for international travel, 2008 edition. Arguin PM, Kozarsky PE, Reed C, editors. Atlanta: Elsevier Mosby; 2007.

Jentes ES, Poumerol G, Gershman MD, Hill DR, Lemarchand J, Lewis R, et al. The revised global yellow fever risk map and recommendations for vaccination, 2010: consensus of the Informal WHO Working Group on Geographic Risk for Yellow Fever. Lancet Infect Dis. 2011;11(8):622–32.

Jentes ES, Lash RR, Johansson MA, Sharp TM, Henry R, Brady OJ, et al. Evidence-based risk assessment and communication: a new global dengue-risk map for travelers and clinicians. J Travel Med. 2016;23(6):taw062.

Lash RR., Walker AT, Lee CV, LaRocque R, Rao SR. Ryan ET, et al. Enabling clinicians to easily find location-based travel health recommendations—is innovation needed? J Travel Med. 2018;25(1):tay035.

1

IMPROVING THE QUALITY OF TRAVEL MEDICINE THROUGH EDUCATION & TRAINING

Suraj Arshanapally, Jessica Allen Tchoukalov

Individuals planning international travel benefit from a pretravel visit dedicated to health-related travel recommendations. Such consultations with clinicians can help travelers remain healthy during and after travel.

Recent outbreaks of infectious diseases (e.g., Zika, coronavirus disease 2019 [COVID-19]) demonstrate the role of international travel in the geographic spread of disease. These outbreaks highlight the need to equip more clinicians with travel medicine training to ensure they can properly educate and advise travelers and prevent travel-related disease spread.

TRAVEL MEDICINE EDUCATION & TRAINING

The pretravel consultation is most effective when the clinician has experience and training related to travel medicine and can provide travelers with up-to-date information and guidance. In the United States, many types of health care professionals, ranging from infectious disease specialists to family medicine practitioners, offer travel medicine care and counseling. Travel medicine professional organizations offer training opportunities and certification programs for clinicians. This training is available via in-person courses or e-learning (e.g., webinars, workshops, online courses). Outlined below are several organizations that provide travel medicine–related trainings and education.

TRAVEL MEDICINE–RELATED PROFESSIONAL ORGANIZATIONS

Aerospace Medical Association

The Aerospace Medical Association (AsMA; www.asma.org) represents professionals in the fields of aviation, space, and environmental medicine who take care of air and space travelers. AsMA publishes the journal *Aviation, Space, and Environmental Medicine*; hosts an annual scientific meeting; and offers continuing medical education and certification in aerospace medicine–related topics.

American Society of Tropical Medicine and Hygiene

Formed in 1951 through the merger of predecessor organizations dating back to 1903, the American Society of Tropical Medicine and Hygiene (ASTMH; www.astmh.org) has a subsection, the American Committee on Clinical Tropical Medicine and Travelers' Health, that focuses exclusively on tropical and travel medicine. ASTMH publishes *The American Journal of Tropical Medicine and Hygiene*, a peer-reviewed scientific journal; hosts the ASTMH annual meeting; hosts an electronic distribution list; and maintains a tropical and travel medicine consultant directory.

In addition, ASTMH offers the CTropMed examination, which leads to a Certificate of Knowledge in Clinical Tropical Medicine and Travelers' Health (www.astmh.org/education-resources/certificate-programs). CTropMed is open to clinicians with a current professional health care license who have passed an ASTMH-approved tropical medicine diploma course or who have sufficient tropical medicine experience. ASTMH also hosts an annual intensive update course in clinical tropical medicine and travelers' health, designed to prepare clinicians planning to take the CTropMed examination.

Infectious Diseases Society of America

The Infectious Diseases Society of America (IDSA; www.idsociety.org) is the largest organization representing infectious disease clinicians in the United States. IDSA has many active members with expertise in tropical and travel medicine. In 2006, IDSA published evidence-based guidelines on the practice of travel medicine in the United States. IDSA publishes travel-related research in 3 journals: *The Journal of Infectious Diseases*, *Clinical Infectious Diseases*, and *Open Forum Infectious Diseases*. IDSA also co-sponsors the annual IDWeek meeting (https://idweek.org) and the online Emerging Infections Network (EIN; https://ein.idsociety.org), a provider-based sentinel network to assist public health authorities with emerging infectious disease surveillance.

International Society for Infectious Diseases

The International Society for Infectious Diseases (ISID; www.isid.org) was organized in 1986 and has approximately 80,000 members in 201 countries. Like IDSA, ISID does not specifically focus on travel medicine. However, its international reach, particularly in low-resource countries, makes travel medicine an important topic in ISID and makes ISID a valuable source of information for infectious diseases clinicians in many overseas travel destinations.

ISID publishes the *International Journal of Infectious Diseases* and hosts the biennial International Congress on Infectious Diseases and the International Meeting on Emerging Diseases and Surveillance. In addition, ISID hosts the Program for Monitoring Emerging Diseases (ProMED; www.promedmail.org)—an open-source electronic system for reporting emerging infectious diseases and toxins, including outbreaks—and the EpiCore (www.epicor.com) global outbreak surveillance system.

International Society of Travel Medicine

The International Society of Travel Medicine (ISTM; www.istm.org) is a multinational organization dedicated to promoting healthy, safe, and responsible travel and movement of all people crossing borders by facilitating advancement of epidemiologic surveillance and research, education, and service in travel and migration medicine. ISTM was founded in 1991 and has over 4,000 members worldwide. ISTM publishes the peer-reviewed *Journal of Travel Medicine* and hosts the TravelMed listserv, where members share information. ISTM also maintains a directory of domestic and international travel medicine clinics affiliated with ISTM members in 90 countries (www.istm.org/AF_CstmClinicDirectory.asp). ISTM hosts committees that address pressing issues in travel medicine (e.g., digital communications and publications); special interest and professional groups, including groups for travel medicine nurses and travel medicine pharmacists; the biennial Conference of the International Society of Travel Medicine; and annual regional sub-meetings.

In addition, ISTM provides an online learning curriculum and offers the Certificate in Travel Health (CTH) Examination (www.istm.org/certificateofknowledge#istmcertintravhealth); passing the examination is one of several required elements for health care professionals (including physicians, nurses, and pharmacists) who provide travel health advice and who participate regularly in travel medicine professional development to receive ISTM certification. ISTM also provides an annual intensive update course in travelers' health designed to prepare clinicians planning to take the CTH exam.

Wilderness Medical Society

Organized in 1983, the Wilderness Medical Society (WMS; www.wms.org) focuses on adventure travel, including wilderness travel and diving. WMS publishes the journal *Wilderness and Environmental Medicine*, and has developed practice guidelines for emergency care in wilderness settings. WMS hosts annual meetings, a world congress, and subspecialty meetings. In addition, WMS offers courses leading to certification in advanced wilderness life support and courses leading to the Diploma in Mountain Medicine (DiMM). WMS also offers a wilderness medical curriculum that, when successfully completed, qualifies members for fellowship in the Academy of Wilderness Medicine.

In addition to the above-mentioned organizations, the World Health Organization maintains a list of regional and national societies of travel medicine on its website (www.who.int/travel-advice/regional-and-national-societies-of-travel-medicine).

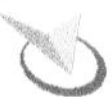

BIBLIOGRAPHY

Chiodini JH, Anderson E, Driver C, Field VK, Flaherty GT, Grieve AM, et al. Recommendations for the practice of travel medicine. Travel Med Infect Dis. 2012;10(3):109–28.

Hill DR, Ericsson CD, Pearson RD, Keystone JS, Freedman DO, Kozarsky PE, et al. The practice of travel medicine: guidelines by the Infectious Diseases Society of America. Clin Infect Dis. 2006;42(12):1499–539.

Kozarsky PE, Steffen R. Travel medicine education—what are the needs? J Travel Med. 2016;23(5):taw039.

LaRocque RC, Jentes ES. Health recommendations for international travel: a review of the evidence base of travel medicine. Curr Opin Infect Dis. 2011;24(5):403–9.

Leder K, Bouchard O, Chen LH. Training in travel medicine and general practitioners: a long-haul journey! J Travel Med. 2015;22(6):357–60.

Ruis JR, van Rijckevorsel GG, van den Hoek A, Koeman SC, Sonder GJ. Does registration of professionals improve the quality of travelers' health advice? J Travel Med. 2009;16(4):263–6.

Schlagenhauf P, Santos-O'Connor F, Parola P. The practice of travel medicine in Europe. Clin Microbiol Infect. 2010;16(3):203–8.

2 Preparing International Travelers

THE PRETRAVEL CONSULTATION

Lin Hwei Chen, Natasha Hochberg

The pretravel consultation offers a dedicated time to prepare travelers for health concerns that might arise during their trips. During the pretravel consultation, clinicians can conduct a risk assessment for each traveler, communicate risk by sharing information about potential health hazards, and manage risk by various means. Managing risk might include giving immunizations, emphasizing to travelers the importance of taking prescribed malaria prophylaxis and other medications (and highlighting the risks of not taking them correctly), and educating travelers about steps they can take to address and minimize travel-associated risks. The pretravel consultation also serves a public health purpose by helping limit the role international travelers could play in the global spread of infectious diseases.

THE TRAVEL MEDICINE SPECIALIST

Travel medicine specialists have in-depth knowledge of immunizations, risks associated with specific destinations, and the implications of traveling with underlying conditions. Therefore, a comprehensive consultation with a travel medicine expert is indicated for all international travelers and is particularly important for those with a complicated health history, anyone taking special risks (e.g., traveling at high elevation, working in refugee camps), or those with exotic or complicated itineraries. Clinicians aspiring to be travel medicine providers can benefit from the resources provided by the International Society of Travel Medicine (ISTM; www.istm.org) and might consider specialty training and certification (see

CDC Yellow Book 2024. Jeffrey Nemhauser, Oxford University Press. © Oxford University Press 2023.
DOI: 10.1093/oso/9780197570944.003.0002

Sec. 1, Ch. 4, Improving the Quality of Travel Medicine Through Education & Training).

COMPONENTS OF A PRETRAVEL CONSULTATION

Effective pretravel consultations require attention to the traveler's health background, and incorporate the itinerary, trip duration, travel purpose, and activities, all of which determine health risks (Table 2-01). The pretravel consultation is the best opportunity to educate the traveler about health risks at the destination and how to mitigate them. The typical pretravel consultation does not include a physical examination, and a separate appointment with the same or a different provider might be necessary to assess fitness for travel. Because travel medicine clinics are not available in some communities, primary care physicians should seek guidance from travel medicine specialists to address areas of uncertainty. The Centers for Disease Control and Prevention (CDC) Travelers' Health website (https://wwwnc.cdc.gov/travel/) also has materials and an interactive web-tool to guide

Table 2-01 **The pretravel consultation: medical history & travel risk assessment**

MEDICAL HISTORY (HEALTH BACKGROUND)	
PAST MEDICAL HISTORY	Age Allergies (especially any pertaining to vaccines, eggs, or latex) Medications Sex Underlying conditions
SPECIAL CONDITIONS	Breastfeeding Cardiopulmonary event (recent) Cerebrovascular event (recent) Disability or handicap Guillain-Barré syndrome (history of) Immunocompromising conditions or medications Older age Pregnancy (including trimester) Psychiatric condition Seizure disorder Surgery (recent) Thymus abnormality
IMMUNIZATION HISTORY	Routine vaccines Travel vaccines
PRIOR TRAVEL EXPERIENCE	High-elevation travel/mountain climbing Malaria chemoprophylaxis Prior travel-related illnesses
TRAVEL RISK ASSESSMENT (TRIP DETAILS)	
ITINERARY	Countries and specific regions, including order of countries visited if >1 country Outbreaks at destination Rural or urban destinations
TIMING	Season of travel Time to departure Trip duration

Table 2-01 The pretravel consultation: medical history & travel risk assessment (continued)

REASON FOR TRAVEL	Adoption Adventure Business Education or research Medical tourism (seeking health care) Pilgrimage Tourism Visiting friends and relatives Volunteer, missionary, or aid work
TRAVEL STYLE	Accommodations (e.g., camping/tent, dormitory, guest house, hostel/budget hotel, local home or host family, tourist/luxury hotel) "Adventurous" eating Independent travel or package tour Level of hygiene at the destination Modes of transportation Traveler risk tolerance Travel with children
SPECIAL ACTIVITIES	Animal interactions (including visiting farms, touring live animal markets) Cruise ship Cycling/motorbiking Disaster relief Diving Extreme sports High elevations Medical care (providing or receiving) Rafting or other water exposure Sexual encounters (planned) Spelunking

primary care physicians through a pretravel consultation.

Personalize travel health advice by highlighting likely exposures and reminding the traveler of ubiquitous risks (e.g., injury, foodborne and waterborne infections, vectorborne diseases, respiratory tract infections—including coronavirus disease 2019 [COVID-19]—and bloodborne and sexually transmitted infections). Balancing cautions with an appreciation of the positive aspects of the journey can lead to a more meaningful pretravel consultation. In addition, pay attention to the cost of recommended interventions. Because some travelers are unable to afford all the recommended immunizations and medications, prioritize interventions (see Sec. 2, Ch. 15, Prioritizing Care for Resource-Limited Travelers).

Assess Individual Risk

Traveler characteristics and destination-specific risk provide the background to assess travel-associated health risks. Such characteristics include personal health background (e.g., past medical history, special conditions, immunization history, medications); prior travel experience; trip details, including itinerary, timing, reason for travel, travel style, and specific activities; and details about the status of COVID-19 and other infectious diseases at the destination.

Certain travelers also might confront special risks. Recent hospitalization for serious problems might lead to a decision to recommend delaying travel. Air travel is contraindicated for patients with certain conditions. For instance, patients should not travel by air <3 weeks after an uncomplicated myocardial infarction or <10 days after thoracic or abdominal surgery. Consult relevant health care providers most familiar with the traveler's underlying illnesses.

Other travelers with specific risks include those who have chronic illnesses, are immunocompromised, or are pregnant. Travelers visiting friends and relatives, long-term travelers, and travelers with small children also face unique risks. More comprehensive discussion on advising travelers with additional health considerations is available in Section 3. Determine whether recent outbreaks or other safety notices have been posted for the traveler's destination by checking information available on CDC Travelers' Health and US Department of State websites and other resources.

In addition to recognizing the traveler's characteristics, health background, and destination-specific risks, discuss anticipated exposures related to special activities. For example, river rafting could expose a traveler to schistosomiasis or leptospirosis, and spelunking in Central America could put the traveler at risk for histoplasmosis. Flying from lowlands to high-elevation areas and trekking or climbing in mountainous regions introduces the risk for altitude illness. Inquire about plans for specific leisure, business, and health care–seeking activities.

Communicate Risk

Once destination-specific risks for a particular itinerary have been assessed, communicate them clearly to the traveler. Health-risk communication is an exchange of information in which the clinician and traveler discuss potential health hazards for the trip and any available preventive measures. Communicating risk is one of the most challenging aspects of a pretravel consultation, because travelers' perception of and tolerance for risk can vary widely. For a more detailed discussion, see Sec. 2, Ch. 2, . . . *perspectives*: Travelers' Perception of Risk.

Manage Risk

VACCINATIONS

Vaccinations are a crucial component of pretravel consultations, and the risk assessment forms the basis of recommendations for travel vaccines. Consider whether the patient has sufficient time to complete a vaccine series before travel; the purpose of travel and specific destination within a country will inform the need for vaccines. At the same time, the pretravel consultation presents an opportunity to update routine vaccines (Table 2-02) and to ensure that eligible travelers are up to date with their COVID-19 vaccinations; see www.cdc.gov/coronavirus/2019-ncov/vaccines/stay-up-to-date.html.

Pay attention to vaccine-preventable diseases for which immunity might have waned over time or after a recent immunocompromising condition (e.g., after a hematopoietic stem cell transplant). Asking whether travelers plan to travel again in the next 1–2 years can help them justify an immunization for travel over several years (e.g., rabies preexposure, Japanese encephalitis) rather than only the upcoming trip. Provide travelers with a record of administered immunizations and instructions to follow up as needed to complete a vaccine series.

MALARIA PREVENTION

Malaria continues to cause substantial morbidity and mortality in travelers. Since 1973, the annual number of US malaria cases reported to CDC has increased; therefore, clinicians must carefully assess travelers' risk for malaria and recommend preventive measures during the pretravel consultation. For travelers going to malaria-endemic countries, discuss malaria transmission, ways to reduce risk including mosquito avoidance, recommendations for prophylaxis, and symptoms of malaria. Additional information on malaria is available in Sec. 2, Ch. 5, Yellow Fever Vaccine & Malaria Prevention Information, by Country, and Sec. 5, Part 3, Ch. 16, Malaria.

SELF-TREATABLE CONDITIONS

Despite health care providers' best efforts, some travelers will become ill. Obtaining reliable and timely medical care during travel can be problematic in many destinations. Consequently, consider prescribing certain medications in advance to enable the traveler to treat common health problems. Box 2-01 provides a list of some of the most

Table 2-02 The pretravel consultation: vaccines to update & consider[1]

ROUTINE VACCINES	
VACCINE	TRAVEL-ASSOCIATED INFECTION OR DISEASE OCCURRENCES & VACCINE RECOMMENDATIONS
COVID-19	International travelers should be fully vaccinated with a COVID-19 vaccine, including all recommended booster doses.
Haemophilus influenzae type b	No reports of travel-related infection; organism ubiquitous worldwide.
Hepatitis B	Recommended for travelers visiting countries where HBsAg prevalence is ≥2%. Vaccination can be considered for all international travelers, regardless of destination, depending upon individual behavioral risk and potential for exposure.
Human papillomavirus (HPV)	No reports of travel-acquired infection; sexual activity during travel might lead to HPV and other sexually transmitted infections.
Influenza	Year-round transmission can occur in tropical areas. Outbreaks have occurred on cruise ships. Novel influenza viruses (e.g., avian influenza viruses H5N1 and H7N9), can be transmitted to travelers visiting areas where these viruses are circulating.
Measles, mumps, rubella	Infections are common in countries and communities that do not immunize children routinely, including parts of Europe. Outbreaks have occurred in the United States because of infection in returning travelers.
Meningococcal (serogroups A, C, W, and Y)	Outbreaks occur regularly in sub-Saharan Africa in the meningitis belt during the dry season, generally December–June, although transmission can occur at other times for those with close contact with local populations. Outbreaks have occurred with Hajj pilgrimage, and the Kingdom of Saudi Arabia requires the quadrivalent vaccine for pilgrims.
Pneumococcal	*Streptococcus pneumoniae* is ubiquitous worldwide; causal relationship to travel is difficult to establish.
Polio	Unimmunized or under-immunized travelers can become infected with either wild poliovirus or vaccine-derived poliovirus. Because the international spread of wild poliovirus in 2014 was declared a Public Health Emergency of International Concern under the International Health Regulations, temporary recommendations for polio vaccination are in place for countries with wild poliovirus circulation for their residents, long-term visitors, and international travelers.
Rotavirus	Common in developing countries, although not a common cause of travelers' diarrhea in adults. The vaccine is only recommended for young children.
Tetanus, diphtheria, pertussis	Rare cases of diphtheria have been attributed to travel. Pertussis has occurred in travelers whose immunity has waned.

(*continued*)

Table 2-02 The pretravel consultation: vaccines to update & consider (continued)

Varicella	Infections are common in countries that do not immunize children routinely, as in most low- and middle-income countries.
Zoster	Travel is a form of stress that might trigger varicella zoster reactivation, but causal relationship is difficult to establish.
TRAVEL VACCINES	
VACCINE	**TRAVEL-ASSOCIATED INFECTION OR DISEASE OCCURRENCES & VACCINE RECOMMENDATIONS**
Cholera	Infections in travelers have been rare. Vaccination can be considered for those participating in humanitarian relief efforts.
Hepatitis A	Hepatitis A is one of the most common vaccine-preventable diseases acquired during travel. Prevaccination serologic testing for hepatitis A immunity before vaccination is not routinely recommended but may be considered in specific settings to reduce costs by not vaccinating people who are already immune.
Japanese encephalitis	Rare cases have occurred, estimated at <1 case/1 million travelers to endemic countries. However, the severe neurologic sequelae and high fatality rate warrant detailed review of trip plans to assess the level of risk.
Rabies	Rabies preexposure immunization simplifies postexposure immunoprophylaxis; rabies immunoglobulin (RIG) might be difficult to obtain in many destinations.
Tick-borne encephalitis (TBE)	Cases have been identified in travelers with an estimated risk of 1/10,000 person-months in travelers. Endemic areas are expanding in Europe. The US Food and Drug Administration has approved the use of TBE vaccine, and the Advisory Committee on Immunization Practices has voted to recommend its use in selected travelers.
Typhoid	The highest risk is for travelers going to Bangladesh (21 cases/100,000 visits), Pakistan (9 cases/100,000 visits), and India (6 cases/100,000 visits), areas where drug-resistant isolates have been increasing.
Yellow fever	Risk occurs mainly in defined areas of sub-Saharan Africa and the Amazonian regions of South America. Some countries require proof of vaccination for entry. For travelers visiting multiple countries, sequence of country entry can affect yellow fever vaccination requirement.

Abbreviations: HBsAg, hepatitis B surface antigen

[1] Based on Advisory Committee on Immunization Practices guidelines, current as of October 21, 2021

common situations for which travelers find self-treatment useful.

Travel health providers need to recognize conditions for which travelers might be at risk and provide information about appropriate self-diagnosis and treatment. Keys to a successful treatment strategy include sharing a simple disease or condition definition, recommending or prescribing treatment, and educating the traveler about the expected outcome of treatment. As an example,

BOX 2-01 The pretravel consultation: self-treatable conditions

The following list includes common situations for which travelers might find self-treatment useful. The extent of self-treatment recommendations offered to travelers should reflect the remoteness and difficulty of travel and the availability of reliable medical care at the destination. Recommended self-treatment options for each of the listed diseases are provided below or in the designated sections of this text.

ALTITUDE ILLNESS: Sec. 4, Ch. 5, High Elevation Travel & Altitude Illness
HIV EXPOSURE (OCCUPATIONAL): Sec. 9, Ch. 4, Health Care Workers, Including Public Health Researchers & Medical Laboratorians
JET LAG: Sec. 8, Ch. 4, Jet Lag
MALARIA: Sec. 5, Part 3, Ch. 16, Malaria
MOTION SICKNESS: Sec. 8, Ch. 7, Motion Sickness
TRAVELERS' DIARRHEA: Sec. 2, Ch. 6, Travelers' Diarrhea
URINARY TRACT INFECTIONS: common among many women; carrying a prescribed antibiotic for empiric treatment can be helpful.
VAGINAL YEAST INFECTIONS: self-treatment course of patient's preferred antifungal medication can be prescribed for people who are prone to infections, sexually active, or who might be receiving antibiotics for other reasons, including doxycycline for malaria chemoprophylaxis.

2

for travelers' diarrhea, inform travelers that most symptoms can be managed with fluid replacement plus loperamide or bismuth subsalicylate; prescribe travelers antibiotics they can carry with them for use in selected cases of incapacitating diarrhea (see Sec. 2, Ch. 6, Travelers' Diarrhea, and Sec. 2, Ch. 7 . . . *perspectives*: Antibiotics in Travelers' Diarrhea—Balancing Benefit & Risk); and tell them to seek medical attention if symptoms persist for 24–36 hours or are particularly severe.

With some activities in remote settings (e.g., trekking), the only alternative to self-treatment would be no treatment. Pretravel counseling might result in a more accurate self-diagnosis and treatment than relying on local medical care in some areas. In addition, the increasing awareness of substandard and counterfeit drugs in pharmacies in certain countries makes it important for travelers to bring quality manufactured drugs with them from a reliable supplier (see Sec. 6, Ch. 3, . . . *perspectives*: Avoiding Poorly Regulated Medicines & Medical Products During Travel).

Encourage travelers to carry a travel health kit with prescription and nonprescription medications and review each traveler's medication list for possible drug–drug interactions. More detailed information for providers and travelers is included in Sec. 2., Ch. 10, Travel Health Kits, and Section 3 has supplementary travel health kit information for travelers who have additional health needs and considerations.

ADDRESS SPECIAL HEALTH RISKS

Travelers with underlying health conditions require additional attention to health issues related to the destination and activities. For instance, travelers with a history of cardiac disease should carry medical reports, including a recent electrocardiogram. Asthma can flare in a traveler visiting a polluted city or from physical exertion during a hike; recommend that travelers discuss with their primary care provider a plan for treatment and carry necessary medication in case of asthma exacerbation.

Instruct travelers on how to obtain travel medical insurance and direct them to resources that provide lists of reputable medical facilities at their destination (e.g., the ISTM website [www.istm.org]; the American Society of Tropical Medicine and Hygiene website [www.astmh.org]; the US Department of State's Your Health Abroad website [https://travel.state.gov/content/travel/en/international-travel/before-you-go/your-health-abroad.html]). Advise travelers to identify any allergies or serious medical conditions on a bracelet or a card to expedite medical care in emergency situations (see Sec. 3, Ch. 4, Highly Allergic Travelers). Section 6 provides more information on preparing for and obtaining health care abroad.

EDUCATE TO CHANGE BEHAVIOR

The pretravel consultation provides another setting to remind travelers of basic health and safety practices during travel, including frequent handwashing, wearing seatbelts, using car seats for infants and children, safe sexual practices, and COVID-19 prevention. Organize topics into a checklist and place priority on the most serious and frequently encountered issues (Table 2-03

2

Table 2-03 The pretravel consultation: key discussion topics

TRAVEL-ASSOCIATED RISK	DISCUSSION POINTS
ALTITUDE ILLNESS	Determine if the itinerary puts the traveler at risk of altitude illness. Discuss preventive measures (e.g., gradual ascent, adequate hydration, medications to prevent and treat).
BLOODBORNE PATHOGENS	Avoid potential exposures (e.g., injections, piercings, tattoos, shared razors). Inform travelers who will provide health care overseas on what to do in case of needlesticks or bloodborne pathogen exposures; discuss use of HIV postexposure prophylaxis. See Box 2-02 for summary on sexual health recommendations for travelers.
DISEASE-SPECIFIC COUNSELING	Advise travelers to prepare for exacerbations or complications of underlying disease(s). Remind travelers to keep medications and supplies in carry-on luggage, to keep medications in their original prescription bottles, and to carry copies of their written prescriptions.
ENVIRONMENTAL HAZARDS	Advise travelers to avoid walking barefoot to reduce their chances of certain parasitic infections. Advise travelers to avoid wading or swimming in freshwater where risk for schistosomiasis or leptospirosis is possible. Caution travelers to avoid contact with animals to reduce the potential for bites and scratches that can transmit rabies. This is particularly important advice for the parents of young children. Remind travelers to apply sunscreen to sun-exposed skin.
IMMUNIZATIONS	Discuss indications for, effectiveness of, and adverse reactions to immunizations. Discuss benefit of antibody titers when past vaccine records are unavailable or unreliable, particularly for hepatitis A, measles, mumps, rubella, and varicella. Review routine immunizations and travel immunizations indicated for the specific itinerary and based on the traveler's medical history. Screen for chronic hepatitis B for people born in countries with HBsAg prevalence ≥2% (see Map 5-07).
MALARIA, YELLOW FEVER & OTHER VECTORBORNE DISEASES	Define vectorborne disease risks at the destination. Discuss personal protective measures and recommended insect bite precautions. For itineraries where malaria transmission is a risk: discuss risks and benefits of malaria chemoprophylaxis and recommended chemoprophylaxis choices. For itineraries where yellow fever virus transmission is a risk (see Sec. 2, Ch. 5, Yellow Fever Vaccine & Malaria Prevention Information, by Country, and Sec. 5, Part 3, Ch. 16, Yellow Fever): assess individual traveler precautions and contraindications for receiving yellow fever vaccine; discuss risks and benefits of vaccination; discuss alternatives to vaccination for travelers at increased risk for adverse events from yellow fever vaccine.

Table 2-03 The pretravel consultation: key discussion topics (continued)

TRAVEL-ASSOCIATED RISK	DISCUSSION POINTS
PERSONAL SAFETY	Advise travelers to look for security bulletins related to their destination and consider areas to avoid. Discuss precautions travelers can take (including avoiding excess alcohol consumption) to minimize risk for traffic accidents, personal assault, robbery, or drowning. Provide information on travel health and medical evacuation insurance.
RESPIRATORY ILLNESSES	Consider influenza self-treatment for high-risk travelers. Discuss diseases and destinations of particular concern.
TRAVELERS' DIARRHEA & OTHER FOOD/WATERBORNE ILLNESSES	Discuss food and water safety. Discuss antibiotics for self-treatment, adjunct medications (e.g., loperamide), and staying hydrated. Recommend strategies to decrease risk of diarrhea.

Abbreviations: HBsAg, hepatitis B surface antigen

and Box 2-02). In addition, address general issues (e.g., preventing injury, sunburn). Written information is essential to supplement oral advice and enables travelers to review the instructions from their clinic visits. CDC's Travelers' Health website (https://wwwnc.cdc.gov/travel/) provides educational material. By giving advice on health risks and self-treatable conditions, clinicians can minimize the traveler's need to seek medical care while abroad and possibly help them return to good health faster.

BOX 2-02 The pretravel consultation: summary of sexual health recommendations for travelers

BEFORE TRAVEL

Get recommended vaccinations, including those that protect against sexually transmitted infections (STIs).
Get recommended tests for HIV and treatable STIs. Be aware of STI symptoms in case any develop.
Obtain condoms to carry on trip.
Consider preexposure prophylaxis medication for HIV for high-risk travelers.
Review local laws about sexual practices and obtain contact information for medical and law enforcement services.
If pregnant or considering pregnancy, review whether Zika virus infection is a risk at destination.

DURING TRAVEL

Use condoms consistently and correctly to decrease the risk of HIV and STIs.
If indicated, be prepared to start taking medications for HIV postexposure prophylaxis or unintended pregnancy within 72 hours after a high-risk sexual encounter.
Never engage in sex with a minor (<18 years old), child pornography, or trafficking activities in any country.
Report suspicious activity to US and local authorities as soon as it occurs.

AFTER TRAVEL

Avoid exposing sexual partners at home. See a clinician to get recommended tests for HIV and STIs.
Get treatment for all diagnosed, treatable STIs.

BIBLIOGRAPHY

Freedman DO, Chen LH. Vaccines for international travel. Mayo Clin Proc. 2019;94(11):2314–39.

Hatz CFR, Chen LH. Pre-travel consultation. In: Keystone JS, Freedman DO, Kozarsky PE, Connor BA, Nothdurft HD, editors. Travel medicine, 4th ed. Philadelphia: Saunders Elsevier; 2019. pp. 25–30.

Hill DR, Ericsson CD, Pearson RD, Keystone JS, Freedman DO, Kozarsky PE, et al. The practice of travel medicine: guidelines by the Infectious Diseases Society of America. Clin Infect Dis. 2006;43(12):1499–539.

International Society of Travel Medicine. The ISTM Body of knowledge for the practice of travel medicine, revised 2017. Atlanta: International Society of Travel Medicine; 2017. Available from: www.istm.org/bodyofknowledge2.

Kozarsky PE, Steffen R. Travel medicine education—what are the needs? J Travel Med. 2016;23(5):taw039.

Leder K, Chen LH, Wilson ME. Aggregate travel vs. single trip assessment: arguments for cumulative risk analysis. Vaccine. 2012;30(15):2600–4.

Leder K, Torresi J, Libman MD, Cramer JP, Castelli F, Schlagenhauf P, et al. GeoSentinel surveillance of illness in returned travelers, 2007–2011. Ann Intern Med. 2013;158(6):456–68.

Leung DT, LaRocque RC, Ryan ET. In the clinic: travel medicine. Ann Intern Med. 2018 Jan 2;168(1):ITC1–16.

Steffen R. Travel vaccine preventable diseases—updated logarithmic scale with monthly incidence rates. J Travel Med. 2018;25(1):tay046.

TRAVELERS' PERCEPTION OF RISK

David Shlim

Travel medicine is based on the concept of risk reduction. In the context of travel medicine, "risk" refers to the possibility of harm occurring during a trip. Some risks are avoidable, while others are not. For example, vaccine-preventable diseases can be mostly avoided, depending on the protective efficacy of the vaccine. Perception of risk is a subjective evaluation of whether a risk is considered large or small; is 1 in 10,000 a large risk or a small risk? Tolerance refers to acknowledging a risk and accepting it; a risk of 1 in 100,000 might be tolerable for one traveler but not for another. The overall perception of risk is based on a combination of likelihood and severity. A low likelihood of a severe and untreatable disease might be perceived as more important than the greater likelihood of a less severe disease.

The rates of diseases (e.g., typhoid fever, malaria, Japanese encephalitis [JE]) in a particular country or location might not suffice for clinicians or travelers to make an individualized decision. Disease risks can range from 1 in 500 (an estimate of the risk for typhoid fever in unvaccinated travelers to Nepal) to 1 in 1,000,000 (an estimate of the risk for JE in travelers to Asia), and travelers need to determine what these statistics mean to them. Additional information to help make an informed decision should, most importantly, include the severity of the disease, how readily the disease can be treated, and the length and type of travel. For example, the disease risks encountered by high-end African safari goers might be quite different than the disease risks for people going to work in resource-poor areas of the same countries.

Even when risk is low, travelers' decisions will still reflect their perception and tolerance of risk. When told that the risk for JE is 1 in 1,000,000, one traveler might reply, "Then I guess I don't have to worry about it," while another might say, "That 1 will be me!" Each traveler will have their own ideas about the risks, benefits, and costs of vaccines and drug prophylaxis; clinicians should discuss these with travelers in detail, with the goal of shared decision-making.

Perception and tolerance of risk are connected to the concept of commitment, particularly in regard to remote, adventurous travel. Commitment refers to the fact that certain parts of a journey might not easily be reversed once entered upon. For example, a traveler trekking into a remote area might need to accept that rescue, if available at all, could be delayed for days. A traveler who has a myocardial infarction in a country with no advanced cardiac services might have a difficult time obtaining definitive medical care. If the traveler has already contemplated and accepted this commitment, they can more appropriately prepare to deal with health concerns if they occur.

The goal of travel medicine should be to help travelers assess the various risks they could face and then educate them on how to manage and minimize, rather than try to eliminate, those risks. Travel medicine practitioners should discuss available risk statistics and discern the traveler's perception and tolerance of risk, including their concerns about the risks from vaccines and prophylactic medications. Once this is done, the provider can then help travelers find their individual comfort level when making decisions about destinations, activities, and prevention measures.

Coronavirus disease 2019 (COVID-19) has had a profound impact on travelers' perception of risk. Every aspect of travel is now colored by the presence of severe acute respiratory syndrome coronavirus 2 (SARS-CoV-2), from the mixing of travelers on the journey itself, to destination

(continued)

TRAVELERS' PERCEPTION OF RISK (CONTINUED)

accommodations and dining venues, to recreation and tourism activities. In addition, now, more than ever before, individual travelers are confronting and addressing their role as potential conduits for the global spread of disease; to minimize the risk of COVID-19 transmission to others, responsible travel currently entails (at a minimum) pretravel vaccination, a negative COVID-19 test result, and posttravel quarantine. The constantly shifting landscape, unprecedented in travel medicine, has upended our understanding and perception of risk. Figuring out whether travel is even safe or wise has become the most prominent decision people must now make, with no easy answers. What is true one week can be completely different a week later.

Risk perception, as it relates to travel in the era of COVID-19, is twofold: the risk of acquiring the disease while traveling, and the risk of being stranded by sudden lockdowns, quarantine, and flight cancellations. Travelers now have to weigh all of these issues well in advance, when planning for the typical overseas journey starts, and try to make guesses about the situation that could exist months into the future. As travel medicine providers, the best guidance we can give to travelers is to refer them to reliable resources of information about the latest conditions at their destination and help them remain flexible and willing to cancel their trip, even at the last moment, if or when the situation at the destination begins to worsen.

. . . *perspectives* chapters supplement the clinical guidance in this book with additional content, context, and expert opinion. The views expressed do not necessarily represent the official position of the Centers for Disease Control and Prevention (CDC).

VACCINATION & IMMUNOPROPHYLAXIS—GENERAL PRINCIPLES

Andrew Kroger, Mark Freedman

The pretravel health consultation is an opportunity to administer routine vaccines that are recommended based on age and other individual characteristics, and travel medicine practitioners should therefore be familiar with the general principles of vaccination and immunoprophylaxis. Routine vaccinations that are usually administered during childhood and adolescence in the United States include diphtheria, tetanus, pertussis (DTaP); *Haemophilus influenzae* type b (Hib); hepatitis A (HepA), hepatitis B (HepB); human papillomavirus (HPV); measles-mumps-rubella (MMR); meningococcal vaccine (MenACWY); pneumococcal disease, including pneumococcal conjugate vaccine (PCV13) and pneumococcal polysaccharide vaccine (PPSV23); poliomyelitis (IPV); rotavirus; and varicella. Influenza vaccine routinely is recommended for all people aged ≥6 months each year. Herpes zoster (shingles) vaccine is recommended for adults aged ≥50 years old. PPSV23 is recommended for all adults ≥65 years old.

Some routine vaccinations are administered at earlier ages for international travelers. For example, measles-mumps-rubella (MMR) vaccine is indicated for infants aged 6–11 months who travel abroad, and hepatitis A vaccine is indicated for some infants aged 6–11 months who travel abroad, whereas these vaccines are not routinely given before age 12 months in the United States.

The Advisory Committee on Immunization Practices (ACIP) website (www.cdc.gov/vaccines/acip/index.html) outlines recommendations, background, adverse reactions, precautions, and contraindications for vaccines and toxoids. For information on vaccinating travelers with altered immune function, see Sec. 3, Ch. 1, Immunocompromised Travelers.

SPACING OF VACCINES & IMMUNOBIOLOGICS

In general, most common vaccines can be given at the same visit, at separate injection sites, without impairing antibody responses or increasing rates of adverse reactions, except as outlined below. Simultaneous administration of indicated vaccines is particularly advantageous for international travelers for whom exposure to several infectious diseases might be imminent. Injectable live vaccines should be administered at intervals of ≥28 days, if not administered simultaneously.

Coronavirus Disease 2019 Vaccines

Coronavirus disease 2019 (COVID-19) vaccines can be administered concomitantly with any other vaccines. For COVID-19 vaccine and immunization information, including interim clinical considerations, see www.cdc.gov/vaccines/covid-19/index.html.

Live-Virus Vaccines

The immune response to an injected or intranasal live-virus vaccine (e.g., MMR, varicella, live attenuated influenza vaccines [LAIV]), might be impaired if administered within 28 days of another live-virus vaccine. Typically, the immune response is impaired only for the second live-virus vaccine administered. Whenever possible, providers should administer injected or intranasal live-virus vaccines on different days ≥28 days apart. If 2 injected or intranasal live-virus vaccines are administered on separate days, but administered <28 days apart, the second vaccine is invalid and should be readministered ≥28 days after the invalid dose.

Measles and other live-virus vaccines can interfere with the response to tuberculin skin testing and the interferon-γ release assay. Tuberculin testing, if otherwise indicated, can be done either on the same day that live-virus vaccines are administered or ≥4 weeks later.

YELLOW FEVER VACCINE

There is no evidence that inactivated vaccines interfere with the immune response to yellow fever vaccine. Therefore, inactivated vaccines can be administered at any time around yellow fever vaccination, including simultaneously. ACIP recommends that yellow fever vaccine be given at the same time as most other live-virus vaccines.

Notwithstanding ACIP's recommendation, limited data suggest that coadministration of yellow fever vaccine with measles-rubella or MMR vaccines might decrease the immune response. One study involving the simultaneous administration of yellow fever and MMR vaccines and a second involving simultaneous administration of yellow fever and measles-rubella vaccines in children demonstrated a decreased immune response against all antigens (except measles) when the vaccines were given on the same day versus 30 days apart. Additional studies are needed to confirm these findings, but the findings suggest that, if possible, yellow fever and MMR vaccines should be given ≥30 days apart.

No data are available on immune response to nasally administered LAIV given simultaneously with yellow fever vaccine. Data from LAIV and MMR vaccines found no evidence of interference, however. If yellow fever vaccine and another injectable live-virus vaccine are not administered simultaneously or ≥30 days apart, providers might consider measuring the patient's neutralizing antibody response to vaccination before travel. Contact the state health department or the Centers for Disease Control and Prevention (CDC) Arboviral Disease Branch (970-221-6400) to discuss serologic testing.

Meningococcal & Pneumococcal Vaccines

In people with conditions that increase the risk for invasive pneumococcal disease (e.g., HIV infection, anatomic or functional asplenia [including sickle-cell disease]), the quadrivalent meningococcal vaccine Menactra (MenACWY-D), should be administered at least 4 weeks after completion of the pneumococcal conjugate vaccine (PCV13) series. Menactra should not be used in children <2 years of age with these risk conditions; MenACWY-CRM (Menveo) can be used instead (see Sec. 5, Part 1, Ch. 13, Meningococcal Disease, for meningococcal vaccine schedules).

Menactra can be administered before or concomitantly with DTaP. If this is not possible, Menactra should be administered 6 months after DTaP in people with HIV infection, anatomic or functional asplenia (including sickle-cell disease), or persistent complement component deficiency, conditions that increase the risk for invasive meningococcal disease.

PCV13 and the pneumococcal polysaccharide vaccine (PPSV23) should be administered at least 8 weeks apart. The minimum interval might be longer than 8 weeks depending on risk-condition and the order in which the vaccines are administered.

Missed Doses & Boosters

In some cases, a scheduled dose of vaccine might not be given on time. Travelers might forget to return to complete a series or receive a booster at a specified time. If this occurs, the dose should be given at the next visit. Available data indicate that intervals longer than those routinely recommended between doses do not affect seroconversion rates or titer when the vaccine schedule is completed. Consequently, an extended interval between doses does not necessitate restarting the series or adding doses of any vaccine. One exception is the preexposure rabies vaccine series. If an extended interval passes between doses of the preexposure rabies vaccine series, clinicians should assess the patient's immune status by serologic testing 7–14 days after the final dose in the series.

Antibody-Containing Blood Products

Antibody-containing blood products from the United States (e.g., immune globulin [IG] products) do not interfere with the immune response to yellow fever vaccine and are not believed to interfere with the response to LAIV or rotavirus vaccines. When MMR and varicella vaccines are given shortly before, simultaneously with, or after an antibody-containing blood product, response to the vaccine can be diminished. The duration of inhibition of MMR and varicella vaccines is related to the dose of IG in the product. MMR and varicella vaccines should either be administered ≥2 weeks before receipt of a blood product or should be delayed 3–11 months after receipt of the blood product, depending on the dose and type of blood product (see Timing and Spacing of Immunobiologics, General Best Practice Guidelines for Immunization: Best Practices Guidance of the Advisory Committee on Immunization Practices; Table 3-6. Recommended intervals between administration of antibody-containing products and measles- or varicella-containing vaccine, by product and indication for vaccination [www.cdc.gov/vaccines/hcp/acip-recs/general-recs/timing.html#t-05]).

If IG administration becomes necessary for another indication after MMR or varicella vaccines have been given, the IG might interfere with the immune response to the MMR or varicella vaccines. Vaccine virus replication and stimulation of immunity usually occur 2–3 weeks after vaccination. If the interval between administration of one of these live vaccines and the subsequent administration of an IG preparation is ≥14 days, the vaccine need not be readministered. If the interval is <14 days, the vaccine should be readministered after the interval shown in Table 3-5 (referenced in the previous paragraph), unless serologic testing indicates that antibodies have been produced. Such testing should be performed after the interval shown in Table 3-5 to avoid detecting antibodies from the IG preparation.

In some circumstances, MMR or varicella vaccine might be indicated for a patient for preexposure (travel) or postexposure prophylaxis. The patient might have received an antibody-containing blood product unrelated to prophylaxis; nevertheless, a potential for vaccine interference exists. Providers can administer MMR or varicella vaccines because the increased risk for disease and the protection afforded by the vaccine outweigh the concern that the vaccine might be less effective because of interference. If the dose is administered, it does not count toward the routine vaccination series and an additional dose of MMR or varicella vaccine should be administered no earlier than the minimum interval for the antibody-containing blood product (highlighted in ACIP's General Best Practice Guidelines for Immunization) applied to the invalid dose of vaccine.

When IG is given with the first dose of hepatitis A vaccine, the proportion of recipients who develop a protective level of antibody is not affected, but antibody concentrations are lower. Because the final concentrations of antibody are still many times higher than those considered protective, the reduced immunogenicity is not expected to be clinically relevant. However, the effect of reduced antibody concentrations on long-term protection is unknown.

IG preparations interact minimally with other inactivated vaccines and toxoids. Other inactivated vaccines can be given simultaneously or at any time interval before or after an antibody-containing blood product is used. However, such vaccines should be administered at different injection sites from the IG.

VACCINATING PEOPLE WITH ACUTE ILLNESSES

Clinicians should take every opportunity to provide needed vaccinations. The decision to delay vaccination because of a current or recent acute illness depends on the severity of the symptoms and their cause. Although a moderate or severe acute illness is sufficient reason to postpone vaccination, minor illnesses (e.g., diarrhea, mild upper respiratory infection with or without low-grade fever, other low-grade febrile illness) are not contraindications to vaccination.

Antimicrobial therapy is not a contraindication to vaccination, except for antiviral agents active against influenza virus (e.g., baloxavir, oseltamivir, peramivir, zanamivir), since these antivirals can interfere with the replication of the live vaccine. If LAIV is administered first, any of these 4 antiviral drugs should be delayed ≥2 weeks, if feasible. Conversely, clinicians should delay LAIV for 48 hours after oseltamivir or zanamivir; for 5 days after peramivir; and for 17 days after baloxavir. Alternatively, clinicians can substitute inactivated influenza vaccine (IIV) for LAIV. Use of antiviral agents active against herpes viruses (e.g., acyclovir), are a precaution against administration of varicella-containing vaccines (varicella, MMRV) because the antiviral agent will interfere with the live vaccine.

Antimicrobial agents can prevent adequate immune response to live attenuated oral typhoid and cholera vaccines.

VACCINATION SCHEDULING FOR SELECTED TRAVEL VACCINES

Table 2-04 lists the minimum ages and minimum intervals between doses for available travel vaccines recommended in the United States. Available travel vaccines, including Japanese encephalitis vaccine, rabies vaccine, inactivated typhoid vaccine, and yellow fever vaccine, do not have routine non-travel recommendations.

ALLERGIES TO VACCINE COMPONENTS

Vaccine components can cause allergic reactions in some recipients. Reactions can be local or systemic and can include anaphylaxis or anaphylactic-like responses. A previous severe allergic reaction to any vaccine, regardless of the component suspected of being responsible for the reaction, is a contraindication to future receipt of the vaccine. Vaccine components responsible for reactions can include adjuvants, animal proteins, antibiotics, the vaccine antigen, preservatives (e.g., thimerosal), stabilizers (e.g., gelatin), or yeast.

Antibiotics & Preservatives

Some vaccines contain trace amounts of antibiotics or preservatives to which people might be allergic. Antibiotics used during vaccine manufacture include gentamicin, neomycin, polymyxin B, and streptomycin. The antibiotics most likely to cause severe allergic reactions (e.g., penicillin, cephalosporins, and sulfa drugs) are not contained in vaccines. Providers administering vaccines should carefully review the prescribing information before deciding if a person with antibiotic allergy should receive the vaccine.

Hepatitis A vaccine, some hepatitis B vaccines, some influenza vaccines, MMR vaccine, IPV, rabies vaccine, smallpox vaccine, and varicella vaccine contain trace amounts of neomycin or other antibiotics; the amount is less than

2

Table 2-04 Recommended & minimum ages, minimum intervals for travel vaccine doses[1]

VACCINE NAME	DOSE	RECOMMENDED AGE	MINIMUM AGE	MINIMUM INTERVAL BETWEEN DOSES
Japanese encephalitis Vero cell (IXIARO)[2]	1	2 months–17 years old 18–65 years old	≥2 months old ≥18 years old	28 days 7 days
	2	2 months–17 years old 18–65 years old	28 days after DOSE 1 7 days after DOSE 1	N/A
Rabies (preexposure)	1		See footnote 3	
	2		7 days after DOSE 1	14 days
	3[4]		21 days–3 years after DOSE 1	N/A
Typhoid Inactivated (ViCPS)		≥2 years	≥2 years	N/A
Typhoid Live attenuated (Ty21a)		≥6 years	≥6 years	See footnote 5
Yellow fever		≥9 months[6]	≥9 months[6]	10 years[7]

Abbreviations: N/A, not applicable; ViCPS, Vi capsular polysaccharide

[1]Adapted from Table 1, Centers for Disease Control and Prevention. General recommendations on immunization: recommendations of the Advisory Committee on Immunization Practices (ACIP). MMWR Recomm Rep. 2011;60(RR-2):1–61.

[2]IXIARO is approved by the US Food and Drug Administration for people aged ≥2 months.

[3]Preexposure immunization for rabies has no minimum age. Reference: Centers for Disease Control and Prevention. Human rabies prevention—United States, 2008: recommendations of the Advisory Committee on Immunization Practices. MMWR Recomm Rep. 2008;57(RR-3):1–28.

[4]Consider administering a third dose of preexposure rabies vaccine to people expecting long-term rabies exposure risks.

[5]Oral typhoid vaccine is recommended to be administered 1 hour before a meal with a cold or lukewarm drink (temperature not to exceed body temperature—98.6°F [37°C]) on alternate days, for a total of 4 doses.

[6]Yellow fever vaccine may be administered to children aged <9 months in certain situations. Reference: Centers for Disease Control and Prevention. Yellow fever vaccine: recommendations of the Advisory Committee on Immunization Practices (ACIP). MMWR Recomm Rep. 2010;59(RR-7):1–27.

[7]Subsequent doses of yellow fever vaccine are recommended for people who previously received vaccine while pregnant, with HIV, or prior to a hematopoietic stem cell transplant (HSCT). Subsequent doses of yellow fever vaccine also are recommended for people at increased risk of contracting yellow fever due to the specific location or duration of travel, or due to virulent virus exposure (e.g., yellow fever laboratory workers). For others, only 1 lifetime dose is recommended.

would normally be used for the skin test to determine hypersensitivity. However, people who have experienced anaphylactic reactions to neomycin generally should not receive these vaccines. Most often, neomycin allergic response is a contact dermatitis—a manifestation of a delayed-type (cell-mediated) immune response—rather than anaphylaxis. A history of delayed-type reactions to neomycin is not a contraindication to receiving these vaccines.

Egg Protein

The most common animal protein allergen is egg protein in vaccines prepared by using embryonated chicken eggs (e.g., yellow fever vaccine, some influenza vaccines).

People who can eat lightly cooked eggs (e.g., scrambled eggs) without a reaction are unlikely to be egg allergic. Egg-allergic people might tolerate egg in baked products (e.g., bread or cake). Tolerance to egg-containing foods does not exclude the possibility of egg allergy. Egg allergy can be confirmed by a consistent medical history of adverse reactions to eggs and egg-containing foods, plus skin or blood testing for immunoglobulin E directed against egg proteins.

People with a history of egg allergy who have experienced only hives after exposure to egg may receive influenza vaccine. Any licensed and recommended influenza vaccine that is otherwise appropriate for the recipient's age and health status may be used.

Those who report having had reactions to egg involving symptoms other than hives (e.g., angioedema, recurrent emesis, lightheadedness, or respiratory distress), or who required epinephrine or another emergency medical intervention, may similarly receive any licensed and recommended influenza vaccine that is otherwise appropriate for the recipient's age and health status. The selected vaccine should be administered in an inpatient or outpatient medical setting, and vaccine administration should be supervised by a health care provider who is able to recognize and manage severe allergic conditions. Cell-culture influenza vaccine (ccIIV4) and recombinant influenza vaccine do not require administration in a supervised setting, since neither vaccine is isolated or grown in eggs nor contains egg protein.

If a person has an egg allergy or a positive skin test to yellow fever vaccine but the vaccination is recommended because of their travel destination–specific risk, desensitization can be performed under direct supervision of a physician experienced in the management of anaphylaxis.

Thimerosal

Thimerosal, an organic mercurial compound in use since the 1930s, has been added to certain immunobiologic products as a preservative for multidose vials. Receiving thimerosal-containing vaccines has been postulated to lead to allergy induction. However, limited scientific evidence is available for this assertion. Allergy to thimerosal usually consists of local delayed-type hypersensitivity reactions. Thimerosal elicits positive delayed-type hypersensitivity to patch tests in 1%–18% of people tested, but these tests have limited or no clinical relevance. Most people do not experience reactions to thimerosal administered as a component of vaccines, even when patch or intradermal tests for thimerosal indicate hypersensitivity. A localized or delayed-type hypersensitivity reaction to thimerosal is not a contraindication to receipt of a vaccine that contains thimerosal.

Since mid-2001, non-influenza vaccines routinely recommended for infants have been manufactured without thimerosal. Vaccines that still contain thimerosal as a preservative include some influenza vaccines, one DT vaccine (www.fda.gov/media/119411/download), and one Td vaccine. Additional information about thimerosal and the thimerosal content of vaccines is available on the US Food and Drug Administration website (www.fda.gov/vaccines-blood-biologics/safety-availability-biologics/thimerosal-and-vaccines).

INJECTION ROUTE & INJECTION SITE

Injectable vaccines are administered by intramuscular and subcutaneous routes. The injection method depends in part on the presence of an adjuvant in some vaccines. Adjuvant refers to a vaccine component, distinct from the antigen, which enhances the immune response to the antigen. Providers should inject vaccines containing an adjuvant (DTaP, DT, HepA, HepB, Hib, HPV, PCV13, Td, Tdap, recombinant zoster vaccine [RZV]) into a muscle mass because subcutaneous or intradermal administration can cause local induration, inflammation, irritation, skin discoloration, and granuloma formation.

Detailed discussion and recommendations about vaccination for people with bleeding disorders or receiving anticoagulant therapy are available in the ACIP's General Best Practices Guidelines for Immunization (www.cdc.gov/vaccines/hcp/acip-recs/general-recs/index.html).

Immunobiologic manufacturers recommend the routes of administration for each product. Deviation from the recommended route of administration can reduce vaccine efficacy or increase local adverse reactions. ACIP publishes detailed recommendations on the route and site for all vaccines. CDC compiled a list of these publications at www.cdc.gov/vaccines/hcp/acip-recs.

POST-IMMUNIZATION ADVERSE EVENT REPORTING

Modern vaccines are safe and effective. Benefits and risks are associated with the use of all immunobiologics. Adverse events after immunization have been reported with all vaccines, ranging from frequent, minor, local reactions (e.g., pain at the injection site), to extremely rare, severe, systemic illness, such as that associated with yellow fever vaccine. Adverse events following specific vaccines and toxoids are discussed in detail in each ACIP statement.

2

In the United States, clinicians are required by law to report selected adverse events occurring after vaccination with any vaccine in the recommended childhood series. In addition, CDC strongly recommends that all vaccine adverse events be reported to the Vaccine Adverse Event Reporting System (VAERS), even if a causal relation to vaccination is not certain. VAERS reporting forms and information are available electronically at www.vaers.hhs.gov or can be requested by telephone at 800-822-7967 (toll-free). Clinicians are encouraged to report electronically at https://vaers.hhs.gov/esub/index.jsp.

BIBLIOGRAPHY

Ezeanolue E, Harriman K, Hunter P, Kroger A, and Pellegrini C. General best practice guidelines for immunization: best practices guidance of the Advisory Committee on Immunization Practices (ACIP) Available from: www.cdc.gov/vaccines/hcp/acip-recs/general-recs/index.html.

Grohskopf LA, Alyanak E, Broder KR, Blanton LH, Fry AM, Jernigan DB, et al. Prevention and control of seasonal influenza with vaccines: recommendations of the Advisory Committee on Immunization Practices—United States, 2020–21 influenza season. MMWR Recomm Rep. 2020;69(8):1–24.

Mbaeyi SA, Bozio CH, Duffy J, Rubin LG, Hariri S, Stephens DS, et al. Meningococcal vaccination: recommendations of the Advisory Committee on Immunization Practices, United States, 2020. MMWR Recomm Rep. 2020;69(9):1–41.

Neunert C, Lim W, Crowther M, Cohen A, Solberg L, Crowther MA. The American Society of Hematology 2011 evidence-based practice guideline for immune thrombocytopenia. Blood. 2011;117(16):4190–207.

Shimabukuro TT, Nguyen M, Martin D, DeStefano F. Safety monitoring in the Vaccine Adverse Event Reporting System (VAERS). Vaccine. 2015;33(36):4398–405.

Staples JE, Bocchini JA Jr., Rubin L, Fischer M. Yellow fever vaccine booster doses: recommendations of the Advisory Committee on Immunization Practices, 2015. MMWR Morb Mortal Wkly Rep. 2015;64(23):647–50.

INTERACTIONS BETWEEN TRAVEL VACCINES & DRUGS

Ilan Youngster, Elizabeth Barnett

During pretravel consultations, travel health providers must consider potential interactions between vaccines and medications, including those already taken by the traveler. A study by S. Steinlauf et al. identified potential drug–drug interactions with travel-related medications in 45% of travelers taking medications for chronic conditions; 3.5% of these interactions were potentially serious.

VACCINE–VACCINE INTERACTIONS

Most common vaccines can be given safely and effectively at the same visit, at separate injection sites, without impairing antibody response or increasing rates of adverse reactions. However, certain vaccines, including pneumococcal and meningococcal vaccines and live virus vaccines, require appropriate spacing; further information about vaccine–vaccine interactions is found in Sec. 2, Ch. 3, Vaccination & Immunoprophylaxis—General Principles.

TRAVEL VACCINES & DRUGS

Live Attenuated Oral Typhoid & Cholera Vaccines

Live attenuated vaccines generally should be avoided in immunocompromised travelers, including those taking antimetabolites, calcineurin inhibitors, cytotoxic agents, immunomodulators, and high-dose steroids (see Table 3-04).

ANTIMALARIAL DRUGS

Chloroquine and atovaquone-proguanil at doses used for malaria chemoprophylaxis can be given concurrently with oral typhoid vaccine. Data from an older formulation of the CVD 103-HgR oral cholera vaccine suggest that the immune response to the vaccine might be diminished when given concomitantly with chloroquine. Administer live attenuated oral cholera vaccine ≥10 days before beginning antimalarial prophylaxis with chloroquine. A study in children using oral cholera vaccine suggested no decrease in immunogenicity when given with atovaquone-proguanil.

ANTIMICROBIAL AGENTS

Antimicrobial agents can be active against the vaccine strains in the oral typhoid and cholera vaccines and might prevent adequate immune response to these vaccines. Therefore, delay vaccination with oral typhoid vaccine by >72 hours and delay oral cholera vaccine by >14 days after administration of antimicrobial agents. Parenteral typhoid vaccine is an alternative to the oral typhoid vaccine for travelers who have recently received antibiotics.

Rabies Vaccine

Concomitant use of chloroquine can reduce the antibody response to intradermal rabies vaccine administered as a preexposure vaccination. Use the intramuscular route for people taking chloroquine concurrently. Intradermal administration of rabies vaccine is not currently approved for use in the United States (see Sec. 5, Part 2, Ch. 19, . . . *perspectives*: Rabies Immunization).

ANTIMALARIAL DRUGS

Any time a new medication is prescribed, including antimalarial drugs, check for known or possible drug interactions (see Table 2-05) and inform the traveler of potential risks. Online clinical decision support tools (e.g., Micromedex) provide searchable databases of drug interactions.

2

Atovaquone-Proguanil

ANTIBIOTICS

Rifabutin, rifampin, and tetracycline might reduce plasma concentrations of atovaquone and should not be used concurrently with atovaquone-proguanil.

ANTICOAGULANTS

Patients on warfarin might need to reduce their anticoagulant dose or monitor their prothrombin time more closely while taking atovaquone-proguanil, although coadministration of these drugs is not contraindicated. The use of novel oral anticoagulants, including dabigatran, rivaroxaban, and apixaban, is not expected to cause significant interactions, and their use has been suggested as an alternative for patients in need of anticoagulation.

ANTIEMETICS

Metoclopramide can reduce bioavailability of atovaquone; unless no other antiemetics are available, this antiemetic should not be used to treat vomiting associated with the use of atovaquone at treatment doses.

ANTIHISTAMINES

Travelers taking atovaquone-proguanil for malaria prophylaxis should avoid using cimetidine (an H2 receptor antagonist) because this medication interferes with proguanil metabolism.

HIV MEDICATIONS

Atovaquone-proguanil might interact with the antiretroviral protease inhibitors atazanavir, darunavir, indinavir, lopinavir, and ritonavir, or the nonnucleoside reverse transcriptase inhibitors (NNRTIs) efavirenz, etravirine, and nevirapine, resulting in decreased levels of atovaquone-proguanil. For travelers taking any of

2

Table 2-05 Drugs & drug classes that can interact with selected antimalarials

ANTIMALARIALS	DRUGS & DRUG CLASSES THAT CAN INTERACT
Atovaquone-proguanil	Cimetidine Fluvoxamine Metoclopromide Rifabutin Rifampin Tetracycline Warfarin
Chloroquine	Ampicillin Antacids Calcineurin inhibitors Cimetidine Ciprofloxacin CYP2D6 enzyme substrates[1] CYP3A4 enzyme inhibitors[2] Digoxin Kaolin Methotrexate QT-prolonging agents[3]
Doxycycline	Antacids Bismuth subsalicylate Barbiturates Calcineurin inhibitors Carbamazepine Iron-containing preparations mTOR inhibitors Penicillin Phenytoin Warfarin
Mefloquine	Antiarrhythmic agents Anticonvulsants Beta blockers Calcineurin inhibitors Calcium channel receptor antagonists CYP3A4 enzyme inducers[4] CYP3A4 enzyme inhibitors[2] H1 receptor antagonists Lumefantrine mTOR inhibitors Phenothiazines Protease inhibitors Tricyclic antidepressants

[1]Examples include flecainide, fluoxetine, metoprolol, paroxetine, and propranolol.
[2]Examples include antiretroviral protease inhibitors (e.g., atazanavir, darunavir, lopinavir, ritonavir, saquinavir); azole antifungals (e.g., itraconazole, ketoconazole, posaconazole, voriconazole); macrolide antibiotics (e.g., azithromycin, clarithromycin, erythromycin); selective serotonin reuptake inhibitors (SSRIs; e.g., fluoxetine, fluvoxamine, sertraline); and cobicistat.
[3]Examples include amiodarone, lumefantrine, and sotalol.
[4]Examples include efavirenz, etravirine, nevirapine, rifabutin, rifampin, and glucocorticoids.

these medications, consider alternative malaria chemoprophylaxis (https://clinicalinfo.hiv.gov/en/table/table-5-significant-pharmacokinetic-interactions-between-drugs-used-treat-or-prevent).

SELECTIVE SEROTONIN REUPTAKE INHIBITORS

Fluvoxamine interferes with the metabolism of proguanil; consider an alternative antimalarial prophylaxis to atovaquone-proguanil for travelers taking this selective serotonin reuptake inhibitor (SSRI).

Chloroquine

ANTACIDS & ANTIDIARRHEALS

Chloroquine absorption might be reduced by antacids or kaolin; travelers should wait ≥4 hours between doses of these medications.

ANTIBIOTICS

Chloroquine inhibits bioavailability of ampicillin, and travelers should wait ≥2 hours between doses of these medications. Chloroquine should not be coadministered with either clarithromycin or erythromycin; azithromycin is a suggested alternative (https://clinicalinfo.hiv.gov/en/table/table-5-significant-pharmacokinetic-interactions-between-drugs-used-treat-or-prevent). Chloroquine also reportedly decreases the bioavailability of ciprofloxacin.

ANTIHISTAMINES

Concomitant use of cimetidine and chloroquine should be avoided because cimetidine can inhibit the metabolism of chloroquine and increase drug levels.

CYP2D6 ENZYME SUBSTRATES

Chloroquine is a CYP2D6 enzyme inhibitor. Monitor patients taking chloroquine concomitantly with other substrates of this enzyme (e.g., flecainide, fluoxetine, metoprolol, paroxetine, propranolol) for side effects.

CYP3A4 ENZYME INHIBITORS

CYP3A4 inhibitors (e.g., erythromycin, ketoconazole, ritonavir) can increase chloroquine levels; concomitant use should be avoided.

DIGOXIN

Chloroquine can increase digoxin levels; additional monitoring is warranted.

IMMUNOSUPPRESSANTS

Chloroquine decreases the bioavailability of methotrexate. Chloroquine also can cause increased levels of calcineurin inhibitors; use caution when prescribing chloroquine to travelers taking these agents.

QT-PROLONGING AGENTS

Avoid prescribing chloroquine to anyone taking other QT-prolonging agents (e.g., amiodarone, lumefantrine, sotalol); when taken in combination, chloroquine might increase the risk for prolonged QTc interval. In addition, the antiretroviral rilpivirine has also been shown to prolong QTc, and clinicians should avoid coadministration with chloroquine.

Doxycycline

ANTACIDS, BISMUTH SUBSALICYLATE, IRON

Absorption of tetracyclines might be impaired by aluminum-, calcium-, or magnesium-containing antacids, bismuth subsalicylate, and preparations containing iron; advise patients not to take these preparations within 3 hours of taking doxycycline.

ANTIBIOTICS

Doxycycline can interfere with the bactericidal activity of penicillin; thus, in general, clinicians should not prescribe these drugs together. Coadministration of doxycycline with rifabutin or rifampin can lower doxycycline levels; monitor doxycycline efficacy closely or consider alternative therapy.

ANTICOAGULANTS

Patients on warfarin might need to reduce their anticoagulant dose while taking doxycycline because of its ability to depress plasma prothrombin activity.

ANTICONVULSANTS

Barbiturates, carbamazepine, and phenytoin can decrease the half-life of doxycycline.

ANTIRETROVIRALS

Doxycycline has no known interaction with antiretroviral agents.

IMMUNOSUPPRESSANTS

Concurrent use of doxycycline and calcineurin inhibitors or mTOR inhibitors (sirolimus) can cause increased levels of these immunosuppressant drugs.

Mefloquine

Mefloquine can interact with several categories of drugs, including anticonvulsants, other antimalarial drugs, and drugs that alter cardiac conduction.

ANTICONVULSANTS

Mefloquine can lower plasma levels of several anticonvulsant medications, including carbamazepine, phenobarbital, phenytoin, and valproic acid; avoid concurrent use of mefloquine with these agents.

ANTIMALARIAL DRUGS

Mefloquine is associated with increased toxicities of the antimalarial drug lumefantrine, which is available in the United States in fixed combination to treat people with uncomplicated *Plasmodium falciparum* malaria. The combination of mefloquine and lumefantrine can cause potentially fatal QTc interval prolongation. Lumefantrine should therefore be avoided or used with caution in patients taking mefloquine prophylaxis.

CYP3A4 ENZYME INDUCERS

CYP3A4 inducers include medications used to treat HIV or HIV-associated infections (e.g., efavirenz, etravirine, nevirapine, rifabutin) and tuberculosis (rifampin). St. John's wort and glucocorticoids are also CYP3A4 inducers. All these drugs (rifabutin and rifampin, in particular) can decrease plasma concentrations of mefloquine, thereby reducing its efficacy as an antimalarial drug.

CYP3A4 ENZYME INHIBITORS

Potent CYP3A4 inhibitors (e.g., antiretroviral protease inhibitors, atazanavir, cobicistat [available in combination with elvitegravir], darunavir, lopinavir, ritonavir, saquinavir); azole antifungals (itraconazole, ketoconazole, posaconazole, voriconazole); macrolide antibiotics (azithromycin, clarithromycin, erythromycin); and SSRIs (fluoxetine, fluvoxamine, sertraline), can increase levels of mefloquine and thus increase the risk for QT prolongation.

Although no conclusive data are available regarding coadministration of mefloquine and other drugs that can affect cardiac conduction, avoid mefloquine use, or use it with caution, in patients taking antiarrhythmic or β-blocking agents, antihistamines (H1 receptor antagonists), calcium channel receptor antagonists, phenothiazines, SSRIs, or tricyclic antidepressants.

IMMUNOSUPPRESSANTS

Concomitant use of mefloquine can cause increased levels of calcineurin inhibitors and mTOR inhibitors (cyclosporine A, sirolimus, tacrolimus).

ANTI-HEPATITIS C VIRUS PROTEASE INHIBITORS

Avoid concurrent use of mefloquine and direct-acting protease inhibitors (boceprevir and telaprevir) used to treat hepatitis C. Newer direct-acting protease inhibitors (grazoprevir, paritaprevir, simeprevir) are believed to be associated with fewer drug–drug interactions, but safety data are lacking; consider alternatives to mefloquine pending additional data.

PSYCHIATRIC MEDICATIONS

Avoid prescribing mefloquine to travelers with a history of mood disorders or psychiatric disease; this information is included in the US Food and Drug Administration boxed warning for mefloquine.

DRUGS USED TO TREAT TRAVELERS' DIARRHEA

Antimicrobials commonly prescribed as treatment for travelers' diarrhea have the potential for interacting with several different classes of drugs (Table 2-06). As mentioned previously, online clinical decision support tools provide searchable databases that can help identify interactions with medications a person may already be taking.

Table 2-06 Drugs & drug classes that can interact with selected antibiotics

ANTIBIOTICS	DRUGS & DRUG CLASSES THAT CAN INTERACT
Azithromycin	Artemether Calcineurin inhibitors HIV medications Warfarin
Fluoroquinolones	Antacids containing magnesium or aluminum hydroxide Sildenafil Theophylline Tizanidine Warfarin
Rifamycins	No clinical drug interactions have been studied; none are expected

2

Azithromycin

ANTICOAGULANTS

Increased anticoagulant effects have been noted when azithromycin is used with warfarin; monitor prothrombin time for people taking these drugs concomitantly.

ANTIMALARIAL DRUGS

Because additive QTc prolongation can occur when azithromycin is used with the antimalarial artemether, avoid concomitant therapy.

HIV MEDICATIONS

Drug interactions have been reported with the macrolide antibiotics, clarithromycin and erythromycin; antiretroviral protease inhibitors; and the NNRTIs, efavirenz and nevirapine. Concomitant use of azithromycin and these drugs can increase the risk of QTc prolongation, but a short treatment course is not contraindicated for those without an underlying cardiac abnormality. When azithromycin is used with the protease inhibitor nelfinavir, advise patients about possible drug interactions.

IMMUNOSUPPRESSANTS

Concurrent use of macrolides with calcineurin inhibitors can cause increased levels of drugs belonging to this class of immunosuppressants.

Fluoroquinolones

ANTACIDS

Concurrent administration of ciprofloxacin and antacids that contain magnesium or aluminum hydroxide can reduce bioavailability of ciprofloxacin.

ANTICOAGULANTS

An increase in the international normalized ratio (INR) has been reported when levofloxacin and warfarin are used concurrently.

ASTHMA MEDICATION

Ciprofloxacin decreases clearance of theophylline and caffeine; clinicians should monitor theophylline levels when ciprofloxacin is used concurrently.

IMMUNOSUPPRESSANTS

Fluoroquinolones can increase levels of calcineurin inhibitors, and doses should be adjusted for renal function.

OTHERS

Sildenafil should not be used by patients taking ciprofloxacin; concomitant use is associated with increased rates of adverse effects. Ciprofloxacin and other fluoroquinolones should not be used in patients taking tizanidine.

2

Rifamycins

RIFAMYCIN SV

No clinical drug interactions have been studied. Because of minimal systemic rifamycin concentrations observed after the recommended dose, clinically relevant drug interactions are not expected.

RIFAXIMIN

Rifaximin is not absorbed in appreciable amounts by intact bowel, and no clinically significant drug interactions have been reported to date with rifaximin except for minor changes in INR when used concurrently with warfarin.

DRUGS USED FOR TRAVEL TO HIGH ELEVATIONS

Before prescribing the carbonic anhydrase inhibitor, acetazolamide, to those planning high elevation travel, carefully review with them the complete list of medications they are already taking (Table 2-07).

Acetazolamide

ACETAMINOPHEN & DICLOFENAC SODIUM

Acetaminophen and diclofenac sodium form complex bonds with acetazolamide in the stomach's acidic environment, impairing absorption. Neither agent should be taken within 30 minutes of acetazolamide. Patients taking acetazolamide also can experience decreased excretion of anticholinergics, dextroamphetamine, ephedrine, mecamylamine, mexiletine, and quinidine.

ANTICONVULSANTS

Acetazolamide should not be given to patients taking the anticonvulsant topiramate because concurrent use is associated with toxicity.

BARBITURATES & SALICYLATES

Acetazolamide causes alkaline urine, which can increase the rate of excretion of barbiturates and salicylates and could cause salicylate toxicity, particularly in patients taking a high dose of aspirin.

Table 2-07 Drugs & drug classes that can interact with selected altitude illness drugs

ALTITUDE ILLNESS DRUG	DRUGS & DRUG CLASSES THAT CAN INTERACT
Acetazolamide	Acetaminophen Anticholinergics Aspirin, high dose Barbiturates Calcineurin inhibitors Corticosteroids Dextroamphetamine Diclofenac sodium Ephedrine Mecamylamine Metformin Mexilitine Quinidine Topiramate
Dexamethasone	Anticholinesterases Anticoagulants Digitalis preparations Hypoglycemic agents Isoniazid Macrolide antibiotics Oral contraceptives Phenytoin

CORTICOSTEROIDS

Hypokalemia caused by corticosteroids could occur when used concurrently with acetazolamide.

DIABETES MEDICATIONS

Use caution when concurrently administering metformin and acetazolamide because of increased risk for lactic acidosis.

IMMUNOSUPPRESSANTS

Monitor cyclosporine, sirolimus, and tacrolimus more closely when given with acetazolamide.

Dexamethasone

Using dexamethasone to treat altitude illness can be lifesaving. Dexamethasone interacts with several classes of drugs, however, including: anticholinesterases, anticoagulants, digitalis preparations, hypoglycemic agents, isoniazid, macrolide antibiotics, oral contraceptives, and phenytoin.

HIV MEDICATIONS

Patients with HIV require additional consideration in the pretravel consultation (see Sec. 3, Ch. 1, Immunocompromised Travelers). A study from Europe showed that ≤29% of HIV-positive travelers disclose their disease and medication status when seeking pretravel advice. Antiretroviral medications have multiple drug interactions, especially through their activation or inhibition of the CYP3A4 and CYP2D6 enzymes.

Several instances of antimalarial prophylaxis and treatment failure in patients taking protease inhibitors and both nucleoside and NNRTIs have been reported. By contrast, entry and integrase inhibitors are not a common cause of drug–drug interactions with commonly administered travel-related medications.

Several potential interactions are listed above, and 2 excellent resources for HIV medication interactions can be found at www.hiv-druginteractions.org and https://clinicalinfo.hiv.gov/en. HIV preexposure prophylaxis with emtricitabine/tenofovir is not a contraindication for any of the commonly used travel-related medications.

HERBAL & NUTRITIONAL SUPPLEMENTS

Up to 30% of travelers take herbal or nutritional supplements. Many travelers consider them to be of no clinical relevance and might not disclose their use unless specifically asked during the pretravel consultation. Clinicians should give special attention to supplements that activate or inhibit CYP2D6 or CYP3A4 enzymes (e.g., ginseng, grapefruit extract, hypericum, St. John's wort). Advise patients against coadministration of herbal and nutritional supplements with medications that are substrates for CYP2D6 or 3A4 enzymes, including chloroquine, macrolides, and mefloquine.

BIBLIOGRAPHY

Frenck RW Jr., Gurtman A, Rubino J, Smith W, van Cleeff M, Jayawardene D, et al. Randomized, controlled trial of a 13-valent pneumococcal conjugate vaccine administered concomitantly with an influenza vaccine in healthy adults. Clin Vaccine Immunol. 2012;19(8):1296–303.

Jabeen E, Qureshi R, Shah A. Interaction of antihypertensive acetazolamide with nonsteroidal anti-inflammatory drugs. J Photochem Photobiol B. 2013;125:155–63.

Kollaritsch H, Que JU, Kunz C, Wiedermann G, Herzog C, Cryz SJ Jr. Safety and immunogenicity of live oral cholera and typhoid vaccines administered alone or in combination with antimalarial drugs, oral polio vaccine, or yellow fever vaccine. J Infect Dis. 1997;175(4):871–5.

Nascimento Silva JR, Camacho LA, Siqueira MM, Freire Mde S, Castro YP, Maia Mde L, et al. Mutual interference on the immune response to yellow fever vaccine and a combined vaccine against measles, mumps and rubella. Vaccine. 2011;29(37):6327–34.

Nielsen US, Jensen-Fangel S, Pedersen G, Lohse N, Pedersen C, Kronborg G, et al. Travelling with HIV: a cross sectional analysis of Danish HIV-infected patients. Travel Med Infect Dis. 2014;12(1):72–8.

Ridtitid W, Wongnawa M, Mahatthanatrakul W, Raungsri N, Sunbhanich M. Ketoconazole increases plasma concentrations of antimalarial mefloquine in healthy human volunteers. J Clin Pharm Ther. 2005;30(3):285–90.

Sbaih N, Buss B, Goyal D, Rao SR, Benefield R, Walker AT, et al. Potentially serious drug interactions resulting from the pre-travel health encounter. Open Forum Infect Dis. 2018;5(11):ofy266.

Stienlauf S, Meltzer E, Kurnik D, Leshem E, Kopel E, Streltsin B, et al. Potential drug interactions in travelers with chronic illnesses: a large retrospective cohort study. Travel Med Infect Dis. 2014;12(5):499–504.

YELLOW FEVER VACCINE & MALARIA PREVENTION INFORMATION, BY COUNTRY

Mark Gershman, Rhett Stoney (Yellow Fever)
Holly Biggs, Kathrine Tan (Malaria)

The following pages present country-specific information on yellow fever (YF) vaccine requirements and recommendations, and malaria transmission information and prevention recommendations. Country-specific maps are included to aid in interpreting the information. The information in this chapter was accurate at the time of publication; however, it is subject to change at any time due to changes in disease transmission or, in the case of YF, changing entry requirements for travelers. Updated information reflecting changes since publication can be found in the online version of this book (www.cdc.gov/yellowbook) and on the Centers for Disease Control and Prevention (CDC) Travelers' Health website (https://wwwnc.cdc.gov/travel). Recommendations for prevention of other travel-associated illnesses can also be found on the CDC Travelers' Health website (https://wwwnc.cdc.gov/travel).

YELLOW FEVER VACCINE

Entry Requirements

Entry requirements for proof of YF vaccination under the International Health Regulations (IHR) differ from CDC's YF vaccination recommendations. Under the IHR, countries are permitted to establish YF vaccine entry requirements to prevent the importation and transmission of YF virus within their boundaries. Certain countries require proof of vaccination from travelers arriving from all countries (Table 5-24); some countries require proof of vaccination only for travelers above a certain age coming from countries with risk for YF virus transmission. The World Health Organization (WHO) defines areas with risk for YF virus transmission as countries or areas where YF virus activity has been reported currently or in the past, and where vectors and animal reservoirs exist.

Unless issued a medical waiver by a yellow fever vaccine provider, travelers must comply with entry requirements for proof of vaccination against YF.

WHO publishes a list of YF vaccine country entry requirements and recommendations for international travelers approximately annually. But because entry requirements are subject to change at any time, health care professionals and travelers should refer to the online version of this book (www.cdc.gov/yellowbook) and the CDC Travelers' Health website (https://wwwnc.cdc.gov/travel) for any updates before departure.

CDC Recommendations

CDC's YF vaccine recommendations are guidance intended to protect travelers from acquiring YF virus infections during international travel. These recommendations are based on a classification system for destination-specific risk for YF virus transmission: endemic, transitional, low potential for exposure, and no risk (Table 2-08). CDC recommends YF vaccination for travel to areas classified as having endemic or transitional risk (Maps 5-10 and 5-11). Because of changes in YF virus circulation, however, recommendations can change; therefore, before departure, travelers and clinicians should check CDC's destination pages for up-to-date YF vaccine information (https://wwwnc.cdc.gov/travel/destinations/list).

Duration of Protection

In 2015, the US Advisory Committee on Immunization Practices published a recommendation that 1 dose of YF vaccine provides long-lasting protection and is adequate for most

Table 2-08 Yellow fever (YF) vaccine recommendation categories[1]

YF VACCINE RECOMMENDATION CATEGORY	RATIONALE
Recommended	Vaccination recommended for all travelers ≥9 months old going to areas with endemic or transitional YF risk, as determined by persistent or periodic YF virus transmission
Generally not recommended	Vaccination generally not recommended for travel to areas where the potential for YF virus exposure is low, as determined by absence of reports of human YF and past evidence suggestive of only low levels of YF virus transmission Vaccination might be considered for a small subset of travelers at increased risk for exposure to YF virus due to prolonged travel, heavy mosquito exposure, or inability to avoid mosquito bites
Not recommended	Vaccination not recommended for travel to areas where there is no risk for YF virus transmission, as determined by absence of past or present evidence of YF virus circulation in the area or environmental conditions not conducive to YF virus transmission

[1]This table is an abbreviated version of Table 1 from: Jentes ES, Poumerol G, Gershman MD, et al. The revised global yellow fever risk map and recommendations for vaccination, 2010: consensus of the Informal WHO Working Group on Geographic Risk for Yellow Fever. Lancet Infect Dis. 2011 Aug;11(8):622–32. The categories of risk of YF virus transmission and corresponding categories of YF vaccine recommendations that appear here are taken unchanged from the referenced article.

travelers. The recommendation also identifies specific groups of travelers who should receive additional doses, and others for whom additional doses should be considered (see Sec. 5, Part 2, Ch. 26, Yellow Fever). In July 2016, WHO officially amended the IHR to stipulate that a completed International Certificate of Vaccination or Prophylaxis is valid for the lifetime of the vaccinee, and YF vaccine booster doses are not necessary. Moreover, countries cannot require proof of revaccination (booster) against YF as a condition of entry, even if the traveler's last vaccination was >10 years ago.

Ultimately, when deciding whether to vaccinate travelers, clinicians should take into account destination-specific risks for YF virus infection, and individual risk factors (e.g., age, immune status) for serious YF vaccine–associated adverse events, in the context of the entry requirements. See Sec. 5, Part 2, Ch. 26, Yellow Fever, for a full discussion of YF disease and vaccination guidance.

MALARIA PREVENTION

The following recommendations to protect travelers from malaria were developed using the best available data from multiple sources. Countries are not required to submit malaria surveillance data to CDC. On an ongoing basis, CDC actively solicits data from multiple sources, including WHO (main and regional offices); national malaria control programs; international organizations; CDC overseas offices; US military; academic, research, and aid organizations; and the published scientific literature. The reliability and accuracy of those data are also assessed.

If the information is available, trends in malaria incidence and other data are considered in the context of malaria control activities within a given country or other mitigating factors (e.g., natural disasters, wars, the coronavirus disease 2019 pandemic) that can affect the ability to control malaria or accurately count and report it. Factors such as the volume of travel to that country and the number of acquired cases reported in the US surveillance system are also examined. In developing its recommendations, CDC considers areas within countries where malaria transmission occurs, substantial occurrences of antimalarial drug resistance, the proportions of species present, and the available malaria prophylaxis options.

2

Clinicians should use these recommendations in conjunction with an individual risk assessment and consider not only the destination but also the detailed itinerary, including specific cities, types of accommodations, season, and style of travel, as well as special health conditions (e.g., pregnancy). Several medications are available for malaria prophylaxis. When deciding which drug to use, consider the itinerary and length of trip, travelers' previous adverse reactions to antimalarials, drug allergies, medical history, and drug costs. For a thorough discussion of malaria and guidance for prophylaxis, see Sec. 5, Part 3, Ch. 16, Malaria.

COUNTRY-SPECIFIC INFORMATION

AFGHANISTAN

YELLOW FEVER VACCINE
Entry requirements: None
CDC recommendation: Not recommended

MALARIA PREVENTION
Transmission areas: All areas <2,500 m (≈8,200 ft) elevation (April–December)
Drug resistance[2]: Chloroquine
Species: *P. vivax* (primarily); *P. falciparum* (less commonly)
Recommended chemoprophylaxis: Atovaquone-proguanil, doxycycline, mefloquine, tafenoquine[3]

ALBANIA

YELLOW FEVER VACCINE
Entry requirements: Required for travelers ≥1 year old arriving from countries with risk for YF virus transmission[1]
CDC recommendation: Not recommended

MALARIA PREVENTION
No malaria transmission

ALGERIA

YELLOW FEVER VACCINE
Entry requirements: Required for travelers ≥9 months old arriving from countries with risk for YF virus transmission; this includes >12-hour airport transits or layovers in countries with risk for YF virus transmission[1]
CDC recommendation: Not recommended

MALARIA PREVENTION
No malaria transmission

AMERICAN SAMOA, UNITED STATES

YELLOW FEVER VACCINE
Entry requirements: None
CDC recommendation: Not recommended

MALARIA PREVENTION
No malaria transmission

ANDORRA

YELLOW FEVER VACCINE
Entry requirements: None
CDC recommendation: Not recommended

MALARIA PREVENTION
No malaria transmission

ANGOLA

YELLOW FEVER VACCINE
Entry requirements: Required for all arriving travelers ≥9 months old
CDC recommended for all travelers ≥9 months old

MALARIA PREVENTION
Transmission areas: All
Drug resistance[2]: Chloroquine
Species: *P. falciparum* (primarily); *P. malariae*, *P. ovale*, and *P. vivax* (less commonly)
Recommended chemoprophylaxis: Atovaquone-proguanil, doxycycline, mefloquine, tafenoquine[3]

ANGUILLA, UNITED KINGDOM

YELLOW FEVER VACCINE
Entry requirements: None
CDC recommendation: Not recommended

MALARIA PREVENTION
No malaria transmission

ANTARCTICA

YELLOW FEVER VACCINE
Entry requirements: None
CDC recommendation: Not recommended

MALARIA PREVENTION
No malaria transmission

ANTIGUA & BARBUDA

YELLOW FEVER VACCINE
Entry requirements: Required for travelers ≥1 year old arriving from countries with risk for YF virus transmission; this includes >12-hour airport transits or layovers in countries with risk for YF virus transmission[1]
CDC recommendation: Not recommended

MALARIA PREVENTION
No malaria transmission

ARGENTINA

YELLOW FEVER VACCINE (MAP 2-01)
Entry requirements: None
CDC recommendations:
Recommended for travelers ≥9 months old going to Corrientes and Misiones Provinces
Generally not recommended for travel to Formosa Province or to designated areas of Chaco, Jujuy, and Salta Provinces
Not recommended for travel limited to provinces and areas not listed above

MALARIA PREVENTION
No malaria transmission

ARMENIA

YELLOW FEVER VACCINE
Entry requirements: None
CDC recommendation: Not recommended

MALARIA PREVENTION
No malaria transmission

MAP

2

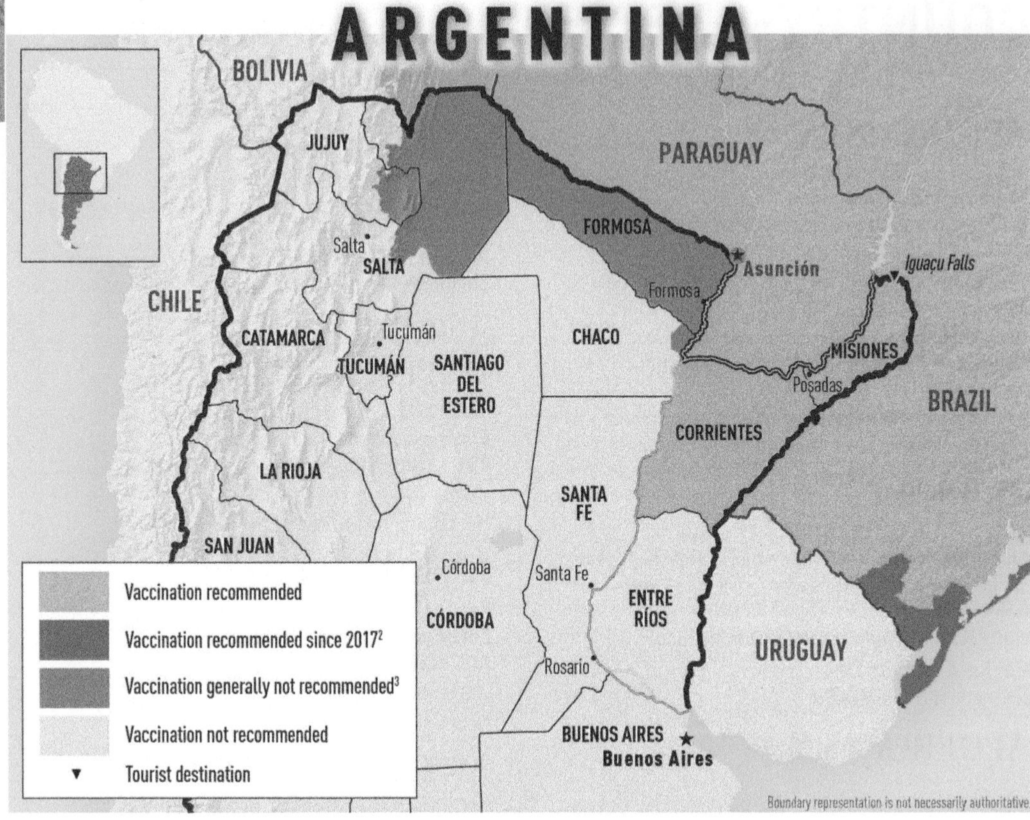

MAP 2-01 Yellow fever vaccine recommendations for Argentina & neighboring countries[1]

[1] For footnotes, see page 84

ARUBA, NETHERLANDS

YELLOW FEVER VACCINE

Entry requirements: Required for travelers ≥9 months old arriving from countries with risk for YF virus transmission; this includes >12-hour airport transits or layovers in countries with risk for YF virus transmission[1]

Entry will be denied if a valid vaccination certificate cannot be provided

CDC recommendation: Not recommended

MALARIA PREVENTION

No malaria transmission

AUSTRALIA

YELLOW FEVER VACCINE

Entry requirements: Required for travelers ≥1 year old arriving from countries with risk for YF virus transmission; this includes >12-hour airport transits or layovers in countries with risk for YF virus transmission[1]

Travelers arriving from the Galápagos Islands of Ecuador are exempt from this requirement

CDC recommendation: Not recommended

MALARIA PREVENTION

No malaria transmission

AUSTRIA

YELLOW FEVER VACCINE

Entry requirements: None

CDC recommendation: Not recommended

MALARIA PREVENTION

No malaria transmission

AZERBAIJAN

YELLOW FEVER VACCINE

Entry requirements: None

CDC recommendation: Not recommended

MALARIA PREVENTION

No malaria transmission

AZORES, PORTUGAL

YELLOW FEVER VACCINE

Entry requirements: None

CDC recommendation: Not recommended

MALARIA PREVENTION

No malaria transmission

BAHAMAS, THE

YELLOW FEVER VACCINE

Entry requirements: Required for travelers ≥1 year old arriving from countries with risk for YF virus transmission; this includes >12-hour airport transits or layovers in countries with risk for YF virus transmission[1]

CDC recommendation: Not recommended

MALARIA PREVENTION

No malaria transmission

BAHRAIN

YELLOW FEVER VACCINE

Entry requirements: Required for travelers ≥9 months old arriving from countries with risk for YF virus transmission; this includes >12-hour airport transits or layovers in countries with risk for YF virus transmission[1]

CDC recommendation: Not recommended

MALARIA PREVENTION

No malaria transmission

BANGLADESH

YELLOW FEVER VACCINE

Entry requirements: Required for travelers ≥1 year old arriving from countries with risk for YF virus transmission; this includes airport transits or layovers in countries with risk for YF virus transmission[1]

CDC recommendation: Not recommended

MALARIA PREVENTION

Transmission areas: Districts of Chittagong Hill Tract (Bandarban, Khagrachari, and Rangamati); and the following districts: Chattogram (Chittagong) and Cox's Bazar (in Chattogram [Chittagong] Division); Mymensingh, Netrakona, and Sherpur (in Mymensingh Division); Kurigram (in Rangpur Division); Habiganj, Moulvibazar, Sunamganj, and Sylhet (in Sylhet Division)
No malaria transmission in Dhaka (the capital)

Drug resistance[2]: Chloroquine

Species: *P. falciparum* (90%); *P. vivax* (10%); *P. malariae* (rare)

Recommended chemoprophylaxis: Atovaquone-proguanil, doxycycline, mefloquine, tafenoquine[3]

BARBADOS

YELLOW FEVER VACCINE

Entry requirements: Required for travelers ≥1 year old arriving from countries with risk for YF virus transmission[1]
Travelers arriving from Guyana or Trinidad & Tobago are exempt from this requirement, unless an outbreak is occurring

CDC recommendation: Not recommended

MALARIA PREVENTION

No malaria transmission

BELARUS

YELLOW FEVER VACCINE

Entry requirements: None

CDC recommendation: Not recommended

MALARIA PREVENTION

No malaria transmission

BELGIUM

YELLOW FEVER VACCINE

Entry requirements: None

CDC recommendation: Not recommended

MALARIA PREVENTION

No malaria transmission

BELIZE

YELLOW FEVER VACCINE

Entry requirements: None

CDC recommendation: Not recommended

MALARIA PREVENTION

Transmission areas: Rare transmission
No malaria transmission in Belize City or on islands frequented by tourists (e.g., Ambergris Caye)

Drug resistance[2]: None

Species: *P. vivax* (primarily)

Recommended chemoprophylaxis: None (insect bite precautions and mosquito avoidance only)[4]

BENIN

YELLOW FEVER VACCINE

Entry requirements: Required for all arriving travelers ≥9 months old

CDC recommended for all travelers ≥9 months old

MALARIA PREVENTION

Transmission areas: All

Drug resistance[2]: Chloroquine

Species: *P. falciparum* (primarily); *P. malariae*, *P. ovale*, and *P. vivax* (less commonly)

Recommended chemoprophylaxis: Atovaquone-proguanil, doxycycline, mefloquine, tafenoquine[3]

BERMUDA, UNITED KINGDOM

YELLOW FEVER VACCINE

Entry requirements: None

CDC recommendation: Not recommended

MALARIA PREVENTION

No malaria transmission

BHUTAN

YELLOW FEVER VACCINE

Entry requirements: None

CDC recommendation: Not recommended

MALARIA PREVENTION

Transmission areas: Rare cases in rural areas <1,700 m (≈5,500 ft) elevation in districts along the southern border shared with India

Drug resistance[2]: Chloroquine

Species: *P. vivax* (primarily); *P. falciparum* (less commonly)

Recommended chemoprophylaxis: None (insect bite precautions and mosquito avoidance only)[4]

2

BOLIVIA

YELLOW FEVER VACCINE (MAP 2-02)

Entry requirements: Required for travelers ≥1 year old arriving from countries with risk for YF virus transmission[1]

CDC recommendations:

Recommended for travelers ≥9 months old going to areas <2,300 m (≈7,550 ft) elevation, east of the Andes Mountains: the entire departments of Beni, Pando, Santa Cruz, and designated areas in the departments of Chuquisaca, Cochabamba, La Paz, and Tarija

Not recommended for travel limited to areas >2,300 m (≈7,550 ft) elevation and any areas not listed above, including the cities of La Paz (administrative capital) and Sucre (constitutional [legislative and judicial] capital)

MALARIA PREVENTION

Transmission areas: All areas <2,500 m (≈8,200 ft) elevation

No malaria transmission in La Paz (administrative capital)

Drug resistance[2]: Chloroquine

Species: *P. vivax* (99%); *P. falciparum* (1%)

Recommended chemoprophylaxis: Atovaquone-proguanil, doxycycline, mefloquine, primaquine,[5] tafenoquine[3]

MAP

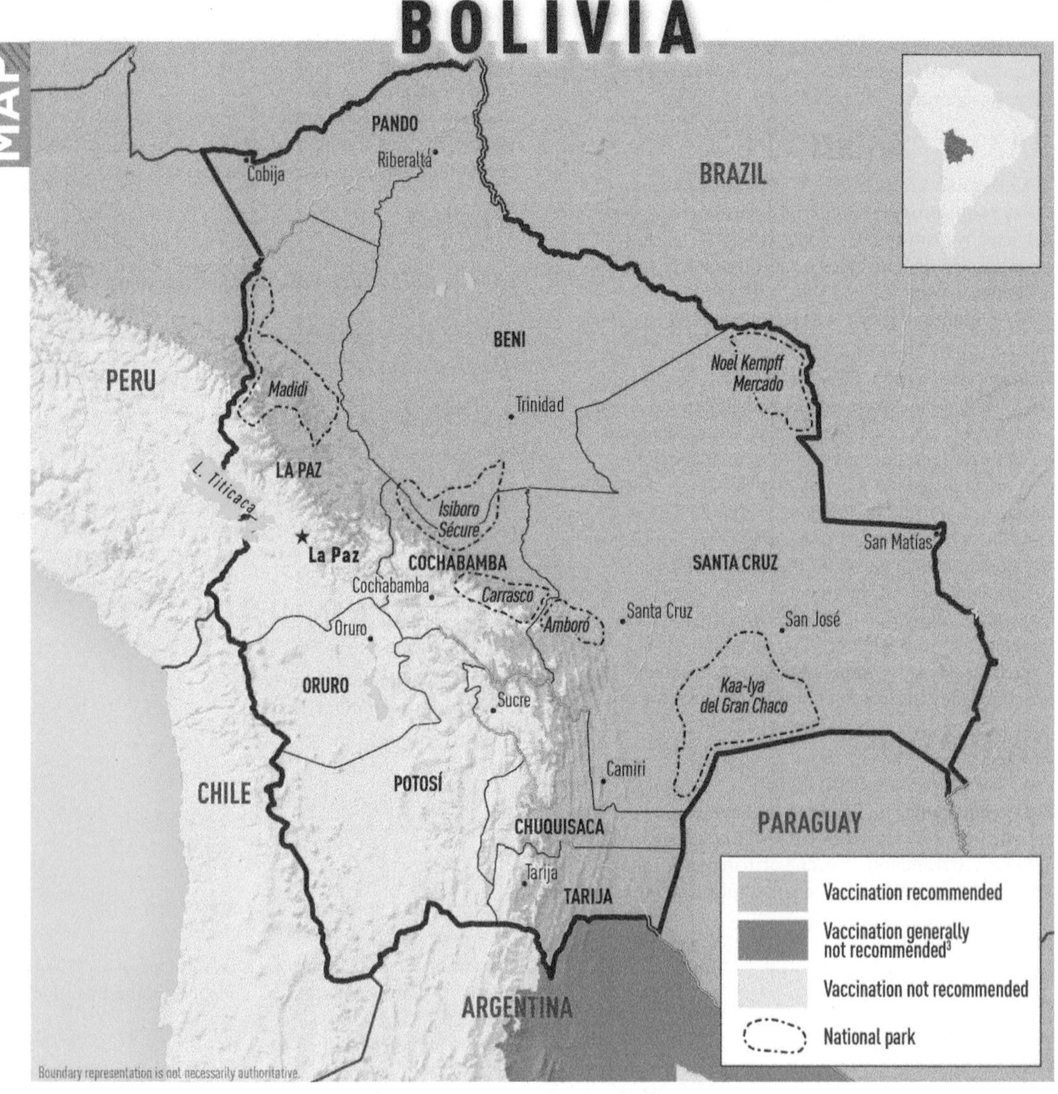

MAP 2-02 Yellow fever vaccine recommendations for Bolivia & neighboring countries[1]

[1] For footnotes, see page 84

BONAIRE, NETHERLANDS

YELLOW FEVER VACCINE

Entry requirements: Required for travelers ≥9 months old arriving from countries with risk for YF virus transmission; this includes >12-hour airport transits or layovers in countries with risk for YF virus transmission[1]

CDC recommendation: Not recommended

MALARIA PREVENTION

No malaria transmission

BOSNIA & HERZEGOVINA

YELLOW FEVER VACCINE

Entry requirements: None

CDC recommendation: Not recommended

MALARIA PREVENTION

No malaria transmission

BOTSWANA

YELLOW FEVER VACCINE

Entry requirements: Required for travelers ≥1 year old arriving from countries with risk for YF virus transmission; this includes transits through countries with risk for YF virus transmission[1]

CDC recommendation: Not recommended

MALARIA PREVENTION

Transmission areas: Districts/subdistricts of Bobirwa, Boteti, Chobe (including Chobe National Park), Ghanzi, Mahalapye, Ngamiland (Ngami), North East (including its capital, Francistown), Okavango, Serowe/Palapye, and Tutume

Rare cases or sporadic foci of transmission in districts/subdistricts of Kgalagadi North, Kgatleng, Kweneng, and Southern

No malaria transmission in Gaborone (the capital)

Drug resistance[2]: Chloroquine

Species: *P. falciparum* (primarily); *P. malariae*, *P. ovale*, and *P. vivax* (less commonly)

Recommended chemoprophylaxis:

Districts/subdistricts of Bobirwa, Boteti, Chobe (including Chobe National Park), Ghanzi, Mahalapye, Ngamiland (Ngami), North East (including its capital, Francistown), Okavango, Serowe/Palapye, and Tutume: Atovaquone-proguanil, doxycycline, mefloquine, tafenoquine[3]

Areas with rare cases or sporadic foci of transmission: no chemoprophylaxis recommended (insect bite precautions and mosquito avoidance only)[4]

BRAZIL

YELLOW FEVER VACCINE (MAP 2-03)

Entry requirements: None

CDC recommendations:

Recommended for travelers ≥9 months old going to the states of Acre, Amapá, Amazonas, Distrito Federal (including the capital city, Brasília), Espírito Santo,* Goiás, Maranhão, Mato Grosso, Mato Grosso do Sul, Minas Gerais, Pará, Paraná,* Piauí, Rio de Janeiro (including the city of Rio de Janeiro and all coastal islands),* Rio Grande do Sul,* Rondônia, Roraima, Santa Catarina,* São Paulo (including the city of São Paulo and all coastal islands),* Tocantins, and designated areas of Bahia*.

Vaccination is also recommended for travelers going to Iguaçu Falls

Not recommended for travel limited to any areas not listed above, including the cities of Fortaleza and Recife

*In 2017, in response to a large YF outbreak in multiple eastern states, CDC expanded its vaccination recommendations for travelers going to Brazil. The expanded YF vaccination recommendations for these states are preliminary. For updates, refer to the CDC Travelers' Health website at https://wwwnc.cdc.gov/travel.

MALARIA PREVENTION (MAP 2-04)

Transmission areas: All areas in the states of Acre, Amapá, Amazonas, Rondônia, and Roraima

Present in the states of Maranhão, Mato Grosso, and Pará, but rare cases in their capital cities (São Luis [capital of Maranhão], Cuiabá [capital of Mato Grosso], Belém [capital of Pará])

Rural and forested areas in the states of Espírito Santo, Goiás, Minas Gerais, Mato Grosso do Sul, Piauí, Rio de Janeiro, São Paolo, and Tocantins

No malaria transmission in the cities of Brasília (the capital), Rio de Janeiro, or São Paolo

No malaria transmission at Iguaçu Falls

Drug resistance[2]: Chloroquine

Species: *P. vivax* (90%); *P. falciparum* (10%)

Recommended chemoprophylaxis:

Transmission areas: Atovaquone-proguanil, doxycycline, mefloquine, tafenoquine[3]

Areas with rare cases: No chemoprophylaxis recommended (insect bite precautions and mosquito avoidance only)[4]

BRITISH INDIAN OCEAN TERRITORY (INCLUDING DIEGO GARCIA), UNITED KINGDOM

YELLOW FEVER VACCINE

Entry requirements: None

CDC recommendation: Not recommended

MALARIA PREVENTION

No malaria transmission

BRUNEI

YELLOW FEVER VACCINE

Entry requirements: Required for travelers ≥9 months old arriving from countries with risk for YF virus transmission; this includes >12-hour airport transits or layovers in countries with risk for YF virus transmission[1]

CDC recommendation: Not recommended

MALARIA PREVENTION

Transmission areas: No human malaria

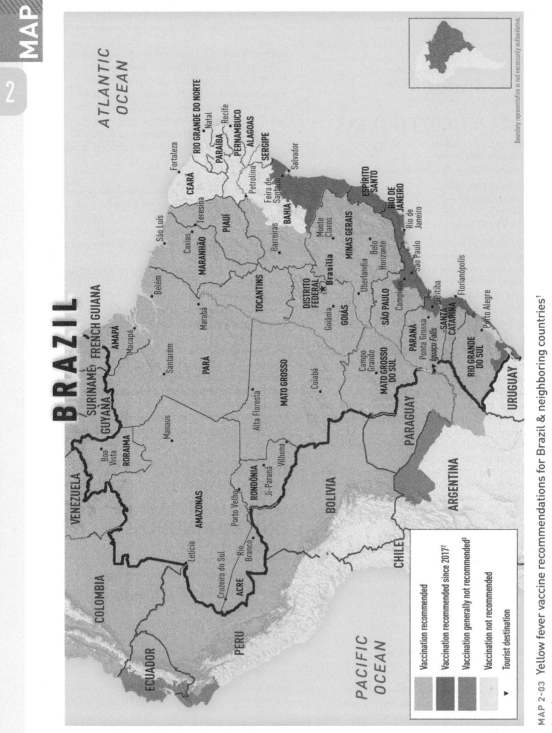

MAP 2-03 Yellow fever vaccine recommendations for Brazil & neighboring countries[1]

[1] For footnotes, see page 84

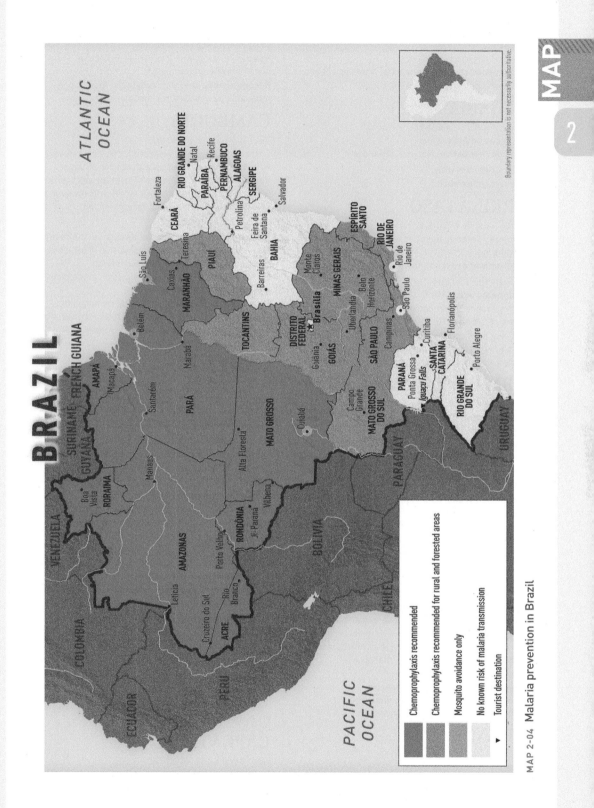

MAP 2-04 Malaria prevention in Brazil

MAP 2

Rare transmission of *P. knowlesi*[6] in primarily forested or forest-fringe areas
Drug resistance: None
Species: *P. knowlesi*[6] (100%)
Recommended chemoprophylaxis: None (insect bite precautions and mosquito avoidance only)[4]

BULGARIA

YELLOW FEVER VACCINE
Entry requirements: None
CDC recommendation: Not recommended

MALARIA PREVENTION
No malaria transmission

BURKINA FASO

YELLOW FEVER VACCINE
Entry requirements: Required for all arriving travelers ≥9 months old
CDC recommended for all travelers ≥9 months old

MALARIA PREVENTION
Transmission areas: All
Drug resistance[2]: Chloroquine
Species: *P. falciparum* (primarily); *P. malariae*, *P. ovale*, and *P. vivax* (less commonly)
Recommended chemoprophylaxis: Atovaquone-proguanil, doxycycline, mefloquine, tafenoquine[3]

BURMA (MYANMAR)

YELLOW FEVER VACCINE
Entry requirements: Required for travelers ≥1 year old arriving from countries with risk for YF virus transmission; this includes >12-hour airport transits or layovers in countries with risk for YF virus transmission[1]
CDC recommendation: Not recommended

MALARIA PREVENTION
Transmission areas: All areas <1,000 m (≈3,300 ft) elevation, including Bagan
Rare transmission in areas >1,000 m (≈3,300 ft) elevation
Drug resistance[2]: Chloroquine and mefloquine
Species: *P. vivax* (60%); *P. falciparum* (40%); *P. knowlesi*,[6] *P. malariae*, and *P. ovale* (rare)
Recommended chemoprophylaxis:
Areas <1,000 m (≈3,300 ft) elevation in the regions of Bago and Tanintharyi, and in the states of Kachin, Kayah, Kayin, and Shan: Atovaquone-proguanil, doxycycline, tafenoquine[3]
Areas <1,000 m (≈3,300 ft) elevation in all other areas: Atovaquone-proguanil, doxycycline, mefloquine, tafenoquine[3]
Areas >1,000 m (≈3,300 ft) elevation: No chemoprophylaxis recommended (insect bite precautions and mosquito avoidance only)[4]

BURUNDI

YELLOW FEVER VACCINE
Entry requirements: Required for all arriving travelers ≥9 months old
CDC recommended for all travelers ≥9 months old

MALARIA PREVENTION
Transmission areas: All
Drug resistance[2]: Chloroquine
Species: *P. falciparum* (primarily); *P. malariae*, *P. ovale*, and *P. vivax* (less commonly)
Recommended chemoprophylaxis: Atovaquone-proguanil, doxycycline, mefloquine, tafenoquine[3]

CAMBODIA

YELLOW FEVER VACCINE
Entry requirements: Required for travelers ≥1 year old arriving from countries with risk for YF virus transmission; this includes >12-hour airport transits or layovers in countries with risk for YF virus transmission[1]
CDC recommendation: Not recommended

MALARIA PREVENTION
Transmission areas: Present throughout the country
No (or negligible) malaria transmission in the cities of Phnom Penh (the capital) and Siem Reap
No (or negligible) malaria transmission at the main temple complex at Angkor Wat
Drug resistance[2]: Chloroquine and mefloquine
Species: *P. vivax* (80%); *P. falciparum* (20%); *P. knowlesi*[6] (rare)
Recommended chemoprophylaxis: Atovaquone-proguanil, doxycycline, tafenoquine[3]

CAMEROON

YELLOW FEVER VACCINE
Entry requirements: Required for all arriving travelers ≥1 year old
CDC recommended for all travelers ≥9 months old

MALARIA PREVENTION
Transmission areas: All
Drug resistance[2]: Chloroquine
Species: *P. falciparum* (primarily); *P. malariae*, *P. ovale*, and *P. vivax* (less commonly)
Recommended chemoprophylaxis: Atovaquone-proguanil, doxycycline, mefloquine, tafenoquine[3]

CANADA

YELLOW FEVER VACCINE
Entry requirements: None
CDC recommendation: Not recommended

MALARIA PREVENTION
No malaria transmission

CANARY ISLANDS, SPAIN

YELLOW FEVER VACCINE
Entry requirements: None
CDC recommendation: Not recommended

MALARIA PREVENTION
No malaria transmission

CAPE VERDE

YELLOW FEVER VACCINE
Entry requirements: Required for travelers ≥1 year old arriving from countries with risk for YF virus transmission[1]
CDC recommendation: Not recommended

MALARIA PREVENTION

Transmission areas: No indigenous cases reported since 2018

Previously, rare cases on Santiago (São Tiago) Island and Boa Vista Island

Drug resistance[2]: Previously, chloroquine

Species: Previously, *P. falciparum* (primarily)

Recommended chemoprophylaxis: None (insect bite precautions and mosquito avoidance only)[4]

CAYMAN ISLANDS, UNITED KINGDOM

YELLOW FEVER VACCINE

Entry requirements: None

CDC recommendation: Not recommended

MALARIA PREVENTION

No malaria transmission

CENTRAL AFRICAN REPUBLIC

YELLOW FEVER VACCINE

Entry requirements: Required for all arriving travelers ≥9 months old

CDC recommended for all travelers ≥9 months old

MALARIA PREVENTION

Transmission areas: All

Drug resistance[2]: Chloroquine

Species: *P. falciparum* (primarily); *P. malariae*, *P. ovale*, and *P. vivax* (less commonly)

Recommended chemoprophylaxis: Atovaquone-proguanil, doxycycline, mefloquine, tafenoquine[3]

CHAD

YELLOW FEVER VACCINE (MAP 5-10)

Entry requirements: Required for travelers ≥9 months old arriving from countries with risk for YF virus transmission[1]

CDC recommendations:

Recommended for travelers ≥9 months old going to areas south of the Sahara Desert

Not recommended for travel limited to areas in the Sahara Desert

MALARIA PREVENTION

Transmission areas: All

Drug resistance[2]: Chloroquine

Species: *P. falciparum* (primarily); *P. malariae*, *P. ovale*, and *P. vivax* (less commonly)

Recommended chemoprophylaxis: Atovaquone-proguanil, doxycycline, mefloquine, tafenoquine[3]

CHILE

YELLOW FEVER VACCINE

Entry requirements: None

CDC recommendation: Not recommended

MALARIA PREVENTION

No malaria transmission

CHINA

YELLOW FEVER VACCINE

Entry requirements: Required for travelers ≥9 months old arriving from countries with risk for YF virus transmission; this includes >12-hour airport transits or layovers in countries with risk for YF virus transmission[1]

Travelers with itineraries limited to Hong Kong Special Administrative Region (SAR) or Macao SAR are exempt from this requirement

CDC recommendation: Not recommended

MALARIA PREVENTION

No malaria transmission

CHRISTMAS ISLAND, AUSTRALIA

YELLOW FEVER VACCINE

Entry requirements: Required for travelers ≥1 year old arriving from countries with risk for YF virus transmission; this includes >12-hour airport transits or layovers in countries with risk for YF virus transmission[1]

Travelers arriving from the Galápagos Islands of Ecuador are exempt from this requirement

CDC recommendation: Not recommended

MALARIA PREVENTION

No malaria transmission

COCOS (KEELING) ISLANDS, AUSTRALIA

YELLOW FEVER VACCINE

Entry requirements: Required for travelers ≥1 year old arriving from countries with risk for YF virus transmission; this includes >12-hour airport transits or layovers in countries with risk for YF virus transmission[1]

Travelers arriving from the Galápagos Islands of Ecuador are exempt from this requirement

CDC recommendation: Not recommended

MALARIA PREVENTION

No malaria transmission

COLOMBIA

YELLOW FEVER VACCINE (MAP 2-05)

Entry requirements: Required for travelers ≥1 year old arriving from Angola, Brazil, Democratic Republic of the Congo, or Uganda; this includes >12-hour airport transits or layovers in any of these countries

CDC recommendations:

Recommended for all travelers ≥9 months old except as follows

Generally not recommended for travel limited to the cities of Barranquilla, Cali, Cartagena, or Medellín

Not recommended for travel limited to areas >2,300 m (≈7,550 ft) elevation, the archipelago department of San Andrés and Providencia, or the city of Bogotá (the capital)

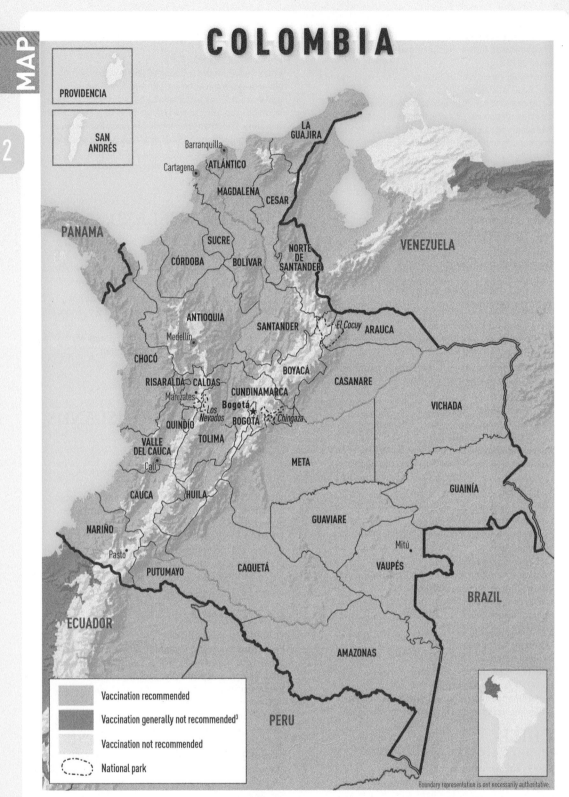

MAP 2-05 Yellow fever vaccine recommendations for Colombia & neighboring countries[1]

[1] For footnotes, see page 84

MALARIA PREVENTION
Transmission areas: All areas <1,700 m (≈5,600 ft) elevation
No malaria transmission in the cities of Bogotá (the capital), Cartagena, or Medellín
Drug resistance[2]: Chloroquine
Malaria species: *P. falciparum* (50%), *P. vivax* (50%)
Recommended chemoprophylaxis: Atovaquone-proguanil, doxycycline, mefloquine, tafenoquine[3]

COMOROS

YELLOW FEVER VACCINE
Entry requirements: None
CDC recommendation: Not recommended

MALARIA PREVENTION
Transmission areas: All
Drug resistance[2]: Chloroquine
Species: *P. falciparum* (primarily); *P. malariae* and *P. vivax* (rare)
Recommended chemoprophylaxis: Atovaquone-proguanil, doxycycline, mefloquine, tafenoquine[3]

CONGO, REPUBLIC OF THE (CONGO-BRAZZAVILLE)

YELLOW FEVER VACCINE
Entry requirements: Required for all arriving travelers ≥9 months old
CDC recommended for all travelers ≥9 months old

MALARIA PREVENTION
Transmission areas: All
Drug resistance[2]: Chloroquine
Species: *P. falciparum* (primarily); *P. malariae*, *P. ovale*, and *P. vivax* (less commonly)
Recommended chemoprophylaxis: Atovaquone-proguanil, doxycycline, mefloquine, tafenoquine[3]

COOK ISLANDS, NEW ZEALAND

YELLOW FEVER VACCINE
Entry requirements: None
CDC recommendation: Not recommended

MALARIA PREVENTION
No malaria transmission

COSTA RICA

YELLOW FEVER VACCINE
Entry requirements: Required for travelers ≥9 months old arriving from countries with risk for YF virus transmission[1]
Included in this requirement are travelers arriving from **Tanzania** and **Zambia**, and designated areas of: **Colombia** (the entire country, *except* the cities of Barranquilla, Bogotá, Cali, Cartagena, and Medellín, and the archipelago department, San Andrés and Providencia); **Ecuador** (the provinces of Morona-Santiago, Napo, Orellana, Pastaza, Sucumbíos, and Zamora-Chinchipe, and excluding the rest of the country); **Paraguay** (the entire country, *except* the city of Asunción); **Peru** (the entire country, *except* the cities of Cusco and Lima, the regions of Cajamarca, Lambayeque, Piura, and Tumbes, and the highland tourist areas of Machu Picchu and the Inca Trail); **Trinidad & Tobago** (the entire country, *except* the urban areas of Port of Spain; travelers with itineraries limited to the island of Tobago, and travelers with airport transits or layovers are also exempt from this requirement)
Travelers arriving from Argentina and Panama are exempt from this requirement
CDC recommendation: Not recommended

MALARIA PREVENTION
Transmission areas: Some transmission in Alajuela Province near the border with Nicaragua
Rare to no transmission in other parts of the country
Drug resistance[2]: None
Species: *P. vivax* (78%); *P. falciparum* (22%)
Recommended chemoprophylaxis:
Alajuela Province near the border with Nicaragua: Atovaquone-proguanil, chloroquine, doxycycline, mefloquine, tafenoquine[3]
All other areas: No chemoprophylaxis recommended (insect bite precautions and mosquito avoidance only)[4]

CÔTE D'IVOIRE (IVORY COAST)

YELLOW FEVER VACCINE
Entry requirements: Required for all arriving travelers ≥9 months old
CDC recommended for all travelers ≥9 months old

MALARIA PREVENTION
Transmission areas: All
Drug resistance[2]: Chloroquine
Species: *P. falciparum* (primarily); *P. malariae*, *P. ovale*, and *P. vivax* (less commonly)
Recommended chemoprophylaxis: Atovaquone-proguanil, doxycycline, mefloquine, tafenoquine[3]

CROATIA

YELLOW FEVER VACCINE
Entry requirements: None
CDC recommendation: Not recommended

MALARIA PREVENTION
No malaria transmission

CUBA

YELLOW FEVER VACCINE
Entry requirements: Required for travelers ≥9 months old arriving from countries with risk for YF virus transmission; this includes >12-hour airport transits or layovers in countries with risk for YF virus transmission[1]
CDC recommendation: Not recommended

MALARIA PREVENTION
No malaria transmission

CURAÇAO, NETHERLANDS

YELLOW FEVER VACCINE

Entry requirements: Required for travelers ≥9 months old arriving from countries with risk for YF virus transmission; this includes >12-hour airport transits or layovers in countries with risk for YF virus transmission[1]

CDC recommendation: Not recommended

MALARIA PREVENTION

No malaria transmission

CYPRUS

YELLOW FEVER VACCINE

Entry requirements: None

CDC recommendation: Not recommended

MALARIA PREVENTION

No malaria transmission

CZECH REPUBLIC

YELLOW FEVER VACCINE

Entry requirements: None

CDC recommendation: Not recommended

MALARIA PREVENTION

No malaria transmission

DEMOCRATIC REPUBLIC OF THE CONGO (CONGO-KINSHASA)

YELLOW FEVER VACCINE

Entry requirements: Required for all arriving travelers ≥9 months old

CDC recommended for all travelers ≥9 months old

MALARIA PREVENTION

Transmission areas: All

Drug resistance[2]: Chloroquine

Species: *P. falciparum* (primarily); *P. malariae*, *P. ovale*, and *P. vivax* (less commonly)

Recommended chemoprophylaxis: Atovaquone-proguanil, doxycycline, mefloquine, tafenoquine[3]

DENMARK

YELLOW FEVER VACCINE

Entry requirements: None

CDC recommendation: Not recommended

MALARIA PREVENTION

No malaria transmission

DJIBOUTI

YELLOW FEVER VACCINE

Entry requirements: Required for travelers ≥1 year old arriving from countries with risk for YF virus transmission; this includes >12-hour airport transits or layovers in countries with risk for YF virus transmission[1]

CDC recommendation: Not recommended

MALARIA PREVENTION

Transmission areas: All

Drug resistance[2]: Chloroquine

Species: *P. falciparum* (60–70%); *P. vivax* (30–40%.); *P. ovale* (rare)

Recommended chemoprophylaxis: Atovaquone-proguanil, doxycycline, mefloquine, tafenoquine[3]

DOMINICA

YELLOW FEVER VACCINE

Entry requirements: Required for travelers ≥1 year old arriving from countries with risk for YF virus transmission; this includes >12-hour airport transits or layovers in countries with risk for YF virus transmission[1]

CDC recommendation: Not recommended

MALARIA PREVENTION

No malaria transmission

DOMINICAN REPUBLIC

YELLOW FEVER VACCINE

Entry requirements: Required for travelers ≥1 year old arriving from the following states in Brazil: Espírito Santo, Mina Gerais, Rio de Janeiro, São Paulo; this includes >12-hour airport transits or layovers in any of these states

CDC recommendation: Not recommended

MALARIA PREVENTION

Transmission areas: Primarily in the provinces near the border with Haiti, and the provinces (including resort areas) of La Altagracia, San Cristóbal, San Juan, and Santo Domingo

In the Distrito Nacional, city of Santo Domingo (the capital), primarily in the La Ciénaga and Los Tres Brazos areas

Rare transmission in other provinces

Drug resistance[2]: None

Species: *P. falciparum* (100%)

Recommended chemoprophylaxis:

Provinces near the border with Haiti, and the provinces (including resort areas) of La Altagracia, San Cristóbal, San Juan, and Santo Domingo: Atovaquone-proguanil, chloroquine, doxycycline, mefloquine, tafenoquine[3]

All other areas: No chemoprophylaxis recommended (insect bite precautions and mosquito avoidance only)[4]

EASTER ISLAND, CHILE

YELLOW FEVER VACCINE

Entry requirements: Easter Island has not stated its YF vaccination certificate requirements

CDC recommendation: Not recommended

MALARIA PREVENTION

No malaria transmission

ECUADOR (INCLUDING THE GALÁPAGOS ISLANDS)

YELLOW FEVER VACCINE (MAP 2-06)

Entry requirements: Required for travelers ≥1 year old arriving from Brazil, Democratic Republic of the Congo, or Uganda; this includes >12-hour airport transits or layovers in any of these countries

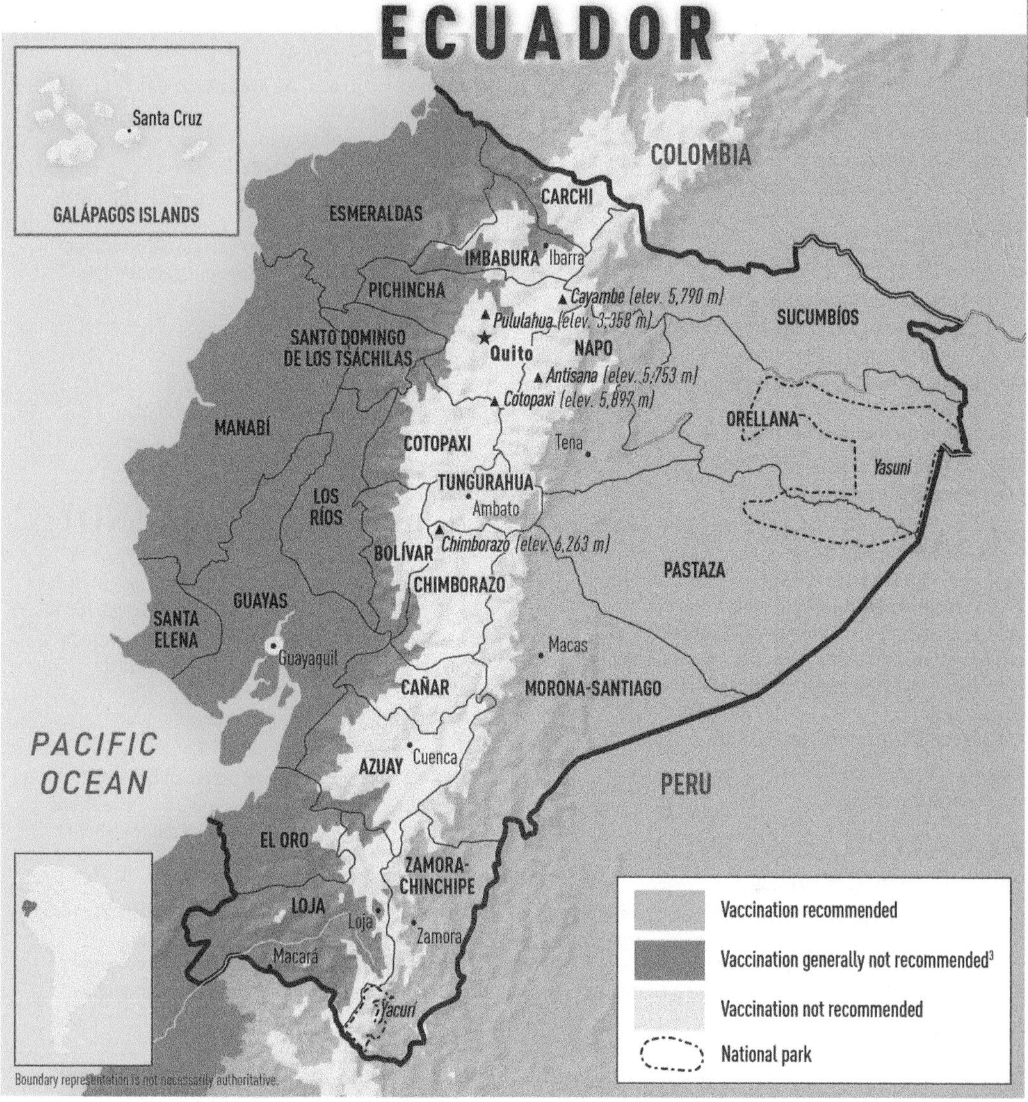

ECUADOR

Santa Cruz
GALÁPAGOS ISLANDS
COLOMBIA
CARCHI
ESMERALDAS
IMBABURA
Ibarra
PICHINCHA
Cayambe (elev. 5,790 m)
Pululahua (elev. 3,358 m)
SUCUMBÍOS
SANTO DOMINGO DE LOS TSÁCHILAS
Quito
NAPO
Antisana (elev. 5,753 m)
Cotopaxi (elev. 5,897 m)
ORELLANA
MANABÍ
COTOPAXI
Tena
Yasuní
TUNGURAHUA
Ambato
LOS RÍOS
BOLÍVAR
Chimborazo (elev. 6,263 m)
PASTAZA
CHIMBORAZO
GUAYAS
SANTA ELENA
Guayaquil
Macas
CAÑAR
MORONA-SANTIAGO
PACIFIC OCEAN
Cuenca
AZUAY
PERU
EL ORO
ZAMORA-CHINCHIPE
LOJA
Loja
Zamora
Macará
Yacurí

Vaccination recommended
Vaccination generally not recommended[3]
Vaccination not recommended
National park

Boundary representation is not necessarily authoritative.

MAP 2-06 **Yellow fever vaccine recommendations for Ecuador & neighboring countries**[1]

[1] For footnotes, see page 84

CDC recommendations:

Recommended for travelers ≥9 months old going to areas <2,300 m (≈7,550 ft) elevation, east of the Andes Mountains, in the provinces of Morona-Santiago, Napo, Orellana, Pastaza, Sucumbíos, Tungurahua,* and Zamora-Chinchipe

Generally not recommended for travel limited to areas <2,300 m (≈7,550 ft) elevation, west of the Andes Mountains, in the provinces of Esmeraldas,* Guayas, Los Ríos, Manabí, Santa Elena, Santo Domingo de los Tsáchilas, and designated areas in the provinces of Azuay, Bolívar, Cañar, Carchi, Chimborazo, Cotopaxi, El Oro, Imbabura, Loja, and Pichincha

Not recommended for travel limited to areas >2,300 m (≈7,550 ft) elevation, the cities of Guayaquil or Quito (the capital), or the Galápagos Islands

*CDC recommendations differ from those published by WHO (www.who.int/travel-advice/vaccines).

MALARIA PREVENTION

Transmission areas: Areas <1,500 m (≈5,000 ft) elevation in the provinces of Carchi, Cotopaxi, Esmeraldas, Morona-Santiago, Orellana, Pastaza, and Sucumbíos

Rare cases <1,500 m (≈5,000 ft) in all other provinces

No malaria transmission in the cities of Guayaquil or Quito (the capital)

No malaria transmission on the Galápagos Islands

Drug resistance[2]: Chloroquine

Species: *P. vivax* (85%); *P. falciparum* (15%)

Recommended chemoprophylaxis:
Transmission areas in the provinces of Carchi, Cotopaxi, Esmeraldas, Morona-Santiago, Orellana, Pastaza, and Sucumbíos: Atovaquone-proguanil, doxycycline, mefloquine, tafenoquine[3]
All other areas with reported malaria transmission: No chemoprophylaxis recommended (insect bite precautions and mosquito avoidance only)[4]

2

EGYPT

YELLOW FEVER VACCINE

Entry requirements: Required for travelers ≥9 months old arriving from countries with risk for YF virus transmission; this includes >12-hour airport transits or layovers in countries with risk for YF virus transmission[1]
CDC recommendation: Not recommended

MALARIA PREVENTION

No malaria transmission

EL SALVADOR

YELLOW FEVER VACCINE

Entry requirements: Required for travelers ≥1 year old arriving from countries with risk for YF virus transmission; this includes >12-hour airport transits or layovers in countries with risk for YF virus transmission[1]
CDC recommendation: Not recommended

MALARIA PREVENTION

No malaria transmission

EQUATORIAL GUINEA

YELLOW FEVER VACCINE

Entry requirements: Required for travelers ≥9 months old arriving from countries with risk for YF virus transmission[1]
CDC recommended for all travelers ≥9 months old

MALARIA PREVENTION

Transmission areas: All
Drug resistance[2]: Chloroquine
Species: *P. falciparum* (primarily); *P. malariae*, *P. ovale*, and *P. vivax* (less commonly)
Recommended chemoprophylaxis: Atovaquone-proguanil, doxycycline, mefloquine, tafenoquine[3]

ERITREA

YELLOW FEVER VACCINE (MAP 5-10)

Entry requirements: Required for travelers ≥9 months old arriving from countries with risk for YF virus transmission[1]
CDC recommendations:
Generally not recommended for travel to the regions of: Anseba, Debub (also known as South or Southern Region), Gash Barka, Ma'ekel (also known as Ma'akel or Central Region), or Semenawi K'eyih Bahri (also known as Northern Red Sea Region)
Not recommended for travel to any areas not listed above, including the Dahlak Archipelago

MALARIA PREVENTION

Transmission areas: All areas <2,200 m (≈7,200 ft) elevation
No malaria transmission in Asmara (the capital)
Drug resistance[2]: Chloroquine
Species: *P. falciparum* (80–85%); *P. vivax* (15–20%); *P. malariae* and *P. ovale* (rare)
Recommended chemoprophylaxis: Atovaquone-proguanil, doxycycline, mefloquine, tafenoquine[3]

ESTONIA

YELLOW FEVER VACCINE

Entry requirements: None
CDC recommendation: Not recommended

MALARIA PREVENTION

No malaria transmission

ESWATINI (SWAZILAND)

YELLOW FEVER VACCINE

Entry requirements: Required for travelers ≥9 months old arriving from countries with risk for YF virus transmission; this includes airport transits or layovers in countries with risk for YF virus transmission[1]
CDC recommendation: Not recommended

MALARIA PREVENTION

Transmission areas: Eastern areas bordering Mozambique and South Africa, including the entire region of Lubombo and the eastern half of Hhohho, Manzini, and Shiselweni Regions
Drug resistance[2]: Chloroquine
Species: *P. falciparum* (primarily); *P. malariae*, *P. ovale*, and *P. vivax* (less commonly)
Recommended chemoprophylaxis: Atovaquone-proguanil, doxycycline, mefloquine, tafenoquine[3]

ETHIOPIA

YELLOW FEVER VACCINE (MAP 2-07)

Entry requirements: Required for travelers ≥9 months old arriving from countries with risk for YF virus transmission; this includes >12-hour airport transits or layovers in countries with risk for YF virus transmission[1]
CDC recommendations:
Recommended for all travelers ≥9 months old except as follows
Generally not recommended for travel limited to the regions of Afar or Somali

MALARIA PREVENTION

Transmission areas: All areas <2,500 m (≈8,200 ft) elevation, except none in Addis Ababa (the capital)
Drug resistance[2]: Chloroquine
Species: *P. falciparum* (80%); *P. vivax* (20%); *P. malariae* and *P. ovale* (rare)

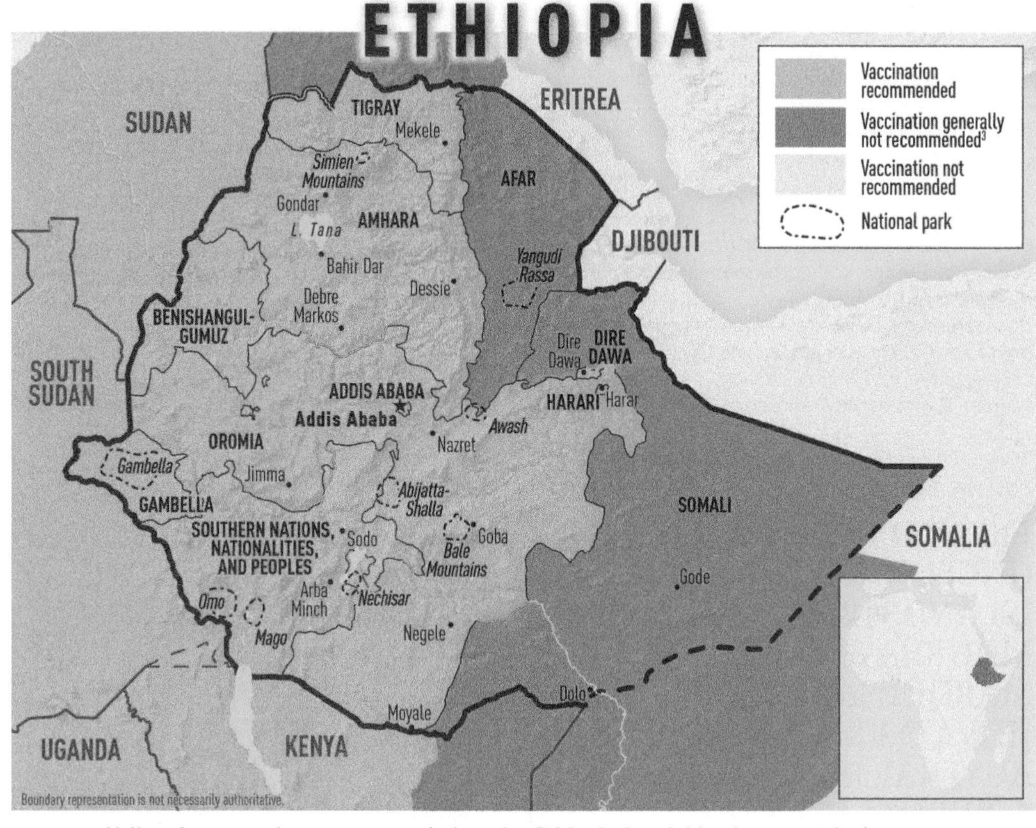

MAP 2-07 Yellow fever vaccine recommendations for Ethiopia & neighboring countries[1]

[1] For footnotes, see page 84

Recommended chemoprophylaxis: Atovaquone-proguanil, doxycycline, mefloquine, tafenoquine[3]

FALKLAND ISLANDS (ISLAS MALVINAS), UK OVERSEAS TERRITORY (ALSO CLAIMED BY ARGENTINA)

YELLOW FEVER VACCINE

Entry requirements: None
CDC recommendation: Not recommended

MALARIA PREVENTION

No malaria transmission

FAROE ISLANDS, DENMARK

YELLOW FEVER VACCINE

Entry requirements: None
CDC recommendation: Not recommended

MALARIA PREVENTION

No malaria transmission

FIJI

YELLOW FEVER VACCINE

Entry requirements: Required for travelers ≥1 year old arriving from countries with risk for YF virus transmission; this includes >12-hour airport transits or layovers in countries with risk for YF virus transmission[1]
CDC recommendation: Not recommended

MALARIA PREVENTION

No malaria transmission

FINLAND

YELLOW FEVER VACCINE

Entry requirements: None
CDC recommendation: Not recommended

MALARIA PREVENTION

No malaria transmission

FRANCE

YELLOW FEVER VACCINE

Entry requirements: None
CDC recommendation: Not recommended

MALARIA PREVENTION

No malaria transmission

2

FRENCH GUIANA

YELLOW FEVER VACCINE

Entry requirements: Required for all arriving travelers ≥1 year old

CDC recommended for all travelers ≥9 months old

MALARIA PREVENTION

Transmission areas: Areas associated with gold mining, primarily the communes near the border with Brazil and Suriname, especially Régina and Saint-Georges-de-l'Oyapock; also, the communes of Kourou, Matoury, and Saint-Élie

No malaria transmission in coastal areas west of Kourou

No malaria transmission in Cayenne City (the capital)

Drug resistance[2]: Chloroquine

Species: *P. vivax* (85%); *P. falciparum* (15%); *P. malariae* (rare)

Recommended chemoprophylaxis: Atovaquone-proguanil, doxycycline, mefloquine, tafenoquine[3]

FRENCH POLYNESIA (INCLUDING THE SOCIETY ISLANDS [BORA-BORA, MOOREA & TAHITI], MARQUESAS ISLANDS [HIVA OA & UA HUKA], AND AUSTRAL ISLANDS [TUBUAI & RURUTU]), FRANCE

YELLOW FEVER VACCINE

Entry requirements: Required for travelers ≥1 year old arriving from countries with risk for YF virus transmission; this includes >12-hour airport transits or layovers in countries with risk for YF virus transmission[1]

CDC recommendation: Not recommended

MALARIA PREVENTION

No malaria transmission

GABON

YELLOW FEVER VACCINE

Entry requirements: Required for all arriving travelers ≥9 months old

CDC recommended for all travelers ≥9 months old

MALARIA PREVENTION

Transmission areas: All

Drug resistance[2]: Chloroquine

Species: *P. falciparum* (primarily); *P. malariae*, *P. ovale*, and *P. vivax* (less commonly)

Recommended chemoprophylaxis: Atovaquone-proguanil, doxycycline, mefloquine, tafenoquine[3]

GAMBIA, THE

YELLOW FEVER VACCINE

Entry requirements: Required for travelers ≥9 months old arriving from countries with risk for YF virus transmission; this includes >12-hour airport transits or layovers in countries with risk for YF virus transmission[1]

CDC recommended for all travelers ≥9 months old

MALARIA PREVENTION

Transmission areas: All

Drug resistance[2]: Chloroquine

Species: *P. falciparum* (primarily); *P. malariae*, *P. ovale*, and *P. vivax* (less commonly)

Recommended chemoprophylaxis: Atovaquone-proguanil, doxycycline, mefloquine, or tafenoquine[3]

GEORGIA

YELLOW FEVER VACCINE

Entry requirements: None

CDC recommendation: Not recommended

MALARIA PREVENTION

No malaria transmission

GERMANY

YELLOW FEVER VACCINE

Entry requirements: None

CDC recommendation: Not recommended

MALARIA PREVENTION

No malaria transmission

GHANA

YELLOW FEVER VACCINE

Entry requirements: Required for all arriving travelers ≥9 months old

CDC recommended for all travelers ≥9 months old

MALARIA PREVENTION

Transmission areas: All

Drug resistance[2]: Chloroquine

Species: *P. falciparum* (primarily); *P. malariae*, *P. ovale*, and *P. vivax* (less commonly)

Recommended chemoprophylaxis: Atovaquone-proguanil, doxycycline, mefloquine, or tafenoquine[3]

GIBRALTAR, UNITED KINGDOM

YELLOW FEVER VACCINE

Entry requirements: None

CDC recommendation: Not recommended

MALARIA PREVENTION

No malaria transmission

GREECE

YELLOW FEVER VACCINE

Entry requirements: None

CDC recommendation: Not recommended

MALARIA PREVENTION

Transmission areas: Rare, local transmission in agricultural areas, associated with imported malaria (May–November)

No malaria transmission in tourist areas

Drug resistance[2]: Not applicable
Species: *P. vivax* (100%)
Recommended chemoprophylaxis: None

GREENLAND, DENMARK

YELLOW FEVER VACCINE

Entry requirements: None
CDC recommendation: Not recommended

MALARIA PREVENTION

No malaria transmission

GRENADA

YELLOW FEVER VACCINE

Entry requirements: Required for travelers ≥1 year old arriving from countries with risk for YF virus transmission; this includes >12-hour airport transits or layovers in countries with risk for YF virus transmission[1]
CDC recommendation: Not recommended

MALARIA PREVENTION

No malaria transmission

GUADELOUPE (INCLUDING MARIE-GALANTE, LA DÉSIRADE & ÎLES DES SAINTES ISLANDS)

YELLOW FEVER VACCINE

Entry requirements: Required for travelers ≥1 year old arriving from countries with risk for YF virus transmission; this includes >12-hour airport transits or layovers in countries with risk for YF virus transmission[1]
CDC recommendation: Not recommended

MALARIA PREVENTION

No malaria transmission

GUAM, UNITED STATES

YELLOW FEVER VACCINE

Entry requirements: None
CDC recommendation: Not recommended

MALARIA PREVENTION

No malaria transmission

GUATEMALA

YELLOW FEVER VACCINE

Entry requirements: Required for travelers ≥1 year old arriving from countries with risk for YF virus transmission; this includes >12-hour airport transits or layovers in countries with risk for YF virus transmission[1]
CDC recommendation: Not recommended

MALARIA PREVENTION

Transmission areas: Primarily in the departments of Alta Verapaz, Escuintla, Izabal, Petén, and Suchitepéquez
Few cases reported in other departments
No malaria transmission in the cities of Antigua or Guatemala City (the capital)
No malaria transmission at Lake Atitlán
Drug resistance[2]: None
Species: *P. vivax* (99%); *P. falciparum* (1%)
Recommended chemoprophylaxis:
Departments of Alta Verapaz, Escuintla, Izabal, Petén, and Suchitepéquez: Atovaquone-proguanil, chloroquine, doxycycline, mefloquine, primaquine,[5] tafenoquine[3]
Other areas with reported malaria transmission: No chemoprophylaxis recommended (insect bite precautions and mosquito avoidance only)[4]

GUINEA

YELLOW FEVER VACCINE

Entry requirements: Required for travelers ≥9 months old arriving from countries with risk for YF virus transmission[1]
CDC recommended for all travelers ≥9 months old

MALARIA PREVENTION

Transmission areas: All
Drug resistance[2]: Chloroquine
Species: *P. falciparum* (primarily); *P. malariae*, *P. ovale*, and *P. vivax* (less commonly)
Recommended chemoprophylaxis: Atovaquone-proguanil, doxycycline, mefloquine, tafenoquine[3]

GUINEA-BISSAU

YELLOW FEVER VACCINE

Entry requirements: Required for all arriving travelers ≥1 year old
CDC recommended for all travelers ≥9 months old

MALARIA PREVENTION

Transmission areas: All
Drug resistance[2]: Chloroquine
Species: *P. falciparum* (primarily); *P. malariae*, *P. ovale*, and *P. vivax* (less commonly)
Recommended chemoprophylaxis: Atovaquone-proguanil, doxycycline, mefloquine, tafenoquine[3]

GUYANA

YELLOW FEVER VACCINE

Entry requirements: Required for travelers ≥1 year old arriving from countries with risk for YF virus transmission; this includes >4-hour airport transits or layovers in countries with risk for YF virus transmission[1]
CDC recommended for all travelers ≥9 months old

MALARIA PREVENTION

Transmission areas: All
Rare cases in the cities of Georgetown (the capital) and New Amsterdam
Drug resistance[2]: Chloroquine
Species: *P. vivax* (60%); *P. falciparum* (40%)
Recommended chemoprophylaxis:

All areas (except the cities of Georgetown and New Amsterdam): Atovaquone-proguanil, doxycycline, mefloquine, tafenoquine[3]
Cities of Georgetown and New Amsterdam: No chemoprophylaxis recommended (insect bite precautions and mosquito avoidance only)[4]

HAITI

YELLOW FEVER VACCINE

Entry requirements: Required for travelers ≥1 year old arriving from countries with risk for YF virus transmission[1]
CDC recommendation: Not recommended

MALARIA PREVENTION

Transmission areas: All (including Labadie, also known as Port Labadee)
Drug resistance[2]: None
Species: *P. falciparum* (99%); *P. malariae* (rare)
Recommended chemoprophylaxis: Atovaquone-proguanil, chloroquine, doxycycline, mefloquine, tafenoquine[3]

HONDURAS

YELLOW FEVER VACCINE

Entry requirements: Required for travelers 1-60 years old arriving from countries with risk for YF virus transmission; this includes >12-hour airport transits or layovers in countries with risk for YF virus transmission[1]
CDC recommendation: Not recommended

MALARIA PREVENTION

Transmission areas:
Throughout the country and on the island of Roatán and other Bay Islands
No malaria transmission in the cities of San Pedro Sula or Tegucigalpa (the capital)
Drug resistance[2]: None
Species: *P. vivax* (93%); *P. falciparum* (7%)
Recommended chemoprophylaxis: Atovaquone-proguanil, chloroquine, doxycycline, mefloquine, tafenoquine[3]

HONG KONG SPECIAL ADMINISTRATIVE REGION, CHINA

YELLOW FEVER VACCINE

Entry requirements: None
CDC recommendation: Not recommended

MALARIA PREVENTION

No malaria transmission

HUNGARY

YELLOW FEVER VACCINE

Entry requirements: None
CDC recommendation: Not recommended

MALARIA PREVENTION

No malaria transmission

ICELAND

YELLOW FEVER VACCINE

Entry requirements: None
CDC recommendation: Not recommended

MALARIA PREVENTION

No malaria transmission

INDIA

YELLOW FEVER VACCINE

Entry requirements: Any traveler ≥9 months old arriving by air or by sea without a YF vaccination certificate will be detained in isolation for ≤6 days if they

- Arrive within 6 days of leaving an area with risk for YF virus transmission, or
- Have been in such an area in transit (exception: passengers and members of flight crews who, while in transit through an airport in an area with risk for YF virus transmission, remained in the airport during their entire stay and the health officer agrees to such an exemption), or
- Arrive on a ship that started from or touched at any port in an area with risk for YF virus transmission ≤30 days before its arrival in India, unless such a ship has been disinsected in accordance with the procedure recommended by the World Health Organization (WHO), or
- Arrive on an aircraft that has been in an area with risk for YF virus transmission and has not been disinsected in accordance with the Indian Aircraft Public Health Rules, 1954, or as recommended by WHO.

The following countries are regarded by the Government of India as areas with risk for YF virus transmission.

- **Africa**: Angola, Benin, Burkina Faso, Burundi, Cameroon, Central African Republic, Chad, Congo, Côte d'Ivoire, Democratic Republic of the Congo, Equatorial Guinea, Ethiopia, Gabon, The Gambia, Ghana, Guinea, Guinea-Bissau, Kenya, Liberia, Mali, Mauritania, Niger, Nigeria, Rwanda, Senegal, Sierra Leone, South Sudan, Sudan, Togo, Uganda
- **Americas**: Argentina, Bolivia, Brazil, Colombia, Ecuador, French Guiana, Guyana, Panama, Paraguay, Peru, Suriname, Trinidad & Tobago (Trinidad only), Venezuela

When a case of YF is reported from any country, the Government of India regards that country as an area with risk for YF virus transmission and adds it to the above list.
CDC recommendation: Not recommended

MALARIA PREVENTION

Transmission areas: Throughout the country, including the cities of Bombay (Mumbai) and New Delhi (the capital)

No malaria transmission in areas >2,000 m (≈6,500 ft) elevation in Himachal Pradesh, Jammu and Kashmir, or Sikkim
Drug resistance[2]: Chloroquine
Species: *P. vivax* (50%); *P. falciparum* (>40%); *P. malariae* and *P. ovale* (rare)
Recommended chemoprophylaxis: Atovaquone-proguanil, doxycycline, mefloquine, tafenoquine[3]

INDONESIA

YELLOW FEVER VACCINE
Entry requirements: Required for travelers ≥9 months old arriving from countries with risk for YF virus transmission[1]
CDC recommendation: Not recommended

MALARIA PREVENTION
Transmission areas: All areas of eastern Indonesia (the provinces of Maluku, North Maluku, East Nusa Tenggara, Papua, and West Papua), including the town of Labuan Bajo and the Komodo Islands in the Nusa Tenggara region
Rural areas of Kalimantan (Borneo), West Nusa Tenggara (includes the island of Lombok), Sulawesi, and Sumatra
Low transmission in rural areas of Java, including Pangandaran, Sukabumi, and Ujung Kulon
No malaria transmission in the cities of Jakarta (the capital) or Ubud
No malaria transmission in the resort areas of Bali or Java, the Gili Islands, or the Thousand Islands (Pulau Seribu)
Drug resistance[2]: Chloroquine (*P. falciparum* and *P. vivax*)
Species: *P. falciparum* (60%); *P. vivax* (40%); *P. knowlesi*,[6] *P. malariae*, and *P. ovale* (rare)
Recommended chemoprophylaxis: Atovaquone-proguanil, doxycycline, mefloquine, tafenoquine[3]

IRAN

YELLOW FEVER VACCINE
Entry requirements: Required for travelers ≥9 months old arriving from countries with risk for YF virus transmission; this includes >12-hour airport transits or layovers in countries with risk for YF virus transmission[1]
CDC recommendation: Not recommended

MALARIA PREVENTION
Transmission areas: No indigenous cases reported since 2017
Previously, in rural areas of the provinces of Fars and Sistan va Baluchestan, and southern, tropical regions of the provinces of Hormozgan and Kerman (March–November)
Drug resistance[2]: Previously, chloroquine
Species: Previously, *P. vivax* (93%) and *P. falciparum* (7%)
Recommended chemoprophylaxis: None (insect bite precautions and mosquito avoidance only)[4]

IRAQ

YELLOW FEVER VACCINE
Entry requirements: None
CDC recommendation: Not recommended

MALARIA PREVENTION
No malaria transmission

IRELAND

YELLOW FEVER VACCINE
Entry requirements: None
CDC recommendation: Not recommended

MALARIA PREVENTION
No malaria transmission

ISRAEL

YELLOW FEVER VACCINE
Entry requirements: None
CDC recommendation: Not recommended

MALARIA PREVENTION
No malaria transmission

ITALY (INCLUDING HOLY SEE [VATICAN CITY])

YELLOW FEVER VACCINE
Entry requirements: None
CDC recommendation: Not recommended

MALARIA PREVENTION
No malaria transmission

JAMAICA

YELLOW FEVER VACCINE
Entry requirements: Required for travelers ≥1 year old arriving from countries with risk for YF virus transmission; this includes >12-hour airport transits or layovers in countries with risk for YF virus transmission[1]
CDC recommendation: Not recommended

MALARIA PREVENTION
No malaria transmission

JAPAN

YELLOW FEVER VACCINE
Entry requirements: None
CDC recommendation: Not recommended

MALARIA PREVENTION
No malaria transmission

JORDAN

YELLOW FEVER VACCINE
Entry requirements: None
CDC recommendation: Not recommended

MALARIA PREVENTION
No malaria transmission

KAZAKHSTAN

YELLOW FEVER VACCINE

Entry requirements: Required for travelers arriving from countries with risk for YF virus transmission; this includes airport transits or layovers in countries with risk for YF virus transmission[1]

CDC recommendation: Not recommended

MALARIA PREVENTION

No malaria transmission

KENYA

YELLOW FEVER VACCINE (MAP 2-08)

Entry requirements: Required for travelers ≥1 year old arriving from countries with risk for YF virus transmission[1]

CDC recommendations:

Recommended for all travelers ≥9 months old except as follows

Generally not recommended for travel limited to: the city of Nairobi (the capital); the counties of the former North Eastern Province (Mandera, Wajir, and Garissa); or the counties (except Taita-Taveta) of the former Coast Province (Kilifi, including the city of Malindi; Kwale; Lamu; Mombasa, including the city of Mombasa; Tana River)

MALARIA PREVENTION (MAP 2-09)

Transmission areas: All areas (including game parks) <2,500 m (≈8,200 ft) elevation, including the city of Nairobi (the capital)

Drug resistance[2]: Chloroquine

Species: *P. falciparum* (primarily); *P. malariae*, *P. ovale*, and *P. vivax* (less commonly)

Recommended chemoprophylaxis: Atovaquone-proguanil, doxycycline, mefloquine, tafenoquine[3]

KIRIBATI (FORMERLY GILBERT ISLANDS; INCLUDING TARAWA, TABUAERAN [FANNING ISLAND] & BANABA [OCEAN ISLAND])

YELLOW FEVER VACCINE

Entry requirements: None

CDC recommendation: Not recommended

MALARIA PREVENTION

No malaria transmission

KOSOVO

YELLOW FEVER VACCINE

Entry requirements: None

CDC recommendation: Not recommended

MALARIA PREVENTION

No malaria transmission

KUWAIT

YELLOW FEVER VACCINE

Entry requirements: None

CDC recommendation: Not recommended

MALARIA PREVENTION

No malaria transmission

KYRGYZSTAN

YELLOW FEVER VACCINE

Entry requirements: None

CDC recommendation: Not recommended

MALARIA PREVENTION

No malaria transmission

LAOS

YELLOW FEVER VACCINE

Entry requirements: None

CDC recommendation: Not recommended

MALARIA PREVENTION

Transmission areas: All, except in Vientiane (the capital) where there is no transmission

Drug resistance[2]: Chloroquine and mefloquine

Species: *P. vivax* (55%); *P. falciparum* (45%); *P. knowlesi*,[6] *P. malariae*, and *P. ovale* (rare)

Recommended chemoprophylaxis:

Areas bordering Burma (the provinces of Bokeo and Luang Namtha), Cambodia; Thailand (the provinces of Champasak and Salavan); and Vietnam: Atovaquone-proguanil, doxycycline, tafenoquine[3]

All other areas with malaria transmission: Atovaquone-proguanil, doxycycline, mefloquine, tafenoquine[3]

LATVIA

YELLOW FEVER VACCINE

Entry requirements: None

CDC recommendation: Not recommended

MALARIA PREVENTION

No malaria transmission

LEBANON

YELLOW FEVER VACCINE

Entry requirements: None

CDC recommendation: Not recommended

MALARIA PREVENTION

No malaria transmission

LESOTHO

YELLOW FEVER VACCINE

Entry requirements: None

CDC recommendation: Not recommended

MALARIA PREVENTION

No malaria transmission

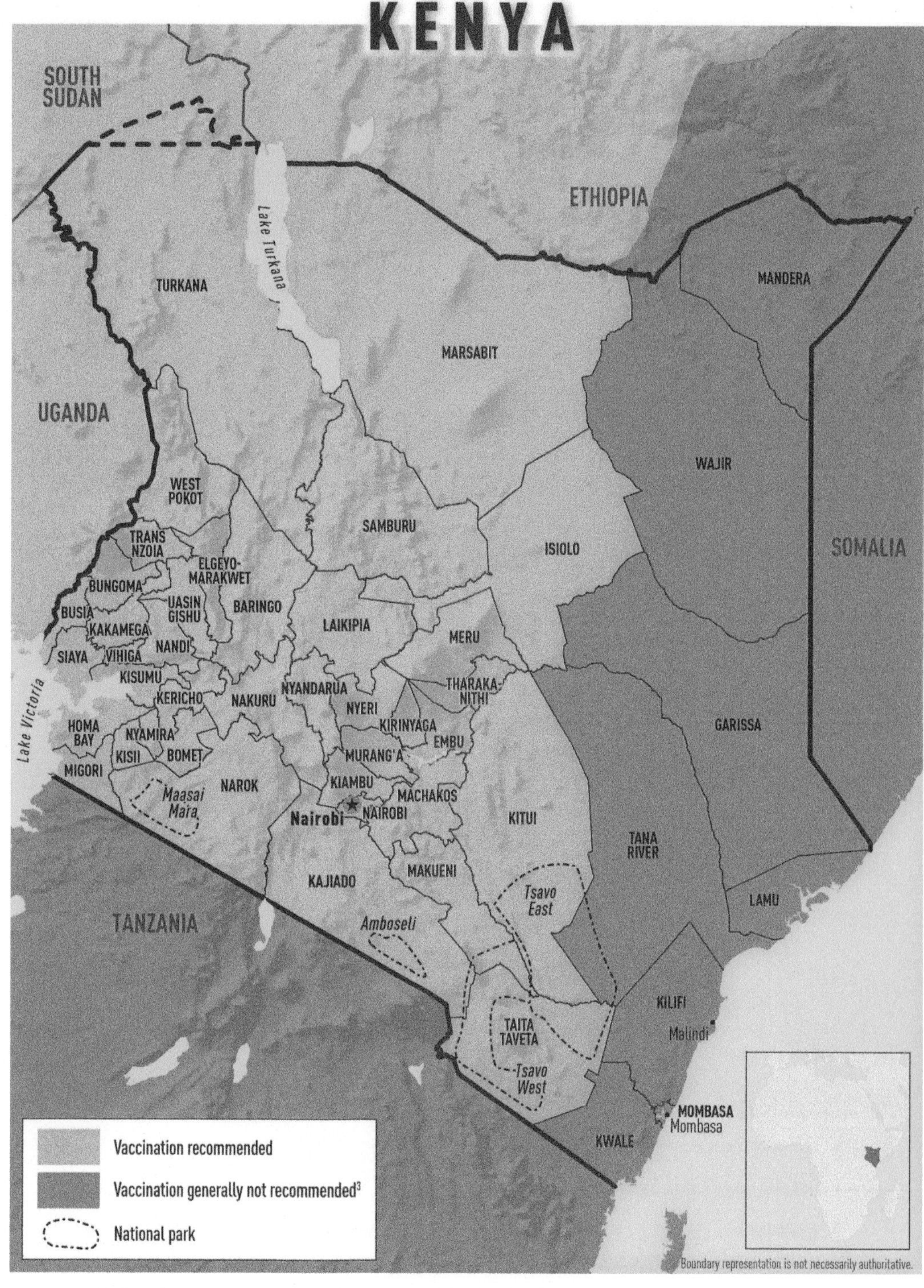

MAP 2-08 Yellow fever vaccine recommendations for Kenya & neighboring countries[1]

[1] For footnotes, see page 84

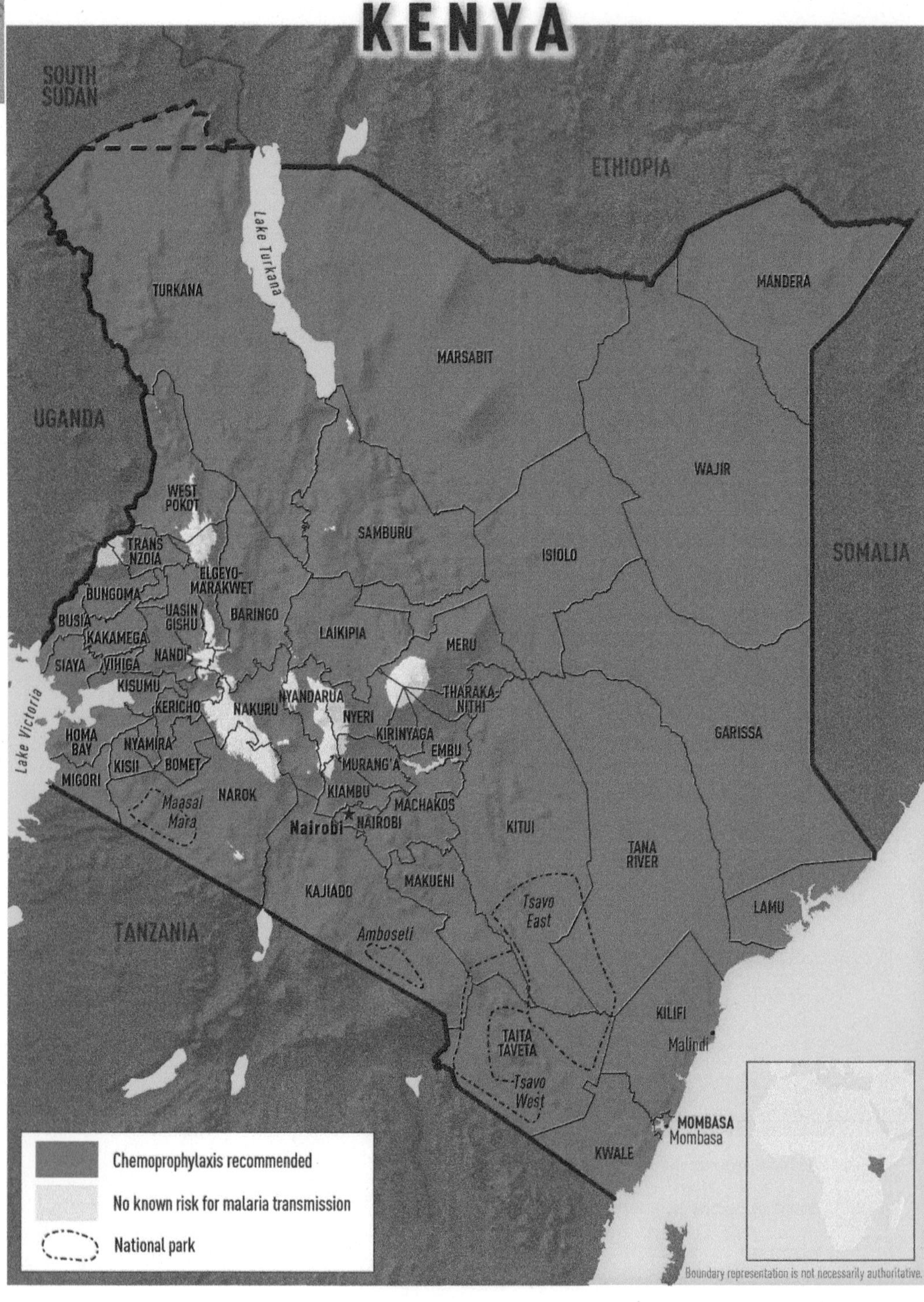
KENYA
SOUTH SUDAN
ETHIOPIA
UGANDA
SOMALIA
TANZANIA
Lake Turkana
Lake Victoria
TURKANA
MARSABIT
MANDERA
WAJIR
WEST POKOT
SAMBURU
ISIOLO
TRANS NZOIA
ELGEYO-MARAKWET
BUNGOMA
UASIN GISHU
BARINGO
BUSIA
KAKAMEGA
LAIKIPIA
MERU
SIAYA
VIHIGA
NANDI
KISUMU
NYANDARUA
THARAKA-NITHI
KERICHO
NAKURU
NYERI
GARISSA
HOMA BAY
NYAMIRA
KIRINYAGA
EMBU
KISII
BOMET
MURANG'A
MIGORI
KIAMBU
Maasai Mara
NAROK
MACHAKOS
Nairobi
NAIROBI
KITUI
TANA RIVER
MAKUENI
KAJIADO
Tsavo East
LAMU
Amboseli
KILIFI
TAITA TAVETA
Malindi
Tsavo West
MOMBASA
Mombasa
KWALE
Chemoprophylaxis recommended
No known risk for malaria transmission
National park
Boundary representation is not necessarily authoritative.

MAP 2-09 Malaria prevention in Kenya

LIBERIA

YELLOW FEVER VACCINE

Entry requirements: Required for travelers ≥9 months old arriving from countries with risk for YF virus transmission[1]

CDC recommended for all travelers ≥9 months old

MALARIA PREVENTION

Transmission areas: All

Drug resistance[2]: Chloroquine

Species: *P. falciparum* (primarily); *P. malariae*, *P. ovale*, and *P. vivax* (less commonly)

Recommended chemoprophylaxis: Atovaquone-proguanil, doxycycline, mefloquine, tafenoquine[3]

LIBYA

YELLOW FEVER VACCINE

Entry requirements: None

CDC recommendation: Not recommended

MALARIA PREVENTION

No malaria transmission

LIECHTENSTEIN

YELLOW FEVER VACCINE

Entry requirements: None

CDC recommendation: Not recommended

MALARIA PREVENTION

No malaria transmission

LITHUANIA

YELLOW FEVER VACCINE

Entry requirements: None

CDC recommendation: Not recommended

MALARIA PREVENTION

No malaria transmission

LUXEMBOURG

YELLOW FEVER VACCINE

Entry requirements: None

CDC recommendation: Not recommended

MALARIA PREVENTION

No malaria transmission

MACAU SPECIAL ADMINISTRATIVE REGION, CHINA

YELLOW FEVER VACCINE

Entry requirements: None

CDC recommendation: Not recommended

MALARIA PREVENTION

No malaria transmission

MADAGASCAR

YELLOW FEVER VACCINE

Entry requirements: Required for travelers ≥9 months old arriving from countries with risk for YF virus transmission; this includes >12-hour airport transits or layovers in countries with risk for YF virus transmission[1]

CDC recommendation: Not recommended

MALARIA PREVENTION

Transmission areas: All; except in Antananarivo (the capital) where malaria transmission is rare

Drug resistance[2]: Chloroquine

Species: *P. falciparum* (primarily); *P. ovale* and *P. vivax* (less commonly)

Recommended chemoprophylaxis:

All areas (except the city of Antananarivo): Atovaquone-proguanil, doxycycline, mefloquine, tafenoquine[3]

Antananarivo: No chemoprophylaxis recommended (insect bite precautions and mosquito avoidance only)[4]

MADEIRA ISLANDS, PORTUGAL

YELLOW FEVER VACCINE

Entry requirements: None

CDC recommendation: Not recommended

MALARIA PREVENTION

No malaria transmission

MALAWI

YELLOW FEVER VACCINE

Entry requirements: Required for travelers ≥1 year old arriving from countries with risk for YF virus transmission; this includes >12-hour airport transits or layovers in countries with risk for YF virus transmission[1]

CDC recommendation: Not recommended

MALARIA PREVENTION

Transmission areas: All

Drug resistance[2]: Chloroquine

Species: *P. falciparum* (primarily); *P. malariae*, *P. ovale*, and *P. vivax* (less commonly)

Recommended chemoprophylaxis: Atovaquone-proguanil, doxycycline, mefloquine, tafenoquine[3]

MALAYSIA

YELLOW FEVER VACCINE

Entry requirements: Required for travelers ≥1 year old arriving from countries with risk for YF virus transmission; this includes >12-hour airport transits or layovers in countries with risk for YF virus transmission[1]

CDC recommendation: Not recommended

MALARIA PREVENTION

Transmission areas: No indigenous cases of human malaria since 2017

Zoonotic transmission of simian malaria occurs in rural, forested areas

No malaria transmission in other areas, including Kuala Lumpur (the capital), in Penang State, on Penang Island, or in George Town (capital of Penang State)

Drug resistance[2]: Previously, chloroquine

Species: *P. knowlesi*[6] (primarily); previously, *P. falciparum*, *P. malariae*, *P. ovale*, and *P. vivax*

Recommended chemoprophylaxis: In rural, forested areas: Atovaquone-proguanil, doxycycline, mefloquine, tafenoquine[3]

MALDIVES

YELLOW FEVER VACCINE

Entry requirements: Required for travelers ≥9 months old arriving from countries with risk for YF virus transmission; this includes >12-hour airport transits or layovers in countries with risk for YF virus transmission[1]

CDC recommendation: Not recommended

MALARIA PREVENTION

No malaria transmission

MALI

YELLOW FEVER VACCINE (MAP 5-10)

Entry requirements: Required for all arriving travelers ≥9 months old

CDC recommendations:

Recommended for travelers ≥9 months old going to areas south of the Sahara Desert

Not recommended for travel limited to areas in the Sahara Desert

MALARIA PREVENTION

Transmission areas: All

Drug resistance[2]: Chloroquine

Species: *P. falciparum* (primarily); *P. malariae*, *P. ovale*, and *P. vivax* (less commonly)

Recommended chemoprophylaxis: Atovaquone-proguanil, doxycycline, mefloquine, tafenoquine[3]

MALTA

YELLOW FEVER VACCINE

Entry requirements: Required for travelers ≥9 months old arriving from countries with risk for YF virus transmission; this includes >12-hour airport transits or layovers in countries with risk for YF virus transmission[1]

CDC recommendation: Not recommended

MALARIA PREVENTION

No malaria transmission

MARSHALL ISLANDS

YELLOW FEVER VACCINE

Entry requirements: None

CDC recommendation: Not recommended

MALARIA PREVENTION

No malaria transmission

MARTINIQUE

YELLOW FEVER VACCINE

Entry requirements: Required for travelers ≥1 year old arriving from countries with risk for YF virus transmission; this includes >12-hour airport transits or layovers in countries with risk for YF virus transmission[1]

CDC recommendation: Not recommended

MALARIA PREVENTION

No malaria transmission

MAURITANIA

YELLOW FEVER VACCINE (MAP 5-10)

Entry requirements: Required for travelers ≥1 year old arriving from countries with risk for YF virus transmission[1]

CDC recommendations:

Recommended for travelers ≥9 months old going to areas south of the Sahara Desert

Not recommended for travel limited to areas in the Sahara Desert

MALARIA PREVENTION

Transmission areas: All; except in the regions of Dakhlet Nouadhibou and Tiris Zemmour where there is no transmission

Drug resistance[2]: Chloroquine

Species: *P. falciparum* (primarily); *P. malariae*, *P. ovale*, and *P. vivax* (less commonly)

Recommended chemoprophylaxis: Atovaquone-proguanil, doxycycline, mefloquine, tafenoquine[3]

MAURITIUS

YELLOW FEVER VACCINE

Entry requirements: None

CDC recommendation: Not recommended

MALARIA PREVENTION

No malaria transmission

MAYOTTE

YELLOW FEVER VACCINE

Entry requirements: Required for travelers ≥1 year old arriving from countries with risk for YF virus transmission; this includes >12-hour airport transits or layovers in countries with risk for YF virus transmission[1]

CDC recommendation: Not recommended

MALARIA PREVENTION

Transmission areas: Rare cases

Drug resistance[2]: Chloroquine

Species: *P. falciparum* (primarily); *P. malariae*, *P. ovale*, and *P. vivax* (less commonly)

Recommended chemoprophylaxis: None (insect bite precautions and mosquito avoidance only)[4]

MEXICO

YELLOW FEVER VACCINE

Entry requirements: None

CDC recommendation: Not recommended

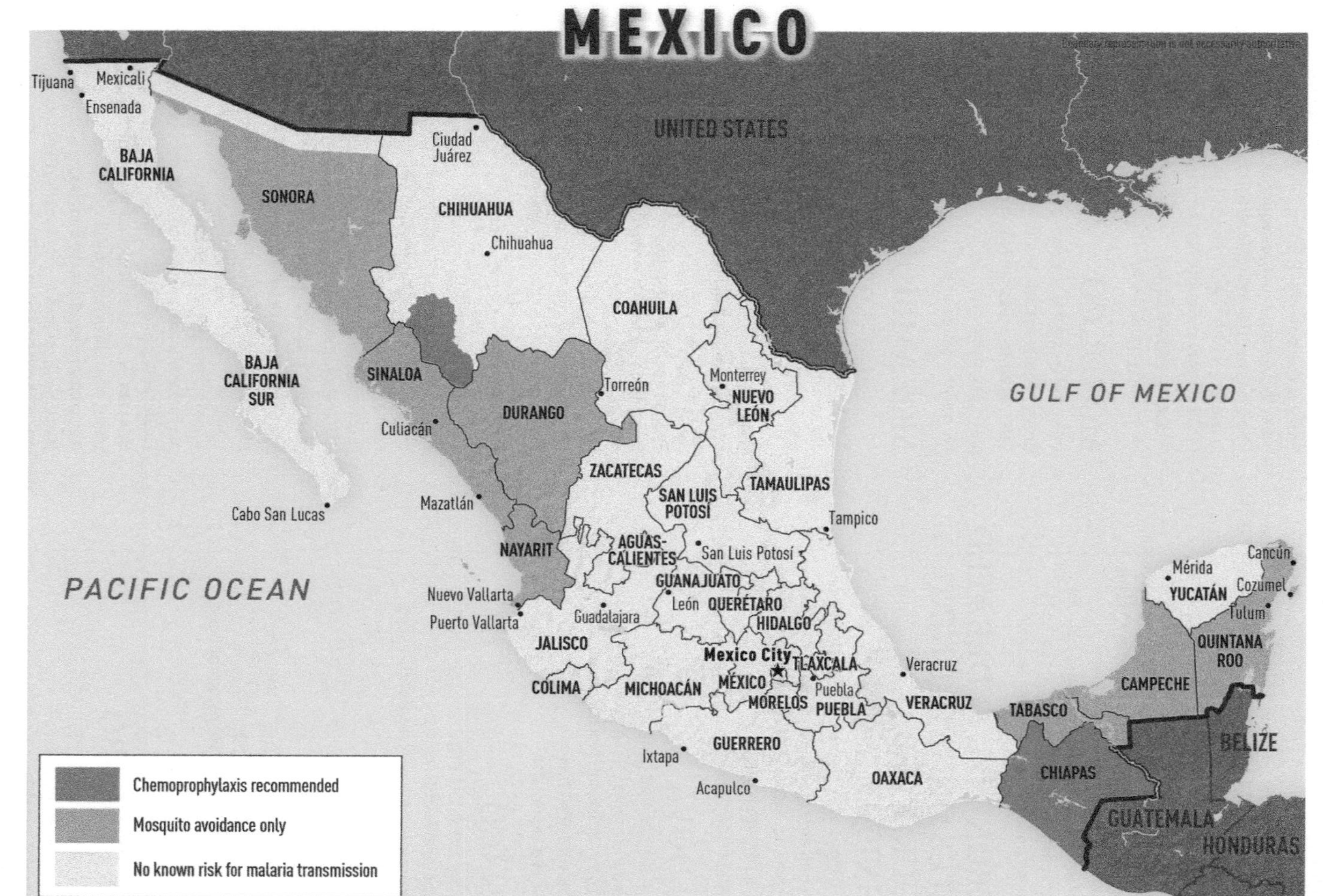

MAP 2-10 Malaria prevention in Mexico

MALARIA PREVENTION
(MAP 2-10)

Transmission areas: Chiapas State and southern part of Chihuahua State
Rare in the states of Campeche, Durango, Nayarit, Quintana Roo, Sinaloa, Sonora, and Tabasco
No malaria transmission along the US–Mexico border
Drug resistance[2]: None
Species: *P. vivax* (100%)
Recommended chemoprophylaxis:
Chiapas State and southern part of Chihuahua State: Atovaquone-proguanil, chloroquine, doxycycline, mefloquine, primaquine,[5] tafenoquine[3]
All other areas with malaria transmission: No chemoprophylaxis recommended (insect bite precautions and mosquito avoidance only)[4]

MICRONESIA, FEDERATED STATES OF (INCLUDING CHUUK, KOSRAE, POHNPEI & YAP)

YELLOW FEVER VACCINE

Entry requirements: None
CDC recommendation: Not recommended

MALARIA PREVENTION

No malaria transmission

MOLDOVA

YELLOW FEVER VACCINE

Entry requirements: None
CDC recommendation: Not recommended

MALARIA PREVENTION

No malaria transmission

MONACO

YELLOW FEVER VACCINE

Entry requirements: None
CDC recommendation: Not recommended

MALARIA PREVENTION

No malaria transmission

MONGOLIA

YELLOW FEVER VACCINE

Entry requirements: None
CDC recommendation: Not recommended

MALARIA PREVENTION

No malaria transmission

MONTENEGRO

YELLOW FEVER VACCINE

Entry requirements: None
CDC recommendation: Not recommended

MALARIA PREVENTION

No malaria transmission

MONTSERRAT, UNITED KINGDOM

YELLOW FEVER VACCINE

Entry requirements: Required for travelers ≥1 year old arriving from countries with risk for YF virus transmission; this includes airport transits or layovers in countries with risk for YF virus transmission[1]
CDC recommendation: Not recommended

MALARIA PREVENTION

No malaria transmission

MOROCCO

YELLOW FEVER VACCINE

Entry requirements: None
CDC recommendation: Not recommended

MALARIA PREVENTION

No malaria transmission

MOZAMBIQUE

YELLOW FEVER VACCINE

Entry requirements: Required for travelers ≥1 year old arriving from countries with risk for YF virus transmission; this includes >12-hour airport transits or layovers in countries with risk for YF virus transmission[1]
CDC recommendation: Not recommended

MALARIA PREVENTION

Transmission areas: All
Drug resistance[2]: Chloroquine
Species: *P. falciparum* (primarily); *P. malariae*, *P. ovale*, and *P. vivax* (less commonly)
Recommended chemoprophylaxis: Atovaquone-proguanil, doxycycline, mefloquine, tafenoquine[3]

NAMIBIA

YELLOW FEVER VACCINE

Entry requirements: Required for travelers ≥9 months old arriving from countries with risk for YF virus transmission; this includes >12-hour airport transits or layovers in countries with risk for YF virus transmission[1]
CDC recommendation: Not recommended

MALARIA PREVENTION

Transmission areas: In the regions of Kavango (East and West), Kunene, Ohangwena, Omaheke, Omusati, Oshana, Oshikoto, Otjozondjupa, and Zambezi
Rare in other parts of the country
No malaria transmission in Windhoek (the capital)
Drug resistance[2]: Chloroquine
Species: *P. falciparum* (primarily); *P. malariae*, *P. ovale*, and *P. vivax* (less commonly)
Recommended chemoprophylaxis:
Kavango (East and West), Kunene, Ohangwena, Omaheke, Omusati, Oshana, Oshikoto, Otjozondjupa, and Zambezi: Atovaquone-proguanil, doxycycline, mefloquine, tafenoquine[3]

All other areas with malaria transmission: No chemoprophylaxis recommended (insect bite precautions and mosquito avoidance only)[4]

NAURU

YELLOW FEVER VACCINE

Entry requirements: None
CDC recommendation: Not recommended

MALARIA PREVENTION

No malaria transmission

NEPAL

YELLOW FEVER VACCINE

Entry requirements: Required for travelers ≥9 months old arriving from countries with risk for YF virus transmission; this includes >12-hour airport transits or layovers in countries with risk for YF virus transmission[1]
CDC recommendation: Not recommended

MALARIA PREVENTION

Transmission areas:
Throughout the country in areas <2,000 m (≈6,500 ft) elevation
No malaria transmission in Kathmandu (the capital) or on typical Himalayan treks
Drug resistance[2]: Chloroquine
Species: *P. vivax* (primarily); *P. falciparum* (<10%)
Recommended chemoprophylaxis: Atovaquone-proguanil, doxycycline, mefloquine, tafenoquine[3]

NETHERLANDS

YELLOW FEVER VACCINE

Entry requirements: None
CDC recommendation: Not recommended

MALARIA PREVENTION

No malaria transmission

NEW CALEDONIA, FRANCE

YELLOW FEVER VACCINE

Entry requirements: Required for travelers ≥1 year old arriving from countries with risk for YF virus transmission; this includes >12-hour airport transits or layovers in countries with risk for YF virus transmission[1]
In the event of an epidemic threat to the territory, a specific vaccination certificate may be required
CDC recommendation: Not recommended

MALARIA PREVENTION

No malaria transmission

NEW ZEALAND

YELLOW FEVER VACCINE

Entry requirements: None
CDC recommendation: Not recommended

MALARIA PREVENTION

No malaria transmission

NICARAGUA

YELLOW FEVER VACCINE

Entry requirements: Required for travelers ≥1 year old arriving from countries with risk for YF virus transmission[1]
CDC recommendation: Not recommended

MALARIA PREVENTION

Transmission areas: Región Autónoma Atlántico Norte (RAAN) and Región Autónoma Atlántico Sur (RAAS)
Rare cases in the departments of Boaco, Chinandega, Estelí, Jinotega, León, Matagalpa, and Nueva Segovia
No malaria transmission in Managua (the capital)
Drug resistance[2]: None
Species: *P. vivax* (80%); *P. falciparum* (20%)
Recommended chemoprophylaxis:
Región Autónoma Atlántico Norte (RAAN) and Región Autónoma Atlántico Sur (RAAS): Atovaquone-proguanil, chloroquine, doxycycline, mefloquine, tafenoquine[3]
All other areas with malaria transmission: No chemoprophylaxis recommended (insect bite precautions and mosquito avoidance only)[4]

NIGER

YELLOW FEVER VACCINE (MAP 5-10)

Entry requirements: Required for all arriving travelers ≥9 months old
CDC recommendations:
Recommended for travelers ≥9 months old going to areas south of the Sahara Desert
Not recommended for travel limited to areas in the Sahara Desert

MALARIA PREVENTION

Transmission areas: All
Drug resistance[2]: Chloroquine
Species: *P. falciparum* (primarily); *P. malariae*, *P. ovale*, and *P. vivax* (less commonly)
Recommended chemoprophylaxis: Atovaquone-proguanil, doxycycline, mefloquine, tafenoquine[3]

NIGERIA

YELLOW FEVER VACCINE

Entry requirements: Required for travelers ≥9 months old arriving from countries with risk for YF virus transmission; this includes airport transits or layovers in countries with risk for YF virus transmission[1]
CDC recommended for all travelers ≥9 months old

MALARIA PREVENTION

Transmission areas: All
Drug resistance[2]: Chloroquine
Species: *P. falciparum* (primarily); *P. malariae*, *P. ovale*, and *P. vivax* (less commonly)

Recommended chemoprophylaxis: Atovaquone-proguanil, doxycycline, mefloquine, tafenoquine[3]

NIUE, NEW ZEALAND

YELLOW FEVER VACCINE

Entry requirements: Required for travelers ≥9 months old arriving from countries with risk for YF virus transmission[1]
CDC recommendation: Not recommended

MALARIA PREVENTION

No malaria transmission

NORFOLK ISLAND, AUSTRALIA

YELLOW FEVER VACCINE

Entry requirements: Required for travelers ≥1 year old arriving from countries with risk for YF virus transmission; this includes >12-hour airport transits or layovers in countries with risk for YF virus transmission[1]
Travelers arriving from the Galápagos Islands of Ecuador are exempt from this requirement
CDC recommendation: Not recommended

MALARIA PREVENTION

No malaria transmission

NORTH KOREA

YELLOW FEVER VACCINE

Entry requirements: Required for travelers ≥1 year old arriving from countries with risk for YF virus transmission[1]
CDC recommendation: Not recommended

MALARIA PREVENTION

Transmission areas: Southern provinces
Drug resistance[2]**:** None
Species: *P. vivax* (100%)
Recommended chemoprophylaxis: Atovaquone-proguanil, chloroquine, doxycycline, mefloquine, primaquine,[5] tafenoquine[3]

NORTH MACEDONIA

YELLOW FEVER VACCINE

Entry requirements: None
CDC recommendation: Not recommended

MALARIA PREVENTION

No malaria transmission

NORTHERN MARIANA ISLANDS (INCLUDING SAIPAN, TINIAN & ROTA), UNITED STATES

YELLOW FEVER VACCINE

Entry requirements: None
CDC recommendation: Not recommended

MALARIA PREVENTION

No malaria transmission

NORWAY

YELLOW FEVER VACCINE

Entry requirements: None
CDC recommendation: Not recommended

MALARIA PREVENTION

No malaria transmission

OMAN

YELLOW FEVER VACCINE

Entry requirements: Required for travelers ≥9 months old arriving from countries with risk for YF virus transmission, with the addition of Rwanda and Tanzania; this includes >12-hour airport transits or layovers in countries with risk for YF virus transmission[1]
CDC recommendation: Not recommended

MALARIA PREVENTION

Transmission areas: Rare sporadic transmission after importation only
Drug resistance[2]**:** Previously, chloroquine
Species: Previously, *P. falciparum* and *P. vivax*
Recommended chemoprophylaxis: None (insect bite precautions and mosquito avoidance only)[4]

PAKISTAN

YELLOW FEVER VACCINE

Entry requirements: Required for travelers ≥1 year old arriving from countries with risk for YF virus transmission; this includes >12-hour airport transits or layovers in countries with risk for YF virus transmission[1]
CDC recommendation: Not recommended

MALARIA PREVENTION

Transmission areas: All areas (including all cities) <2,500 m (≈8,200 ft) elevation
Drug resistance[2]**:** Chloroquine
Species: *P. vivax* (80%); *P. falciparum* (20%)
Recommended chemoprophylaxis: Atovaquone-proguanil, doxycycline, mefloquine, tafenoquine[3]

PALAU

YELLOW FEVER VACCINE

Entry requirements: None
CDC recommendation: Not recommended

MALARIA PREVENTION

No malaria transmission

PANAMA

YELLOW FEVER VACCINE (MAP 2-11)

Entry requirements: Required for travelers ≥1 year old arriving from countries with risk for YF virus transmission[1]
CDC recommendations:
Recommended for travelers ≥9 months old going to all mainland areas east of the Canal Zone including Darién Province, the indigenous provinces (comarcas indígena) of Emberá and Kuna Yala (also spelled Guna Yala), and areas of the provinces of Colón and Panamá, east of the Canal Zone

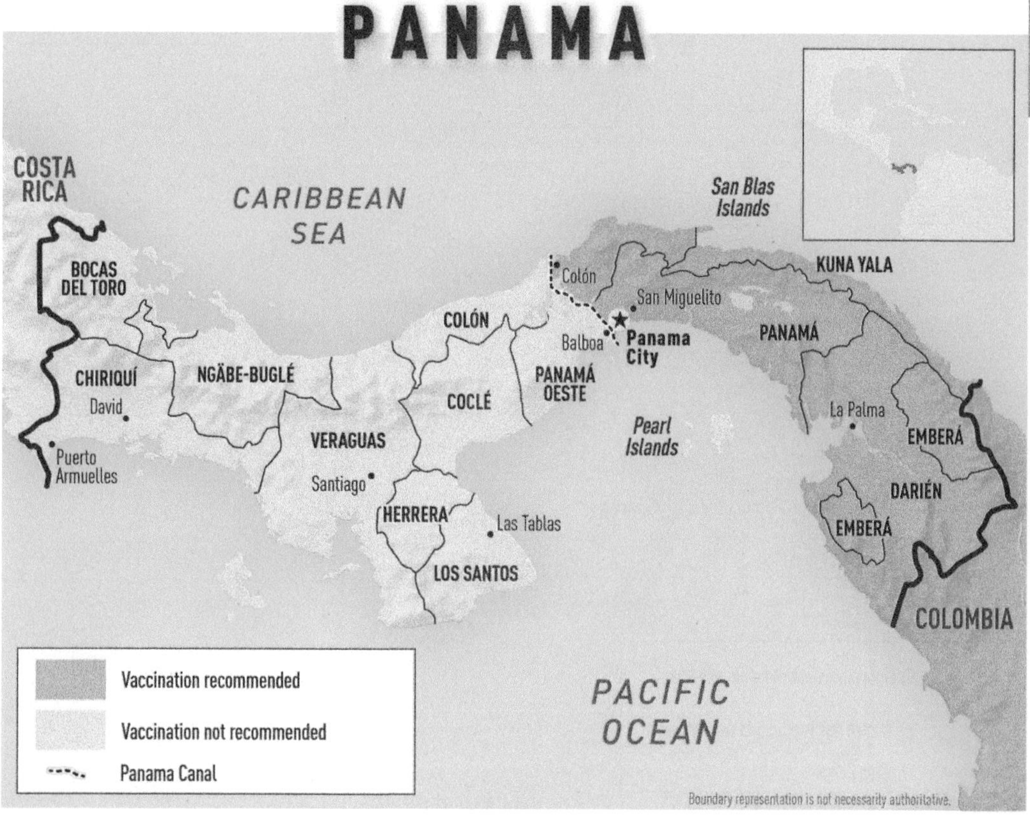

PANAMA

MAP 2-11 Yellow fever vaccine recommendations for Panama & neighboring countries[1]

[1] For footnotes, see page 84

Not recommended for travel limited to the Canal Zone; areas west of the Canal Zone; Panama City (the capital); Balboa district (Pearl Islands) of Panamá Province; or the San Blas Islands of Kuna Yala Province

MALARIA PREVENTION (MAP 2-12)

Transmission areas: The provinces of Bocas del Toro, Chiriquí, Colón, Darién, Panamá, and Veraguas

The indigenous provinces (*comarcas indígena*) of Emberá, Kuna Yala (also spelled Guna Yala), and Ngäbe-Buglé

No malaria transmission in the province of Panamá Oeste, in the Canal Zone, or in Panama City (the capital)

Drug resistance[2]: Chloroquine (east of the Panama Canal)

Species: *P. vivax* (97%); *P. falciparum* (3%)

Recommended chemoprophylaxis:

Darién, Emberá, Kuna Yala, and eastern Panamá Provinces: Atovaquone-proguanil, doxycycline, mefloquine, primaquine,[5] tafenoquine[3]

Bocas del Toro, Chiriquí, Colón, Veraguas, and Ngäbe-Buglé Provinces: Atovaquone-proguanil, chloroquine, doxycycline, mefloquine, primaquine,[5] tafenoquine[3]

PAPUA NEW GUINEA

YELLOW FEVER VACCINE

Entry requirements: Required for travelers ≥1 year old arriving from countries with risk for YF virus transmission; this includes airport transits or layovers in countries with risk for YF virus transmission[1]

CDC recommendation: Not recommended

MALARIA PREVENTION

Transmission areas: Throughout the country in areas <2,000 m (≈6,500 ft) elevation

Drug resistance[2]: Chloroquine (both *P. falciparum* and *P. vivax*)

Species: *P. falciparum* (75%); *P. vivax* (25%); *P. malariae* and *P. ovale* (rare)

Recommended chemoprophylaxis: Atovaquone-proguanil, doxycycline, mefloquine, tafenoquine[3]

PARAGUAY

YELLOW FEVER VACCINE

Entry requirements: Required for travelers ≥1 year old arriving from Bolivia, Brazil, Peru, or Venezuela; this includes this includes >24-hour transits or layovers in those countries[1]

MAP

2

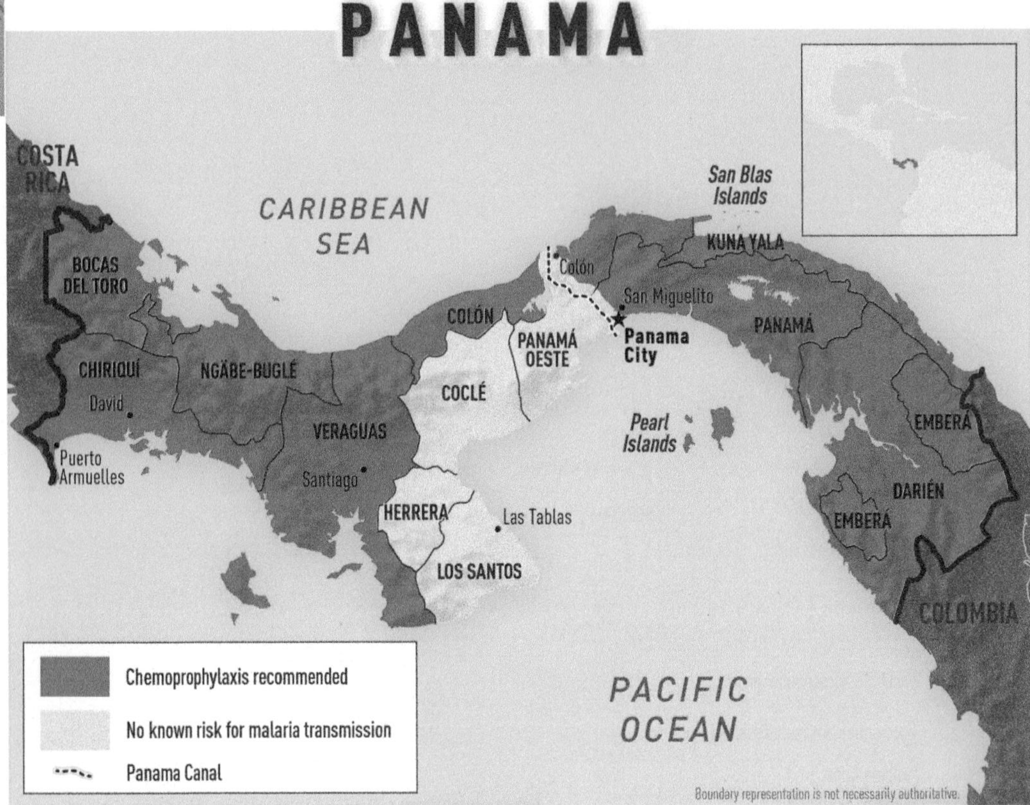

MAP 2-12 Malaria prevention in Panama

CDC recommendations:
Recommended for all travelers ≥9 months old except as follows
Generally not recommended for travel limited to the city of Asunción (the capital)

MALARIA PREVENTION
No malaria transmission

PERU

YELLOW FEVER VACCINE (MAP 2-13)
Entry requirements: None
CDC recommendations:
Recommended for travelers ≥9 months old going to areas <2,300 m (≈7,550 ft) elevation in the regions of Amazonas, Cusco, Huánuco, Junín, Loreto, Madre de Dios, Pasco, Puno, San Martín, and Ucayali, and designated areas of Ancash (far northeast), Apurímac (far north), Ayacucho (north and northeast), Cajamarca (north and east), Huancavelica (far north), La Libertad (east), and Piura (east)
Generally not recommended for travel limited to the following areas west of the Andes: the regions of Lambayeque and Tumbes, and designated areas of Cajamarca (west-central), and Piura (west)
Not recommended for travel limited to areas >2,300 m (≈7,550 ft) elevation, areas west of the Andes not listed above, the city of Lima (the capital), and the highland tourist areas (the city of Cusco, the Inca Trail, and Machu Picchu)

MALARIA PREVENTION (MAP 2-14)
Transmission areas: All areas of the country <2,500 m (≈8,200 ft) elevation, including the cities of Iquitos and Puerto Maldonado, and only the remote eastern areas in the regions of La Libertad and Lambayeque
No malaria transmission in the following areas: Lima Province; the cities of Arequipa, Ica, Moquegua, Nazca, Puno, or Tacna; the highland tourist areas (the city of Cusco, Machu Picchu, Lake Titicaca); along the Pacific Coast
Drug resistance[2]: Chloroquine
Species: *P. vivax* (80%); *P. falciparum* (20%)
Recommended chemoprophylaxis: Atovaquone-proguanil, doxycycline, mefloquine, tafenoquine[3]

PHILIPPINES

YELLOW FEVER VACCINE
Entry requirements: Required for travelers ≥9 months old arriving from countries with risk for YF virus transmission; this includes >12-hour airport transits or layovers in countries with risk for YF virus transmission[1]
CDC recommendation: Not recommended

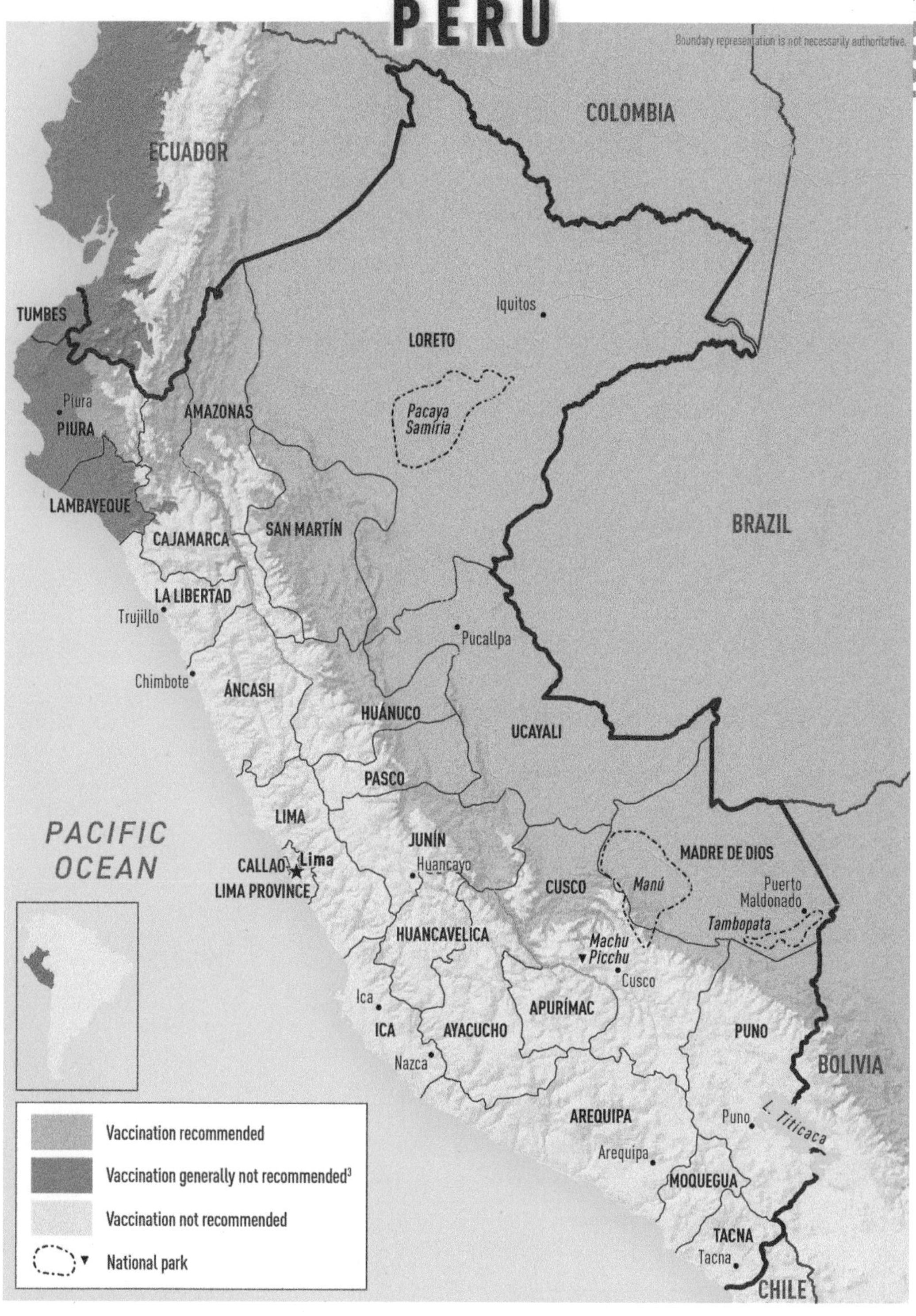

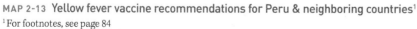

MAP 2-13 Yellow fever vaccine recommendations for Peru & neighboring countries[1]

[1] For footnotes, see page 84

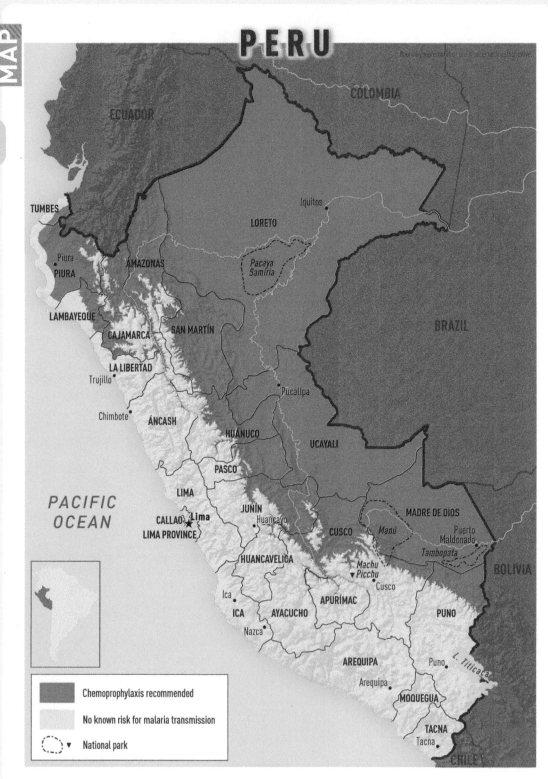

MAP 2-14 Malaria prevention in Peru

MALARIA PREVENTION

Transmission areas: Palawan and Mindanao Islands
No malaria transmission in metropolitan Manila (the capital) or other urban areas
Drug resistance[2]: Chloroquine
Species: *P. falciparum* (85%); *P. vivax* (15%); *P. knowlesi*,[6] *P. malariae*, and *P. ovale* (rare)
Recommended chemoprophylaxis: Atovaquone-proguanil, doxycycline, mefloquine, tafenoquine[3]

PITCAIRN ISLANDS, UNITED KINGDOM

YELLOW FEVER VACCINE

Entry requirements: Required for travelers ≥1 year old arriving from countries with risk for YF virus transmission[1]
CDC recommendation: Not recommended

MALARIA PREVENTION

No malaria transmission

POLAND

YELLOW FEVER VACCINE

Entry requirements: None
CDC recommendation: Not recommended

MALARIA PREVENTION

No malaria transmission

PORTUGAL

YELLOW FEVER VACCINE

Entry requirements: None
CDC recommendation: Not recommended

MALARIA PREVENTION

No malaria transmission

PUERTO RICO, UNITED STATES

YELLOW FEVER VACCINE

Entry requirements: None
CDC recommendation: Not recommended

MALARIA PREVENTION

No malaria transmission

QATAR

YELLOW FEVER VACCINE

Entry requirements: Required for travelers ≥9 months old arriving from countries with risk for YF virus transmission[1]
CDC recommendation: Not recommended

MALARIA PREVENTION

No malaria transmission

RÉUNION

YELLOW FEVER VACCINE

Entry requirements: None
CDC recommendation: Not recommended

MALARIA PREVENTION

No malaria transmission

ROMANIA

YELLOW FEVER VACCINE

Entry requirements: None
CDC recommendation: Not recommended

MALARIA PREVENTION

No malaria transmission

2

RUSSIA

YELLOW FEVER VACCINE

Entry requirements: None
CDC recommendation: Not recommended

MALARIA PREVENTION

No malaria transmission

RWANDA

YELLOW FEVER VACCINE

Entry requirements: Required for travelers ≥1 year old arriving from countries with risk for YF virus transmission[1]
CDC recommendation: Generally not recommended for travel to Rwanda

MALARIA PREVENTION

Transmission areas: All
Drug resistance[2]: Chloroquine
Species: *P. falciparum* (primarily); *P. malariae*, *P. ovale*, and *P. vivax* (less commonly)
Recommended chemoprophylaxis: Atovaquone-proguanil, doxycycline, mefloquine, tafenoquine[3]

SABA, NETHERLANDS

YELLOW FEVER VACCINE

Entry requirements: None
CDC recommendation: Not recommended

MALARIA PREVENTION

No malaria transmission

SAINT BARTHELEMY, FRANCE

YELLOW FEVER VACCINE

Entry requirements: Required for travelers ≥1 year old arriving from countries with risk for YF virus transmission; this includes >12-hour airport transits or layovers in countries with risk for YF virus transmission[1]
CDC recommendation: None

MALARIA PREVENTION

No malaria transmission

SAINT HELENA,* UNITED KINGDOM

YELLOW FEVER VACCINE

Entry requirements: Required for travelers ≥1 year old arriving from countries with risk for YF virus transmission[1]

CDC recommendation: Not recommended
*For YF vaccine entry requirements and recommendations and malaria prevention information for Ascension Island and Tristan da Cunha archipelago, see: UNITED KINGDOM (including CHANNEL ISLANDS, ISLE OF MAN, ASCENSION ISLAND & TRISTAN DA CUNHA ARCHIPELAGO)

MALARIA PREVENTION
No malaria transmission

SAINT KITTS (SAINT CHRISTOPHER) & NEVIS

YELLOW FEVER VACCINE
Entry requirements: Required for travelers ≥1 year old arriving from countries with risk for YF virus transmission[1]
CDC recommendation: Not recommended

MALARIA PREVENTION
No malaria transmission

SAINT LUCIA

YELLOW FEVER VACCINE
Entry requirements: Required for travelers ≥9 months old arriving from countries with risk for YF virus transmission[1]
CDC recommendation: Not recommended

MALARIA PREVENTION
No malaria transmission

SAINT MARTIN, FRANCE

YELLOW FEVER VACCINE
Entry requirements: Required for travelers ≥1 year old arriving from countries with risk for YF virus transmission; this includes >12-hour airport transits or layovers in countries with risk for YF virus transmission[1]
CDC recommendation: Not recommended

MALARIA PREVENTION
No malaria transmission

SAINT PIERRE & MIQUELON, FRANCE

YELLOW FEVER VACCINE
Entry requirements: None
CDC recommendation: Not recommended

MALARIA PREVENTION
No malaria transmission

SAINT VINCENT & THE GRENADINES

YELLOW FEVER VACCINE
Entry requirements: Required for travelers ≥1 year old arriving from countries with risk for YF virus transmission[1]
CDC recommendation: Not recommended

MALARIA PREVENTION
No malaria transmission

SAMOA (FORMERLY WESTERN SOMOA)

YELLOW FEVER VACCINE
Entry requirements: Required for travelers ≥1 year old arriving from countries with risk for YF virus transmission; this includes >12-hour airport transits or layovers in countries with risk for YF virus transmission[1]
CDC recommendation: Not recommended

MALARIA PREVENTION
No malaria transmission

SAN MARINO

YELLOW FEVER VACCINE
Entry requirements: None
CDC recommendation: Not recommended

MALARIA PREVENTION
No malaria transmission

SÃO TOMÉ & PRÍNCIPE

YELLOW FEVER VACCINE
Entry requirements: Required for travelers ≥1 year old arriving from countries with risk for YF virus transmission; this includes airport transits or layovers in countries with risk for YF virus transmission[1]
CDC recommendation: Generally not recommended for travel to São Tomé & Príncipe

MALARIA PREVENTION
Transmission areas: All
Drug resistance[2]: Chloroquine
Species: *P. falciparum* (primarily); *P. malariae*, *P. ovale*, and *P. vivax* (less commonly)
Recommended chemoprophylaxis: Atovaquone-proguanil, doxycycline, mefloquine, tafenoquine[3]

SAUDI ARABIA

YELLOW FEVER VACCINE
Entry requirements: Required for travelers ≥9 months old arriving from countries with risk for YF virus transmission; this includes >12-hour airport transits or layovers in countries with risk for YF virus transmission[1]
CDC recommendation: Not recommended

MALARIA PREVENTION
Transmission areas: Asir and Jazan (also spelled Jizan) Regions near the Yemen border only
No malaria transmission in the cities of Jeddah, Mecca, Medina, Riyadh (the capital), or Ta'if
Drug resistance[2]: Chloroquine
Species: *P. falciparum* (primarily); *P. vivax* (rare)
Recommended chemoprophylaxis: Atovaquone-proguanil, doxycycline, mefloquine, tafenoquine[3]

SENEGAL

YELLOW FEVER VACCINE
Entry requirements: Required for travelers ≥9 months old arriving from countries with risk for YF virus transmission; this includes airport transits

or layovers in countries with risk for YF virus transmission[1]
CDC recommended for all travelers ≥9 months old

MALARIA PREVENTION
Transmission areas: All
Drug resistance[2]: Chloroquine
Species: *P. falciparum* (primarily); *P. malariae*, *P. ovale*, and *P. vivax* (less commonly)
Recommended chemoprophylaxis: Atovaquone-proguanil, doxycycline, mefloquine, tafenoquine[3]

SERBIA

YELLOW FEVER VACCINE
Entry requirements: None
CDC recommendation: Not recommended

MALARIA PREVENTION
No malaria transmission

SEYCHELLES

YELLOW FEVER VACCINE
Entry requirements: Required for travelers ≥1 year old arriving from countries with risk for YF virus transmission; this includes airport transits or layovers in countries with risk for YF virus transmission[1]
CDC recommendation: Not recommended

MALARIA PREVENTION
No malaria transmission

SIERRA LEONE

YELLOW FEVER VACCINE
Entry requirements: Required for all arriving travelers
CDC recommended for all travelers ≥9 months old

MALARIA PREVENTION
Transmission areas: All
Drug resistance[2]: Chloroquine
Species: *P. falciparum* (primarily); *P. malariae*, *P. ovale*, and *P. vivax* (less commonly)
Recommended chemoprophylaxis: Atovaquone-proguanil, doxycycline, mefloquine, tafenoquine[3]

SINGAPORE

YELLOW FEVER VACCINE
Entry requirements: Required for travelers ≥1 year old arriving from countries with risk for YF virus transmission; this includes >12-hour airport transits or layovers in countries with risk for YF virus transmission[1]
CDC recommendation: Not recommended

MALARIA PREVENTION
No malaria transmission

SINT EUSTATIUS, NETHERLANDS

YELLOW FEVER VACCINE
Entry requirements: Required for travelers ≥6 months old arriving from countries with risk for YF virus transmission[1]
CDC recommendation: Not recommended

MALARIA PREVENTION
No malaria transmission

SINT MAARTEN, NETHERLANDS

YELLOW FEVER VACCINE
Entry requirements: Required for travelers ≥9 months old arriving from countries with risk for YF virus transmission[1]
CDC recommendation: Not recommended

MALARIA PREVENTION
No malaria transmission

SLOVAKIA

YELLOW FEVER VACCINE
Entry requirements: None
CDC recommendation: Not recommended

MALARIA PREVENTION
No malaria transmission

SLOVENIA

YELLOW FEVER VACCINE
Entry requirements: None
CDC recommendation: Not recommended

MALARIA PREVENTION
No malaria transmission

SOLOMON ISLANDS

YELLOW FEVER VACCINE
Entry requirements: Required for travelers ≥9 months old arriving from countries with risk for YF virus transmission[1]
CDC recommendation: Not recommended

MALARIA PREVENTION
Transmission areas: All
Drug resistance[2]: Chloroquine
Species: *P. vivax* (70%); *P. falciparum* (30%); *P. ovale* (<1%)
Recommended chemoprophylaxis: Atovaquone-proguanil, doxycycline, mefloquine, tafenoquine[3]

SOMALIA

YELLOW FEVER VACCINE (MAP 5-10)
Entry requirements: None
CDC recommendations:
Generally not recommended for travel to the regions of Bakool, Banaadir, Bay, Galguduud, Gedo, Hiiraan (also spelled Hiran), Lower Juba (also known as Jubbada Hoose), Middle Juba (also known as Jubbada Dhexe), Lower Shabelle (also known as Shabeellaha Hoose), or Middle Shabelle (also known as Shabeellaha Dhexe)
Not recommended for travel to areas not listed above

MALARIA PREVENTION

Transmission areas: All

Drug resistance[2]: Chloroquine

Species: *P. falciparum* (90%); *P. vivax* (5–10%); *P. malariae* and *P. ovale* (rare)

Recommended chemoprophylaxis: Atovaquone-proguanil, doxycycline, mefloquine, tafenoquine[3]

2

SOUTH AFRICA

YELLOW FEVER VACCINE

Entry requirements: Required for travelers ≥1 year old arriving from countries with risk for YF virus transmission; this includes >12-hour airport transits or layovers in countries with risk for YF virus transmission[1]

CDC recommendation: Not recommended

MALARIA PREVENTION (MAP 2-15)

Transmission areas: Along the border with Mozambique and Zimbabwe

KwaZulu-Natal Province: uMkhanyakude District; the districts of King Cetshwayo and Zululand (few cases)

Limpopo Province: the districts of Mopani and Vhembe; the districts of Capricorn, Greater Sekhukhune, and Waterberg (few cases)

Mpumalanga Province: Ehlanzeni District

Kruger National Park

Drug resistance[2]: Chloroquine

Species: *P. falciparum* (primarily); *P. malariae*, *P. ovale*, and *P. vivax* (less commonly)

Recommended chemoprophylaxis:

KwaZulu-Natal Province (uMkhanyakude District); Limpopo Province (the districts of Mopani and Vhembe); Mpumalanga Province (Ehlanzeni District); and Kruger National Park: Atovaquone-proguanil, doxycycline, mefloquine, tafenoquine[3]

All other areas with malaria transmission (including the districts of King Cetshwayo and Zululand in KwaZulu-Natal Province, and the districts of Capricorn, Greater Sekhukhune, and Waterberg in Limpopo Province): No chemoprophylaxis recommended (insect bite precautions and mosquito avoidance only)[4]

MAP

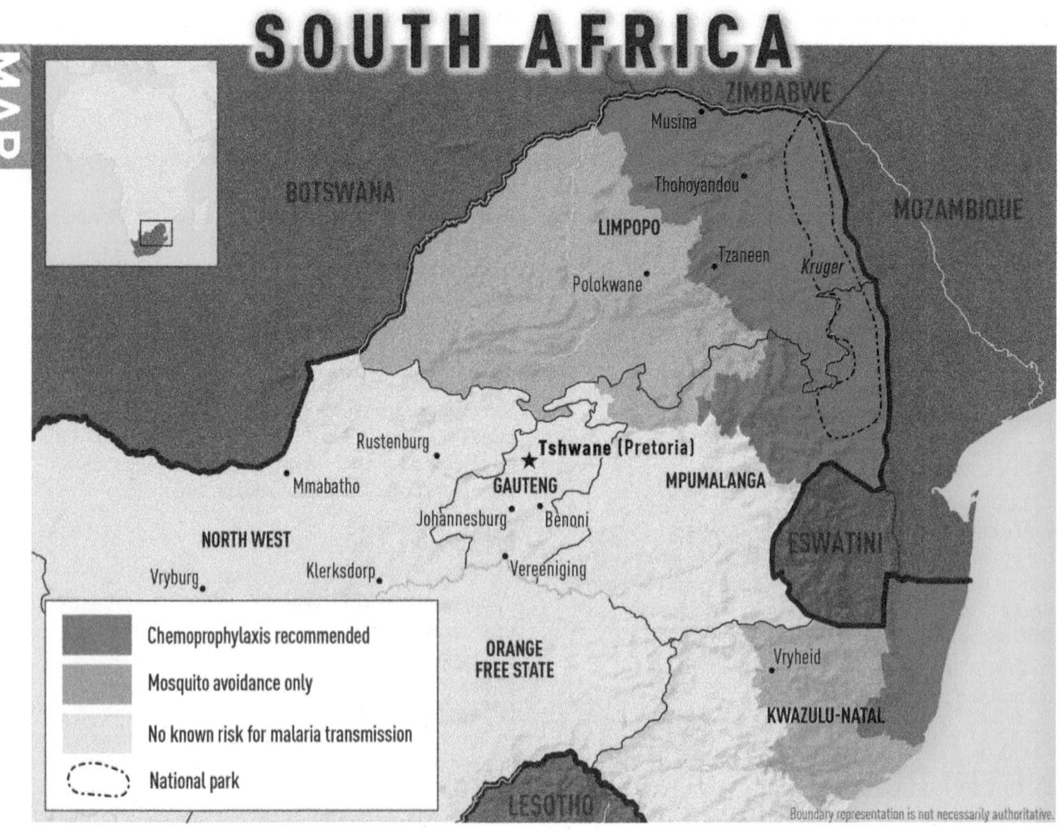

MAP 2-15 Malaria prevention in South Africa

SOUTH GEORGIA & THE SOUTH SANDWICH ISLANDS, UK OVERSEAS TERRITORY (ALSO CLAIMED BY ARGENTINA)

YELLOW FEVER VACCINE

Entry requirements: South Georgia & the South Sandwich Islands has not stated its YF vaccination certificate requirements

CDC recommendation: Not recommended

MALARIA PREVENTION

No malaria transmission

SOUTH KOREA

YELLOW FEVER VACCINE

Entry requirements: None

CDC recommendation: Not recommended

MALARIA PREVENTION

Transmission areas: Limited to the months of March–December in rural areas in the northern parts of the provinces of Inch'ŏn (also spelled Incheon), Kangwŏn (also spelled Gangwon), and Kyŏnggi (also spelled Gyeonggi), including the demilitarized zone (DMZ)

Drug resistance[2]: None

Species: *P. vivax* (100%)

Recommended chemoprophylaxis: Atovaquone-proguanil, chloroquine, doxycycline, mefloquine, primaquine,[5] or tafenoquine[3]

SOUTH SUDAN

YELLOW FEVER VACCINE

Entry requirements: Required for all arriving travelers ≥9 months old

CDC recommended for all travelers ≥9 months old

MALARIA PREVENTION

Transmission areas: All

Drug resistance[2]: Chloroquine

Species: *P. falciparum* (primarily); *P. malariae*, *P. ovale*, and *P. vivax* (less commonly)

Recommended chemoprophylaxis: Atovaquone-proguanil, doxycycline, mefloquine, tafenoquine[3]

SPAIN

YELLOW FEVER VACCINE

Entry requirements: None

CDC recommendation: Not recommended

MALARIA PREVENTION

No malaria transmission

SRI LANKA

YELLOW FEVER VACCINE

Entry requirements: Required for travelers ≥9 months old arriving from countries with risk for YF virus transmission; this includes >12-hour airport transits or layovers in countries with risk for YF virus transmission[1]

CDC recommendation: Not recommended

MALARIA PREVENTION

No malaria transmission

SUDAN

YELLOW FEVER VACCINE (MAP 5-10)

Entry requirements: None

CDC recommendations:

Recommended for travelers ≥9 months old going to areas south of the Sahara Desert

Not recommended for travel limited to areas in the Sahara Desert or the city of Khartoum (the capital)

MALARIA PREVENTION

Transmission areas: All

Drug resistance[2]: Chloroquine

Species: *P. falciparum* (90%); *P. vivax* (5–10%); *P. malariae* and *P. ovale* (rare)

Recommended chemoprophylaxis: Atovaquone-proguanil, doxycycline, mefloquine, tafenoquine[3]

SURINAME

YELLOW FEVER VACCINE

Entry requirements: Required for travelers ≥1 year old arriving from countries with risk for YF virus transmission; this includes >12-hour airport transits or layovers in countries with risk for YF virus transmission[1]

CDC recommended for all travelers ≥9 months old

MALARIA PREVENTION

Transmission areas: Primarily in Sipaliwini District, near the border with French Guiana

Limited transmission in the districts of Brokopondo, Marowijne, and Para (near the border with French Guiana)

No malaria transmission in districts along the Atlantic Coast or in Paramaribo (the capital)

Drug resistance[2]: Chloroquine

Species: *P. vivax* (70%); *P. falciparum* (30%)

Recommended chemoprophylaxis:

Sipaliwini District near the border with French Guiana: Atovaquone-proguanil, doxycycline, mefloquine, tafenoquine[3]

All other areas with malaria transmission: No chemoprophylaxis recommended (insect bite precautions and mosquito avoidance only)[4]

SWEDEN

YELLOW FEVER VACCINE

Entry requirements: None

CDC recommendation: Not recommended

MALARIA PREVENTION

No malaria transmission

2

SWITZERLAND

YELLOW FEVER VACCINE

Entry requirements: None
CDC recommendation: Not recommended

MALARIA PREVENTION

No malaria transmission

SYRIA

YELLOW FEVER VACCINE

Entry requirements: None
CDC recommendation: Not recommended

MALARIA PREVENTION

No malaria transmission

TAIWAN

YELLOW FEVER VACCINE

Entry requirements: None
CDC recommendation: Not recommended

MALARIA PREVENTION

No malaria transmission

TAJIKISTAN

YELLOW FEVER VACCINE

Entry requirements: None
CDC recommendation: Not recommended

MALARIA PREVENTION

Transmission areas: No indigenous cases reported since 2014
Drug resistance[2]: Previously, chloroquine
Species: Previously, *P. vivax* (90%) and *P. falciparum* (10%)
Recommended chemoprophylaxis: None (insect bite precautions and mosquito avoidance only)[4]

TANZANIA

YELLOW FEVER VACCINE

Entry requirements: Required for travelers ≥1 year old arriving from countries with risk for YF virus transmission; this includes >12-hour airport transits or layovers in countries with risk for YF virus transmission[1]
CDC recommendation: Generally not recommended for travel to Tanzania

MALARIA PREVENTION

Transmission areas: All areas <1,800 m (≈5,900 ft) elevation
Drug resistance[2]: Chloroquine
Species: *P. falciparum* (primarily); *P. malariae* and *P. ovale* (less commonly); *P. vivax* (rare)
Recommended chemoprophylaxis: Atovaquone-proguanil, doxycycline, mefloquine, tafenoquine[3]

THAILAND

YELLOW FEVER VACCINE

Entry requirements: Required for travelers ≥9 months old arriving from countries with risk for YF virus transmission; this includes >12-hour airport transits or layovers in countries with risk for YF virus transmission[1]
CDC recommendation: Not recommended

MALARIA PREVENTION
(MAP 2-16)

Transmission areas: Primarily the provinces that border Burma, Cambodia (few cases in Buri Ram Province), and Malaysia (few cases in Satun Province)
Also, the provinces of Phitsanulok and Ubon Ratchathani (bordering Laos), and Surat Thani (especially in the rural forest and forest-fringe areas of these provinces)
Rare to few cases in other parts of Thailand, including the cities of Bangkok (the capital), Chiang Mai, and Chiang Rai, or on the islands of Koh Pha Ngan, Koh Samui, or Phuket
No malaria transmission on the islands of Krabi Province (Ko Lanta, Koh Phi, Koh Yao Noi, Koh Yao Yai) or in Pattaya City
Drug resistance[2]: Chloroquine and mefloquine
Species: *P. vivax* (80%); *P. falciparum* (<20%); *P. knowlesi*,[6] *P. malariae*, and *P. ovale* (rare)
Recommended chemoprophylaxis:
Provinces that border Burma, Cambodia (except Buri Ram Province), and Malaysia (except Satun Province); the provinces of Phitsanulok, Ubon Ratchathani, and Surat Thani: Atovaquone-proguanil, doxycycline, tafenoquine[3]
All other areas with malaria transmission (including the provinces of Buri Ram and Satun): No chemoprophylaxis recommended (insect bite precautions and mosquito avoidance only)[4]

TIMOR-LESTE

YELLOW FEVER VACCINE

Entry requirements: None
CDC recommendation: Not recommended

MALARIA PREVENTION

Transmission areas: Rare cases; outbreak in Indonesia border area in mid-2020
Drug resistance[2]: Previously, chloroquine
Species: Previously, *P. falciparum* (50%), *P. vivax* (50%), *P. ovale* (<1%), and *P. malariae* (<1%)
Recommended chemoprophylaxis: None (insect bite precautions and mosquito avoidance only)[4]

TOGO

YELLOW FEVER VACCINE

Entry requirements: Required for all arriving travelers ≥9 months old
CDC recommended for all travelers ≥9 months old

MALARIA PREVENTION

Transmission areas: All
Drug resistance[2]: Chloroquine
Species: *P. falciparum* (primarily); *P. malariae*, *P. ovale*, and *P. vivax* (less commonly)
Recommended chemoprophylaxis: Atovaquone-proguanil, doxycycline, mefloquine, tafenoquine[3]

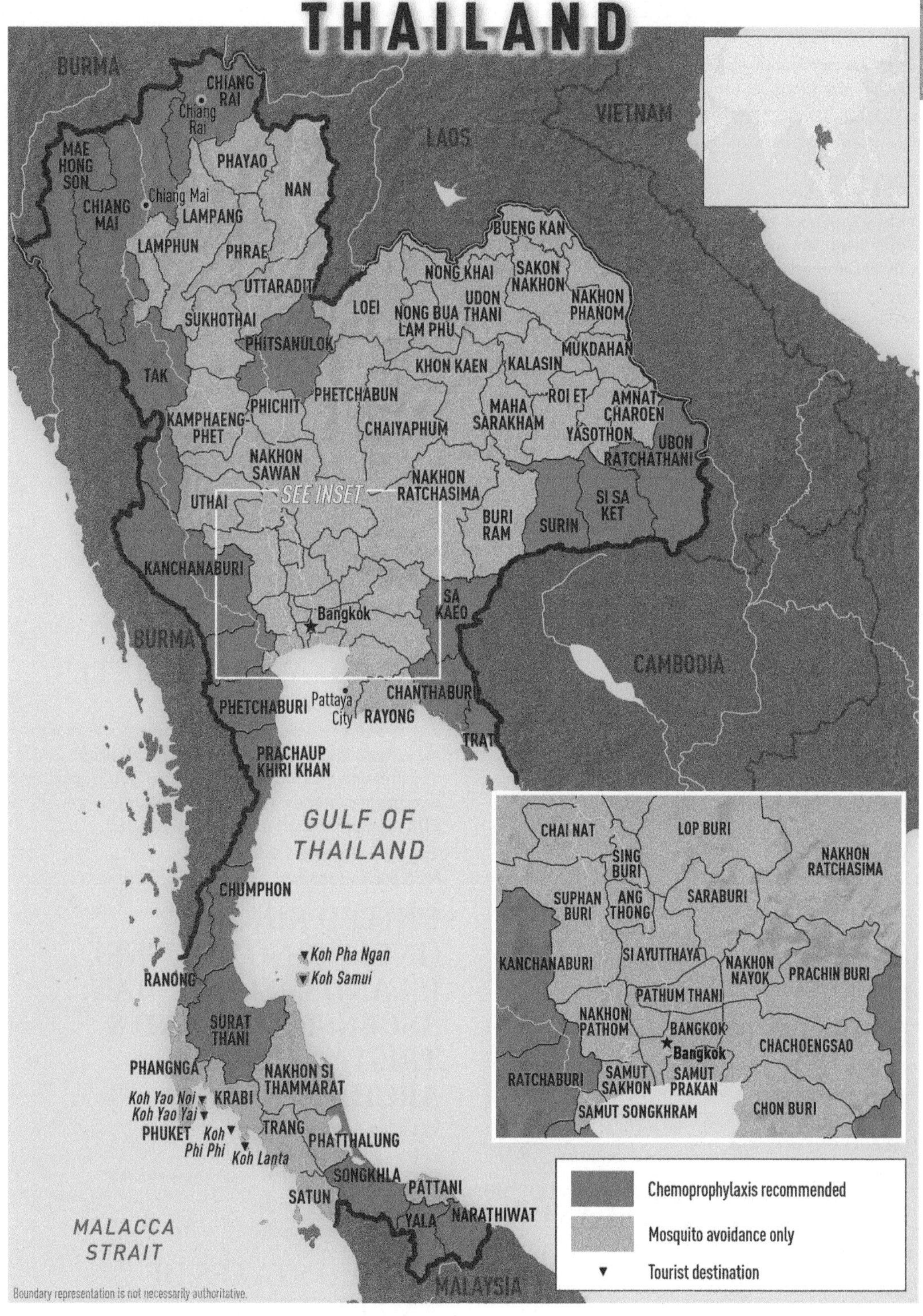
THAILAND
BURMA
CHIANG RAI
Chiang Rai
MAE HONG SON
PHAYAO
NAN
CHIANG MAI
Chiang Mai
LAMPANG
LAMPHUN
PHRAE
UTTARADIT
SUKHOTHAI
PHITSANULOK
TAK
LAOS
VIETNAM
BUENG KAN
NONG KHAI
SAKON NAKHON
UDON THANI
NAKHON PHANOM
LOEI
NONG BUA LAM PHU
MUKDAHAN
KHON KAEN
KALASIN
PHETCHABUN
ROI ET
AMNAT CHAROEN
KAMPHAENG PHET
PHICHIT
MAHA SARAKHAM
CHAIYAPHUM
YASOTHON
UBON RATCHATHANI
NAKHON SAWAN
NAKHON RATCHASIMA
SEE INSET
UTHAI
SI SA KET
BURI RAM
SURIN
KANCHANABURI
SA KAEO
Bangkok
BURMA
CAMBODIA
PHETCHABURI
Pattaya City
CHANTHABURI
RAYONG
TRAT
PRACHAUP KHIRI KHAN
GULF OF THAILAND
CHUMPHON
Koh Pha Ngan
Koh Samui
RANONG
SURAT THANI
PHANGNGA
NAKHON SI THAMMARAT
Koh Yao Noi
Koh Yao Yai
KRABI
PHUKET
Koh Phi Phi
Koh Lanta
TRANG
PHATTHALUNG
SONGKHLA
PATTANI
SATUN
YALA
NARATHIWAT
MALACCA STRAIT
MALAYSIA
CHAI NAT
LOP BURI
SING BURI
NAKHON RATCHASIMA
SUPHAN BURI
ANG THONG
SARABURI
KANCHANABURI
SI AYUTTHAYA
NAKHON NAYOK
PRACHIN BURI
PATHUM THANI
NAKHON PATHOM
BANGKOK
Bangkok
CHACHOENGSAO
RATCHABURI
SAMUT SAKHON
SAMUT PRAKAN
SAMUT SONGKHRAM
CHON BURI
Chemoprophylaxis recommended
Mosquito avoidance only
Tourist destination
Boundary representation is not necessarily authoritative.

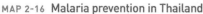

MAP 2-16 Malaria prevention in Thailand

TOKELAU, NEW ZEALAND

YELLOW FEVER VACCINE

Entry requirements: None
CDC recommendation: Not recommended

MALARIA PREVENTION

No malaria transmission

TONGA

YELLOW FEVER VACCINE

Entry requirements: None
CDC recommendation: Not recommended

MALARIA PREVENTION

No malaria transmission

TRINIDAD & TOBAGO

YELLOW FEVER VACCINE

Entry requirements: None
CDC recommendations:
Recommended for travelers ≥9 months old going to densely forested areas on Trinidad
Not recommended for cruise ship passengers, airplane passengers in transit, or travel limited to Tobago

MALARIA PREVENTION

No malaria transmission

TUNISIA

YELLOW FEVER VACCINE

Entry requirements: None
CDC recommendation: Not recommended

MALARIA PREVENTION

No malaria transmission

TURKEY

YELLOW FEVER VACCINE

Entry requirements: None
CDC recommendation: Not recommended

MALARIA PREVENTION

No malaria transmission

TURKMENISTAN

YELLOW FEVER VACCINE

Entry requirements: None
CDC recommendation: Not recommended

MALARIA PREVENTION

No malaria transmission

TURKS & CAICOS ISLANDS, UNITED KINGDOM

YELLOW FEVER VACCINE

Entry requirements: None
CDC recommendation: Not recommended

MALARIA PREVENTION

No malaria transmission

TUVALU

YELLOW FEVER VACCINE

Entry requirements: None
CDC recommendation: Not recommended

MALARIA PREVENTION

No malaria transmission

UGANDA

YELLOW FEVER VACCINE

Entry requirements: Required for all arriving travelers ≥1 year old
CDC recommended for all travelers ≥9 months old

MALARIA PREVENTION

Transmission areas: All
Drug resistance[2]: Chloroquine
Species: *P. falciparum* (primarily); *P. malariae*, *P. ovale*, and *P. vivax* (less commonly)
Recommended chemoprophylaxis: Atovaquone-proguanil, doxycycline, mefloquine, tafenoquine[3]

UKRAINE

YELLOW FEVER VACCINE

Entry requirements: None
CDC recommendation: Not recommended

MALARIA PREVENTION

No malaria transmission

UNITED ARAB EMIRATES

YELLOW FEVER VACCINE

Entry requirements: Required for travelers ≥9 months old arriving from countries with risk for YF virus transmission; this includes >12-hour airport transits or layovers in countries with risk for YF virus transmission[1]
CDC recommendation: Not recommended

MALARIA PREVENTION

No malaria transmission

UNITED KINGDOM (INCLUDING CHANNEL ISLANDS, ISLE OF MAN, ASCENSION ISLAND & TRISTAN DA CUNHA ARCHIPELAGO)

YELLOW FEVER VACCINE

Entry requirements: None
CDC recommendation: Not recommended

MALARIA PREVENTION

No malaria transmission

UNITED STATES OF AMERICA

YELLOW FEVER VACCINE

Entry requirements: None
CDC recommendation: Not recommended

MALARIA PREVENTION
No malaria transmission

URUGUAY

YELLOW FEVER VACCINE
Entry requirements: None
CDC recommendation: Not recommended

MALARIA PREVENTION
No malaria transmission

UZBEKISTAN

YELLOW FEVER VACCINE
Entry requirements: None
CDC recommendation: Not recommended

MALARIA PREVENTION
No malaria transmission

VANUATU

YELLOW FEVER VACCINE
Entry requirements: None
CDC recommendation: Not recommended

MALARIA PREVENTION
Transmission areas: All
Drug resistance[2]: Chloroquine
Species: *P. vivax* (75%–90%); *P. falciparum* (10-25%); *P. ovale* (<1%)
Recommended chemoprophylaxis: Atovaquone-proguanil, doxycycline, mefloquine, tafenoquine[3]

VENEZUELA

YELLOW FEVER VACCINE (MAP 2-17)
Entry requirements: Required for travelers ≥1 year old arriving from Brazil; this includes >12-hour airport transits or layovers in Brazil

VENEZUELA

Vaccination recommended
Vaccination generally not recommended[3]
Vaccination not recommended
National park

Boundary representation is not necessarily authoritative.

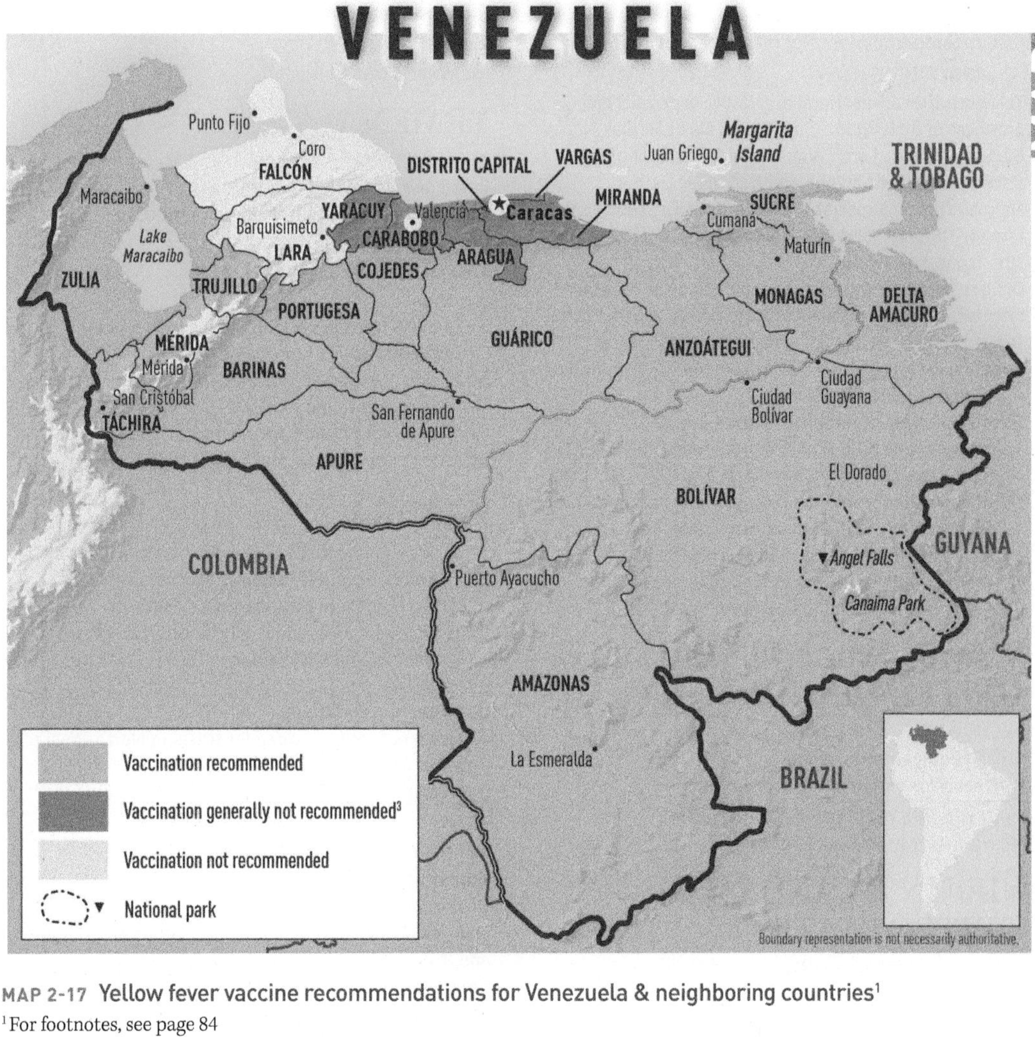

MAP 2-17 Yellow fever vaccine recommendations for Venezuela & neighboring countries[1]

[1] For footnotes, see page 84

CDC recommendations:
Recommended for all travelers ≥9 months old except as follows
Generally not recommended for travel limited to the Distrito Capital or the states of Aragua, Carabobo, Miranda, Vargas, or Yaracuy
Not recommended for travel limited to areas >2,300m (≈7,550 ft) elevation in the states of Mérida, Táchira, or Trujillo; the states of Falcón or Lara; Margarita Island; or the cities of Caracas (the capital) or Valencia

MALARIA PREVENTION
Transmission areas: All areas <1,700 m (≈5,600 ft) elevation and Angel Falls
Drug resistance[2]: Chloroquine
Species: *P. vivax* (75%); *P. falciparum* (25%)
Recommended chemoprophylaxis: Atovaquone-proguanil, doxycycline, mefloquine, tafenoquine[3]

VIETNAM

YELLOW FEVER VACCINE
Entry requirements: None
CDC recommendation: Not recommended

MALARIA PREVENTION
Transmission areas: Rural areas only, especially the provinces of Bình Phước, Bình Thuận, Đắk Lắk, Đăk Nông, Gia Lai, Lai Châu, Lâm Đồng, Phú Yên, and Quảng Nam. Rare cases in the Mekong and Red River Deltas
No malaria transmission in the cities of Da Nang, Hai Phong, Hanoi (the capital), Ho Chi Minh City (Saigon), Nha Trang, Quy Nhon
Drug resistance[2]: Chloroquine and mefloquine resistance reported. Emerging resistance to artemisinin in Bình Phước, Đắk Lắk, Đăk Nông, Gia Lai, Khánh Hòa, Ninh Thuận.
Species: *P. vivax* (55%); *P. falciparum* (44%); *P. knowlesi*,[6] *P. malariae*, and *P. ovale* (rare)
Recommended chemoprophylaxis:
The provinces of Bình Phước, Bình Thuận, Đắk Lắk, Đăk Nông, Gia Lai, Lai Châu, Lâm Đồng, Phú Yên, and Quảng Nam: Atovaquone-proguanil, doxycycline, tafenoquine[3]
All other areas with malaria transmission (including provinces in the Mekong and Red River Deltas): No chemoprophylaxis recommended (insect bite precautions and mosquito avoidance only)[4]

VIRGIN ISLANDS (BRITISH), UNITED KINGDOM

YELLOW FEVER VACCINE
Entry requirements: None
CDC recommendation: Not recommended

MALARIA PREVENTION
No malaria transmission

VIRGIN ISLANDS (US), UNITED STATES

YELLOW FEVER VACCINE
Entry requirements: None
CDC recommendation: Not recommended

MALARIA PREVENTION
No malaria transmission

WAKE ISLAND, UNITED STATES

YELLOW FEVER VACCINE
Entry requirements: None
CDC recommendation: Not recommended

MALARIA PREVENTION
No malaria transmission

WALLIS & FUTUNA, FRANCE

YELLOW FEVER VACCINE
Entry requirements: Required for travelers ≥1 year old arriving from countries with risk for YF virus transmission; this includes >12-hour airport transits or layovers in countries with risk for YF virus transmission[1]
CDC recommendation: Not recommended

MALARIA PREVENTION
No malaria transmission

YEMEN

YELLOW FEVER VACCINE
Entry requirements: None
CDC recommendation: Not recommended

MALARIA PREVENTION
Transmission areas: All areas <2,000 m (≈6,500 ft) elevation
No malaria transmission in Sana'a (the capital)
Drug resistance[2]: Chloroquine
Species: *P. falciparum* (primarily); *P. malariae*, *P. ovale*, and *P. vivax* (less commonly)
Recommended chemoprophylaxis: Atovaquone-proguanil, doxycycline, mefloquine, tafenoquine[3]

ZAMBIA

YELLOW FEVER VACCINE
Entry requirements: Required for travelers ≥1 year of age arriving from countries with risk for YF virus transmission; this includes >12-hour airport transits or layovers in countries with risk for YF virus transmission[1]
CDC recommendations:
Generally not recommended for travel to North-Western Province or Western Province
Not recommended for travel to any areas not listed above

MALARIA PREVENTION
Transmission areas: All
Drug resistance[2]: Chloroquine
Species: *P. falciparum* (primarily); *P. malariae*, *P. ovale*, and *P. vivax* (less commonly)
Recommended chemoprophylaxis: Atovaquone-proguanil, doxycycline, mefloquine, tafenoquine[3]

ZIMBABWE

YELLOW FEVER VACCINE

Entry requirements: Required for travelers ≥9 months old arriving from countries with risk for YF virus transmission; this includes >12-hour airport transits or layovers in countries with risk for YF virus transmission[1]

CDC recommendation: Not recommended

MALARIA PREVENTION

Transmission areas: All.

Drug resistance[2]: Chloroquine

Species: *P. falciparum* (primarily); *P. malariae*, *P. ovale*, and *P. vivax* (less commonly)

Recommended chemoprophylaxis: Atovaquone-proguanil, doxycycline, mefloquine, tafenoquine[3]

2

FOOTNOTES

Yellow Fever Vaccine

[1]Current as of November 2022. This is an update of the 2010 map created by the Informal WHO Working Group on the Geographic Risk of Yellow Fever.

Malaria Prevention

2

[2]Refers to *Plasmodium falciparum* malaria, unless otherwise noted.

[3]Tafenoquine can cause potentially life-threatening hemolysis in people with glucose-6-phosphate-dehydrogenase (G6PD) deficiency. Rule out G6PD deficiency with a quantitative laboratory test before prescribing tafenoquine to patients.

[4]Mosquito avoidance includes applying topical mosquito repellant, sleeping under an insecticide-treated mosquito net, and wearing protective clothing (e.g., long pants and socks, long-sleeve shirt). For additional details on insect bite precautions, see Sec. 4, Ch. 6, Mosquitoes, Ticks & Other Arthropods.

[5]Primaquine can cause potentially life-threatening hemolysis in people with G6PD deficiency. Rule out G6PD deficiency with a quantitative laboratory test before prescribing primaquine to patients.

[6]*P. knowlesi* is a malaria species with a simian (macaque) host. Human cases have been reported from most countries in Southwest Asia and are associated with activities in forest or forest-fringe areas. *P. knowlesi* has no known resistance to antimalarials.

Yellow Fever Maps

[1]Current as of November 2022. This is an update of the 2010 map created by the Informal WHO Working Group on the Geographic Risk of Yellow Fever.

[2]In 2017, the Centers for Disease Control and Prevention (CDC) expanded its YF vaccination recommendations for travelers going to Brazil because of a large YF outbreak in multiple states in that country. Please refer to the CDC Travelers' Health website (https://wwwnc.cdc.gov/travel/) for more information and updated recommendations.

[3]YF vaccination is *generally not recommended* for travel to areas where the potential for YF virus exposure is low. Vaccination might be considered, however, for a small subset of travelers going to these areas who are at increased risk for exposure to YF virus due to prolonged travel, heavy exposure to mosquitoes, or inability to avoid mosquito bites. Factors to consider when deciding whether to vaccinate a traveler include destination-specific and travel-associated risks for YF virus infection; individual, underlying risk factors for having a serious YF vaccine–associated adverse event; and destination entry requirements.

TRAVELERS' DIARRHEA

Bradley Connor

Travelers' diarrhea (TD) is the most predictable travel-related illness. Attack rates range from 30%–70% of travelers during a 2-week period, depending on the destination and season of travel. Traditionally, TD was thought to be prevented by following simple dietary recommendations (e.g., "boil it, cook it, peel it, or forget it"), but studies have found that people who follow these rules can still become ill. Poor hygiene practices in local restaurants and underlying hygiene and sanitation infrastructure deficiencies are likely the largest contributors to the risk for TD.

TD is a clinical syndrome that can result from a variety of intestinal pathogens. Bacteria are the predominant enteropathogens and are thought to account for ≥80%–90% of cases. Intestinal viruses account for at least 5%–15% of illnesses, although the use of multiplex molecular diagnostic assays demonstrates that their contribution to the overall burden of TD disease is probably greater than previously estimated. Infections with protozoal pathogens are slower to manifest symptoms and collectively account for ≈10% of diagnoses in longer-term travelers (see Sec. 11, Ch. 7, Persistent Diarrhea in Returned Travelers).

What is commonly known as "food poisoning" involves the ingestion of infectious agents that release toxins (e.g., *Clostridium perfringens*) or consumption of preformed toxins (e.g., *Staphylococcal* food poisoning). In toxin-mediated illness, both vomiting and diarrhea can be present; symptoms usually resolve spontaneously within 12–24 hours.

INFECTIOUS AGENTS

Bacteria

Bacteria are the most common cause of TD. Overall, the most common pathogen identified is enterotoxigenic *Escherichia coli*, followed by *Campylobacter jejuni*, *Shigella* spp., and *Salmonella* spp. Enteroaggregative and other *E. coli* pathotypes also are commonly found in cases of TD. Surveillance also points to *Aeromonas* spp., *Plesiomonas* spp., and newly recognized pathogens (*Acrobacter*, enterotoxigenic *Bacteroides fragilis*, *Larobacter*) as potential causes of TD.

Viruses

Viral diarrhea can be caused by several pathogens, including astrovirus, norovirus, and rotavirus.

Protozoal Parasites

Giardia is the main protozoal pathogen found in TD. *Entamoeba histolytica* and *Cryptosporidium* are relatively uncommon causes of TD. The risk for *Cyclospora* is highly geographic and seasonal: the most well-known risks are in Guatemala, Haiti, Nepal, and Peru. *Dientamoeba fragilis* is a flagellate occasionally associated with diarrhea in travelers. Several pathogens are discussed in their own chapters in Section 5.

RISK FOR TRAVELERS

TD occurs equally in male and female travelers; it is more common in young adult travelers than in older travelers. In short-term travelers, bouts of TD do not appear to protect against future attacks, and >1 episode of TD can occur during a single trip. A cohort of expatriates residing in Kathmandu, Nepal, experienced an average of 3.2 episodes of TD per person during their first year. In more temperate regions, seasonal variations in diarrhea risk can occur. In South Asia, for example, much higher TD attack rates are reported during the hot months preceding the monsoon.

Particularly in locations where large numbers of people lack plumbing or latrine access, stool contamination in the environment will be greater and more accessible to disease-transmitting vectors (e.g., flies). Inadequate electrical capacity leading to frequent blackouts or poorly functioning refrigeration can result in unsafe food storage and an additional increased risk for disease. Lack of safe, potable water contributes to food and drink contamination, as do unhealthful shortcuts in cleaning hands, countertops, cutting boards, utensils, and foods (e.g., fruits and vegetables). In some places, handwashing might not be a social norm and could represent an extra expense; thus, adequately equipped handwashing stations might not be available in food preparation areas.

Where provided, effective food handling courses have been shown to decrease the risk for TD. However, even in high-income countries, food handling and preparation in restaurants has been linked to TD caused by pathogens such as *Shigella sonnei*.

2

CLINICAL PRESENTATION

The incubation period between exposure and clinical presentation can provide clues to etiology. Toxin-mediated illness, for example, generally causes symptoms within a few hours. By contrast, bacterial and viral pathogens have an incubation period of 6–72 hours. In general, protozoal pathogens have longer incubation periods (1–2 weeks), rarely presenting in the first few days of travel. An exception is *Cyclospora cayetanensis*, which can present quickly in areas of high risk.

Bacterial and viral TD present with the sudden onset of bothersome symptoms that can range from mild cramps and urgent loose stools to severe abdominal pain, bloody diarrhea, fever, and vomiting; with norovirus, vomiting can be more prominent. Diarrhea caused by protozoa (e.g., *E. histolytica*, *Giardia duodenalis*) generally has a more gradual onset of low-grade symptoms, with 2–5 loose stools per day.

Untreated, bacterial diarrhea usually lasts 3–7 days. Viral diarrhea generally lasts 2–3 days. Protozoal diarrhea can persist for weeks to months without treatment. An acute bout of TD can lead to persistent enteric symptoms, even in the absence of continued infection. This presentation is commonly referred to as postinfectious irritable bowel syndrome (see Sec. 11, Ch. 7, Persistent Diarrhea in Returned Travelers). Other postinfectious sequelae can include reactive arthritis and Guillain-Barré syndrome.

PREVENTION

Vaccines are not available in the United States for pathogens that commonly cause TD. Traveler adherence to recommended approaches can, however, help reduce, although never fully eliminate, the risk for illness. These recommendations include making careful food and beverage choices, using agents other than antimicrobial medications for prophylaxis, and carefully washing hands with soap whenever available. When handwashing is not possible, small containers of hand sanitizer containing ≥60% alcohol can make it easier for travelers to clean their hands before eating. Refer to the relevant chapters in Section 5 (Cholera, Hepatitis A, and Typhoid & Paratyphoid Fever) for details regarding vaccines to prevent other foodborne and waterborne infections to which travelers are susceptible.

Food & Beverage Selection

Care in selecting food and beverages can help minimize the risk for acquiring TD. See Sec. 2, Ch. 8, Food & Water Precautions, for detailed food and beverage recommendations. Although food and water precautions are recommended, travelers are not always able to adhere to the advice. Furthermore, food safety factors (e.g., restaurant hygiene) are out of the traveler's control.

Non-Antimicrobial Drugs for Prophylaxis

BISMUTH SUBSALICYLATE

The primary agent studied for prevention of TD, other than antibiotics, is bismuth subsalicylate (BSS), the active ingredient in adult formulations of Pepto-Bismol. Studies from Mexico have shown that this agent, taken either as 2 oz. of liquid or 2 chewable tablets 4 times per day, reduces the incidence of TD by approximately 50%. BSS commonly causes blackening of the tongue and stool and can cause constipation, nausea, and rarely tinnitus.

CONTRAINDICATIONS & SAFETY

Travelers with aspirin allergy, gout, or renal insufficiency, and those taking anticoagulants, methotrexate, or probenecid should not take BSS. In travelers taking aspirin or salicylates for other reasons, concomitant use of BSS can increase the risk of developing salicylate toxicity.

BSS is not generally recommended for children aged <12 years; some clinicians use it off-label, however, with caution to avoid administering BSS to children aged ≤18 years with viral infections (e.g., influenza, varicella), because of the risk for Reye's syndrome. BSS is not recommended for children aged <3 years or pregnant people.

Studies have not established the safety of BSS use for >3 weeks. Because of the number of tablets required and the inconvenient dosing, BSS is not commonly used as TD prophylaxis.

PROBIOTICS

Probiotics (e.g., *Lactobacillus* GG, *Saccharomyces boulardii*) have been studied in small numbers of people as TD prevention, but results are inconclusive, partly because standardized preparations of these bacteria are not reliably available. Studies of probiotics to prevent TD are ongoing, but data are insufficient to recommend their use (see the Sec. 2, Ch. 14, Complementary & Integrative Health Approaches to Travel Wellness).

Anecdotal reports claim beneficial outcomes after using bovine colostrum as a daily prophylaxis agent for TD. However, commercially sold preparations of bovine colostrum marketed as dietary supplements are not approved by the US Food and Drug Administration (FDA). Because no data from rigorous clinical trials demonstrate efficacy, insufficient information is available to recommend the use of bovine colostrum to prevent TD.

Prophylactic Antibiotics

Older controlled studies showed that use of antibiotics reduced diarrhea attack rates by 90%. For most travelers, though, the risks associated with the use of prophylactic antibiotics (see below) do not outweigh the benefits. Prophylactic antibiotics might rarely be considered for short-term travelers who are high-risk hosts (e.g., immunocompromised people or people who have significant medical comorbidities).

The prophylactic antibiotic of choice has changed over the past few decades as resistance patterns have evolved. Historically, fluoroquinolones have been the most effective antibiotics for prophylaxis and treatment of bacterial TD pathogens, but resistance among *Campylobacter* and *Shigella* species globally now limits their use. In addition, fluoroquinolones are associated with tendinitis, concerns for QT interval prolongation, and an increased risk for *Clostridioides difficile* infection. Current guidelines discourage their use for prophylaxis. Alternative considerations include rifaximin and rifamycin SV.

ANTIMICROBIAL RESISTANCE & OTHER ADVERSE CONSEQUENCES

Prophylactic antibiotics are not recommended for most travelers. Prophylactic antibiotics afford no protection against nonbacterial pathogens and can remove normally protective microflora from the bowel, increasing the risk for infection with resistant bacterial pathogens. Travelers can become colonized with extended-spectrum β-lactamase-producing Enterobacteriaceae (ESBL-PE), a risk that is increased by exposure to antibiotics while abroad (see Sec 2, Ch. 17, . . . *perspectives*: Antibiotics in Travelers' Diarrhea—Balancing Benefit & Risk, and Sec. 11, Ch. 5, Antimicrobial Resistance).

Use of prophylactic antibiotics limits therapeutic options if TD occurs; a traveler relying on prophylactic antibiotics will need to carry an alternative antibiotic to use if severe diarrhea develops. Additionally, use of antibiotics has been associated with allergic and other adverse reactions.

TREATMENT

Antibiotics

The effectiveness of a particular antimicrobial drug depends on the etiologic agent and its antibiotic sensitivity (Table 2-09). If tolerated, single-dose regimens are equivalent to multidose regimens and might be more convenient for the traveler.

AZITHROMYCIN

Azithromycin is an alternative to fluoroquinolones (see below), although enteropathogens with decreased azithromycin susceptibility have been documented in several countries. The simplest azithromycin treatment regimen is a single dose of 1,000 mg, but side effects (mainly nausea) can limit the acceptability of this large dose; taking the medication as 2 divided doses on the same day can help.

Table 2-09 Acute diarrhea antibiotic treatment recommendations[1]

ANTIBIOTIC	DOSE	DURATION
Azithromycin[2,3]	1,000 mg 500 mg QD	Single or divided dose[4] 3 days
Ciprofloxacin	750 mg 500 mg BID	Single dose[4] 3 days
Levofloxacin	500 mg QD	1–3 days[4]
Ofloxacin	400 mg BID	1–3 days[4]
Rifamycin SV[5]	388 mg BID	3 days
Rifaximin[5]	200 mg TID	3 days

Abbreviations: BID, twice daily; QD, once daily; TID, three times a day
[1]Antibiotic regimens can be combined with loperamide 4 mg, initially, followed by 2 mg after each loose stool, not to exceed 16 mg in a 24-hour period.
[2]Use empirically as first-line treatment for travelers' diarrhea in Southeast Asia or other areas if fluoroquinolone-resistant bacteria are suspected.
[3]Preferred treatment for dysentery or febrile diarrhea.
[4]If symptoms are not resolved after 24 hours, continue daily dosing for up to 3 days.
[5]Do not use if clinical suspicion for *Campylobacter*, *Salmonella*, *Shigella*, or other causes of invasive diarrhea. Use may be reserved for patients unable to receive azithromycin or fluoroquinolones.

FLUOROQUINOLONES

Fluoroquinolones (e.g., ciprofloxacin, levofloxacin) have traditionally been the first-line antibiotics for empiric therapy of TD or to treat specific bacterial pathogens. Increasing microbial resistance to fluoroquinolones, however, especially among *Campylobacter* isolates, limits their usefulness in many destinations, particularly South and Southeast Asia, where both *Campylobacter* infection and fluoroquinolone resistance are prevalent. Increasing fluoroquinolone resistance has been reported from other destinations and in other bacterial pathogens, including in *Salmonella* and *Shigella*. Furthermore, fluoroquinolones now carry a black box warning from the FDA regarding multiple adverse reactions including aortic tears, hypoglycemia, mental health side effects, and tendinitis and tendon rupture.

RIFAMYCINS

RIFAMYCIN SV

A new therapeutic option is rifamycin SV, approved by the FDA in November 2018 to treat TD caused by noninvasive strains of *E. coli* in adults. Rifamycin SV is a nonabsorbable antibiotic in the ansamycin class of antibacterial drugs formulated with an enteric coating that targets delivery of the drug to the distal small bowel and colon. Two randomized clinical trials showed that rifamycin SV was superior to placebo and noninferior to ciprofloxacin in the treatment of TD. As with rifaximin (see below), travelers would need to carry a separate antibiotic (e.g., azithromycin) in case of infection due to an invasive pathogen.

RIFAXIMIN

Rifaximin has been approved to treat TD caused by noninvasive strains of *E. coli*. Since travelers likely cannot distinguish between invasive and noninvasive diarrhea, however, and since they would have to carry a backup drug in the event of invasive diarrhea, the overall usefulness of rifaximin as empiric self-treatment remains undetermined.

ANTIMICROBIAL RESISTANCE & OTHER ADVERSE CONSEQUENCES

Antibiotics are effective in reducing the duration of diarrhea by ≈1–2 days in cases caused by bacterial pathogens susceptible to the antibiotic prescribed. However, concerns about the adverse consequences of using antibiotics to treat TD remain. Travelers who take antibiotics are at risk of becoming colonized by drug-resistant organisms (e.g., ESBL-PE), resulting in potential harm to travelers—particularly immunocompromised people and people prone to urinary tract infections—and the possibility of introducing resistant bacteria into the community.

In addition, antibiotic use can affect the travelers' own microbiota and increase the potential for *C. difficile* infection. These concerns must be weighed against the consequences of TD and the role of antibiotics in shortening the acute illness and possibly preventing postinfectious sequelae. Primarily because of these concerns, an expert advisory panel was convened in 2016 to prepare consensus guidelines on the prevention and treatment of TD. The advisory panel suggested a classification of TD using functional impact for defining severity (Box 2-03) rather than the frequency-based algorithm used traditionally. The guidelines suggest an approach that matches therapeutic intervention with severity of illness, in terms of both safety and effectiveness (Box 2-04).

Antimotility Agents

Antimotility agents provide symptomatic relief and are useful therapy in TD. Synthetic opiates (e.g., diphenoxylate, loperamide) can reduce frequency of bowel movements and therefore enable travelers to ride on an airplane or bus. Loperamide appears to have antisecretory properties as well. The safety of loperamide when used along with an antibiotic has been well established, even in cases of invasive pathogens; however, acquisition of ESBL-PE might be more common when loperamide and antibiotics are coadministered.

Antimotility agents alone are not recommended for patients with bloody diarrhea or those who have diarrhea and fever. Loperamide can be used in children, and liquid formulations are available. In practice, however, these drugs are rarely given to children aged <6 years.

Oral Rehydration Therapy

Fluids and electrolytes are lost during TD, and replenishment is important, especially in young children, older adults, and adults with chronic medical illness. In otherwise healthy adult travelers, severe dehydration from TD is unusual unless vomiting is prolonged. Nonetheless, replacement of fluid losses is key to diarrhea therapy and helps the traveler feel better more quickly. Travelers should remember to use only beverages that are sealed, treated with chlorine, boiled, or are otherwise known to be purified (see Sec. 2, Ch. 9, Water Disinfection).

For severe fluid loss, replacement is best accomplished with oral rehydration solution (ORS) prepared from packaged oral rehydration salts (e.g., those provided by the World Health

BOX 2-03 Acute travelers' diarrhea: functional definitions

MILD DIARRHEA
Tolerable, not distressing, does not interfere with planned activities

MODERATE DIARRHEA
Distressing or interferes with planned activities

SEVERE DIARRHEA
Incapacitating or completely prevents planned activities
All dysentery is considered severe

BOX 2-04 Acute travelers' diarrhea: treatment recommendations

MILD DIARRHEA

Antibiotic treatment not recommended

Consider treatment with bismuth subsalicylate or loperamide

MODERATE DIARRHEA

Antibiotics can be used for treatment

- Azithromycin
- Fluoroquinolones
- Rifaximin (for moderate, noninvasive diarrhea)

Antimotility drugs

- Consider loperamide for use as monotherapy or as adjunctive therapy

SEVERE DIARRHEA

Antibiotic treatment is advised (single-dose regimens may be used)

- Azithromycin is preferred
- Fluoroquinolones or rifaximin[1] can be used for severe, non-dysenteric diarrhea

Antimotility drugs

- Consider loperamide for use as adjunctive therapy
- Not recommended as monotherapy for patients with bloody diarrhea or diarrhea and fever

[1]Treatment recommendations developed prior to the approval of rifamycin SV in the United States; because rifamycin SV is in the same antimicrobial drug category as rifaximin and because both have the same mechanism of action, rifamycin SV can be considered an alternative therapy.

Organization). ORS is widely available at stores and pharmacies in most low- and middle-income countries. ORS is prepared by adding 1 packet to the indicated volume of boiled or treated water—generally 1 liter. Due to their saltiness, travelers might find most ORS formulations relatively unpalatable. In mild cases, rehydration can be maintained with any preferred liquid (including sports drinks), although overly sweet drinks (e.g., sodas) can cause osmotic diarrhea if consumed in quantity.

Travelers' Diarrhea Caused by Protozoa

The most common parasitic cause of TD is *Giardia duodenalis*, and treatment options include metronidazole, nitazoxanide, and tinidazole (see Sec. 5, Part 3, Ch.12, Giardiasis). Amebiasis (see Sec. 5, Part 3, Ch. 1, Amebiasis) should be treated with metronidazole or tinidazole, then treated with a luminal agent (e.g., iodoquinol or paromomycin). Although cryptosporidiosis is usually a self-limited illness in immunocompetent people, clinicians can consider nitazoxanide as a treatment option (see Sec. 5, Part 3, Ch. 3, Cryptosporidiosis). Cyclosporiasis should be treated with trimethoprim-sulfamethoxazole but not trimethoprim alone (see Sec. 5, Part 3, Ch. 5, Cyclosporiasis).

Travelers' Diarrhea in Children

Children who accompany their parents on trips to high-risk destinations can contract TD, and their risk is elevated if they are visiting friends and family. Causative organisms include bacteria responsible for TD in adults, as well as viruses (e.g., norovirus, rotavirus). The main treatment for TD in children is ORS. Infants and younger children with TD are at greater risk for dehydration, which is best prevented by the early initiation of oral rehydration.

Consider recommending empiric antibiotic therapy for bloody or severe watery diarrhea or evidence of systemic infection. In older children and teenagers, treatment guidelines follow those for adults, with possible adjustments in the dose of medication. Among younger children, macrolides (e.g., azithromycin) are considered first-line antibiotic therapy. Rifaximin is approved for use in children aged ≥12 years. Rifamycin SV is approved for use only in adults.

Breastfed infants should continue to nurse on demand, and bottle-fed infants can continue to drink formula. Older infants and children should be encouraged to eat and should consume a regular diet. Children in diapers are at risk for developing diaper rash on their buttocks in response to liquid stool. Barrier creams (e.g., zinc oxide, petrolatum) could be applied at the onset of diarrhea to help prevent and treat rash; hydrocortisone cream is the best treatment for an established rash. More information about diarrhea and dehydration is discussed in Sec. 7, Ch. 3, Traveling Safely with Infants & Children.

BIBLIOGRAPHY

Black RE. Epidemiology of travelers' diarrhea and relative importance of various pathogens. Rev Infect Dis. 1990;12(Suppl 1):S73–9.

DeBruyn G, Hahn S, Borwick A. Antibiotic treatment for travelers' diarrhea. Cochrane Database Syst Rev. 2000;3:1–21.

Eckbo EJ, Yansouni CP, Pernica JM, Goldfarb DM. New tools to test stool: managing travelers' diarrhea in the era of molecular diagnostics. Infect Dis Clin N Am. 2019;33(1):197–212.

Kantele A, Lääveri T, Mero S, Vilkman K, Pakkanen S, Ollgren J, et al. Antimicrobials increase travelers' risk of colonization by extended-spectrum beta lactamase producing Enterobacteriaceae. Clin Infect Dis. 2015;60(6):837–46.

Kendall ME, Crim S, Fullerton K, Han PV, Cronquist AB, Shiferaw B, et al. Travel-associated enteric infections diagnosed after return to the United States, Foodborne Diseases Active Surveillance Network (FoodNet), 2004–2009. Clin Infect Dis. 2012;54(Suppl 5):S480–7.

McFarland LV. Meta-analysis of probiotics for the prevention of travelers' diarrhea. Travel Med Infect Dis. 2007;5(2):97–105.

Riddle MS, Connor BA, Beeching NJ, DuPont HL, Hamer DH, Kozarsky PE, et al. Guidelines for the prevention and treatment of travelers' diarrhea: a graded expert panel report. J Travel Med. 2017;24(Suppl 1):S2–19.

Riddle MS, DuPont HL, Connor BA. ACG clinical guideline: diagnosis, treatment, and prevention of acute diarrheal infections in adults. Am J Gastroenterol. 2016;111(5):602–22.

Schaumburg F, Correa-Martinez CL, Niemann S, Köck R, Becker K. Aetiology of traveller's diarrhea: a nested case-control study. Travel Med Infect Dis. 2020;37:101696.

Schaumburg F, Sertic SM, Correa-Martinez C, Mellmann A, Kock R, Becker K. Acquisition and colonization dynamics of antimicrobial-resistant bacteria during international travel: a prospective cohort study. Clin Microbiol Infect. 2019;25(10):e1–1287.e7.

Shlim DR. Looking for evidence that personal hygiene precautions prevent travelers' diarrhea. Clin Infect Dis. 2005;41(Suppl 8):S531–5.

Steffen R, Hill DR, DuPont HL. Traveler's diarrhea: a clinical review. JAMA. 2015;313(1):71–80.

Youmans BP, et al. Characterization of the human gut microbiome during travelers' diarrhea. Gut Microbes. 2015;6(2):110–9.

Zboromyrska Y, Hurtado JC, Salvador P, Alvarez-Martinez MJ, Valls ME, Marcos MA, et al. Aetiology of travelers' diarrhea: evaluation of a multiplex PCR tool to detect different enteropathogens. Clin Microbiol Infect. 2014;20:O753–9.

2

ANTIBIOTICS IN TRAVELERS' DIARRHEA—BALANCING BENEFIT & RISK

Mark Riddle, Bradley Connor

BENEFIT

For the past 30 years, randomized controlled trials have consistently and clearly demonstrated that antibiotics shorten the duration of illness and alleviate the disability associated with travelers' diarrhea (TD). Treatment with an effective antibiotic shortens the average duration of a TD episode by 1–2 days, and if the traveler combines an antibiotic with an antimotility agent (e.g., loperamide), duration of illness is shortened even further. Emerging data on the potential long-term health consequences of TD (e.g., chronic constipation, dyspepsia, irritable bowel syndrome) might suggest a benefit of early antibiotic therapy given the association between more severe and longer disease and risk for postinfectious consequences.

RISK

Antibiotics commonly used to treat TD have side effects, some of which are severe but rare. Perhaps of greater concern is the recent understanding that antibiotics used by travelers can contribute to changes in the host microbiome and to the acquisition of multidrug-resistant bacteria. Multiple observational studies have found that travelers (in particular, travelers to South and Southeast Asia) who develop TD and take antibiotics are at risk for colonization with extended-spectrum β-lactamase–producing Enterobacteriaceae (ESBL-PE).

The direct effect of colonization on the average traveler appears limited; carriage is most often transient, but it does persist in a small percentage of colonized persons. Elderly travelers (because of the serious consequences of bloodstream infections in this population) and those with a history of recurrent urinary tract infections (because *Escherichia coli* is a common cause) might be at an increased risk for health consequences from ESBL-PE colonization. At a minimum, clinicians should make these travelers aware of the risk and counsel them to convey their travel exposure history to their treating providers if they become ill after travel. Of broader importance, international travel has been associated with subsequent ESBL-PE colonization among close-living contacts, suggesting potentially wider public health consequences from ESBL-PE acquisition during travel.

THE CHALLENGE

The challenge providers and travelers face is how to balance the health benefit of short-course antibiotic treatment of TD with the risk for colonization and global spread of resistance. The role played by travelers in the translocation of infectious disease and resistance cannot be ignored, but the ecology of ESBL-PE infections is complex and includes diet, environment, immigration, and local nosocomial transmission dynamics. ESBL-PE infections are an emerging health threat, and addressing this complex problem will require multiple strategies, including antibiotic stewardship.

AN APPROACH

Health care providers need to have conversations with travelers about the multilevel (individual, community, global) and multifactorial risks of developing TD: travel, individual behaviors (e.g., hand hygiene), diet (e.g., safe selection of foods and beverages), and other risk avoidance measures. But then, knowing it is often difficult to prevent or even reduce the risk for TD through behaviors and diet alone, what is the most reasonable way to prepare travelers for empiric TD self-treatment before a trip? Clinicians can strongly emphasize reserving antibiotics for moderate to severe TD and using antimotility agents for self-treatment of mild TD.

When it comes to managing TD, we expect the traveler to be both diagnostician and health care provider. For even the most astute traveler, making an appropriately informed decision about their own health can be challenged by the anxiety-provoking onset of that first abdominal cramp in sometimes austere and inconvenient settings. Given that TD counseling is competing with numerous other pretravel health topics that need to be covered, travel medicine providers might want to develop and implement simple messaging, handouts, or easy-to-access electronic health guidance. Providing travelers with clear written guidance about TD prevention and step-by-step instructions about how and when to use medications for TD is crucial.

Though further studies are needed (and many are under way), a rational approach involves using a single-dose regimen of an antibiotic that minimizes microbiome disruption and risk for colonization. Additionally, as travel and untreated TD independently increase the risk for ESBL-PE colonization, nonantibiotic chemoprophylactic strategies (e.g., self-treatment with bismuth subsalicylate), can decrease both the acute and posttravel risk concerns. Strengthening the resilience of the host microbiota to prevent infection and unwanted colonization, as with the use of prebiotics or probiotics, are promising potential strategies but need further investigation.

BIBLIOGRAPHY

Arcilla MS, van Hattem JM, Haverkate MR, Bootsma MCJ, van Genderen PJJ, Goorhuis A, et al. Import and spread of extended-spectrum β-lactamase-producing Enterobacteriaceae by international travellers (COMBAT study): a prospective, multicentre cohort study. Lancet Infect Dis. 2017;17(1):78–85.

Riddle MS, Connor BA, Beeching NJ, DuPont HL, Hamer DH, Kozarsky P, et al. Guidelines for the prevention and treatment of travelers' diarrhea: a graded expert panel report. J Travel Med. 2017;24 (Suppl 1):S57–74.

... *perspectives* chapters supplement the clinical guidance in this book with additional content, context, and expert opinion. The views expressed do not necessarily represent the official position of the Centers for Disease Control and Prevention (CDC).

FOOD & WATER PRECAUTIONS

Brigette Gleason, Vincent Hill, Patricia Griffin

2

Contaminated food and water pose a risk for travelers. Many infectious diseases associated with contaminated food and water are caused by pathogens transmitted via the fecal–oral route. Additional information on pathogens associated with travelers' diarrhea, prophylaxis, and treatment options can be found in Sec. 2, Ch. 6, Travelers' Diarrhea.

FOOD

Travelers should select food with care. Travelers should follow food safety practices recommended in the United States while abroad (www.cdc.gov/foodsafety/keep-food-safe.html). Raw food is especially likely to be contaminated. Raw or undercooked meat, fish, shellfish, and produce can be contaminated with pathogens, and some fish harvested from tropical waters can transmit toxins that survive cooking (see Sec. 4, Ch. 10, Food Poisoning from Marine Toxins).

In areas where hygiene and sanitation are inadequate or unknown, travelers should avoid consuming salads, uncooked vegetables, raw unpeeled fruits, and unpasteurized fruit juices. Fruits that can be peeled are safest when peeled by the person who eats them. Advise travelers to rinse produce with safe water (see Sec. 2, Ch. 9, Water Disinfection); washing with water alone, however, does not remove all pathogens from produce. Foods of animal origin, including meat and eggs, should be cooked thoroughly (www.cdc.gov/foodsafety/keep-food-safe.html), and travelers should select pasteurized milk and milk products, including soft cheeses. In restaurants, inadequate refrigeration and lack of food safety training among staff can result in transmission of pathogens or their toxins. Consumption of food and beverages obtained from street vendors increases the risk of illness. In general, fully cooked foods that are served hot and foods that travelers carefully prepare themselves are safest.

Travelers should not bring perishable food from high-risk areas back to their home country without refrigeration. Moreover, travelers should exercise the same cautions about food and water served on flights as they do for restaurants.

Clinicians should advise travelers to wash their hands with soap and water before preparing or eating food, after using the bathroom or changing diapers, before and after caring for someone who is ill, and after contact with animals or animal environments. When soap and water are not available, travelers should use an alcohol-based hand sanitizer containing ≥60% alcohol, then wash hands with soap and water as soon as possible. Hand sanitizer is not as effective as handwashing for removing some germs, like *Cryptosporidium* or norovirus, and does not work well when hands are visibly dirty or greasy. The Centers for Disease Control and Prevention (CDC) website Handwashing: Clean Hands Save Lives (www.cdc.gov/handwashing) provides additional information.

Feeding Infants

BREASTFEEDING

For infants aged <6 months, the safest way to feed is to breastfeed exclusively. Practicing careful hygiene when using a breast pump can reduce the risk of getting germs into the milk. For details, see How to Keep Your Breast Pump Kit Clean: The Essentials (www.cdc.gov/healthywater/hygiene/healthychildcare/infantfeeding/breastpump.html). For information on malaria prophylaxis for breastfeeding patients see Sec. 5, Part 3, Ch. 16, Malaria, and Sec. 7, Ch. 2, Travel & Breastfeeding.

FORMULA

For infants who get formula, parents should consider using liquid, ready-to-feed formula, which is sterile. When preparing formula from commercial powder, following the manufacturers' instructions usually is sufficient. Although no powdered formula is sterile, travelers should consider packing enough for their trip because manufacturing standards vary widely around the world.

Formula safety can be increased by reconstituting powder using hot water (≥158°F; ≥70°C); instruct travelers to pack a food thermometer to test water temperature, especially for infants <3 months of age and those with weakened immune systems. Prepared formula should be used within 2 hours of preparation or refrigerated for a maximum of 24 hours. After feeding, any remaining liquid or prepared formula should be discarded.

For more on infant feeding hygiene, see How to Clean, Sanitize, and Store Infant Feeding Items (www.cdc.gov/healthywater/hygiene/healthychildcare/infantfeeding/cleansanitize.html) and *Cronobacter*: Prevention & Control (www.cdc.gov/cronobacter/prevention.html).

WATER

Swallowing, inhaling aerosols of, and having contact with contaminated water can transmit pathogens that cause diarrhea, vomiting, or ear, eye, skin, respiratory, or nervous system infections. Travelers should follow safe water practices recommended in the United States while abroad (www.cdc.gov/healthywater).

Drinking Water & Other Beverages

In many parts of the world, particularly where water treatment, sanitation, and hygiene are inadequate, tap water can contain disease-causing agents, including bacteria, viruses, parasites, or chemical contaminants. Consequently, tap water might be unsafe for drinking, preparing food and beverages, making ice, cooking, and brushing teeth. Infants, young children, pregnant people, older people, and immunocompromised people (e.g., those with HIV or on chemotherapy or certain medications) might be especially susceptible to illness.

Travelers should avoid drinking or putting tap water into their mouths unless they are reasonably certain the water is safe. Similarly, travelers should avoid ice since it may have been prepared with tap water. Box 2-05 provides tips and recommendations of other safe water and beverage practices for travelers.

BOX 2-05 Safe water & beverage practices: a checklist of recommendations for travelers

- ☐ Many people choose to disinfect or filter their water when traveling to destinations where safe tap water might not be available (for details and proper techniques, see Sec. 2, Ch. 9, Water Disinfection).
- ☐ Beverages made with water that has just been boiled (e.g., tea, coffee), generally are safe to drink.
- ☐ Unless further disinfected, tap water safe for drinking is not sterile and should not be used for sinus or nasal irrigation or rinsing, including use in neti pots and for ritual ablution. Never use tap water to clean or rinse contact lenses. Avoid getting tap water in your mouth when showering or bathing.
- ☐ Water that looks cloudy or discolored could be contaminated with chemicals and will not be made safe by boiling or disinfection. In these situations, use bottled water.
- ☐ In areas where tap water could be unsafe, use only commercially bottled water from an unopened, factory-sealed container, or water that has been adequately disinfected for drinking, preparing food and beverages, making ice, cooking, and brushing teeth.
- ☐ When served in unopened, factory-sealed cans or bottles, carbonated beverages, commercially prepared fruit drinks, water, alcoholic beverages, and pasteurized drinks generally can be considered safe. Because surfaces on the outside of cans and bottles might be contaminated, these surfaces should be wiped clean and dried before opening or drinking directly from the container.
- ☐ Beverages that might not be safe for consumption include iced drinks and fountain drinks or other drinks made with tap water. Because ice might be made from contaminated water, ask that all beverages be served without ice.
- ☐ The alcohol content of alcoholic beverages will not kill bacteria in ice made from contaminated water.

Recreational Water

Pathogens that cause gastrointestinal, respiratory, skin, ear, eye, and neurologic illnesses can be transmitted via contaminated recreational freshwater or marine water. Water from inadequately treated pools, hot tubs, spas, or water playgrounds, including splash pads or spray parks, can also be contaminated. Recreational water contaminated by human feces from swimmers, animal waste, sewage, or wastewater runoff can appear clear but still contain disease-causing infectious or chemical agents. Ingesting even small amounts of such water can cause illness. Infectious pathogens (e.g., *Cryptosporidium*) can survive for days, even in well-maintained and safely operated pools, water playgrounds, and hot tubs and spas. To protect other people, children and adults with diarrhea should not enter recreational water.

Maintaining proper pH and free chlorine or bromine concentration is necessary for preventing transmission of most infectious pathogens in water in pools, water playgrounds, and hot tubs or spas. If travelers would like to test recreational water before use, CDC recommends pH 7.2–7.8 and a free available chlorine concentration of 3–10 parts per million (ppm) in hot tubs and spas (4–8 ppm if bromine is used) and 1–10 ppm in pools and water playgrounds (2–10 ppm for aquatic venues using cyanuric acid as a chlorine stabilizer). Travelers can purchase test strips at most superstores, hardware stores, and pool supply stores.

Pseudomonas, which can cause "hot tub rash" or "swimmer's ear," and *Legionella* (see Sec. 5, Part 1, Ch. 9, Legionnaires' Disease & Pontiac Fever) can multiply in hot tubs and spas in which chlorine or bromine concentrations are not adequately maintained. Travelers at increased risk for legionellosis (e.g., people ≥50 years of age, those with immunocompromising conditions), should avoid entering or walking near higher-risk areas (e.g., hot tubs, spas). Travelers also should avoid pools, water playgrounds, and hot tubs or spas where bather limits are not enforced or where the water is cloudy. Additional guidance can be found at CDC's Healthy Swimming website (www.cdc.gov/healthywater/swimming).

Travelers should not swim or wade near storm drains; in water that could be contaminated with human or animal feces, sewage, or wastewater runoff; in lakes or rivers after heavy rainfall; in water that smells bad, looks discolored, or has algal mats, foam, or scum on the surface; in freshwater streams, canals, or lakes in schistosomiasis-endemic areas of Africa, Asia, the Caribbean, and South America (see Sec. 5, Part 3, Ch. 20, Schistosomiasis); in water that might be contaminated with urine from animals infected with *Leptospira* (see Sec. 5, Part 1, Ch. 10, Leptospirosis); or in warm seawater or brackish water (mixture of fresh and sea water), particularly when they have wounds.

Travelers with open wounds should consider avoiding all water contact. Seawater and brackish water can contain pathogens (e.g., *Vibrio* spp.) that can cause wound infections and sepsis. If a sore or open wound comes into contact with untreated recreational water, it should be washed thoroughly with soap and water to reduce the chance of infection. If travelers with wounds do plan water contact, they should cover the wound with a water-repellent bandage.

Naegleria fowleri (www.cdc.gov/parasites/naegleria) is a parasite found around the world in warm freshwater, including lakes, rivers, ponds, hot springs, and locations with water warmed by discharge from power plants and industrial complexes. To help prevent a rare but fatal infection caused by this parasite, travelers should hold their noses shut or wear a nose clip when swimming, diving, or participating in similar activities in warm freshwater. Travelers also should avoid digging in or stirring up sediment, especially in warm water. Clinicians should inform travelers that *Naegleria fowleri* infection also has been linked to use of contaminated tap water for sinus or nasal irrigation.

BIBLIOGRAPHY

Centers for Disease Control and Prevention. Cronobacter: Prevention & Control. Available from: www.cdc.gov/cronobacter/prevention.html.

Centers for Disease Control and Prevention. Drinking water: camping, hiking, travel. Available from: www.cdc.gov/healthywater/drinking/travel/index.html.

Centers for Disease Control and Prevention. Food safety. Available from: www.cdc.gov/foodsafety/index.html.

Centers for Disease Control and Prevention. Global Water, Sanitation & Hygiene (WASH): Travelers' Health. Available from: www.cdc.gov/healthywater/global/traveler_health.html.

Centers for Disease Control and Prevention. Healthy swimming: hot tub rash (Pseudomonas/Folliculitis). Available from: www.cdc.gov/healthywater/swimming/swimmers/rwi/rashes.html.

Centers for Disease Control and Prevention. Healthy swimming: swimming and ear infections. Available from: www.cdc.gov/healthywater/swimming/swimmers/rwi/ear-infections.html.

Centers for Disease Control and Prevention. *Legionella* (Legionnaires' disease and Pontiac fever). Available from: www.cdc.gov/legionella/index.html.

Centers for Disease Control and Prevention. Parasites—*Naegleria fowleri*—primary amebic meningoencephalitis (PAM)—amebic encephalitis. Available from: www.cdc.gov/parasites/naegleria/index.html.

Eberhart-Phillips J, Besser RE, Tormey MP, Koo D, Feikin D, Araneta MR, et al. An outbreak of cholera from food served on an international aircraft. Epidemiol Infect. 1996;116(1):9–13.

WATER DISINFECTION

Howard Backer, Vincent Hill

Waterborne diseases are a risk for international travelers who visit countries where access to safe water, adequate sanitation, and proper hygiene is limited, and for wilderness visitors who rely on surface water in any country, including the United States. In both high-income and low- and middle-income countries, lack of potable water is one of the most immediate public health problems faced after natural disasters (e.g., earthquakes, hurricanes, tsunamis), or in refugee camps. The list of potential waterborne pathogens is extensive and includes bacteria, viruses, protozoa, and parasitic helminths.

Most of the organisms that cause travelers' diarrhea can be waterborne. Many types of bacteria and viruses can cause intestinal (enteric) infection through drinking water. Common waterborne protozoa include *Cryptosporidium*, *Entamoeba histolytica* (the cause of amebic dysentery), and *Giardia*. Parasitic worms are not commonly transmitted through drinking water, but drinking water is a potential means of transmission for some. Respiratory viruses, including coronaviruses like severe acute respiratory syndrome coronavirus 2 (SARS-CoV-2), can be passed in feces, but the risk for fecal transmission, including through water, is considered low; for more details, see the US Centers for Disease Control and Prevention (CDC) website on the National Wastewater Surveillance System (NWSS) (www.cdc.gov/healthywater/surveillance/wastewater-surveillance/wastewater-surveillance.html).

International travelers and wilderness visitors have no reliable resources to evaluate local water system quality. Substantial progress has been made toward the goal of safe drinking water and sanitation worldwide, particularly in Asia and Latin America. Seven hundred and eighty million people (11% of the world's population), however, still lack a safe water source; 2.5 billion people lack access to improved sanitation, and >890 million people still practice open defecation.

Where treated tap water is available, aging or inadequate water treatment infrastructure might not effectively disinfect water or maintain water quality during distribution. Some larger hotels and resorts might use additional onsite water treatment to generate potable water. Where untreated surface or well water is used, and no sanitation infrastructure exists, the risk for waterborne infection is high.

All international travelers—especially long-term travelers and expatriates—should become familiar with and use simple methods to ensure safe drinking water. Bottled water has become the convenient solution for most travelers, but in some places, bottled water might not be superior to tap water. Moreover, plastic bottles create an ecological problem because most low- and middle-income countries do not recycle them. Water disinfection methods that can be applied in the field include use of heat, clarification, filtration, chemical disinfection, and ultraviolet radiation (UVR). Several of these methods are scalable, and some can be improvised from local resources, allowing adaptation to disaster relief and refugee situations. Table 2-10 compares the advantages and disadvantages of the different methods. Additional information on water treatment and disinfection methods can be found at CDC's Water Treatment Options when Hiking, Camping, or Traveling website (www.cdc.gov/healthywater/drinking/travel).

FIELD TECHNIQUES FOR WATER TREATMENT

Heat

Common intestinal pathogens are readily inactivated by heat. Microorganisms are killed in a shorter time at higher temperatures, but temperatures as low as 140°F (60°C) are effective when a longer contact time is used. Pasteurization uses this principle to kill foodborne enteric pathogens and spoilage-causing organisms at temperatures between 140°F (60°C) and 158°F (70°C), well below the boiling point of water (212°F [100°C]).

Boiling is not necessary to kill common intestinal pathogens, but boiling is the only easily recognizable end point that does not require a thermometer. All organisms, except bacterial spores (which are rarely waterborne enteric pathogens), are killed within seconds at boiling temperature. In addition, the time required to heat the water from 140°F (60°C) to boiling works toward heat disinfection. Any water brought to a boil should be adequately disinfected; if fuel supplies are adequate, however, CDC recommends that travelers boil water for a full minute to account for user variability in identifying boiling points and to add a margin of safety.

Although the boiling point for water decreases with increasing elevation, at common terrestrial travel elevations, the temperature needed to achieve boiling is still well above the temperature required to inactivate enteric pathogens. For example, at 16,000 ft (≈4,900 m) elevation, the boiling temperature of water is 182°F (≈83°C). In hot climates with sunshine, a water container placed in a simple reflective solar oven can reach pasteurization temperatures of 150°F (≈65°C).

Travelers with access to electricity can bring a small electric heating coil, and many hotels have electric water pots to brew tea or coffee. When possible, travelers should avoid using water from the hot water tap for drinking or food preparation, because hot tap water can contain higher levels of metals, like copper and lead, that leach from the building's water heater and pipes.

Clarification

Clarification refers to techniques that reduce the cloudiness (turbidity) of water caused by the presence of natural organic and inorganic material. Clarification can markedly improve both the appearance and taste of the water. Decreasing turbidity is an indicator that microbiological contamination will also be reduced, but not enough to ensure water potability; clarification techniques facilitate disinfection by filtration or chemical treatment.

COAGULATION & FLOCCULATION

Large particles like silt and sand will settle by gravity (sedimentation). Cloudiness due to dissolved substances or smaller particles that remain suspended in water can be improved by using chemical products that coagulate and flocculate (i.e., cause clumping). This process removes many, but not all, microorganisms unless the product also contains a disinfectant.

Alum, an aluminum salt widely used in food, cosmetic, and medical applications, is the principal agent for coagulation/flocculation. Travelers should add one-fourth teaspoon (1/4 tsp) of alum powder to 1 quart (32 oz; .95 L) of cloudy water; stir frequently for a few minutes and add more powder as necessary until clumps form. Allow the clumped material to settle into the bottom of the container, and then pour the water through a coffee filter or clean, fine cloth to remove the sediment. Since most microbes are removed but not all, travelers must use a second disinfection step.

Table 2-10 Water disinfection techniques: advantages & disadvantages

TECHNIQUE	ADVANTAGES	DISADVANTAGES
HEAT	Does not impart additional taste or color. Single-step process that inactivates all enteric pathogens. Efficacy not compromised by contaminants or particles in the water.	Does not improve taste, odor, or appearance of water. Fuel sources might be scarce, expensive, or unavailable. No residual protection; does not prevent stored water from recontamination.
FILTRATION	Simple to operate. Does not require holding time for treatment; water can be consumed immediately after filtering. Many commercial product designs available. Adds no unpleasant taste; often improves water taste and appearance. Can be combined with chemical disinfection to increase microbe removal.	Adds bulk and weight to baggage. Many filters do not reliably remove viruses. More expensive than chemical treatment. Eventually clogs from suspended particulate matter and might require some field maintenance or repair. No residual protection; does not prevent stored water from recontamination.
CHEMICAL DISINFECTION: HALOGENS & ELECTROLYTIC SOLUTIONS	Inexpensive. Widely available in liquid or tablet form. Bad taste can be removed by simple techniques. Flexible dosing. Equally easy to treat large and small volumes. Residual protection; can prevent stored water from recontamination.	Imparts taste and odor to water. Flexible dosing requires understanding of principles of chemical disinfection. Iodine is physiologically active and has potential adverse health effects. Not readily effective against *Cryptosporidium* oocysts. Efficacy decreases with cloudy water. Liquid disinfectants are corrosive and can stain clothing.
CHEMICAL DISINFECTION: CHLORINE DIOXIDE	Low doses impart no taste or color to water. Simple to use and available in liquid or tablet form. More potent than equivalent doses of chlorine. Effective against all waterborne pathogens, including *Cryptosporidium.*	Volatile and sensitive to sunlight; do not expose tablets to air; rapidly use chlorine dioxide solutions. No residual protection; does not prevent stored water from recontamination. Requires several hours contact time for disinfection.
ULTRAVIOLET RADIATION (UVR)	Imparts no taste, odor, or color to water. Portable battery-operated devices are available. Effective against all waterborne pathogens. Extra doses of UVR can be used for added assurance and with no side effects.	Requires clear (not cloudy or turbid) water. Does not improve taste or appearance of water. Relatively expensive, except solar disinfection (SODIS) method. Requires batteries or power source (except SODIS). Cannot know if devices are delivering required UVR doses. No residual protection; does not prevent stored water from recontamination.

Some commercially available tablets or powder packets combine a flocculant with a chemical disinfectant. Travelers should check their product to determine whether they need additional disinfection.

Filtration

2

Portable hand-pump or gravity-drip filters with various designs and types of filter media are commercially available to international travelers. Filter pore size is the primary determinant of a filter's effectiveness (see Figure 2-01). Manufacturers claiming a US Environmental Protection Agency (EPA) designation of water "purifier" for their products must conduct their own testing to demonstrate their filters can remove at least 10^6 bacteria (99.9999%), 10^4 viruses (99.99%), and 10^3 *Cryptosporidium* oocysts or *Giardia* cysts (99.9%). The EPA does not independently test the validity of these claims.

FILTER PORE SIZE

Most portable filters are microfilters with a pore size <1 μm, which should readily remove bacteria and protozoan parasites like *Cryptosporidium* and *Giardia.* Travelers should not expect portable microfilters to effectively remove enteric viruses (e.g., norovirus) with an average size of 0.03 μm (see Table 2-11).

For areas with high levels of human and animal activity in the watershed or in places with poor sanitation, travelers should use higher levels of filtration or other techniques to remove viruses. If using a microfilter, travelers can pretreat water with chlorine to remove viruses. Progressively finer levels of filtration, known as ultrafiltration, nanofiltration, and reverse osmosis, all can remove viruses (see Figure 2-01). Ultrafilters with pore size of 0.01 μm should be effective for removing viruses, bacteria, and parasites. Other available portable ultrafilters use hollow-fiber

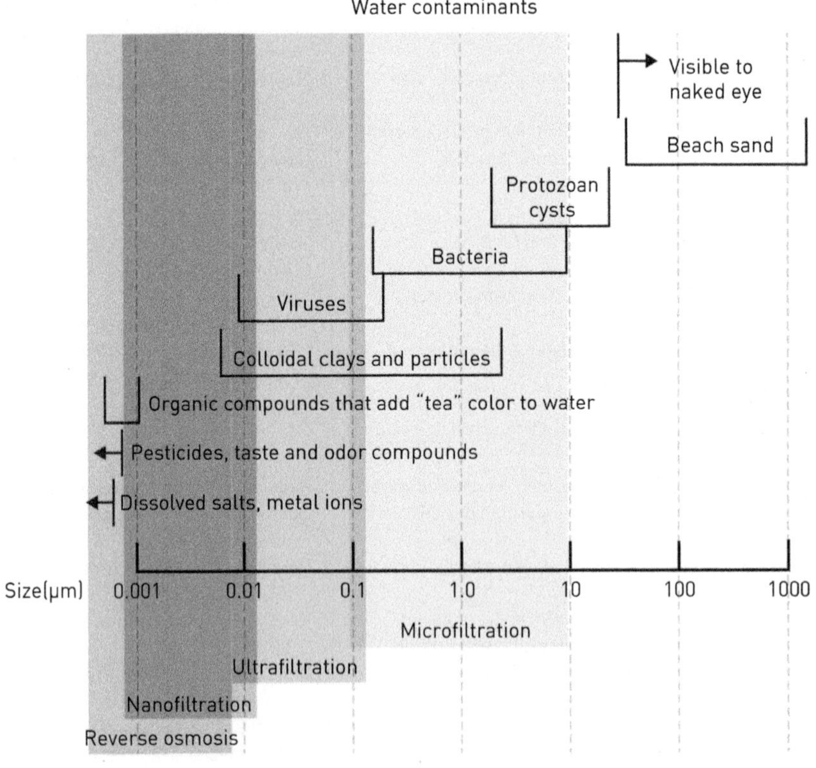

FIGURE 2-01. **Water contaminants: particle sizes & filtration methods**

Source: Auerbach PS, ed. Wilderness Medicine, 7th edition. Philadelphia: Elsevier; 2017.

Table 2-11 Waterborne pathogens (average sizes) & filter pore size needed to achieve disinfection

WATERBORNE PATHOGEN	AVERAGE SIZE (μM)	FILTER PORE SIZE NEEDED (μM)	FILTER CLASS
Viruses	0.03	Not specified (optimally ≤0.01)	Ultrafilter
Enteric bacteria (e.g., *Escherichia coli*)	0.5 × 2–8	≤0.2–0.4	Microfilter
Cryptosporidium oocysts	4–6	≤1	Microfilter
Giardia cysts	8 × 19	≤3.0–5.0	Microfilter
Helminth eggs	30 × 60	Not specified	Any
Schistosome larvae	50 × 100	Not specified	Any

technology that operate by gravity, hand-pump, or drink-through methods. Nanofilters have rated pore sizes of 0.001 μm and will remove chemicals and organic molecules from water. Reverse osmosis filters have a pore size of ≤0.0001 μm (0.1 nm) and will remove monovalent salts and dissolved metals, achieving water desalination. Progressively smaller pore size filters are available; however, these filters are both more costly and require greater pressures to push water through the filter, often at a slower rate. For these reasons, small hand-pump reverse osmosis units can be a challenge for land-based travelers to use, but they are a viable survival aid for ocean voyagers; military and refugee camps use larger, powered devices.

ACTIVATED CHARCOAL, CLAY, SAND & GRAVEL

Many household and field filters include granular activated charcoal (GAC), which further treats water by adsorbing organic and inorganic chemicals, including chlorine and iodine compounds, and most heavy metals, thereby improving odor, taste, and safety. GAC filters trap, but do not kill, microorganisms, and they are generally not rated for microbe removal.

In resource-limited international settings, communities and households might use filters made from ceramic clay or simple sand and gravel (slow sand or biosand). When no other means of disinfection is available in remote or austere situations, travelers and wilderness visitors can improvise an emergency gravel and sand filter using a 20-liter (≈5.5 gallon) bucket (see Figure 2-02).

Chemical Disinfection

HALOGENS

CHLORINE COMPOUNDS & IODINE

Chemical disinfectants for drinking water treatment, including chlorine compounds, iodine, and chlorine dioxide, commonly are available as commercial products. Sodium hypochlorite, the active ingredient in common household bleach, has been used for over a century and is the primary disinfectant promoted by CDC and the World Health Organization (WHO). Other chlorine-containing compounds, widely available in granular or tablet formulations (e.g., calcium hypochlorite and sodium dichloroisocyanurate), are equally effective for water treatment.

An advantage of chemical water disinfection products is flexible dosing that enables their use by individual travelers, small or large groups, or communities. In emergency situations, or when other commercial chemical disinfection water treatment products are not available, household bleach can be used with flexible dosing based on water volume and clarity. Refer to CDC recommendations at www.cdc.gov/healthywater/emergency/drinking/making-water-safe.html.

2

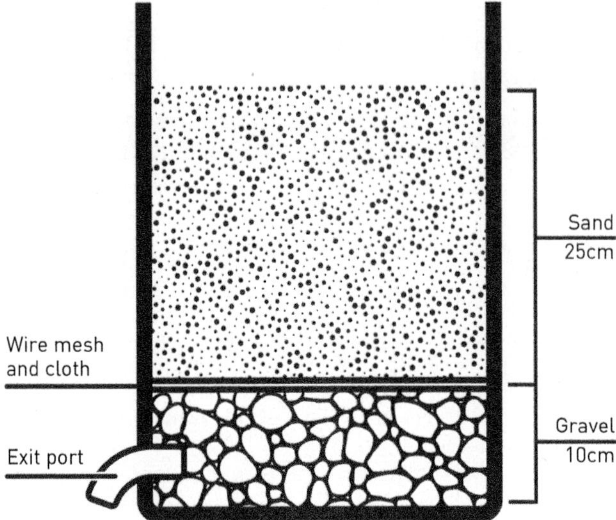

FIGURE 2-02. **Emergency gravel and sand filter**

Gravel and sand filters are constructed by forming layers of aggregate increasing from very fine sand at the top to large gravel at the bottom near the exit port. An emergency sand filter can be made in a 20 L (≈5 gal) bucket, composed of a 10-centimeter (≈4 inch) layer of gravel beneath a 25-centimeter (≈10 inch) layer of sand; a layer of cotton cloth, sandwiched between two layers of wire mesh, separates the sand and gravel layers.

Given adequate concentrations and length of exposure (contact time), chlorine and iodine have similar activity and are effective against bacteria and viruses (see Effect of Chlorination on Inactivating Selected Pathogens, www.cdc.gov/safewater/effectiveness-on-pathogens.html). Although *Giardia* cysts are more resistant than other bacteria and viruses to chemical disinfection, field-level concentrations of chlorine and iodine are effective against this parasite when longer contact times are used. For this reason, dosing and concentrations of chemical disinfection products are generally targeted at *Giardia* cysts.

Another common protozoan parasite, *Cryptosporidium*, is poorly inactivated by chlorine- or iodine-based disinfection at practical concentrations, even with extended contact times. Chemical disinfection can be supplemented with filtration to remove these resistant oocysts from drinking water.

Cloudy water contains disinfectant-neutralizing substances and requires higher concentrations or contact times with chemical disinfectants. Advise travelers to clarify cloudy water using settling, coagulation/flocculation, or filtration (described above) before adding the disinfectant.

Because iodine has physiologic activity, WHO recommends limiting drinking iodine-disinfected water to a few weeks. People with unstable thyroid disease or known iodine allergy should not use iodine for chemical disinfection. In addition, pregnant people should not use iodine to disinfect water for prolonged periods of time because of potential adverse effects on the fetal thyroid. Advise pregnant travelers to use an alternative method of water disinfection (e.g., heat, chlorination, filtration).

Taste preference for iodine over chlorine is individual; neither is particularly palatable in doses recommended for field use. The taste of halogen-treated water can be improved by running the water through a filter containing GAC, by adding a pinch of powdered ascorbic acid (vitamin C), or by adding 5–10 drops of 3% hydrogen peroxide per quart (32 oz; ≈1 L) of water, then stirring or shaking, which can be repeated until the taste of chlorine or iodine is gone.

CHLORINE DIOXIDE

Chlorine dioxide (ClO_2) kills most waterborne pathogens, including *Cryptosporidium* oocysts, at practical doses and contact times. Several commercial ClO_2 products are available in liquid or tablet form, but relatively few data are available on testing of these products for different water conditions.

SALT (SODIUM CHLORIDE) ELECTROLYSIS

Electrolytic water purifiers generate a mixture of oxidants, including hypochlorite, by passing an electrical current through a simple brine salt solution. Commercially available small units use salt, water, and a 12-volt DC (automobile) battery to quickly create a chlorine solution that can be used treat ≤200 liters of water.

SILVER & OTHER PRODUCTS

Silver ion has bactericidal effects in low doses; attractive features include lack of color, taste, and odor, and the ability of a thin coating on a container to maintain a steady, low concentration in water. Silver ion concentration in water can be strongly affected by adsorption onto the surface of the container, and limited testing on viruses and cysts has been performed. Silver is widely used by European travelers as a drinking water disinfectant, but in the United States, silver is approved only for maintaining microbiologic quality of stored water. Silver is available alone or in combination with chlorine in tablet formulation.

Several other common products, including hydrogen peroxide, citrus juice, and potassium permanganate, have antibacterial effects in water and are marketed in commercial products for travelers. However, none has sufficient data to recommend them for water disinfection at low doses in the field.

Ultraviolet Radiation

Ultraviolet radiation (UVR) kills bacteria, viruses, and *Cryptosporidium* oocysts in water; efficacy depends on dose and exposure time. Moreover, because suspended particles can shield microorganisms from UVR, UVR units have limited effectiveness in disinfecting water with high levels of suspended solids and turbidity.

In the field, portable battery-operated units capable of delivering a metered, timed dose of UVR are an effective way to disinfect 1–2 liters of clear water at a time. Larger units with greater outputs are available for use in places where a power source is available.

SOLAR IRRADIATION

Using sunlight to irradiate water (solar disinfection or SODIS) can improve the microbiologic quality of water and can be used in austere emergency situations. Because UVR is blocked by particles, travelers should clarify highly

Table 2-12 Field water disinfection techniques: effectiveness against waterborne pathogens

TECHNIQUE	BACTERIA	VIRUSES	PROTOZOAN CYSTS (e.g., *GIARDIA*, AMEBAS)	*CRYPTOSPORIDIUM*	HELMINTHS & SCHISTOSOMES
HEAT	+	+	+	+	+
FILTRATION[1]	+	+/–	+	+	+
HALOGENS[2,3]	+	+	+	–	+/–
CHLORINE DIOXIDE	+	+	+	+	+

[1]Many filters make no claims for viruses. Hollow-fiber filters with ultrafiltration pore size of 0.01 μm and reverse osmosis are effective.
[2]Higher concentrations and longer contact time are required to disinfect waterborne protozoan cysts than bacteria or viruses.
[3]Helminth eggs are not very susceptible to chlorine or iodine, but risk for waterborne transmission is very low.

turbid water first. The optimal procedure is to use transparent bottles (e.g., clear plastic beverage bottles) laid on their side and exposed to sunlight for a minimum of 6 hours with intermittent agitation. Under cloudy weather conditions, water must be placed in the sun for 2 consecutive days. The Swiss Federal Institute of Aquatic Sciences and Technology provides more details on SODIS (see www.sodis.ch/index_EN for more details).

2

CHOOSING A DISINFECTION TECHNIQUE

Table 2-12 summarizes advantages and disadvantages of field water disinfection techniques and their microbicidal efficacy. Travelers can use a UVR-generating device or liquid bleach (1–2 drops of per quart [liter] of water) to disinfect tap water. Trekkers or campers might prefer to use filters rated to remove viruses. Advise travelers to practice disinfection methods before leaving for their destination.

BIBLIOGRAPHY

Backer HD. Field water disinfection. In: Auerbach PS, editor. Wilderness medicine, 7th edition. Philadelphia: Elsevier; 2017. pp. 1985–2030.

Backer HD, Derlet RW, Hill VR. Wilderness Medical Society clinical practice guidelines for water disinfection for wilderness, international travel, and austere situations. Wilderness Environ Med. 2019;30(4S):S100–20.

Centers for Disease Control and Prevention. Safe water system. Available from: www.cdc.gov/safewater/index.html.

Sobsey MD, Stauber CE, Casanova LM, Brown JM, Elliott MA. Point of use household drinking water filtration: a practical, effective solution for providing sustained access to safe drinking water in the developing world. Environ Sci Technol. 2008;42(12):4261–7.

Swiss Federal Institute of Aquatic Science and Technology. SODIS method. Dübendorf, Switzerland: Swiss Federal Institute of Aquatic Science and Technology; 2012. Available from: www.sodis.ch/index_EN.html.

Wilhelm N, Kaufmann A, Blanton E, Lantagne D. Sodium hypochlorite dosage for household and emergency water treatment: updated recommendations. J Water Health. 2018;16:112–25.

World Health Organization. Boil water technical brief 2015. Available from: www.who.int/publications/i/item/WHO-FWC-WSH-15.02.

World Health Organization. Guidelines for drinking-water quality, 4th edition; 2017. Available from: www.who.int/publications/i/item/9789241549950.

TRAVEL HEALTH KITS

Aisha Rizwan

Regardless of their destination, international travelers should assemble and carry a travel health kit. Travelers should tailor the contents to their specific needs, the type and length of travel, and their destination(s). Kits can be assembled at home or purchased at a local store, pharmacy, or online. Travel health kits can help to ensure travelers have supplies they need to manage preexisting medical conditions and treat any exacerbations of these conditions, prevent illness and injury related to traveling, and take care of minor health problems as they occur.

TRAVELING WITH MEDICATIONS

Instruct international travelers to carry all medications in their original containers with clear labels that easily identify the contents, the patient's name, and dosing regimen information. Although travelers might prefer packing their medications into small bags, pillboxes, or daily-dose containers, officials at ports of entry might require that medications be in their original prescription containers.

Travelers should carry copies of all prescriptions, including generic names, preferably translated into the local language of the destination. For controlled substances and injectable medications, travelers should carry a note on letterhead stationery from the prescribing clinician or travel clinic. Translating the letter into the local language at the destination and attaching the translation to the original document could prove helpful if the document is needed during the trip. Some countries do not permit certain medications. For questions about medication restrictions, particularly regarding controlled substances, travelers should contact the US embassy or consulate of the destination country (www.usembassy.gov).

A travel health kit is useful only when it is easily accessible. Travelers should always carry the kit with them (e.g., in a carry-on bag); sharp objects like scissors and fine splinter tweezers must remain in checked luggage, however. Travelers should make sure that any liquid or gel-based items packed in carry-on bags do not exceed size limits, although exceptions are made for certain medical reasons. For more information, call the Transportation Security Administration (TSA) at 866-289-9673 (toll-free, Monday–Friday, 8 a.m. to 11 p.m., and weekends and holidays 9 a.m. to 8 p.m.) or see the TSA Customer Service webpage (www.tsa.gov/contact/customer-service). The US embassy or consulate at the destination country can also provide details.

SUPPLIES FOR PREEXISTING MEDICAL CONDITIONS

Travelers with preexisting medical conditions should carry enough medication for the duration of their trip and an extra supply in case the trip extends for any reason. If additional supplies (e.g., glucose monitoring items) or medications are needed to manage exacerbations of existing medical conditions, these should be carried as well (see Sec. 3, Ch. 3, Travelers with Chronic Illnesses). People with preexisting conditions (e.g., allergies, diabetes), should consider wearing an alert bracelet. Needles and syringes can be difficult to purchase in some locations, so travelers should take more than needed for the length of the trip. In addition, travelers needing needles and syringes will also be required to carry a letter from the prescribing clinician on letterhead stationery.

GENERAL TRAVEL HEALTH KIT SUPPLIES

Boxes 2-06, 2-07, 2-08, 2-09, and 2-10 provide sample checklists of items travelers might consider including in their basic travel health kits. Provide travelers with needed details and instructions about any prescribed medications, including antibiotics for self-treatment of diarrhea, medications to treat altitude illness, and malaria chemoprophylaxis. Relevant chapters of this book offer additional suggestions for travel health kit contents depending on underlying health issues,

BOX 2-06 Sample travel health kit checklist for travelers: prescription medicines & medical supplies

- ☐ Antibiotics for self-treatment of moderate to severe travelers' diarrhea (if prescribed)
- ☐ Antihistamines, epinephrine auto-injectors (e.g., an EpiPen 2-Pak), short course of oral steroid medications (for travelers, including children, with a history of severe allergic reactions or anaphylaxis)
- ☐ Antimalarial medication (if prescribed)
- ☐ Insulin and diabetes testing supplies
- ☐ Medicine to prevent or treat altitude illness (if prescribed)
- ☐ Needles or syringes (plus extras) for injectable medicines
- ☐ Prescription glasses/contact lenses (consider packing an extra pair of each)
- ☐ Prescription medicines taken regularly at home
- ☐ Sleep aids (if prescribed)

Pack all prescription medicines (+ a copy of the prescription) and any necessary medical supplies in a carry-on bag. Medicines should be in their original containers with labels that clearly identify contents, patient name, and dosing information. Consider wearing a medical alert bracelet or necklace if you have chronic illnesses or underlying health conditions.

2

BOX 2-07 Sample travel health kit checklist for travelers: over-the-counter medications

- ☐ Over-the-counter medicines taken regularly at home
- ☐ Medicines for pain or fever, for example:
  - ○ Acetaminophen
  - ○ Aspirin
  - ○ Ibuprofen
- ☐ Medicines (not antibiotics) for stomach upset or diarrhea, for example:
  - ○ Antidiarrheal medication (e.g., loperamide [Imodium] or bismuth subsalicylate [Pepto-Bismol])
  - ○ Packets of oral rehydration salts for dehydration
  - ○ Mild laxatives
  - ○ Antacids
- ☐ Medicines for mild upper respiratory conditions, for example:
  - ○ Antihistamine
  - ○ Decongestant, alone or in combination with antihistamine
  - ○ Cough suppressant or expectorant
  - ○ Cough drops
- ☐ Medicines for motion sickness
- ☐ Sleep aids (non-prescription)
- ☐ Eye drops
- ☐ Nose drops or spray

BOX 2-08 Sample travel health kit checklist for travelers: basic first aid

- ☐ Adhesive bandages and tape, multiple sizes
- ☐ Antifungal and antibacterial spray or creams
- ☐ Anti-itch gel or cream for insect bites and stings
- ☐ Antiseptic wound cleanser
- ☐ Commercial suture kit (for travel to remote areas)
- ☐ Cotton swabs
- ☐ Digital thermometer
- ☐ Disposable latex-free gloves
- ☐ Elastic/compression bandage wrap for sprains and strains
- ☐ First aid quick reference card
- ☐ Gauze
- ☐ Hydrocortisone cream (1%)
- ☐ Moleskin or molefoam for blister prevention and treatment
- ☐ Safety pins
- ☐ Scissors (pack sharp metal objects in checked baggage; small, rounded tip bandage scissors might be available for purchase in certain stores or online)
- ☐ Triangular bandage to wrap injuries and to make an arm or shoulder sling
- ☐ Tweezers (pack sharp metal objects in checked baggage)

BOX 2-09 Sample travel health kit checklist for travelers: supplies to prevent illness & injury

- ☐ Antibacterial hand wipes or an alcohol-based hand sanitizer containing ≥60% alcohol
- ☐ Ear plugs
- ☐ Face masks
- ☐ Insect repellents for skin and clothing
- ☐ Latex condoms
- ☐ Mosquito net (for protection against insect bites while sleeping; can be pretreated with insect repellent)
- ☐ Personal safety equipment (for example, child safety seats, bicycle or motorcycle helmets)
- ☐ Sun protection (for example, protective clothing, sunglasses, sunscreen)
- ☐ Water purification method(s) if visiting remote areas, camping, or staying in areas where access to clean water is limited

BOX 2-10 Sample travel health kit checklist for travelers: documents

- ☐ Contact information card (carry at all times) that includes the street addresses, telephone numbers, and email addresses of:
  - Family member or close contact remaining in the United States
  - Health care provider(s) at home
  - Hospitals or clinics (including emergency services) at your destination(s)
  - Insurance policy information
  - Lodging at the destination(s)
  - US embassy or consulate address and telephone number in your destination country or countries
- ☐ Copies of all prescriptions for medications, eyeglasses/contacts, and other medical supplies, including generic names; preferably translated into the local language of the destination
- ☐ Documentation of preexisting conditions (for example, diabetes or allergies) in English and preferably translated into the local language of the destination
- ☐ Electrocardiogram (EKG) if you have existing heart disease, including any known abnormal heart rhythms (arrhythmias)
- ☐ Health insurance, supplemental travel health insurance, medical evacuation insurance, and travel insurance policy numbers, carrier contact information, and copies of claim forms
- ☐ International Certificate of Vaccination or Prophylaxis (ICVP) card showing proof of vaccination, or an appropriate medical waiver, for travel to destinations where vaccinations are required by the country for entry

In addition to bringing the medical documents on this list, be sure to leave copies with a family member or close contact who will remain in the United States (in case of an emergency). Consider having electronic copies of documents, as well.

itinerary, and planned activities or intended reasons for travel.

TRAVEL KITS WHEN TRAVELING WITH CHILDREN

Box 2-11 provides a checklist of items travelers might consider bringing if they are traveling with children.

COMMERCIAL MEDICAL KITS

Travelers can obtain commercial medical kits for a wide range of circumstances, from basic first aid to advanced emergency life support. Companies also manufacture advanced medical kits for adventure travelers, customizing them based on specific travel needs. In addition, specialty kits are available for travelers managing diabetes, dealing with dental emergencies, and participating in aquatic activities. Many pharmacy, grocery, retail, and outdoor sporting goods stores, as well as online retailers, sell their own basic first aid kits. Travelers who choose to purchase a preassembled kit should review the contents of the kit carefully to ensure that it has everything needed; any necessary additional items should be added.

BOX 2-11 Sample travel health kit checklist for travelers: supplies for children

- ☐ Baby wipes
- ☐ Change mat
- ☐ Children's medicine for pain or fever
- ☐ Diapers
- ☐ Insect repellent (avoid using products containing oil of lemon eucalyptus [OLE] or para-menthane-3,8-diol [PMD] on children <3 years old)
- ☐ Medicines taken regularly at home
- ☐ Motor vehicle restraints (for example, stroller, seatbelts, or car seat)
- ☐ Rash cream
- ☐ Sterilizing equipment for baby bottles
- ☐ Sun protection
- ☐ Thermometer

BIBLIOGRAPHY

Goodyer L and Gibbs J. Travel medical kits. In: Keystone JS, Kozarsky PE, Connor BA, Nothdurft HD, Mendelson M, Leder K, editors. Travel medicine, 4th edition. Philadelphia: Saunders Elsevier; 2019. pp. 61–4.

Harper LA, Bettinger J, Dismukes R, Kozarsky PE. Evaluation of the Coca-Cola company travel health kit. J Travel Med. 2002;9(5):244–6.

2

LAST-MINUTE TRAVELERS

Gail Rosselot

It is never too late for a pretravel consultation. Although travelers are encouraged to access pretravel care ≥1 month before departure, clinicians can provide services within days or even hours of departure. As defined by the World Health Organization, the last-minute traveler (LMT) is anyone departing for an international destination on short notice, typically ≤2 weeks. Some reports suggest LMTs comprise up to 16% of a clinic population and include business travelers, relief workers, students, travelers visiting friends and relatives, travelers who planned a trip for some time but delayed seeking pretravel care, or travelers unsuccessful at obtaining an earlier appointment. Regardless of the reason or time constraints, clinicians should offer all travelers support for their upcoming trips.

PRETRAVEL VISIT PRIORITIES

Delivering pretravel services to LMTs can be challenging. Typically, LMTs only have time for a single encounter. During the last-minute pretravel consultation, consider what risk-reduction strategies might be necessary to address the following.

Clinic availability. For last-minute appointments, telemedicine services might be an option (for more details, see Sec. 2, Ch. 16, Telemedicine).

Time until departure. Weeks? Days? Hours?

Itinerary vaccinations. What is current vaccine availability? How long before post-vaccination immunity is achieved (e.g., ≥10 days after receiving yellow fever [YF] vaccine)? What are the destination's vaccine requirements (e.g., YF or meningococcal)? What is the recommendation for vaccines requiring multiple doses?

Traveler's health status and immunizations. Does the traveler have any preexisting health problems? Do they need booster vaccinations or to complete an unfinished vaccination series?

Resources at destination. What items does the traveler need to carry with them (e.g., adequate medication supply, travel kit items, illness self-treatment options)?

Coronavirus disease 2019. What are the destination requirements for coronavirus disease 2019 (COVID-19) testing or vaccination documentation?

Vaccinations

Consider each traveler's itinerary, trip activities, risk for infection at the destination, and cumulative risk associated with repeat travel. Educate travelers about the value and safety of vaccinations; emphasize preventive behaviors for travelers who might not be adequately protected if they are vaccinated immediately before travel or who do not have sufficient time to complete a vaccine series.

ROUTINE VACCINES

Most travelers who attended school in the United States received routine vaccinations as children. For travelers who are not up to date on vaccinations, provide first or additional vaccine doses, including influenza vaccine, according to Advisory Committee on Immunization Practices (ACIP) schedules, and arrange for return visits as needed.

RECOMMENDED VACCINES: SINGLE-DOSE PROTECTION

Even with limited time before departure, research supports the use of certain single-dose vaccines, if indicated, to initiate protection in LMTs. These include cholera for selected travelers, hepatitis A (monovalent), meningococcal (quadrivalent, ACWY), polio booster (inactivated), and typhoid (injectable) vaccines. Chapters on the respective diseases in Section 5 provide indications and dosing.

RECOMMENDED VACCINES: MULTIPLE DOSES NEEDED

LMTs often cannot complete the schedule of vaccines requiring multiple doses to induce full protection. Carefully evaluate the need for these vaccines, factoring in destination, incidence, and disease severity. If a traveler needs protection against hepatitis B, Japanese encephalitis (JE), or rabies, consider alternative approaches, including use of an approved, accelerated schedule or, depending on expected duration of stay and level of risk, identifying vaccination resources for the traveler at the destination. Travelers should be aware that vaccines received in some countries might be of substandard quality (see Sec. 6, Ch. 3, . . . *perspectives*: Avoiding Poorly Regulated Medicines & Medical Products During Travel). Because travelers' level of protection will be unclear if they do not complete a full series of multidose vaccination, provide preventive behavior counseling.

HEPATITIS B

A shortened schedule of 2 doses (at 0 and 28 days) of Heplisav-B vaccine is approved for adults ≥18 years of age. For LMTs with imminent exposure (e.g., disaster relief workers), clinicians can use an accelerated vaccination schedule with Twinrix, the combination hepatitis A and hepatitis B vaccine at 0, 7, and 21–30 days, plus a 12-month booster. Arrange a follow-up visit(s) for short-term travelers to complete the series, and help extended-stay travelers identify resources at their destination to complete the schedule.

JAPANESE ENCEPHALITIS

In the United States, the JE vaccine, IXIARO, has been approved for use with an accelerated schedule (0, 7 days). For at-risk LMTs who cannot complete the full primary vaccine series ≥1 week before travel, counsel them to strictly adhere to insect precautions. Alternatively, help travelers identify reliable sources for IXIARO vaccination at their destination, or with internationally (but not domestically) available, single-dose JE vaccines, (e.g., Imojev [Sanofi Pasteur] or live attenuated SA 14-14-2 JE vaccine [Chengdu Institute of Biological Products]).

RABIES

In the United States, rabies preexposure vaccination previously consisted of a series of 3 intramuscular injections of a rabies vaccine given on days 0, 7, and 21 or 28. The ACIP recently revised its recommendations for rabies preexposure vaccination and approved a 2-dose preexposure regimen given on days 0 and 7. This revised schedule has the advantage of being both less expensive and easier to complete prior to travel. There is, however, an absence of data on how long this 2-dose series provides protection against rabies virus exposure. As a result, travelers with a sustained risk for rabies exposure should either have a titer drawn or receive a third dose of vaccine within 3 years of the initial series.

For travelers who started, but did not complete, a rabies preexposure vaccination series and had a potential rabies exposure, provide the same postexposure prophylaxis as for a completely unimmunized person. Regardless of whether travelers are vaccinated or not, emphasize animal avoidance (see Sec. 4, Ch. 7, Zoonotic Exposures: Bites, Stings, Scratches & Other Hazards, Sec 5, Part 2, Ch. 18, Rabies, and Sec 5, Part 2, Ch. 19, . . . *perspectives*: Rabies Immunization). Encourage travelers to purchase insurance for evacuation or urgent postexposure treatment (see Sec. 6, Ch. 1, Travel Insurance, Travel Health Insurance & Medical Evacuation Insurance). As warranted, offer longer-stay travelers the option to receive the rabies vaccine series at their destination.

2

REQUIRED VACCINES

CORONAVIRUS DISEASE 2019

The Centers for Disease Control and Prevention (CDC) advises all eligible international travelers to be up to date with their COVID-19 vaccinations (primary series and booster[s]) before travel; see www.cdc.gov/coronavirus/2019-ncov/vaccines/stay-up-to-date.html. Travelers should also check to confirm the latest COVID-19 entry requirements at their destination.

MENINGOCOCCAL

Quadrivalent (ACWY) meningococcal vaccine is required for adults and children >2 years of age traveling to Saudi Arabia for religious pilgrimage. Hajj visas cannot be issued without proof that applicants received meningococcal conjugate vaccine ≥10 days and ≤5 years before arriving in Saudi Arabia.

YELLOW FEVER

Travelers who receive YF vaccine <10 days before entering a risk area are at risk of infection with YF virus. Documentation of vaccination against YF becomes valid 10 days after administration. When proof of vaccination against YF is required by a country on the traveler's itinerary, and the LMT is planning to arrive before 10 days have elapsed, clinicians can suggest the traveler rearrange the order of travel or reschedule the trip. Otherwise, the traveler risks being denied entry, quarantined, or revaccinated at the border. In travelers for whom YF vaccine is contraindicated, YF vaccine Uniform Stamp Owners (clinicians designated by their state or territorial health department to administer YF vaccine) can issue a medical waiver letter in lieu of vaccination. See Sec. 5, Part 2, Ch. 26, Yellow Fever, for more details.

Malaria & Other Mosquito-Borne Illnesses

Clinicians must factor in time until departure and local pharmacy supply when considering malaria chemoprophylaxis choices for LMTs, in addition to the usual considerations of cost, drug resistance at destination, itinerary, medical contraindications, and patient preference. For travelers departing in ≤2 weeks, options for malaria chemoprophylaxis include atovaquone-proguanil or doxycycline in addition to education about mosquito avoidance and follow-up for fever. Consider primaquine or tafenoquine only if time allows for glucose-6-phosphate-dehydrogenase (G6PD) screening; do not prescribe either of these drugs without first knowing the traveler's G6PD status (see Sec. 5, Part 3, Ch. 16, Malaria). Educating travelers about insect avoidance can help them to avoid Zika, dengue, and chikungunya infections at their destination and help to prevent local disease transmission (see Sec. 4, Ch. 6, Mosquitoes, Ticks & Other Arthropods).

Risk-Management Health Counseling

Pretravel counseling is critical for LMTs. Determine travelers' knowledge and experience in managing travel health risks, and focus on major risks of the trip and special issues for LMTs (see Box 2-12). LMTs benefit most when provided with simple, prioritized messages about prevention and self-care.

SPECIAL CHALLENGES

Travelers Leaving in Less Than 48 Hours

If travel is imminent, clinicians can still provide telehealth or secure digital messaging for prevention counseling and recommendations for services at the destination. During the consultation, emphasize and reassure the LMT that many travel health risks can be prevented by adhering to healthy behaviors.

Travelers with Preexisting Medical Conditions

LMTs with preexisting conditions might be at increased risk for acute episodes of comorbid conditions (see Sec. 3, Ch. 3, Travelers with Chronic Illnesses). These travelers should carry a portable medical record, know reliable sources for medical care at their destination, and purchase travel health insurance, trip insurance, and medical evacuation insurance. In addition, encourage these travelers to schedule a pretravel appointment or conversation with their treating clinician. Some conditions (e.g., immunosuppression, pregnancy), often require additional discussion or advanced planning and could warrant delaying departure (see Sec. 3, Ch. 1, Immunocompromised Travelers, and Sec. 7, Ch. 1, Pregnant Travelers).

BOX 2-12 Last-minute travelers (LMTs): supplemental counseling topics

GENERAL PREVENTION MESSAGES

For general prevention messages, see Sec. 2, Ch. 1, The Pretravel Consultation.

REASSURANCE

Address concerns that "last-minute" consultation visits are "too late."

Assure travelers that vaccinations, regardless of when they are given, have value, and protective immunity continues to develop.

Although high-risk exposures are possible on arrival to the destination, educate travelers about cumulative risk associated with repeat travel.

ONLINE RESOURCES

Inform travelers where online they can find information on destination medical services:

- US Department of State (www.travel.state.gov)
- International Society of Travel Medicine clinic directory (www.istm.org)

Provide resources for health information for international travel:

- CDC Travelers' Health (https://wwwnc.cdc.gov/travel)
- Heading Home Healthy (www.headinghomehealthy.org)
- Pre-Travel Providers' Rapid Evaluation Portal (www.gten.travel/prep/prep)

Encourage LMTs to obtain travel health and medical evacuation insurance.

TRAVEL HEALTH KITS

Educate LMTs that drugs and health kit products purchased abroad might be counterfeit or substandard.

Encourage LMTs to purchase and pack medications for travelers' diarrhea or altitude illness, over-the-counter drugs, first aid supplies, insect repellent, sunscreen, condoms, and thermometers before leaving the United States (see Sec. 2, Ch. 10, Travel Health Kits).

Inform travelers to check 24-hour pharmacies, airport clinics, and online companies offering overnight or expedited shipping to obtain needed kits or supplies.

POSTTRAVEL APPOINTMENT

Have the LMT return to the clinic after travel to complete any unfinished vaccine series.

Initiate preparation in advance of the next spur-of-the-moment travel.

Extended-Stay Travelers

A last-minute consultation will not provide adequate time for a full medical and psychological evaluation or additional education for an expatriate. Advise extended-stay travelers to arrange an early consultation with a qualified clinician at their destination.

Traveler Requests: Carrying Vaccines or Off-Label Dosing

Because of time constraints, some LMTs might ask to carry a vaccine abroad or for a vaccine to be administered off-label (e.g., different schedule, double dosing). Due to cold chain concerns, it is rarely advisable to provide travelers with a supplied vaccine. Clinicians who administer a vaccine in a nonstandard manner can face medical-legal issues and induce a false sense of protection in the traveler.

Recurring Last-Minute Travelers

Clinics that frequently see LMTs might want to address this as an administrative issue. The clinical practice could build flexibility into the schedule and proactively identify groups likely to travel last minute (e.g., college students, corporate employees, relief workers). For these travelers, the clinic might consider routine pretravel visits or preemptive vaccinations for certain itineraries.

BIBLIOGRAPHY

Centers for Disease Control and Prevention. Epidemiology and prevention of vaccine-preventable diseases, 13th edition. Hamborsky J, Kroger A, Wolfe S, editors. Washington DC: Public Health Foundation; 2015.

Chen LH, Leder K, Wilson ME. Business travelers: vaccination considerations for this population. Expert Rev Vaccines. 2013;12(4):453–66.

Cramer JP, Jelninek T, Paulke-Korinek M, Reisinger EC, Dieckmann S, Alberer M, et al. One-year immunogenicity kinetics and safety of a purified chick embryo cell rabies vaccine and inactivated Vero cell-derived Japanese encephalitis vaccine administered concomitantly according to a new, 1-week, accelerated primary series. J Trav Med. 2016;23(3):1–8.

Flaherty GT, Hasnol MH, Sulaiman LH. Better late than never—an analysis of last-minute travelers attending a specialist travel medicine clinic in Ireland. Int J Trav Med Glob Health. 2019;7(4):123–28.

Sanford CA, d Jong EC. Immunizations. Med Clin N Am. 2016;100:247–59.

Soentjens P. Improved information tools and measures are needed for the last-minute traveller. J Trav Med. 2020;27(2):taz097.

Wong C, Scotland L. The last minute traveller. In: Shaw M, Wong C, editors. The practical compendium of immunisations for international travel. Auckland (NZ): Adis; 2015. pp. 117–23.

World Health Organization. International travel and health 2012. Available from: www.who.int/publications/i/item/9789241580472.

Yates JA, Rao SR, Walker AT, Esposito DH, Sotir M, LaRocque RC, et al.; Global TravEpiNet Consortium. Characteristics and preparation of the last-minute traveler: analysis of vaccine usage in the Global TravEpiNet Consortium. J Trav Med. 2019;26(6):taz031.

Zuckerman JN, Van Damme P, Van Herck K, Loscher T. Vaccination options for last-minute travellers in need of travel-related prophylaxis against hepatitis A and B and typhoid fever: a practical guide. Trav Med Infect Dis. 2003;1(4):219–26.

2

MENTAL HEALTH

Thomas Valk

International travel is stressful. Stressors vary to some extent with the type of travel: short-term tourist travel likely creates the least stress, whereas frequent travel, humanitarian and disaster work, and expatriation cause the most. The stressors of travel can cause preexisting psychiatric disorders to recur, latent or undiagnosed problems to become apparent, and new problems to arise. In addition, jet lag, fatigue, travel during a pandemic, and work or family pressures can trigger anxiety and aggravate depressive symptoms in short-term travelers.

OCCURRENCE OF MENTAL HEALTH PROBLEMS IN TRAVELERS

Data on the rate at which mental health problems occur in travelers are non-existent. Few data from clinical populations include a study of British diplomats, in which 11% of medical evacuations were nonphysical, or psychological in nature. In this study, among people evacuated for psychological reasons, 71% were in their 20s; the overall incidence for psychological evacuations was 0.3%, 41% of which were for depression. In a study of the US Foreign Service from 1982 through 1986, the incidence of psychiatric evacuations was 0.2%. Of these, 50% were for substance use or affective disorder, and evacuations for mania and hypomanic states accounted for 3%.

A study of psychiatric emergencies in travelers to Hawaii estimated a rate of 0.2% for tourists and 2% for transient travelers (those arriving in Hawaii with no immediate plans to leave) versus 1% for residents. The study listed diagnoses in this population, in order of decreasing frequency, as schizophrenia, alcohol abuse, anxiety reaction, and depression. Finally, researchers in a landscape analysis of travel-related psychosis generated a rough calculation of incidence rate for psychiatric hospitalization of tourists to a destination of high religious significance (Jerusalem) and noted 19.7 cases per 100,000; ≥3.5% of these were psychotic episodes without prior psychiatric history.

THE PRETRAVEL CONSULTATION & MENTAL HEALTH EVALUATION

Travel health providers should include mental health screening in any pretravel consultation. Some groups especially warrant mental health screening, including people planning extended or frequent travel; participants in humanitarian or disaster relief work; and anyone intending to take up long-term or semipermanent residence in another country. Because travel medicine specialists rarely have mental health credentials, they should use a brief inquiry aimed at eliciting previously diagnosed psychiatric disorders. To introduce this portion of the consultation and to elicit the most cooperation, practitioners can enumerate that international travel is stressful for everyone and has been associated with the emergence or reemergence of mental health problems; the availability of culturally compatible mental health services varies widely; and laws regarding the use of illicit substances can be severe in some countries.

Ask travelers about indicators of overt or underlying mental health problems. Some areas to cover include whether the traveler previously experienced, was treated for, or was diagnosed with a psychiatric disorder, including any associated with prior travel, and the type of treatment (inpatient, outpatient, or medications) involved, if any. Also inquire about current psychiatric disorders and treatment and whether any members of their immediate family have serious mental health problems. In addition, ask travelers about current or past use of illicit substances and whether they have a formally diagnosed substance use disorder or if health care providers, friends, or family have suggested that the traveler might be using alcohol or other substances to excess.

In general, any history of inpatient treatment, psychotic episodes, violent or suicidal behavior, affective disorder (including mania, hypomania, or major depression), any treatment for substance use problems, and any current treatments warrant further evaluation by a mental health professional, preferably one experienced in handling problems related to international travel. On occasion, a patient's mental status during the pretravel consultation will be notably abnormal, which also should prompt a referral to a mental health professional for further evaluation.

CHALLENGES & BARRIERS TO HEALTHY TRAVEL

People with mental health issues might face several challenges and barriers to healthy travel. Be prepared to discuss and help the traveler manage the many of the following situations.

Contraindicated Medications

Mefloquine can cause neuropsychiatric side effects. Avoid prescribing mefloquine for malaria prophylaxis to patients with mental health issues. Please see the discussion of mefloquine in Sec. 5, Part 3, Ch. 16, Malaria.

Laboratory Monitoring of Medication Levels

For travelers who need routine laboratory testing to measure levels of lithium or other mood-stabilizing medications, clinicians should make them aware that they could face challenges in locating in-country laboratory facilities capable of this testing. Inform travelers that medication levels might fluctuate, particularly in environments with high ambient temperatures, because increased perspiration can lead to lithium toxicity, even on a consistent dose.

Medical Evacuation Insurance

Encourage travelers with mental health issues to consider purchasing international travel health and medical evacuation insurance policies that include coverage for psychiatric emergencies. Caution the traveler that many medical evacuation policies exclude psychiatric emergencies or evacuation for preexisting conditions. See Sec. 6, Ch. 1, Travel Insurance, Travel Health Insurance & Medical Evacuation Insurance, for details.

Mental Health Treatment

Long-term travelers or expatriates might have difficulty finding culturally compatible mental health treatment in the destination country. Counsel these travelers to seek assistance from a mental health professional with overseas experience.

Refilling Prescriptions

Long-term travelers and expatriates might have difficulty obtaining refills of psychotropic medications while living overseas because availability, or even legality, of these drugs varies from country to country. Travelers should check with the country's embassy or with a reputable in-country pharmacy or health care provider. As permitted by local laws, long-term travelers can have visiting friends or relatives, or other members of their company or organization, bring additional medication.

Support Groups

Currently sober travelers with substance use disorders might want to attend Alcoholics Anonymous (AA), Narcotics Anonymous (NA), or comparable meetings while overseas. AA and NA websites provide lists of meetings by country (see Sec. 3, Ch. 5, Substance Use & Substance Use Disorders, for more details). Travelers should confirm availability and language of meetings in advance.

Traveling with Psychotropic Medications

Customs regulations in some countries prohibit importation of medications used to treat mental health disorders. Customs officials might confiscate Schedule II drugs (www.dea.gov/drug-information/drug-scheduling) commonly used to treat attention deficit disorder (e.g., narcotics or stimulants, including amphetamines and methylphenidate). Rules vary by country, and travelers should check with the host country's embassy before traveling. Health care providers, including pharmacists, in the destination country might be able to provide guidance to colleagues about medication restrictions.

Advise travelers to carry medications in their original containers, along with a letter from the prescribing physician indicating the medical reason for the prescription. Remind them that customs officials might seize their medication even if they adhere to these guidelines.

STRESSORS & COUNTERMEASURES

Culture Shock

Nearly anyone visiting a foreign culture can experience culture shock. With culture shock, travelers lose their sense of mastery over their environment, and even routine tasks of everyday life become a challenge. Separation from family and support systems, unfamiliar behavior and language, and new threats to health and safety can aggravate culture shock. Foreknowledge of the phenomenon will help minimize the stress experienced, as will advance study of the culture, language, and health and security threats and possible countermeasures.

For most travelers, culture shock is a limited syndrome that does not usually go beyond variations in mood, energy, sleep, and attitudes toward the host country culture, like an adjustment disorder. Advise travelers that symptoms lasting >12 months could require assessment. In addition, suggest regular exercise, moderation in intoxicant use, adequate sleep and nutrition, and relaxation techniques (e.g., meditation, yoga, biofeedback) to help reduce the stress associated with international travel.

Jet Lag

Jet lag is a common, manageable stressor for most international travelers. Travelers and travel health providers can find more details about this condition and what to do about it in Sec. 8, Ch. 4, Jet Lag.

Travel During a Pandemic

The coronavirus disease 2019 (COVID-19) pandemic has exacerbated travel-associated stress and concerns over becoming a possible conduit for disease transmission. Any steps travelers can take (see Box 2-13) to gain some measure of control over their personal health and to mitigate COVID-19–related risk factors might help assuage some of this stress. Recommended information resources for travelers include the Centers for Disease Control and Prevention website (www.cdc.gov/coronavirus/2019-ncov/travelers/); the US Department of State website (https://travel.state.gov/content/travel/en/traveladvisories/COVID-19-Country-Specific-Information.html); and/or the embassy or ministry of health website for the traveler's destination.

Advise travelers to review a variety of travel health insurance options and to consider purchasing policies that cover cancellations of travel and that provide for emergency medical care and medical evacuations due to COVID-19. Remind travelers that their travel experience could differ from what they had planned or expected; to have

BOX 2-13 Addressing potential stressors associated with travel during the coronavirus disease 2019 (COVID-19) pandemic: a checklist for travelers

- ☐ Be up to date with your COVID-19 vaccinations (including all recommended boosters) at least 2 weeks before travel.
- ☐ Do your research. Be prepared to comply with all requirements (e.g., pretravel vaccination and testing, post-arrival quarantine and providing contact information) for your international travel destination and for the United States; be aware that requirements can change between when you book your travel and when travel takes place.
- ☐ Get tested for COVID-19 before departure if required by your destination or recommended by current guidance.
- ☐ Obtain accepted formats for demonstrating proof of vaccination and negative test results; be prepared to provide before departure or on arrival.
- ☐ Identify (before travel, if possible) COVID-19 testing locations at your destination.
- ☐ Have contingency plans (e.g., alternative housing arrangements, reserve budget) in case of travel delays, cancellations, or itinerary modifications.
- ☐ Use personal protective measures (e.g., mask wearing) throughout your journey, including at places of congregation (e.g., airports, bus stations, train stations), on various modes of transportation (e.g., airplanes, buses, ships, trains), and at your destination.

contingency plans in place in case of travel delays or interruptions; and to avoid crowded places, particularly in destinations where vaccine coverage is low or case rates and hospitalizations due to COVID-19 are high. For travelers with a low level of risk tolerance, those whose underlying health conditions place them at greater risk for severe COVID-19, or those who are considering travel with young, vaccine-ineligible children, it also might be appropriate to discuss and counsel delaying travel until some future date.

POSTTRAVEL MENTAL HEALTH ISSUES

Travelers who witness or who are directly involved in traumatic or life-threatening events can experience acute stress disorder (ASD) or posttraumatic stress disorder (PTSD). Examples of such events include motor vehicle accidents, assault or rape, terrorist incidents, natural disasters, or war. The work performed by humanitarian aid workers, disaster relief workers, and war correspondents increases their risk of developing subclinical or overt ASD or PTSD. For travelers who have had traumatic experiences, clinicians should inquire about recurrent, intrusive recollections, distressing dreams, and feeling as if the event is happening repeatedly; avoiding thoughts, feelings, activities, places, or people that lead to memories of the event; diminished interest in activities, inability to experience positive emotions, or an inability to remember significant details of the event; and difficulty sleeping or concentrating, irritability, or an exaggerated startle response.

Symptoms of PTSD can occur months or even years after an event. Thus, clinicians should educate returning travelers about the possibility of having such symptoms in the future. If there is concern about a traveler's possible reaction to a traumatic event, refer them to a mental health professional.

People who have lived away from their home culture for extended periods of time (e.g., expatriate employees and their families) can experience reverse culture shock, which includes symptoms and a clinical course like that of culture shock. For example, first-year college students who spent their high school years abroad might find their "home" culture strange, compared with their fellow students who could be uninterested in their overseas experiences. Adults returning from abroad can experience a decreased standard of living or can find their "home" culture changed in unanticipated ways.

BIBLIOGRAPHY

Airault R, Valk TH. Travel-related psychosis (TrP): a landscape analysis. J Travel Med. 2018;25(1):1–7.

American Psychiatric Association. Diagnostic and statistical manual of mental disorders, 5th edition. DSM-5. Arlington, VA: American Psychiatric Association; 2013.

Benedek DM, Wynn GH. Clinical manual for management of PTSD. Arlington, VA: American Psychiatric Publishing; 2011.

Bonny-Noach H, Sagiv-Alayoff M. Rescuing Israeli travellers: effects of substance abuse, mental health, geographic region of rescue, gender and age of rescuees. J Travel Med. 2017;24(5):tax045.

Feinstein A, Owen J, Blair N. A hazardous profession: war, journalists, and psychopathology. Am J Psychiatry. 2002;159(9):1570–5.

Felkai P, Kurimay T. Patients with mental problems—the most defenseless travellers. J Travel Med. 2017;24(5):tax005.

Liese B, Mundt KA, Dell LD, Nagy L, Demure B. Medical insurance claims associated with international business travel. Occup Environ Med. 1997;54(7):499–503.

Patel D, Easmon CJ, Dow C, Snashall DC, Seed PT. Medical repatriation of British diplomats resident overseas. J Travel Med. 2000;7(2):64–9.

Streltzer J. Psychiatric emergencies in travelers to Hawaii. Compr Psychiatry. 1979;20(5):463–8.

Valk, TH. Mental health issues of travelers. In Keystone J, Kozarsky P, Connor, B, Nothdurft H, Mendelson M, Leder K, editors. Travel medicine, 4th edition. London: Elsevier; 2018. pp. 463–8.

LGBTQ+ TRAVELERS

Patricia Walker

Lesbian, gay, bisexual, transgender, queer (LGBTQ+) travelers share many of the same hopes and desires as other people when traveling: to have a safe, happy, and memorable trip. LGBTQ+ travelers have similar risk-taking behaviors as other travelers, which are influenced more by age, gender, socioeconomic status, mental health considerations, and substance use, rather than sexual attraction or identity. LGBTQ+ travelers face some unique risks, however, and clinicians counseling them should tailor their advice accordingly.

OVERVIEW

LGBTQ+ travelers contribute greatly to economic development and can convey powerful positive messages related to human rights worldwide. The United Nations World Trade Organization Second Global Report on LGBTQ+ Tourism in 2017 acknowledged that LGBTQ+ persons travel more frequently, demonstrate higher than average spending patterns, and demonstrate brand awareness and loyalty. LGBTQ+ travelers have long been aware of gay-friendly destinations in the United States, including Provincetown, Massachusetts, and Fire Island, New York; and in Europe, including Mykonos, Greece, and Sitges, Spain. Human rights have improved in some countries, and the international tourism industry has become more responsive to LGBTQ+ travelers; many international travel destinations are now recognized as gay friendly.

Open for Business is a coalition of leading global companies dedicated to LGBTQ+ inclusion, and recognizes the powerful advantages of inclusive, diverse societies that improve economic, business, and individual performance. The travel industry has long recognized that marketing to the LGBTQ+ community makes economic sense; the International Gay and Lesbian Travel Association was founded in 1983, and provides free travel resources and information, while working to promote quality and safety for LGBTQ+ travelers worldwide.

LGBTQ+ travelers are as diverse as other travelers in terms of how, where, and with whom they prefer to travel; risk-taking behavior; gender expression; skin color; citizenship; and income. In a 2015 study conducted by Global Marketing, behavior of gay men travelers differed from lesbian travelers in several ways: gay men were more likely to travel with other adults, visit gay bars, and have more disposable time and income; lesbian travelers were more likely to travel with family, be more interested in child-friendly rather than LGBTQ+ friendly environments, and have travel preferences and budget constraints more closely aligned to people who are not LGTBQ+ than to gay men. People who are transgender might be more likely to travel for medical reasons, seeking high-quality and affirmational medical and surgical care.

Technology also has changed how LGBTQ+ travelers interact with others while traveling. In one study, 31% of gay men use dating apps while traveling, compared with 4% of lesbian travelers and 15% of all Americans. Men who used the internet to set up dates prior to travel reported far more sexual partners and were much more likely to report having sex with a new partner.

There is no single standard message for counseling the LGBTQ+ traveler (see Box 2-14). During the pretravel consultation with LGBTQ+ travelers, include routine travel advice and specific counseling tailored to the itinerary and planned activities (see Sec. 2, Ch. 1, The Pretravel Consultation). Focused counseling for the LGBTQ+ traveler should include, at a minimum, a discussion of infectious disease risks, legal considerations, safety and security issues, and screening and counseling for potential mental health problems and substance use disorders.

INFECTIOUS DISEASE COUNSELING

A paucity of research data on LGBTQ+ travelers has been published; a 2021 English language, no date filter, PubMed search found only 41 articles, 30 of which focused on men who have sex with men (MSM) and 2 of which were case reports concerning transgender travelers (1 on genital dermatitis, the other on deep venous thrombosis). Studies have been reported on MSM from Australia, Belgium, Canada, China, Denmark, India, Sweden, Vietnam and those going to Mardi Gras in New Orleans or Key West, Florida, but no studies specific to lesbian travelers have been published.

A 2019 review article on MSM who travel provides advice for clinicians counseling this specific patient population. Studies on MSM behavior while traveling show mixed results—some engage in more high-risk sexual behavior during travel, and some less. A greater risk for acquisition of sexually transmitted infections (STIs) has been shown in MSM who travel, use social apps or illicit drugs, engage in unprotected anal intercourse, join mass gatherings (including Gay Pride), and engage in circuit parties.

In a meta-analysis of foreign travel and sexual behavior, the pooled rate of casual sex was 19.5% for all women and 24.8% for all men. In the same analysis, the rate of unprotected intercourse among women who had casual travel sex was 62.1% and 62.3% among men.

The US Preventive Services Taskforce recommends behavioral counseling for all sexually active adolescents and for adults who are at increased

BOX 2-14 Counseling LGBTQ+ travelers: a checklist for clinicians

- ☐ Assess each patient's travel-related risk behaviors
- ☐ Ask direct questions regarding sexual identity and behavior
- ☐ Consider screening people at risk for hepatitis B virus, hepatitis C virus, and HIV infection per national guidelines
- ☐ Discuss diseases specific to sexual practices and use of gloves and dental dams
- ☐ Provide clear counseling and online resources (Table 2-13) regarding legal, cultural, and safety issues
- ☐ Provide direct advice on safer sex and sexually transmitted infection prevention, including consistent condom use and HIV preexposure and postexposure prophylaxis
- ☐ Provide nonjudgmental and detailed counseling specific to LGBTQ+ travelers' risks
- ☐ Update vaccines per schedules, including hepatitis A, hepatitis B, human papillomavirus, and others, as appropriate

risk for STIs. Provide nonjudgmental counseling to LGBTQ+ travelers. The Gay and Lesbian Medical Association has resources to assist clinicians counseling LGTBQ+ patients.

Counsel travelers that safe sex is proven to reduce the risk of receiving or transmitting chlamydia, gonorrhea, hepatitis A and B, HIV, human papillomavirus (HPV), pubic lice, and syphilis. Depending on a patient's sexual risk behavior, counsel them on the use of condoms, dental dams, and gloves to reduce risk for STIs. See Sec. 9, Ch. 12, Sex & Travel, for general counseling recommendations on sex and travel.

Enteric Infections

Patients who engage in oral–anal sex might be unaware of their risk for acquiring enteric infections, both bacterial (e.g., *Salmonella, Shigella*) and parasitic (e.g., *Blastocystis* spp., *Dientamoeba fragilis, Giardia*). Counsel patients on use of dental dams and careful washing of hands and genitalia, before and after sex. Offer typhoid vaccination per national guidelines (see Sec. 5, Part 1, Ch. 24, Typhoid & Paratyphoid Fever).

Hepatitis A

Hepatitis A virus (HAV) is transmitted via the fecal–oral route during person-to-person sexual contact and from contaminated food and water. Hepatitis A outbreaks have been reported among MSM. Counsel LGBTQ+ travelers on safer sex, including the use of dental dams, and recommend HAV vaccination.

Hepatitis B

Hepatitis B virus (HBV) is transmitted via percutaneous or mucus membrane exposure to body fluids infected with HBV. MSM have a higher seroprevalence of HBV; offer vaccination to this group irrespective of travel plans. Consider screening for HBV infection in high-risk, previously unvaccinated travelers, including MSM.

Hepatitis C

Hepatitis C virus is generally transmitted via parenteral routes but can be transmitted sexually. Hepatitis C outbreaks have been reported among MSM and have been associated with unprotected anal intercourse, genital ulcerative disease, and traumatic sexual practices (e.g., fisting [inserting a hand in the rectum]). Counsel patients on safer sex practices, including the use of condoms and gloves.

HIV

Assess sexual risk behavior and counsel travelers, including people at risk for sexual assault, on use of preexposure prophylaxis (PrEP) and postexposure prophylaxis (PEP). Remind patients that long-term travel, particularly for work, might require HIV testing. Countries might deny entry to people with evidence of HIV infection, and carrying PrEP might be mistaken as evidence of such. See Sec. 5, Part 2, Ch. 11, Human Immunodeficiency Virus / HIV, and Sec. 3, Ch. 1, Immunocompromised Travelers, for additional information.

Human Papillomavirus

Human papillomavirus (HPV) is highly prevalent among MSM. HPV infection is associated with penile, anal, and oropharyngeal cancers and precancers. Offer HPV vaccination per national guidelines.

Invasive Meningococcal Disease

Invasive meningococcal disease (IMD) is a risk for travelers going to the African meningitis belt and among Hajj pilgrims (see Sec. 5, Part 1, Ch. 13, Meningococcal Disease). Another, less well-known group at risk for IMD are MSM, who may have higher carriage rates for *Neisseria meningitidis*. Potential risk behaviors for IMD include regularly visiting crowded venues; traveling to mass gatherings (e.g., Gay Pride festivals); using illegal drugs; and having multiple sexual partners. Recommend vaccination for HIV-positive travelers. Some local public health authorities have also recommended routine vaccination against meningococcal disease for MSM.

LEGAL CONSIDERATIONS

LGBTQ+ travelers face unique legal issues and risks while traveling abroad. Many countries have made strides toward combating discrimination against LGBTQ+ persons, but many other countries continue to discriminate against and abuse LGBTQ+ persons. Over 70 countries still consider consensual same-sex sexual relations a crime that can carry severe punishment, including the death penalty. Many countries do not legally recognize same-sex marriage or allow or recognize LGBTQ+ adoptions. Attitudes, even within countries with legal protections, will vary among people and communities where LGBTQ+ persons travel.

The United Nations (UN) has been addressing human rights abuses of the LGBTQ+ community since the 1990s. In a 2015 speech, UN Deputy Commissioner for Human Rights Flavia Pansieri summarized the abuses of the LGBTQ+ community, including murder, rape, mob attacks, abuse by police and prison officials, criminal sanctions, arrest and imprisonment, blackmail and harassment, forced medications and surgeries in medical settings to try to change sexual orientation, forced sterilization of people who are transgender, humiliation, discrimination, job loss, evictions, and refusal of medical treatment. Such issues are a reality in many countries, and clinicians should offer LGBTQ+ travelers resources on differing international laws, attitudes, and customs, and emphasize the realities of behavior constraints that can make a trip safer (Table 2-13).

Travel health providers also should remind LGBTQ+ travelers that they are subject to the

Table 2-13 Online resources for LGBTQ+ travelers

ORGANIZATION	RESOURCE	AVAILABLE FROM
EQUALDEX	Explore the progress of LGBTQ+ rights across the world	www.equaldex.com
Gay and Lesbian Medical Association	Resources for patients	www.glma.org/index.cfm?fuseaction=Page.viewPage&pageId=938&parentID=534
International Gay and Lesbian Travel Association		www.iglta.org
ILGA World: International Lesbian, Gay, Bisexual, Trans and Intersex Association		https://ilga.org
National Alliance on Mental Illness	LGBTQI	www.nami.org/Your-Journey/Identity-and-Cultural-Dimensions/LGBTQI
National Center for Transgender Equality	Issues: Travel	https://transequality.org/issues/travel
The Trevor Project: Saving Young LGBTQ Lives		www.thetrevorproject.org
US Department of State	Country Reports on Human Rights Practices	www.state.gov/reports-bureau-of-democracy-human-rights-and-labor/country-reports-on-human-rights-practices/
	Country Information	https://travel.state.gov/content/travel/en/international-travel/International-Travel-Country-Information-Pages.html
	LGBTI Family Travel Tips	https://travel.state.gov/content/dam/NEWTravelAssets/pdfs/LGBTI%20Pocket%20Card-Pride%20Weekend_FINAL.pdf
	LGBTI Travelers	https://travel.state.gov/content/travel/en/international-travel/before-you-go/travelers-with-special-considerations/lgbti.html

laws of any country to which they are traveling, and encourage travelers to read about their destinations before departure. The US Department of State annually publishes Country Reports on Human Rights Practices, which includes a detailed, country-by-country report of issues pertinent to the LGBTQ+ community and offers the printable LGBTQ+ Family Travel Tips pocket card at their website (see Table 2-13 for the website address).

2

SAFETY & SECURITY

A general approach to travel safety and security is outlined in Sec. 4, Ch. 11, Safety & Security Overseas. As with many travelers, the joy of feeling more freedom to express oneself while traveling, coupled with substance use, could result in behaviors that put travelers at risk. Each traveler's perception of and willingness to accept risk also varies (see Sec. 2, Ch. 2, . . . *perspectives*: Travelers' Perception of Risk).

LGBTQ+ travelers should be aware that gay-friendly neighborhoods might not reflect societal acceptance and safety in a country overall. LGBTQ+ persons have a lifetime of experience assessing situations to determine whether they can safely be themselves. When traveling, LGBTQ+ persons should be aware of sociocultural differences that can affect their true situational safety. The US Department of State notes that authorities in some countries could be involved in entrapment campaigns, with law enforcement monitoring websites, mobile phone apps, or meeting places. Counsel patients to be cautious connecting with the local community. The US Department of State offers tips for the LGBTQ+ community for staying safe while abroad, including researching destinations, updating passports, packing important documents, living abroad with a foreign national spouse or partner, visa issues, and adoption issues.

Advise transgender travelers that the Transportation Security Administration (TSA) offers specific screening considerations for transgender passengers, including information on reporting prostheses or discrimination at screening checkpoints, at the TSA website, www.tsa.gov/transgender-passengers.

Although published data are lacking, media reports suggest that people who are openly lesbian, whether single or coupled, and people who are transgender might be at greater risk for physical and sexual assault worldwide. LGBTQ+ travelers should contact the nearest US embassy or consulate (www.usembassy.gov) if they have troubles while abroad; the Department of State website assures travelers that consular officers will protect their privacy and will not generalize, make assumptions, or pass judgment.

MENTAL HEALTH & SUBSTANCE USE

LGBTQ+ identity can be a source of strength and courage for many, but the lack of acceptance, overt discrimination, rejection, and denial of rights can lead to or exacerbate mental health issues among this population. Lesbian, gay, and bisexual adults are more than twice as likely as other adults to experience a mental health condition, and people who are transgender are >4 times more likely to experience a mental health condition than people who are cisgender (persons whose gender identity corresponds with their birth sex). Adolescents and young adults are at particularly high risk for suicide, and LGBTQ+ youth are more than twice as likely to experience persistent feelings of sadness and hopelessness than their peers who are not LGTBQ+. Transgender youth face further disparities and are twice as likely to experience depressive symptoms, seriously consider suicide, and attempt suicide compared with cisgender lesbian, gay, bisexual, queer, and questioning youth.

LGBTQ+ adults are twice as likely to experience a substance use disorder, and people who are transgender are 4 times as likely. Heavy drinking, binge drinking, tobacco use, and use of illicit drugs, including amyl nitrate (known as poppers), cannabis, MDMA (known as ecstasy or Molly), and amphetamines are more common in segments of the LGBTQ+ community. Several studies outline the association of recreational drug use with riskier sexual behavior during travel, including unprotected anal intercourse in MSM.

As outlined in Sec. 2, Ch. 12, Mental Health, travel medicine providers should screen for depression and anxiety in people planning extended or frequent travel; participants in humanitarian or disaster relief work; and anyone intending to take up long-term or semipermanent residence in another country. Little research and no published guidelines are available on LGBTQ+ travelers and mental health or substance abuse outcomes during and after travel, but the available data on prevalence of mental health issues and substance use suggest screening is appropriate for all LGBTQ+ travelers, including adolescents, for both mental health and substance use or abuse concerns.

2

BIBLIOGRAPHY

Aguero F, Masuet-Aumatell C, Morchon S, Ramon-Torrell JP. Men who have sex with men: a group of travelers with special needs. Travel Med Infect Dis. 2019;28:74–80.

Gay and Lesbian Medical Association. Guidelines for care of lesbian, gay, bisexual and transgender patients. San Francisco: GLMA; 2006. Available from: http://glma.org/_data/n_0001/resources/live/GLMA%20guidelines%202006%20FINAL.pdf.

Pansieri F. Keynote address by United Nations Deputy High Commissioner for Human Rights at the panel, Human Rights for All: Protection and promotion of the human rights of LGBTI individuals—From local communities to global organizations, November 20, 2015. Available from: www.ohchr.org/EN/NewsEvents/Pages/DisplayNews.aspx?NewsID=16798&LangID=E.

US Department of State. Country information. Available from: https://travel.state.gov/content/travel/en/international-travel/International-Travel-Country-Information-Pages.html.

US Department of State. Country reports on human rights practices. Available from: www.state.gov/reports-bureau-of-democracy-human-rights-and-labor/country-reports-on-human-rights-practices.

US Department of State. LGTBI family travel tips. Available from: https://travel.state.gov/content/dam/NEWTravelAssets/pdfs/LGBTI%20Pocket%20Card-Pride%20Weekend_FINAL.pdf.

Vivancos R, Abubakar I, Hunter PR. Foreign travel, casual sex, and sexually transmitted infections: systematic review and meta-analysis. Int J Infect Dis. 2010;14(10):e842–51.

COMPLEMENTARY & INTEGRATIVE HEALTH APPROACHES TO TRAVEL WELLNESS

David Shurtleff, Kathleen Meister, Shawn Stout

Travelers often ask their health care providers about the use of complementary or integrative health approaches for travel-related illnesses and conditions. Claims made about dietary supplements, herbal products (see Box 2-15), and other complementary approaches for travel-related health problems may not be supported by evidence. Be prepared to discuss what is known about the reported benefits of complementary and integrative health approaches and to counsel travelers on their possible side effects or interactions with prescribed vaccines or medications.

CLAIMS VERSUS SCIENCE

Altitude Illness

Many natural products, including coca leaf, garlic, *Ginkgo biloba*, and vitamin E, have been promoted for preventing or treating altitude illness. For more information on altitude illness, see Sec. 4, Ch. 5, High Elevation Travel & Altitude Illness.

COCA LEAF

Coca leaf, chewed or made into tea, has been used for altitude illness, but no strong evidence has shown that it works or that it has adverse effects.

BOX 2-15 Dietary supplements & unproven therapies

- Unproven therapies are discussed in this chapter only for educational purposes and are not recommended for use. The Centers for Disease Control and Prevention only endorses therapies approved by the US Food and Drug Administration (FDA).
- FDA regulates dietary supplements, but the regulations are generally less strict than those for prescription or over-the-counter drugs. Learn more at www.nccih.nih.gov/health/supplements/wiseuse.htm.
- Clinicians and travelers should consult the FDA's safety advisories to learn the latest regarding product recalls and safety alerts: www.fda.gov/food/recalls-outbreaks-emergencies/alerts-advisories-safety-information.
- Two major safety concerns about dietary supplements are potential drug interactions and product contamination. Analyses of supplements sometimes find differences between labeled and actual ingredients. For example, products marketed as dietary supplements have been found to contain illegal hidden ingredients, such as prescription drugs.

Travelers should be aware that using coca leaf will cause a positive drug test result for cocaine metabolites.

GARLIC

No evidence supports claims that garlic helps reduce altitude illness. Garlic supplements appear safe for most adults. Possible side effects include breath and body odor, heartburn, and upset stomach. Some people have allergic reactions to garlic. Short-term use of most commercially available garlic supplements poses only a limited risk for drug interactions.

GINKGO BILOBA

Studies of *Ginkgo biloba* for preventing altitude illness are inadequate to justify recommendations about its use. Products made from standardized ginkgo leaf extracts appear to be safe when used as directed. However, ginkgo can increase the risk of bleeding in some people and interact with anticoagulants. In addition, studies by the National Toxicology Program showed that rodents developed liver and thyroid tumors after being given a ginkgo extract for up to 2 years.

VITAMIN E

One study investigated vitamin E, in combination with other antioxidants, for altitude illness; no significant benefit was observed.

Colds & Flu

Although colds and flu are not uniquely travel-related hazards, many people try to avoid these illnesses during a trip. Complementary health approaches that have been advocated for preventing or treating colds or influenza include echinacea, garlic and other herbs, nasal saline irrigation, probiotics, vitamin C, zinc products, and others.

ECHINACEA

Numerous studies have tested the herb echinacea to see whether it can prevent colds or relieve cold symptoms. A 2014 systematic review concluded that echinacea has not been convincingly shown to be effective; however, a weak effect was not ruled out.

GARLIC & OTHER HERBS

No strong evidence supports claims that garlic, Chinese herbs, oil of oregano, or eucalyptus essential oil prevent or treat colds, or that the homeopathic product Oscillococcinum prevents or treats influenza or influenza-like illness.

NASAL SALINE IRRIGATION

Nasal saline irrigation (e.g., use of neti pots), can be useful and safe for chronic sinusitis. Nasal saline irrigation also can help relieve the symptoms of acute upper respiratory tract infections, but the evidence is not definitive. Even in places where tap water is safe to drink, people should use only sterile, distilled, boiled-then-cooled, or specially filtered water for nasal irrigation to avoid the risk of introducing waterborne pathogens.

PROBIOTICS

Probiotics might reduce susceptibility to colds or other upper respiratory tract infections and the duration of the illnesses, but the quality of the evidence is low or very low.

VITAMIN C

Taking vitamin C supplements regularly reduces the risk of catching a cold among people who perform intense physical exercise, but not in the general population. Taking vitamin C on a regular basis might lead to shorter-duration colds, but taking it only after cold symptoms appear does not. Vitamin C supplements appear to be safe, even at high doses.

ZINC

Zinc taken orally, often in the form of lozenges, within 24 hours of symptom onset might reduce the duration of a cold. No firm recommendation currently can be made, however, regarding prophylactic zinc supplementation because of insufficient data. When taken in large doses, side effects from zinc can include nausea and diarrhea, copper deficiency, and decreased absorption of some medications. Intranasal use of zinc can cause anosmia (loss of sense of smell), which can be long-lasting or permanent.

Coronavirus Disease 2019

A variety of dietary supplements, including elderberry, melatonin, colloidal silver, vitamin C, vitamin D, and zinc have each been suggested to prevent or treat coronavirus disease 2019 (COVID-19). Except for colloidal silver (for which no plausible mechanism of action exists), the listed supplements have theoretical applications in preventing or treating COVID-19; evidence of efficacy from clinical trials is limited, however, and without clear demonstration of benefit.

In addition, use of colloidal silver and zinc carries health and safety concerns. Colloidal silver (and other silver products) can cause argyria, a permanent blue-gray discoloration of the skin and other organs. High-dose supplementation with zinc can cause nausea and diarrhea, copper deficiency, and decreased absorption of some medications. The National Institutes of Health (NIH) COVID-19 Treatment Guidelines (www.covid19treatmentguidelines.nih.gov) recommend against supplementation with zinc above the recommended dietary allowance because of these risks and the lack of evidence of clinical benefit.

The NIH COVID-19 Treatment Guidelines provide up-to-date guidance on dietary supplements and COVID-19 for health care providers and travelers. For additional information on COVID-19 prevention and treatment, see Sec. 5, Part 2, Ch. 3, COVID-19.

Homeopathic Vaccines

Proponents of homeopathy claim that products called nosodes, or homeopathic vaccines, are effective substitutes for conventional immunizations. No credible scientific evidence or plausible scientific rationale supports these claims. For more information on travel vaccines, see Sec. 2, Ch. 3, Vaccination & Immunoprophylaxis—General Principles.

Insect Repellents

Many products are promoted as "natural" insect repellents, and their use can appeal to people who prefer not to use synthetic products. Products promoted as natural mosquito repellents include citronella products, neem oil (a component of agricultural insecticide products promoted on some websites for home use), and oil of lemon eucalyptus (OLE). Essential oils and other natural products are promoted to repel bed bugs. Travelers should use only Environmental Protection Agency (EPA)–registered insect repellents; more information is available at the EPA website (www.epa.gov/insect-repellents/find-repellent-right-you).

BOTANICALS

Laboratory-based studies found that botanicals, including citronella products, worked for shorter periods than products containing DEET (N,N-diethyl-m-toluamide or N,N-diethyl-3-methyl-benzamide). For people who choose to use botanicals, the Centers for Disease Control and Prevention (CDC) recommends EPA-registered products containing OLE (oil of lemon eucalyptus). Limited evidence suggests that neem oil could be beneficial as a natural repellent. For more information on insect repellents, see Sec. 4, Ch. 6, Mosquitoes, Ticks & Other Arthropods).

2

BED BUG REPELLENTS

No evidence supports effectiveness of natural products marketed to repel bed bugs. Instead, encourage travelers to follow steps to detect and avoid bed bugs (e.g., inspecting mattresses, keeping their luggage off the floor or bed). More information is available at CDC's Parasites website (www.cdc.gov/parasites/bedbugs) and in Section 4, Box 4-10, Recommended protective measures to avoid or reduce bed bug exposure.

Jet Lag & Sleep Problems

Complementary approaches suggested for jet lag or other sleep problems include aromatherapy and herbs (e.g., chamomile, kava, valerian); the dietary supplement melatonin; and relaxation techniques. See Sec. 8, Ch. 4, Jet Lag, for more information.

AROMATHERAPY

Very little evidence supports the belief that aromatherapy or the herbs chamomile or valerian help with insomnia. Major side effects are uncommon, but chamomile can cause allergic reactions. Another herb, kava, also is promoted for sleep, but good research on its effectiveness is lacking. More importantly, kava supplements have been linked to a risk of severe liver damage.

MELATONIN

Some evidence suggests that melatonin supplements can help with sleep problems caused by jet lag in people traveling either east or west. Melatonin is sold as a dietary supplement; dietary supplements are less strictly regulated than drugs. The amounts of ingredients in dietary supplements can vary, and product contamination is a potential concern. A 2017 analysis of melatonin supplements sold in Canada found that their actual melatonin content ranged from <83% to >478% of the labeled content and that substantial lot-to-lot variation was evident. Also, 26% of products contained serotonin as a contaminant.

Melatonin supplements appear to be safe for most people who use them for discrete periods of time; an absence of studies examining the effects associated with continued use makes it challenging to know with certainty its long-term safety and tolerability. In a 2019 systematic review of mostly short-term trials of melatonin for sleep problems, the most frequently reported adverse events were daytime sleepiness (1.66%), dizziness (0.74%), headache (0.74%), other sleep-related adverse events (0.74%), and hypothermia (0.62%). Almost all adverse events were considered mild–moderate in severity and tended to resolve either spontaneously or after discontinuing treatment.

Caution people with epilepsy or who take an oral anticoagulant against using melatonin without medical supervision. In addition, advise travelers not to take melatonin early in the day, because it can cause sleepiness and delay adaptation to local time.

RELAXATION TECHNIQUES

Relaxation techniques (e.g., progressive relaxation and other mind and body practices, including mindfulness-based stress reduction) can help with insomnia, but their effectiveness for jet lag has not been established.

Malaria

Many consumer websites promote "natural" ways to prevent or treat malaria, which often involve dietary changes or herbal products (e.g., quinine from the cinchona tree [*Cinchona* spp.]) or extracts and material from the artemisia plant (*Artemisia annua* L. or sweet wormwood). Strongly urge patients to follow official recommendations, including the use of malaria chemoprophylaxis, and not to rely on unproven "natural" approaches to prevent or treat such a serious disease. Recommended drugs to prevent and treat malaria are described in Sec. 5, Part 3, Ch. 16, Malaria.

Motion Sickness

Complementary approaches advocated for preventing or treating motion sickness include acupressure and magnets, ginger, homeopathic remedies, and pyridoxine (vitamin B_6).

ACUPRESSURE & MAGNETS

Research does not support the use of acupressure or magnets for motion sickness.

GINGER

Although some studies have shown that ginger might ease pregnancy-related nausea and vomiting, no strong evidence shows that it helps with motion sickness. In some people, ginger can have mild side effects (e.g., abdominal discomfort). Research has not definitively shown whether ginger interacts with medications, but concerns have been raised that it could interact with anticoagulants. The effect of using ginger supplements with common over-the-counter drugs for motion sickness (e.g., dimenhydrinate [Dramamine]) is unknown.

HOMEOPATHIC REMEDIES

No evidence supports claims that homeopathic products prevent or alleviate motion sickness.

PYRIDOXINE (VITAMIN B_6)

Although an American Congress of Obstetrics and Gynecology 2015 Practice Bulletin Summary recommends pyridoxine (vitamin B_6) alone or in combination with doxylamine (an antihistamine) as a safe and effective treatment for nausea and vomiting associated with pregnancy, no evidence supports claims that pyridoxine prevents or alleviates motion sickness. Taking excessive doses of pyridoxine supplements for long periods of time can affect nerve function.

Sun Protection

Many "natural sunscreen" products are promoted online, as are recipes for homemade sunscreen and advice on consuming dietary supplements or drinking teas to protect against sun damage. No studies have proven that any dietary supplement or herbal product, including aloe vera, beta carotene, epigallocatechin gallate (EGCG; a green tea extract), or selenium reduces the risk for skin cancer or sun damage. For more information, see Sec. 4, Ch. 1, Sun Exposure.

Travelers' Diarrhea

A variety of products, including activated charcoal, goldenseal, grapefruit seed extract, and probiotics are claimed to prevent or treat travelers' diarrhea (TD). Counsel travelers about food and water safety precautions. For more information, see Sec. 2, Ch. 8, Food & Water Precautions.

ACTIVATED CHARCOAL

No solid evidence supports claims that activated charcoal helps with TD, bloating, stomach cramps, or gas. The side effects of activated charcoal have not been well documented but were mild when it was tested on healthy people. Children should not be given activated charcoal for diarrhea and dehydration because it can absorb nutrients, enzymes, and antibiotics in the intestine and mask the severity of fluid loss.

GOLDENSEAL

No high-quality research has been published on goldenseal for TD. Studies show that goldenseal inhibits cytochrome P450 enzymes, raising concerns that goldenseal might increase the toxicity or alter the effects of some drugs.

GRAPEFRUIT SEED EXTRACT

Claims that grapefruit seed extract can prevent bacterial foodborne illnesses are not supported by research. People who need to avoid grapefruit because it interacts with medicine they are taking should also avoid grapefruit seed extract.

PROBIOTICS

To date, insufficient evidence exists to draw definite conclusions about the efficacy of probiotics for the prevention of TD. Although some studies have had promising results, meta-analyses have reached conflicting conclusions. Interpretation of the evidence is difficult because studies have used a variety of microbial strains, some studies were not well controlled, and the optimal doses and duration of use have not been defined. For more information, see Sec. 2, Ch. 6, Travelers' Diarrhea.

UNTESTED THERAPIES USED IN OTHER COUNTRIES

CDC does not recommend traveling to other countries for untested medical interventions or to buy medications that are not approved in the United States. For more information see the chapters in Section 6, Health Care Abroad.

2

TALKING TO TRAVELERS ABOUT COMPLEMENTARY HEALTH APPROACHES

Given the vast number of complementary or integrative interventions and the wealth of potentially misleading information about them that can be found on the internet, discussing the use of these approaches with patients can seem daunting. Be proactive, though, because surveys show that many patients are reluctant to raise the topic with health care providers. Federal agencies (e.g., the National Center for Complementary and Integrative Health [NCCIH]) offer evidence-based resources (www.nccih.nih.gov/health/providers) to help providers and their patients have meaningful discussions about complementary approaches.

ACKNOWLEDGMENTS

The authors thank Mr. Philip Kibak of ICF for his editorial assistance.

BIBLIOGRAPHY

Bauer I. Travel medicine, coca and cocaine: demystifying and rehabilitating Erythroxylum—a comprehensive review. Trop Dis Travel Med Vaccines. 2019 Nov 26;5:20.

Besag FMC, Vasey MJ, Lao KSJ, Wong ICK. Adverse events associated with melatonin for the treatment of primary or secondary sleep disorders: a systematic review. CNS Drugs. 2019;33(12):1167–86.

Erland LA, Saxena PK. Melatonin natural health products and supplements: presence of serotonin and significant variability of melatonin content. J Clin Sleep Med. 2017;13(2):275–81.

Karsch-Völk M, Barrett B, Kiefer D, Bauer R, Ardjomand-Woelkart K, Linde K. Echinacea for preventing and treating the common cold. Cochrane Database Syst Rev. 2014(2):CD000530.

Molano Franco D, Nieto Estrada VH, Gonzalez Garay AG, Martí-Carvajal AJ, Arevalo-Rodriguez I. Interventions for preventing high altitude illness: part 3. Miscellaneous and non-pharmacological interventions. Cochrane Database Syst Rev. 2019(4):CD013315.

US Food and Drug Administration. Is it really "FDA approved?" Available from: www.fda.gov/consumers/consumer-updates/it-really-fda-approved.

US Food and Drug Administration. Is rinsing your sinuses with neti pots safe? Available from: www.fda.gov/consumers/consumer-updates/rinsing-your-sinuses-neti-pots-safe.

Wang C, Lü L, Zhang A, Liu C. Repellency of selected chemicals against the bed bug (Hemiptera: Cimicidae). J Econ Entomol. 2013;106(6):2522–9.

Zhao Y, Dong BR, Hao Q. Probiotics for preventing acute upper respiratory tract infections. Cochrane Database Syst Rev. 2022(8):CD006895.pub4.

PRIORITIZING CARE FOR RESOURCE-LIMITED TRAVELERS

Zoon Wangu, Elizabeth Barnett

Travelers seen in pretravel clinic consultations often have financial constraints and must pay out of pocket for pretravel care, because many health insurance plans provide no or limited coverage for travel immunizations and prophylactic medications. Optimizing care for travelers without adequate insurance coverage or with only modest means can challenge the abilities of even the savviest travel medicine clinician. As an example, the estimated cost of a pretravel consultation for a backpacker from the United States planning a 4-week trip to West Africa could easily exceed $1,000 for the initial consultation and vaccinations, excluding malaria prophylaxis.

Travelers on a limited budget might be at increased risk for travel-associated infections because they are more likely to visit remote areas, stay in more modest accommodations, and eat in restaurants with lower hygiene standards. However, the total cost of hospitalization, treatment, and lost wages after becoming ill with a vaccine- or prophylaxis-preventable disease can easily exceed the upfront cost of vaccination and prophylaxis, making the pretravel consultation particularly important. Travelers also must consider the cost and benefit of purchasing travel health insurance and medical evacuation insurance before travel (see Sec. 6, Ch. 1, Travel Insurance, Travel Health Insurance & Medical Evacuation Insurance). Use the pretravel consult as an opportunity to help guide travel health recommendations for travelers with financial constraints.

VACCINES

Required Travel Vaccines

Only meningococcal and yellow fever vaccines are required categorically, and then only for some travelers: meningococcal vaccine for pilgrims traveling to Mecca during the Hajj, and yellow fever vaccine for travelers to certain countries in Africa and South America (see Sec. 2, Ch. 5, Yellow Fever Vaccine & Malaria Prevention Information, by Country). Prioritize administration and documentation of these vaccines; travelers without them could be denied entry to their destination. Be aware that even travelers staying only briefly in a yellow fever-endemic country (e.g., during an airport layover) might still need evidence of vaccination to be permitted entry to other countries on their itinerary.

In a few specific circumstances, travelers to polio-affected countries might be asked to show proof of polio vaccination before departure if their stay is >4 weeks (see Sec. 5, Part 2, Ch. 17, Poliomyelitis). Travelers and clinicians should check the Centers for Disease Control and Prevention (CDC) Travelers' Health website (https://wwwnc.cdc.gov/travel/destinations/list/) for the latest recommendations for their destinations.

Routine Vaccines

All travelers should be current with routine vaccines before international travel, regardless of destination. The benefits of routine vaccines extend beyond the travel period, and many provide lifelong immunity. Because these vaccines are mass-produced as part of scheduled national childhood and adult vaccination programs, associated costs generally are low, and many insurance companies reimburse the patient for the cost of administration. Travelers also can obtain these vaccines in a health department or primary care setting, where costs might be lower than at a travel clinic.

For travelers not up to date with routine vaccines, prioritize administration of those that protect against diseases for which the traveler is most likely to be at general risk (e.g., hepatitis A, influenza, and measles). Children in the United States routinely receive hepatitis A vaccine, but it is not included in the adult immunization schedule. Some travelers might be immune to diseases for which travel medicine providers would consider immunization; pretravel antibody testing might be covered by insurance when vaccines are not. Assess the time to departure to decide whether to test rather than vaccinate.

Recommended Travel Vaccines

When prioritizing recommended vaccines, consider time until departure (see Last-Minute Travelers, Sec. 2, Ch. 11), risk for disease at the destination, effectiveness and safety of the vaccine, and likelihood of future benefit because of repeat travel. As previously noted, hepatitis A vaccine is not currently listed as a routine vaccine for US adults; however, this vaccine can provide lifelong immunity and clinicians should consider administering it to any traveler not previously vaccinated. Hepatitis B vaccine is recommended for all US adults under age 60; since hepatitis B acquisition is not frequently associated with travel, however, vaccination against hepatitis B might be a lower priority for travelers with limited resources, unless their destinations are areas of high disease incidence or they plan to engage in activities that place them at increased risk of exposure to bloodborne pathogens (see Sec. 5, Part 2, Ch. 8, Hepatitis B).

Typhoid vaccine is ≈50%–80% effective in preventing disease, and protection is not long-lasting. Thus, typhoid vaccine is more critical for travelers to higher-risk destinations where acquiring typhoid is more likely, and to areas where typhoid is harder to treat because of multidrug resistance (e.g., Southeast Asia and the Indian subcontinent).

CORONAVIRUS DISEASE 2019

Clinicians should discuss and recommend vaccination against severe acute respiratory syndrome coronavirus 2 (SARS-CoV-2), regardless of destination (see Sec. 5, Part 2, Ch. 3, COVID-19).

JAPANESE ENCEPHALITIS

Review the traveler's itinerary in detail to determine the need for Japanese encephalitis (JE) vaccine (see Sec. 5, Part 2, Ch. 13, Japanese Encephalitis). Some travelers might be able to obtain the single-dose JE vaccine, which is much less expensive and is available outside the United States, but bear in mind (and educate travelers about) issues surrounding quality of vaccines in many countries (see Sec. 6, Ch. 3, . . . *perspectives*: Avoiding Poorly Regulated Medicines & Medical Products During Travel). Whether or not travelers accept the JE vaccine, provide instructions for when and how to use insect repellents and other measures to prevent mosquito bites (see Sec. 4, Ch. 6, Mosquitoes, Ticks & Other Arthropods).

RABIES

When considering rabies vaccine for resource-limited travelers, factor in the risk for animal exposure, access to local health care, and availability of rabies immune globulin and rabies vaccine at the traveler's destination (see Sec. 5, Part 2, Ch. 18, Rabies). Advise travelers who decline preexposure immunization to devise a plan of action in case an exposure occurs. In many areas, rabies vaccine or rabies immune globulin are difficult or impossible to obtain, and travelers might need to be medically evacuated to receive full and proper postexposure prophylaxis.

MALARIA PROPHYLAXIS

Every pretravel consultation should include detailed advice about preventing mosquito bites (see Sec. 4, Ch. 6, Mosquitoes, Ticks & Other Arthropods). Malaria risk varies widely depending on destination, accommodations, and activities during travel. Costs associated with the different regimens vary widely. Providers should stay up to date on the cost of antimalarial medications in their region and at pharmacies, so they can recommend the most cost-effective drug based on the traveler's planned itinerary. If travelers ask whether they can purchase antimalarial drugs at their destination, advise them about the risk of inappropriate, substandard, and counterfeit medications and discourage them from this practice (see Sec. 6, Ch. 3, . . . *perspectives*: Avoiding Poorly Regulated Medicines & Medical Products During Travel).

TRAVELERS' DIARRHEA

Travelers' diarrhea (TD) is among the most common travel-related illnesses. Consider prescribing antibiotics to travelers to treat incapacitating diarrhea. Prophylaxis is indicated only in select patients at high risk for complications from TD (Sec. 2, Ch. 6, Travelers' Diarrhea). As with antimalarial drugs purchased at the destination, advise travelers about the risk of purchasing counterfeit antibiotics overseas.

PREVENTIVE BEHAVIORS

For each traveler, weigh the potential severity of illness against the affordability and availability of immunization or prophylaxis, as well as the level of protection provided. In cases where a disease is potentially deadly but where affordable, effective chemoprophylaxis options exist (e.g., malaria), work with the traveler to identify an acceptable prescribed chemoprophylaxis regimen and emphasize the importance of not eschewing medication due to cost.

In addition, educate all travelers about the importance of employing preventive behaviors that can serve to reduce their exposure risks: avoiding animals, using insect bite precautions, following safe sex practices, washing their hands or using alcohol-based hand sanitizer frequently, and observing food and water precautions to the best of their ability. Strongly advise all travelers, and especially those unable to afford some of the more costly immunizations or prophylactic medications, to practice these behaviors. In the era of the COVID-19 pandemic, offer advice about mask use, encourage travelers to take note of the level of SARS-CoV-2 infection at their destination, and to be mindful about avoiding large gatherings. Reassure travelers that the actions they take to avoid preventable health risks also can protect against travel-associated conditions that are more prevalent than certain vaccine-preventable diseases.

BIBLIOGRAPHY

Adachi K, Coleman MS, Khan N, Jentes ES, Arguin P, Rao SR, et al. Economics of malaria prevention in US travelers to West Africa. Clin Infect Dis. 2014;58(1):11–21.

IBM Micromedex. RED BOOK System. Truven Health Analytics, Greenwood Village, Colorado, USA. Available from: www.ibm.com/watson/health/provider-client-training/micromedex-red-book.

Jentes ES, Blanton JD, Johnson KJ, Petersen BW, Lamias MJ, Robertson K, et al. The global availability of rabies immune globulin and rabies vaccine in clinics providing indirect care to travelers. J Travel Med. 2014;21(1):62–6.

Johnson DF, Leder K, Torresi J. Hepatitis B and C infection in international travelers. J Travel Med. 2013;20(3):194–202.

Mangtani P, Roberts JA. Economic evaluations of travelers' vaccinations. In: Zuckerman JN, Jong EC, editors. Travelers' vaccines, 2nd edition. Shelton, CT: People's Medical Publishing House; 2010. pp. 553–67.

Riddle MS, Connor BA, Beeching NJ, DuPont HL, Hamer DH, Kozarsky P, et al. Guidelines for the prevention and treatment of travelers' diarrhea: a graded expert panel report. J Travel Med. 2017;24(1):S63–80.

Wu D, Guo CY. Epidemiology and prevention of hepatitis A in travelers. J Travel Med. 2013;20(6):394–9.

2

TELEMEDICINE

Taylan Bozkurt, José F. Flórez-Arango, Matt Levi, Scott Norton

Telemedicine means "practicing medicine at a distance," but in common usage it refers to providing diagnostic and therapeutic services via electronic transfer of medical information. Telemedicine encounters can be as simple as patients asking providers health-related questions via the telephone or secure email or as complex as real-time monitoring of the health of astronauts at the International Space Station.

Many analyses of telemedicine programs focus on cost savings for medical organizations or on the benefits provided to distinct population subsets such as underserved urban populations or populations for whom transportation is difficult (e.g., patients in nursing homes, correctional facilities, remote areas). Few analyses have looked at total costs across the entire health care system.

BENEFITS OF TELEMEDICINE

Benefits of telemedicine include expanding access to specialty care, expediting delivery of care (minimizing wait times), and providing opportunities to confirm or obviate the need for someone to see a provider in person—an advantage for individuals or populations for whom an in-person visit is impractical, inconvenient, arduous, or costly.

Telemedicine has several unique uses for the practice of travel medicine. For instance, telemedicine can be used as an alternative to the in-person pretravel consultation. Moreover, travelers can use telemedicine to maintain continuity of care for existing conditions, enabling them to travel farther and longer by extending the interval between in-person visits. Notably, travelers who develop acute illnesses or injuries, have exacerbations of existing conditions, experience high-risk exposures, or need to seek medical advice while abroad can use telemedicine platforms to discuss issues with a trusted provider.

Travel health providers also benefit from using telemedicine. When a traveler seeks medical care in the country they are visiting, the local provider can use telemedicine to obtain additional information from the patient's regular providers or health records. Clinicians who conduct posttravel evaluations can obtain prompt consultative support when travelers present with unusual clinical findings.

2

CONDUCTING A REMOTE PRETRAVEL CONSULTATION

Telemedicine provides a convenient way to deliver pretravel consultations with the same elements as an in-person visit. Providers should continue to follow the same professional standards used during in-person consultations, including adherence to a code of ethics, security and privacy practices, and clinical guidelines. What can and cannot be done in a remote consultation varies by state; clinicians should check with their state's medical board about any restrictions. Furthermore, the policies and practices of telehealth programs underwent major changes during the coronavirus disease 2019 (COVID-19) pandemic and will continue to change; providers will need to remain current with what is and is not permissible. A valuable resource on telemedicine, including requirements by state, is prognoCIS (https://prognocis.com/wp-content/uploads/2017/01/Telemedicine-Whitepaper.pdf), and many additional online resources related to telemedicine standards, guidelines, and practice are available (Table 2-14).

Table 2-14 Online telemedicine resources

ORGANIZATION OR SOURCE	RESOURCE	AVAILABLE FROM
American Medical Association	AMA Telehealth Quick Guide	www.ama-assn.org/practice-management/digital/ama-telehealth-quick-guide
	Digital Health Payment	www.ama-assn.org/practice-management/digital/digital-health-payment
American Telemedicine Association	ATA's CDC Yellowbook page	www.americantelemed.org/resource/cdc-yellowbook/
	Resources	www.americantelemed.org/resource/
	Telehealth. Is. Health	www.americantelemed.org
Center for Connected Health Policy	Resources & Reports	www.cchpca.org/resources/
Federation of State Medical Boards	The Appropriate Use of Telemedicine Technologies in the Practice of Medicine (2022)	www.fsmb.org/siteassets/advocacy/policies/fsmb-workgroup-on-telemedicineapril-2022-final.pdf
The National Academy of Medicine	The Role of Telehealth in an Evolving Health Care Environment (Workshop Summary, 2012)	www.nap.edu/catalog/13466/the-role-of-telehealth-in-an-evolving-health-care-environment
prognoCIS	The Physician's Guide to Telemedicine in 2018	https://prognocis.com/wp-content/uploads/2019/01/Telemedicine-Whitepaper.pdf

Table 2-14 Online telemedicine resources (continued)

ORGANIZATION OR SOURCE	RESOURCE	AVAILABLE FROM
US Department of Health and Human Services: Centers for Medicare & Medicaid Services	COVID-19 Emergency Declaration Blanket Waivers for Health Care Providers	www.cms.gov/files/document/summary-covid-19-emergency-declaration-waivers.pdf
	General Provider Telehealth and Telemedicine Tool Kit	www.cms.gov/files/document/general-telemedicine-toolkit.pdf
	Medicare Coverage and Payment of Virtual Services (video)	https://youtu.be/Bsp5tlFnYHk
	Medicare Telemedicine Health Care Provider Fact Sheet	www.cms.gov/newsroom/fact-sheets/medicare-telemedicine-health-care-provider-fact-sheet
	Telehealth	www.cms.gov/Medicare/Medicare-General-Information/Telehealth
	Medicare Learning Network Fact Sheet: Telehealth Services	www.cms.gov/Outreach-and-Education/Medicare-Learning-Network-MLN/MLNProducts/downloads/TelehealthSrvcsfctsht.pdf
US Department of Health and Human Services: Health Resources & Services Administration	Learn More about Telehealth: for Providers	www.telehealth.hhs.gov/providers/
US Department of Health and Human Services: Office for Civil Rights	Health Information Privacy	www.hhs.gov/hipaa/index.html
World Health Organization: Pan American Health Organization	Teleconsultations during a Pandemic	https://www3.paho.org/ish/images/docs/covid-19-teleconsultations-en.pdf

Medical practices should provide patients with a resource that outlines the expectations and outcomes of telemedicine before they schedule a consultation, including the limitations of a remote consultation. For example, the ability to conduct a complete physical examination is limited, but current technology can help replicate a near in-person quality of inspection, auscultation, palpation, and various other core elements of a physical examination. Intake information, including medical history, prior medical records, and diagnostic information can all be requested from patients and made available to providers in advance of the consultation. Encourage patients to set up and test their connections to the telemedicine software or equipment before the encounter.

At the time of the consultation, establish informed consent with the patient and ensure that the patient is in an appropriate care setting. Depending on state regulations, a patient might need to be in a location where the provider is licensed to practice medicine at the time of the consultation (see Legal Issues: Privacy & Security, later in this chapter). Depending on circumstances, a telepresenter (e.g., another health care provider or translator) might need to be with the patient to assist with the intake and exam.

Prescribing Medications & Vaccines

Depending on state and country-specific regulations, medications and vaccines can be prescribed during a telemedicine encounter. Where applicable, pharmacies or other allied health care providers can receive certain prescriptions electronically or over the phone, and eligible providers can dispense the medications or administer vaccines.

2

Yellow fever vaccine is available only at designated yellow fever vaccine clinics, and travelers might need to schedule a separate visit to receive it. For medications (e.g., malaria prophylaxis) and vaccines not routinely stocked at a local pharmacy, the traveler should allow time for the pharmacy to order them.

WHEN A TRAVELER IS ABROAD

US-based health care providers, regardless of their level of expertise in travel medicine, might be asked to provide a consultation for someone traveling outside the United States. The provider's willingness, comfort, and ability to provide a remote consultation under these circumstances will vary with the type of question or nature of the problem, their ability to charge for services, the technical quality of the communication, and perhaps the time of day. Providers must remember that the same security and privacy practices apply during a telemedicine consult as in a conventional, in-person, domestic consultation.

The Centers for Disease Control and Prevention (CDC) does not endorse procuring medication or filling prescriptions abroad because of the risk for counterfeit drugs (see Sec. 6, Ch. 3, . . . *perspectives*: Avoiding Poorly Regulated Medicines & Medical Products During Travel). In an emergency, however, such as when a traveler's medication is lost or stolen, a provider might be able to help locate local, reputable sources for replacement.

LEGAL ISSUES: PRIVACY & SECURITY

US Federal Law & International Law

Telemedicine consultations must comply with state and federal privacy and security laws, including the Health Insurance Portability and Accountability Act (HIPAA). In addition, providers should investigate specific legal requirements of the country where the traveler is located; some countries have strict requirements related to the transfer of personal health data, and even a patient's written consent might not be sufficient to allow this.

Communicating with patients abroad deserves a careful assessment of data and protection laws relative to the originating (i.e., overseas) location, type of service, and means of electronic transmission. Providers must ensure that the technology and video software chosen to conduct remote pretravel consultations and telemedicine encounters, whether store-and-forward (asynchronous) or live interactive video (synchronous), is HIPAA-compliant and meets the privacy and data security requirements of the countries involved. Although encryption is not specifically addressed under HIPAA, ensuring technology is encrypted will help providers safeguard patient health information.

Providers should communicate with at-home patients via an established patient portal or other HIPAA-compliant method. In urgent or unexpected situations, however, patients often will communicate via their personal email accounts, many of which are not encrypted. Remember that no data storage system or transmission of data over the internet, or any other public network, is guaranteed to be secure.

US State Laws & Regulations

In the United States, each state has its own telemedicine laws and regulations, most of which address reimbursement issues (e.g., informing providers and insurance carriers which telemedicine services are reimbursed) but not the practice of telemedicine. Therefore, providers must perform due diligence to ensure that they conduct telemedicine encounters in accordance with the laws and regulations applicable in their local jurisdiction.

In response to the COVID-19 pandemic, some states modified licensure requirements to support cross-state telemedicine. Providers should check with the Federation of State Medical Boards to ensure they are following all state and federal policies (see Table 2-14). Without appropriate licensing, some states do not permit providers to practice telemedicine or to prescribe certain medications across state lines. Therefore, travel medicine clinics and providers must carefully read medical board regulations before embarking on telemedicine consults across state lines. No state prohibits the practice of telemedicine across state lines, but many do require providers to have required licensure. For example, a provider living in State A conducting a telemedicine encounter with a patient in State B would need to be licensed in both states. The standards for maintaining privacy and security during an international telemedicine consult are the same as for domestic consults.

In addition, providers—particularly solo practitioners or those not part of a larger health care network or system—should explore whether a business associate agreement or contract is needed. When working with international partners (e.g., companies based outside the country in which the provider practices), additional legal issues can arise and should be considered.

TECHNOLOGY ISSUES

Providers should consider the bandwidth and connectivity needed for live interactive video telemedicine encounters. Connectivity can be inadequate in some places, and website accessibility can be made difficult because of internal firewalls. Mobile hotspots can be used in some situations in lieu of dial-up or Ethernet connections.

Some telemedicine vendors have optimized software to work in low-bandwidth settings; others have focused on markets where high-bandwidth networks are more widely available. Providers should have their technology vendor provide information about minimum bandwidth requirements that they can review with patients to ensure a seamless telemedicine encounter.

BOX 2-16 PHOTOGRAPHS IN TELEMEDICINE: ADVICE FOR TRAVELERS

One of the most common ways that travelers use telemedicine is by sending photographs of travel-associated rashes and minor injuries to their home providers with implicit requests for a diagnosis and for treatment recommendations. Nowadays, most such photos are digital images taken with smart phones. Although the cameras on smart phones are seemingly simple to use, travel medicine providers often find these photographs blurry (due to poor focusing, motion artifact, or improper depth of field), poorly lit, or marred by distracting objects in the foreground or background. Even with well-focused, well-lit photographs, discerning which body part is being shown or which lesion is the one in question can be difficult. The following recommendations can help travelers take more useful, information-laden photographs.

PICTURES SHOULD SHOW

- Distribution (i.e., the parts of the body that are involved)
- Configuration and arrangement of lesions with respect to one another (grouping)
- A primary lesion (e.g., an undamaged blister)
- Lesions with secondary changes (e.g., an open or eroded blister)

MARK THE LESION

- If several lesions are present, or if the lesion is subtle, indicate the specific lesion using a marking pen or (for digital images) editing software.

USE GOOD LIGHTING

- Take pictures in a well-lit room, or outdoors in a shaded area.

TAKE SEVERAL PICTURES

- An orientation view should show the entire body or affected body part; the location of the lesion should be obvious in the picture.
- A mid-distance view should center on the lesion and show an anatomical landmark (e.g., belly button, armpit) for orientation and size.
- A close-up view can be physically close (under 18") using the camera's macro function or from farther away if using a zoom lens.
- Take pictures both straight-on and from different angles.
- Make sure the lesion is in the center of the picture; the lesion should fill most of frame but also include some normal skin around it.
- Include a scale/size comparison in the picture (use either a ruler or measuring tape or a standard object like a pencil, paper clip, or US coin).
- Show the normal opposite side for comparison (e.g., a swollen elbow and the uninvolved elbow).
- For lesions on the head, neck, and face, remove jewelry; and for hair problems, focus on scalp.
- Take as many pictures as necessary; send sharply focused, well-lit photos only; blurry pictures are not helpful, even if they are 5MB.

Although not required, providers also should recommend that patients use private, secure connections and avoid using public Wi-Fi such as that available in hotels, internet cafes, and airports, because these connections can pose privacy and security risks.

2

REIMBURSEMENT

Much like reimbursement for face-to-face encounters, providers need to ensure that their clinic meets certain legal requirements and payer guidelines. In the United States, the pretravel consultation might not be reimbursed by health insurance companies, so a telemedicine practice might be primarily fee-for-service. If corporate personnel are traveling for work and their companies are paying for the associated health care they receive, providers should make certain the company permits their employees to engage in telemedicine and will reimburse for this service.

BIBLIOGRAPHY

Kennedy KM, Flaherty GT. Medico-legal risk, clinical negligence and the practice of travel medicine. J Travel Med. 2016;23(5).

Rokosh RS, Lewis II WC, Chaikof EL, Kavraki LE. 2021. How should we prepare for the post-pandemic world of telehealth and digital medicine? NAM Perspect. Washington, DC: National Academy of Medicine; 2021. Available from: https://nam.edu/how-should-we-prepare-for-the-post-pandemic-world-of-telehealth-and-digital-medicine/.

RISK MANAGEMENT ISSUES IN TRAVEL MEDICINE

Andrés Henao-Martínez, Carlos Franco-Paredes

Travel medicine providers, just as practitioners in other medical specialties, are at risk for legal action. Claims for medical negligence could involve failure of duty of care; failure to uphold the standard of practice; care resulting in physical, financial, or psychological loss; and loss caused directly by the failure to reach the standard of care.

Although travel medicine practitioners come from many backgrounds, in the travel medicine arena they are preventive medicine specialists. As such, in giving advice, travel medicine practitioners provide education and not generally "hands on" patient care. Although misunderstandings and legal action might occur despite best efforts, certain guidance is helpful.

Communication. The likelihood of a lawsuit is lessened by good communication between the provider and the traveler. Providers should verbally cover all elements of a pretravel consultation during the visit or provide written material for the patient to take home. Because time is a limitation, clinics should provide handouts on how to avoid common health problems not discussed during the consultation. Written information about medications being given or prescribed also is helpful.

Documentation. Clinics should have a method for documenting all aspects of the consultation and include an area within the record for the provider to comment on the patient's questions or responses to recommendations. Many electronic medical records enable the provider to add items unique to travel health and to add comments regarding the consultation.

Identification of problems. Providers should consult with their risk management personnel or legal advisors in the event of a contentious office visit or exchange after the visit. Nonjudgmental documentation of all communications between traveler and provider is critical.

EXAMPLES OF RISK MANAGEMENT ISSUES IN TRAVEL MEDICINE

Prescription Medications

FLUOROQUINOLONES

Fluoroquinolone use can be associated with central nervous system adverse events, peripheral neuropathy, and tendinopathies (e.g., tendinitis, tendon rupture). Lawsuits regarding these problems occur, and whether a single dose of a fluoroquinolone used for the self-treatment of travelers' diarrhea can lead to such events is unknown. Thus, even though prescriptions come from pharmacies with directions and adverse event information, discuss these potential adverse events with patients.

MEFLOQUINE

Mefloquine can cause serious neuropsychiatric adverse events, including visual hallucinations, psychosis, insomnia, seizures, dizziness, nightmares, and motor and sensory neuropathies. These adverse events can persist after the drug is discontinued. Do not prescribe mefloquine to patients with a seizure disorder or a psychiatric disorder (e.g., depression, generalized anxiety disorder, psychosis, schizophrenia). The Centers for Disease Control and Prevention (CDC) also recommends against mefloquine use in patients with cardiac conduction abnormalities.

(continued)

RISK MANAGEMENT (CONTINUED)

2

Travelers receiving a prescription for mefloquine should receive a copy of the US Food and Drug Administration (FDA) medication guide (www.accessdata.fda.gov/drugsatfda_docs/label/2008/019591s023lbl.pdf).

Because of its low cost and convenient weekly dosing, however, mefloquine remains an attractive option for some travelers. Therefore, when recommending mefloquine for malaria prophylaxis, document clearly and carefully the reasons for selecting this drug over other antimalarial drugs. Review the medical history for potential contraindications and include a note to that effect in the patient's record.

PRIMAQUINE & TAFENOQUINE

Primaquine and tafenoquine can cause potentially fatal hemolysis in glucose-6-phosphate dehydrogenase (G6PD)-deficient patients. Screen for G6PD deficiency in anyone receiving a prescription for either of these medications. People who are pregnant or lactating should not receive primaquine or tafenoquine.

DRUG-DRUG INTERACTIONS

Drug-drug interactions can occur among medications prescribed for travelers, and clinicians should include medication reconciliation as an essential part of the traveler's history. Electronic medical records and other pharmacy aids are useful to alert clinicians of drug interactions when they are making decisions about travel medication prescriptions. Use caution when prescribing fluoroquinolones and macrolides for travelers taking other QT interval-prolonging agents. Concurrent use of antibiotics with cholera or oral typhoid vaccines can diminish the body's immune response to the vaccine. Antibody-containing products might affect live attenuated vaccines.

OFF-LABEL USE

Providers sometimes find it useful to recommend medications to travelers that are not approved by the FDA for the specified purpose. Examples include use of primaquine alone for malaria prophylaxis and rifaximin to prevent travelers' diarrhea. Providers will sometimes recommend medications for uses other than those considered standard of care; document the discussion with the traveler prior to prescribing, along with the traveler's acceptance.

Vaccine Side Effects & Contraindications

To deliver effective and safe vaccinations, carefully review the patient's past medical history, allergies, and vaccination history. Failure to administer a vaccine correctly can cause an adverse event or result in a traveler acquiring a preventable disease abroad. If a patient refuses a vaccine, discuss with them the reasons why and then document any relevant conversations regarding the risk of acquiring a disease. Counsel travelers known to be immunocompromised, or whose immune status precludes a protective antibody response to vaccination, about the possibility of decreased vaccine-related immunity.

Serious vaccine-associated adverse events could be due to a variety of causes. Allergic reactions to vaccine components are possible. Immunocompromised travelers might suffer adverse events after receiving live vaccines. Inquire about the traveler's allergies, history of pregnancy, breastfeeding status, immunosuppressive medications, and immunocompromised status—information that is crucial to minimizing vaccine-associated adverse events. Have vaccine information statements available, and provide these to each vaccinated traveler (www.cdc.gov/vaccines/hcp/vis/index.html).

Document each patient's history and the data used to make decisions, especially when a vaccine is not given or when administering a vaccine despite precautions about its use. Make certain patients understand any risks associated with deviating from Advisory Committee for Immunization Practices-recommended dosing schedules (e.g., those used for the accelerated delivery of some vaccines). Document the discussion in the patient's record.

Deep Vein Thrombosis

Long-distance air travel increases the risk for deep vein thrombosis (DVT) and pulmonary embolism by approximately 3-fold. The association is stronger with flights of longer duration. Counsel patients about DVT, recommend measures to decrease risk for DVT (e.g., occasional walking, selecting an aisle seat, exercises), and document this discussion in the medical record (see Sec. 8, Ch. 3, Deep Vein Thrombosis & Pulmonary Embolism).

Medical Clearance for International Assignments

Providers should be aware of the potential legal entanglements incurred when a prospective international business traveler who is unfit for international assignment is cleared, and then a negative outcome ensues. See a more complete discussion of this topic in Sec. 9, Ch. 1, The International Business Traveler.

SUMMARY & RECOMMENDATIONS

Maintaining a standard of care in one's practice is important protection for both patient and health care provider. Clinic providers should have adequate training in travel medicine and engage in continuing education. Travel medicine clinics should have at least 1 provider who has earned the Certificate in Travel Health (CTH) awarded by the International Society of Travel Medicine (ISTM) upon successful completion of the CTH examination. Providers also should remain current in the field of travel medicine by accessing continuing education programs offered by CDC and ISTM (see Sec. 1, Ch. 4, Improving the Quality of Travel Medicine Through Education & Training). Following standards of care and the recommendations in this chapter could help reduce the risk for legal action against the provider and the travel medicine clinic.

BIBLIOGRAPHY

Burton B. Australian army faces legal action over mefloquine. BMJ. 2004;329(7474):1062.

Hinrichs-Krapels S, Bussmann S, Dobyns C, Kácha O, Ratzmann N, Holm Thorvaldsen J, et al. Key considerations for an economic and legal framework facilitating medical travel. Front Public Health. 2016;4:47.

Kennedy KM, Flaherty GT. Medico-legal risk, clinical negligence and the practice of travel medicine. J Travel Med. 2016;23(5):taw048.

Lapostolle F, Surget V, Borron SW, Desmaizières M, Sordelet D, Lapandry C, et al. Severe pulmonary embolism associated with air travel. N Engl J Med. 2001;345(11):779–83.

. . . *perspectives* chapters supplement the clinical guidance in this book with additional content, context, and expert opinion. The views expressed do not necessarily represent the official position of the Centers for Disease Control and Prevention (CDC).

3 Travelers with Additional Considerations

IMMUNOCOMPROMISED TRAVELERS

Camille Kotton, Andrew Kroger, David Freedman

Immunocompromised people make up 1%–2% of patients seen in US travel clinics, and they largely pursue itineraries like those of immunocompetent travelers. Pretravel preparation for people with a suppressed immune status, whether due to a health condition, medication, or other treatment, is complex. During the pretravel consult for an immunocompromised traveler, consider additional issues (e.g., the patient's increased risk for travel-associated infections and diseases, the effects travel can have on the patient's underlying condition, and the patient's response or adverse reactions to pretravel vaccines and travel medications). Key points to emphasize with immunocompromised travelers during a pretravel visit are summarized in Box 3-01.

For more information on altered immunocompetence and vaccine administration, see the Advisory Committee on Immunization Practices (ACIP) General Best Guidelines for Immunization: Altered Immunocompetence

CDC Yellow Book 2024. Jeffrey Nemhauser, Oxford University Press. © Oxford University Press 2023.
DOI: 10.1093/oso/9780197570944.003.0003

BOX 3-01 Key patient education points for immunocompromised travelers

DEVELOP A PLAN IN CASE OF ILLNESS

Identify clinics or hospitals in the destination country capable of providing care to immunocompromised patients

Know how to access and use US embassy resources

Purchase supplemental insurance to cover trip cancellation due to illness, the cost of health care received abroad, and medical evacuation

FOOD & WATER PRECAUTIONS

Follow safe food and water precautions (see Sec. 2, Ch. 8, Food & Water Precautions)

Pack and regularly use antibacterial hand wipes or an alcohol-based hand sanitizer containing ≥60% alcohol

MULTIDRUG-RESISTANT ORGANISMS

Immunocompromised people have an augmented risk for infection with multidrug-resistant organisms

Alert your health care provider(s) about any post-travel illness and provide travel information details

MEDICATIONS

Bring extra medications in case of travel delays; ensure medications are labeled and in original packaging

Avoid taking medications purchased at destination due to potential drug–drug interactions

Drugs purchased at destination might also be counterfeit, falsely labeled, falsified, spurious, or substandard (see Sec. 6, Ch. 3, . . . *perspectives*: Avoiding Poorly Regulated Medicines & Medical Products During Travel)

SUN PROTECTION

Immunocompromised people have dramatically increased rates of skin cancer

Some medications used by immunocompromised people increase their risk of photosensitivity

Use sun protection regularly (see Sec. 4, Ch. 1, Sun Exposure)

BRING A TRAVEL HEALTH/FIRST AID KIT (see Sec. 2, Ch. 10, Travel Health Kits)

(www.cdc.gov/vaccines/hcp/acip-recs/general-recs/immunocompetence.pdf).

PRETRAVEL CONSIDERATIONS

Guidance regarding travel-related prophylaxis and vaccination for immunocompromised individuals is less evidence-based than routine guidance for travelers; the recommendations included here are based on the best available data and the practices of experienced clinicians.

Causes of Immunosuppression. Clinicians should recognize that different underlying conditions and medications produce varying degrees of immunocompromise.

Consultation with Other Providers. With permission, consider consulting with the traveler's primary or specialty care provider(s) to identify whether the underlying medical condition is stable, to discuss fitness for travel, and to verify medications and doses. Travel medicine providers also can use such a consultation to evaluate whether any travel-related disease-prevention measures could destabilize the underlying medical condition, either directly or through drug interactions.

Contraindications & Other Health Risks. Providers should assess whether the traveler's conditions, medications, and treatments constitute contraindications to, decrease the effectiveness of, or increase the risk for adverse events from any of the disease-prevention measures recommended for the proposed trip. Depending on the destination, prevention measures might include immunizations or medications for malaria chemoprophylaxis and/or self-treatment for travelers' diarrhea. Providers also should assess whether health hazards at the destination could exacerbate any underlying conditions or cause more severe health outcomes in an immunocompromised traveler, and determine whether specific interventions are available to mitigate these risks.

Emergency Planning. All international travelers should have plans in place in the event they become ill overseas; this is an even more critical component of pretravel preparation for immunocompromised travelers. An immunocompromised traveler should have a plan for when and how to seek care overseas, including a plan for medical evacuation, if necessary, and a plan for how to pay for it. For more details, see the chapters in Sec. 6, Ch. 1, Travel Insurance, Travel Health Insurance & Medical Evacuation Insurance, and Sec. 6, Ch. 2, Obtaining Health Care Abroad.

Immune Status & Vaccinations. The traveler's immune status is particularly relevant to vaccinations. Overall considerations for vaccine recommendations (e.g., destination, likely risk for exposure to disease) are the same for immunocompromised travelers as for other travelers. Providers should weigh the risk for severe illness or death from a vaccine-preventable disease against potential adverse events from administering a live vaccine to an immunocompromised patient. In some cases, an immunocompromised traveler might be unable to tolerate recommended immunizations, in which case the traveler should consider changing the itinerary, altering the planned travel activities, or deferring the trip.

APPROACH TO IMMUNIZATIONS

Take a careful history and consider the nature of underlying diseases when preparing anyone for international travel. Keep in mind that not all medical conditions necessitate special considerations for pretravel immunizations (see Table 3-01). Recommend and provide all appropriate travel vaccines to those with chronic health conditions. Two categories of travelers requiring special consideration with regard to immunizations are those with limited immune deficits and those with severe immune compromise. Vaccine recommendations for different categories of immunocompromised adults are listed in Table 3-02 and Table 3-03.

Table 3-01 Health conditions & treatments that do not require specialized immunization precautions at the pretravel visit

HEALTH CONDITION OR TREATMENT	CIRCUMSTANCES UNDER WHICH NO SPECIALIZED PRECAUTIONS ARE REQUIRED
Cancer History	Received last chemotherapy treatment ≥3 months previously and malignancy in remission. For patients receiving immunotherapy agents (e.g., checkpoint inhibitors), discuss all travel and vaccination plans directly with the oncologist; waiting times for vaccination can be longer.
Corticosteroid treatments	Short- or long-term daily or alternate-day therapy with <20 mg of prednisone or equivalent. Maintenance steroids at physiologic doses (replacement therapy). Steroid inhalers or topical steroids (i.e., skin, ears, or eyes). Intraarticular, bursal, or tendon steroid injections. >1 month since high-dose (≥20 mg/day of prednisone or equivalent for ≥2 weeks) steroid use.[1]
Hematopoietic stem cell transplant recipients or CAR-T cell recipients	Meets all criteria: >2 years posttransplant; not on immunosuppressive drugs; no evidence of ongoing malignancy; and without graft-versus-host disease.
Multiple sclerosis or autoimmune disease (e.g., inflammatory bowel disease, rheumatoid arthritis, systemic lupus erythematosus)	Not receiving immunosuppressive or immunomodulatory drug therapy, although definitive data are lacking

[1]After short-term (<2 weeks) therapy with daily or alternate-day dosing of ≥20 mg of prednisone or equivalent, some experts will wait ≥2 weeks before administering live vaccines.

Table 3-02 Immunization of immunocompromised adults: live vaccines*

LIVE VACCINES	HIV INFECTION CD4 COUNT ≥200/ML	HIV INFECTION CD4 COUNT <200/ML	SEVERE IMMUNOSUPPRESSION (NON-HIV)	ASPLENIA	RENAL FAILURE
Bacillus Calmette-Guérin (BCG)	CONTRAINDICATED	CONTRAINDICATED	CONTRAINDICATED	USE AS INDICATED	USE AS INDICATED
Cholera[1]	NO DATA	NO DATA	NO DATA	USE AS INDICATED	USE AS INDICATED
Ebola[2]	CONSIDER	CONSIDER	CONSIDER	USE AS INDICATED	USE AS INDICATED
Influenza, live attenuated	CONTRAINDICATED	CONTRAINDICATED	CONTRAINDICATED	CONTRAINDICATED	PRECAUTION
Measles-mumps-rubella[3]	RECOMMENDED	CONTRAINDICATED	CONTRAINDICATED	USE AS INDICATED	USE AS INDICATED
Smallpox/monkeypox[4] (JYNNEOS)	NO DATA	NO DATA	NO DATA	NO DATA	NO DATA
Typhoid, Ty21a	CONTRAINDICATED	CONTRAINDICATED	CONTRAINDICATED	USE AS INDICATED	USE AS INDICATED
Varicella (adults)[5]	CONSIDER	CONTRAINDICATED	CONTRAINDICATED	USE AS INDICATED	USE AS INDICATED
Yellow fever[6]	PRECAUTION	CONTRAINDICATED	CONTRAINDICATED	USE AS INDICATED	OTHER CONSIDERATIONS[7]

*A determination that a vaccine is *contraindicated* or has a *precaution* is based on Advisory Committee on Immunization Practices (ACIP) recommendations. *Use as indicated* means the vaccine should be used the same in travelers as in non-travelers with this condition. *Recommended* means the vaccine is recommended for all patients in this category.

[1]No safety or efficacy data exist regarding use of the current formulation of CVD 103-HgR vaccine in HIV-positive adults or people with severe immunosuppression. Limited data from an older formulation of the CVD 103-HgR suggest no association between the vaccine and serious or systemic adverse events, and slightly lower immunogenicity of the vaccine in HIV-positive versus HIV-negative adults.

[2]Providers need to weigh the risk associated with vaccination against the risk for Ebola disease in HIV-positive and severely immunosuppressed patients.

[3]Measles-mumps-rubella (MMR) vaccination is recommended for all HIV-infected patients aged ≥12 months with (for patients aged <6 years) CD4+ T-lymphocyte count ≥15% or (for patients aged ≥6 years) CD4+ T-lymphocyte count ≥15% and CD4+ T-lymphocyte counts ≥200/mL for ≥6 months, if they are without evidence of measles immunity. IG can be administered for short-term protection of people facing high risk of measles and for whom MMR vaccine is contraindicated. Additional guidance is available from www.cdc.gov/mmwr/preview/mmwrhtml/rr6204a1.htm.

[4]Some experts would consider JYNNEOS a non-live vaccine since it is replication-incompetent.

[5]Varicella vaccine should not be administered to people who have cellular immunodeficiencies, but people with impaired humoral immunity (including congenital or acquired hypoglobulinemia or dysglobulinemia) can be vaccinated. HIV-positive adults with CD4+ T-lymphocyte counts ≥200 cells/mL can receive 2 doses of vaccine spaced at 3-month intervals. VariZIG (varicella zoster–specific immune globulin) is recommended for people exposed to varicella or herpes zoster if they do not have evidence of varicella immunity and have contraindications to vaccination.

[6]For details, see Sec. 5, Part 2, Ch. 26, Yellow Fever. Yellow fever (YF) vaccination is a precaution for asymptomatic HIV-infected people with CD4+ T-lymphocyte counts of 200–499/mL. YF vaccination is not a precaution for people with asymptomatic HIV infection and CD4+ T-lymphocyte counts ≥500/mL. ACIP also considers YF vaccine contraindicated for symptomatic HIV patients without AIDS and with CD4+ T-lymphocyte counts <200/mL.

[7]No data suggest increased risk of serious adverse events after use of YF vaccine in people with renal failure; varying degrees of immune deficit might be present, however, and providers should carefully weigh vaccine risks and benefits before deciding to vaccinate people with this condition.

Table 3-03 Immunization of immunocompromised adults: non-live vaccines*

NON-LIVE VACCINES	HIV INFECTION CD4 COUNT ≥200/ML	HIV INFECTION CD4 COUNT <200/ML	SEVERE IMMUNOSUPPRESION (NON-HIV)	ASPLENIA	RENAL FAILURE
COVID-19	USE AS INDICATED	USE AS INDICATED	USE AS INDICATED	USE AS INDICATED	USE AS INDICATED
DTaP	USE AS INDICATED	USE AS INDICATED	USE AS INDICATED	USE AS INDICATED	USE AS INDICATED
Haemophilus influenzae type b (Hib)	USE AS INDICATED	USE AS INDICATED	OTHER CONSIDERATIONS[1]	RECOMMENDED[2]	USE AS INDICATED
Hepatitis A[3]	RECOMMENDED	RECOMMENDED	USE AS INDICATED	USE AS INDICATED	USE AS INDICATED
Hepatitis B[4]	RECOMMENDED	RECOMMENDED	USE AS INDICATED	USE AS INDICATED	RECOMMENDED[5]
Human papillomavirus[6]	USE AS INDICATED	USE AS INDICATED	USE AS INDICATED	USE AS INDICATED	USE AS INDICATED
Influenza, inactivated or recombinant	RECOMMENDED	RECOMMENDED	RECOMMENDED	RECOMMENDED	RECOMMENDED
Japanese encephalitis[7]	NO DATA	NO DATA	NO DATA	NO DATA	NO DATA
Meningococcal conjugate (ACWY)[8]	RECOMMENDED	RECOMMENDED	USE AS INDICATED	RECOMMENDED	USE AS INDICATED
Meningococcal group B	USE AS INDICATED	USE AS INDICATED	USE AS INDICATED	RECOMMENDED	USE AS INDICATED
PCV15 followed by PPSV23[9]	RECOMMENDED	RECOMMENDED	RECOMMENDED	RECOMMENDED	RECOMMENDED
PCV20[9]	RECOMMENDED	RECOMMENDED	RECOMMENDED	RECOMMENDED	RECOMMENDED
Polio (IPV)	USE AS INDICATED	USE AS INDICATED	USE AS INDICATED	USE AS INDICATED	USE AS INDICATED
Rabies	USE AS INDICATED	OTHER CONSIDERATIONS[10]	OTHER CONSIDERATIONS[10]	USE AS INDICATED	USE AS INDICATED

(continued)

Table 3-03 Immunization of immunocompromised adults: non-live vaccines (continued)

NON-LIVE VACCINES	HIV INFECTION CD4 COUNT ≥200/ML	HIV INFECTION CD4 COUNT <200/ML	SEVERE IMMUNOSUPPRESION (NON-HIV)	ASPLENIA	RENAL FAILURE
Td or Tdap	USE AS INDICATED	USE AS INDICATED	USE AS INDICATED	USE AS INDICATED	USE AS INDICATED
Tick-borne encephalitis	NO DATA	NO DATA	NO DATA	NO DATA	NO DATA
Typhoid, Vi	USE AS INDICATED	USE AS INDICATED	USE AS INDICATED	USE AS INDICATED	USE AS INDICATED
Zoster, recombinant (RZV)[11]	RECOMMENDED	RECOMMENDED	RECOMMENDED	USE AS INDICATED	USE AS INDICATED

Abbreviations: COVID-19, coronavirus disease; PCV13, 13-valent pneumococcal conjugate vaccine; PPSV23, 23-valent pneumococcal polysaccharide vaccine.

**Use as indicated* means the vaccine should be used the same in travelers as in non-travelers with this condition. *Recommended* means the vaccine is recommended for all patients in this category.

[1]Recipients of a hematopoietic stem cell transplant should be vaccinated with a 3-dose regimen 6–12 months after a successful transplant, regardless of vaccination history; administer doses ≥4 weeks apart.

[2]In adults, Hib is recommended for people with asplenia only if they have not previously received Hib vaccine.

[3]Routinely indicated for all men who have sex with men, patients with chronic hepatitis, patients with HIV infection, injection drug users, and others.

[4]Hepatitis B vaccination is indicated for people at risk for infection by sexual exposure, including sex partners of hepatitis B surface antigen (HBsAg)-positive people, sexually active people who are not in a long-term mutually monogamous relationship, people seeking evaluation or treatment for a sexually transmitted disease, men who have sex with men, people at risk for infection by percutaneous or mucosal exposure to blood, current or recent injection drug users, household contacts of HBsAg-positive people, residents and staff of facilities for developmentally disabled people, health care and public safety workers with reasonably anticipated risk for exposure to blood or blood-contaminated body fluids, people with end-stage renal disease, international travelers to regions with high or intermediate levels (HBsAg prevalence >2%) of endemic hepatitis B virus infection (see Map 5-07), people with chronic liver disease, people <60 years of age with diabetes, and people with HIV infection.

[5]Adult patients ≥20 years old receiving hemodialysis or with other immunocompromising conditions should receive 1 dose of 40 µg/mL Recombivax HB administered on a 3-dose schedule at 0, 1, and 6 months or 2 doses of 20 µg/mL, or (Engerix-B) administered simultaneously on a 4-dose schedule at 0, 1, 2, and 6 months. Test for antibodies to hepatitis B virus surface antigen serum after vaccination, and revaccinate if initial antibody response is absent or suboptimal (<10 mIU/mL). HIV-infected nonresponders might react to a subsequent vaccine course if CD4+ T-lymphocyte counts rise to 500/mL after institution of highly active antiretroviral therapy. Heplisav-B (HepB-CpG) is a non-aluminum adjuvanted vaccine and should be administered as 2 doses, 1 month apart, in people ≥18 years of age, including hemodialysis and immunocompromised people. Postvaccination serologic testing is recommended. See text for discussion of other immunocompromised groups.

[6]Human papillomavirus (HPV) vaccine (3 dose schedule at 0, 1–2, and 6 months) is recommended through age 26 years.

[7]No safety or efficacy data exist regarding the use of IXIARO in immunocompromised people. In general, inactivated vaccines can be administered safely to people with altered immunocompetence, using the usual doses and schedules, but the effectiveness might be suboptimal. The inactivated, Vero cell–derived Japanese encephalitis vaccine, IXIARO, is the only Japanese encephalitis vaccine available in the United States; other types of Japanese encephalitis vaccines, including live vaccines, are available internationally but are not included here.

[8]Refer to Table 5-03. Meningococcal vaccines licensed & available in the United States: recommendations for travelers to or residents of countries where meningococcal disease is hyperendemic or epidemic

[9]On October 20, 2021, the ACIP approved recommendations to use PCV20 alone, or PCV15 in series with PPSV23, for all adults aged ≥65 years and for adults aged 19–64 years with underlying medical conditions who have not previously received a pneumococcal conjugate vaccine or whose vaccination history is unknown. Official guidance on use of these vaccines is being developed.

[10]For postexposure prophylaxis, both vaccine (5 doses at day 0, 3, 7, 14, 28) and immune globulin should be given to immunocompromised people regardless of previous vaccination status.

[11]For patients with altered immunocompetence, RZV is recommended for people ≥18 years old. RZV is recommended for people ≥50 years old without altered immunocompetence. Patients with renal disease or asplenia who are taking immunosuppressive medication should receive RZV beginning at 18 years of age.

Preparing Travelers with Limited Immune Deficits

ASPLENIA

Asplenia is associated with varying degrees of immune deficit. For vaccination purposes, people with asplenia generally are not considered immunocompromised, and live vaccines are not contraindicated. People with anatomic or functional asplenia (including those with sickle cell disease or complement deficiency) and people taking eculizumab or ravulizumab (complement inhibitors used to treat paroxysmal nocturnal hemoglobinuria and atypical hemolytic uremic syndrome) are susceptible to overwhelming and rapidly progressive sepsis with certain bacterial pathogens, despite indicated immunizations.

Although response to vaccines might be diminished compared with people who have a functioning spleen, immunization against *Haemophilus influenzae* type b, and meningococcal (MenACWY and MenB) and pneumococcal disease, is recommended for patients with asplenia, regardless of travel plans. Because age-appropriate dosing and schedules for this population differ from competent hosts, consult the recommended immunization schedules (www.cdc.gov/vaccines/schedules/hcp/index.html) and the guidelines in Table 3-02 and Table 3-03.

Advise asplenic travelers to seek immediate medical attention if they develop a fever and to be prepared to initiate broad-spectrum antibiotic self-treatment. Moreover, people with asplenia should consider avoiding travel to destinations lacking immediate access to high-standard medical care.

ASYMPTOMATIC HIV INFECTION

Asymptomatic adults with HIV and CD4+ T-lymphocyte counts of 200–499/mL are considered to have limited immune deficits and should be vaccinated according to the guidelines in Table 3-02 and Table 3-03. To categorize risk in people living with HIV, use CD4+ T-lymphocyte counts performed while the patient is receiving antiretroviral drugs, rather than nadir counts. The Advisory Committee on Immunization Practices (ACIP) recommends hepatitis A (HepA), hepatitis B (HepB), meningococcal (MenACWY), and pneumococcal vaccines for all HIV-positive patients, regardless of travel plans. Live attenuated influenza vaccine (LAIV) is contraindicated in all patients with HIV, regardless of CD4+ T-lymphocyte count.

The Infectious Diseases Society of America (IDSA) has identified a knowledge gap in the optimal time to initiate vaccination after starting antiretroviral therapy. Many clinicians advise a 3-month delay after immune reconstitution (usually 6 months after initiation of antiretroviral therapy) if possible, before immunizations are administered in order to maximize the immune response to vaccination. Although seroconversion rates and geometric mean titers of antibody response to vaccines might be less than those measured in healthy controls, most vaccines can elicit protective antibody levels in HIV-infected patients in this category.

Transient increases in HIV viral load, which return quickly to baseline, have been observed after administration of several different vaccines; this generally does not occur in patients whose viral loads are well controlled on antiretroviral therapies. The clinical significance of these increases is not known, but the increases do not preclude the use of any vaccine.

HEPATITIS A VACCINE

Because response to HepA vaccine might be reduced in people with HIV infection, perform postvaccination serologic testing on all people with HIV infection ≥1 month after they complete the HepA vaccine series. Consider repeating the vaccine series for patients with poor immune response (i.e., hepatitis A virus [HAV] IgG titer <10 mIU/mL), particularly those who later demonstrate improved immune status (e.g., increased CD4+ T-lymphocyte counts, decreased HIV viral load). If HAV IgG titers are still <10 mIU/mL ≥1 month after the revaccination series, additional vaccination is not recommended; instead, counsel the person on the need to receive HepA immune globulin after an exposure or for higher-risk travel.

HEPATITIS B VACCINE

In a study of people infected with HIV who had no immune response to 1 or 2 courses of recombinant HepB vaccine, 2 doses of adjuvanted vaccine (Heplisav-B) were 87% effective in achieving seroprotection.

INTRAVENOUS IMMUNOGLOBULIN

People with HIV might receive periodic doses of intravenous immunoglobulin (IVIG), which can interfere with the immune response to MMR and varicella vaccine. If considering vaccination with MMR or varicella vaccine, administer the vaccines ≈14 days before the next scheduled IVIG dose.

MEASLES-MUMPS-RUBELLA VACCINE

Two doses of measles-mumps-rubella (MMR) vaccine are recommended for all HIV-infected individuals aged ≥12 months who do not have evidence of current severe immunosuppression (i.e., individuals aged ≤5 years must have CD4+ T-lymphocyte percentages ≥15% for ≥6 months; individuals aged >5 years must have CD4+ T-lymphocyte percentages ≥15% and CD4+ T-lymphocyte counts ≥200 lymphocytes/mL for ≥6 months). Specific recommendations are available for MMR vaccine in people living with HIV (see www.cdc.gov/vaccines/hcp/acip-recs/general-recs/immunocompetence.pdf).

CHRONIC DISEASES

Factors to consider when assessing the level of immune competence of patients with chronic diseases include clinical stability, comorbidities, complications, duration, severity, and any potentially immunosuppressing treatment (see Sec. 3, Ch. 3, Travelers with Chronic Illnesses). The pretravel health consultation is an opportunity to ensure that these individuals are vaccinated with recommended routine vaccinations (e.g., HepB and pneumococcal vaccines).

COMPLEMENT DEFICIENCIES

Patients with complement deficiencies can receive any live or inactivated vaccine.

DYSGAMMAGLOBULINEMIAS

Many people with hypogammaglobulinemia or dysgammaglobulinemia receive periodic doses of IVIG, which can interfere with the immune response to MMR and varicella vaccine. If considering vaccination MMR or varicella vaccine, administer the vaccines ≈14 days before the next scheduled IVIG dose.

MULTIPLE SCLEROSIS

Modern multiple sclerosis (MS) therapy often includes aggressive and early immunomodulatory therapy, even for patients with stable disease. Inactivated vaccines, including HepB, human papillomavirus, influenza, tetanus, and recombinant zoster vaccines generally are considered safe for people with MS. In the event of a clinical relapse, however, delay vaccination until patients have stabilized or begun to improve, typically 4–6 weeks after the relapse began. Although safety and efficacy data are lacking, inactivated vaccines are theoretically safe for people with MS being treated with interferon medication, glatiramer acetate, mitoxantrone, fingolimod, or monoclonal antibody class drugs (e.g., natalizumab, ocrelizumab, rituximab). Published studies are lacking on the safety and efficacy of other vaccines (e.g., HepA, meningococcal, pertussis, pneumococcal, polio, typhoid).

LIVE VACCINES

Do not administer live vaccines to people with MS during therapy with immunosuppressant drugs (e.g., azathioprine, cladribine, cyclophosphamide, methotrexate, mitoxantrone, ponesimod, teriflunomide); during chronic corticosteroid therapy; or during therapy with any immunosuppressive biologic agents, including alemtuzumab, natalizimab, ocrelixumab, ocrelizumab, ofatumumab, ozanimod, rituximab, and siponimod. Although definitive studies of glatiramer acetate and interferon therapy are lacking, MS experts generally do not classify them as immunosuppressive medications, and their use does not preclude live vaccine administration. Published studies suggest that live viral MMR and varicella vaccines are safe for people with stable MS if administered 1 month before starting, or at the appropriate interval after discontinuing, immunosuppressive therapy (see Vaccine Considerations for Travelers with Severe Immune Compromise, later in this chapter).

YELLOW FEVER VACCINE

A small case series published in 2011 reported worsening of MS symptoms and plaques in 5 of 7 patients with relapsing-remitting MS who received yellow fever (YF) vaccine. In contrast, two other studies (published in 2020 and 2021) identified no exacerbations among 55 people with MS who received YF vaccine at different stages of their disease and who were taking a wide variety of medications. Before administering YF vaccine to people with MS who are receiving disease-modifying therapy or nataluzimab, consider the risk of YF virus infection at the destination, as well as potential vaccine-associated risks. Because the effects of YF vaccination in patients receiving disease-modifying therapy or nataluzimab have not been fully studied, decisions about YF vaccination should be made in consultation with the patient's neurologist. For brief exposures (e.g., only a few days in a YF endemic area) vaccinating travelers with MS against YF likely should be avoided. Weigh the risks and benefits of vaccination for travelers anticipating more prolonged exposures.

Preparing Travelers with Severe Immune Compromise

SEVERELY IMMUNOCOMPROMISING CONDITIONS

Severely immunocompromised people include those with aplastic anemia, graft-versus-host disease, symptomatic HIV/AIDs, some congenital immunodeficiencies, active leukemia or lymphoma, or generalized malignancy. Others with severe immune compromise include people who recently received radiation therapy or checkpoint inhibitor treatment (therapy of autoimmune complications of treatment is immunosuppressive); people receiving active immunosuppression for solid organ transplants; and both chimeric antigen receptor (CAR)-T cell and hematopoietic stem cell transplant (HSCT) recipients (≤2 years of transplantation or still taking immunosuppressive drugs).

In most cases, severely immunocompromised people should not receive live vaccines, and inactivated vaccines will likely be less effective. These patients should consider postponing travel until their immune function improves. For people likely to travel in the future, usual travel-related vaccines can be initiated before beginning immunosuppressive therapies, if feasible. Whenever possible, administer inactivated vaccines ≥2 weeks and live vaccines ≥4 weeks before immunosuppression.

SYMPTOMATIC HIV/AIDS

Clinicians need to know an HIV-infected traveler's current CD4+ T-lymphocyte count for the pretravel consultation. People with HIV and CD4+ T-lymphocyte counts <200/mL, a history of an AIDS-defining illness without immune reconstitution, or clinical manifestations of symptomatic HIV are considered to have severe immunosuppression (see Sec. 5, Part 2, Ch. 11, Human Immunodeficiency Virus / HIV), and they should not receive live viral or live bacterial vaccines because of the risk that the vaccine could cause serious systemic disease. For MMR vaccine, severe immunosuppression is defined as CD4+ T-lymphocyte percentages <15% in any age group or CD4+ T-lymphocyte counts <200/mL in people >5 years old (see www.cdc.gov/mmwr/preview/mmwrhtml/rr6204a1.htm).

Recommend that newly diagnosed, treatment-naïve patients with CD4+ T-lymphocyte counts <200/mL delay travel pending reconstitution of CD4+ T-lymphocyte counts with antiretroviral therapy and, ideally, complete suppression of detectable viral replication. Delaying travel helps minimize the risk for infection and avoid immune reconstitution illness while away.

CHRONIC LYMPHOCYTIC LEUKEMIA & HEMATOPOIETIC STEM CELL TRANSPLANT

People with chronic lymphocytic leukemia have poor humoral immunity, even early in the disease course, and rarely respond to vaccines. Hematopoietic stem cell transplant (HSCT) recipients who received vaccines before their transplant should be revaccinated routinely afterward, regardless of the source of the transplanted stem cells. Begin complete revaccination with standard childhood vaccines 6 months after HSCT, with the caveat that MMR and varicella vaccines should be administered 24 months after transplant and only if the recipient is immunocompetent. Thus, HSCT recipients ideally should delay travel ≥2 years after transplant to allow for full revaccination.

Administer inactivated influenza vaccine beginning ≥6 months after HSCT and annually thereafter. A dose of inactivated influenza vaccine can be given ≥4 months after transplant if there is a community outbreak.

SOLID ORGAN TRANSPLANT RECIPIENTS

For solid organ transplant recipients, the risk for infection is greatest in the first year after transplant; recommend to travelers that they should postpone trips to high-risk destinations until after that time.

MEDICATIONS THAT COMPROMISE THE IMMUNE SYSTEM

3

A variety of medications and biologic agents compromise the immune system. Regard anyone taking these medications as severely immunocompromised. Doses of inactivated vaccines received while receiving immunosuppressive medications or during the 2 weeks before starting such medications should not be counted toward a primary vaccination series or relied upon to induce adequate immune responses. Patients should be revaccinated with all indicated inactivated vaccines at least 3 months after potent immunosuppressive therapy is discontinued.

ALKYLATING AGENTS

Regard anyone taking alkylating agents (e.g., cyclophosphamide) as severely immunocompromised.

ANTIMETABOLITES

Regard anyone taking antimetabolites (e.g., 6-mercaptopurine, azathioprine, methotrexate) as severely immunocompromised.

BIOLOGIC AGENTS

Immunosuppressive or immunomodulatory biologic agents can produce immunocompromise by the mechanisms outlined in Table 3-04. B cell–depleting agents (cladribine, ocrelizumab, ofatumumab, ozanimod, rituximab, siponimod) and lymphocyte-depleting agents (alemtuzumab, thymoglobulin) induce major immunosuppression. Consideration of the clinical context in which these were given is important, especially in hematologic malignancies.

CANCER CHEMOTHERAPEUTIC AGENTS

Cancer chemotherapeutic agents are classified as severely immunosuppressive, as demonstrated by increased rates of opportunistic infections and blunting of responses to certain vaccines among patient groups. Some of these agents are less immunosuppressive than others (e.g., tamoxifen and trastuzumab, given to breast cancer patients, are less immunosuppressive than alkylating agents or antimetabolites), but clinical data to support safety with live vaccines are lacking. Vaccination following immunotherapies (e.g., checkpoint inhibitors, CAR-T cell treatments) has not been well studied, and until additional data are available, avoid vaccinating patients receiving these treatments with live attenuated vaccines for 3–6 months after treatment or until they have had immune reconstitution.

HIGH-DOSE CORTICOSTEROIDS

Most clinicians consider a dose of >2 mg/kg of body weight or ≥20 mg per day of prednisone (or its equivalent) in people who weigh >10 kg, when administered for ≥2 weeks, as sufficiently immunosuppressive to raise concern about the safety of vaccination with live vaccines. Furthermore, the immune response to vaccines could be impaired. Clinicians should wait ≥1 month after discontinuation of high-dose systemic corticosteroid therapy before administering a live-virus vaccine.

TRANSPLANT-RELATED IMMUNOSUPPRESSIVE DRUGS

Regard anyone receiving transplant-related immunosuppressive drugs as severely immunocompromised. Examples of transplant-related immunosuppressive drugs include azathioprine, belatacept, cyclosporine, everolimus, mycophenolate mofetil, prednisone, sirolimus, and tacrolimus.

TUMOR NECROSIS FACTOR BLOCKERS

Tumor necrosis factor (TNF) blockers (e.g., adalimumab, certolizumab pegol, etanercept, golimumab, infliximab) blunt the immune response to certain chronic infections and certain vaccines. When used alone or in combination regimens with other disease-modifying agents to treat rheumatoid disease, TNF blockers are associated with an impaired response to HepA, influenza, and pneumococcal vaccines, suggesting that for better protection, all doses in the HepA and pneumococcal series should be given before travel. The use of live vaccines is contraindicated for most people receiving these therapies.

Table 3-04 Immunosuppressive & immunomodulatory biologic agents that preclude use of live vaccines[1]

GENERIC NAME	TRADE NAME	MECHANISM OF ACTION
Abatacept	Orencia	Binds CD80 and CD86, thereby blocking interaction with CD28
Acalabrutinib	Calquence	Tyrosine kinase inhibitor
Adalimumab	Humira	Binds and blocks TNF-α
Alemtuzumab	Campath	Binds CD52 antigen
Anakinra	Kineret	Blocks IL-1
Atezolizumab	Tecentriq	Blocks Programmed Cell Death Ligand 1 (PD-L1)
Avelumab	Bavencio	Blocks Programmed Cell Death Ligand 1 (PD-L1)
Basiliximab	Simulect	Blocks the IL-2Ra receptor chain
Belatacept	Nulojix	Binds CD80 and CD86, thereby blocking interaction with CD28
Bevacizumab	Avastin	Binds VEGF
Certolizumab pegol	Cimzia	Blocks TNF-α
Cetuximab	Erbitux	Binds to EGFR, and inhibits the binding of EGF and TGF-α
Dasatinib	Sprycel	Bcr-Abl tyrosine kinase inhibitor
Dimethyl fumarate	Tecfidera	Activates the nuclear erythroid 2-related factor 2 transcriptional pathway
Etanercept	Enbrel	Blocks TNF-α
Fingolimod	Gilenya	Sphingosine 1-phosphate receptor modulator
Glatiramer acetate	Copaxone	Immunomodulatory; target unknown
Golimumab	Simponi	Blocks TNF-α
Ibritumomab tiuxetan	Zevalin	Binds to CD20 cells
Ibrutinib	Imbruvica	Tyrosine kinase inhibitor
Imatinib mesylate	Gleevec, STI 571	Signal transduction inhibitor/protein-tyrosine kinase inhibitor
Infliximab	Remicade	Blocks TNF-α
Interferon α	Pegasys, PegIntron	Immunomodulatory

(continued)

Table 3-04 Immunosuppressive & immunomodulatory biologic agents that preclude use of live vaccines (continued)

GENERIC NAME	TRADE NAME	MECHANISM OF ACTION
Interferon beta-1a	Avonex, Rebif	Immunomodulatory; target unknown
Interferon beta-1b	Betaseron	Immunomodulatory; target unknown
Lenalidomide	Revlimid	Immunomodulatory
Natalizumab	Tysabri	Binds α4-integrin on leukocytes, which inhibits adhesion
Nivolumab	Opdivo	Activates CD8 cells by targeting the PD-1 pathway
Ocrelizumab	Ocrevus	Binds CD20
Ofatumumab	Arzerra	Binds CD20
Panitumumab	Vectibix	Binds EGFR, inhibiting the binding of other ligands
Pembrolizumab	Keytruda	Activates CD8 cells by targeting the PD-1 pathway
Rilonacept	Arcalyst	Binds and blocks IL-1
Rituximab	Rituxan	Binds CD20
Sarilumab	Kevzara	Binds IL-6
Secukinumab	Cosentyx	Selectively binds to the interleukin-17A (IL-17A) cytokine
Sunitinib malate	Sutent	Multikinase inhibitor
Tocilizumab	Actemra	Binds IL-6
Tofacitinib	Xeljanz	JAK kinase inhibitor
Trastuzumab	Herceptin	Binds to the Human EGFR 2 (HER2)
Ustekinumab	Stelara	Binds to IL-12 and IL-23
Vedolizumab	Entyvio	Binds integrin $\alpha_4\beta_7$
Zanubrutinib	Brukinsa	Tyrosine kinase inhibitor

Abbreviations: CD, cluster of differentiation; CTLA, cytotoxic T-lymphocyte antigen; EGFR, epidermal growth factor receptor; IL, interleukin; PD, programmed cell death protein; TGF, transforming growth factor; TNF, tumor necrosis factor; VEGF, vascular endothelial growth factor.

[1]This table is based primarily on conservative expert opinion, given the lack of clinical data. Numerous agents often are given in combination with other agents (especially chemotherapy) and are immunosuppressive when given together. The list provides examples but is not inclusive of all biologic agents that suppress or modulate the immune system. Not all therapeutic monoclonal antibodies or other biologic agents result in immunosuppression; details of individual agents not listed here must be reviewed before determining whether live viral vaccines can be given. Interferon and glatiramer acetate given to patients with multiple sclerosis (MS) are immunomodulators and are generally not classified by MS experts as immunosuppressive so do not preclude live vaccine administration (except perhaps yellow fever vaccine), but clinical data to support safety with live vaccines are lacking.

VACCINE CONSIDERATIONS FOR TRAVELERS WITH SEVERE IMMUNE COMPROMISE

Inform severely immunocompromised people that their response to vaccination might be muted. The immunosuppressive regimen does not predict the decrease in response to vaccination. No basis exists for interpreting laboratory studies of general immune parameters to predict vaccine safety or efficacy. Recent data in solid organ transplant recipients vaccinated before transplant suggest that a prolonged phase of protective antibody titers can exist after transplant. In general, serologic testing for response to most travel-related vaccines is not clinically recommended.

The length of time clinicians should wait after discontinuation of immunosuppressive therapies before administering a live vaccine is not uniform and depends on the therapy. For cancer chemotherapy, radiation therapy, and highly immunosuppressive medications (exclusive of lymphocyte-depleting agents and organ transplant immunosuppression), the waiting period is 3 months. For lymphocyte-depleting agents (alemtuzumab, rituximab), the waiting period is ≥6 months, although IDSA guidelines suggest that the waiting period should be ≥1 year. For immunosuppressive corticosteroid regimens, the waiting period is 1 month.

Restarting immunosuppression after live vaccination has not been studied, but some experts would recommend waiting ≥1 month. Special considerations for travelers with severe immune compromise apply for several travel-related vaccines.

CHOLERA

The safety and effectiveness of the oral live attenuated bacterial cholera vaccine, Vaxchora, has not been established in immunocompromised people. An older formulation of CVD 103-HgR vaccine was not associated with serious or systemic adverse events in patients with HIV, although the data are limited.

EBOLA

Safety and efficacy of Ebola Zaire live recombinant vaccine (ERVEBO, rVSV-ZEBOV vaccine [Merck Sharp & Dohme Corp.]) has not been adequately assessed in immunocompromised adults. A small number of adults living with HIV have been vaccinated with ERVEBO, and additional studies are ongoing to investigate its use in people living with HIV without severe immune compromise. The risk from vaccination with ERVEBO in immunocompromised people should be weighed against the risk for Ebola virus disease.

HEPATITIS A

Data indicate that immunocompromised people, notably those being treated with immunosuppressive drugs, can have inadequate or slow seroconversion after a single dose of HepA vaccine. Limited data also suggest that modified dosing regimens, including a doubling of the standard antigen dose or administration of additional doses prior to travel, might increase response rates.

Solid organ transplant candidates who are unvaccinated, undervaccinated, or seronegative for HepA should receive a 2-dose HepA vaccine series. People with immunocompromising conditions should start a 2-dose HepA vaccine series as soon as travel is considered. Immunocompromised people traveling in <2 weeks should simultaneously receive the initial dose of HepA vaccine and HepA immune globulin (IG); administer the vaccine and the IG in separate limbs. Testing for the presence of HAV antibody after vaccination is recommended for immunocompromised people whose subsequent clinical management depends on knowledge of their immune status and people for whom revaccination might be indicated. Because response to HepA vaccine might be reduced in people with HIV infection, perform postvaccination serologic testing on all people with HIV infection ≥1 month after they complete the HepA vaccine series.

HEPATITIS B

The humoral immune response to HepB vaccine is reduced in immunocompromised children and adults. Limited data indicate that modified dosing regimens could increase response rates. As with dialysis patients, use a 3-dose series of 40 μg Recombivax HB at 0, 1, and 6 months, or a 4-dose series of 40 μg Engerix-B at 0, 1, 2, and 6 months. Heplisav-B (HepB-CpG) is an adjuvanted vaccine and is administered as 2 doses, 1 month apart, in people ≥18 years old. Postvaccination serologic testing after any HepB vaccination series is recommended to confirm response and guide the need for revaccination in immunocompromised people.

JAPANESE ENCEPHALITIS

Although recommended for numerous destinations (see Sec. 5, Part 2, Ch. 13, Japanese Encephalitis), no data are available on the safety or efficacy of Japanese encephalitis (JE) vaccines in immunocompromised patients. JE vaccine should be given to at-risk travelers. As with other vaccines, immunocompromised patients likely will have decreased intensity and durability of protection, and more frequent booster doses might be indicated.

RABIES

Immunocompromised people deemed at risk for vaccine-preventable rabies should receive a 3-dose series of vaccine on days 0, 7, and 21 or 28, but not the 2-dose series (day 0 and day 7) recommended in 2021 for immunocompetent people. Furthermore, administer the vaccine as an intramuscular injection, not as an intradermal injection as recommended by some authorities outside the United States. Serologic postvaccination testing might be indicated. For postexposure rabies prophylaxis, all severely immunocompromised people should generally receive rabies vaccine at days 0, 3, 7, 14, and 28, plus human rabies immune globulin, regardless of previous vaccination history.

SMALLPOX / MONKEYPOX

JYNNEOS (Imvamune, Imvanex) is an approved by the US Food and Drug Administration (FDA) vaccine for prevention of smallpox and monkeypox, but it is not commercially available. JYNNEOS is a live, attenuated, nonreplicating, virus-derived vaccine that is indicated for first responders participating in smallpox or monkeypox outbreaks. Unlike the live, replication-competent smallpox vaccine (ACAM2000), JYNNEOS is not contraindicated for use in immunocompromised people and should be safe. Immunocompromised people might, however, have a diminished immune response to the vaccine.

TICK-BORNE ENCEPHALITIS

Immunocompromised people might have a diminished immune response to killed tick-borne encephalitis vaccine, which is FDA-approved and safe for this population.

TYPHOID FEVER

CDC recommends administering injectable Vi capsular polysaccharide vaccine (Typhim Vi, ViCPS) rather than live, oral *Salmonella typhi* vaccine Ty21A (Vivotif) for at-risk, immunocompromised patients. Data on the safety and efficacy of typhoid vaccines in immunocompromised patients are lacking.

YELLOW FEVER

CONTRAINDICATIONS

In general, strongly discourage unvaccinated travelers with severe immune compromise from traveling to destinations where infection with YF virus is a risk. Severe immunosuppression is a contraindication to YF vaccination because these patients are at increased risk of developing a serious adverse event (e.g., life-threatening YF vaccine–associated viscerotropic disease, YF vaccine–associated neurologic disease). Additionally, YF vaccination is contraindicated in people with a history of a thymus disorder associated with abnormal immune cell function (e.g., myasthenia gravis or thymoma); this contraindication applies regardless of whether the person has undergone therapeutic thymectomy (see Sec. 5, Part 2, Ch. 26, Yellow Fever). No data are available to support IgA deficiency as a contraindication to YF vaccination.

If patients are unable to avoid travel to areas where YF vaccination is recommended (see Maps 5-10 and 5-11) and the immunocompromised traveler is previously unvaccinated, inform them of YF risk, carefully instruct them in methods to avoid mosquito bites, and provide them with a vaccination medical waiver in their International Certificate of Vaccination or Prophylaxis (see https://wwwnc.cdc.gov/travel/page/icvp, and Sec. 5, Part 2, Ch. 26, Yellow Fever). Travelers falling into this category might choose to travel during periods of lower disease activity. Warn travelers that some countries with YF vaccine entry requirements might not honor YF vaccination waiver documents and that the traveler might be refused entry or quarantined.

PRECAUTIONS (RELATIVE CONTRAINDICATIONS)

ACIP considers certain conditions with limited immune deficits (e.g., asymptomatic HIV infection) to be precautions (as opposed to contraindications) to administration of YF vaccine. For these patients, offer YF vaccine if travel to YF-endemic areas is unavoidable, and monitor vaccine recipients closely for possible adverse effects. If country entry requirements, and not true exposure risk, are the only reasons to vaccinate a traveler with asymptomatic HIV infection or a limited immune deficit, the physician should provide a waiver (see https://wwwnc.cdc.gov/travel/page/icvp, and Sec. 5, Part 2, Ch. 26, Yellow Fever).

Studies show that higher CD4+ T-lymphocyte counts and suppressed HIV viral loads seem to be the key determinants for developing protective neutralizing antibodies after YF vaccination. Patients with undetectable viral loads respond well to YF vaccination regardless of CD4+ T-lymphocyte counts, although data are limited in those with CD4+ T-lymphocyte counts <200/mL. Because vaccine response might be suboptimal, such vaccinees are candidates for serologic testing 1 month after vaccination. For information about serologic testing, contact the state health department or CDC's Division of Vector-Borne Diseases at 970-221-6400. Current data from clinical and epidemiologic studies are insufficient to evaluate the actual risk for severe adverse effects associated with YF vaccine among recipients with limited immune deficits.

BOOSTER DOSES

Because a single dose of YF vaccine provides long-lasting protection, ACIP no longer recommends booster doses for most travelers. Additional doses of YF vaccine are recommended, however, for some people who might not have as robust or sustained immune response to YF vaccine.

People who received HSCT after receiving a dose of YF vaccine and who are sufficiently immunocompetent to be safely vaccinated should be revaccinated if travel puts them at risk for YF. People infected with HIV when they received their last dose of YF vaccine should receive a dose every 10 years if they continue to be at risk for YF and if their current CD4+ T-lymphocyte counts do not indicate precautions or contradictions. Recent data suggest that YF vaccination before solid organ transplant, even long before transplant, generally provides protective antibody levels after transplant.

ZOSTER

Although no extra pretravel indication exists, many travel clinics administer zoster vaccines. In 2021, the FDA approved the use of recombinant zoster vaccine (RZV), now the only available preparation in the United States, for all immunocompromised people ≥18 years of age.

ACIP recommends 2 doses of recombinant zoster vaccine for all adults ≥19 years old who are or who will be immunodeficient or immunosuppressed due to disease or therapy, regardless of travel plans. Qualifying underlying conditions include, but are not limited to, HSCT or solid organ transplant recipients, hematologic and or generalized cancer, HIV, and people receiving immunosuppressive therapy.

HOUSEHOLD CONTACTS

Routine Vaccines

Three live vaccines (MMR, rotavirus, and varicella) should be administered to susceptible household contacts and other close contacts of immunocompromised patients when indicated. If a varicella vaccine recipient has a rash after vaccination, direct contact with susceptible household contacts with altered immunocompetence should be avoided until the rash resolves. Educate immunocompromised patients about the risk for fecal–oral transmission of poliovirus in countries where the oral polio vaccine is used, since there have been reports of reversion to wild type virus with associated clinical disease.

For influenza vaccination, choose inactive influenza vaccine (IIV); household and other close contacts of mildly or moderately immunocompromised patients can safely receive LAIV if they are unable to receive IIV. LAIV is contraindicated in close contacts and caregivers of severely immunocompromised people who require a protected environment.

Smallpox / Monkeypox Vaccine

ACAM2000 is a live, replicating smallpox vaccine, indicated for use in military personnel and laboratory workers with potential exposure to the virus. Recipients of the vaccine can transmit the virus to household and intimate contacts; therefore, vaccinated family or household members should implement infection control measures, particularly those with immunocompromise. JYNNEOS is an FDA-approved but not commercially available live nonreplicating smallpox/monkeypox vaccine that would not be contraindicated in immunocompromised individuals or their contacts.

Yellow Fever Vaccine

Yellow fever vaccine can be administered to household contacts when indicated.

MALARIA PROPHYLAXIS & TREATMENT

Malaria infection and the drugs used to treat it can exacerbate an immunocompromised traveler's underlying condition. Moreover, asplenia, HIV, and some immunosuppressive regimens can predispose travelers to more serious malaria infection. For these reasons, stress the need for malaria prophylaxis and strict adherence to mosquito bite avoidance to immunocompromised travelers to malaria-endemic areas (see Sec. 2, Ch. 5, Yellow Fever Vaccine and Malaria Prevention Information, by Country; Sec. 4, Ch. 6, Mosquitoes, Ticks & Other Arthropods; and Sec. 5, Part 3, Ch. 16, Malaria).

People Infected with HIV

Malaria is more severe in people infected with HIV; malaria infection increases HIV viral load and could exacerbate disease progression. In addition, take extra care when researching potential drug interactions in people with HIV who are receiving antiretroviral therapy. The University of Liverpool offers an interactive web-based resource for assessing possible drug interactions (www.hiv-druginteractions.org; a mobile application also is available).

CHEMOPROPHYLAXIS

Some older maintenance regimens for HIV have been noted to interact with drugs used for malaria chemoprophylaxis. Notably, chloroquine, mefloquine, and primaquine can interact with older maintenance regimens for HIV, particularly those containing protease inhibitors (PIs). Efavirenz lowers serum levels of both atovaquone and proguanil, but no evidence suggests clinical failure of these agents when used concurrently. Efavirenz also potentially can increase the production of hemotoxic primaquine metabolites.

Most current first-line regimens for HIV (integrase and entry inhibitors) have few drug interactions. Commonly used integrase inhibitors (bicetegravir, cabotegravir, dolutegravir, elvitegravir, raltegravir), and nucleoside/nucleotide reverse transcriptase inhibitor (NRTI) combinations (brand names include Descovy-Tivicay, Truvada-Tivicay) have no known interactions with CDC-recommended malaria chemoprophylactic drugs; the cobicistat booster co-formulated with elvitegravir (Stribild, Genvoya) theoretically could increase mefloquine levels. The emtricitabine, rilpivirine, tenofovir alafenamide (TAF)/tenofovir disoproxil fumarate (TDF) combinations (Odefsey and Complera) similarly have no interactions with antimalarial drugs.

TREATMENT

Malaria treatment regimens, including artemisinin derivatives, quinine/quinidine, lumefantrine (part of the artemether/lumefantrine combination, Coartem), and atovaquone and proguanil potentially could have interactions with many non-nucleoside reverse transcriptase inhibitors (NNRTIs), PIs, and the CCR5 receptor antagonist, maraviroc. Seek advice from CDC or other malaria experts when treating patients for malaria who are also on antiretrovirals.

Organ Transplant Recipients

In organ transplant recipients, atovaquone-proguanil might be the most appropriate malaria prophylactic agent because other antimalarials can interact with calcineurin inhibitors and mTor inhibitors (cyclosporine, everolimus, sirolimus, tacrolimus). Chloroquine, doxycycline mefloquine, and primaquine can elevate calcineurin inhibitor levels. Chloroquine and mefloquine can interact with calcineurin inhibitors to prolong the QT interval. Some travel-related medications need to be dose-adjusted according to altered hepatic or renal function.

ENTERIC INFECTIONS

Many foodborne and waterborne infections (e.g., those caused by *Campylobacter, Cryptosporidium, Giardia, Listeria, Salmonella*, or *Shigella*) can be severe or become chronic in immunocompromised people. Provide all travelers with instruction on safe food and beverage precautions; travelers' diarrhea can occur despite strict adherence. Meticulous hand hygiene, including frequent and thorough handwashing with soap and water, is the best prevention against gastroenteritis. Travelers should wash hands after contact with public surfaces, after any contact with animals or their living areas, and before preparing or eating food.

Travelers' Diarrhea

Selecting antimicrobial drugs for appropriate self-treatment of travelers' diarrhea (see Sec. 2, Ch. 6, Travelers' Diarrhea) requires special consideration of potential drug interactions in patients already taking medications for chronic medical conditions. Fluoroquinolones, rifaximin, and rifamycin SV are active against several enteric bacterial pathogens and are not known to have major interactions with highly active antiretroviral therapy (HAART) drugs. Macrolide antibiotics can, however, interact with HAART drugs. Fluoroquinolones and azithromycin are generally well tolerated in combination with calcineurin inhibitors and mTor inhibitors, but in rare instances increase a prolonged QT interval (caution in those >500 ms).

Waterborne Diseases

To reduce the risk for cryptosporidiosis, giardiasis, and other waterborne infections, immunocompromised travelers should avoid swallowing water during swimming and other water-based recreational activities and should not swim in water that might be contaminated with sewage or animal waste. Travelers with liver disease should consider avoiding direct exposure to salt water because of the risk for *Vibrio* spp. exposure, and all immunocompromised people should avoid raw seafood. Patients and clinicians should be aware of the risk for infection or colonization with multidrug-resistant organisms during travel; remind immunosuppressed travelers who become ill to report recent travel to their doctors.

REDUCING RISK FOR OTHER DISEASES

3

Geographically focal infections that pose an increased risk for severe outcomes for immunocompromised people include visceral leishmaniasis (see Sec. 5, Part 3, Ch. 15, Visceral Leishmaniasis) and inhaled fungal infections such as *Talaromyces marneffei* (formerly *Penicillium marneffei*) in Southeast Asia, and coccidioidomycosis (see Sec. 5. Part 4, Ch. 1, Coccidioidomycosis / Valley Fever) and histoplasmosis (see Sec. 5, Part 4, Ch. 2, Histoplasmosis) in the Americas.

Coronavirus Disease 2019

People with immunocompromising conditions or who are on immunosuppressive therapy are at increased risk for severe illness, hospitalization, and death if infected with severe acute respiratory syndrome coronavirus 2 (SARS-CoV-2), the virus that causes coronavirus disease 2019 (COVID-19). Moreover, moderately or severely immunocompromised people might routinely shed infectious virus for ≤20 days (see Sec. 5, Part 2, Ch. 3, COVID-19).

Counsel moderately and severely immunocompromised people to be up to date with their COVID-19 vaccinations (www.cdc.gov/coronavirus/2019-ncov/vaccines/recommendations/immuno.html) before travel. Because people who are immunocompromised might have a less robust immune response to COVID-19 vaccines, even those whose vaccinations are up to date should maintain awareness of the COVID-19 situation at their destination. In the pretravel consultation, discuss the possible options of reconsidering travel or delaying travel to destinations where COVID-19 transmission is currently high and risk for infection is greater.

CDC also provides COVID-19 cruise ship information at www.cdc.gov/coronavirus/2019-ncov/travelers/cruise-travel-during-covid19.

html. SARS-CoV-2 spreads easily on cruise ships; outbreaks can overwhelm onboard medical capacity, and ship-to-shore medical evacuations can be challenging (see Sec. 8, Ch. 6, Cruise Ship Travel).

In addition to helping ensure that moderately and severely immunocompromised travelers are up to date with their COVID-19 vaccinations, provide information on the importance of taking protective measures (e.g., wearing a well-fitting mask or respirator while in public indoor spaces, avoiding spending time in poorly ventilated indoor locations). Suggest to immunocompromised travelers that they also consider wearing a well-fitting mask or respirator when outdoors during sustained close contact with others. Advise close contacts (e.g., household members, caregivers) of immunocompromised people to adhere to the same precautions. For the latest guidance and recommendations regarding COVID-19 vaccinations, boosters, and therapeutic options, see www.cdc.gov/coronavirus/2019-nCoV/index.html.

3

Tuberculosis

Establishing the tuberculosis status of immunocompromised travelers going to regions endemic for tuberculosis can be helpful in the evaluation of subsequent illness (see Sec. 5, Part 1, Ch. 23, . . . *perspectives*: Testing Travelers for *Mycobacterium tuberculosis* Infection). Depending on the traveler's degree of immune suppression, the baseline tuberculosis status might be assessed by a tuberculin skin test, *Mycobacterium tuberculosis* antigen–specific interferon-γ assay (i.e., QuantiFERON-TB Gold or T-SPOT TB, both generally more sensitive in immunocompromised patients than skin testing), or chest radiograph. The need for posttravel testing (often 3 months after travel) depends on exposure risk during the trip, medical conditions, and other factors.

People with HIV and transplant recipients might require primary or secondary prophylaxis for opportunistic infections (e.g., *Mycobacterium*, *Pneumocystis*, and *Toxoplasma* spp.). Adherence to all indicated prophylactic regimens should be confirmed before travel.

BIBLIOGRAPHY

Agarwal N, Ollington K, Kaneshiro M, Frenck R, Melmed GY. Are immunosuppressive medications associated with decreased responses to routine immunizations? A systematic review. Vaccine. 2012;30(8):1413–24.

Barte H, Horvath TH, Rutherford GW. Yellow fever vaccine for patients with HIV infection. Cochrane Database Syst Rev. 2014;(1):CD010929.

Buchan CA, Kotton CN; AST Infectious Diseases Community of Practice. Travel medicine, transplant tourism, and the solid organ transplant recipient—Guidelines from the American Society of Transplantation Infectious Diseases Community of Practice. Clin Transplant. 2019;33(9):e13529.

Dekkiche S, de Valliere S, D'Acremont V, Genton B. Travel-related health risks in moderately and severely immunocompromised patients: a case-control study. J Travel Med. 2016;23(3):taw001.

Farez MF, Correale J. Yellow fever vaccination and increased relapse rate in travelers with multiple sclerosis. Arch Neurol. 2011;68(10):1267–71.

Garcia Garrido HM, Wieten RW, Grobusch MP, Goorhuis A. Response to hepatitis A vaccination in immunocompromised travelers. J Infect Dis. 2015;212(3):378–85.

Huttner A, Eperon G, Lascano AM, Roth S, et al. Risk of MS relapse after yellow fever vaccination: A self-controlled case series. Neurol Neuroimmunol Neuroinflamm. 2020;7(4):e726.

Infectious Disease Society of America. Guidelines for the prevention and treatment of opportunistic infections in adults and adolescents with HIV. Available from: www.idsociety.org/practice-guideline/prevention-and-treatment-of-opportunistic-infections-among-adults-and-adolescents.

Kroger A, Bahta L, Hunter P. General best practice guidelines for immunization. Best practices guidance of the Advisory Committee on Immunization Practices (ACIP) [updated May 4, 2021]. Available from: www.cdc.gov/vaccines/hcp/acip-recs/general-recs/downloads/general-recs.pdf.

Loebermann M, Winkelmann A, Hartung HP, Hengel H, Reisinger EC, Zettl UK. Vaccination against infection in patients with multiple sclerosis. Nat Rev Neurol. 2011;8(3):143–51.

Luks AM, Swenson ER. Evaluating the risks of high altitude travel in chronic liver disease patients. High Alt Med Biol. 2015;16(2):80–8.

Pacanowski J, Lacombe K, Campa P, Dabrowska M, Poveda JD, Meynard JL, et al. Plasma HIV-RNA is the key determinant of long-term antibody persistence after yellow fever immunization in a cohort of 364 HIV-infected patients. J Acquir Immune Defic Syndr. 2012;59(4):360–7.

Papeix C, Mazoyer J, Maillart E, Bensa C, et al. Multiple sclerosis: Is there a risk of worsening after yellow fever vaccination? Multiple Sclerosis J. 2021;27(14):2280–3.

Perry RT, Plowe CV, Koumare B, Bougoudogo F, Kotloff KL, Losonsky GA, et al. A single dose of live oral cholera vaccine CVD 103-HgR is safe and immunogenic in HIV-infected and HIV-noninfected adults in Mali. Bull World Health Organ. 1998;76(1):63–71.

Rubin LG, Levin MJ, Ljungman P, Davies EG, Avery R, Tomblyn M, et al. 2013 IDSA clinical practice guideline for vaccination of the immunocompromised host. Clin Infect Dis. 2014;58(3):309–18.

Schwartz BS, Rosen J, Han PV, Hynes NA, Hagmann SH, Rao SR, et al. Immunocompromised travelers: demographic characteristics, travel destinations, and pretravel health care from the U.S. Global TravEpiNet Consortium. Am J Trop Med Hyg. 2015;93(5):1110–6.

Visser LG. TNF-α antagonists and immunization. Curr Infect Dis Rep. 2011;13(3):243–7.

Wieten RW, Goorhuis A, Jonker EF, de Bree GJ, de Visser AW, van Genderen PJ, et al. 17D yellow fever vaccine elicits comparable long-term immune responses in healthy individuals and immune-compromised patients. J Infect. 2016;72(6):713–22.

Wyplosz B, Burdet C, Francois H, Durrbach A, Duclos-Vallee JC, Mamzer-Bruneel MF, et al. Persistence of yellow fever vaccine-induced antibodies after solid organ transplantation. Am J Transplant. 2013;13(9):2458–61.

TRAVELERS WITH DISABILITIES

Jasmine Owens, Eric Cahill

The Americans with Disabilities Act (www.dol.gov/general/topic/disability/ada) defines an individual with a disability as a person who has a physical or mental impairment that substantially limits ≥1 major life activity, has a record of such an impairment, or is regarded as having such an impairment.

According to the World Health Organization, an activity limitation can include difficulty seeing, hearing, walking, or problem-solving. With proper preparation, many travelers with disabilities can travel internationally. The following guidelines can help support safe, accessible travel for people with various disabilities:

Assess. Assess each international itinerary individually, in consultation with travel agencies or tour operators that provide services to people with disabilities.

Review. Review (and refer travelers to) online resources for additional information (Table 3-05).

Suggest. Suggest that travelers ensure necessary accommodations are available throughout the entire trip.

Recommend. Recommend travelers enroll in the US Department of State's Smart Traveler Enrollment Program (https://step.state.gov/step) to receive security messages and to make it easier for the US embassy or consulate to assist in an emergency.

HUMAN RIGHTS

Each country has its own standard of accessibility for people with disabilities. Unlike the United States, many countries do not legally require accommodations for people with disabilities. Several websites can help the traveler answer questions about accessibility for a specific destination or provide support if an emergency occurs. Travel agents, hotels, airlines, or cruise ship companies can also serve as sources for information about services available during the trip and at the destination, including for service animals. Table 3-06 includes resources for travelers with disabilities to help them gather information about accommodations and human rights frameworks at their destination.

AIR TRAVEL REGULATIONS & STANDARDS

Air Carrier Access Act

In 1986, Congress passed the Air Carrier Access Act (ACAA) to ensure that people with disabilities are treated without discrimination in a way

Table 3-05 Online resources for travelers with disabilities or chronic illnesses[1]

ORGANIZATION / SOURCE	RESOURCE	AVAILABLE FROM
American Council of the Blind	Travel Resources	https://acb.org/content/travel-resources
Autism Speaks	Traveling with Autism	www.autismspeaks.org/traveling-autism
Christopher & Dana Reeve Foundation	Traveling with your wheelchair	www.christopherreeve.org/living-with-paralysis/home-travel/traveling-with-your-wheelchair
Disabled World	Travel: Accessible Disability Travel Information	www.disabled-world.com/travel/
Epilepsy Foundation	Air Travel and Epilepsy	www.epilepsy.com/sites/core/files/atoms/files/Air%20Travel%20Factsheet_0.pdf
Federal Aviation Administration	Acceptance Criteria for Portable Oxygen Concentrators	www.faa.gov/about/initiatives/cabin_safety/portable_oxygen
Federal Maritime Commission	Cruise Vacations: Know Before You Go	www.fmc.gov/wp-content/uploads/2018/09/PVO2014-508.pdf
International Civil Aviation Organization	Air Transport Accessibility	www.icao.int/safety/iStars/Pages/Air-Transport-Accessibility.aspx
National Association of the Deaf	Cruise Lines	www.nad.org/resources/transportation-and-travel/cruise-lines/
	Transportation and Travel	www.nad.org/resources/transportation-and-travel/
New Directions Travel		www.newdirectionstravel.org/
Society for Accessible Travel & Hospitality		https://sath.org/
USA.gov	Your Legal Disability Rights	www.usa.gov/disability-rights#item-213969
US Department of Homeland Security, Transportation Security Administration	Disabilities and Medical Conditions	www.tsa.gov/travel/special-procedures
	Disability Notification Card	www.tsa.gov/sites/default/files/disability_notification_card_508.pdf
	Request for TSA Cares Assistance	www.tsa.gov/contact-center/form/cares
	What Can I Bring?	www.tsa.gov/travel/security-screening/whatcanibring/medical

Table 3-05 Online resources for travelers with disabilities or chronic illnesses (continued)

ORGANIZATION / SOURCE	RESOURCE	AVAILABLE FROM
US Department of State	Travelers with Disabilities	https://travel.state.gov/content/travel/en/international-travel/before-you-go/travelers-with-special-considerations/traveling-with-disabilties.html
US Department of Transportation	Guide: Air Travelers with Developmental Disabilities	www.transportation.gov/sites/dot.gov/files/docs/Developmental_Disabilities_Guide.pdf
	Service Animals (Including Emotional Support Animals)	www.transportation.gov/individuals/aviation-consumer-protection/service-animals-including-emotional-support-animals
	Traveling with a Disability	www.transportation.gov/individuals/aviation-consumer-protection/traveling-disability
	What Airline Employees, Airline Contractors, and Air Travelers with Disabilities Need to Know About Access to Air Travel for Persons with Disabilities – July 15, 2005	www.transportation.gov/individuals/aviation-consumer-protection/what-airline-employees-airline-contractors-and-air
	Wheelchairs and Other Assistive Devices	www.transportation.gov/individuals/aviation-consumer-protection/wheelchairs-and-other-assistive-devices
WheelchairTravel.org	Wheelchair Users' Guide to Air Travel	https://wheelchairtravel.org/air-travel/

[1]Some travelers with disabilities or chronic illnesses might need additional attention and adaptation of transportation services. This table is not intended to be an exhaustive list of resources.

consistent with the safe carriage of all air passengers. These regulations were established by the US Department of Transportation (DOT) and apply to all flights provided by US airlines and flights to or from the United States by foreign carriers.

ACAA ensures carriers cannot refuse transportation based on a disability. The ACAA has a few exceptions, however; for example, the carrier can refuse transportation if the person with a disability would endanger the health or safety of other passengers or if transporting the person would be a violation of Federal Aviation Administration safety rules. Travelers and their clinicians can learn more about exceptions and other aspects of the ACAA by reviewing What Airline Employees, Airline Contractors, and Air Travelers with Disabilities Need to Know about Access to Air Travel for Persons with Disabilities (see Table 3-05 for link).

Air carriers are also obliged to accept a declaration by travelers with disabilities that they are self-reliant. A medical certificate (a written statement from the traveler's health care provider saying that the traveler can complete the flight safely without requiring extraordinary medical care or endangering other travelers) might be required in specific situations. Examples of specific situations include a person intending to travel with a possible communicable disease, a person requiring a stretcher or oxygen, or a person whose medical condition can be reasonably expected to affect the operation of the flight.

Table 3-06 Accommodations & human rights frameworks for people with disabilities: information sources for travelers

ORGANIZATION/SOURCE	RESOURCE	AVAILABLE FROM	NOTES
US Department of State	International Travel	https://travel.state.gov/content/travel/en/international-travel.html	To find information on accessibility for travelers with mobility limitations, enter a country or area in the search bar titled: *Learn about your destination*. Information on accessibility can be found in the section: *Local Laws and Special Circumstances*
	Country Reports on Human Rights Practices (Human Rights Reports)	www.state.gov/reports/2019-country-reports-on-human-rights-practices	Select a year and country, then read section 6 of the report for information about the human rights and social service framework protecting citizens with disabilities in the destination country

Under the guidelines of the ACAA, when a traveler with disability requests assistance, the airline is obliged to meet certain accessibility requirements. For example, carriers must provide access to the aircraft door (preferably by a level entry bridge), an aisle seat, and a seat with removable armrests. However, aircraft with <30 seats generally are exempt from these requirements. Any aircraft with >60 seats must have an onboard wheelchair, and personnel must help move the onboard wheelchair from a seat to the lavatory area upon request. Only wide-body aircraft with ≥2 aisles are required to have fully accessible lavatories.

Airline personnel are not required to assist with feeding, visiting the lavatory, or dispensing medication to travelers. Travelers with disabilities who require this type of assistance should travel with a companion or attendant. DOT maintains a toll-free hotline (800-778-4838 [voice] or 800-455-9880 [TTY]), available 9 a.m. to 5 p.m. Eastern Time, Monday–Friday, except federal holidays, to provide general information to consumers about the rights of air travelers with disabilities and to assist air travelers with time-sensitive disability-related issues.

Many non–US airlines voluntarily adhere to codes of practice that are similar to US legislation based on guidelines from the International Civil Aviation Organization (ICAO; see Table 3-05). These guidelines are not identical to those outlined in US legislation, however, and the degree of implementation can vary by airline and location. Travelers planning to fly between foreign countries or within a foreign country while abroad should check with the overseas airlines to ensure that the carriers adhere to accessibility standards adequate for their needs. ICAO (see Table 3-05) also provides accessibility scores for airports across the world that can aid in travel planning.

Assistive Devices

Assistive devices can make traveling more accessible for people with disabilities. Travelers and their health care providers can consult the DOT and Transportation Security Administration (TSA) websites (see Table 3-05) for information on traveling with an assistive device. Travelers should check for specific policies for assistive devices, including wheelchairs, portable machines, batteries, respirators, and portable oxygen concentrators.

In-Flight Services

Airlines are not permitted to require travelers to provide advance notice of a disability. Airlines might require up to 48 hours advance notice and 1-hour advance check-in, however, for certain accommodations that require preparation time for services (if they are available on the flight), such as medical oxygen for use on board the aircraft, carriage of an incubator, hook-up for a respirator to the aircraft electrical power supply, accommodation for a passenger who must travel in a stretcher, transport of a battery-powered wheelchair on an aircraft with <60 seats, provision by the airline of hazardous material packaging for batteries used in wheelchairs or other assistive devices, accommodation for ≥10 people with disabilities who travel as a group, or provision of an onboard wheelchair for use on an aircraft that does not have an accessible lavatory.

All audiovisual displays played on aircraft for safety and informational purposes must use captioning or a sign language interpreter as part of the video presentation. The captioning must be in the predominant languages in which the carrier communicates with passengers on the flight. The current ACAA rule does not require the captioning of in-flight entertainment.

AIRPORT ACCOMMODATIONS

Security Screening

The TSA has established a program for screening travelers with disabilities and their equipment, mobility aids, and devices. TSA permits prescription liquid medications and other liquids needed by people with disabilities and medical conditions. Travelers with disabilities or medical conditions that affect TSA screening might use a TSA Notification Card to communicate with screening officers; they can also learn more about TSA guidelines for disabilities and medical conditions online (see Table 3-05).

As with other people with disabilities or medical conditions, travelers with hearing loss (i.e., individuals who are deaf or who are hard of hearing) can provide the TSA officer with a notification card or other medical documentation that describes their condition and informs the officer about the need for assistance with the screening process. Travelers are not required to remove any hearing aids or external cochlear implant devices. Additional screening, including a pat-down or device inspection, might be required if assistive devices alarm security technology.

Travelers with disabilities or medical conditions can call the TSA helpline toll free at 855-787-2227, federal relay 711, or check TSA's website (www.tsa.gov/travel/special-procedures) for answers to questions about screening policies, procedures, and the security checkpoints.

Closed Captioning

As part of the ACAA, DOT rules require any airport terminal facility that receives federal financial assistance to enable or ensure high-contrast captioning at all times on televisions and other audiovisual displays. Captioning is required on televisions and other audiovisual displays located in any common area of the terminal to which passengers have access, including the gate area, ticketing area, passenger lounges, and leased commercial shop and restaurant spaces.

Telecommunication Devices

Current ACAA rules require people with hearing loss to self-identify to airline carrier personnel to ensure their receipt of accessible information. Passenger information, including information about flight schedule changes, connections, gate assignments, and baggage claim must be transmitted in a timely manner through an accessible method of communication to those who have identified themselves as having hearing loss.

Passengers with hearing loss must identify themselves to carrier personnel at the gate area or the customer service desk even if they have already done so at the ticketing area. The ACAA rules do not require a sign language interpreter to ensure that a passenger with hearing loss receives all pertinent information. If an airline carrier provides telephone reservation and information service to the public, these services must be available to people with hearing loss through a telecommunications device for the deaf (TDD), telecommunications relay services, or other technology.

Wheelchairs

Travelers can decide to rent wheelchairs and medical equipment at their destination. Research on renting wheelchairs might include checking the availability of wheelchair and medical equipment providers. In addition, organizations such as Mobility International USA (www.miusa.org) have information about overseas medical equipment providers. The country voltage, type of electrical plug, and reliability of the electrical infrastructure at the destination country might make one type of wheelchair preferable over another. In some cases, a manual instead of a power wheelchair is the preferred assistive device.

BOARDING & DEPLANING WITH A WHEELCHAIR

3

Smaller airplanes might not have a jetway, and travelers who use wheelchairs might need to be manually lifted or carried down the stairs. Some airports have adapted hoists or lifts. An aisle chair is usually required to board and deplane an airplane. Travelers should be sure to mention they need an aisle chair, both when reserving tickets and when checking in at the airport. Additional wheelchair traveling tips are available through Wheelchair Travel's Wheelchair Users' Guide to Air Travel (https://wheelchairtravel.org/air-travel).

SERVICE ANIMALS

Some travelers require a service animal for travel support. Travelers who require service animals, including emotional support animals, should check with the airline and the destination country to ensure that both will permit the animal and that the traveler obtains all required documentation (see Sec. 7, Ch. 6, Traveling with Pets & Service Animals). Clinicians can use the following recommendations to assist travelers with service animals. Travelers can contact the foreign embassy or consulate of the destination country for information on possible restrictions and cultural norms about service animals. Travelers should find out about any required quarantine, vaccination, and documentation for the service animal; consult their veterinarian for tips about traveling with service animals; and contact destination hotels to make certain they will accommodate service animals.

CRUISE SHIPS

Companies or entities conducting programs or tours on cruise ships that dock at US ports have obligations regarding access for travelers with disabilities, even if the ship itself is of foreign registry, as outlined in Title III of the Americans with Disabilities Act (www.ada.gov/regs2010/titleIII_2010/titleIII_2010_regulations.htm). All travelers with disabilities should check with cruise lines regarding availability of requested or needed items before booking. Cruise ship operators and travel agents that cater to travelers with special needs also exist.

BOX 3-02 Managing chronic health conditions during international travel: a checklist for travelers

BEFORE TRAVEL

- ☐ Contact your health insurance carrier or review your health insurance plan. If your insurance does not provide overseas coverage, the US Department of State strongly recommends purchasing supplemental medical insurance and medical evacuation plans.
- ☐ Visit the US Department of State's Your Health Abroad webpage (https://travel.state.gov/content/travel/en/international-travel/before-you-go/your-health-abroad.html).
- ☐ Visit the Centers for Disease Control and Prevention, Travelers' Health website (https://wwwnc.cdc.gov/travel/) for health actions before, during, and after travel.

DURING TRAVEL

- ☐ Carry medical alert information and a letter from your health care provider describing medical conditions, medications, potential complications, and other pertinent medical information.
- ☐ Carry enough prescription medication to last the entire trip, including extra medicine in case of delay. Carry prescriptions in their labeled containers, not in a pill pack.
- ☐ Some prescription medications that are legal in the United States are illegal in other countries. Contact the US embassy or consulate at your destination (www.usembassy.gov) to learn more about bringing prescription medicines overseas.

MEDICAL CONSIDERATIONS

Some travelers can have both a disability and an underlying health condition. Box 3-02 provides a list of suggestions the travel health provider can use to help the traveler plan to manage their condition while abroad. For more details, refer to Sec. 3, Ch. 3, Travelers with Chronic Illnesses.

BIBLIOGRAPHY

Barnett S. Communication with deaf and hard-of-hearing people: a guide for medical education. Acad Med. 2002 Jul; 77(7):694–700.

Bauer I. When travel is a challenge: travel medicine and the "dis-abled" traveler. Travel Med Infect Dis. 2018:22;66–72.

International Civil Aviation Organization. Manual on access to air transport by persons with disabilities. Montréal: International Civil Aviation Organization; 2013. Available from: www.skywisesolutions.com/files/manual_on_access_to_air_transport_by_persons_with_disabilities_-_icao.pdf.

The National Association of the Deaf. Legal rights, 6th edition: The guide for deaf and hard of hearing people. Washington, DC: Gallaudet University Press; 2015.

US Department of Transportation. Nondiscrimination on the basis of disability in air travel. Available from: www.govinfo.gov/content/pkg/FR-2018-05-23/pdf/2018-10814.pdf.

World Health Organization. International Classification of Functioning, Disability and Health (ICF). Geneva: The Organization; 2001. Available from: www.who.int/standards/classifications/international-classification-of-functioning-disability-and-health.

TRAVELERS WITH CHRONIC ILLNESSES

Noreen Hynes

Although traveling abroad can be relaxing and rewarding, the physical demands of travel can be stressful, particularly for travelers with underlying chronic illnesses. With adequate preparation, however, these travelers can have safe and enjoyable trips. For more detailed information on assisting immunocompromised travelers, travelers with disabilities, highly allergic travelers, and travelers with substance use disorders prepare for international travel, see the respective chapters in this section.

Patients should see their established health care providers well in advance of travel to ensure that all chronic conditions are controlled, and management is optimized. Clinicians should encourage patients to seek pretravel consultation prior to paying for nonrefundable trips, and at least 4–6 weeks before departure to ensure adequate time to respond to immunizations, try new medications before travel, or redefine the itinerary based upon pretravel consultation recommendations.

GENERAL APPROACH

Advising Travelers

Adequate preparation for patients with chronic illnesses for international travel requires the active participation of both the traveler and the travel health provider. Box 3-03 includes a checklist of pretravel activities for travelers with chronic illnesses.

Health Care Provider Roles & Responsibilities

Health care providers play a critical role in helping patients with chronic underlying conditions travel safely. Ask patients about previous health-related issues encountered during travel (e.g., complications during air travel). In addition to sharing the advice found in Box 3-03, ensure the traveler has sufficient medication (and proper storage conditions) for the

BOX 3-03 A checklist for travelers with chronic illnesses preparing for international travel

- ☐ Carry copies of all prescriptions.
- ☐ Check with the foreign embassy or consulate for your destination country in the United States to clarify whether any medication restrictions exist. Some countries do not allow visitors to bring certain medications into the country, especially narcotics and psychotropic medications.
- ☐ Favor travel to destinations that have access to quality care for your condition (see Sec. 6, Ch. 2, Obtaining Health Care Abroad)
- ☐ Obtain an established provider letter. The letter should be on office letterhead stationery and outline existing medical conditions, medications prescribed (including generic names), and any equipment required to manage the condition. By law, some states do not permit a travel health specialist to furnish such a letter if the specialist is not also the primary care provider or established provider of record.
- ☐ Pack a travel health kit (see Sec. 2, Ch. 10, Travel Health Kits). Take health kits on board as carry-on luggage, and bring all necessary medications and medical supplies (e.g., pouching for ostomies) in their original containers.
- ☐ Select a medical assistance company that allows you to store your medical history so it can be accessed worldwide.
- ☐ Sign up for the Smart Traveler Enrollment Program (https://step.state.gov/step), a free service of the US Department of State to US citizens and permanent residents, to receive destination-specific travel and security updates. This service also allows the Department of State to contact international travelers during emergencies.
- ☐ Stay hydrated, wear loose-fitting clothing, and walk and stretch at regular intervals during long-distance travel (see Sec. 8, Ch. 3, Deep Vein Thrombosis & Pulmonary Embolism).
- ☐ Wear a medical alert bracelet or carry medical information on your person. Various brands of jewelry or tags, even electronic ones, are available.

3

entire trip, plus extra in case of unexpected delays. Because medications should be taken based on elapsed time and not time of day, offering travelers guidance on scheduling when to take medications during and after crossing time zones might be needed.

Educate travelers on possible drug interactions (see Sec. 2, Ch. 4, Interactions Between Travel Vaccines & Drugs). Some medications used to treat chronic medical illnesses (e.g., warfarin) can interact with prescribed self-treatment for travelers' diarrhea or malaria chemoprophylaxis. Discuss all medications patients use, including medications taken daily, those taken on an as-needed basis, and dietary supplements or herbal products.

In addition, discuss supplemental insurance options for travelers, including policies that cover trip cancellation in the event of illness, supplemental medical insurance, and medical evacuation insurance. Supplemental medical insurance can reimburse travelers for money paid for health care abroad; most medical insurance policies do not cover the cost of health care received in other countries. Medical evacuation insurance covers moving the person from the place of illness or injury to a place where they can receive definitive care. Travelers might need assistance to identify supplemental insurance plans that will cover costs for preexisting conditions (see Sec. 6, Ch. 1, Travel Insurance, Travel Health Insurance & Medical Evacuation Insurance).

Help patients devise a Personal Travel Health Plan. This plan should give instructions for managing minor problems or exacerbations of underlying illnesses and should include information about medical facilities available in the destination country (see Sec. 6, Ch. 2, Obtaining Health Care Abroad).

SPECIFIC CHRONIC MEDICAL CONDITIONS

Chronic illness or acute illness affecting underlying chronic disease might affect the recommendations clinicians make to a traveler after completing the risk assessment conducted as part of the pretravel consultation (see Sec. 2, Ch. 1, The Pretravel Consultation). Some online resources for travelers who have ≥1 chronic medical conditions can be found in Table 3-05 (in Sec. 3, Ch. 2, Travelers with Disabilities) and Table 3-07.

Chronic conditions include those affecting the cardiovascular, endocrine, gastrointestinal, genitourinary, hematological, hepatic, neurologic, and respiratory systems. Table 3-08 addresses issues and recommendations related to specific chronic medical illnesses and should be used in

3

Table 3-07 **Online resources for travelers with chronic illnesses: disease & condition-specific**

DISEASE/CONDITION	ORGANIZATION/SOURCE	RESOURCE	AVAILABLE FROM
ANTICOAGULATION	Anticoagulation Forum	Centers of Excellence Resource Center	https://acforum-excellence.org/Resource-Center
CANCER	American Cancer Society	Eat Right and Stay Active while Traveling	www.cancer.org/latest-news/eat-right-and-stay-active-while-traveling.html
CELIAC DISEASE	National Celiac Association	Eating GF when traveling abroad	https://nationalceliac.org/celiac-disease-questions/eating-gf-when-traveling-abroad
CHRONIC PAIN	International Pain Foundation	Top Tips for Traveling Abroad with Chronic Pain	https://internationalpain.org/top-tips-for-traveling-abroad-with-chronic-pain
DIABETES	American Diabetes Association	Air Travel and Diabetes	www.diabetes.org/resources/know-your-rights/discrimination/public-accommodations/air-travel-and-diabetes
EPILEPSY	Epilepsy Foundation	Travel and Holidays	www.epilepsy.com
	Epilepsy Society (UK)		https://epilepsysociety.org.uk/living-epilepsy/travel
HEART CONDITIONS	American Heart Association	Healthy Travel	www.heart.org/en/healthy-living/healthy-lifestyle/mental-health-and-wellbeing/healthy-travel
INFLAMMATORY BOWEL DISEASE	Crohn's & Colitis Foundation	Traveling with IBD	www.crohnscolitisfoundation.org/what-is-ibd/traveling-with-ibd

(continued)

Table 3-07 **Online resources for travelers with chronic illnesses: disease & condition-specific (continued)**

DISEASE/CONDITION	ORGANIZATION/SOURCE	RESOURCE	AVAILABLE FROM
KIDNEY DISEASE	American Association of Kidney Patients (AAKP)	International Travel while on Dialysis	https://aakp.org/international-travel-while-on-dialysis
	National Kidney Foundation	Foreign Travel Tips for Dialysis Patients	www.kidney.org/newsletter/foreign-travel
	Global Dialysis (UK)	Travel Advice	www.globaldialysis.com/component/content/article/30/75-travel-advice.html
LUNGS & CHEST	American Lung Association	Traveling with Oxygen	www.lung.org/lung-health-diseases/lung-procedures-and-tests/oxygen-therapy/traveling-with-oxygen
MULTIPLE SCLEROSIS	Multiple Sclerosis Foundation	Tips for Traveling Abroad with MS	https://msfocus.org/Magazine/Magazine-Items/Posted/Tips-for-Traveling-Abroad-with-MS.aspx
SLEEP APNEA	American Sleep Association	Travel: CPAP Machines	www.sleepassociation.org/sleep-apnea/cpap-machines/travel
	American Sleep Apnea Association	US Travel Tips for CPAP Users	www.sleepapnea.org/treat/cpap-therapy/us-travel-tips-for-cpap-users/

conjunction with the other recommendations given throughout this book.

Travelers also might want to investigate international health care accreditation agencies to identify health care facilities at the travel destination that have received recognition or accreditation for high care standards and good patient safety records. If travelers or their health care providers have concerns about fitness for air travel or the need to obtain a medical certificate before travel, the medical unit affiliated with the specific airline is a valuable source for information.

Travelers who require service animals, including emotional support animals, should check with the airline and the destination country to ensure both the air carrier and the country will allow the animal; documentation and permits might also be required (see Sec. 7, Ch. 6, Traveling with Pets & Service Animals). Travelers planning to use supplemental oxygen on the aircraft or needing other equipment (e.g., a wheelchair) must inform the airline far in advance of planned travel. The Transportation Security Administration (TSA) Cares Helpline (toll-free at 855-787-2227) or TSA Cares online assistance (www.tsa.gov/contact-center/form/cares) also can provide information on how to prepare for the airport security screening process for a particular disability or medical condition.

Table 3-08 Special considerations for travelers with chronic illnesses

CONDITION	CONTRAINDICATIONS TO & TIMING OF AIRLINE TRAVEL	PRETRAVEL RECOMMENDATIONS & CONSIDERATIONS	IMMUNIZATION CONSIDERATIONS	ADDITIONAL CONSIDERATIONS & GUIDANCE
GENERAL CONSIDERATIONS	Travelers unlikely to survive the flight due to preexisting condition Any traveler with serious and acute contagious disease (e.g., acute, untreated tuberculosis; COVID-19)			
AUTOIMMUNE & RHEUMATOLOGIC DISEASES	None	Baseline TST or IGRA before starting TNF blockers	Immunosuppressive medications including TNF blockers might alter response to immunizations Live attenuated vaccines might be contraindicated	Emphasize safe food and water precautions and good hand hygiene
CANCER	Anemia, severe (Hgb <8.5 g/dL) Cardiovascular, gastrointestinal, or pulmonary/respiratory complications (see below for details) Cerebral edema due to intracranial tumor	Emphasize safe food and water precautions Plan for self-management of dehydration DVT precautions Supplemental oxygen Wear loose-fitting clothing to prevent worsening of lymphedema	Immunosuppressive medications might alter response to travel vaccines Live attenuated vaccines might be contraindicated Revaccination might be necessary after cancer treatment	Check for medication restrictions at the destination (e.g., pain relief/control) See Sec. 3, Ch. 1, Immunocompromised Travelers, for additional recommendations

(continued)

Table 3-08 Special considerations for travelers with chronic illnesses (continued)

CONDITION	CONTRAINDICATIONS TO & TIMING OF AIRLINE TRAVEL	PRETRAVEL RECOMMENDATIONS & CONSIDERATIONS	IMMUNIZATION CONSIDERATIONS	ADDITIONAL CONSIDERATIONS & GUIDANCE
CARDIOVASCULAR & OTHER CIRCULATORY DISORDERS[a]	Angina, unstable Arrhythmia, uncontrolled CHF, severe or decompensated Eisenmenger Syndrome Hypertension, uncontrolled Post-acute coronary syndrome *Low risk*: minimum 3 days before travel *Moderate risk*: minimum 10 days before travel *High risk* or awaiting further intervention or treatment: defer air travel until disease is stabilized Post-CABG: minimum 10 days, and improving, before travel Post-percutaneous coronary intervention (elective): minimum 2 days, and no complications, before travel Post-percutaneous pacemaker or implanted defibrillator placement: minimum 2–3 days, if uncomplicated, before travel Post-sickle cell crisis: minimum 10 days post-event, and improving, before travel Valvular heart disease, severe, symptomatic	Supplemental oxygen Plan for self-management of dehydration and volume overload; may include adjusting medications Bring copy of recent ECG Bring pacemaker or AICD card DVT precautions	Influenza Pneumococcal	Have sublingual nitroglycerin available in carry-on bag Mefloquine[b] (antimalarial prophylaxis) not recommended for people with cardiac conduction abnormalities, particularly those with ventricular arrhythmias Provider primarily responsible for prescribing anticoagulation should tailor INR self-monitoring and management regimen
CNS & PNS DISORDERS	Neurologic process, unstable Post-CVA: minimum 10–14 days, and improving, before travel Post-TIA: minimum 3 days, and no recurrence, before travel Post-cranial surgery: minimum 7–14 days, and improving, before travel Seizure disorder, poorly controlled	Mefloquine antimalarial chemoprophylaxis is contraindicated in travelers with underlying seizure disorder; check for drug-drug interactions		Patients with myasthenia gravis: mefloquine & chloroquine antimalarial chemoprophylaxis, and YF vaccine are all generally contraindicated

DIABETES MELLITUS	None	Plan for self-management of dehydration, diabetic foot, and pressure sores Insulin adjustments Check FSBG at 4–6-hour intervals during air travel Discuss changes in insulin or oral agent regimen with diabetes specialist Provide physician's letter stating need for all equipment, including syringes, glucose meter, and supplies	Influenza Pneumococcal Hepatitis B	Keep insulin and all glucose meter supplies in carry-on bag Bring food and supplies needed to manage hypoglycemia during travel Check feet daily for pressure sores For guidance re: YF vaccine, see Approach to Immunizations: Preparing Travelers with Severe Immune Compromise: Vaccine Considerations for Travelers with Severe Immune Compromise: Yellow Fever, in Sec. 3, Ch. 1, Immunocompromised Travelers
GASTROINTESTINAL DISORDERS (INCLUDING LIVER DISEASE)	Bowel obstruction GI bleed, active or recurrent Liver failure, uncompensated Post–major abdominal surgery: minimum 10–14 days, and improving, before travel Post–colonoscopy (uncomplicated): minimum 24 hours before travel Post–laparoscopic surgery: minimum 3–5 days, and improving, before travel	Emphasize safe food and water precautions For travelers with chronic liver disease, cirrhosis, or heavy alcohol use, advise against eating raw or undercooked shellfish, due to possible overwhelming *Vibrio vulnificus* sepsis Consider prescribing prophylactic antibiotics for TD	Influenza Pneumococcal Hepatitis A Hepatitis B	Increased colostomy output might occur during air travel Patients with cirrhosis and history of hepatopulmonary syndrome or portopulmonary hypertension might be at increased risk for clinical deterioration with travel to high elevations H2-receptor antagonists and PPIs increase susceptibility to TD Use mefloquine with caution in travelers with chronic liver disease
RENAL FAILURE & CHRONIC RENAL INSUFFICIENCY	None	Emphasize safe food and water precautions Plan for self-management of dehydration, which can worsen renal function Arrange dialysis abroad, if needed Adjust medications for CrCl	Influenza Pneumococcal Hepatitis B	Know pre-departure HIV, hepatitis C, and hepatitis B status Atovaquone-proguanil (Malarone) contraindicated when CrCl <30 mL/min AAKP and Global Dialysis (see Table 3-07) can help locate dialysis centers; check accreditation

(continued)

Table 3-08 Special considerations for travelers with chronic illnesses (continued)

CONDITION	CONTRAINDICATIONS TO & TIMING OF AIRLINE TRAVEL	PRETRAVEL RECOMMENDATIONS & CONSIDERATIONS	IMMUNIZATION CONSIDERATIONS	ADDITIONAL CONSIDERATIONS & GUIDANCE
				CKD can predispose patients to increased risk of DVTs and altitude sickness For guidance re: YF vaccine, see Approach to Immunizations: Preparing Travelers with Severe Immune Compromise: Vaccine Considerations for Travelers with Severe Immune Compromise: Yellow Fever, in Sec. 3, Ch. 1, Immunocompromised Travelers
RESPIRATORY TRACT DISORDERS	Asthma, severe or labile Bullous lung disease Lower respiratory tract infection, active Post–major chest surgery: minimum 10–14 days, and improving, before travel Post–PTX (spontaneous): minimum 7 days after full inflation before travel Post–PTX (traumatic): minimum 14 days after full inflation, before travel Pulmonary hypertension, severe Supplemental oxygen requirements: high, rapidly fluctuating, or increasing	Supplemental oxygen Discuss with airline need for other equipment on plane (e.g., nebulizer) Plan for self-management of exacerbations (including asthma, COPD) DVT precautions	Influenza Pneumococcal	Consider carrying a short course of antibiotics and steroids for exacerbations Consider taking an inhaler in a carry-on bag, even if not used routinely

Abbreviations: AAKP, American Association of Kidney Patients; AICD, automatic implantable cardioverter defibrillator; CABG, coronary artery bypass graft; CHF, congestive heart failure; CKD, chronic kidney disease; CNS, central nervous system; COPD, chronic obstructive pulmonary disease; COVID-19, coronavirus disease; CrCl, creatinine clearance; CVA, cerebrovascular accident; DVT, deep vein thrombosis; ECG, electrocardiogram; FSBG, fingerstick blood glucose; GI, gastrointestinal; Hgb, hemoglobin; HIV, human immunodeficiency virus; IGRA, interferon-γ release assay; INR, international normalized ratio; PNS, peripheral nervous system; PPIs, proton-pump inhibitors; PTX, pneumothorax; TD, travelers' diarrhea; TIA, transient ischemic attack; TNF, tumor necrosis factor; TST, tuberculin skin test; YF, yellow fever.

[a]There is a spectrum of airline travel–related risk that depends on the cardiovascular disorder, the defined risk group within the disorder, and the time since the acute event (if applicable). Evidence basis for recommendations is suboptimal, however.

[b]See Sec. 5, Part 3, Ch. 16, Malaria, for additional details.

BIBLIOGRAPHY

Aisporna C, Erickson-Hurt C. End-of-life travel: A bucket list desire for patients with life limiting illnesses. J Hospice Pall Nursing. 2019;21(5):397–403.

Furuto Y, Kawamura M, Namikawa A, Takahashi H, Shibuya Y. Health risk of travel for chronic kidney disease patients. J Res Med Sci. 2020;25:22.

Heng S, Hughes B, Hibbert M, Khasraw M, Lwin Z. Traveling with cancer: A guide for oncologists in the modern world. J Glob Oncol. 2019;5:1–10.

International Air Transport Association. Medical manual, 12th edition; July 2020. Available from: www.iata.org/en/publications/medical-manual.

Josephs LK, Coker RK, Thomas M; British Thoracic Society Air Travel Working Group. Managing patients with stable respiratory disease planning air travel: a primary care summary of the British Thoracic Society recommendations. Prim Care Respir J. 2013;22(2):234–8.

McCarthy AE, Burchard GD. The travelers with pre-existing disease. In: Keystone JS, Kozarsky PE, Connor BA, Nothdurft HD, Mendelson M, Leder K, editors. Travel medicine, 4th edition. Philadelphia: Saunders Elsevier; 2018. pp. 263–6.

Pinsker JE, Becker E, Mahnke CB, Ching M, Larson NS, Roy D. Extensive clinical experience: a simple guide to basal insulin adjustments for long-distance travel. J Diabetes Metab Disord. 2013;12(1):59.

Ringwald J, Strobel J, Eckstein R. Travel and oral anticoagulation. J Travel Med. 2009;16(4):276–83.

Smith D, Toff W, Joy M, Dowdall N, Johnston R, Clark L, et al. Fitness to fly for passengers with cardiovascular disease. Heart. 2010;96(Suppl_2):ii1–16.

US Department of Justice. Exemption from import or export requirements for personal medical use. Title 21 CFR §1301.26. 2004 Sep 14. Available from: www.deadiversion.usdoj.gov/fed_regs/rules/2004/fr0914.htm.

HIGHLY ALLERGIC TRAVELERS

Sue Ann McDevitt, Gail Rosselot

Allergies are the 6th leading cause of chronic illness in the United States, and >50 million Americans experience allergies each year. Food allergies affect 8%–11% of children and adults in the United States; other major allergen categories include dust, insect venom, latex rubber, medications, mold, pets, and pollen. Highly allergic travelers might experience severe allergic reactions that could interrupt or alter planned activities or require emergency medical care during travel. Pay special attention to travelers with a history of anaphylaxis (see Box 3-04).

Travelers with severe allergies face health and safety risks during their journeys, and international itineraries expose travelers to numerous possible allergy triggers. Comprehensive lists of transportation-related and country-specific triggers are not typically available, and language barriers, lack of 9-1-1–like emergency services, and unfamiliar environments and menu items can

BOX 3-04 Anaphylaxis: key points for travelers & health care providers

- Anaphylaxis is an acute, life-threatening systemic allergic reaction; it can have a wide range of clinical manifestations, including cardiac (heart), dermatologic (skin), gastrointestinal (digestive tract), and respiratory (lungs)
- Main risks for anaphylaxis in adults: medications and stinging insect venom
- Main risks for anaphylaxis in children and adolescents: foods and stinging insect venom
- Among patients with a history of severe allergic reactions, approximately 1 in 4 have never had a specialist consult
- Although the first-line medication for anaphylaxis is epinephrine, auto-injectors are available in only approximately 1 in 3 countries around the world
- The lifetime risk for anaphylaxis is 1%–5%; studies suggest increasing incidence

compound the risk. Any environmental or food allergy can affect the success or pleasure of a trip, but severe reactions can be trip-altering and life-threatening.

Help travelers reduce their chances of being exposed to allergy triggers and having a (severe) reaction by emphasizing proactive communication and providing pretravel services that include careful assessment and prevention counseling. Assist highly allergic travelers in creating a written emergency action plan, a critical element of their pretravel preparation. Even during the shortest office visit, confirm allergies and provide guidance to help travelers respond appropriately to severe reactions. Early recognition of anaphylaxis and prompt self-administration of epinephrine and other medications can be lifesaving.

PRETRAVEL ASSESSMENT

During the pretravel assessment, routinely ask travelers about vaccine and vaccine-component, medication, food, and environmental allergies. At each visit, inquire about all drugs, including prescribed, over-the-counter, herbal, recreational, and international brands. Patients' allergies can worsen or improve over time, and new allergies might develop. Check vaccine ingredients listed in the manufacturer's product insert to appropriately care for individuals with history of allergic reactions.

Asthma and food and insect venom allergies are as likely to occur among international travelers as they are among the general population. Review the nature and extent of any reported allergy and the traveler's experience with allergies and self-care management skills.

PREPARATION

Travelers with severe allergies might need extra pretravel preparation. Clinicians can provide customized self-care plans that include suggestions for extra travel medical kit items, travel medical insurance recommendations, country-specific information (where available), guidelines for communication about severe allergies, and referral to a specialist, if warranted (see Box 3-05).

BOX 3-05 Allergy self-care management plan: a checklist for travelers

- ☐ Identify allergy triggers and learn how to avoid them.
- ☐ If you have a history of anaphylaxis, see an allergy specialist before you travel.
- ☐ Research emergency services at your destination: where are they located, how to contact them.
- ☐ Anticipate and research dietary and environmental allergy triggers for airplanes, cruise ships, and trains.
- ☐ Ask about airline allergy policies in advance of travel; alert gate and onboard personnel about specific allergy triggers.
- ☐ Bring along allergy-safe food and snacks, if indicated.
- ☐ Bring several copies of a written emergency action plan for preventing and responding to reactions; keep a copy with you at all times. Consider having a copy translated into the destination language.
- ☐ Buy travel medical assistance insurance and confirm coverage for medical and emergency services overseas.
- ☐ Check your prescriptions, confirm expiration dates, and carry extra medical supplies of all self-care therapies (e.g., antihistamines, inhalers, prednisone) in your carry-on luggage; medically necessary liquids and medications in excess of Transportation Security Administration (TSA) limits are allowed.
- ☐ Epinephrine
  - o Keep your epinephrine auto-injector supply (2 or more) on your person, not in overhead bins.
  - o Never rely on an airline having epinephrine readily available.
  - o Recognize signs of a severe allergic reaction and know when to use medications and epinephrine auto-injectors; get additional training if needed.
  - o If you use epinephrine to self-treat an allergic reaction, you must go to an emergency room for evaluation and monitoring until you are fully stable.
- ☐ Share action plans with guides and traveling companions; never be too embarrassed or hesitant to alert others about a severe allergy.
- ☐ Wear a medical identification bracelet; carry a card or electronic equivalent listing all medical conditions and medications.

BOX 3-06 Food allergies: a checklist for travelers

- ☐ Ask about menu items, ingredients, and preparations; sauces are often a cause of reaction due to hidden ingredients.
- ☐ Bring along nonperishable food supply in case safe food cannot be located during travel.
- ☐ Carry "chef cards" (www.foodallergy.org/diningout) or equivalents (www.allergytranslation.com; www.selectwisely.com) in English and the languages of destination countries to communicate food allergies to all restaurant staff.
- ☐ Carry a supply of sanitary wipes to clean hands and wipe down tray tables and eating utensils.
- ☐ Consider staying in accommodations that provide small refrigerators or kitchens for self-catering.
- ☐ Dietary vigilance is critical; when in doubt, avoid a food item.
- ☐ European Union countries and some others mandate menu labeling for 8–14 different allergens (e.g., shellfish, soy, tree nuts, wheat).
- ☐ FARE's website (www.foodallergy.org) has food allergy guidelines for 13 countries.
- ☐ International travel raises the risk for trying foods that could contain allergy triggers; avoid "street food" and consider eating at chain restaurants where ingredients and food preparation are more standardized.
- ☐ Main food allergens: dairy products and milk; eggs; fish and shellfish; peanuts; sesame; soy; tree nuts; wheat.
- ☐ Research destinations for in-country allergy websites and "allergy aware" restaurants and grocery stores.
- ☐ When purchasing food during travel, read food labels carefully, and seek language assistance, if needed.

3

BOX 3-07 Airborne allergies: a checklist for travelers

- ☐ Review Box 3-05 (Allergy self-care management plan: a checklist for travelers).
- ☐ Consider packing pillow and mattress covers.
- ☐ Use a well-fitting face mask to minimize particulate matter exposure.
- ☐ Ensure easy cancellation policies with your host or property owner in advance; on arrival you might find your accommodations put you at increased risk for exposure to airborne allergens (e.g., tiled or wood flooring is preferable to carpeting to minimize dust allergen reactions).
- ☐ Identify and reserve smoke free (pet free) accommodations and restaurants when possible.
- ☐ If you have asthma, pack all equipment including spacers, nebulizers, and peak flow meters.
- ☐ Minimize outdoor activity when air quality is poor, or pollen count is very high.
- ☐ Research air quality and pollen counts at destinations.
  - Air quality: www.waqi.info
  - Pollen counts: https://patients.eaaci.org/worldwide-map-of-pollen-monitoring-stations/

BOX 3-08 Skin & contact allergies: a checklist for travelers

- ☐ Hiking boots and backpacks can have allergens or irritants in the manufacture or gluing process.
  - Try out equipment before departure to see if you have a reaction.
- ☐ Test any product applied to the skin (e.g., insecticides, repellents, and sunscreens) before travel.
  - Try on all clothing items pretreated with these products to see if you have a reaction.

Suggest travelers view information from organizations with resources that promote safe international travel for people with allergies, such as the American Academy of Allergy, Asthma, and Immunology (AAAAI; www.aaaai.org), Asthma and Allergy Foundation of America (AAFA; www.aafa.org/page/traveling-with-asthma-allergies.aspx), and the Food Allergy and Research Foundation (FARE; www.foodallergy.org). These organizations publish websites, educational materials, template allergy action plans, and communication tools that can help travelers reduce their chances of exposure to allergic triggers.

3

Encourage travelers with severe allergies to seek pretravel care well in advance of departure. In particular, consider providing a specialist referral to any traveler with a history of idiopathic anaphylaxis, new severe allergies, and recent or recurrent severe allergic reactions; help travelers understand that a specialist might generate additional recommendations that could delay or reroute their travel.

BIBLIOGRAPHY

American Academy of Allergy, Asthma & Immunology. School tools: anaphylaxis and food allergy resources for professionals. Available from: www.aaaai.org/Tools-for-the-Public/School-Tools.

Cardona V, Ansotegui IJ, Ebisawa M, El-Gamal Y, Fernandez Rivas M, Fineman S, et al. World Allergy Organization anaphylaxis guidance 2020. World Allergy Organ J. 2020;13(10):100472.

Food Allergy Research & Education (FARE). Food allergy and anaphylaxis plan. Available from: www.foodallergy.org/living-food-allergies/food-allergy-essentials/food-allergy-anaphylaxis-emergency-care-plan.

Shaker MS, Wallace DV, Golden DBK, Oppenheimer J, Bernstein JA, Campbell RL, et al. Anaphylaxis—a 2020 practice parameter update, systematic review, and Grading of Recommendations, Assessment, Development and Evaluation (GRADE) analysis. J Allergy Clin Immunol. 2020;145:1082–1123.

Wang J. Sicherer SH; American Academy of Pediatrics, Section on Allergy and Immunology. Guidance on completing a written allergy and anaphylaxis emergency plan. Pediatrics. 2017;139(3):e20164005.

SUBSTANCE USE & SUBSTANCE USE DISORDERS

W. Robert Lange, Lara DePadilla, Erin Parker, Kristin Holland

In 2020, 40.3 million people aged 12 or older in the United States (14.5% of this population) reportedly had a substance use disorder (SUD) in the past year (www.samhsa.gov/data/report/2020-nsduh-annual-national-report). The prevalence of SUDs underlines the need to ensure that people who use drugs, those experiencing SUD, and those recovering from SUD have access to information that can reduce their risk of harms (e.g., overdose) and support recovery efforts. Travel, for business or pleasure, can exacerbate SUDs, cause clinical deterioration in people with a chemical dependence disorder, and impede participation in recovery support systems (e.g., 12-step groups) that help people maintain abstinence from substance use.

Travelers should be aware of policies and risks associated with substance use in nations where they are traveling. Substances that are legal in the United States, including medications used to treat SUDs, might be illegal in other countries. In addition, travelers could encounter substances in other countries that are less common in the United States, or substances that are more potent or adulterated in unexpected ways. Finally, traveling to places where substance and alcohol use regulations and policies differ from the traveler's home (e.g., countries or states where cannabis use is legal or countries where the legal drinking age is lower than in the United States) could provide opportunities for people who otherwise do not use substances, including alcohol, to use them; such use could be associated with negative health consequences and other risky behaviors.

Most psychoactive products can complicate the physiologic adjustments associated with international travel (e.g., adaptation to different climates, elevations, time zones). Alcohol and drug use also can cause deterioration of clinical conditions during travel and can precipitate other medical problems associated with travel, including diarrheal diseases, heat-related illness, and motion sickness. Furthermore, alcohol and drugs are major contributors to unintentional injury, near-drowning, violence, arrest or detention, repatriation, and death while traveling.

ALCOHOL

Some people identify travel as an opportunity for increased alcohol consumption. Discuss with them that adults of legal drinking age can choose not to drink, or to drink in moderation by limiting intake to ≤2 drinks in a day for men or ≤1 drink in a day for women. Drinking less alcohol is better for health than drinking more, and individuals who do not drink should not start. People of legal drinking age who should not drink at all include those with certain medical conditions, those taking medications that can interact with alcohol, and those unable to control the amount they drink or who are recovering from alcohol use disorder. See the Dietary Guidelines for Americans (www.cdc.gov/alcohol/fact-sheets/moderate-drinking.htm) for more information.

On its own, excessive alcohol use can produce undesirable effects for travelers (see Table 3-09). In addition, even small amounts of alcohol can interact with medications specifically prescribed for travel, creating adverse reactions leading to unwanted visits to unfamiliar health care providers. Alert travelers about the risks associated with drinking in other countries. In many places, alcohol concentrations in beverages exceed those found in the United States. In some countries, alcohol use is illegal in certain settings; policies can vary. Remind all travelers not to drink and drive; each country sets its own legal maximum blood alcohol concentration; in some countries, the level is below that in the United States.

Excessive Alcohol Use

Excessive alcohol use includes binge drinking, heavy drinking, and any drinking by pregnant women or people younger than the legal drinking age. Binge drinking, the most common form of excessive drinking, is defined as consuming 4 or more drinks during a single occasion (for women), and 5 or more drinks during a single occasion (for men). Although most people who binge drink do not have a severe alcohol use disorder, binge

Table 3-09 Adverse clinical effects associated with alcohol consumption during international travel

DURING TRAVEL	Barotrauma Dehydration Hypoxemia Intoxication Motion sickness Sedation
AT THE DESTINATION	Unintentional injury or death (e.g., dive-related injuries, drowning, falls, motor vehicle crashes) Acclimatization (including heat exhaustion and heat stroke, hypothermia, and frostbite) Altitude Illness / Acute Mountain Sickness Gastrointestinal disturbances (including travelers' diarrhea) Jet lag

drinking is a harmful risk behavior associated with serious injuries and multiple diseases.

Excessive alcohol use, including binge drinking, is associated with short-term (e.g., alcohol poisoning, overdoses, injuries, violence) and long-term (e.g., liver disease, cancer, heart disease, hypertension) health conditions. Excessive alcohol use increases a person's chances of engaging in risky sexual activity including unprotected sex, sex with multiple partners, or sex with a partner at risk for sexually transmitted infections (STIs). It is also associated with unintentional injuries (e.g., motor vehicle crashes, falls, burns, alcohol poisoning); violence (e.g., homicide, suicide, intimate partner violence, sexual assault); and STIs.

Tips for drinking less include setting limits, counting drinks, managing triggers (certain people, places, or activities might tempt the traveler to drink more than planned), and being around people who support moderation in or abstinence from drinking. For more details on excessive alcohol use and its effects on health, see www.cdc.gov/alcohol/index.htm.

Alcohol Use Disorder

Excessive drinking is also associated with an increased risk for alcohol use disorder, a chronic medical condition (www.niaaa.nih.gov/publications/brochures-and-fact-sheets/understanding-alcohol-use-disorder). Options and strategies for people with alcohol use disorder to avoid alcohol during travel are presented in Box 3-09; Alcoholics Anonymous (www.aa.org) provides information on meetings occurring domestically and internationally. Suggest travelers use the acronym HALT (Hungry, Angry, Lonely, Tired) to remind them

BOX 3-09 Strategies for people with alcohol use disorder to avoid alcohol during travel

BEFORE LEAVING

Connect or reconnect with

- A counselor/sponsor/mentor
- Support groups (e.g., Alcoholics Anonymous, Narcotics Anonymous)

Select

- Destinations and season wisely (e.g., avoid gatherings associated with alcohol, such as Octoberfest festivals)
- Direct flights to avoid layovers and long travel times
- Travel agencies/resorts that specialize in alcohol-free travel

Consider

- How to avoid people and places that trigger cravings and return to use
- Traveling with a trusted friend

Plan ahead

- Call ahead to have mini bar/alcohol removed from room
- Discuss disulfiram with your healthcare provider
- Pack favorite audio materials, books, journals
- Research support groups at destination (www.aa.org)
- Research other potential treatment/support services

WHILE AWAY

Healthy behaviors

- Attend support group meetings (as appropriate) at destination
- For business meetings/events: "be discreet, meet and greet, then retreat"
- Participate in spa/gym/athletic activities
- Remain connected with counselor/sponsor/mentor and home network
- Request that the mini bar/alcohol be removed from the room if not already done so
- Stick to your routine; avoid blocks of idle time; meditate
- Use technology (e.g., Zoom, chat rooms) whenever in-person support group meeting attendance is not possible

Avoid

- Alcohol (e.g., bourbon, whiskey, wine) tasting events
- Happy Hours and open bars; use caution when attending "team building" events
- Low alcohol and "alcohol-free" beer
- People/places that could trigger cravings
- Wine-pairing suppers or events
- Winery or microbrewery tours

of the triggers for drinking and the need to take appropriate avoidance measures.

Pharmacologic options are available to assist in treating alcohol use disorder, including acamprosate, disulfiram, and naltrexone. Advise travelers taking disulfiram to avoid "alcohol-free" beers because these products can contain ≤0.5% alcohol, enough to produce a reaction. Moreover, it is inadvisable to initiate first-time pharmacologic intervention at the onset of an international trip.

CANNABIS

The cannabis plant contains more than 100 compounds (or cannabinoids). Cannabis (marijuana, weed, pot, dope) refers to the dried flowers, leaves, stems, and seeds of the cannabis plant, as well as concentrates, edibles, extracts, tinctures, vape cartridges, and other products that contain Δ-9-tetrahydrocannabinol, the main psychoactive ingredient of the plant. Because cannabinoid use policies vary from country to country, travelers should review the policies and regulations around transport, possession, and use of cannabis or cannabinoids in the countries to which they are traveling and passing through. In many countries, possession and use of cannabis can result in severe criminal penalties, including imprisonment.

Cannabis has been legalized in some US states for medical or nonmedical adult use, and although its use and possession at some airports might be allowed, cannabis remains categorized as a Schedule I substance (www.dea.gov/drug-information/drug-scheduling) in the United States and is illegal at the federal level. Cruise lines follow federal law; federal scheduling of cannabis as a Schedule I substance also prohibits use and possession on cruise ships.

OPIOIDS

According to the National Survey on Drug Use and Health (https://nsduhweb.rti.org), in 2020, 9.5 million people aged >12 years reported misusing prescription opioids or using heroin within the past 12 months, and 2.7 million reported having an opioid use disorder (OUD). OUD is not uncommon in the United States, and travel medicine providers likely will encounter patients experiencing, or in recovery for, this condition. Preparing travelers with OUD to travel internationally requires additional planning.

Illicit opioid use and misuse of prescription opioids are factors that increase risk for overdose. Evidence-based strategies for reducing the risk for overdose associated with illicit opioid use include use of fentanyl test strips (FTS) and access to naloxone. FTS are used to determine whether fentanyl has been mixed with drugs; naloxone can reverse an overdose from opioids, including fentanyl, heroin, and prescription opioid medications.

Medications for Treating Opioid Use Disorder

Medications are available to effectively prevent overdose, treat OUD, and sustain recovery; these medications might be restricted or prohibited in other countries, however. Examples of medications used to treat OUD include buprenorphine and methadone, which act as opioid agonists. These medications reduce cravings and withdrawal symptoms and block the effects of other opioids (e.g., heroin). The opioid antagonist naltrexone works by blocking the effects of opioids.

The Transportation Security Administration (TSA), US Department of State, and US Centers for Disease Control and Prevention (CDC) provide guidance for traveling with prescription medications, including medications used to treat substance use disorders. Travelers should check with the US embassy (www.usembassy.gov) located in the country they plan to visit or travel through to make certain their medications are allowed in that country and determine whether they need any documentation to bring medications. The International Narcotics Control Board provides information on country regulations for travelers carrying medications containing controlled substances at www.incb.org/incb/en/travellers/country-regulations.html.

Travelers should carry all medications in their original labeled container with a copy of the prescription printed on the container and a statement from the medical director of the clinic or prescribing physician on letterhead detailing the care being provided. The name listed on prescriptions, medication bottles, and letters from health care providers should match the name on the traveler's passport. Although medications can be packed in carry-on or checked baggage, traveling with prescriptions in carry-on luggage can help to ensure ready access to medications in an emergency or if checked luggage is lost.

METHADONE

In the United States, methadone treatment programs are strictly regulated by the federal government, and methadone treatment for OUD can only be dispensed by federally certified opioid treatment programs (OTPs); regulations include prerequisites to be eligible for take-home medication. Most methadone treatment programs dispense the medication daily in person, and a patient must complete continuous treatment in an OTP for >12 months before being permitted to take home >1 week's supply of methadone. A maximum of 1 month's (31 days) supply of methadone can be provided to patients who have completed 2 years of continuous treatment.

Recovery Support Services

Encourage patients with OUD to review information about recovery support services in other countries, such as information provided on the Narcotics Anonymous website (www.na.org). In addition, global advocacy and support groups are available for people taking methadone and other treatments for OUD. For instance, the German organization INDRO e.V. operates the Coordinating and Information Resource Center for International Travel by Patients Receiving Methadone and other Substitution Treatments for Opiate Addiction (https://indro-online.de/en/the-coordinating-and-information-resource-center-for-international-travel) and publishes International Travel Regulations for Patients Participating in Drug Substitution Treatment (https://indro-online.de/en/travel-regulations-for-patients-participating-in-drug-substitution-treatment) and the Methadone Worldwide Travel Guide (https://indro-online.de/en/methadone-worldwide-travel-guide).

SUBSTANCE USE DISORDER TREATMENT

A subtype of "medical tourism" (see Sec. 6, Ch. 4, Medical Tourism) involves travel to another country for SUD treatment and rehabilitation care ("rehab tourism"). Box 3-10 lists some pros and cons of tourism for substance use disorder treatment. Travelers exploring this option might be seeking a greater range of treatment options at less expense than what is available domestically.

Before a traveler selects an international program for SUD treatment, encourage them to review information that can help them better understand proposed treatments. Evidence-based guidance is available from the Substance Abuse and Mental Health Services Administration (www.samhsa.gov/medication-assisted-treatment;

BOX 3-10 Pros & cons of international substance use disorder treatment

PROS	CONS
Treatment and accommodations might be more affordable	Difficult for family to visit or have an active role in treatment process
Privacy and seclusion might better afford anonymity	Difficult to arrange follow-up care; might be unable to liaise with local (at-home) support systems and services
Separation from triggers, stressors, sources of drugs, friends/family/acquaintances not supportive of recovery	Language or communication challenges
Potentially wider range of treatment alternatives	Differences in customs, attitudes, treatment plans
Combining vacation with treatment	Potential issues involving payment options, coverage, and reimbursement with standard medical insurance; not covered by travel health insurance
	Uncertainty about treatment modalities, quality of care, success rates

www.samhsa.gov/medication-assisted-treatment/medications-counseling-related-conditions/co-occurring-disorders; www.samhsa.gov/resource/ebp/treatment-stimulant-use-disorders) and CDC (www.cdc.gov/drugoverdose/featured-topics/evidence-based-strategies.html).

BIBLIOGRAPHY

Bergman BG, Hoeppner BB, Nelson LM, Slaymaker V, Kelly JF. The effects of continuing care on emerging adult outcomes following residential addiction treatment. Drug Alcohol Depend. 2015;153:207–14.

Centers for Disease Control and Prevention (CDC). Vital signs: overdoses of prescription opioid pain relievers—United States, 1999–2008. MMWR MorbMortal Wkly Rep. 2011;60(43):1487–92.

Centers for Disease Control and Prevention. Recovery is possible: treatment for opioid addiction. Available from: www.cdc.gov/drugoverdose/featured-topics/treatment-recovery.html.

Centers for Disease Control and Prevention. Traveling abroad with medicine. Available from: https://wwwnc.cdc.gov/travel/page/travel-abroad-with-medicine.

Paz A, Sadetzki S, Potasman I. High rates of substance abuse among long-term travelers to the tropics: an interventional study. J Travel Med. 2004;11(2):75–81.

Rundle AG, Revenson TA, Friedman M. Business travel and behavioral and mental health. J Occup Environ Med. 2018;60(7):612–6.

Substance Abuse and Mental Health Services Administration. Federal guidelines for opioid treatment programs. HHS publication no. (SMA) PEP15-FEDGUIDEOTP. Rockville, MD: The Administration; 2015. Available from: https://store.samhsa.gov/sites/default/files/d7/priv/pep15-fedguideotp.pdf.

Transportation Service Administration. Travel tips: Can you pack your meds in a pill case and more questions answered. Available from: www.tsa.gov/travel/travel-tips/can-you-pack-your-meds-pill-case-and-more-questions-answered.

Wackernah RC, Minnick MJ, Clapp P. Alcohol use disorder: pathophysiology, effects, and pharmacologic options for treatment. Subst Abuse Rehabil. 2014;23(5):1–12.

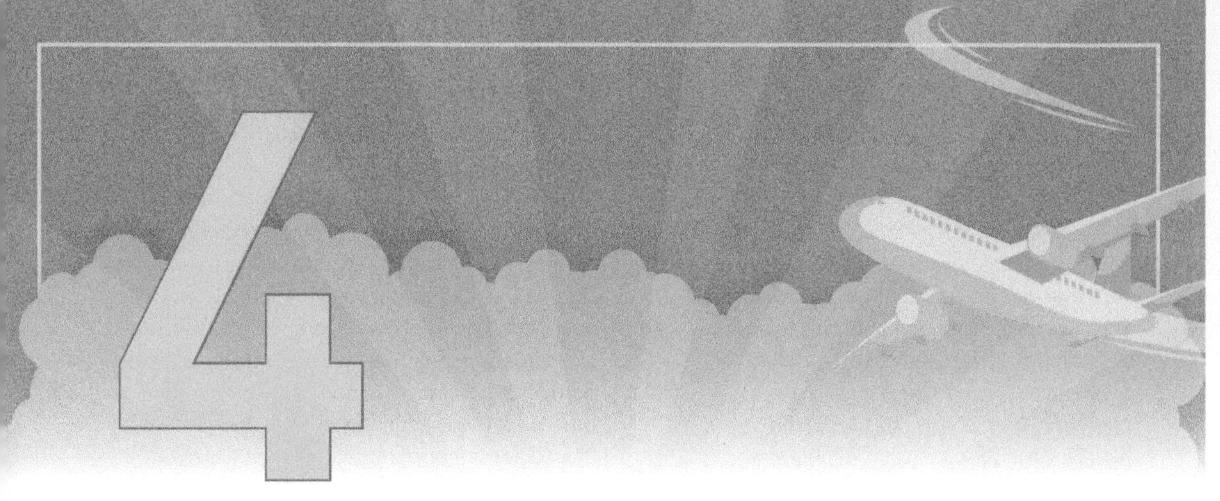

4 Environmental Hazards & Risks

SUN EXPOSURE

Karolyn Wanat, David Fivenson, Scott Norton

When international travelers engage in outdoor activities, they might be exposed to more ultraviolet (UV) radiation (UVR) than they are accustomed to, particularly if travel takes them to sunnier locations, lower latitudes, or higher elevations. Even winter activities (e.g., snow skiing) can result in significant UVR exposure. Short bursts of high-intensity UVR (e.g., infrequent beach vacations), as well as frequent, prolonged, cumulative UVR exposure can cause acute effects (e.g., sunburn and phototoxic medication reactions) and delayed effects from chronic exposure (e.g., sun damage, premature aging, skin cancers).

RISK FACTORS

Time of year, time of day, and location influence a traveler's UVR exposure. Most UVR reaches the earth's surface during summer months. Ultraviolet B (UVB), which is more carcinogenic than ultraviolet A (UVA), is most intense from 10 a.m.–4 p.m. at higher elevations and in locations closer to the equator. Snow and sand reflect UVR, thereby increasing UVB exposure. Although UVA is less carcinogenic than UVB, UVA occurs at high intensity throughout daylight hours. UVA causes more acute photosensitivity reactions than UVB, and it contributes more to premature aging.

Ultraviolet Index

The US National Weather Service prepares a daily Ultraviolet Index (UVI) for most zip codes. The UVI is calculated by a computer model that couples solar energy delivered at ground level with the ozone forecast and adjusts for elevation, atmospheric aerosol properties, and cloud conditions. The globally accepted UVI scale ranges from

CDC Yellow Book 2024. Jeffrey Nemhauser, Oxford University Press.
DOI: 10.1093/oso/9780197570944.003.0004

0 (at night or under a smoke-filled sky) to 16 (at high elevation in the tropics with no cloud cover). Higher UVIs indicate greater risks for skin- and eye-damaging UVR.

Daily UVIs for US locations are available at www.weather.gov/rah/uv. Global data for many sites outside the United States are available at the WHO website, www.who.int/news-room/q-a-detail/radiation-the-ultraviolet-(uv)-index.

Underlying Medical Conditions

People with certain medical conditions are at increased risk for adverse effects of UV exposure. Solid-organ transplant recipients, for example, are at much greater risk for UVB-induced skin cancers. People with autoimmune connective tissue diseases (e.g., systemic lupus erythematosus) exhibit heightened photosensitivity. Counsel these patients on how to protect themselves during hours of maximal exposure.

Photosensitizing Medications

Many medications, including several prescribed specifically for travelers, can lead to photosensitivity reactions. Examples include:

Antibiotics, including doxycycline (and other tetracyclines to a lesser degree), fluoroquinolones, sulfonamides.

Many types of cancer therapies (e.g., chemotherapeutic agents, radiation therapy, some immunomodulators) can be sun sensitizers during treatment, and effects can linger even after completion of therapy.

Nonsteroidal anti-inflammatory drugs (NSAIDs), especially ibuprofen, ketoprofen, naproxen, piroxicam.

Other common medications (e.g., furosemide, methotrexate, sulfonylureas, thiazide diuretics, retinoids).

CONSEQUENCES

Sunburn

Sunburn is a common and self-limited condition caused by UVA or UVB. Clinical features vary from mild pink to painful red skin with swelling and blistering on exposed surfaces. Systemic symptoms can include headache, fever, chills, nausea, vomiting, and muscle aches. Sunburn is preventable and travelers should not regard it as an inevitable part of vacation.

Sunburn management consists of symptomatic pain relief. People rarely notice they are developing a sunburn while the burn is occurring. When discomfort begins, people can take cool baths or apply wet compresses and bland topical emollients (e.g., petrolatum, zinc oxide). Refrigerating topical emollients before application can provide added relief. Aloe vera commonly is used as a sunburn remedy, but studies regarding its benefit are equivocal.

Intact blisters should not be ruptured intentionally. Topical corticosteroids (e.g., hydrocortisone 1% cream or ointment) or diclofenac gel can decrease pain and inflammation. Sunburn patients typically benefit from rest in a cool setting, extra fluids, and oral pain relievers (e.g., acetaminophen, ibuprofen, naproxen). Systemic steroids do not improve symptoms or hasten recovery.

For severe blistering cases, clinicians might need to hospitalize patients for fluid replacement (oral or intravenous) and pain control and treat them as they would burn patients, maintaining clean skin by gentle cleansing and treatment with emollients. Tense or painful blisters can be sterilely drained, but the blister roof should remain intact to serve as a sterile dressing.

Sun Damage & Skin Cancer

High-intensity or chronic exposure to UVR (particularly UVA) causes permanent loss of skin elasticity, wrinkling, and solar lentigines (brown macules with irregular borders), especially in people with fair skin. Avoiding sun overexposure and preventing sunburn are the best ways to avoid these skin changes.

The World Health Organization (WHO) characterizes UVR as a carcinogen with the potential to induce skin cancers via DNA damage. In addition, skin cancers are the most common malignancies in the United States, and basal and squamous cell carcinomas (BCCs and SCCs) are linked closely to UV exposure. BCCs typically appear as pearly, red papules that might bleed, ulcerate, or grow into nodules; they appear often on sun-exposed areas. BCCs rarely metastasize and are generally cured with excision or other local treatments.

SCCs present as scaling or bleeding papules or plaques on sun-exposed areas. Advanced or long-standing SCCs are 10× more likely to metastasize than BCCs. Solid-organ transplant patients who are on immunosuppressive therapy and patients with chronic lymphocytic leukemia are at increased risk for SCCs.

Melanoma is the most serious of the UV-associated skin cancers; it is also the least common, but its incidence is increasing among most populations. Risk factors for melanoma include fair skin, genetic susceptibility, and a history of blistering sunburns before the age of 18. Melanomas have a variety of clinical presentations, the most common of which is an irregularly bordered, darkly pigmented flat or raised spot on the skin that changes in size, shape, or both over time. For clinical suspicion for melanoma, clinicians should refer the patient for prompt evaluation and possible biopsy. Of the skin cancers, melanomas have the greatest morbidity and mortality; in 2018, the latest year for which incidence data are available, ≈84,000 new cases of melanoma of the skin were reported in the United States, and ≈8,200 people died from this cancer. Early detection and treatment (simple excision with margins) lead to complete recovery in most cases. Depending on the tumor stage, patients might need additional surgeries, evaluations, treatment with chemotherapeutic or biological agents, and regular monitoring.

While some reports describe an association between chronic and cumulative sun exposure and SCC, and intermittent intense sun exposure and blistering sunburns with BCC and melanoma, the evidence for this in the literature is mixed.

Other Photosensitivity Disorders

Increased exposure to sunlight, particularly UVA, can exacerbate existing skin conditions and can unmask photosensitivity disorders, such as autoimmune connective tissue diseases (e.g., dermatomyositis or systemic lupus erythematosus), phototoxic medication reactions, polymorphous light eruption, porphyrias, and solar urticaria. A person experiencing prolonged or severe symptoms after sun exposure (e.g., arthralgias, fever, pruritus, swelling) should seek medical evaluation.

PHOTO-ONYCHOLYSIS

Photo-onycholysis is a separation or lifting of the nail plate from the nail bed in people taking an oral photosensitizing agent, usually a medication, in association with intense sun exposure. The most common setting is someone taking doxycycline for malaria prophylaxis during a trip to a tropical location.

PHYTOPHOTODERMATITIS

Phytophotodermatitis is a noninfectious condition that results from action of UVA radiation on naturally occurring photosensitizing compounds, furocoumarins, that occur in several plant families. In the tropics, the most common source is the photosensitizing juice of certain types of limes, often called Persian, wild, or key limes; in northern temperate regions, the most common source is giant hogweed (*Heracleum mentagazzium*). The interaction of UV light and the furocoumarins causes an exaggerated sunburn that creates a painful line of blisters where the juice was on the skin, followed by linear, brown, hyperpigmented patches that take weeks or months to resolve.

PREVENTION

Travelers should prepare and plan to prevent sun overexposure. To encourage safe sun behaviors, clinicians can remind travelers that UVB radiation is highest during midday, that UV exposure still occurs in cooler weather and on overcast days, and that UVR increases with travel to lower latitudes (closer to the equator) and higher elevations.

Sun Avoidance

If possible, travelers can decrease UV exposure by avoiding direct sun during peak hours, 10 a.m. to 4 p.m. Travelers can seek shade under trees, umbrellas, or other structures to reduce UV exposure; UV rays can still reflect off surfaces, however, including snow and sand. Studies show that concomitantly using shade and sunscreen is more effective than reliance on a single method to protect people from excessive UVR.

Sunscreens

Sunscreens are topical preparations containing substances that reflect or absorb light in the

BOX 4-01 Choosing a sunscreen

The most effective sunscreens are broad-spectrum, combining agents capable of filtering (either by absorbing or reflecting) both ultraviolet A and B (UVA and UVB) radiation.

The American Academy of Dermatology Practice Safe Sun guidelines (Box 4-05) recommend using products with a sun protection factor (SPF) ≥30.

Current labeling guidelines adopted by the US Food and Drug Administration (FDA) in 2010 indicate that broad-spectrum sunscreen products with an SPF ≥15 may state: If used as directed with other sun-protection measures, [this product] decreases the risk of skin cancer and early skin aging caused by the sun.

The same labeling guidelines do not permit manufacturers to claim that products are waterproof or sweatproof; sunscreens may be labeled "water resistant" for up to either 40 or 80 minutes.

CHOOSING A SUNSCREEN OUTSIDE THE UNITED STATES

Sunscreens sold outside the United States contain a much wider variety of UV filters.

The UV filters listed below have lower reported environmental toxicity, but none have yet come up for review before the FDA.

The FDA process for UV filter approval is under review and will most likely begin with systematic human toxicity testing of the currently allowed UV filters before agents in use elsewhere in the world are included.

In Europe, Japan, and Australia, commonly available UV filters in sunscreens include the following:

Mexoryl XL (drometrizole trisiloxane)
Neo Heliopan AP (bisdisulizole disodium)
Neo Heliopan E1000 (amiloxate)
Parsol 5000 (enzacamene, 4-MBC)
Tinsorb A2B (tris-biphenyl triazine)
Tinsorb M (bisoctrizole)
Tinsorb S (bemotrizinol)
Tinsorb S Aqua (polysilicone-15)
Uvasorb HEB (iscotrizinol)
Uvinul A Plus (diethylamino, hydroxybenzoyl hexyl benzoate)
Uvinul T 150 (octyl triazone)

In South America, commonly available UV filters in sunscreens include the following:

Mexoryl SL (benzylidene camphor sulfonic acid)
Mexoryl SO (camphor benzalkonium)
Mexoryl SW (polyacryamidomethylbenzylidene camphor)
PEG-25 PABA (ethoxylated ethyl-4-aminobenzoate)

UV wavelengths and reduce the amount of UVR that reaches the skin. There are two classes of active ingredients, known as UV filters, in sunscreen products: chemical (sometimes referred to as organic) and physical (sometimes referred to as mineral or inorganic). Sunscreen products can contain chemical or physical filters, or both, and might include >1 of each type. FDA regulates sunscreens and their filtering agents in the United States, but some other countries permit the use of chemical filtering agents not approved by the FDA. See Box 4-01 for filtering agents in sunscreen products from different countries.

CHOOSING A SUNSCREEN

Travelers can use many criteria when selecting a sunscreen, but in practical terms, the best sunscreens are those that people choose to use consistently. See Box 4-01 for additional details on choosing sunscreens.

SUN PROTECTION FACTOR

The US Food and Drug Administration (FDA) uses a strict protocol to determine a product's sun protection factor (SPF): how much UVB radiation is required to cause a sunburn on skin protected by topical sunscreen products versus the amount of UVB required to cause a sunburn on unprotected skin (see Box 4-02). SPF measures protection from UVB only, not UVA. Most people know that the higher the SPF, the greater degree of protection from UVB and from sunburn.

In theory, an SPF of 30 means that only 1/30th of the UVB reaches the skin—or that a person can remain in the sun 30× as long—when the sunscreen is applied. To achieve the desired SPF, however, a person must apply an adequate amount of sunscreen, avoid rinsing or rubbing or sweating it off, and reapply it every 2 hours. From a mathematical perspective, sunscreens rated as SPF 30 block 97% of UVB, SPF 50 block 98%, and SPF 100

BOX 4-02 US Food and Drug Administration (FDA) sunscreen definitions

SUN PROTECTION FACTOR (SPF)

A measure of how much solar energy (UVB radiation) is required to produce sunburn on protected skin (i.e., in the presence of sunscreen) relative to the amount of solar energy required to produce sunburn on unprotected skin. As the SPF value increases, sunburn protection increases.

BROAD SPECTRUM

The FDA permits a sunscreen to be labeled as "broad spectrum" if it provides adequate protection from both UVA and UVB radiation.

WATER RESISTANT

Claims of water resistance on a sunscreen's label must indicate whether the sunscreen remains effective for 40 minutes or 80 minutes while swimming or sweating, based on standard testing. Sunscreens that do not meet this standard must include a direction instructing consumers to use a water-resistant sunscreen when swimming or sweating.

The FDA does not define, nor does it use, the following terms: baby-safe, reef-safe, anti-aging, sport, kid-friendly, dermatologist-tested, all natural, sweat-proof, or waterproof.

block 99%. The FDA discourages claims of SPF >50 on a product's label because it is meaningless.

CHEMICAL (ORGANIC) UV FILTERS

Sunscreens with chemical UV filters are absorbed into the skin and work like a sponge to absorb the sun's rays. Chemical UV filters currently approved for use in the United States include avobenzone, cinoxate, ecamsule, homosalate, octinoxate, octisalate, octocrylene, and oxybenzone. Less commonly used filters include dioxybenzone, ensulizole, meradimate, padimate O, and sulisobenzone. Products containing chemical UV filters can be easier to apply and are less likely to leave a white residue than physical UV filters. People with naturally dark skin might be averse to using certain sunscreens because they leave a whitish appearance or ashy look; however, people with dark skin also need protection against the short- and long-term effects of UVR described above. Box 4-03 provides information on some possible

BOX 4-03 Risks associated with sunscreen use: human

CHEMICAL (ORGANIC) ULTRAVIOLET (UV) FILTERS

Contact dermatitis, both allergic and irritant.

Sun sensitivity (associated with avobenzone, cinoxate, octocrylene).

Several studies show that chemical UV filtering agents can be absorbed across the skin and reach detectable levels in human blood and tissues. Chemical UV filters have been widely detected in urine, blood, and breast milk. Many of these compounds are being studied as possible endocrine disruptors, which means they might interfere with hormones doing their normal bodily functions. The effects, if any, that chemical UV filters have on hormones like thyroid, estrogen, and testosterone in humans, marine or aquatic organisms, or ecosystems are unclear. In experimental animal studies, where much higher amounts of UV filter have been used, reports of significant changes in thyroid and sex hormones and potential effects on fertility and fetal development have been reported.

Recent reports of potential carcinogenicity of sunscreens were the result of poor manufacturing practices that allowed contaminants (e.g., benzene) to taint the products and were not due to intrinsic carcinogenicity of the sunscreen agents.

PHYSICAL (INORGANIC) UV FILTERS

Rarely, cause skin irritation.

People should avoid using as sprays, because inhaling metallic nanoparticles can be harmful to the lungs.

BOX 4-04 Risks associated with sunscreen use: environmental

Among the most concerning reports about sunscreens is that ultraviolet (UV) filters might harm marine ecosystems. This is a complex and unresolved point, because coral is damaged by a variety of environmental changes, especially cycles of increased ocean water temperatures. Laboratory evidence suggests that high concentrations of certain UV filters damage the symbiotic algae, known as zooxanthellae, that live within the live tips of coral, causing a loss of color known as "coral bleaching." Repeated cycles of bleaching can kill living coral. Many other marine and aquatic organisms are also being studied for possible effects caused by chemical sunscreens. Overall, less evidence shows that physical UV filters (zinc oxide and titanium dioxide) pose toxicity to humans, animals, or the environment.

Clinicians should suggest that travelers choose sunscreens that are the least harmful for marine ecosystems. Several states and nations have legislation prohibiting the use of chemical (organic) sunscreens in favor of products containing physical (inorganic) UV filters, zinc oxide or titanium oxide. Many ocean resort destinations have banned some of the chemical UV filters; these include Hawaii, the US Virgin Islands, Palau, Bonaire, Aruba, Mexico, Brazil, and numerous locations in the European Union. Travelers should check regulations in effect at their destination prior to departure.

When selecting sunscreens that contain chemical UV filters, travelers should choose products that contain less than 3% avobenzone, 3% cinoxate, 3% ecamsule, 10% homosalate, 5% octinoxate, 5% octisalate, 5% octocrylene, or 5% oxybenzone.

Good sources of independent information for consumers and travelers on ever-changing sunscreen information include Consumer Reports (www.consumerreports.org) and the Environmental Working Group (www.ewg.org), both of which regularly review and rate sunscreen products and their components.

The National Oceanographic and Atmospheric Administration (NOAA) provides a useful infographic on this topic (https://oceanservice.noaa.gov/news/sunscreen-corals.html).

4

health risks associated with use of chemical UV filters.

PHYSICAL (INORGANIC) UV FILTERS

Physical, or inorganic, UV filters reflect both UVA and UVB from the skin's surface. Worldwide, only 2 products are used as physical filters: zinc oxide and titanium dioxide. These metallic oxides are pulverized into microparticle or nanoparticle size, then mixed with a vehicle or emollient that permits them to be applied smoothly to the skin. Sunscreens might contain none, one, or both agents.

Physical sunscreens pose very little risk of causing allergic or irritant contact dermatitis (see Box 4-03). They can, however, leave a thin, white film or cast on the skin. Nevertheless, current products are cosmetically more acceptable than the older thick, opaque pastes.

Travelers also might opt for or be required to use sunscreens with physical UV filters due to reported adverse environmental effects of chemical UV filter–containing sunscreens (see Box 4-04). Some locations that require physical UV filters include Aruba, Bonaire, parts of Mexico, Palau, and the US Virgin Islands. In 2018, Hawaii passed a law banning sunscreens containing octinoxate and oxybenzone in response to evidence of their toxicity to coral marine life.

SUNSCREENS FOR CHILDREN

Parents or guardians should protect children <6 months old from direct sun exposure, opt for shade, and dress children in lightweight long-sleeved shirts, long pants, wide-brimmed hats, and sunglasses. They can protect infants by using covered strollers or perambulators, umbrellas or parasols, and hats, rather than by applying sunscreen.

For children >6 months of age, parents or guardians should use sunscreens with physical UV filters (titanium dioxide or zinc oxide) rather than chemical UV filters; physical UV filters are less likely to irritate young children's sensitive skin. Teens might want an oil-free sunscreen for the face to help avoid exacerbations of acne due to thicker, oily preparations. Adults can safely use sunscreen marketed for children.

BOX 4-05 Recommendations for safe sun exposure for travelers

Avoid direct sun exposure between 10 a.m. and 4 p.m. when ultraviolet (UV) rays are strongest.
When going outside, opt for shady areas, such as the full shade provided by natural or man-made fixed objects. Trees provide varying degrees of sun protection depending on the density of the foliage.
Consider using portable shade shelters (e.g., awnings, canopies, umbrellas and parasols, beach tents, similar shade structures). Look for items made with fabrics having a UV protection factor (UPF) >30.
Wear lightweight long-sleeved garments made of fabric with a UPF >30.
Wear a hat with circumferential brim ≥3 inches wide that shades the face, neck, and ears. Do not rely on standard baseball caps; opt for sun-specific caps that include ear and neck flaps, many of which are made of UPF fabrics.
Wear sunglasses to protect eyes from UV radiation.
Remember that UV light reflected off water, snow, or sand can amplify UV radiation received.
Apply a broad-spectrum sunscreen daily, ≥15 minutes before going outside to allow absorption in the skin's outermost layer.
Choose a sunscreen that protects against UVA and UVB rays. Use products with a sun protection factor (SPF) ≥30; to adequately cover the body, apply ≥1 fluid ounce (equivalent to 2 tablespoons or a shot glass) of sunscreen.
Reapply sunscreen every 2–4 hours, more frequently when sweating or after being in water. Be sure to apply sunscreen to commonly missed areas (e.g., ears, tops of the feet).
Apply a lip balm with SPF ≥30. Remember that many lip balms are simply petrolatum-based moisturizers for chapped lips; look specifically for products labeled as SPF 30 or more.

Source: Adapted from the American Academy of Dermatology Association's Practice Safe Sun guidelines. Available from www.aad.org/public/everyday-care/sun-protection/shade-clothing-sunscreen/practice-safe-sun.

APPLYING SUNSCREEN

Guidelines for sunscreen use recommend regular application of lotions or cream-based broad-spectrum UVA and UVB blocking (SPF ≥30) products (see Box 4-05). People should reapply sunscreen to all exposed areas every 2–4 hours. The average adult needs 1 fluid ounce (1 shot glass full) for each application. People should gently and evenly spread sunscreen, not rub in, on all exposed skin ≥15 minutes prior to going outside to allow UVR blocking effects to penetrate the outer skin layers. Stick or roll-on sunscreens are easy to apply, but people often apply these unevenly, leading to sunburned areas missed during application. If travelers choose to use these products, they should gently spread the product after application.

SPRAY SUNSCREENS

People often apply spray sunscreens unevenly, especially under breezy conditions. Consumer Reports (July 2020) recommends holding the spray nozzle 1 inch from the skin and spraying until the skin glistens uniformly, then gently spreading the product to evenly coat the skin, even if the product claims to be "no rub." Some environmental health organizations discourage use of spray sunscreens because the contents are as likely to get into the environment as they are to get onto a person's skin.

People should avoid spraying the sunscreen on or near the face, because the particulate components can injure the eyes or damage lung tissue if inhaled. People should spray their palms and then apply the sunscreen to their faces. Similarly, parents or guardians should avoid spray products for small children due to risks for inhalation and getting product in children's eyes; adults should spray product on their own hands and then apply onto the child's skin.

Protective Clothing

Sun-protective garments (e.g., pants, long-sleeved shirts, hats) protect against UVR, but efficacy depends on the fabric. Thicker fabrics with tighter or denser weaves (e.g., denim), offer higher UV Protection Factor (UPF). Like SPF, the UPF of a fabric or material represents the fraction of UVR that penetrates the material. UPF 50, for example, means only 1/50th of the UVR gets through the fabric; 98% of UVR is blocked. A UPF rating of 15–24 is considered good, 25–39 is very good, and ≥40 is excellent. Many outdoor clothing and active wear manufacturers now use densely woven, lightweight, quick drying, synthetic UPF fabrics to make extremely comfortable shirts, pants, and hats.

Many companies also use UPF fabric to make swim-shirts, also called rash guards. Swim-shirts are available with short or long sleeves or with built-in hoods. Because UPF 50 fabric blocks 98% of UVR, a person does not need to apply sunscreen to surfaces covered by the shirts, and parents might choose these for young children who dislike having sunscreen applied. Surfers, lap swimmers, and open-water swimmers might prefer smaller, tighter sizes for a streamlined (hydrodynamic) feel in the water.

HATS

The ideal hat has a circumferential brim ≥3 inches wide that shades the face, neck, and ears. People should not rely on standard baseball caps for sun protection, because these do not protect the ears or neck. Instead, people should opt for sun-specific caps that include ear and neck flaps, many of which are made of UPF fabrics. These can be quite effective, especially for children.

SUNGLASSES

UVR exposure can have short- and long-term damaging effects on the eyes. UVA can harm central vision by damaging the macula. UVB can damage the anterior eye (cornea and lens); acute exposure can lead to corneal burns, and extended exposure can lead to cataracts. UVR can penetrate clouds and haze, so people should protect their eyes regardless of atmospheric conditions.

Excessive UVB exposure, even over several hours, can cause a corneal sunburn, also called photokeratitis or snow blindness. Photokeratitis causes extremely painful sensitivity to light, often causing a person to keep their eyes closed for several hours or more. Snow blindness can occur when UVR reflected off snow nearly doubles the UV exposure to the eye. Other symptoms include copious tearing (watery eyes), injected sclerae (noninfectious pink eye), or a gritty foreign-body sensation of the eye. These symptoms are usually temporary and rarely cause permanent damage to the eyes.

Long-term UVR exposure can lead to cataract formation, age-related macular degeneration, benign conjunctival growths (called pterygium and pinguecula), and cancers of the eyelids or even the conjunctivae.

Sunglasses provide UV protection for the eyes. Wrap-around sunglasses or those with sun-blocking sidepieces provide the best UV protection. People should choose close-fitting frames that contour to the shape of the face to prevent exposure to direct and reflected UVR from all sides and angles.

People also should choose sunglasses that are rated UV 400; these block nearly 100% of damaging UVR. Lenses should have a uniform tint throughout; although gray tints offer the best color fidelity, tint color (e.g., amber, gray, green) does not affect sun protection efficacy. Polarized or mirrored lenses are not more effective at protecting against UVR. Inexpensive, non-branded sunglasses rated UV 400 are just as effective as expensive, designer-label sunglasses. Parents or guardians should provide appropriate eye protection for children. Some contact lenses offer a modicum of UV protection, but people should also wear sunglasses with contact lenses.

The American Academy of Ophthalmology and the American Optometry Association provide recommendations and information on gradient, transitional, and prescription sunglasses at these websites: Tips for Choosing the Best Sunglasses (www.aao.org/eye-health/glasses-contacts/sunglasses-3); Recommended Types of Sunglasses (www.aao.org/eye-health/glasses-contacts/sunglasses-recommended-types); and Ultraviolet (UV) Protection (www.aoa.org/healthy-eyes/caring-for-your-eyes/uv-protection).

Beach Umbrellas & Sunshade Shelters

Several types of shade shelters are available: umbrellas, canopies, and tents. Many shelters marketed for sunshade combine several features. People should choose a shelter made with a fire-resistant UPF 50 fabric, usually nylon or polyester, and a durable but lightweight frame. Additional features travelers should consider are the size needed to accommodate number of people who will use the shelter at once; the weight and ability to collapse and easily transport the shelter; water-resistant fabric for rain squalls; open or mesh sides that allow adequate air circulation; ability to securely anchor the shelter to the ground with stakes, fillable sandbags, or a combination; and easy assembly, ideally by 1 person. Standard camping tents generally are unsuitable for sun shelters.

Travelers should select beach umbrellas with ample diameter and directional tilt, so the protective field can be adjusted as the sun rises and crosses the sky. Tall umbrellas with a small surface area lose their protective benefits when the sun is at a low angle. Wind gusts can uproot and launch umbrellas, posing a safety hazard. Therefore, people should select an umbrella with parts that can be attached securely to each other and placed firmly in the ground. Screw-type bases can anchor an umbrella in the sand, but usually are sold separately. Travelers should be aware that some public beaches limit the size of shade shelters that can be used.

SUNLESS TANNING

Topical sunless tanning products are a safer way people can gain a tanned look. Although these products make the skin appear darker, they do not provide photoprotection, and travelers should still use sunscreen when exposed to UVR. Sunless tanning products can produce streaking when people sweat or go swimming and can generate an unnatural orange hue on areas of the skin where applied.

Many people believe that getting a pre-vacation tan by using tanning beds will help protect them from vacation sunburns. However, tanning bed lights rely on UVA, which is associated with premature aging. Tanning by this method is roughly equivalent to using an SPF 4 sunscreen, which will not prevent sunburns or other forms of solar damage.

ADDITIONAL SOURCES OF INFORMATION

Consumer Reports (CR) and the Environmental Working Group (EWG) review and rate sunscreen products and their components annually. In general, CR ratings (www.consumerreports.org/products/sunscreens-34523/sunscreen-33614/view2) emphasize human safety, ease of use, truth in advertising, cost, and performance, while the EWG (www.ewg.org/sunscreen) emphasizes environmental safety. Both identify sunscreens by brand name.

4

BIBLIOGRAPHY

American Cancer Society. Skin cancer. Available from: www.cancer.org/cancer/skin-cancer.html.

Diaz JH, Nesbitt Jr. T. Sun exposure behavior and protection: recommendations for travelers. J Travel Med. 2013;20(2):108–18.

Fivenson D, Sabzevari N, Qiblawi S, Blitz J, Norton BB, Norton SA. Sunscreens: UV filters to protect us. Part 2: Increasing awareness of UV filters and their potential toxicities to us and our environment. Int J Womens Dermatol. 2020;7(1):45–69.

Mitchelmore CL, Burns EE, Conway A, Heyes A, Davies IA. A critical review of organic ultraviolet filter exposure, hazard, and risk to corals. Environ Toxicol Chem. 2021;40(4):967–88.

Monteiro AF, Rato M, Martins C. Drug-induced photosensitivity: photoallergic and phototoxic reactions. Clin Dermatol. 2016;34:571.

Religi A, Backes C, Moccozet L, Vuilleumier L, Vernez D, Bulliard JL. Body anatomical UV protection predicted by shade structures: a modeling study. Photochem Photobiol. 2018;94(6):1289–96.

Sabzevari N, Qiblawi S, Norton SA, Fivenson D. Sunscreens: UV filters to protect us. Part 1: Changing regulations and choices for optimal sun protection. Int J Womens Dermatol. 2021;7(1):28–44.

Skin Cancer Foundation. Sun protection: your daily sun protection guide. Available from: www.skincancer.org/prevention/sun-protection.

Suh S, Pham C, Smith J, Mesinkovska NA. The banned sunscreen ingredients and their impact on human health: a systematic review. Int J Dermatol. 2020;59(9):1033–42.

US Preventive Services Task Force; Grossman DC, Curry SJ, Owens DK, Barry MJ, Caughey AB, Davidson KW, et al. Behavioral counseling to prevent skin cancer: US Preventive Services Task Force recommendation statement. JAMA. 2018;319(11):1134–42.

Wood C. Sun and skin: is travel health advice needed? Travel Med Infect Dis. 2013;11(6):438–9.

Young AR, Claveau J, Rossi AB. Ultraviolet radiation and the skin: photobiology and sunscreen photoprotection. J Am Acad Dermatol 2017;76:S100.

EXTREMES OF TEMPERATURE

Howard Backer, David Shlim

4

International travelers encounter extremes of climate to which they might not be accustomed. Exposure to heat and cold can result in serious injury or death. Travelers should investigate the climate extremes they will face during their journey and prepare themselves with knowledge, proper clothing, and equipment to prevent problems. Travelers should also be aware that climate change is expanding the range and severity of exposure to heat across many travel destinations. Regions with wide temperature fluctuation present risk for both heat and cold problems.

HEAT-RELATED ILLNESS

Risk for Travelers

Heat-related illness is most often seen in occupational, military, and competitive sport activities, but also can occur from recreational activities. Many of the most popular travel destinations are hot tropical or arid areas. Travelers who sit on the beach or by the pool and do only short walking tours incur minimal risk for heat-related illness. People participating in more strenuous activities (e.g., hiking or biking) in hot environments are at greater risk, especially those coming from cool or temperate climates who are not in good physical condition and who are unacclimatized to heat.

Physiology

Unlike in the cold, where adaptive behaviors play a more important role in body heat conservation, tolerance to heat depends largely on physiologic factors. Heat regulation depends on a combination of physiological and environmental factors. The major means of heat dissipation are radiation while at rest and evaporation of sweat during exercise, both of which become minimal when air temperatures are above 95°F (35°C) and humidity is high.

Cardiovascular status and conditioning are the major physiologic variables affecting the response to heat stress at all ages. Two major organ systems are most critical in temperature regulation: the cardiovascular system, which must increase blood flow to shunt heat from the core to the surface while meeting the metabolic demands of exercise; and the skin, where sweating and heat exchange take place. Many chronic illnesses limit tolerance to heat and predispose people to heat-related illness, most importantly, cardiovascular disease, diabetes, renal disease, certain medications, and extensive skin disorders or scarring that limit sweating.

Apart from environmental conditions and intensity of exercise, dehydration is the most important predisposing factor in heat-related illness. Dehydration reduces exercise performance, decreases time to exhaustion, and increases internal heat load. Temperature and heart rate increase in direct proportion to the level of dehydration. Sweat is a hypotonic fluid containing sodium and chloride. Sweat rates commonly reach 1 liter per hour or more, resulting in substantial fluid and sodium loss.

Clinical Presentations

MILD

Mild heat-related problems can be treated in the field and usually do not require medical evaluation or evacuation.

Heat cramps are painful muscle contractions that begin ≥1 hours after stopping exercise and most often involve heavily used muscles in the calves, thighs, and abdomen. Rest and passive stretching of the muscle, supplemented by commercial rehydration solutions or water and salt, rapidly relieve symptoms. Drinking water and eating a salty snack also is sufficient. Travelers can make a simple oral salt solution, as described for heat exhaustion.

Heat edema, another mild heat-related illness, occurs more frequently in women than in men. Characterized by mild swelling of the hands and feet during the first few days of heat exposure, this condition typically resolves spontaneously. Travelers should not treat heat edema with diuretics, which can delay heat acclimatization and cause dehydration.

Prickly heat (miliaria or heat rash) manifests as small, red, raised itchy bumps on the skin and is caused by obstruction of the sweat ducts. Prickly heat resolves spontaneously, aided by relief from heat and avoiding continued sweating. Travelers can best prevent prickly heat by wearing light, loose clothing and avoiding heavy, continuous sweating.

MODERATE

Moderate and severe heat-related illnesses present with collapse (syncope) or inability to continue exertion in heat and are treated similarly with rest, removal from heat or direct sun, and administering fluids and salt.

HEAT SYNCOPE

Heat syncope—sudden fainting caused by vasodilation—occurs in unacclimated people standing in the heat or after 15–20 minutes of exercise. Consciousness rapidly returns when the patient is supine. Rest, relief from heat, and oral rehydration are mainstays of treatment.

HEAT EXHAUSTION

Most people who experience symptoms associated with exercise in the heat or the inability to continue exertion in the heat are suffering from heat exhaustion. The presumed cause of heat exhaustion is loss of fluid and electrolytes, but there are no objective markers to define the syndrome. Transient mental changes (e.g., irritability, confusion, irrational behavior) might be present in heat exhaustion, but major neurologic signs (e.g., seizures, coma) indicate heat stroke or profound hyponatremia. Body temperature could be normal or mildly to moderately elevated. Heat exhaustion also can develop over several days in unacclimatized people and often is misdiagnosed as "summer flu" because of findings of weakness, fatigue, headache, dizziness, anorexia, nausea, vomiting, and diarrhea.

Most cases of heat exhaustion can be treated with supine rest in the shade or other cool place and oral water or fluids containing glucose and salt; subsequently, spontaneous cooling occurs, and patients recover within hours. Travelers can prepare a simple oral salt solution by adding one-fourth to one-half teaspoon (1/4–1/2 tsp) of table salt (or two 1-g salt tablets) to 1 liter (33 oz) of water. To improve taste, add a few teaspoons of sugar or orange or lemon juice to the mixture. Commercial sports-electrolyte drinks also are effective. Plain water plus salty snacks might be more palatable and equally effective. Without cessation of activity and passive or active cooling measures (see below), heat exhaustion can progress to heat stroke.

SEVERE

Severe heat-related illness requires medical evacuation and emergency medical attention.

HEAT STROKE

Heat stroke is a medical emergency requiring aggressive cooling measures and hospitalization for support. Heat stroke is the only form of heat-related illness in which the mechanisms for thermal homeostasis have failed, and the body does not spontaneously restore the temperature to normal. Uncontrolled fever and circulatory collapse cause organ damage to the brain, kidneys, liver, and heart. Damage is related to duration and peak elevation of body temperature.

Onset of heat stroke can be acute or gradual. Acute (also known as exertional) heat stroke is characterized by collapse while exercising in the heat, usually with profuse sweating. It can affect healthy, physically fit people. By contrast, gradual or nonexertional (referred to sometimes as classic or epidemic) heat stroke occurs in chronically ill people experiencing passive exposure to heat over several days. Sufferers of nonexertional heat stroke might not perspire. Victims of both exertional and nonexertional heat stroke demonstrate altered mental status and markedly elevated body temperature.

Early symptoms are similar to those of heat exhaustion, including confusion or change in personality, loss of coordination, dizziness, headache, and nausea, but these progress to more severe symptoms. A presumptive diagnosis of heat stroke is made in the field when people have body temperature ≥104°F (≥41°C) and marked alteration of mental status, including delirium, convulsions, and coma; even without a thermometer, people

BOX 4-06 Heat stroke management

In the field, maintain the airway if victim is unconscious, and immediately institute cooling measures by these methods, if available:

Move the victim to the shade or some cool place out of the sun.

Use evaporative cooling: remove excess clothing to maximize skin exposure, spray tepid water on the skin, and maintain air movement over the body by fanning. Alternatively, place cool or cold wet towels over the body and fan to promote evaporation.

Apply ice or cold packs to the neck, axilla, groin, and as much of the body as possible. Vigorously massage the skin to limit constriction of blood vessels and to prevent shivering, which will increase body temperature.

Immerse the victim in cool or cold water (e.g., a nearby pool, natural body of water, bath). An ice bath cools fastest. Always attend and hold the person while in the water.

Encourage rehydration for those able to take oral fluids.

with heat stroke will feel hot to the touch. If a thermometer is available, a rectal temperature is the safest and most reliable way to check the temperature of someone with suspected heat stroke; an axillary temperature might give a reasonable estimation. See Box 4-06 for additional guidance on managing heat stroke.

Heat stroke is life threatening, and many complications occur in the first 24–48 hours, including liver or kidney damage and abnormal bleeding. Most victims have significant dehydration, and many require hospital intensive care management to replace fluid losses. If evacuation to a hospital is delayed, patients should be monitored closely for several hours for temperature swings.

EXERCISE-ASSOCIATED HYPONATREMIA

Hyponatremia occurs in both endurance athletes and recreational hikers due to physiologic mechanisms that result in failure of the kidneys to correct salt and fluid imbalances properly. Excess fluid retention occurs when antidiuretic hormone (secreted inappropriately) influences the kidneys to both retain water and excrete sodium. Sodium losses through sweat also contribute to hyponatremia.

In the field setting, altered mental status in a patient with normal body temperature and a history of taking in large volumes of water suggests hyponatremia. Excessive water ingestion is also a major contributor to exercise-associated hyponatremia; the recommendation to force fluid intake during prolonged exercise and the attitude that "you can't drink too much" is outdated and dangerous. Prevention includes drinking only enough to relieve thirst. During prolonged exercise (>12 hours) or heat exposure, people should take supplemental sodium. Most sports-electrolyte drinks do not contain sufficient sodium to prevent hyponatremia; on the other hand, salt tablets often cause nausea and vomiting. For recreational athletes, food is the most efficient vehicle for salt replacement. Snacks should include not just sweets, but salty foods (e.g., trail mix, crackers, pretzels).

Symptoms of heat exhaustion and early exercise-associated hyponatremia are similar, including anorexia, nausea, emesis, headache, muscle weakness, and lethargy; hyponatremia symptoms can, however, progress to confusion and seizures, and coma. Severe hyponatremia can be distinguished from other heat-related illnesses by persistent alteration of mental status without elevated body temperature, delayed onset of major neurologic symptoms, or deterioration hours after cessation of exercise and removal from heat. Where medical care and clinical laboratory resources are available, clinicians can measure the patient's serum sodium to diagnose hyponatremia and guide treatment.

Treating clinicians should restrict fluid if hyponatremia is suspected (neurologic symptoms in the absence of hyperthermia or other diagnoses). If the patient is conscious and can tolerate oral intake, clinicians should give salty snacks with sips of water or a solution of concentrated broth (2–4 bouillon cubes in 1/2 cup of water). Obtunded hyponatremic patients require hypertonic saline.

Prevention

CLOTHING

Travelers should wear lightweight, loose, light-colored clothing that allows maximum air circulation for evaporation but also gives protection from the sun (see Sec. 4, Ch. 1, Sun Exposure). In addition, travelers can wear a wide-brimmed hat, which can markedly reduce radiant heat exposure.

FLUID & ELECTROLYTE REPLACEMENT

During exertion, fluid intake improves performance and decreases the likelihood of illness. Reliance on thirst alone is not sufficient to prevent mild dehydration, and forcing a person who is not thirsty to drink water increases the risk of hyponatremia. During mild to moderate exertion, electrolyte replacement offers no advantage over plain water. A person exercising for many hours in the heat should replace salt by eating salty snacks or by lightly salting mealtime food or fluids. Salt tablets swallowed whole can cause gastrointestinal irritation and vomiting; tolerability can be improved by dissolving tablets in 1 L of water. Using urine volume and color to monitor fluid needs is most accurate in the morning.

HEAT ACCLIMATIZATION

Heat acclimatization is a process of physiologic adaptation that occurs in residents of and visitors to hot environments. Increased sweating that contains less salt, and decreased energy expenditure with lower rise in body temperature for a given workload, is the result. Only partial adaptation occurs from passive exposure to heat. Full acclimatization, especially cardiovascular, requires 1–2 hours of exercise in the heat each day. With a suitable amount of daily exercise, most acclimatization changes occur within 10 days. Decay of acclimatization occurs within days to weeks if there is no heat exposure.

PHYSICAL CONDITIONING

If possible, all travelers should acclimatize before departing for hot climates by exercising ≥1 hour daily in the heat. Physically fit travelers have improved exercise tolerance and capacity but still benefit from acclimatization. If this is not possible, clinicians should advise travelers to limit exercise intensity and duration during their first week of travel. Travelers also should try to conform to the local practice in most hot regions and avoid strenuous activity during the hottest part of the day.

COLD-RELATED ILLNESS & INJURY

Risk for Travelers

Travelers do not have to be in an arctic or high-elevation environment to encounter problems with cold. Humidity, rain, and wind can produce hypothermia with temperatures around 50°F (10°C). Even in temperate climates, people can rapidly become hypothermic in water. Although reports of severe hypothermia in international travelers are rare, people planning trips to wilderness areas should be familiar with the major mechanisms of heat loss (convection, conduction, and radiation) and how to mitigate them by taking shelter from the wind, getting and staying dry, and keeping warm by building a fire.

Being caught without shelter in a wilderness environment represents a significant risk for accidental hypothermia. Many high-elevation travel destinations, however, are not wilderness areas. Local inhabitants and villages offer shelter and protection from extreme cold weather. In Nepal, for example, trekkers almost never experience hypothermia except in rare instances in which they get lost in a storm.

Clinical Presentations

HYPOTHERMIA

Hypothermia is defined as a core body temperature <95°F (<35°C). When people are faced with an environment in which they cannot keep warm, they first feel chilled, then they shiver, and eventually they stop shivering because their metabolic reserves are exhausted. Body temperature continues to decrease, depending on ambient temperatures. As core body temperature falls, neurologic function decreases; almost all hypothermic people with a core temperature of ≤86°F (≤30°C) are comatose. The record low core body temperature in an adult who survived is 56°F (13°C).

Travelers heading to cold climates should ask questions and research clothing and equipment. Modern clothing, gloves, and particularly footwear have greatly decreased the chances of suffering cold injury in extreme climates. Cold-related illness and injury occurs more often after accidents (e.g., avalanches, unexpected nights outside) than during normal recreational activities.

People engaging in recreational activities or working around cold water face a different sort of risk. Within 15 minutes, immersion hypothermia can render a person unable to swim or float. In these cases, a personal flotation device is critical, as is knowledge about self-rescue and righting a capsized boat.

Other medical conditions associated with cold affect mainly the skin and the extremities. These can be divided into nonfreezing cold injuries and freezing injuries (frostbite).

NONFREEZING COLD INJURY

Nonfreezing cold-related injuries include trench foot (immersion foot), pernio (chilblains), and cold urticaria. Trench foot is caused by prolonged immersion of the feet in cold water (32°F–59°F; 0°C–15°C). The damage is mainly to nerves and blood vessels, and the result is pain aggravated by heat and a dependent position of the limb. Severe cases can take months to resolve. Unlike frostbite, avoid rapid rewarming of trench foot, which can make the damage much worse.

Pernio are localized, inflammatory lesions occurring mainly on the hands after exposure to only moderately cold weather. The bluish-red lesions are thought to be caused by prolonged, cold-induced vasoconstriction. Rapid rewarming makes the pain worse; slow rewarming is preferred. Nifedipine can be an effective treatment.

Cold urticaria are localized or general wheals with itching. The rate of change of temperature, not the absolute temperature, induces this form of skin lesion. If cold urticaria occur regularly in a traveler, they can be prevented or ameliorated by prior treatment with antihistamines.

FREEZING COLD INJURY

Frostbite describes tissue damage caused by direct freezing of the skin. Once severe tissue damage occurs, little can be done. Fortunately, modern equipment and clothing are available to protect adventure tourists from frostbite. The condition now occurs mainly as the result of accidents, severe unexpected weather, or failure to plan appropriately.

Frostbite is usually graded like burns. First-degree frostbite involves reddening of the skin without deeper damage. The prognosis for complete healing is virtually 100%. Second-degree frostbite involves blister formation. Blisters filled with clear fluid have a better prognosis than blood-tinged blisters. Third-degree frostbite represents full-thickness injury to the skin and possibly the underlying tissues. No blisters form, the skin darkens over time and might turn black. If the tissue is completely devascularized, amputation will be necessary.

Severely frostbitten skin is numb and appears whitish or waxy. The generally accepted method for treating a frozen digit or limb is rapid rewarming in water heated to 104°F–108°F (40°C–42°C). Immerse the frozen area completely in the heated water. Use a thermometer to ensure the water is kept at the correct temperature. Rewarming can be associated with severe pain, so analgesics should be given if needed. Once rewarmed, protect frostbitten skin against freezing again. It is better to keep digits frozen a little longer and rapidly rewarm them than to allow them to thaw out slowly or to thaw and refreeze. A cycle of freeze-thaw-refreeze is devastating to tissue, often resulting in amputation.

Once the area has rewarmed, examine for blisters, and note whether the blisters extend to the end of the digit. Proximal blisters usually mean that the tissue distal to the blister has suffered full-thickness damage. For treatment, avoid further mechanical trauma to the area and prevent infection. In the field, wash the area thoroughly with a disinfectant (e.g., povidone iodine), put dressings between the toes or fingers to prevent maceration, use fluffs (expanded gauze sponges) for padding, and cover with a roller gauze bandage. These dressings can be left on safely for up to 3 days at a time. Prophylactic antibiotics are not needed in most situations.

In the rare situation in which a foreign traveler suffers frostbite and can be evacuated to an advanced medical setting within 24–72 hours, there may be a role for thrombolytic agents (e.g., prostacyclin, recombinant tissue plasminogen activator). Clinicians managing a case of frostbite within the first 72 hours should carefully consider the risks and benefits of using these drugs; consultation with an expert is strongly recommended. Beyond 72 hours after thawing, these interventions probably are not beneficial.

Once a patient with frostbite has reached a definitive medical setting, clinicians should not rush to do surgery. The usual time from injury to surgery is 4–5 weeks. Clinicians can use technetium-99m (Tc-99m) scintigraphy and magnetic resonance imaging to define the extent of the damage. Once the delineation between dead and viable tissue becomes clear, clinicians can plan surgery that preserves the remaining digits.

BIBLIOGRAPHY

Aleeban M, Mackey TK. Global health and visa policy reform to address dangers of Hajj during summer seasons. Front Public Health. 2016;4:280.

Armstrong LE, Casa DJ, Millard-Stafford M, Moran DS, Pyne SW, Roberts WO. American College of Sports Medicine position stand. Exertional heat illness during training and competition. Med Sci Sports Exerc. 2007;39(3):556–72.

Asplund CA, O'Connor FG, Noakes TD. Exercise-associated collapse: an evidence-based review and primer for clinicians. Br J Sports Med. 2011;45(14):1157e62.

Bennett BL, Hew-Butler T, Rosner MH, Myers T, Lipman GS. Wilderness Medical Society clinical practice guidelines for the management of exercise-associated hyponatremia: 2019 update. Wilderness Environ Med. 2020;31(1)50–62.

Cauchy E, Cheguillaume B, Chetaille E. A controlled trial of a prostacyclin and rt-PA in the treatment of severe frostbite. N Engl J Med. 2011;364(2):189–90.

Epstein Y, Moran DS. Extremes of temperature and hydration. In: Keystone JS, Kozarsky PE, Connor BA, Nothdurft HD, Mendelson M, Leder K, editors. Travel medicine 4th edition. Philadelphia: Elsevier; 2019. pp. 407–16.

Freer L, Handford C, Imray CHE. Frostbite. In: Auerbach PS, editor. Wilderness medicine, 7th edition. Philadelphia: Elsevier; 2017. pp. 197–221.

Hadad E, Rav-Acha M, Heled Y, Epstein Y, Moran DS. Heat stroke: a review of cooling methods. Sports Med. 2004;34(8):501–11.

Lipman GS, Gaudio FG, Eifling KP, Ellis MA, Otten EM, Grissom CK. Wilderness Medical Society clinical practice guidelines for the prevention and treatment of heat illness: 2019 update. Wilderness Environ Med. 2019;30(4S):S33–46.

McDermott BP, Anderson SA, Armstrong LE, Casa DJ, Cheuvront SN, Cooper L, et al. National Athletic Trainers' Association position statement: fluid replacement for the physically active. J Athl Train. 2017;52(9):877–895.

O'Brien KK, Leon LR, Kenefick RW, O'Connor FG. Clinical management of heat-related illnesses. In: Auerbach PS, editor. Wilderness medicine, 7th edition. Philadelphia: Elsevier; 2019. pp. 267–75.

AIR QUALITY & IONIZING RADIATION

Audrey Pennington, Armin Ansari

Although air pollution has decreased in many parts of the world, it represents a major and growing health problem for the residents of some cities in certain industrializing countries. Polluted air can be difficult or impossible for travelers to avoid; the risk is generally low, however, for otherwise healthy people who have only limited exposure. Conversely, those with preexisting heart and lung disease, children, and older adults have an increased risk for adverse health effects from even short-term exposure to air pollution.

AIR QUALITY

Travelers, particularly people with underlying cardiorespiratory disease, should investigate the air quality at their destination. The AirNow website (http://airnow.gov) provides basic information about local air quality by using the Air Quality

4

Table 4-01 Air quality index levels

AIR QUALITY INDEX LEVELS	AIR QUALITY INDEX VALUES	DESCRIPTION
Good	0–50	Satisfactory air quality Air pollution poses little or no risk
Moderate	51–100	Acceptable air quality Some pollutants could represent a moderate health concern for members of sensitive groups
Unhealthy for sensitive groups	101–150	Members of sensitive groups might experience health effects General public not likely to be affected
Unhealthy	151–200	Everyone could begin to experience health effects Sensitive groups might experience more serious health effects
Very unhealthy	201–300	Health alert: everyone might experience more serious health effects
Hazardous	301–500	Health warnings of emergency conditions Entire population is more likely to be affected

Source: Air Quality Index Basics. Available from: www.airnow.gov/aqi/aqi-basics.

Index (AQI) (Table 4-01). The World Air Quality Index (https://waqi.info) project shows real-time air quality and air pollution data for >10,000 air stations in >80 countries around the world, and the World Health Organization posts historical data on outdoor air pollution in urban areas (http://gamapserver.who.int/gho/interactive_charts/phe/oap_exposure/atlas.html).

Dust masks, surgical masks, and bandanas offer limited protection against severely polluted air. When air is severely polluted (e.g., during wildland fires), the best protection strategies are to avoid prolonged time spent outdoors and to be aware of guidance or directives from local health or emergency management officials (see Wildfire Smoke Factsheet: Protect Your Lungs from Wildfire Smoke or Ash, www.epa.gov/sites/default/files/2018-11/documents/respiratory_protection-no-niosh-5081.pdf). Respirators are specifically designed to remove contaminants from the air or to provide clean respirable air from another source. The National Institute for Occupational Safety and Health (NIOSH) provides a testing, approval, and certification program for respirators (www.cdc.gov/niosh/npptl/topics/respirators/cel/default.html). Parents should be aware that NIOSH does not currently certify respirators for children.

Travelers should be mindful of, and limit exposures to, outdoor and indoor air pollution and carbon monoxide (Table 4-02). Secondhand smoke from smoking tobacco is a primary contributor to indoor air pollution. Other potential sources of indoor air pollutants include cooking or combustion sources (e.g., kerosene, coal, wood, animal dung). Major sources of indoor carbon monoxide include methane gas ranges and ovens, unvented gas or kerosene space heaters, and coal- or wood-burning stoves. Ceremonial incense and candles are asthma triggers that often are not recognized.

Mold

Travelers might visit flooded areas as part of emergency, medical, or humanitarian relief missions. Water damage to buildings can lead to mold contamination. Mold is a more serious health hazard for immunocompromised people and for those who have respiratory problems (e.g., asthma). To prevent exposures that could result in adverse health effects, travelers should avoid areas where mold contamination is obvious, and use personal protective equipment (PPE) such as gloves,

Table 4-02 Strategies to mitigate adverse health effects of air pollution

ENVIRONMENTAL SOURCE	POLLUTANTS	TRAVELER CATEGORY	MITIGATION STRATEGIES
Indoor air	High levels of smoke (e.g., from cooking and combustion sources, tobacco, incense, and candles)	Long-term travelers and expatriates	Consider purchasing indoor air filtration system
		All travelers	Avoidance
Outdoor air	Poor air quality (high levels of air pollution) or areas potentially affected by wildland fires	Travelers with preexisting asthma, chronic obstructive pulmonary disease, heart disease	Limit strenuous or prolonged outdoor activity
		All travelers	Facemasks (offer limited protection)

4

goggles, waterproof boots, and NIOSH-approved N95 or higher respirators when working in moldy environments. To learn more about mold and respirators, see the Centers for Disease Control and Prevention (CDC) website, Respiratory Protection for Residents Reentering and/or Cleaning Homes that Were Flooded (www.cdc.gov/disasters/disease/respiratory.html). Travelers should anticipate the environment to which they are traveling and bring enough PPE, because supplies might be scarce or unavailable in the countries visited. Travelers should keep hands, skin, and eyes clean and free from mold-contaminated dust. For additional information, review CDC recommendations, Mold Cleanup and Remediation, at www.cdc.gov/mold/cleanup.htm.

RADIATION

Background radiation levels can vary substantially from region to region, but these variations are natural and do not represent a health concern. Several regions in the world have high natural background radiation, including Guarapari (Brazil), Kerala (India), Ramsar (Iran), and Yangjiang (China), but traveling to these areas does not pose a threat to health. By contrast, travelers should be aware of and avoid regions known to be contaminated with radioactive materials (e.g., areas surrounding the Chernobyl nuclear power plant in Ukraine and the Fukushima Daiichi nuclear power plant in Japan). These areas have radiation levels that greatly exceed background levels and represent a substantial health and safety risk.

The Chernobyl nuclear power plant is located 100 km (62 miles) northwest of Kyiv. The 1986 incident that occurred at that facility contaminated regions in 3 republics—Ukraine, Belarus, and Russia—but the highest radioactive ground contamination is ≤30 km (19 miles) of Chernobyl.

The Fukushima Daiichi plant is located 240 km (150 miles) north of Tokyo. After the accident in 2011, the area within a 20-km (12-mile) radius of the plant was evacuated. Japanese authorities also advised evacuation from locations farther away to the northwest of the plant. Because Japanese authorities continue to clean the affected areas and monitor the situation, access requirements and travel advisories change. The US Department of State recommends against all unnecessary travel to areas designated by the Japanese government to be restricted because of radioactive contamination. For up-to-date safety information or current travel advisories for any country, see the US Department of State's website (https://travel.state.gov/content/travel/en/traveladvisories/traveladvisories.html) or check with the US embassy or consulate in that country.

In most countries, areas of known radioactive contamination are fenced or marked with signs. Any traveler seeking long-term (more than a few months) residence near a known or suspected contaminated area should consult with staff of the nearest US embassy, and inquire about any advisories regarding drinking water quality or purchase of meat, fruit, and vegetables from local farmers.

Radiation emergencies are rare. In case of such an emergency, travelers should follow instructions provided by local authorities. If such information is not forthcoming, US travelers should seek advice from the nearest US embassy or consulate.

Natural disasters (e.g., floods) might displace industrial or clinical radioactive sources. In all circumstances, travelers should exercise caution when they encounter unknown objects or equipment, especially if the objects have the basic radiation trefoil symbol or other radiation signs (for examples, see https://remm.hhs.gov/radsign.htm). Travelers who encounter a questionable object should avoid touching or moving it, and notify local authorities as quickly as possible.

4

BIBLIOGRAPHY

Ansari A. Radiation threats and your safety: a guide to preparation and response for professionals and community. Boca Raton, FL: Chapman & Hall/CRC; 2009.

Brandt M, Brown C, Burkhart J, Burton N, Cox-Ganser J, Damon S, et al. Mold prevention strategies and possible health effects in the aftermath of hurricanes and major floods. MMWR Recomm Rep. 2006;55(RR-8):1–27.

Brook RD, Rajagopalan S, Pope CA 3rd, Brook JR, Bhatnagar A, Diez-Roux AV, et al. Particulate matter air pollution and cardiovascular disease: an update to the scientific statement from the American Heart Association. Circulation. 2010;121(21):2331–78.

Cohen AJ, Brauer M, Burnett R, Anderson HR, Frostad J, Estep K, et al. Estimates and 25-year trends of the global burden of disease attributable to ambient air pollution: an analysis of data from the global burden of diseases study 2015. Lancet. 2017;389(10082):1907–18.

Eisenbud M, Gesell TF. Environmental radioactivity: from natural, industrial, and military sources, 4th edition. San Diego: Academic Press; 1997.

Guarnieri M, Balmes JR. Outdoor air pollution and asthma. Lancet. 2014;383(9928):1581–92.

Shaffer R, Cichowicz J, Chew G, Hsu J. Non-occupational uses of respiratory protection—what public health organizations and users need to know. NIOSH Science blogs. January 4, 2018. Available from: https://blogs.cdc.gov/niosh-science-blog/2018/01/04/respirators-public-use.

US Environmental Protection Agency. Wildfire smoke: a guide for public health officials. Research Triangle Park, NC: EPA-452/R-19-901; 2019.

SCUBA DIVING: DECOMPRESSION ILLNESS & OTHER DIVE-RELATED INJURIES

Daniel Nord, Gregory Raczniak, James Chimiak

Published estimates report anywhere from 0.5 million to 4 million people in the United States participate in recreational diving; many travel to tropical areas of the world to dive. Divers face a variety of medical challenges, but because dive injuries generally are rare, few clinicians are trained to prevent, diagnose, or treat them. Recreational divers should assess potential risks before diving, be prepared to recognize signs of injury, and seek qualified dive medicine help promptly when needed.

PREPARING FOR DIVE TRAVEL

When assisting patients who are planning dive-related travel, take into consideration chronic health conditions, any recent changes in health (e.g., injuries, pregnancy, surgeries), and medication use. Underlying respiratory conditions (e.g., asthma, chronic obstructive pulmonary disease, infections, history of spontaneous pneumothorax) can challenge the breathing capacity required of divers. Mental health disorders (e.g., anxiety, claustrophobia, substance abuse) and disorders affecting central nervous system higher function and consciousness (e.g., seizures) raise special concerns about diving fitness. While it is important to review patient medications for their compatibility with diving, usually the primary concern is the underlying condition for which the patient takes medication.

People with known risk factors for coronary artery disease, including but not limited to diabetes, elevated blood pressure, family history, an abnormal lipid profile, and smoking history, who wish to either begin a dive program or continue diving, should undergo a physical examination to assess their cardiovascular fitness. This examination might include an electrocardiogram, exercise treadmill test, or echocardiogram. Diving is a potentially strenuous activity that can put substantial demands on the cardiovascular system. Serious injury and death are associated with poor physical conditioning; regular aerobic exercise should already be part of a diver's routine before arriving for their dive physical and subsequent diving.

During the travel medicine examination, remind divers (and would-be divers) of actions they can take in advance to reduce or eliminate risks. Identifying and assessing potential hazards (e.g., environment, water and weather conditions, planned depth and bottom time) can help divers make decisions about acceptable risk. Preparing for a safe dive also includes having an up-to-date emergency action plan, on-hand first aid supplies (with ample oxygen), and reliable communication devices. Using correct and well-maintained protective equipment, diving with supervision, and ensuring that medical care is available in the event of an emergency are other controls divers can implement. A diver should never feel compelled to make a dive, especially if feeling unwell.

Of special note, many dive operators routinely screen clients by requiring a medical statement signed by the diver's physician with approval to dive. Divers should communicate with their dive operator ahead of travel to acquire the necessary form to share with their personal physician. By being prepared with properly signed documentation upon arrival at their dive destination, the traveling diver can forestall denial of dive privileges.

DIVING DISORDERS

Barotrauma

Barotrauma is an injury to soft tissues resulting from a pressure differential between an airspace in the body and the ambient pressure. The resultant expansion or contraction of that space can cause injury.

EAR & SINUS

The most common injury in divers is ear barotrauma (Box 4-07). On descent, failure to equalize pressure changes within the middle ear space creates a pressure gradient across the eardrum. As the middle ear tissues swell with edema—a consequence of the increased pressure—the pressure difference across the eardrum pushes it into the middle ear space, causing it to bleed and possibly rupture.

Forceful equalization under these conditions can increase the pressure differential between the inner ear and the middle ear, resulting in round window rupture with perilymph leakage and inner ear damage. To avoid these pathologic processes, divers must learn proper equalization techniques. Health care providers can coach this effort by

BOX 4-07 Symptoms of ear barotrauma

Decreased hearing
Pain
Sensation of fullness
Sensation of "water in the ear" (serous fluid/blood accumulation in the middle ear)
Tinnitus (ringing in the ears)
Vertigo (dizziness or sensation of spinning)

observing movement of the tympanic membrane using simple otoscopy.

Paranasal sinuses, because of their relatively narrow connecting passageways, are especially susceptible to barotrauma, generally on descent. With small changes in pressure (depth), symptoms are usually mild and subacute but can be exacerbated by continued diving. Larger pressure changes can be more injurious, especially with forceful attempts at equilibration (e.g., the Valsalva maneuver). Additional risk factors for ear and sinus barotrauma include:

- Use of solid earplugs.
- Medication (e.g., overuse or prolonged use of decongestants leading to rebound congestion).
- Ear or sinus surgery.
- Nasal deformity or polyps.
- Chronic nasal and sinus disease that interferes with equilibration during the large barometric pressure changes encountered while diving.

Divers who suspect they have ear or sinus barotrauma should discontinue diving and seek medical attention.

PULMONARY

Scuba divers reduce the risk for lung overpressure problems by breathing normally and ascending slowly when breathing compressed gas. Overexpansion of the lungs can result if a scuba diver ascends toward the surface without exhaling, which can happen, for example, when a novice diver panics and kicks back toward the surface. During ascent, compressed gas trapped in the lung increases in volume until the expansion exceeds the elastic limit of lung tissue, causing damage and allowing gas bubbles to escape into 3 possible locations: the pleural space, mediastinum, or pulmonary vasculature. Gas entering the pleural space can cause lung collapse or pneumothorax. Gas entering the mediastinum (the space around the heart, trachea, and esophagus) causes mediastinal emphysema and frequently tracks under the skin (subcutaneous emphysema) or into the tissue around the larynx, sometimes precipitating a change in voice characteristics. Gas rupturing the alveolar walls can enter the pulmonary capillaries and pass via the pulmonary veins to the left side of the heart, resulting in arterial gas embolism (AGE).

Mediastinal or subcutaneous emphysema might resolve spontaneously, but pneumothorax generally requires specific treatment to remove the air and reinflate the lung. AGE is a medical emergency, requiring urgent intervention with hyperbaric oxygen therapy (recompression treatment).

Lung overinflation injuries from scuba diving can range from mild to dramatic and life threatening. Although pulmonary barotrauma is uncommon in divers, prompt medical evaluation is necessary, and clinicians must rule out this condition in patients presenting with post-dive respiratory or neurologic symptoms.

Decompression Illness

Decompression illness (DCI) describes bubble-related dysbaric injuries, including AGE and decompression sickness (DCS). Because scientists consider these 2 conditions to result from separate causes, they are described here separately. From a clinical and practical standpoint, however, distinguishing between them in the field might be impossible and unnecessary, because the initial treatment is the same for both (Table 4-03). DCI can occur even in divers who have carefully followed the standard decompression tables and the principles of safe diving. Serious permanent injury or death can result from AGE or DCS.

ARTERIAL GAS EMBOLISM

Gas entering the arterial blood through ruptured pulmonary vessels can distribute bubbles into the body tissues, including the heart and brain, where they can disrupt circulation or damage vessel walls. The clinical presentation of arterial gas embolism (AGE) ranges from minimal neurologic findings to dramatic symptoms requiring urgent and aggressive treatment.

In general, suspect AGE in any scuba diver who surfaces unconscious or loses consciousness within 10 minutes after surfacing. Initiate basic life support, including administration of the

Table 4-03 Decompression illness syndromes: clinical findings

ARTERIAL GAS EMBOLISM	DECOMPRESSION SICKNESS
Ataxia Blurred vision Chest pain or bloody sputum Loss of consciousness Convulsions Dizziness Muscular weakness Numbness or paresthesia Paralysis Personality change, difficulty thinking, or confusion	Loss of bowel or bladder function Collapse or unconsciousness Coughing spasms or shortness of breath Dizziness Unusual fatigue Itching Joint aches or pain Mottling or marbling of skin Numbness or tingling Paralysis Personality changes Staggering, loss of coordination, or tremors Weakness

4

highest fraction of oxygen. Because relapses can and do occur, divers suffering AGE should be rapidly evacuated to a hyperbaric oxygen treatment facility even if they appear to have recovered fully.

DECOMPRESSION SICKNESS ("THE BENDS")

Breathing air under pressure causes excess inert gas (usually nitrogen) to dissolve in and saturate body tissues. The amount of gas dissolved is proportional to, and increases with, the total depth and time a diver is below the surface. As the diver ascends, the excess dissolved gas must be cleared through respiration. Depending on the amount of gas dissolved and the rate of ascent, some gas can supersaturate tissues, where it separates from solution to form bubbles, interfering with blood flow and tissue oxygenation.

Other Conditions Related to Diving

DROWNING

Any incapacitation while underwater can result in drowning (see Sec. 4, Ch. 12, Injury & Trauma).

HAZARDOUS MARINE LIFE

Oceans and waterways are filled with marine animals, most of which are generally harmless unless threatened. Most injuries among divers are the result of chance encounters or defensive maneuvers of marine life. Wounds from marine life have many common characteristics, including bacterial contamination, foreign bodies, bleeding, and occasionally venom. See Sec. 4, Ch. 7, Zoonotic Exposures: Bites, Stings, Scratches & Other Hazards, for prevention and injury management recommendations.

IMMERSION (INDUCED) PULMONARY EDEMA

The normal hemodynamic effects of water immersion account for a shift of fluid from peripheral to central circulation that can result in higher pressures within the pulmonary capillary bed, forcing excess fluid into the lungs. Cold water can cause peripheral vasoconstriction and augment this central fluid shift. Symptoms and signs of immersion (induced) pulmonary edema (IPE) generally begin on descent or at depth and include chest pain, dyspnea, wheezing, and productive cough with frothy, sometimes pink-tinged sputum. Although not entirely well understood, age, overhydration, overexertion, negative inspiratory pressure, and left ventricular hypertrophy are believed to increase IPE risk in otherwise healthy divers. Anyone experiencing acute pulmonary edema while diving requires a work-up to rule out myocardial ischemia, evaluation of left ventricular function, hypertrophy, and valvular integrity.

NITROGEN NARCOSIS

At increasing depths, generally >100 ft (≈30 m), the partial pressure of nitrogen within the breathing gas increases, causing narcosis in all recreational divers. Nitrogen narcosis can be life threatening when it impairs a diver's ability to make appropriate and proper decisions while under water. This narcosis quickly clears on ascent and is not seen on the surface after a dive, which helps differentiate this condition from AGE.

OXYGEN TOXICITY

At increasing partial pressures of oxygen, levels in the blood become high enough to cause seizures. This condition is not seen when diving on compressed air within recreational depth limits.

4

DIVING & AIR TRAVEL

Flying after Diving

The risk of developing decompression sickness increases when divers go to increased altitude too soon after a dive. Commercial aircraft cabins are generally pressurized to the equivalent of 6,000–8,000 ft (≈1,830–2,440 m) above sea level. Instruct asymptomatic divers to wait before flying at an altitude or cabin pressure >2,000 ft (610 m) for

- ≥12 hours after surfacing from a single no-decompression dive;
- ≥18 hours after multiple dives or multiple days of diving; or
- 24–48 hours after a dive that required decompression stops.

These recommended preflight surface intervals reduce, but do not eliminate, risk for DCS. Longer surface intervals further reduce this risk.

Diving after Flying

There are no guidelines for diving after flying. Divers should wait a sufficient period to acclimate mentally and physically to their new location to focus solely on the dive.

PREVENTING DIVING DISORDERS

Recreational divers should dive conservatively and well within the no-decompression limits of their dive tables or computers. When multiple dives are planned, strict guidelines, known as surface intervals, are prescribed to allow adequate time for dissolved inert gas to drop to acceptable levels before the next dive. Tables derived from man-tested algorithms have traditionally been used by divers to manually calculate dive times and surface intervals. Dive computers possess the reliability and computing power to use the same algorithms and compute individual guidance based on real-time depth and time inputs. Dive computers have largely replaced the use of tables for the manual process of dive planning.

Risk factors for DCI are primarily dive depth, dive time, and rates of ascent. Additional factors, such as altitude exposure soon after a dive, difficult diving conditions (e.g., colder water, currents, decreased visibility, wave action), dives to depths >60 ft (18 m), multiple consecutive days of diving or repetitive dives, overhead situations (e.g., diving in underwater caves or wrecks), strenuous exercise, and certain physiologic variables (e.g., dehydration), also increase risk. Caution divers to stay well hydrated and rested and dive within the limits of their training. Diving is a skill that requires training and certification and should be done with a well-trained, attentive companion (dive buddy).

TREATMENT OF DIVING DISORDERS

Definitive treatment of DCI begins with early recognition of symptoms, followed by recompression with hyperbaric oxygen. Be suspicious of any unusual symptoms occurring soon after a dive, especially neurological symptoms, and evaluate these properly. Provide a high concentration (100%) of supplemental oxygen; surface-level oxygen given for first aid might relieve the signs and symptoms of DCI and should be administered as soon as possible.

Because of either incidental causes, immersion, or DCI itself, which can cause capillary leakage, divers often are dehydrated. In most cases, treatment includes administering isotonic glucose-free intravenous fluids. Oral rehydration fluids also can be helpful, provided they can be administered safely (i.e., if the diver is conscious and can maintain their airway).

The definitive treatment of DCI is recompression and oxygen administration in a hyperbaric chamber. Stable or remitting symptoms of mild DCI (e.g., constitutional symptoms, some cutaneous sensory changes, limb pain, or rash) in divers reporting from remote locations without a hyperbaric facility might not require recompression. Medical management decisions made with the assistance of a qualified dive medicine physician also should account for the prevailing circumstances, logistics and hazards of evacuation, and the implications of failing to recompress. Serial neurologic exams are essential to the decision-making process.

Divers Alert Network (DAN) maintains 24-hour emergency consultation and evacuation assistance at +1-919-684-9111 (collect calls accepted). DAN can help with the medical management of injured divers by deciding if recompression is needed, providing the location of the closest recompression facility, and arranging patient transport. Divers and health care providers also can contact DAN for routine, nonemergency consultation by telephone at 919-684-2948, extension 6222, or by accessing the DAN website (https://dan.org/).

Travelers who plan to scuba dive might want to ascertain whether recompression facilities are available at their destination before embarking on their trip.

4

BIBLIOGRAPHY

Brubakk AO, Neuman TS, Bennett PB, Elliott DH. Bennett and Elliott's physiology and medicine of diving, 5th edition. London: Saunders; 2003.

Chapter 6: Pulmonary and Venous Disorders. In: J. Chimiak, editor. The heart & diving. Durham (NC): Divers Alert Network. Available from: https://dan.org/wp-content/uploads/2020/07/the-heart-and-diving-dan-dive-medical-reference.pdf.

Dear G, Pollock NW. DAN America dive and travel medical guide, 5th edition. Durham, NC: Divers Alert Network; 2009.

Divers Alert Network. Flying after diving. 2003. Available from: https://dan.org/research-reports/research-studies/flying-after-diving.

Mitchell SJ, Doolette DJ, Wachholz, CJ, Vann RD, editors. Management of mild or marginal decompression illness in remote locations. Sydney, Australia: Undersea and Hyperbaric Medical Society; 2004.

Moon RE. Treatment of decompression illness. In: Bove AA, Davis JC, editors. Bove and Davis' diving medicine, 4th edition. Philadelphia: WB Saunders; 2004. pp. 195–223.

Neuman TS, Thom SR. Physiology and medicine of hyperbaric oxygen therapy. Philadelphia, PA: Saunders; 2008.

US Navy. The Navy diving manual revision 7. USA: Carlisle Military Library; 2018.

HIGH ELEVATION TRAVEL & ALTITUDE ILLNESS

Peter Hackett, David Shlim

Typical high-elevation travel destinations include Colorado ski resorts with lodgings at 8,000–10,000 ft (≈2,440–3,050 m); Cusco, Peru (11,000 ft; ≈3,350 m); La Paz, Bolivia (12,000 ft; ≈3,650 m); Lhasa, Tibet Autonomous Region (12,100 ft; ≈3,700 m); Everest base camp, Nepal (17,700 ft; ≈5,400 m); and Mount Kilimanjaro, Tanzania (19,341 ft; ≈5,900 m). High-elevation environments expose travelers to cold, low humidity, increased ultraviolet radiation, and decreased air pressure, all of which can cause health problems. The biggest concern, however, is hypoxia, due to the decreased partial pressure of oxygen (PO_2). At 10,000 ft (≈3,050 m), for example, the inspired PO_2 is only 69% of that at sea level; acute exposure to this reduced PO_2 can lower arterial oxygen saturation to 88%–91%.

The magnitude and consequences of hypoxic stress depend on the elevation, rate of ascent, and duration of exposure; host genetic factors may also contribute. Hypoxemia is greatest during sleep; day trips to high-elevation destinations with an evening return to a lower elevation are much less stressful on the body. Because of the key role of ventilation, travelers must avoid taking respiratory depressants at high elevations.

ACCLIMATIZATION

The human body can adjust to moderate hypoxia at elevations ≤17,000 ft (≈5,200 m) but requires time to do so. Some acclimatization to high elevation continues for weeks to months, but the acute process, which occurs over the first 3–5 days following ascent, is crucial for travelers. The acute phase is associated with a steady increase in ventilation, improved oxygenation, and changes in cerebral blood flow. Increased red cell production does not play a role in acute acclimatization, although a decrease in plasma volume over the first few days does increase hemoglobin concentration.

Altitude illness can develop before the acute acclimatization process is complete, but not afterwards. In addition to preventing altitude illness, acclimatization improves sleep, increases comfort and sense of well-being, and improves submaximal endurance; maximal exercise performance at high elevation will always be reduced compared to that at low elevation.

Travelers can optimize acclimatization by adjusting their itineraries to avoid going "too high too fast" (see Box 4-08). Gradually ascending to elevation or staging the ascent provides crucial time for the body to adjust. For example, acclimatizing for a minimum of 2–3 nights at 8,000–9,000 ft (≈2,450–≈2,750 m) before proceeding to a higher elevation is markedly protective against acute mountain sickness (AMS). The Wilderness Medical Society recommends avoiding ascent to a sleeping elevation of ≥9,000 ft (≈2,750 m) in a single day; ascending at a rate of no greater than 1,650 ft (≈500 m) per night in sleeping elevation once above 9,800 ft (≈3,000 m); and allowing an extra night to acclimatize for every 3,300 ft (≈1,000 m) of sleeping elevation gain. These reasonable recommendations can still be too fast for some travelers and annoyingly slow for others.

ALTITUDE ILLNESS

Risk to Travelers

Susceptibility and resistance to altitude illness are, in part, genetically determined traits, but there are no simple screening tests to predict risk. Training or physical fitness do not affect risk. A traveler's sex plays a minimal role, if any, in determining predisposition. Children are as susceptible as adults; people aged >50 years have slightly less risk. Any unacclimatized traveler proceeding to a sleeping elevation of ≥8,000 ft (≈2,450 m)—and sometimes lower—is at risk for altitude illness. In addition, travelers who have successfully adjusted to one elevation are at risk when moving to higher sleeping elevations, especially if the elevation gain is >2,000–3,000 ft (600–900 m).

How a traveler previously responded to high elevations is the most reliable guide for future trips, but only if the elevation and rate of ascent are similar, and even then, this is not an infallible predictor. In addition to underlying, inherent baseline susceptibilities, a traveler's risk for developing altitude illness is influenced by 3 main factors: elevation at destination, rate of ascent, and exertion (Table 4-04). Creating an itinerary to avoid any occurrence of altitude illness is difficult because of variations in individual

BOX 4-08 Acclimatization tips: a checklist for travelers

- ☐ Ascend gradually.
- ☐ Avoid going directly from low elevation to >9,000 ft (2,750 m) sleeping elevation in 1 day.
- ☐ Once above 9,000 ft (≈2,750 m), move sleeping elevation by no more than 1,600 ft (≈500 m) per day, and plan an extra day for acclimatization every 3,300 ft (≈1,000 m).
- ☐ Consider using acetazolamide to speed acclimatization if abrupt ascent is unavoidable.
- ☐ Avoid alcohol for the first 48 hours at elevation.
- ☐ If a regular caffeine user, continue using to avoid a withdrawal headache that could be confused with an altitude headache.
- ☐ Participate in only mild exercise for the first 48 hours at elevation.
- ☐ A high-elevation exposure (> 9,000 ft [≈2,750 m]) for ≥2 nights, within 30 days before the trip, is useful, but closer to the trip departure is better.

Table 4-04 Risk categories for developing acute mountain sickness (AMS)

RISK CATEGORY	DESCRIPTION	PROPHYLAXIS RECOMMENDATIONS
Low	People with no prior history of altitude illness ascending to <9,000 ft (2,750 m) People taking ≥2 days to arrive at 8,200–9,800 ft (≈2,500–3,000 m), with subsequent increases in sleeping elevation <1,600 ft (≈500 m) per day, and an extra day for acclimatization every 3,300 ft (1,000 m) increase in elevation	Acetazolamide prophylaxis generally not indicated
Moderate	People with prior history of AMS ascending to 8,200–9,200 ft (≈2,500–2,800 m) elevation (or above) in 1 day People with no history of AMS ascending to >9,200 ft (2,800 m) elevation in 1 day All people ascending >1,600 ft (≈500 m) per day (increase in sleeping elevation) at elevations >9,800 ft (3,000 m), but with an extra day for acclimatization every 3,300 ft (1,000 m)	Acetazolamide prophylaxis would be beneficial and should be considered
High	People with a history of AMS ascending to >9,200 ft (≈2,800 m) in 1 day All people with a prior history of HAPE or HACE All people ascending to >11,400 ft (≈3,500 m) in 1 day All people ascending >1,600 ft (≈500 m) per day (increase in sleeping elevation) at elevations >9,800 ft (≈3,000 m), without extra days for acclimatization People making very rapid ascents (e.g., <7-day ascent of Mount Kilimanjaro)	Acetazolamide prophylaxis strongly recommended

Abbreviations: HACE, high-altitude cerebral edema; HAPE, high-altitude pulmonary edema

susceptibility, as well as in starting points and terrain. The goal for the traveler might not be to avoid all symptoms of altitude illness but to have no more than mild illness, thereby avoiding itinerary changes or the need for medical assistance or evacuation.

Destinations of Risk

Some common high-elevation destinations require rapid ascent by a non-pressurized airplane to >11,000 ft (≈3,400 m), placing travelers in a high-risk category for AMS. A common travel medicine question is whether to recommend acetazolamide for travelers when gradual or staged acclimatization is not feasible. With rates of altitude illness approaching 30%–40% in these situations, a low threshold for chemoprophylaxis is advised. In some cases (e.g., Cusco and La Paz), travelers can descend to elevations much lower than the airport to sleep for 1–2 nights and then begin their ascent, perhaps obviating the need for medication.

Itineraries along some trekking routes in Nepal, particularly Everest base camps, push the limits of many people's ability to acclimatize. Even on standard schedules, incidence of altitude illness can approach 30% at the higher elevations. Whenever possible, adding extra days to the trek can make for a more enjoyable and safer climb.

Altitude Illness Syndromes

Altitude illness is divided into 3 syndromes: acute mountain sickness (AMS), high-altitude cerebral edema (HACE), and high-altitude pulmonary edema (HAPE). Some clinicians consider high-altitude headache a separate entity because isolated headache can occur without the combined symptoms that define AMS.

ACUTE MOUNTAIN SICKNESS

AMS is the most common form of altitude illness, affecting 25% of all visitors sleeping at elevations >8,000 ft (≈2,450 m) in Colorado.

DIAGNOSIS

Diagnosis of AMS is based on a history of recent ascent to high elevation and the presence of subjective symptoms. AMS symptoms are like those of an alcohol hangover; headache is the cardinal symptom, usually accompanied by ≥1 of the following: anorexia, dizziness, fatigue, nausea, or, occasionally, vomiting. Uncommonly, AMS presents without headache. Symptom onset is usually 2–12 hours after initial arrival at a high elevation or after ascent to a higher elevation, and often during or after the first night. Preverbal children with AMS can develop loss of appetite, irritability, and pallor. AMS generally resolves within 12–48 hours if travelers do not ascend farther.

The condition is typically self-limited, developing and resolving over 1–3 days. Symptoms starting after 3 days of arrival to high elevation and without further ascent should not be attributed to AMS. AMS has no characteristic physical findings; pulse oximetry is usually within the normal range for the elevation, or slightly lower than normal.

The differential diagnosis of AMS is broad; common considerations include alcohol hangover, carbon monoxide poisoning, dehydration, drug intoxication, exhaustion, hyponatremia, and migraine. Travelers with AMS will improve rapidly with descent ≥1,000 ft (≈300 m), and this can be a useful indication of a diagnosis of AMS.

TREATMENT

Although rarely available, supplemental oxygen at 1–2 liters per minute will relieve headaches within about 30 minutes and resolve other AMS symptoms over hours. The popular small, handheld cans of compressed oxygen can provide brief relief, but contain too little oxygen (5 liters at most) for sustained improvement. Travelers with AMS but without HACE or HAPE (both described below) can remain safely at their current elevation and self-treat with non-opiate analgesics (e.g., ibuprofen 600 mg or acetaminophen 500 mg every 8 hours) and antiemetics (e.g., ondansetron 4 mg orally disintegrating tablets).

Acetazolamide speeds acclimatization and resolves AMS, but is more commonly used and better validated for use as prophylaxis. Dexamethasone is more effective than acetazolamide at rapidly relieving the symptoms of moderate to severe AMS. If symptoms worsen while the traveler is at the same elevation, or despite supplemental oxygen or medication, descent is mandatory.

HIGH-ALTITUDE CEREBRAL EDEMA

As an encephalopathy, HACE is considered "end stage" AMS. Fortunately, HACE is rare, especially at elevations <14,000 ft (≈4,300 m). HACE is often a secondary consequence of the severe hypoxemia that occurs with HAPE.

DIAGNOSIS

Unlike AMS, HACE presents with neurological findings, particularly altered mental status, ataxia, confusion, and drowsiness, similar to alcohol intoxication. Focal neurologic findings and seizures are rare in HACE; their presence should lead to suspicion of an intracranial lesion, a seizure disorder, or hyponatremia. Other considerations for the differential diagnosis include carbon monoxide poisoning, drug intoxication, hypoglycemia, hypothermia, and stroke. Coma can ensue within 24 hours of onset.

TREATMENT

In populated areas with access to medical care, HACE can be treated with supplemental oxygen and dexamethasone. In remote areas, initiate descent for anyone suspected of having HACE, in conjunction with dexamethasone and oxygen, if available. If descent is not feasible, supplemental oxygen or a portable hyperbaric device, in addition to dexamethasone, can be lifesaving. Coma is likely to ensue within 12–24 hours of the onset of ataxia in the absence of treatment or descent.

HIGH-ALTITUDE PULMONARY EDEMA

HAPE can occur by itself or in conjunction with AMS and HACE; incidence is roughly 1 per 10,000 skiers in Colorado, and ≤1 per 100 climbers at >14,000 ft (≈4,300 m).

DIAGNOSIS

Early diagnosis is key; HAPE can be more rapidly fatal than HACE. Initial symptoms include chest congestion, cough, exaggerated dyspnea on exertion, and decreased exercise performance. If unrecognized and untreated, HAPE progresses to dyspnea at rest and frank respiratory distress, often with bloody sputum. This typical progression over 1–2 days is easily recognizable as HAPE, but the condition sometimes presents only as central nervous system dysfunction, with confusion and drowsiness.

Rales are detectable in most victims. Pulse oximetry can aid in making the diagnosis; oxygen saturation levels will be at least 10 points lower in HAPE patients than in healthy people at the same elevation. Oxygen saturation values of 50%–70% are common. The differential diagnosis for HAPE includes bronchospasm, myocardial infarction, pneumonia, and pulmonary embolism.

TREATMENT

In most circumstances, descent is urgent and mandatory. Administer oxygen, if available, and exert the patient as little as possible. If immediate descent is not an option, use of supplemental oxygen or a portable hyperbaric chamber is critical.

Patients with mild HAPE who have access to oxygen (e.g., at a hospital or high-elevation medical clinic) might not need to descend to a lower elevation and can be treated with oxygen over 2–4 days at the current elevation. In field settings, where resources are limited and there is a lower margin for error, nifedipine can be used as an adjunct to descent, oxygen, or portable hyperbaric oxygen therapy. A phosphodiesterase inhibitor can be used if nifedipine is not available, but concurrent use of multiple pulmonary vasodilators is not recommended. Descent and oxygen are much more effective treatments than medication.

MEDICATIONS

Recommendations for use and dosages of medications to prevent and treat altitude illness are outlined in Table 4-05.

Acetazolamide

MECHANISM OF ACTION

When taken preventively, acetazolamide hastens acclimatization to high-elevation hypoxia, thereby reducing occurrence and severity of AMS. It also enhances recovery if taken after symptoms have developed. The drug works primarily by inducing a bicarbonate diuresis and metabolic acidosis, which stimulates ventilation and increases alveolar and arterial oxygenation. By using acetazolamide, high-elevation ventilatory acclimatization that normally takes 3–5 days takes only 1 day. Acetazolamide also eliminates central sleep apnea, or periodic breathing, which is common at high elevations, even in those without a history of sleep disorder breathing.

DOSE

An effective dose for prophylaxis that minimizes the common side effects of increased urination and paresthesia of the fingers and toes is 125 mg every 12 hours, beginning the day before ascent and continuing the first 2 days at elevation, and longer if ascent continues. Acetazolamide can also be taken episodically for symptoms of AMS, as needed. To date, the only dose studied for treatment is 250 mg (2 doses taken 8 hours apart), although the lower dosage used for prevention has anecdotally been successful. The pediatric dose is 5 mg/kg/day in divided doses, up to 125 mg, twice a day.

ADVERSE & ALLERGIC REACTIONS

Allergic reactions to acetazolamide are uncommon. Since acetazolamide is a sulfonamide derivative, cross-sensitivity between acetazolamide, sulfonamides, and other sulfonamide derivatives is possible.

Dexamethasone

Dexamethasone is effective for preventing and treating AMS and HACE and might prevent HAPE as well. Unlike acetazolamide, if the drug is discontinued at elevation before acclimatization, mild rebound can occur. Acetazolamide is preferable to prevent AMS while ascending, and dexamethasone generally should be reserved for treatment, usually as an adjunct to descent. The adult dose is 4 mg every 6 hours; rarely is it needed

Table 4-05 Recommended medication dosing to prevent & treat altitude illness

MEDICATION	INDICATION	ROUTE	DOSE
Acetazolamide	AMS, HACE prevention	PO	125 mg twice a day; 250 mg twice a day if >100 kg body weight Pediatric: 2.5 mg/kg every 12 hours, up to 125 mg
	AMS treatment	PO	250 mg twice a day[1]
Dexamethasone	AMS, HACE prevention	PO	2 mg every 6 hours or 4 mg every 12 hours Pediatric: do not use for prophylaxis
	AMS, HACE treatment	PO, IV, IM	AMS: 4 mg every 6 hours HACE: 8 mg once, then 4 mg every 6 hours Pediatric: 0.15 mg/kg/dose every 6 hours up to 4 mg
Nifedipine	HAPE prevention	PO	30 mg SR version every 12 hours or 20 mg SR version every 8 hours
	HAPE treatment	PO	30 mg SR version every 12 hours or 20 mg SR version every 8 hours
Salmeterol[2]	HAPE prevention	Inhaled	125 μg twice a day
Sildenafil	HAPE prevention	PO	50 mg every 8 hours
Tadalafil	HAPE prevention	PO	10 mg twice a day

Abbreviations: AMS, acute mountain sickness; HACE, high-altitude cerebral edema; HAPE, high-altitude pulmonary edema; IM, intramuscular; IV, intravenous; PO, by mouth; SR, sustained release.

[1]This dose can also be used as an adjunct to dexamethasone for HACE treatment; dexamethasone remains the primary treatment for HACE.

[2]Use only in conjunction with oral medications and not as monotherapy for HAPE prevention.

for more than 1–2 days. An increasing trend is to use dexamethasone for "summit day" on high peaks (e.g., Aconcagua and Kilimanjaro) to prevent abrupt altitude illness.

Ibuprofen

Recent studies have shown that taking ibuprofen 600 mg every 8 hours helps prevent AMS, although not quite as effectively as acetazolamide. Ibuprofen is, however, available over the counter, inexpensive, and well tolerated.

Nifedipine

Nifedipine both prevents and ameliorates HAPE. For prevention, nifedipine is generally reserved for people who are particularly susceptible to the condition. The adult dose for prevention or treatment is 30 mg of extended release every 12 hours, or 20 mg every 8 hours.

Phosphodiesterase-5 Inhibitors

Phosphodiesterase-5 inhibitors selectively lower pulmonary artery pressure, with less effect on systemic blood pressure than nifedipine. Tadalafil, 10 mg taken twice a day during ascent, can prevent HAPE. It is also being studied as a possible treatment.

PREVENTING SEVERE ALTITUDE ILLNESS OR DEATH

The main point of instructing travelers about altitude illness is not to eliminate the possibility of mild illness but to prevent death or evacuation. Because the onset of symptoms and the clinical course are sufficiently slow and predictable, there is no reason for anyone to die from altitude illness unless they are trapped by weather or geography in situations where descent is impossible. Travelers can adhere to 3 rules to help prevent death or serious consequences from altitude illness:

- Know the early symptoms of altitude illness and be willing to acknowledge when symptoms are present.
- Never ascend to sleep at a higher elevation when experiencing symptoms of altitude illness, no matter how minor the symptoms seem.
- Descend if the symptoms become worse while resting at the same elevation.

For trekking groups and expeditions going into remote high-elevation areas, where descent to a lower elevation could be problematic, a pressurization bag (e.g., the Gamow bag) can be beneficial. A foot pump produces an increased pressure of 2 lb/in^2, mimicking a descent of 5,000–6,000 ft (≈1,500–1,800 m) depending on the starting elevation. The total packed weight of bag and pump is about 14 lb (6.5 kg).

Preexisting Medical Conditions

Travelers with preexisting medical conditions must optimize their treatment and have their conditions stable before departure. In addition, these travelers should have plans for dealing with exacerbation of their conditions at high elevations. Travelers with underlying medical conditions (e.g., coronary artery disease, any form of chronic pulmonary disease or preexisting hypoxemia, obstructive sleep apnea [OSA], or sickle cell trait)—even if well controlled—should consult a physician familiar with high-elevation medical issues before undertaking such travel (Table 4-06).

Table 4-06 Ascent risk associated with various underlying medical conditions & risk factors

LIKELY NO EXTRA RISK	CAUTION REQUIRED[1]	ASCENT CONTRAINDICATED
Asthma (well-controlled)	Angina (stable)	Angina (unstable)
Children and adolescents	Arrhythmias (poorly controlled)	Asthma (unstable, poorly controlled)
Chronic obstructive pulmonary disease (mild)	Chronic obstructive pulmonary disease (moderate)	Cerebral space-occupying lesions
Coronary artery disease (following revascularization)	Cirrhosis	Cerebral vascular aneurysms or arteriovenous malformations (untreated, high-risk)
Diabetes mellitus	Coronary artery disease (nonrevascularized)	Chronic obstructive pulmonary disease (severe/very severe)
Elderly	Cystic fibrosis (FEV_1 30%–50% predicted)	Cystic fibrosis (FEV_1 <30% predicted)
Hypertension (controlled)	Heart failure (compensated)	Heart failure (decompensated)
Neoplastic diseases	Hypertension (poorly controlled)	Myocardial infarction or stroke (<90 days before ascent)
Obesity (Class 1/Class 2)[2]	Infants <6 weeks old	Pregnancy (high-risk)
Obstructive sleep apnea (mild/moderate)	Obesity (Class 3)[3]	Pulmonary hypertension (pulmonary artery systolic pressure >60 mm Hg)
Pregnancy (low-risk)	Obstructive sleep apnea (severe)	Sickle cell anemia
Psychiatric disorders (stable)	Pulmonary hypertension (mild)	
Sedentary	Radial keratotomy surgery	
Seizure disorder (controlled)	Seizure disorder (poorly controlled)	
	Sickle cell trait	

Abbreviations: FEV_1, forced expiratory volume in 1 second

[1]Travelers with these conditions most often require consultation with a physician experienced in high-altitude medicine and a comprehensive management plan.
[2]Class 1 obesity: Body Mass Index (BMI) of 30 to <35; Class 2 obesity: BMI of 35 to <40.
[3]Class 3 obesity: BMI of ≥40.

Clinicians advising travelers should know that in most high-elevation resorts and cities, "home" oxygen is readily available. In North America, this requires a prescription that the traveler can carry, or oxygen can be arranged beforehand. Supplemental oxygen, whether continuous, episodic, or nocturnal, depending on the circumstances, is very effective at restoring oxygenation to low elevation values and eliminates the risk for altitude illness and exacerbation of preexisting medical conditions.

DIABETES MELLITUS

Travelers with diabetes can travel safely to high elevations, but they must be accustomed to exercise if participating in strenuous activities at elevation and carefully monitor their blood glucose. Diabetic ketoacidosis can be triggered by altitude illness and can be more difficult to treat in people taking acetazolamide. Not all glucose meters read accurately at high elevations.

OBSTRUCTIVE SLEEP APNEA

Travelers with sleep disordered breathing who are planning high-elevation travel should receive acetazolamide. Those with mild to moderate OSA who are not hypoxic at home might do well without a continuous positive airway pressure (CPAP) device, while those with severe OSA should be advised to avoid high-elevation travel unless they receive supplemental oxygen in addition to their CPAP. Oral appliances for OSA can be useful adjuncts when electrical power is unavailable.

PREGNANCY

There are no studies or case reports describing fetal harm among people who briefly travel to high elevations during their pregnancy. Nevertheless, clinicians might be prudent to recommend that pregnant people do not stay at sleeping elevations >10,000 ft (≈3,050 m). Travel to high elevations during pregnancy warrants confirmation of good maternal health and verification of a low-risk gestation. Advise pregnant travelers of the dangers of having a pregnancy complication in remote, mountainous terrain.

RADIAL KERATOTOMY

Most people do not have visual problems at high elevations. At very high elevations, however, some people who have had radial keratotomy procedures might develop acute farsightedness and be unable to care for themselves. LASIK and other newer procedures may produce only minor visual disturbances at high elevations.

BIBLIOGRAPHY

Bartsch P, Swenson ER. Acute high-altitude illnesses. N Engl J Med. 2013;369(17):1666–7.

Hackett PH, Luks AM, Lawley JS, Roach RC. High-altitude medicine and pathophysiology. In: Auerbach PS, editor. Wilderness medicine, 7th edition. Philadelphia: Elsevier; 2017. pp. 8–28.

Hackett PH, Roach RC. High altitude cerebral edema. High Alt Med Biol. 2004;5(2):136–46.

Luks AM, Auerbach PS, Freer L, Grissom CK, Keyes LE, McIntosh SE, et al. Wilderness Medical Society clinical practice guidelines for the prevention and treatment of acute altitude illness: 2019 update. Wilderness Environ Med. 2019;30(4S):S3–18.

Luks AM, Hackett PH. High altitude and preexisting medical conditions. In: Auerbach PS, editor. Wilderness medicine, 7th edition. Philadelphia: Elsevier; 2017. pp. 29–39.

Luks AM, Hackett PH. Medical conditions and high-altitude travel. N Engl J Med. 2022;386(4):364–73.

Luks AM, Swenson ER. Medication and dosage considerations in the prophylaxis and treatment of high-altitude illness. Chest. 2008;133(3):744–55.

Meier D, Collet TH, Locatelli I, Cornuz J, Kayser B, Simel DL, Sartori C. Does this patient have acute mountain sickness? The rational clinical examination systematic review. JAMA. 2017;318(18):1810–19.

Roach RC, Lawley JS, Hackett PH. High-altitude physiology. In: Auerbach PS, editor. Wilderness medicine, 7th edition. Philadelphia: Elsevier; 2017. pp. 2–8.

Woolcott OO. The Lake Louise Acute Mountain Sickness score: still a headache. High Alt Med Biol. 2021;22(4):351–2.

MOSQUITOES, TICKS & OTHER ARTHROPODS

John-Paul Mutebi, John Gimnig

Vectorborne diseases are found at almost every travel destination. Because few vaccines are available to protect travelers, the best way to prevent vectorborne diseases is to avoid being bitten by ticks and insects, including mosquitoes, fleas, chiggers, and flies, that transmit pathogens that cause disease. Travel health practitioners should advise travelers to use repellents and take other precautions to prevent bites.

VACCINE OPTIONS & MALARIA PROPHYLAXIS

Vaccines are currently available to protect against 3 vectorborne diseases in US travelers: Japanese encephalitis, tick-borne encephalitis, and yellow fever (see the respective chapters in Section 5 for details). No vaccines or prophylactic drugs are available in the United States for other mosquito-borne diseases (e.g., chikungunya, filariasis, West Nile encephalitis, Zika); tick-borne diseases (e.g., Lyme borreliosis, relapsing fever); sand fly–borne diseases (e.g., cutaneous or visceral leishmaniasis); or blackfly–borne diseases (e.g., onchocerciasis [river blindness]).

In June 2021, Dengvaxia was recommended by the Advisory Committee on Immunization Practices (ACIP) to prevent dengue in children aged 9–16 years who had laboratory-confirmed previous dengue virus infection and who live in dengue-endemic areas. Dengue is endemic to the US territories of American Samoa, Puerto Rico, and US Virgin Islands, and to freely associated states including the Federated States of Micronesia, the Republic of Marshall Islands, and the Republic of Palau. The dengue vaccine will not be available for use in travelers not living in dengue-endemic areas in the US territories, however.

Prophylactic drugs are available to protect against malaria; however, the effectiveness of malaria prophylaxis is variable, depending on patterns of drug resistance, bioavailability, individual behavior, and compliance with medication (see Sec. 2, Ch. 5, Yellow Fever Vaccine & Malaria Prevention Information, by Country, and www.cdc.gov/malaria/travelers/country_table/a.html).

INSECT REPELLENTS

When used as directed, insect repellents registered by the Environmental Protection Agency (EPA) have been proven safe and effective, even for pregnant and breastfeeding people. The Centers for Disease Control and Prevention (CDC) has evaluated information published in peer-reviewed scientific literature and data available from EPA to identify several types of EPA-registered products that safely and effectively prevent insect bites. Products containing the following active ingredients typically provide reasonably long-lasting protection:

DEET (chemical name: N,N-diethyl-m-toluamide or N,N-diethyl-3-methyl-benzamide). Products containing DEET include, but are not limited to, Off!, Cutter, Sawyer, and Ultrathon.

PICARIDIN (KBR 3023 [Bayrepel] and icaridin outside the United States; chemical name: 2-[2-hydroxyethyl]-1-piperidinecarboxylic acid 1-methylpropyl ester). Products containing picaridin include, but are not limited to, Cutter Advanced, Skin So Soft Bug Guard Plus, and Autan (outside the United States).

OIL OF LEMON EUCALYPTUS (OLE) or **PMD** (chemical name: para-menthane-3,8-diol, the synthesized version of OLE). Products containing OLE and PMD include, but are not limited to, Repel and Off! Botanicals. CDC does not recommend using "pure" oil of lemon eucalyptus (an essential oil that is not formulated) as a repellent, because it has not undergone validated testing for safety and efficacy and is not registered with EPA as an insect repellent. In general, parents should not use products containing OLE or PMD on children <3 years old to avoid potential allergic skin reactions.

IR3535 (chemical name: 3-[N-butyl-N-acetyl]-aminopropionic acid, ethyl ester). Products containing IR3535 include, but are not limited to, Skin So Soft Bug Guard Plus Expedition and SkinSmart.

2-UNDECANONE (chemical name: methyl nonyl ketone). The product BioUD contains 2-undecanone.

EPA characterizes the active ingredients DEET and picaridin as "conventional" repellents. The biopesticide repellents (OLE, PMD, IR3535, and 2-undecanone) are derived from, or are synthetic versions of, natural materials.

4

Travelers can find the right insect repellent for their needs by searching the EPA website Find the Repellent that is Right for You (www.epa.gov/insect-repellents/find-repellent-right-you) and the National Pesticide Information Center website, Choosing and Using Insect Repellents (http://npic.orst.edu/ingred/ptype/repel.html). Recommendations from these websites are based on peer-reviewed journal articles and scientific studies and data submitted to regulatory agencies.

Ideally, travelers should purchase repellents before departing the United States. A wide variety of repellents are available at camping, sporting goods, and military surplus stores. When purchasing repellents overseas, travelers should look for the active ingredients specified above on the product labels; some names of products available internationally also are provided above.

Efficacy

Published data indicate that repellent efficacy and duration of protection vary considerably among products and among arthropod species. Product efficacy and duration of protection are also markedly affected by ambient temperature, level of activity, amount of perspiration, exposure to water, being rubbed off during activities, and other factors.

In general, higher concentrations of active ingredients provide longer duration of protection, regardless of the active ingredient. Products with <10% active ingredient might offer only limited protection, often 1–2 hours. Products that offer sustained-release or controlled-release (microencapsulated) formulations, even with lower active ingredient concentrations, might provide longer protection times. Studies suggest that DEET efficacy tends to peak at a concentration of ≈50%, and that concentrations above that do not offer a marked increase in protection time against mosquitoes. Regardless of the product used, if travelers start getting bitten they should reapply, but not more often than the label allows.

The effectiveness of non–EPA-registered insect repellents, including some natural repellents, is unknown, and travelers should avoid using them (see www.epa.gov/insect-repellents).

Repellents & Sunscreen

Repellents applied according to label instructions can be used with sunscreen with no reduction in repellent activity. However, limited data show that DEET-containing insect repellents applied over sunscreen decrease the sun protection factor (SPF) of the sunscreen by one-third.

Travelers should avoid products that combine sunscreen with repellents because sunscreen might need to be reapplied more often and in larger amounts than what is needed for the repellent component to provide protection from biting insects. In general, travelers should use separate products, apply sunscreen first, and then apply the repellent. Because SPF decreases when a DEET-containing insect repellent is used, travelers might need to reapply sunscreen more frequently. Travelers must remember to use both sunscreen and insect repellents according to the manufacturer's instructions for each.

Use on Clothing & Gear

Travelers can treat clothing, hats, shoes, mosquito nets, outwear, and camping gear with permethrin for added protection. Permethrin is a highly effective insecticide, acaricide (pesticide that kills ticks and mites), and repellent. At a concentration of 0.5%, permethrin-treated clothing repels and kills ticks, chiggers, mosquitoes, and other biting and nuisance arthropods. Clothing and other items must be treated 24–48 hours before packing for travel to allow them to dry. As with all pesticides, travelers should always follow the label instructions.

Products such as Permanone and Sawyer, Permethrin, Repel, and Ultrathon Permethrin

Clothing Treatment are registered with the EPA specifically for use by consumers to treat clothing and gear. Alternatively, clothing pretreated with permethrin is commercially available and marketed to consumers in the United States as Insect Shield, BugsAway, or Insect Blocker.

Permethrin-treated materials retain repellency or insecticidal activity after repeated launderings, but should be retreated as described on the product label to provide continued protection. Clothing treated before purchase is labeled for efficacy through many launderings. Clothing treated with the other repellent products described above (e.g., DEET) provides protection from biting arthropods but will not last through washing and will require more frequent application.

Precautions

Box 4-09 contains precautions clinicians can share with travelers regarding the use of insect repellents. Severe reactions to insect repellents are rare. If a traveler experiences a rash or other reaction (e.g., itching, swelling) from a repellent, they should wash off the product using mild soap and water and discontinue its use. Travelers seeking health care because of a reaction to a repellent should take the product container with them to the doctor's office. Reactions associated with insect repellent use are outlined in MedlinePlus (https://medlineplus.gov/ency/article/002763.htm).

Permethrin should never be applied to the skin but only to clothing, mosquito nets, or other fabrics as directed on the product label.

Children & Pregnant People

Certain insect repellent products containing OLE as their sole active ingredient at concentrations of ≤30% can be used on children <3 years of age; parents should always read the product label before use. Insect repellents containing DEET, Picaridin, IR3535, and 2-undecanone can be used on children without age restriction (see www.epa.gov/insect-repellents/using-insect-repellents-safely-and-effectively#children). Travelers can protect infants from insect bites by dressing them in clothing that covers their arms and legs, by covering strollers and baby carriers with mosquito netting, and by using appropriate insect repellent. Other than the safety tips listed above, EPA does not recommend any additional precautions for using registered repellents on children or on people who are pregnant or lactating.

INSECT BITE PREVENTION

Travelers can reduce their risk for bites from mosquitoes, ticks, fleas, sand flies, and other arthropods by using EPA-registered insect repellents. Travelers should also minimize areas of exposed skin by wearing long-sleeved shirts, long pants, boots, and hats. Tucking in shirts, tucking pants into socks, and wearing closed shoes instead of

BOX 4-09 Precautions when using insect repellents: guidance for travelers

Apply repellents only to exposed skin or clothing, as directed on the product label. Do not apply to skin covered by clothing.

Never use repellents on cuts, wounds, or irritated skin.

When using sprays, do not spray directly on the face—spray product on hands first and then apply to face. Do not apply to eyes or mouth; apply only sparingly around ears.

Wash hands after application to avoid accidental ingestion or exposure to eyes.

Children should not handle repellents. Instead, adults should apply repellent to their own hands first and then gently spread product on the child's exposed skin. Avoid applying repellents to children's hands. After returning indoors, wash children's treated skin and clothing with soap and water or give the child a bath.

Use just enough repellent to cover exposed skin or clothing. Heavy application and saturation are generally unnecessary for effectiveness. If biting insects do not respond to a thin film of repellent, apply a bit more.

After returning indoors, wash repellent-treated skin with soap and water, or bathe.

Follow instructions on the product label for handling repellent-treated clothing.

sandals also might help reduce risk. Application of repellents or insecticides (e.g., 0.5% permethrin) to clothing and gear can provide an added layer of protection. Remind travelers to always follow instructions on the label when applying repellents or insecticides. Additional prevention techniques are provided below.

Mosquitoes

More than 3,000 different mosquito species live worldwide, and each has specific biting behaviors; some species have local and regional variations, meaning biting behaviors might not be uniform throughout the distribution range of a specific species. Mosquitoes bite throughout the day and night, although each species tends to have peak activity at certain times.

4

The peak biting activity of *Aedes aegypti* (the primary vector for chikungunya, dengue, Mayaro, yellow fever, and Zika) is after sunrise (dawn) and at sunset (dusk). By contrast, peak biting activity for *Culex quinquefasciatus* (a vector for filariasis; Japanese, St. Louis, and West Nile encephalitis; and Usutu) is typically after sunset, usually between 10–11 p.m. The biting activity of *Anopheles* mosquitoes, the primary vectors for malaria worldwide, varies with the species. Peak biting activity for *Anopheles gambiae*, for example, the primary malaria vector in Africa, is between 3–6 a.m. Peak biting activity for *Anopheles albimanus*, an important malaria vector in Central and South America, is between 10–11 p.m.

Avoiding peak biting activity periods minimizes the chances of vectorborne disease. Although some mosquito species can roughly be described as day-biters and others as nocturnal feeders, regional variations and overlap in feeding times means that travelers need to be cautious about mosquito bites at all times of day and night in regions where mosquito-borne diseases are a risk.

As much as possible, travelers should avoid visiting areas with active outbreaks of mosquito-borne diseases. The CDC Travelers' Health website (https://wwwnc.cdc.gov/travel/) provides updates on regional disease transmission patterns and outbreaks. For more on mosquito bite prevention techniques, see Prevent Mosquito Bites (www.cdc.gov/mosquitoes/mosquito-bites/prevent-mosquito-bites.html).

SPATIAL REPELLENTS

Spatial repellents, including aerosol insecticide sprays, vaporizing mats, and mosquito coils, contain active ingredients (e.g., metofluthrin, allethrin) people can use to protect against insect bites. Spray aerosols can help clear mosquitoes from larger spaces, while coils and spatial repellents repel mosquitoes from more circumscribed areas.

Although many of these products have repellent or insecticidal activity under certain conditions, they have not yet been adequately evaluated in peer-reviewed studies for efficacy in preventing vectorborne diseases. Travelers should supplement use of these products with an EPA-registered repellent on skin or clothing and by using mosquito nets in areas where vectorborne diseases are a risk or biting arthropods are noted.

Some products available internationally might contain pesticides that are not registered for use in the United States. Conversely, travelers intending to bring their own spatial repellents should make sure the repellents are legal for use at their destination. Travelers should consult the US embassy website in the destination country. Advise travelers to use spatial repellents with caution and to avoid direct inhalation of spray or smoke.

Ticks

Hiking, camping, and hunting are examples of activities that could bring travelers in close contact with ticks. Travelers should avoid wooded and brushy areas with high grass and leaf litter, and stay in the center of hiking trails. For more on tick bite prevention techniques, see Preventing Tick Bites (www.cdc.gov/ticks/avoid/on_people.html).

Figure 4-01 provides instructions on how to remove attached ticks. Counsel travelers who develop rash or fever within several weeks of removing a tick to see a doctor; travelers should

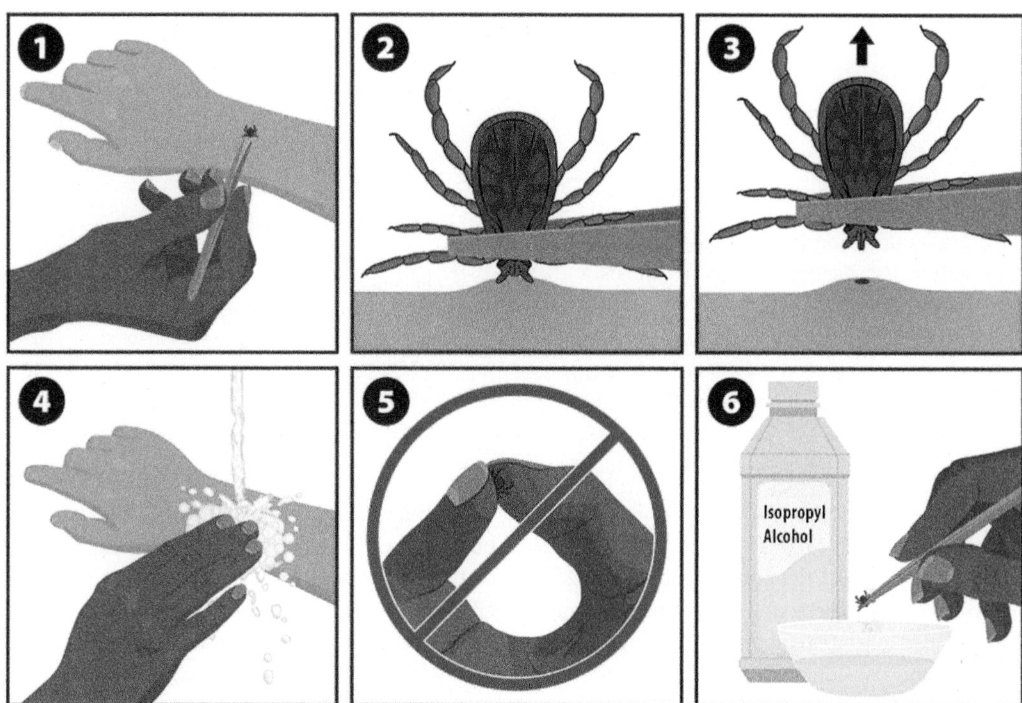

FIGURE 4-01 **How to remove a tick: instructions for travelers**

If a tick is attached to the skin, remove it as soon as possible.
Several tick removal devices are available on the market, but a plain set of fine-tipped tweezers work very well.
Using fine-tipped tweezers, grasp the tick as close to the surface of the skin as possible.
Pull upward with steady, even pressure without twisting or jerking the tick; twisting or jerking can cause the mouthparts of the tick to break off in the skin.
If the mouthparts of the tick break off in the skin, and they can be removed easily, remove them with tweezers.
If the mouthparts cannot be removed easily, leave them alone and allow the skin to heal.
After removing the tick, thoroughly clean the bite area and your hands with rubbing alcohol or soap and water.
Never crush a tick with your fingers.
Dispose of live ticks by placing them in alcohol or a sealed bag/container, wrapping them tightly with tape, or flushing them down the toilet.

provide details (if known) about the bite, including when and where it occurred.

Fleas

Flea bites often occur on the lower legs and feet. Travelers can protect these areas of the body by wearing long socks and pants. In addition, travelers should not feed or pet stray or wild animals. For more on flea bite prevention techniques, see Preventing Flea Bites (www.cdc.gov/fleas/avoid/on_people.html). For more on the importance of avoiding animals while traveling, see Sec. 4, Ch. 7, Zoonotic Exposures: Bites, Stings, Scratches & Other Hazards.

Sand Flies

Sand flies are most active during dawn and dusk. If possible, travelers should limit outdoor activities during those times.

BED BUGS

Bed bugs have not been shown to transmit disease to humans. A recent surge in bed bug infestations worldwide, particularly in high-income countries, is thought to be related to international travel, changes in pest control strategies in travel lodgings, and insecticide resistance. Bed bug infestations have been reported in hotels, theaters, and locations where people

BOX 4-10 Recommended protective measures to avoid or reduce bed bug exposure

INSPECT THE PREMISES

Look carefully for bed bugs on mattresses, box springs, bedding, and furniture, particularly built-in furniture with the bed, desk, and closets as a continuous structural unit. Bed bug eggs and nymphs are very small and can be easily overlooked.

SEEK ALTERNATIVE LODGING

Travelers who observe evidence of bed bug activity—whether it be the bugs themselves or physical signs (e.g., blood-spotting on linens)—should seek alternative lodging.

PRACTICE LUGGAGE PRECAUTIONS

Keep suitcases off the floor. Keep suitcases closed when not in use. Remove clothing and needed items (e.g., toiletry bags and shaving kits) from the suitcase only as necessary. Carefully inspect all clothing and other items before returning them to the suitcase.

4

congregate, even in the workplace, dormitories, and schools.

Bed bugs are small, flat insects that are reddish-brown in color, wingless, and range from 1–7 mm in length. Bed bug bites can produce strong allergic reactions and considerable emotional stress. Bed bugs can be transported in luggage and on clothing and by transporting personal belongings in contaminated transport vehicles.

Travelers can take measures to avoid bed bug bites and avoid transporting them in luggage and clothing (Box 4-10). Prevention is by far the most effective and inexpensive way to protect oneself from these pests. The cost associated with ridding a personal residence of bed bugs is considerable, and efforts at controlling bed bugs are often not immediately successful, even when conducted by professionals.

BIBLIOGRAPHY

Barnard DR, Xue RD. Laboratory evaluation of mosquito repellents against *Aedes albopictus*, *Culex nigripalpus*, and *Ochlerotatus triseriatus* (Diptera: Culicidae). J Med Entomol. 2004;41(4):726–30.

Fradin MS, Day JF. Comparative efficacy of insect repellents against mosquito bites. N Engl J Med. 2002;347(1):13–8.

Goodyer LI, Croft AM, Frances SP, Hill N, Moore SJ, Onyango SP, et al. Expert review of the evidence base for arthropod bite avoidance. J Travel Med. 2010;17(3):182–92.

Lupi E, Hatz C, Schlagenhauf P. The efficacy of repellents against *Aedes*, *Anopheles*, *Culex* and *Ixodes* spp.—a literature review. Travel Med Infect Dis. 2013;11(6):374–411.

Montemarano AD, Gupta RK, Burge JR, Klein K. Insect repellents and the efficacy of sunscreens. Lancet. 1997;349(9066):1670–1.

Murphy ME, Montemarano AD, Debboun M, Gupta R. The effect of sunscreen on the efficacy of insect repellent: a clinical trial. J Am Acad Dermatol. 2000;43(2 Pt 1):219–22.

Pages F, Dautel H, Duvallet G, Kahl O, de Gentile L, Boulanger N. Tick repellents for human use: prevention of tick bites and tick-borne diseases. Vector Borne Zoonotic Dis. 2014;14(2): 85–93.

Strickman D, Frances, SP, Debboun M. Prevention of bug bites, stings, and disease. Florida Entomologist. 2009;92(4):677–8.

US Environmental Protection Agency. Using insect repellents safely and effectively. Available from: www.epa.gov/insect-repellents/using-insect-repellents-safely-and-effectively.

ZOONOTIC EXPOSURES: BITES, STINGS, SCRATCHES & OTHER HAZARDS

Kendra Stauffer, Ryan Wallace, G. Gale Galland, Nina Marano

International travelers might encounter familiar animals (e.g., dogs and cats) that demonstrate unfamiliar behavior, and unfamiliar animals that can be venomous, toxic, or aggressive. People coming from areas where dangerous reptiles do not exist, for example, do not necessarily recognize the risk posed when they visit places where reptiles can threaten human health.

Animals do not have to be sick to be a risk to humans. The normal flora of poultry, reptiles, and ruminants can cause serious infections in humans, and rodents, bats, and nonhuman primates can be carriers of disease. Any animal (domestic or wild) can attack if it feels threatened, is protecting its young or territory, or is injured or ill. Free-roaming (stray) dogs are also common in many destinations and do not behave like pet dogs. Travelers should be aware that attacks by domestic animals are far more common than attacks by wildlife, and secondary infections of wounds can result in serious illness or death. Table 4-07 highlights groups of animals that are common reservoirs and routes of transmission of zoonotic diseases.

BITES & SCRATCHES

Bites from certain mammals encountered during foreign travel (bats, cats, dogs, monkeys, and rodents) present a risk for serious infection. Saliva from these animals can be contaminated so heavily with pathogens that a bite might not be required to cause human infection, and exposures can occur through cuts, scratches, or mucous membranes. For example, a 60-year-old man visiting Morocco was scratched on the face by a dog, became sick with rabies, and died.

Prevention

ANIMAL ADOPTION

Travelers should avoid the temptation to adopt stray animals from abroad, because the animals' medical history often is unknown, behavioral screening is incomplete or inaccurate, and the animal might be infected or incubating a disease not found in the United States. See Sec. 4, Ch. 9, Bringing Animals & Animal Products into the United States, for more details.

ANIMAL AVOIDANCE

Advise travelers to never pet, handle, or feed unfamiliar animals, domestic or wild, even in captive settings (e.g., game ranches, petting zoos), particularly in areas where rabies is enzootic. Safaris and ecotours may encourage up-close contact with animals; these animals are wild, however, often have unpredictable behavior, and associate humans with food. Travelers should exercise caution to avoid bites, scratches, and exposure to infectious materials.

Animals in some areas have learned that plastic or paper lunch bags, often placed in backpacks, are a food source. Monkeys are notorious for climbing into vehicles and opening backpacks to get food. Remind travelers to keep food items separated from personal effects in the vehicle. Travelers also should remove shiny or flashy jewelry, because these can attract attention from monkeys. Monkey bites are common in India, Thailand, Indonesia, and Bali, and most injuries occur when people try to touch or feed these animals.

When navigating cities, travelers should move wide around corners or blind spots, and check under restaurant tables, food stalls, and parked

Table 4-07 Animal reservoirs & mechanisms / routes of human exposure to zoonotic diseases & pathogens[1]

ANIMAL RESERVOIR	BITES & SCRATCHES	INHALATION & INGESTION
Bats	**BACTERIAL**	
		Leptospira spp. *Pasteurella* spp. Salmonellosis Yersiniosis
	VIRAL	
	Rabies	>200 bat-associated viruses (almost all RNA) Hemorrhagic fever viruses Paramyxoviruses (parainfluenza type 2 virus, Mapuera, Menangle, Nipah, Hendra) Coronaviruses (SARS-CoV-1, SARS-CoV-2, MERS)
	FUNGAL	
		Blastomycosis Cryptococcosis Histoplasmosis
Birds	**BACTERIAL**	
	Psittacosis	Avian mycobacteriosis Psittacosis Salmonellosis
	VIRAL	
		Avian influenza (highly pathogenic) in humans
	FUNGAL	
		Histoplasmosis
Cats & dogs	**BACTERIAL**	
	Capnocytophaga canimorsus Plague Tularemia	*Bartonella* spp. *Brucella* spp. *Campylobacter* spp. *Leptospira* spp. *Pasteurella* spp.
	VIRAL	
	Rabies	

Table 4-07 Animal reservoirs & mechanisms / routes of human exposure to zoonotic diseases & pathogens (continued)

ANIMAL RESERVOIR	BITES & SCRATCHES	INHALATION & INGESTION
Monkeys	**BACTERIAL**	
		Campylobacter spp. Salmonellosis Shigellosis
	VIRAL	
	B virus Rabies Simian retroviruses	
Rodents	**BACTERIAL**	
		Leptospira spp.[2] Salmonellosis[2]
	VIRAL	
	Lymphocytic choriomeningitis virus Monkeypox Rat-bite fever Viral hemorrhagic fevers	Arenavirus[2] Hantavirus[2] Hemorrhagic fever with renal syndrome[2] Lassa fever[2] Lymphocytic choriomeningitis virus[2] Monkeypox[3] Viral hemorrhagic fevers[2]
Rodent fleas, ticks & mites	**BACTERIAL**	
	Bartonella spp. Lyme disease Plague Rickettsial infections Tularemia	
	VIRAL	
	Tick-borne encephalitis	

[1]See Healthy Pets, Healthy People: Diseases That Can Spread Between Animals and People (www.cdc.gov/healthypets/diseases/index.html).
[2]Transmitted through inhalation or ingestion of rodent feces or urine.
[3]Transmitted through direct rodent contact.

vehicles, because cats, dogs, and monkeys tend to rest in these places. Startling one of these animals might result in a bite or scratch. Advise parents traveling with young children to watch them carefully around unfamiliar animals, because children are more likely to be bitten or scratched and to sustain more severe injuries.

PRETRAVEL VACCINES

Before departure, travelers should have a current tetanus vaccination or documentation of a booster vaccination in the previous 10 years (see Sec. 5, Part 1, Ch. 21, Tetanus). Travel health providers also should assess a traveler's need for preexposure rabies vaccine (see Sec. 5, Part 2, Ch. 18, Rabies).

Management

HIGH-RISK EXPOSURES

A high-risk exposure is an animal bite or scratch that was unprovoked or that came from an animal that appeared ill. Provoked bites and scratches are often inflicted when a person attempts to feed or handle an otherwise healthy-appearing animal. Unprovoked bites and scratches increase the likelihood that the animal might be sick and possibly infectious for certain zoonotic diseases (e.g., rabies). Travelers with high-risk exposures should seek professional medical care immediately, and not wait until they return to their home country.

4

B VIRUS

If bitten or scratched by a monkey, travelers should be evaluated for B virus postexposure prophylaxis (PEP; see Sec. 5, Part 2, Ch. 1, B Virus). B virus is enzootic in macaque monkeys (e.g., crab-eating macaques, rhesus macaques) found in North Africa and Gibraltar, and in Asia. Although B virus infections in humans are rare, and no reports of infection in travelers have been documented, the death rate in infected humans is high. Travelers should properly clean the wound after being bitten; prophylactic antiviral treatment with acyclovir or ganciclovir might be indicated in some cases.

RABIES

A health care professional should evaluate travelers bitten or scratched by any animal to assess the need for rabies PEP (see Sec. 5, Part 2, Ch. 18, Rabies). If a suspected rabies exposure has occurred, travelers should stop their journey and travel to a reliable place where they can obtain appropriate PEP; this could require traveling to another country. During the pretravel consultation, suggest countries where PEP is available and most accessible (see www.cdc.gov/rabies/resources/countries-risk.html).

Rabies exposures are relatively common among travelers and are positively correlated with length of stay. One study estimated travelers' rabies exposure incidence at 0.4% per month of stay, and other studies have shown that most exposures occur within the first 2 weeks of travel, indicating that even short-term travel can pose a risk for exposure.

Bats, a reservoir for rabies and rabies-related viruses globally, have very small, sharp teeth that might not leave discernable bite marks; travelers might not recognize or might trivialize bat exposure and not seek care. In many countries, bats, cats, dogs, and terrestrial carnivores are the most commonly reported rabid animals. Rabies is comparatively rare in primates and rodents. Rodent exposures should not constitute a rabies exposure with very rare exceptions.

TETANUS

Travelers with high-risk exposures, including animal bites and scratches, who were not recently vaccinated for tetanus will require a dose of tetanus toxoid–containing vaccine (Tdap, Td, or DTaP). This applies to people who received their most recent tetanus toxoid–containing vaccine >5 years before their exposure and to people who have not received ≥3 doses of tetanus toxoid–containing vaccines (see Sec. 5, Part 1, Ch. 21, Tetanus).

WOUND CARE

If a traveler receives a bite or scratch wound, they should clean the wound as soon as possible by washing with soap and running water for ≥20 minutes to prevent infections (e.g., B virus, rabies). Where possible, health care professionals should promptly clean and debride wounds contaminated with necrotic tissue, dirt, or other foreign materials. Often, a course of antibiotics is appropriate after animal bites or scratches because such wounds can lead to local or systemic infections. Some bite or scratch wounds might need to be left open to heal by secondary intention.

STINGS & ENVENOMATIONS

Snakes, insects, marine fish, and invertebrates are hazards to humans in many locations. Snakebites usually occur in areas where human populations coexist with dense snake populations (e.g., Southeast Asia, sub-Saharan Africa, Australia, tropical areas in the Americas). Of the 3,000 species of snakes, 600 species are venomous, and only 200 species can kill or significantly wound a human. One study showed that 25%–40% of venomous snakebites result in negligible or trivial envenomation.

Bites and stings from spiders and scorpions can be painful and can result in illness and death, particularly among infants and children. Other insects and arthropods (e.g., mosquitoes, ticks) can transmit infections (see Sec 4, Ch. 6, Mosquitoes, Ticks & Other Arthropods).

Most injuries from marine fish and invertebrates occur from chance encounters or defensive maneuvers. Resulting wounds have many common characteristics: bacterial contamination, foreign bodies, and occasionally venom. The incidence of venomous injuries from marine fish and invertebrates is rising as the popularity of surfing, scuba diving, and snorkeling increases. Most species responsible for human injuries, including jellyfish, scorpionfish, stingrays, stonefish, and sea urchins, live in tropical coastal waters.

Prevention

SITUATIONAL AWARENESS

Most stings and envenomation result from startling, stepping on, handling, attempting to feed, or otherwise harassing an animal. Before engaging in recreational activities, travelers should try to learn about the animals they might encounter, including their characteristics and habitats. Travelers should be especially aware of their surroundings at night and during warm weather, when snakes tend to be more active. The same caveat (awareness of surroundings) applies when conditions involve poor visibility, rough water, or confined areas.

PROTECTIVE CLOTHING

Travelers planning hikes in outdoor areas possibly inhabited by venomous snakes or biting insects should wear heavy, ankle-high or taller boots, and long sleeves and pants (see Sec. 4, Ch. 6, Mosquitoes, Ticks & Other Arthropods, for information on proper insect repellent use). Advise travelers going surfing, diving, or snorkeling to wear rash guards and swim boots, or other protective footwear.

Management

Instruct travelers to seek immediate medical attention any time a sting or envenomation occurs. Lifeguard stations at beaches or local clinics might have treatment kits for common stings or envenomations. In case of injury, species identification can help direct the best course of treatment. If possible, travelers or their companions should provide photographs of the animal to aid medical personnel. Travelers or their companions can immobilize an affected limb and apply a pressure bandage that does not restrict blood flow as first aid measures during transport to a medical facility.

Victims or their companions should not make incisions at bite sites or use tourniquets to restrict blood flow to affected extremities. Snakebite care is controversial and is best left to local emergency medical personnel. Specific antivenoms are available for some snakes in some areas; knowing the species of snake involved might prove critical to management. Consultation with a herpetologist can be beneficial.

If the traveler does not see or recognize the animal, health care providers will need to base treatment on the nature of the injury and the clinical effects. Bear in mind that—in some cases, at least—signs and symptoms might not appear for hours after contact. Symptoms can range from localized mild swelling and redness to more severe clinical findings (e.g., difficulty breathing or swallowing, chest pain, intense pain at the sting or bite site). Medical management will vary according to the severity of symptoms; therapy could include diphenhydramine, steroids, pain medication, and antibiotics.

INHALATION & INGESTION

The normal flora in the saliva, urine, and feces of many animals are pathogenic for humans. Exposure to animal body fluids is not always obvious or recognized, however. For example, water contaminated with animal urine or feces might be used to wash food items. In 2008, an indirect (inhalation) exposure to Marburg virus occurred in 2 tourists who visited a cave inhabited by bats, Python Cave in western Uganda. One case was fatal, and neither person reported a bite or scratch from a bat. Caves and mines also have other inhalation and ingestion hazards, such as fungi (see Sec. 5, Part 4, Ch. 2, Histoplasmosis).

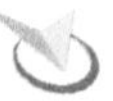

Prevention

To help prevent inhalation of aerosolized urine or feces, discourage travelers from going into densely populated animal habitats (e.g., caves, corrals, mines, tunnels) housing large populations of animals. Travelers planning to enter densely populated animal habitats (e.g., bat caves) should don protective equipment (e.g., face shield, respirator, gloves) and clothing. Upon leaving the area, travelers should appropriately doff dirty equipment and clothing and wash or bathe as soon as possible. Travelers also should plan to remove all food and drink from their backpacks before entering populated animal habitats.

Management

Illness related to animal excreta might not appear for hours or even weeks after exposure. Health care providers must take highly detailed travel histories that include all activities that could result in exposure to or contact with animals and their habitats.

4

BIBLIOGRAPHY

Daly RF, House J, Stanek D, Stobierski MG. Compendium of measures to prevent disease associated with animals in public settings. J Am Vet Med Assoc. 2017;251(11):1268–92.

Diaz JH. The global epidemiology, syndromic classification, management, and prevention of spider bites. Am J Trop Med Hyg. 2004;71(2):239–50.

Gauthier P, Bellanger A-P, Bozon F, Lepiller Q, Chirouze C, Marguet P. A survey investigating the current practice of French health professionals regarding infection risk after monkey bites. Zoonoses Public Health. 2020;67(2):193–7.

Gautret P, Harvey K, Pandey P, Lim PL, Leder K, Piyaphanee W, et al. Animal-associated exposure to rabies virus among travelers, 1997–2012. Emerg Infect Dis. 2015;21(4):569–77.

Han BA, Kramer AM, Drake JM. Global patterns of zoonotic disease in mammals. Trends Parasitol. 2016;32(7):565–77.

Hifumi T, Sakai A, Kondo Y, Yamamoto A, Morine N, Ato M, et al. Venomous snake bites: clinical diagnosis and treatment. J Intensive Care. 2015;3(16):1–9.

Meerburg BG, Singleton GR, Kijlstra A. Rodent-borne diseases and their risks for public health. Crit Rev Microbiol. 2009;35(3):221–70.

Wieten RW, Tawil S, van Vugt M, Goorhuis A, Grobusch MP. Risk of rabies exposure among travelers. Neth J Med. 2015;73(5):219–26.

World Health Organization. WHO expert consultation on rabies, second report. World Health Organ Tech Rep Ser. 2013;982:1–139.

Wu AC, Rekant SI, Baca ER, Jenkins RM, Perelygina LM, Hilliard JK, et al. Notes from the field: monkey bite in a public park and possible exposure to herpes B virus – Thailand, 2018. MMWR, 2020;69(9):247–8.

ZOONOSES—THE ONE HEALTH APPROACH

Ria Ghai, Casey Barton Behravesh

The One Health approach recognizes that the health of people is closely connected to the health of animals and our shared environment. This concept is not new but has been increasingly recognized in recent years as an effective way to address health issues at the human–animal–environment interface. One Health issues include zoonotic diseases, emerging infectious diseases like coronavirus disease 2019 (COVID-19), antimicrobial resistance, food safety and food security, and other shared health threats at the human–animal–environment interface.

Because no single person, organization, or sector can address challenges at the human–animal–environment interface, successful public health interventions require the cooperation of many partners. Professionals in human health (epidemiologists, nurses, physicians, public health practitioners), animal health (agricultural workers, paraprofessionals, veterinarians), environment (climate scientists, ecologists, wildlife experts), and other areas of expertise need to communicate, collaborate on, and coordinate activities based on a common, overarching goal: to achieve optimal health outcomes for people, animals, plants, and our shared environment.

Numerous benefits of One Health collaboration have been documented. For example, rabies is fatal in >99% of human cases and causes ≈59,000 human deaths annually around the world. Most (>99%) deaths are associated with exposure to rabid dogs. Preventing rabies in canines through annual or biannual mass dog vaccination campaigns has effectively prevented human-associated mortality. To be most successful, this strategy requires a One Health approach that includes partnership between human, animal, and environmental health professions at the programmatic and policy levels.

ZOONOTIC DISEASES

Zoonotic diseases are diseases that can be transmitted between animals. Zoonotic diseases require a One Health approach for effective prevention, detection, and response. Approximately 60% of all known human infectious disease agents originate in animals, including *Brucella*, HIV, *Salmonella*, and rabies virus. Most new or emerging infectious diseases in humans are zoonotic (e.g., COVID-19, Ebola, and highly pathogenic avian influenza). Furthermore, 80% of diseases with bioterrorism potential are zoonotic (e.g., anthrax, plague).

ONE HEALTH & TRAVEL MEDICINE

International travelers can be at risk for zoonotic diseases through various types of exposures, not just direct or indirect contact with wild or domestic animals or arthropod vectors. Contaminated environmental surfaces, freshwater sources (e.g., ponds, rivers), and food and beverages have been implicated as sources of zoonotic illness in humans. Failure to identify sources of exposure associated with a traveler's destination, itinerary, and activities can delay correct diagnosis and treatment and potentially increase the risk for further transmission of disease.

Patients benefit when health care providers use a One Health approach. In pretravel consultations, ensure travelers are aware of zoonotic and other infectious disease risks in areas where they are traveling, and encourage them to take measures to prevent or reduce those risks. For example, advise travelers to avoid settings with elevated zoonotic disease transmission risks like wildlife markets and farms. Consider administering rabies vaccine or offer prophylactic medications (e.g., antibiotics), as appropriate, to travelers for whom visiting high-risk zoonotic transmission settings is unavoidable.

In the posttravel setting, ask questions about interactions with animals, including domestic animals like companion and production animals and wildlife, both free-ranging and captive. Inquire about the apparent health of these animals and about animal habitats encountered during travel. Occasionally, health care providers and other zoonotic disease experts (e.g., veterinarians) might need to consult on a patient with a suspected zoonotic disease.

DIRECT & INDIRECT ANIMAL CONTACT

Travelers should be aware of the risks associated with animal contact. Direct contact with the saliva, blood, urine, mucus, feces, or other body fluids of an infected animal increases the risk for exposure to zoonotic pathogens; common routes of contact include petting or handling animals and being bitten or scratched (see Sec. 4, Ch. 7, Zoonotic Exposures: Bites, Stings, Scratches & Other Hazards). Additionally, visits to locations that pose a heightened risk of contact with animals that can carry diseases, such as wet markets where animals and their products are sold, or caves inhabited by bats, are best avoided when possible.

Because knowing which animals could be carrying pathogenic organisms can be difficult, especially because animal carriers often appear healthy, recommend that travelers avoid contact with unfamiliar animals and their products, including gifts or souvenirs made of animal products that might not have been treated to ensure their safety. If contact with live animals or animal products cannot be avoided, travelers should ensure they seek medical care immediately if they are bitten, scratched, or develop signs of illness following animal interactions, and report their animal interactions to the health care provider.

ZOONOTIC DISEASE VECTORS

Plague (*Yersinia pestis* infection), rickettsial diseases, and yellow fever are examples of zoonotic diseases transmitted by insect vectors. Travelers can minimize exposure to vectors by adhering to insect precautions and regularly performing tick checks on people and any traveling pets (see Sec. 4, Ch. 6, Mosquitoes, Ticks & Other Arthropods).

ZOONOTIC FOODBORNE EXPOSURES

4

Because many foodborne pathogens have an animal reservoir, consuming raw or undercooked animal parts or products exposes travelers to zoonotic pathogens. In many developing countries, for example, unpasteurized milk, or dairy products made from unpasteurized milk, such as cheese, could put travelers at risk for *Brucella*, *Campylobacter*, *Cryptosporidium*, *Listeria*, and other pathogens. Travelers should avoid eating bushmeat—raw, smoked, or partially processed meat from bats, nonhuman primates, rodents, or other wild animals. Advise travelers to eat only fully cooked meat, eggs, fish, shellfish, and other foods, and to drink only pasteurized milk and dairy products, to reduce the risk for foodborne illness while traveling (see Sec. 2, Ch. 8, Food & Water Precautions, for more details).

BIBLIOGRAPHY

Angelo KM, Barbre K, Shieh WJ, Kozarsky PE, Blau DM, Sotir MJ, Zaki SR. International travelers with infectious diseases determined by pathology results, Centers for Disease Control and Prevention—United States, 1995–2015. Trav Med Infect Dis. 2017;19:8–15.

Centers for Disease Control and Prevention. Healthy pets, healthy people. Available from: www.cdc.gov/healthypets.

Centers for Disease Control and Prevention. One Health. Available from: www.cdc.gov/onehealth/index.html.

Daly RF, House J, Stanek D, Stobierski MG. Compendium of measures to prevent disease associated with animals in public settings, 2017. J Am Vet Med Assoc. 2017;251(11):1269–92.

Day M. Human-animal health interactions: the role of One Health. Am Fam Phys. 2016;93(5):344–6.

Food and Agriculture Organization of the United Nations, World Organization for Animal Health, and World Health Organization. Taking a multisectoral, One Health approach: a tripartite guide to addressing zoonotic diseases in countries. Geneva: The Organizations; 2019.

Hurley JW, Friend M. Zoonoses and travel. In: Friend M, editor. Disease emergence and resurgence: the wildlife-human connection. Reston (VA): US Geological Survey; 2006. pp. 191–206.

BRINGING ANIMALS & ANIMAL PRODUCTS INTO THE UNITED STATES

G. Gale Galland, Emily Pieracci, Kendra Stauffer

The Centers for Disease Control and Prevention (CDC) restricts the importation of any animals or animal products into the United States that might pose a public health threat. Any animal or animal product can be restricted from entry if CDC has reasonable knowledge or suspicion that it poses a human health risk. CDC currently has explicit restrictions for specific animals, including bats, cats, civets, dogs, insects and other non-animal vectors, nonhuman primates, African rodents, and some turtles, as well as products made from these animals. Importers must comply with CDC requirements to bring these animals or items into the United States.

Any animal, including service and emotional support animals, that leaves the United States must meet all entry requirements to reenter the United States, even if the animal previously lived in the United States (see Sec. 7, Ch. 6, Traveling with Pets & Service Animals). Many animals also are regulated by other federal agencies or by state governments. Therefore, travelers should check with the US Department of Agriculture (USDA), the US Fish and Wildlife Service (FWS), and the destination state and territorial health authorities for specific rules about importation.

Animal import and reentry requirements vary depending on the countries visited while abroad. Travelers should check entry requirements provided by CDC (www.cdc.gov/importation/bringing-an-animal-into-the-united-states/index.html), USDA (www.aphis.usda.gov/aphis/pet-travel/bring-pet-into-the-united-states), and FWS (www.fws.gov/international/Permits/by-activity/personal-pets.html). Travelers also should check USDA requirements for interstate transport of animals in US states and territories (www.aphis.usda.gov/aphis/pet-travel/interstate-pet-travel).

ANIMAL HEALTH CERTIFICATES

CDC does not require general health certificates for animals entering the United States. Some states or territories might require health certificates for entry, however, and some airlines might require these certificates for transport. Before departure, travelers should check with the departments of health and agriculture at the destination, and with the airline, for any health certificate requirements. The department of environmental protection or department of natural resources of some states and local governments might have additional requirements.

INTERNATIONAL PET RESCUE & ADOPTION

Although often done with the best of intentions, rescuing and importing stray animals from foreign countries can create human health risks when those animals are introduced into the United States. Travelers are at an increased risk for bites and scratches from fearful and stressed animals, which could result in injury or exposure to infectious diseases (e.g., rabies). Animals infected with zoonotic diseases might not show outward signs of being ill, but can still spread these diseases to people. Therefore, all rescued animals should be examined by a licensed veterinarian before departure from the country of origin and after arrival into the United States. Travelers who intend on rescuing animals should visit a travel medicine clinic prior to departure to discuss rabies preexposure prophylaxis.

In July 2021, CDC implemented a temporary suspension for the importation of dogs from countries with a high risk of dog-maintained rabies virus variant (DMRVV; see Bringing a Dog into the United States, www.cdc.gov/dogtravel). During the suspension period, dogs rescued or adopted from high-risk countries must enter the United States through a CDC-approved port of entry (Atlanta, Los Angeles, Miami, or New York) and undergo examination and revaccination against rabies immediately upon arrival (www.cdc.gov/importation/bringing-an-animal-into-the-united-states/approved-care-facilities.html). Dogs that do not meet CDC's entry requirements will be denied entry and returned to the country of departure at the importer's expense.

IMPORTING LIVE ANIMALS

Bats

Bats are reservoirs of many viruses that can infect humans; examples include filoviruses, Nipah, rabies, and severe acute respiratory syndrome (SARS) coronaviruses. To reduce the risk of introducing these viruses, CDC requires a permit for importation of all live bats and does not allow bats to be imported as pets. Bat import permit applications must be submitted electronically at www.cdc.gov/cpr/ipp/applications/index.htm. Many bat species require additional FWS permits.

Cats

Cats are subject to inspection at US ports of entry and can be denied entry if there is evidence of infection with a disease of public health concern. If a cat appears ill, examination by a licensed veterinarian at the owner's expense might be required before entry is permitted. CDC does not require cats to have proof of rabies vaccination for importation into the United States, but does recommend vaccination. In addition, many states and territories have rabies vaccination requirements for cats. Importers should check with state and territorial health authorities at the destination to determine whether state or territorial agencies require rabies vaccinations for cats (see www.cdc.gov/importation/bringing-an-animal-into-the-united-states/cats.html).

Civets & Related Animals

To reduce the risk of introducing severe acute respiratory syndrome (SARS) coronavirus, the United States does not allow importation of civets and related animals in the family Viverridae. With permission from CDC, however, exceptions can be made for animals imported for science, education, or exhibition (see www.cdc.gov/importation/bringing-an-animal-into-the-united-states/civets.html). People who want to import civets and related animals should check with the USDA and FWS for additional requirements.

Dogs

Dogs are subject to inspection upon entry into the United States if they have evidence of infection with a communicable disease or if they have not been vaccinated against rabies. If a dog appears ill, examination by a licensed veterinarian, at the owner's expense, might be required before entry is permitted.

Rabies vaccination is required for all dogs, including service animals and emotional support animals, entering the United States from a country that is considered at high risk for DMRVV, as determined by CDC rabies experts. Dogs from high-risk countries must be accompanied by a current, valid rabies vaccination certificate that includes the following information:

- Name and address of owner
- Breed, sex, age, color, markings, and other identifying information for the dog
- Date of rabies vaccination and vaccine product information
- Date of expiration of vaccination
- Name, license number, address, and signature of administering veterinarian

Rabies certificates have expiration dates ranging from 1–3 years from the date of vaccination, depending on the type of vaccine. All dogs must be ≥12 weeks (84 days) old before receiving their first rabies vaccination. Rabies vaccinations must occur ≥28 days before arrival in the United States, because it takes 28 days for full vaccine effectiveness. Additional requirements apply during the period of CDC's temporary suspension on the importation of dogs from high-risk countries.

CDC recommends, and most US state and local authorities require, routine rabies vaccination of dogs. Importers should check with state and local authorities at the final destination to determine requirements for rabies vaccination.

STATES & TERRITORIES WITH ADDITIONAL REQUIREMENTS

All dogs and cats arriving in the state of Hawaii or the territory of Guam, even those arriving from the US mainland, are subject to locally imposed quarantine requirements. For more information about animal importation into Hawaii, see http://hdoa.hawaii.gov/ai/aqs. For more information about animal importation into Guam, see https://doag.guam.gov/animal-health-animal-control.

Insects

Importation of insect vectors and infectious biologic agents are regulated under the same program as bats. In some circumstances, known vectors of human disease (e.g., ticks, mosquitoes), can be imported into the United States with a permit from CDC (at www.cdc.gov/cpr/ipp/index.htm).

Primates

Nonhuman primates can transmit a variety of serious diseases to humans, including Ebola virus disease and tuberculosis. Nonhuman primates can be imported into the United States only by a CDC-registered importer and only for scientific, educational, or exhibitory purposes. All nonhuman primates are considered endangered or threatened, and they also require FWS permits for importation.

Nonhuman primates cannot be imported as pets. Nonhuman primates kept as pets in the United States that travel outside the country will not be allowed to reenter the United States as pets (see www.cdc.gov/importation/bringing-an-animal-into-the-united-states/monkeys.html).

Rodents

African rodents are a known source of communicable diseases (e.g., monkeypox) that can be transferred to humans. CDC does not allow the importation of these animals. Exceptions might be made for animals imported for science, education, or exhibition, with permission from CDC. Importers should check with USDA and FWS for additional requirements to import African rodents (see www.cdc.gov/importation/bringing-an-animal-into-the-united-states/african-rodents.html).

Turtles

Turtles often are kept as pets but can transmit *Salmonella* to humans. CDC restricts the importation of some turtles. A person can import ≤6 viable turtle eggs or live turtles with a shell length <4 inches (10 cm) for noncommercial purposes. More live turtles or viable turtle eggs can be imported with CDC permission, but only for science, education, or exhibition. CDC does not restrict the importation of live turtles with a shell length ≥4 inches (see www.cdc.gov/importation/bringing-an-animal-into-the-united-states/turtles.html). Importers should check with USDA and FWS for additional requirements to import turtles.

Other Animals

Travelers planning to import horses, poultry or other birds, ruminants, swine, or dogs used for handling livestock or for commercial resale or adoption should contact the National Import Export Services, a part of the USDA Animal and Plant Health Inspection Service, at 301-851-3300, or visit www.aphis.usda.gov/aphis/ourfocus/animalhealth/animal-and-animal-product-import-information to learn about additional requirements.

Travelers planning to import bears, wild birds, wild members of the cat family, fish, rabbits, reptiles, spiders, or other wild or endangered animals should contact FWS at 800-344-9453 (toll-free general number) or 703-358-1949 (FWS Office of Law Enforcement), or visit www.fws.gov/program/office-of-law-enforcement/information-importers-exporters.

IMPORTING ANIMAL PRODUCTS

Bushmeat

Imported animal products often include items intended for human consumption. Bushmeat, generally raw, smoked, or partially processed meat from wild animals, might harbor infectious or zoonotic agents that can cause human or animal disease. As people have migrated around the world, bushmeat has become a growing commodity in the global wildlife trade.

CDC prohibits importation of bushmeat from CDC-restricted species into the United States. Bushmeat from other species also is restricted under USDA or FWS regulations. In addition to the human and animal health risks, many of the wild animals commonly hunted for bushmeat are threatened or endangered species protected by international wildlife laws and treaties (e.g., the Convention on International Trade of Endangered Species [CITES]).

For additional information about importing animals and animal products into the United States and for permit applications, travelers should visit www.cdc.gov/importation/index.html or contact 1-800-CDC INFO (1-800-232-4636). To request CDC permission to import a CDC-regulated animal or product, send an email to CDCanimalimports@cdc.gov.

Trophies & Other Animal Products

Travelers often want to import animal skins, hunting trophies, or other items made from animals when returning from a trip. These items must either be rendered noninfectious (see www.cdc.gov/importation/animal-products.html) or be accompanied by an import permit. CDC restricts products made from bats, nonhuman primates, African rodents, and civets and related animals in the family Viverridae. These products also might be regulated by other US federal agencies.

CDC has the right to restrict other items known to carry infectious diseases. For example, CDC restricts bringing souvenirs made from goat hide (e.g., goatskin drums) into the United States because they have been associated with cases of anthrax in humans. Travelers who want to import hunting trophies or other products made from animals should check with CDC, USDA, and FWS to make sure they comply with federal regulations.

BIBLIOGRAPHY

Allocati, N, Petrucci, AG, DiGiovanni, P, Masulli, M, DiIlio, C KeLaurenzi, VE. Bat–man disease transmission: zoonotic pathogens from wildlife reservoirs to human populations. Cell Death Discov. 2016;2:16048.

Centers for Disease Control and Prevention. Multistate outbreak of monkeypox—Illinois, Indiana, and Wisconsin, 2003. MMWR Morb Mortal Wkly Rep. 2003;52(23):537–40.

Centers for Disease Control and Prevention. Multistate outbreak of Salmonella infections associated with exposure to turtles—United States, 2007–2008. MMWR Morb Mortal Wkly Rep. 2008;57(3):69–72.

DeMarcus TA, Tipple MA, Ostrowski SR. US policy for disease control among imported nonhuman primates. J Infect Dis. 1999;179 Suppl 1:S281–2.

Jansen W, Merkle M, Daun A, Flor M, Grabowski NT, Klein G. The quantity and quality of illegally imported products of animal origin in personal consignments into the European Union seized at two German airports between 2010 and 2014. Plos One. 2016;11(2):1–14.

Pieracci EG, Pearson CM, Wallace RM, Blanton JD, Whitehouse ER, Ma X, et al. Vital signs: trends in human rabies deaths and exposures—United States, 1938–2018. MMWR Morb Mortal Wkly Rep. 2019;68(23):524–8.

Murphy J, Sirfri, CD, Pruitt R, Hornberger M, Bonds D, Blanton J, et al. Human rabies—Virginia, 2017. MMWR Morb Mortal Wkly Rep. 2019;67(5152):1410–4.

National Association of State Public Health Veterinarians, Compendium of Animal Rabies Prevention and Control Committee; Brown CM, Slavinski S, Ettestad P, Sidwa TJ, Sorhage FE. Compendium of animal rabies prevention and control, 2016. J Am Vet Med Assoc. 2016;248(5):505–17.

Wu D, Tu C, Xin C, Xuan H, Meng Q, Liu Y, et al. Civets are equally susceptible to experimental infection by two different severe acute respiratory syndrome coronavirus isolates. J Virol. 2005;79(4):2620–5.

FOOD POISONING FROM MARINE TOXINS

Vernon Ansdell

Poisoning from ingesting marine toxins is an underrecognized hazard for travelers, particularly in the tropics and subtropics. Climate change, coral reef damage, expanding international trade and tourism, growing seafood consumption, and spread of toxic algal blooms are all contributing to an increasing risk (Map 4-01).

CIGUATERA FISH POISONING

Ciguatera fish poisoning occurs after eating reef fish contaminated with toxins like ciguatoxin or maitotoxin. These potent toxins originate from *Gambierdiscus toxicus*, a small marine organism (dinoflagellate) that grows on and around coral reefs. Dinoflagellates are ingested by herbivorous fish. The toxins produced by *G. toxicus* are then modified and concentrated as they pass up the marine food chain to carnivorous fish and finally to humans. Ciguatoxins are concentrated in fish liver, intestines, roe, and heads.

G. toxicus might proliferate on dead coral reefs more effectively than other dinoflagellates. The risk for ciguatera poisoning is likely to increase as coral reefs deteriorate because of climate change, ocean acidification, offshore construction, and nutrient runoff.

Risk to Travelers

Approximately 50,000 cases of ciguatera poisoning are reported worldwide annually, but because the disease is underrecognized and underreported, reports are likely grossly underestimated. The incidence in travelers to highly endemic areas has been estimated as high as 3 per 100. Ciguatera is widespread in tropical and subtropical waters, usually between the latitudes of 35°N and 35°S, and is particularly common in the Pacific and Indian Oceans and the Caribbean Sea. The incidence and geographic distribution of ciguatera poisoning are increasing. Newly recognized areas of risk include Madeira and the Canary Islands, parts of the Mediterranean, and the western Gulf of Mexico. Be aware that travelers with ciguatera fish poisoning might seek care after returning home to

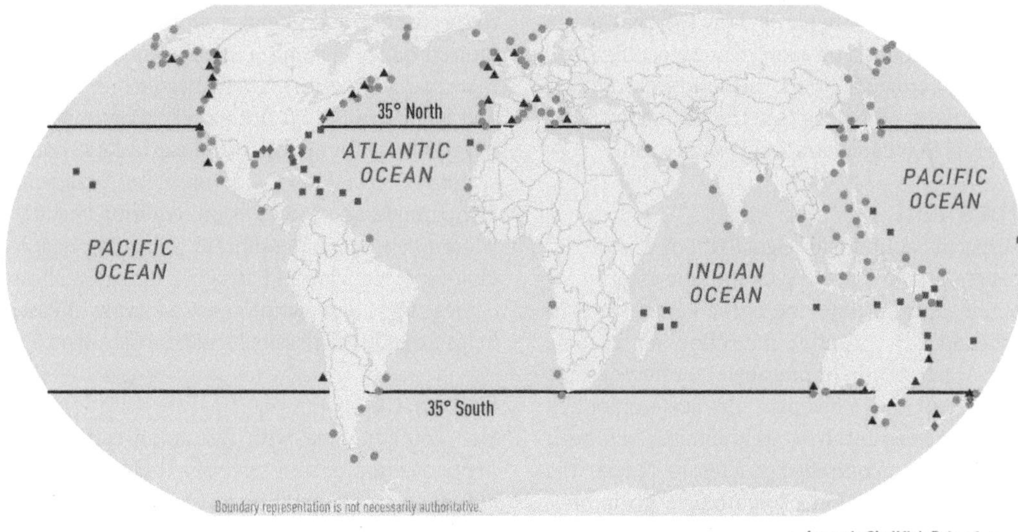

MAP 4-01 **Worldwide distribution of selected seafood poisonings**

Source: US National Office for Harmful Algal Blooms, Woods Hole Oceanographic Institution, Woods Hole, MA: 2016. Available from: https://hab.whoi.edu/maps/regions-world-distribution/. Harmful algal blooms (HABs) occur widely and contribute to seafood toxicity. Risk for human poisoning depends on the particular seafood consumed, where it was caught or harvested, and—in some instances—the exposure of that seafood to an HAB.

nonendemic (temperate) areas. In addition, cases of ciguatera fish poisoning are seen with increasing frequency in nonendemic areas because of the increasing global trade in seafood products.

Fish most likely to cause ciguatera poisoning are large carnivorous reef fish (e.g., amberjack, barracuda, grouper, moray eel, sea bass, sturgeon). Omnivorous and herbivorous fish (e.g., parrot fish, red snapper, surgeonfish) also can be a risk.

Clinical Presentation

Ciguatera poisoning can cause cardiovascular, gastrointestinal, neurologic, and neuropsychiatric illness. The first symptoms usually develop within 3–6 hours after eating contaminated fish but can be delayed up to 30 hours. General signs and symptoms include fatigue, general malaise, and insomnia. Cardiovascular signs and symptoms include bradycardia, heart block, or hypotension. Gastrointestinal signs and symptoms include diarrhea, nausea, vomiting, and abdominal pain. Neurologic and neuropsychiatric signs and symptoms include paresthesia, weakness, pain in the teeth or a sensation that the teeth are loose, a burning or metallic taste in the mouth, generalized itching, sweating, and blurred vision. Cold allodynia (abnormal sensation when touching cold water or objects) has been a reported characteristic, but acute sensitivity to both heat and cold can be present. Neurologic symptoms usually last a few days to several weeks but can persist for months or even years.

The overall death rate from ciguatera poisoning is <0.1% but varies according to the toxin dose and availability of medical care to deal with complications. The diagnosis of ciguatera poisoning is based on the characteristic signs and symptoms and a history of eating fish species known to carry ciguatera toxin. The US Food and Drug Administration (FDA) can test fish in their laboratory at Dauphin Island, Alabama. No test for ciguatera toxins in human clinical specimens is readily available.

Prevention

Ciguatera toxins do not affect the texture, taste, or smell of fish, nor are they destroyed by canning, cooking, freezing, pickling, salting, or smoking, or by gastric acid. To prevent ciguatera fish poisoning, travelers should avoid or limit consumption of reef fish, particularly fish that weigh >5 pounds; counsel travelers to never eat high-risk fish (e.g., barracuda, moray eel) and to avoid eating the parts of the fish (e.g., the head, intestines, liver, roe) that concentrate ciguatera toxin.

Treatment

No specific antidote for ciguatoxin or maitotoxin poisoning is available. Symptomatic treatments include amitriptyline for chronic paresthesias, depression, or pruritus; fluoxetine for chronic fatigue; gabapentin or pregabalin for neuropathic symptoms; and nifedipine or acetaminophen for headaches. Intravenous mannitol has been reported in uncontrolled studies to reduce the severity and duration of neurologic symptoms, particularly if given ≤48 hours of symptom onset; give mannitol only to hemodynamically stable, well-hydrated patients.

After recovery, advise patients to avoid consuming alcohol, caffeine, fish, and nuts for ≥6 months because these might cause symptom relapse.

SCOMBROID

Scombroid is caused by eating fish that contain high levels of histamine. Bacteria convert histidine, an essential amino acid found in the flesh of the fish, to histamine. The process of histidine conversion can be mitigated by inhibiting bacterial growth through proper storage of freshly caught fish by refrigeration or icing. Conversely, when fish are improperly stored after capture, bacterial overgrowth can occur, facilitating and accelerating histamine production.

One of the most common fish poisonings, scombroid occurs worldwide in both temperate and tropical waters. Fish typically associated with scombroid have naturally high levels of histidine in their flesh and include amberjack, anchovies, bluefish, herring, mackerel, mahi mahi (dolphin fish), marlin, sardines, and tuna. Histamine and other scombrotoxins are resistant to canning, cooking, freezing, and smoking.

Clinical Presentation

Scombroid poisoning resembles an acute allergic reaction and usually appears 10–60 minutes after a person eats contaminated fish. Signs and symptoms include abdominal cramps and diarrhea, blurred vision, flushing of the face and upper body resembling sunburn, severe headaches, itching, and palpitations. Left untreated, symptoms usually resolve within 12 hours but can last ≤48 hours.

Rarely, respiratory compromise, malignant arrhythmias, and hypotension requiring hospitalization can occur. Scombroid poisoning has no long-term sequelae and usually is diagnosed from clinical signs and symptoms. Clustering of cases helps exclude the possibility of true fish allergy.

Prevention

Fish contaminated with histamine can have a peppery, sharp, or salty taste or a "bubbly" feel, but will usually look, smell, and taste normal. The key to prevention is to make sure fish are properly iced or refrigerated at temperatures <38°F (<3.3°C) or immediately frozen after being caught. Canning, cooking, freezing, or smoking will not destroy histamine in contaminated fish.

Treatment

Scombroid poisoning usually responds well to antihistamines, typically H1-receptor antagonists, although H2-receptor antagonists also might provide some benefit.

SHELLFISH POISONING

Shellfish, including crustaceans (Dungeness crab, lobster, and shrimp), filter-feeding bivalve mollusks (clams, cockles, mussels, oysters, and scallops), and gastropod mollusks (abalone, moon snails, and whelks) can harbor toxins that result in several different poisoning syndromes. Toxins originate in small marine organisms (diatoms or dinoflagellates) ingested and concentrated by shellfish.

Risk to Travelers

Contaminated (toxic) shellfish can be found in temperate and tropical waters, typically during or after phytoplankton blooms, also called harmful algal blooms (HABs). One example of a HAB is the Florida red tide caused by *Karenia brevis*.

Clinical Presentation

Poisoning results in gastrointestinal and neurologic illness of varying severity. Symptoms typically appear 30–60 minutes after a person ingests toxic shellfish but can be delayed for several hours. Diagnosis is usually through exclusion, and typically is made clinically in patients with a history of having recently eaten shellfish.

AMNESIC SHELLFISH POISONING

Amnesic shellfish poisoning (ASP) is a rare form of shellfish poisoning caused by eating shellfish contaminated with domoic acid, produced by diatoms of the *Pseudonitzchia* spp. Outbreaks of ASP have been reported in the Americas (Canada, Chile), Europe (Belgium, France, Ireland, Portugal, Scotland, Spain), and the Pacific (Australia, New Zealand). Implicated shellfish include razor clams, mussels, scallops, and other crustaceans.

In most cases, gastrointestinal symptoms (e.g., abdominal pain, diarrhea, vomiting) develop within 24 hours of eating toxic shellfish, followed by headache, cognitive impairment, and memory loss. Symptoms usually resolve within hours to days after shellfish ingestion. Hypotension, arrhythmias, ophthalmoplegia, coma, and death have been reported in severe cases. Survivors might exhibit severe anterograde, short-term memory deficits.

DIARRHEIC SHELLFISH POISONING

Diarrheic shellfish poisoning (DSP) results from eating shellfish contaminated with toxins (e.g., okadaic acid). DSP occurs worldwide, and outbreaks have been reported in the Americas (Canada, Chile, United States, and Uruguay), Asia (China, Japan), and Europe (Belgium, France, Ireland, Scandinavia, Spain).

Most cases result from eating toxin-containing bivalve mollusks (e.g., mussels, scallops). Symptoms usually occur within 2 hours of consumption and include abdominal pain, chills, diarrhea, nausea, and vomiting. Symptoms usually resolve within 2–3 days. No deaths from DSP have been reported.

NEUROTOXIC SHELLFISH POISONING

Neurotoxic shellfish poisoning (NSP) is caused by eating shellfish contaminated with brevetoxins produced by the dinoflagellate *K. brevis.* NSP is predominately an illness of the Western Hemisphere (the Caribbean, Gulf of Mexico, southeastern coast of the United States), but the disease also has been reported from New Zealand.

NSP usually presents as a gastroenteritis accompanied by neurologic symptoms resembling mild ciguatera or paralytic shellfish poisoning (described below), 30 minutes to 3 hours after a person eats shellfish. Aerosolized red tide respiratory irritation (ARTRI) also can occur when people inhale aerosolized brevetoxins in sea spray, and has been reported in association with a red tide (*K. brevis* HAB) in Florida. ARTRI can induce bronchoconstriction and cause acute, temporary respiratory discomfort in healthy people. People with asthma might experience more severe and prolonged respiratory effects.

PARALYTIC SHELLFISH POISONING

Paralytic shellfish poisoning (PSP) is the most common and most severe form of shellfish poisoning. PSP is caused by eating shellfish contaminated with saxitoxins. These potent neurotoxins are produced by various dinoflagellates. A wide range of shellfish can cause PSP, but most cases occur after people eat clams or mussels.

PSP occurs worldwide but is most common in temperate waters off the Atlantic and Pacific coasts of North America, including Alaska. Other countries in the Americas (Chile), as well as countries in Asia (China, the Philippines), Europe (Ireland, Scotland), and the Pacific (Australia, New Zealand) have also reported cases.

Symptoms usually appear 30–60 minutes after a person eats toxic shellfish and include numbness and tingling of the face, lips, tongue, arms, and legs. Patients also might have diarrhea and vomiting, headache, and nausea. Severe cases are associated with ingestion of large doses of toxin and clinical features such as ataxia, dysphagia, flaccid paralysis, mental status changes, and respiratory failure. The case-fatality ratio depends on the availability of modern medical care, including mechanical ventilation; rates of death among children can be particularly high.

Prevention

Shellfish poisoning can be prevented by avoiding potentially contaminated shellfish, which is particularly important in areas during or shortly after algal blooms, locally referred to as "red tides" or "brown tides." Consuming shellfish also carries a very high risk for infection from various viral (e.g., hepatitis A virus, norovirus) and bacterial (e.g., *Salmonella*, *Shigella*, *Vibrio parahaemolyticus*, and *V. vulnificus*) pathogens. Ideally, travelers to developing countries should consider avoiding eating shellfish. Marine shellfish toxins cannot be destroyed by cooking or freezing.

Treatment

Treatment is symptomatic and supportive. Severe cases of paralytic shellfish poisoning might require mechanical ventilation.

BIBLIOGRAPHY

Chan TY. Ciguatera fish poisoning in East Asia and Southeast Asia. Mar Drugs. 2015;13(6):3466–78.

Friedman MA, Fleming LE, Fernandez M et al. Ciguatera fish poisoning: treatment, prevention and management. Mar Drugs. 2008;6:456–79.

Hungerford JM. Scombroid poisoning: a review. Toxicon. 2010;56(2):231–43.

Isbister GK, Kiernan MC. Neurotoxic marine poisoning. Lancet Neurol. 2005;4(4):219–28.

Palafox NA, Buenoconsejo-Lum LE. Ciguatera fish poisoning: review of clinical manifestations. J Toxicol Toxin Rev. 2001;20(2):141–60.

Schnorf H, Taurarii M, Cundy T. Ciguatera fish poisoning: a double-blind randomized trial of mannitol therapy. Neurology. 2002;58(6):873–80.

Sobel J, Painter J. Illnesses caused by marine toxins. Clin Infect Dis. 2005;41(9):1290–6.

4

SAFETY & SECURITY OVERSEAS

Virginia Lehner

US citizens traveling abroad face a wide range of risks not generally prevalent in the United States. These risks include sanitation issues (e.g., non-potable water), increased risk for traffic accidents due to poor road conditions and unfamiliarity with local norms, local insectborne illness or disease vectors, injury from adventure tourism or overexposure to unfamiliar climates, and violence ranging from petty theft to terrorism.

Travelers going overseas, particularly tourists, can also face additional challenges in seeking help when they find themselves in distress. Language, culture, and local laws can be barriers, and travelers might not have an immediately accessible network of friends or family to assist them in an emergency. Local government responses to accidents or crime might not be what travelers expect; in some instances, an effective local government might not even exist to respond. Travelers should research conditions at their destination before departure to learn what risks they could likely face and make plans to mitigate those risks abroad.

INFORMED TRAVEL

As indicated above, travelers should make informed decisions prior to departure, based on clear, timely, and reliable safety and security information. The Bureau of Consular Affairs (CA) within the US Department of State (the organization charged with protecting US citizens abroad) provides would-be travelers with a broad range of information for every country in the world through its webpages, Travel.State.Gov (https://travel.state.gov/content/travel.html) and US Embassy and Consulate (www.usembassy.gov/websites).

Travel Advisories & Travel to High-Risk Areas

At the broadest level, CA assigns every country a metrics-based travel advisory level ranging from 1: Exercise normal precautions to 4: Do not travel. Travelers can see travel advisories at Travel.State.Gov (https://travel.state.gov/content/travel/en/traveladvisories/traveladvisories.html); accompanying country information pages describe the risks and conditions and the actions travelers should take to mitigate risks in each country. Country information pages provide extensive travel information, including details about entry and exit requirements, local laws and customs, health conditions, accessibility for travelers with disabilities and for other key groups, typical scams and other crimes, transportation safety, and other relevant topics. The Department of State also warns people not to visit certain high-risk countries or areas because of local conditions and limited ability to provide consular services in those places (see https://travel.state.gov/content/travel/en/international-travel/before-you-go/travelers-with-special-considerations/high-risk-travelers.html).

US embassies and consulates abroad also issue event-based alerts to inform US citizens of specific safety, security, or health concerns that put travelers at immediate risk (e.g., civil aviation risks, crime threats, demonstrations, health events, weather events). For more information, see http://travel.state.gov/travelsafely.

Smart Traveler Enrollment Program (STEP)

Advise US citizen travelers to enroll with the Department of State's Smart Traveler Enrollment Program (STEP; https://step.state.gov/step). A free service, STEP allows enrollees to receive information and alerts from local US embassies or consulates about safety, security, or health conditions at their destination. STEP can also help the local embassy or consulate locate missing US citizens or contact them in an emergency (e.g., civil unrest, a family emergency, natural disasters).

Preparing Friends & Family

The Department of State advises travelers to share their itinerary with friends and family, including the names and contact information for travel agencies, planned tours, and lodging. Travelers should establish reasonable expectations for "check-in" communications with family and friends. In addition to having their own copies, travelers also should provide trusted friends and family with copies of important documents like passports, visas, health insurance cards, and credit cards in case any of these items are lost or stolen.

Medical Insurance

The US government does not provide medical insurance for US travelers overseas and will not pay costs for travelers receiving international medical care. Medicare and Medicaid do not cover these costs, nor do many private domestic health insurance plans. Thus, travelers should purchase supplemental insurance prior to travel (see Sec. 6, Ch. 1, Travel Insurance, Travel Health Insurance & Medical Evacuation Insurance). Because travel insurance policy coverages vary, travelers should carefully read the terms to make sure the policy fits their needs. Travelers might need additional insurance coverage to cover the costs of emergency medical care, medical transport back to the United States, travel and accommodation costs in the event of interrupted or delayed travel, 24-hour contact services, and treatment received overseas for any preexisting conditions, including pregnancy.

LOCAL LAWS

US citizens are subject to local laws during travel abroad. Travelers who violate those laws—even unknowingly—can face arrest, imprisonment, or deportation. In addition, some crimes are prosecutable both in the United States and in the country where the crime was committed. US citizens arrested or detained abroad should ask local law enforcement or prison officials to notify the US embassy or consulate immediately.

Faith-Based Travelers

Faith-based travel encompasses a wide range of activities (e.g., attending pilgrimages, participating in service projects, conducting missionary work, taking part in faith-based tours). Millions of faith-based travelers participate safely in some type of religious travel every year. In addition to being aware of basic country conditions that impact all travelers, US faith-based travelers should know that in some countries, conducting religious activities without proper registration, or at all, is a crime (see https://travel.state.gov/content/travel/en/international-travel/before-you-go/travelers-with-special-considerations/faith-based-travel.html).

LGBTQ+ Travelers

Lesbian, gay, bisexual, transgender, queer, and intersex (LGBTQ+) travelers face unique challenges when traveling abroad (see Sec. 2, Ch. 13, LGBTQ+ Travelers, and https://travel.state.gov/content/travel/en/international-travel/before-you-go/travelers-with-special-considerations/lgbti.html). Laws and attitudes in some countries might negatively affect safety and ease of travel for LGBTQ+ persons, and legal protections vary between countries. Many countries do not legally recognize same-sex marriage and >70 countries criminalize consensual same-sex sexual relations, sometimes with severe punishment. Travelers should review the Human Rights Report (www.state.gov/reports-bureau-of-democracy-human-rights-and-labor/country-reports-on-human-rights-practices) for further details before travel.

Travelers with Disabilities

Each country has its own laws regarding accessibility for, or discrimination against, people with physical, sensory, intellectual, or mental disabilities. Enforcement of accessibility and other laws relating to people with disabilities is inconsistent (see Sec. 3, Ch. 2, Travelers with Disabilities, and https://travel.state.gov/content/travel/en/international-travel/before-you-go/travelers-with-special-considerations/traveling-with-disabilties.html).

Travelers with Dual Nationality

Countries have different regulations for dual nationals; some do not permit dual nationality, while others infer dual nationality based on the birthplace of a traveler's parent. US citizens should check with the embassy of any country for relevant nationality laws before travel (see https://travel.state.gov/content/travel/en/international-travel/before-you-go/travelers-with-special-considerations/Dual-Nationality-Travelers.html).

CRIME, CRISES & TERRORISM

Crime

Crime is one of the most common threats to the safety of US citizens abroad. Travelers should research crime trends and patterns at their destination using the Overseas Security Advisory Council Country Security Reports (www.osac.gov), which provide baseline security information for every country around the world. Although strategies to avoid becoming a crime victim are, for the most part, the same everywhere, travel health providers should stress the following points with international travelers:

- Avoid accommodations on the ground floor or immediately next to the stairs, and lock all windows and doors.
- Do not wear expensive clothing or accessories.
- If confronted in a robbery, give up all valuables and do not resist attackers. Resistance can escalate to violence and result in injury or death.
- Limit travel at night; travel with a companion, and vary routine travel habits.
- Take only recommended, safe modes of local transportation.

Crime victims should contact the local authorities and the nearest US embassy, consulate, or consular agency for assistance. The Department of State can help replace stolen passports, contact family and friends, identify health care providers, explain the local criminal justice process, and connect victims of crime with available resources, including a list of local attorneys and medical providers. The Department of State does not have the legal authority to conduct a criminal investigation, prosecute crimes, or provide legal advice or counsel.

Crises

Whether traveling or living outside the United States, US citizens should prepare for potential crises (see https://travel.state.gov/content/travel/en/international-travel/before-you-go/crisis-abroad--be-ready.html). The Department of State is committed to assisting US citizens who become victims of crime, who need assistance during a crisis or a natural disaster, or who need consular services (e.g., replacing a lost or stolen passport, providing a loan to return to the United States). The Department of State also can attempt to locate missing US citizens abroad. Nevertheless, US citizens should proactively research resources available for the country or countries where they are traveling or residing, stay connected with the nearest US embassy or consulate, and create personal safety plans.

Terrorism

Despite being a worldwide threat and cause for concern, terrorist attacks have involved relatively few international travelers. Past attacks have included assassinations, bombings, hijackings, kidnappings, and suicide operations. Bombings are typically conducted with the use of improvised explosive devices (IEDs), but biological and chemical attacks remain a concern in some high-threat countries. Potential targets include business offices, clubs, hotels, houses of worship, public transportation systems, residential areas, restaurants, schools, shopping malls, high-profile sporting events, and other tourist destinations where people gather in large numbers (see https://travel.state.gov/content/travel/en/international-travel/emergencies/terrorism.html). To reduce their chances of becoming victims of terrorism, travelers should be cautious of unexpected packages; avoid wearing clothing that identifies them as a tourist (e.g., a T-shirt bearing the US flag or the logo of a favorite US-based sports team); look out for unattended bags or packages in public places and other crowded areas; and try to blend in with the locals. These strategies incorporate the same defensive alertness and good judgment that people should use to prevent becoming victims of crime. Awareness is key, and travelers should be knowledgeable of their surroundings and adopt protective measures.

4

BIBLIOGRAPHY

Federal Aviation Administration. Prohibitions, restrictions and notices. Available from: www.faa.gov/air_traffic/publications/us_restrictions.

US Department of State. Country information. Available from: https://travel.state.gov/content/travel/en/international-travel/International-Travel-Country-Information-Pages.html.

US Department of State. Country reports on human rights practices. Available from: www.state.gov/j/drl/rls/hrrpt.

US Department of State. Crisis abroad: be ready. Available from: https://travel.state.gov/content/travel/en/international-travel/before-you-go/crisis-abroad--be-ready.html.

US Department of State. Travel.State.Gov. Available from: https://travel.state.gov/content/travel.html.

INJURY & TRAUMA

Michael Ballesteros, Erin Sauber-Schatz

In 2017 and 2018, >1,500 US citizens died from nonnatural causes in foreign countries, excluding deaths in the wars in Iraq and Afghanistan. Motor vehicle crashes—not crime or terrorism—are the number 1 cause of nonnatural deaths among US citizens living, working, or traveling abroad (Figure 4-02). In 2017 and 2018, 431 Americans died in vehicle crashes in foreign countries (28% of nonnatural deaths). Another 291 were victims of homicide (19%), 266 drowned or died as a result of a boating incident (17%), and 218 died of suicide (14%).

Travel destinations might lack emergency care that approximates US standards; trauma centers capable of providing care for serious injuries are uncommon outside urban areas, if they exist at all. Make travelers aware of their increased risk for injuries when traveling or

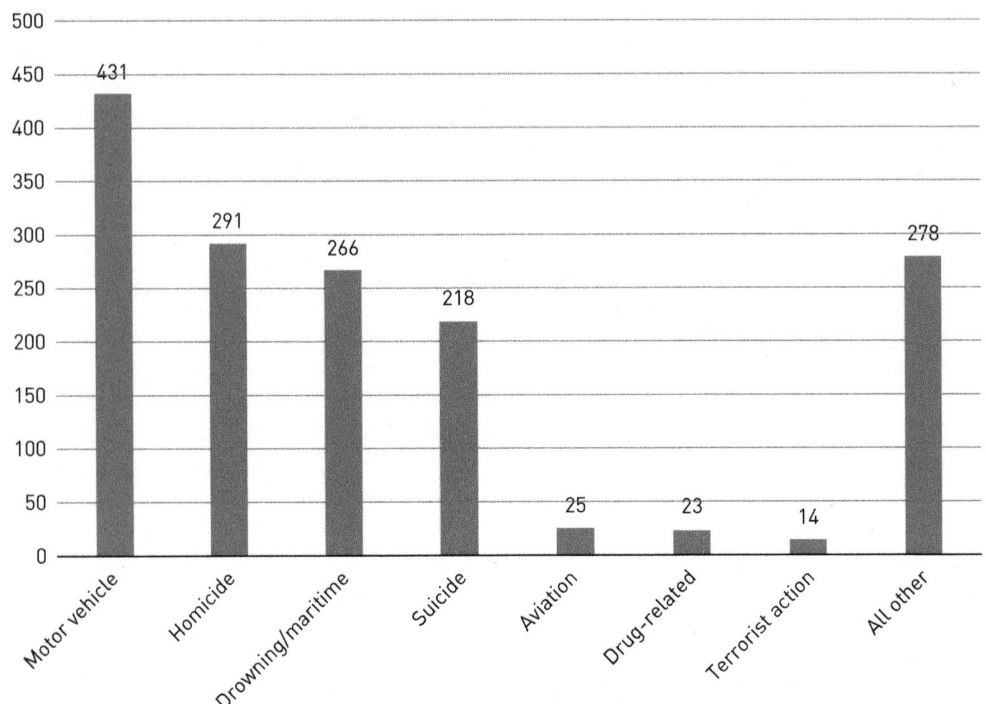

4

FIGURE 4-02 Leading causes of injury death for U.S. citizens in foreign countries, 2016 & 2017[1,2,3,4]

[1]Data from U.S. Department of State. Deaths of US citizens in foreign countries by nonnatural causes. Washington, DC: US Department of State. Available from: https://travel.state.gov/content/travel/en/international-travel/while-abroad/death-abroad1/death-statistics.html.

[2]Excludes deaths of US citizens fighting wars in Afghanistan or Iraq, and deaths not reported to the US embassy or consulate.

[3]Motor Vehicle includes deaths classified as "vehicle accidents," including the following subcategories: auto, bus, motorcycle, pedestrian, train, and other.

[4]All Other includes deaths classified as armed conflict, natural disaster, other accident, and undetermined/unknown.

residing internationally, particularly in low- and middle-income countries, and to take preventive steps to reduce the chances of serious injury.

ROAD TRAFFIC INJURIES

Globally, approximately 3,700 people are killed each day in motor vehicle crashes involving bicycles, buses, cars, motorcycles, trucks, and pedestrians. In 2017 and 2018, among the 431 US citizen road traffic deaths abroad, 62% were among drivers and occupants of passenger vehicles (e.g., cars, trucks, sport utility vehicles), and 21% were people on motorcycles. The countries with the most US citizen road traffic deaths were Mexico (n=126; 29%), Thailand (n=29; 7%), and Vietnam (n=17; 4%). For information on motor vehicle crashes and road safety, see Sec. 8, Ch. 5, Road & Traffic Safety.

VIOLENCE

Violence, including suicide and homicide, is a leading worldwide public health problem that affects US citizens traveling, working, or residing internationally. Each year, >1.6 million people lose their lives to violence, and only one-fifth of that total is due to armed conflict. Rates of violent deaths in low- and middle-income countries are 3 times those in higher-income countries, although variations exist within countries. For longer-term travelers, social isolation and substance abuse might increase the risk for depression and suicide; these risks might be amplified in areas with poverty and rigid gender roles. See Sec. 2, Ch. 12, Mental Health, for more detailed information on suicide prevention.

Mexico, the Philippines, Haiti, and Jamaica have the highest number of homicide deaths among US citizens abroad; Mexico accounts for 52% of all homicide deaths in US citizens living or traveling in foreign countries. Criminals might view US travelers as wealthy, naïve targets, inexperienced and unfamiliar with the culture, and less able to seek assistance once victimized. Traveling in high-poverty areas or regions of civil unrest, using alcohol or drugs, and visiting unfamiliar environments, particularly at night, increase the likelihood of a traveler becoming a victim of violence (see Sec. 4, Ch. 11, Safety & Security Overseas, for more information).

WATER & AQUATIC INJURIES

Drowning is often the leading cause of injury death to US citizens visiting countries where water recreation is a major activity. Although risk factors are not clearly defined, lack of familiarity with local water currents and conditions, inability to swim, and absence of lifeguards on duty likely contribute to drowning deaths. Rip currents can be especially dangerous. Diving into shallow water is a risk factor for head and spinal cord injuries, and young men are affected disproportionately. In some cases of aquatic injuries, alcohol or drug use is a factor.

Boating can be a hazard, especially if boaters are unfamiliar with the equipment they are using, do not know proper boating etiquette or rules for watercraft navigation, or are new to the water environment in a foreign country. Many boating fatalities result from inexperience or failure to wear a personal flotation device (lifejacket); boaters should have enough lifejackets on board for all passengers. Children and weak swimmers should always wear a lifejacket whenever boating. Advise travelers not to ride in boats operated by obviously inexperienced, uncertified, or intoxicated drivers.

Scuba diving is a frequent pursuit of travelers to coastal destinations. Researchers estimate the death rate among divers worldwide is ≈16 deaths per 100,000 divers per year. Travelers should either be experienced divers or dive with a reputable dive shop and instructors. See the Sec. 4, Ch. 4, Scuba Diving: Decompression Illness & Other Dive-Related Injuries, for a more detailed discussion about diving risks and preventive measures.

Travelers should not swim alone or in unfamiliar waters and should wear appropriately sized, US Coast Guard–approved lifejackets whenever participating in water recreation activities (e.g., sailboarding, water skiing, whitewater boating or rafting, or operating personal watercraft). If travel includes planned water activities, travelers should consider bringing their own lifejackets. Travelers also can increase the likelihood of survival in an emergency by improving their swimming skills, learning safe rescue techniques (e.g., use of poles or ropes as rescue aids so responders can avoid entering the water), and taking cardiopulmonary resuscitation (CPR) classes prior to traveling.

If overseas with children, an adult with swimming skills should be within arm's length when infants and toddlers are in or around pools and other bodies of water; even with older children and better swimmers, the supervising adult should focus on the child and not engage in any distracting activities. Travelers with children should remain vigilant, because swimming pools and ponds might not have fences around them to keep children safe. See the World Health Organization drowning resources (www.who.int/violence_injury_prevention/drowning/en) and the International Life Saving Federation (https://ilsf.org) for more information.

OTHER UNINTENTIONAL INJURIES

Adventure Activities

Adventure activities (e.g., kayaking, mountain biking and climbing, off-roading, whitewater rafting, skiing, skydiving, snowboarding) are popular among travelers. A lack of rapid emergency trauma response, inadequate trauma care in remote locations, and sudden, unexpected weather changes can compromise safety and hamper rescue efforts, delay care, and reduce survivability (see Sec. 9, Ch. 11, Adventure Travel). For recreational activities with a risk for falling, encourage travelers to use a helmet and to bring their own from home if helmets are unlikely to be available at the destination.

Aircraft Crashes

In 2017 and 2018, 25 US citizens abroad died in aircraft crashes. Travel by local, lightweight

BOX 4-11 Additional travel preparation tips for mitigating injury & trauma: a checklist for travelers

- ☐ Purchase special travel health and medical evacuation insurance if destinations include countries where access to good medical care might not be available (see Sec. 6, Ch. 1, Travel Insurance, Travel Health Insurance & Medical Evacuation Insurance).
- ☐ Learn basic first aid and CPR before traveling internationally with another person.
- ☐ Bring a travel health kit, customized to anticipated itinerary and activities.
- ☐ Review US Department of State travel advisories and alerts (www.travel.state.gov/destination) and check the US embassy or consulate (www.usembassy.gov) for country-specific personal security risks and safety tips.
- ☐ Enroll in the US Department of State's Smart Traveler Enrollment Program (https://step.state.gov/step). Enrolled travelers receive emails about safety conditions at their destination and direct embassy contact in case of natural disasters and man-made emergencies (e.g., political unrest, rioting, terrorist activity).

aircraft can be risky in many countries. Travel on unscheduled flights, in small aircraft, at night, in inclement weather, and with inexperienced pilots carries the greatest risks. Travelers should avoid using local, unscheduled, small aircraft, and refrain from flying in bad weather and at night, if possible. If available, travelers should choose larger aircraft (>30 seats), because these are more likely to have undergone stricter and more regular safety inspections. Larger aircraft also provide more protection in a crash.

Carbon Monoxide Poisoning

Carbon monoxide (CO) inhalation, poisoning, and death can occur during fires, but also can result from exposure to improperly vented heating devices. Travelers might want to bring a personal CO detector that can sound an alert in the presence of this lethal gas. Engine exhaust is a dangerous, unanticipated source of CO poisoning; remind travelers to avoid diving and swimming off the back of boats where exhaust fumes typically discharge.

Fires

In developing countries where building codes are not enforced or do not exist, fires represent a risk to traveler health and safety. Many locations have no smoke alarms or access to emergency services, and the fire department's focus is on putting out fires rather than on fire prevention or victim rescue.

To prevent fire-related injuries, travelers should select accommodations no higher than the 6th floor (fire ladders generally cannot reach higher than the 6th floor) and confirm that hotels have smoke alarms and, preferably, sprinkler systems. Suggest to travelers that they might want to bring their own smoke alarms with them, and that they should always identify ≥2 escape routes from buildings. Crawling low under smoke and covering one's mouth with a wet cloth are helpful for escaping a fire. Families should agree on a meeting place outside the building in case of a fire. The National Fire Protection Association has additional guidance (Hotel & Motel Safety) that could be useful internationally (see www.nfpa.org/-/media/Files/Public-Education/Resources/Safety-tip-sheets/HotelMotelSafety.ashx).

TRAVEL PREPARATION TIPS

When planning or arranging for a trip outside the United States, health care providers, vendors of travel services, and travelers themselves should consider taking the additional actions listed in Box 4-11.

BIBLIOGRAPHY

Balaban V, Sleet DA. Pediatric travel injuries: risk, prevention, and management. In: Kamat DM, Fischer PR, editors. American Academy of Pediatrics textbook of global child health, 2nd edition. Elk Grove Village (IL): American Academy of Pediatrics; 2015:315–38.

Cortés LM, Hargarten SW, Hennes HM. Recommendations for water safety and drowning prevention for travelers. J Travel Med. 2006;13(1):21–34.

Denny SA, Quan L, Gilchrist J, McCallin T, Shenoi R, Yusuf S, et al. Prevention of drowning. Pediatrics. 2019;143(5):e20190850.

Guse CE, Cortes LM, Hargarten SW, Hennes HM. Fatal injuries of US citizens abroad. J Travel Med. 2007;14(5):279–87.

Krug EG, Mercy JA, Dahlberg LL, Zwi AB. The world report on violence and health. Lancet. 2002;360(9339):1083–8.

McInnes RJ, Williamson LM, Morrison A. Unintentional injury during foreign travel: a review. J Travel Med. 2002;9:297–307.

US Department of State. Traveler's checklist. Available from: https://travel.state.gov/content/travel/en/international-travel/before-you-go/travelers-checklist.html.

Vann RD, Lang MA, editors. Recreational diving fatalities. Proceedings of the Divers Alert Network 2010 April 8–10 workshop. Durham (NC): Divers Alert Network; 2011.

World Health Organization. Global health estimates 2016: deaths by cause, age, sex, by country and by region, 2000–2016. Geneva: The Organization; 2018.

World Health Organization. Global report on drowning: preventing a leading killer. Geneva: The Organization; 2014. Available from: www.who.int/violence_injury_prevention/global_report_drowning/en.

4

DEATH DURING TRAVEL

Francisco Alvarado-Ramy, Kendra Stauffer

Death of a friend, relative, or coworker can be immensely distressing. The situation is aggravated when the death occurs abroad, where grieving individuals might be unfamiliar with local laws, language, culture, and processes for investigation and release of the body. Whether dealing with the death locally or from their home country, next of kin could face large, unanticipated costs and labor-intensive administrative requirements.

Depending on the circumstances surrounding the death, some countries require an autopsy. For travel companions of the deceased, in addition to friends and relatives, sources of support might include the US consulate or embassy, a travel insurance provider (particularly if coverage included repatriation of remains), the airline, a tour operator, faith-based and aid organizations, or the deceased person's employer. Official identification of the body will likely be needed, and official documents likely will need to be issued by the consular office. A body can be identified by witness statements of those who knew the person well, by analyzing DNA samples, by checking fingerprints, by reviewing dental radiographs, or by inspecting surgical implants.

DEATH ONBOARD A CONVEYANCE

Federal regulations require that all deaths aboard commercial flights and ships destined for the United States be reported to the Centers for Disease Control and Prevention (CDC). For details, see Guidance for Airlines on Reporting Onboard Deaths or Illnesses to CDC (www.cdc.gov/quarantine/air/reporting-deaths-illness/guidance-reporting-onboard-deaths-illnesses.html) and Guidance for Cruise Ships: How to Report Onboard Death or Illness to CDC (www.cdc.gov/quarantine/cruise/reporting-deaths-illness/guidance-how-report-onboard-death-illness.html).

Commercial Aircraft

The Federal Aviation Administration requires that flight attendants receive training in cardiopulmonary resuscitation (CPR) and in proper use of an automated external defibrillator (AED) at least once every 2 years. Under US laws, Good Samaritan laws offer protections for actions brought in a federal or state court that result from acts or omissions when people assist in a medical emergency during flight, unless there is gross negligence or willful misconduct.

If CPR is performed in an aircraft cabin for ≥30 minutes with no signs of life, and no shocks advised by an AED, the person can be presumed dead and resuscitation efforts halted. Airlines can choose to specify additional criteria for presuming death, depending on the availability of ground-to-air medical consultation services or a physician aboard the flight (see Sec. 8, Ch. 2, . . . *perspectives*: Responding to Medical Emergencies when Flying). In these cases, the body should be secured and covered for the remainder of the flight.

Cruise Ships

If death occurs on a cruise ship, the crew are usually able to provide logistical support to repatriate the body. Cruise ships are equipped with morgues and body bags and are staffed with health care professionals capable of providing clinical care. Any death involving an accident, violence, or foul play will require more extended and complicated processes. US consular officials will be able to provide general guidance and legal aid resource options (see https://travel.state.gov/content/travel/en/legal/travel-legal-considerations/internl-judicial-asst/Retaining-Foreign-Attorney.html). Some travel insurance products cover legal services abroad. Travelers should be aware of exclusions and limitations of travel insurance products prior to purchasing.

OBTAINING US DEPARTMENT OF STATE ASSISTANCE

When a US citizen dies outside the United States, the deceased person's next of kin or legal representative should notify US consular officials at the Department of State. Consular personnel are available 24 hours a day, 7 days a week, to assist US citizens during overseas emergencies.

If the next of kin or legal representative is in the foreign country with the deceased US citizen, that person should contact the nearest US embassy or consulate for assistance. Contact information for US embassies and consulates overseas can be found at the Department of State website (www.usembassy.gov).

Family members, domestic partners, or legal representatives who are in a different country from the deceased should call the Department of State's Office of Overseas Citizens Services in Washington, DC, from 8 a.m. to 5 p.m. Eastern time, Monday through Friday, at 888-407-4747 (toll-free) or 202-501-4444. For emergency assistance after working hours or on weekends and holidays, call the Department of State switchboard at 202-647-4000 and ask to speak with the Overseas Citizens Services duty officer. In addition, the US embassy closest to or in the country where the US citizen died can provide support (www.usembassy.gov).

The Department of State has no funds to assist in the return of remains of US citizens who die abroad. US consular officers assist the next of kin by conveying instructions to the appropriate offices within the foreign country and providing information to the family on how to send the necessary private funds to cover the costs of preparing and repatriating the deceased person's remains. Upon issuance of a local (foreign) death certificate, the nearest US embassy or consulate can prepare a consular report of the death of an American abroad. Copies of that report are provided to the next of kin or legal representative and can be used in US courts to settle estate matters. If the deceased person has no next of kin or legal representative in-country, a consular officer will act as a provisional conservator of the deceased person's personal effects.

IMPORTING HUMAN REMAINS FOR BURIAL, ENTOMBMENT, OR CREMATION

CDC regulates the importation of human remains and provides guidance for their importation. The requirements are more stringent if the person died from a disease classified as quarantinable in the United States (www.cdc.gov/quarantine/human-remains.html).

Except for cremated remains, human remains intended for burial, entombment, or cremation after entry into the United States must be accompanied by a death certificate stating the cause of death. A death certificate is an official government document that certifies that a death has occurred and provides identifying information about the deceased, including (at a minimum) name, age, and sex. The document must also certify the time, place, and cause of death, if known. If the official government document is not written in English, it must be accompanied by an English language translation of the official government document, the authenticity of which must be attested to by a person licensed to perform acts in legal affairs in the country where the death occurred.

In lieu of a death certificate, a copy of the Consular Mortuary Certificate and the Affidavit of Foreign Funeral Director and Transit Permit together constitute acceptable identification of human remains. If a death certificate is not available in time for returning the remains, the US embassy or consulate should provide a Consular Mortuary Certificate stating whether the person died from a disease classified as quarantinable in the United States (www.cdc.gov/quarantine/aboutlawsregulationsquarantineisolation.html). A person transporting human remains must also meet requirements of the country of origin, air carrier, the Transportation Security Administration, and Customs and Border Protection.

EXPORTING HUMAN REMAINS

CDC does not regulate the exportation of human remains outside the United States, although other state and local regulations might apply. The United States Postal Service is the only courier legally allowed to ship cremated remains. Exporters of human remains and travelers taking human remains out of the United States should be aware that they must meet the importation requirements of the destination country. Information regarding these requirements can be obtained from the foreign embassy or consulate (see https://travel.state.gov/content/travel/en/consularnotification/ConsularNotificationandAccess.html). Air carriers also might have their own requirements, of which individuals transporting remains outside of the United States should be aware (see www.tsa.gov/travel/security-screening/whatcanibring/items/cremated-remains).

4

BIBLIOGRAPHY

Bureau of Consular Affairs, US State Department. Death abroad. Available from: https://travel.state.gov/content/passports/en/abroad/events-and-records/death.html.

Bureau of Consular Affairs, US State Department. Return of remains of deceased US citizens. Available from: https://travel.state.gov/content/travel/en/international-travel/while-abroad/death-abroad1/return-of-remains-of-deceased-us-citizen.html.

Centers for Disease Control and Prevention. Importation of human remains into the United States for burial, entombment, or cremation. Available from: www.cdc.gov/importation/human-remains.html.

Centers for Disease Control and Prevention. Importation of human remains final rule. Specific laws and regulations governing the control of communicable diseases. Available from: www.cdc.gov/importation/laws-and-regulations/human-remains-importation-requirements.html.

Centers for Disease Control and Prevention. Quarantine station contact list, map, and fact sheets. Available from: www.cdc.gov/quarantine/quarantinestationcontactlistfull.html

Connolly R, Prendiville R, Cusack D, Flaherty G. Repatriation of human remains following death in international travelers. J Travel Med. 2017;24(2):1–6.

International Air Transport Association. Death on board; 2018. Available from: www.iata.org/contentassets/ccbdc54681c24574bebf2db2b18197a5/death-on-board-guidelines.pdf.

National Funeral Directors Association. International shipping regulations. Available from: www.nfda.org/resources/operations-management/shipping-remains/international-shipping-regulations.

US Customs and Border Protection. What is the process for bringing bodies in coffins/ashes in urns into the United States? Available from: https://help.cbp.gov/s/article/Article-237?language=en_US.

5

Travel-Associated Infections & Diseases

CDC Yellow Book 2024. Jeffrey Nemhauser, Oxford University Press. © Oxford University Press 2023.
DOI: 10.1093/oso/9780197570944.003.0005

PART 1: BACTERIAL

5

Table 5-01 Vaccine-Preventable Diseases: Bacterial

VACCINE	TRADE NAME (MANUFACTURER)	DESCRIPTION[1] & ROUTE OF ADMINISTRATION	AGE LIMITS	DOSES	PRESCRIBING & BOOSTER INFORMATION, RECOMMENDATIONS & RESTRICTIONS
Anthrax	BioThrax (Emergent BioSolutions)	Cell-free filtrates of avirulent *Bacillus anthracis*, IM or SC (SC preferred)	18–65 y	3	www.fda.gov/vaccines-blood-biologics/vaccines/biothrax www.cdc.gov/vaccines/hcp/acip-recs/vacc-specific/anthrax.html
Cholera	VAXCHORA (Emergent BioSolutions)	Live-attenuated, PO	50 mL 2 to <6 y	1	www.fda.gov/vaccines-blood-biologics/vaccines/vaxchora www.cdc.gov/vaccines/hcp/acip-recs/vacc-specific/cholera.html
			100 mL ≥6–64 y	1	
Diphtheria	For all diphtheria vaccines licensed for use in the United States, see: www.fda.gov/vaccines-blood-biologics/vaccines/vaccines-licensed-use-united-states				
	Adacel (TDaP) (Sanofi Pasteur)	Tetanus, diphtheria toxoids + acellular pertussis antigens, IM	10–64 y	1	www.fda.gov/vaccines-blood-biologics/vaccines/adacel www.cdc.gov/vaccines/hcp/acip-recs/vacc-specific/dtap.html
	BOOSTRIX (TDaP) (GlaxoSmithKline)	Tetanus, diphtheria toxoids + pertussis antigens, IM	≥10 y	1	www.fda.gov/vaccines-blood-biologics/vaccines/boostrix www.cdc.gov/vaccines/hcp/acip-recs/vacc-specific/dtap.html
	TDVAX (MassBiologics)	Tetanus, diphtheria toxoids, IM	≥7 y	3 (primary series) + 1 (booster)	www.fda.gov/vaccines-blood-biologics/vaccines/tdvax www.cdc.gov/vaccines/hcp/acip-recs/vacc-specific/dtap.html
	TENIVAC (Td) (Sanofi Pasteur)	Tetanus, diphtheria toxoids, IM	≥7 y	3 (primary series) + 1 (booster)	www.fda.gov/vaccines-blood-biologics/vaccines/tenivac www.cdc.gov/vaccines/hcp/acip-recs/vacc-specific/dtap.html

Meningococcal (Quadrivalent, ACWY)	Menactra (Sanofi Pasteur)	Conjugate, IM	9–23 mo	2	www.fda.gov/vaccines-blood-biologics/vaccines/menactra www.cdc.gov/vaccines/hcp/acip-recs/vacc-specific/mening.html
			≥2 y	1	
	MenQuadfi (Sanofi Pasteur)	Conjugate, IM	≥2 y	1	www.fda.gov/vaccines-blood-biologics/menquadfi www.cdc.gov/vaccines/hcp/acip-recs/vacc-specific/mening.html
	MENVEO (GlaxoSmithKline)	Conjugate, IM	2 mo	4	www.fda.gov/vaccines-blood-biologics/vaccines/menveo www.cdc.gov/vaccines/hcp/acip-recs/vacc-specific/mening.html
			3–6 mo	Depends on age at 1st vaccination	
			7–23 mo	2	
			≥2 y	1	
Meningococcal (Monovalent, B)	BEXSERO (GlaxoSmithKline)	Recombinant, IM	10–25 y	2	www.fda.gov/vaccines-blood-biologics/vaccines/bexsero www.cdc.gov/vaccines/hcp/acip-recs/vacc-specific/mening.html
	TRUMENBA (Pfizer)	Recombinant, IM	10–25 y	2	www.fda.gov/vaccines-blood-biologics/vaccines/trumenba www.cdc.gov/vaccines/hcp/acip-recs/vacc-specific/mening.html
Pertussis	For all pertussis vaccines licensed for use in the United States, see: www.fda.gov/vaccines-blood-biologics/vaccines/vaccines-licensed-use-united-states				
	Adacel (TDaP) (Sanofi Pasteur)	Tetanus, diphtheria toxoids + acellular pertussis antigens, IM	10–64 y	1	www.fda.gov/vaccines-blood-biologics/vaccines/adacel www.cdc.gov/vaccines/hcp/acip-recs/vacc-specific/dtap.html
	BOOSTRIX (TDaP) (GlaxoSmithKline)	Tetanus, diphtheria toxoids + pertussis antigens, IM	≥10 y	1	www.fda.gov/vaccines-blood-biologics/vaccines/boostrix www.cdc.gov/vaccines/hcp/acip-recs/vacc-specific/dtap.html

(*continued*)

Table 5-01 Vaccine-Preventable Diseases: Bacterial (continued)

VACCINE	TRADE NAME (MANUFACTURER)	DESCRIPTION[1] & ROUTE OF ADMINISTRATION	AGE LIMITS	DOSES	PRESCRIBING & BOOSTER INFORMATION, RECOMMENDATIONS & RESTRICTIONS
Plague	Discontinued in 1999; newer vaccines in development, none commercially available or FDA-approved				
Pneumococcal	PREVNAR 13 (Wyeth)	Conjugate, IM	6 wk to <6 y	4	www.fda.gov/vaccines-blood-biologics/vaccines/prevnar-13 www.cdc.gov/vaccines/hcp/acip-recs/vacc-specific/pneumo.html
			6 y to <18 y	1	
	VAXNEUVANCE (Merck)	Conjugate, IM	≥18 y	1	www.fda.gov/vaccines-blood-biologics/vaccines/vaxneuvance www.cdc.gov/vaccines/hcp/acip-recs/vacc-specific/pneumo.html
	PREVNAR 20 (Wyeth)	Conjugate, IM	≥18 y	1	www.fda.gov/vaccines-blood-biologics/vaccines/prevnar-20 www.cdc.gov/vaccines/hcp/acip-recs/vacc-specific/pneumo.html
	PNEUMOVAX 23 (Merck)	Polysaccharide, IM or SC	≥50 y	1	www.fda.gov/vaccines-blood-biologics/vaccines/pneumovax-23-pneumococcal-vaccine-polyvalent www.cdc.gov/vaccines/hcp/acip-recs/vacc-specific/pneumo.html
Q Fever	Available in Australia only				
Tetanus	For all tetanus vaccines licensed for use in the United States, see: www.fda.gov/vaccines-blood-biologics/vaccines/vaccines-licensed-use-united-states				
	Adacel (TDaP) (Sanofi Pasteur)	Tetanus, diphtheria toxoids + acellular pertussis antigens, IM	10–64 y	1	www.fda.gov/vaccines-blood-biologics/vaccines/adacel www.cdc.gov/vaccines/hcp/acip-recs/vacc-specific/dtap.html
	BOOSTRIX (TDaP) (GlaxoSmithKline)	Tetanus, diphtheria toxoids + pertussis antigens, IM	≥10 y	1	www.fda.gov/vaccines-blood-biologics/vaccines/boostrix www.cdc.gov/vaccines/hcp/acip-recs/vacc-specific/dtap.html

	TDVAX (MassBiologics)	Tetanus, diphtheria toxoids, IM	≥7 y	3 (primary series) + 1 (booster)	www.fda.gov/vaccines-blood-biologics/vaccines/tdvax www.cdc.gov/vaccines/hcp/acip-recs/vacc-specific/dtap.html
	TENIVAC (Td) (Sanofi Pasteur)	Tetanus, diphtheria toxoids, IM	≥7 y	3 (primary series) + 1 (booster)	www.fda.gov/vaccines-blood-biologics/vaccines/tenivac www.cdc.gov/vaccines/hcp/acip-recs/vacc-specific/dtap.html
Tuberculosis	bacillus Calmette-Guérin (BCG) is no longer commercially available in the United States				
Typhoid fever	Typhim Vi (Sanofi Pasteur)	Polysaccharide, IM	≥2 y	1	www.fda.gov/vaccines-blood-biologics/vaccines/typhim-vi www.cdc.gov/vaccines/hcp/acip-recs/vacc-specific/typhoid.html
	Vivotif (Emergent BioSolutions)	Live-attenuated, PO	≥6 y	4	https://vivotif.com/downloads/Vivotif_Prescribing_Information_2017.pdf www.cdc.gov/vaccines/hcp/acip-recs/vacc-specific/typhoid.html

Abbreviations: IM, intramuscular; PO, orally; SC, subcutaneously
[1]For an overview and description of vaccine types, see: www.hhs.gov/immunization/basics/types/index.html

ANTHRAX

Kate Hendricks, Antonio Vieira, Rita Traxler, Chung Marston

5

INFECTIOUS AGENT: *Bacillus anthracis*	
ENDEMICITY	Enzootic and endemic to agricultural regions in sub-Saharan Africa, Central and South America, central and southwestern Asia, and southern and eastern Europe Enzootic but not endemic to the United States, Canada, and western Europe
TRAVELER CATEGORIES AT GREATEST RISK FOR EXPOSURE & INFECTION	Adventure tourists Immigrants and refugees Military personnel Scientists conducting anthrax fieldwork
PREVENTION METHODS	In enzootic areas, avoid direct or indirect contact with animals and animal products, trophies, souvenirs Comply with regulations and restrictions against importing prohibited animal products, trophies, and souvenirs Scientists conducting anthrax fieldwork should obtain preexposure vaccination and use personal protective equipment
DIAGNOSTIC SUPPORT	A clinical laboratory certified in high complexity testing; state health department; CDC's Bacterial Special Pathogens Branch (bspb@cdc.gov); or CDC Emergency Operations Center (770-488-7100)

INFECTIOUS AGENT

Anthrax is caused by aerobic, gram-positive, encapsulated, spore-forming, nonmotile, nonhemolytic, rod-shaped bacterium, *Bacillus anthracis*.

TRANSMISSION

Most human infections with *B. anthracis* result from handling *B. anthracis*–infected animals or their carcasses, meat, hides, or wool. Products derived from infected animals (e.g., drumheads, wool clothing) are additional documented sources of human infection.

Anthrax infection can occur via cutaneous, ingestion, injection, and inhalation routes. Spores introduced through the skin can result in cutaneous anthrax; breaks in the skin increase susceptibility. Eating meat from infected animals can result in ingestion (also called gastrointestinal) anthrax. Since 2000, injection transmission has been reported in cases of *B. anthracis* soft-tissue infections among intravenous heroin users in northern Europe. Aerosolized spores from contaminated hides or wool can cause inhalation anthrax. Anthrax in humans generally is not considered contagious; person-to-person transmission of cutaneous anthrax has been reported only rarely and only in instances of extremely close contact with an infected person (e.g., breastfeeding, dressing a wound, direct skin contact with the blood from a patient with anthrax).

EPIDEMIOLOGY

Anthrax is a zoonotic disease primarily affecting ruminant herbivores (e.g., antelope, cattle, deer, goats, sheep) that become infected by ingesting vegetation, soil, or water that has been contaminated with *B. anthracis* spores; humans are generally incidental hosts. Anthrax is most common in agricultural regions in sub-Saharan Africa, Central and South America, central and southwestern Asia, and southern and eastern Europe. Although outbreaks still occur in livestock and wild herbivores in Canada, the United States, and western Europe, human anthrax in these areas is now rare.

Worldwide, the most reported form of anthrax in humans is cutaneous anthrax (95%–99%). Anthrax can occur after playing or handling drums made from contaminated goatskins. Although the risk of acquiring anthrax from drums imported from anthrax-endemic countries appears low, life-threatening or fatal disease is possible. Cases of cutaneous (n=4), ingestion (n=1), and inhalation (n=3) anthrax have been reported in people who have handled, played, or made such drums; bystanders to such indoor activities have rarely been infected.

Outbreaks of cutaneous and ingestion anthrax have been associated with handling infected animals and butchering and eating meat from those animals. Most of these outbreaks have occurred in endemic areas in Africa and Asia. A handful of cutaneous cases have been reported in travelers with direct or indirect contact with animals or their byproducts. One instance occurred in a tourist who traveled to Namibia, Botswana, and South Africa in 2006; another, in a traveler to Turkey in 2018. A third case happened in a scientist who was conducting anthrax fieldwork in Namibia, also in 2018.

Severe soft-tissue infections, including cases complicated by sepsis and systemic infection, are suspected to be due to recreational use of heroin contaminated with *B. anthracis* spores. No associated cases have been identified in people who have not injected heroin.

Inhalation exposure was historically associated with the industrial processing of hides or wool. More recently, bioterrorist activities directed toward the American public were implicated as a source of inhalation exposure. Occasional anthrax cases have occurred in the United States and elsewhere, in which the exposure source remains unidentified.

Travelers are at greatest risk for infection in areas where the disease is more prevalent. Destination categories that increase risk for infection include safari areas where direct contact with animals or carcasses might occur; regions with limited meat inspections and processing capacity; and areas where travelers are exposed to livestock byproducts (e.g., souvenirs). Immigrants and refugees in areas of low socioeconomic development and limited food availability also might be at increased risk of contracting anthrax due to lack of proper inspection of meat and animal products.

CLINICAL PRESENTATION

Anthrax has 4 main clinical presentations—cutaneous, ingestion, injection, and inhalation. Anthrax meningitis can complicate any of the 4 main clinical presentations and can occur with no obvious portal of entry, in which case it is called primary anthrax meningitis.

Cutaneous Anthrax

Cutaneous anthrax usually develops 1–7 days after exposure, but incubation periods up to 17 days have been reported. Before antimicrobial therapy became available, almost a quarter of patients with cutaneous anthrax died. The case-fatality ratio is <2% with antimicrobial therapy.

Localized itching, followed by development of a painless papule, heralds cutaneous anthrax. The papule then turns into a vesicle that enlarges and ulcerates, ultimately becoming a depressed black eschar 7–10 days after the appearance of the initial lesion. Edema around lesions is characteristic, sometimes with secondary vesicles, hyperemia, and regional lymphadenopathy. Head, neck, forearms, and hands are the most common sites affected. Patients might have malaise and headache; about one-third are febrile.

Ingestion Anthrax

Ingestion anthrax usually develops 1–7 days after eating contaminated meat; incubation periods up to 16 days have been reported, however. Left untreated, more than half of cases will die; with treatment, the case-fatality ratio decreases slightly, to <40%. Ingestion anthrax has 2 main types: oropharyngeal and intestinal. Patients with either form usually have fever and chills.

Oropharyngeal anthrax is characterized by severe sore throat, difficulty swallowing, swelling of the neck, and regional lymphadenopathy; airway compromise and death can occur. Nausea, vomiting, and diarrhea, which might be bloody, are more typical of intestinal anthrax; marked ascites or coagulopathy also can develop. Later symptoms can include shortness of breath and altered mental status, with shock and death occurring 2–5 days after disease onset.

Injection Anthrax

Anthrax in injection drug users usually develops within 1–4 days of exposure; death occurs in more than a quarter of confirmed cases. Case-patients present with severe soft-tissue infection manifested by swelling, erythema, and excessive bruising at the injection site; pain might be less than anticipated for the degree of swelling. Most patients become septic.

Inhalation Anthrax

Inhalation anthrax usually develops within a week after exposure, but the incubation period could be prolonged, up to 2 months. Before 2001, fatality ratios for inhalation anthrax were 90%; since then, ratios have fallen to 45% with improved treatment. During the first few days of illness (the prodromal period), most patients exhibit fever, chills, and fatigue. These symptoms can be accompanied by cough, shortness of breath, chest pain, and nausea or vomiting, making inhalation anthrax difficult to distinguish from influenza, coronavirus disease 2019 (COVID-19), or community-acquired pneumonia.

5

Over the next day or so, shortness of breath, cough, and chest pain become more common, and nonthoracic complaints (e.g., nausea, vomiting, altered mental status, diaphoresis, headache) develop in a third or more of patients. Upper respiratory tract symptoms occur in only a quarter of patients, and myalgias are rare. Altered mental status or shortness of breath generally brings patients to the attention of the medical establishment and heralds the fulminant phase of illness.

Anthrax Meningitis

Anthrax meningitis can develop from hematogenous spread of any of the clinical forms of anthrax, or it can occur alone; half of all reported cases are sequelae of cutaneous anthrax. The condition should be suspected in patients with anthrax who have severe headache, altered mental status (including confusion), meningeal signs, or neurologic deficits of any kind. Intracranial bleeding occurs in about two-thirds of patients with anthrax meningitis. Most cases of anthrax meningitis are fatal.

DIAGNOSIS

Include anthrax in the differential diagnosis of travelers returning with unexplained fevers or new skin lesions. Ask about recent travel to anthrax-endemic areas (www.cdc.gov/anthrax/specificgroups/travelers.html) and inquire about activities, such as direct contact with animals and animal products, drumming, and souvenir purchases, including animal-hide drums, leather, and hides.

Any of several methods can be used to make a laboratory diagnosis of anthrax infection: bacterial culture with isolation of *B. anthracis*; detection of bacterial DNA, antigens, or toxins; or detection of a host immune response to *B. anthracis*. Although lethal toxin can be detected in a single acute-phase serum, detection of a host immune response requires paired acute- and convalescent-phase serum samples.

In the United States, anthrax is a nationally notifiable disease. Laboratory Response Network reference laboratories can perform confirmatory testing (e.g., isolate identification). Laboratories at the Centers for Disease Control and Prevention (CDC) can perform isolate identification and conduct other complex tests (e.g., mass spectrometry for toxin, quantitative serology, antigen detection in tissues). Internationally, relevant national reference laboratories should perform testing.

For diagnostic support and specimen submission guidance, contact the state, local, territorial, or tribal public health department. Public health departments should urgently notify CDC of any suspected anthrax cases through the CDC Emergency Operations Center (770-488-7100). CDC's Bacterial Special Pathogens Branch can coordinate testing needs in conjunction with the public health department and other CDC programs; specimen collection and submission guidelines and algorithms for laboratory diagnosis are available at www.cdc.gov/anthrax/lab-testing/index.html. Collect specimens for culture before initiating antimicrobial therapy.

Diagnostic procedures for inhalation anthrax include thoracic imaging studies to detect a widened mediastinum or pleural effusion. Drainage of pleural effusions can be useful for diagnosis and can increase survival because it removes a nidus for toxin. Regardless of route of infection, patients with systemic anthrax should have a diagnostic evaluation to rule out meningitis.

TREATMENT

Treat naturally occurring localized or uncomplicated cutaneous anthrax with 7–10 days of a single oral antibiotic. First-line agents include ciprofloxacin (or levofloxacin or moxifloxacin) or doxycycline; clindamycin is an alternative, as is penicillin if the bacterial isolate is penicillin-susceptible. Pending results of confirmatory testing, treat systemic anthrax with combination broad-spectrum intravenous antimicrobial drugs and one of the anthrax antitoxins approved for use by the US Food and Drug Administration (www.phe.gov/about/barda/anthrax/Pages/antitoxins.aspx); delays in initiating therapy can be fatal. Online recommendations for the treatment and prevention of anthrax are available for the following groups:

- Adults: https://wwwnc.cdc.gov/eid/article/20/2/13-0687_article
- People who are pregnant, postpartum, and lactating: https://wwwnc.cdc.gov/eid/article/20/2/13-0611_article
- Children: http://pediatrics.aappublications.org/content/133/5/e1411

PREVENTION

In 2019, CDC published updated recommendations from the Advisory Committee on Immunization Practices (ACIP) for preexposure use of anthrax vaccine and for postexposure management of previously unvaccinated people (www.cdc.gov/mmwr/volumes/68/rr/rr6804a1.htm). Vaccination against anthrax is not recommended for most travelers, except for researchers working in anthrax-endemic areas who could be at high risk for direct contact with animals and animal products. Vaccine is also recommended to members of the military traveling to these areas.

To prevent anthrax exposures while visiting anthrax-endemic countries, travelers should avoid direct and indirect contact with animal carcasses and should not eat meat from animals butchered after having been found dead or ill. Cooking contaminated meats does not eliminate the risk of contracting anthrax. Thus, travelers should determine the provenance of the meat they are being served in rural areas, and ask for meat that has been inspected by health authorities.

No tests are available to determine if animal byproducts are free from *B. anthracis* spore contamination; travelers should be aware of regulations concerning and restrictions against the importation of prohibited animal products, trophies, and souvenirs. Additional information regarding import regulations can be found in Sec. 4, Ch. 9, Bringing Animals & Animal Products into the United States; at the US Department of Agriculture, Animal and Plant Health Inspection Service website, Import-Export Regulations (www.aphis.usda.gov/aphis/ourfocus/importexport); and the World Organization for Animal Health website, Terrestrial Animal Health Code, Anthrax (www.oie.int/en/disease/anthrax).

CDC website: www.cdc.gov/anthrax

BIBLIOGRAPHY

Beatty ME, Ashford DA, Griffin PM, Tauxe RV, Sobel J. Gastrointestinal anthrax. Arch Int Med. 2003;163:2527–31.

Bower WA, Schiffer J, Atmar RL, Keitel WA, Friedlander AM, Liu L, et al.; ACIP Anthrax Vaccine Work Group. Use of anthrax vaccine in the United States: recommendations of the Advisory Committee on Immunization Practices, 2019. MMWR Recomm Rep. 2019;68(4):1–14.

Bradley JS, Peacock G, Krug S, et al. Pediatric anthrax clinical management. Pediatrics. 2014;133(5):e1411–36.

Centers for Disease Control and Prevention. Gastrointestinal anthrax after an animal-hide drumming event—New Hampshire and Massachusetts, 2009. MMWR Morb Mortal Wkly Rep. 2010;59(28):872–7.

Hendricks KA, Wright ME, Shadomy SV, Bradley JS, Morrow MG, Pavia AT, et al. Centers for Disease Control and Prevention expert panel meetings on prevention and treatment of anthrax in adults. Emerg Infect Dis. 2014;20(2):e130687.

Holty JEC, Bravata DM, Liu H, Olshen RA, McDonald KM, Owens DK. Systematic review: a century of inhalational anthrax cases from 1900 to 2005. Ann Intern Med. 2006;144:270–80.

Katharios-Lanwermeyer S, Holty JE, Person M, Sejvar J, Haberling D, Tubbs H, et al. Identifying meningitis during an anthrax mass casualty incident: systematic review of systemic anthrax since 1880. Clin Infect Dis. 2016;62(12):1537–45.

Meaney-Delman D, Zotti ME, Creanga AA, Misegades LK, Wako E, Treadwell TA, et al.; Workgroup on Anthrax in

Pregnant and Postpartum Women. Special considerations for prophylaxis for and treatment of anthrax in pregnant and postpartum women. Emerg Infect Dis. 2014;20(2):e130611.

National Anthrax Outbreak Control Team. An outbreak of anthrax among drug users in Scotland, December 2009 to December 2010. Health Protection Scotland, 2011. Available from: https://hpspubsrepo.blob.core.windows.net/hps-website/nss/2327/documents/1_anthrax-outbreak-report-2011-12.pdf.

Van den Enden E, Van Gompel A, Van Esbroeck M. Cutaneous anthrax, Belgian traveler. Emerg Infect Dis. 2006;12(3):523–5.

BARTONELLA INFECTIONS

Christina Nelson

5

BARTONELLA QUINTANA INFECTION

INFECTIOUS AGENT: *Bartonella quintana*	
ENDEMICITY	Worldwide, wherever human body lice are found
TRAVELER CATEGORIES AT GREATEST RISK FOR EXPOSURE & INFECTION	Humanitarian aid workers Immigrants and refugees in crowded conditions
PREVENTION METHODS	Bathe and launder clothes regularly Avoid overcrowding and sharing clothes or bedding
DIAGNOSTIC SUPPORT	A clinical laboratory certified in high complexity testing, or contact CDC's Division of Vector-Borne Diseases (970-221-6400)

CARRIÓN DISEASE

INFECTIOUS AGENT: *Bartonella bacilliformis*	
ENDEMICITY	South America, Andes Mountains at 1,000–3,000 m (≈3,300–9,800 ft) elevation
TRAVELER CATEGORIES AT GREATEST RISK FOR EXPOSURE & INFECTION	Adventure tourists
PREVENTION METHODS	Avoid insect bites
DIAGNOSTIC SUPPORT	A clinical laboratory certified in high complexity testing, or contact CDC's Division of Vector-Borne Diseases (970-221-6400)

CAT SCRATCH DISEASE

INFECTIOUS AGENT: *Bartonella henselae*	
ENDEMICITY	Worldwide, wherever cat fleas are found
TRAVELER CATEGORIES AT GREATEST RISK FOR EXPOSURE & INFECTION	Travelers who encounter cats
PREVENTION METHODS	Avoid kittens and stray cats Control fleas on felines
DIAGNOSTIC SUPPORT	A clinical laboratory certified in high complexity testing, or contact CDC's Division of Vector-Borne Diseases (970-221-6400)

INFECTIOUS AGENT

Several gram-negative bacteria in the genus *Bartonella* cause human disease through various transmission routes. Human illness primarily is caused by *B. quintana* (known historically as "trench fever"), *B. bacilliformis* (Carrión disease), and *B. henselae* (cat scratch disease [CSD]). A variety of *Bartonella* spp. can cause subacute, culture-negative endocarditis; other clinical syndromes (e.g., encephalitis, ocular disease, osteomyelitis) due to *Bartonella* spp. have been reported. Additional *Bartonella* spp. that cause human illness have been described recently.

TRANSMISSION

B. quintana is transmitted by the human body louse; *B. bacilliformis* is transmitted by infected phlebotomine sand flies of the genus *Lutzomyia*; and *B. henselae* is transmitted through scratches from domestic or feral cats, particularly kittens. Direct transmission of *B. henselae* to humans by the bite of infected cat fleas likely can occur but has not yet been proven.

EPIDEMIOLOGY

B. quintana and CSD infections occur worldwide. *B. quintana* infections typically occur in populations that lack access to proper hygiene, (e.g., refugees living in crowded conditions, people experiencing homelessness). Minimal data are reported on CSD among travelers, but in the United States, CSD is more common in children, in southern states, and during the months August–January.

Carrión disease has limited geographic distribution; transmission occurs in the Andes Mountains at 1,000–3,000 m (≈3,300–9,800 ft) elevation. Most cases are reported in Peru, but cases have also occurred in Bolivia, Chile, Colombia, and Ecuador. Short-term travelers to endemic areas are likely at low risk.

CLINICAL PRESENTATION

Bartonella quintana Infection

Symptoms of *B. quintana* infection include fever, headache, transient rash, and bone pain, mainly in the shins, neck, and back.

Carrión Disease

Carrión disease has 2 distinct phases: an acute phase (Oroya fever) characterized by fever, myalgia, headache, and anemia; and an eruptive phase (verruga peruana) characterized by red-to-purple nodular skin lesions.

Cat Scratch Disease

CSD typically manifests as a papule or pustule at the inoculation site and enlarged, tender lymph nodes that develop proximal to the inoculation site 1–3 weeks after exposure. *B. henselae* infections also can cause prolonged fever. Atypical manifestations include follicular conjunctivitis, encephalitis, neuroretinitis, osteomyelitis, or infection of the liver or spleen.

Bacillary Angiomatosis

Bacillary angiomatosis can present as skin, subcutaneous, or bone lesions, and is caused by *B. henselae* or *B. quintana*; peliosis hepatis manifests as liver lesions and is caused by *B. henselae*. Both occur primarily in people infected with HIV.

DIAGNOSIS

Bartonella quintana Infection

B. quintana infection can be diagnosed by serology, polymerase chain reaction (PCR) testing, or blood culture. Endocarditis caused by *Bartonella* spp. can be diagnosed by elevated serology and by PCR or culture of excised heart valve tissue.

Carrión Disease

Oroya fever is typically diagnosed via blood culture or direct observation of the bacilli in peripheral blood smears, but sensitivity of these methods is low. PCR and serologic testing also might aid diagnosis. Clinicians can contact CDC's Division of Vector-Borne Diseases for diagnostic consultation by calling 970-221-6400.

Cat Scratch Disease

CSD can be diagnosed presumptively in patients with typical presentation and a compatible exposure history. Serology can confirm the diagnosis, although cross-reactivity might limit interpretation in some circumstances. Serology is available from large commercial laboratories. *B. henselae* also can be detected by PCR or culture of lymph node aspirates by using special techniques. Some specialized laboratories offer *Bartonella* testing with novel techniques, but lack adequate clinical validation data; clinicians should consider these options with caution.

TREATMENT

Each variation of Bartonella infection has distinct recommended treatments.

Bartonella quintana Infection

Doxycycline plus gentamicin is the recommended treatment for *B. quintana* bacteremia and associated symptoms (e.g., fever and rash).

5

Carrión Disease

Treat Oroya fever using chloramphenicol or ciprofloxacin.

Cat Scratch Disease

Antibiotics may not be necessary for the treatment of typical CSD, since it can resolve without treatment. Consider prescribing azithromycin for patients with extensive lymphadenopathy or to shorten the course of disease.

A small percentage of people will develop disseminated disease with severe complications. The effect of antibiotic treatment in reducing risk of progression to atypical disease is unknown. Doxycycline plus rifampin appears to promote disease resolution for *B. henselae* neuroretinitis; regimens and duration of treatment might vary by clinical presentation.

PREVENTION

Travelers should protect themselves from bites of body lice and sand flies (see Sec. 4, Ch. 6, Mosquitoes, Ticks & Other Arthropods). People, especially those who are immunocompromised, should avoid kittens and stray cats; rough play with associated scratches is a particular risk. People can reduce the risk for cats to carry *B. henselae* by controlling fleas and limiting cats' outdoor roaming. People also should wash their hands promptly after handling cats.

CDC website: www.cdc.gov/bartonella

BIBLIOGRAPHY

Angelakis E, Raoult D. Pathogenicity and treatment of *Bartonella* infections. Int J Antimicrob Agents. 2014;44(1):16–25.

Eremeeva ME, Gerns HL, Lydy SL, Goo JS, Ryan ET, Mathew SS, et al. Bacteremia, fever, and splenomegaly caused by a newly recognized *Bartonella* species. N Engl J Med. 2007;356(23):2381–7.

Florin TA, Zaoutis TE, Zaoutis LB. Beyond cat scratch disease: widening spectrum of *Bartonella henselae* infection. Pediatrics. 2008;121(5):e1413–25.

Lydy SL, Eremeeva ME, Asnis D, Paddock CD, Nicholson WL, Silverman DJ, et al. Isolation and characterization of *Bartonella bacilliformis* from an expatriate Ecuadorian. J Clin Microbiol. 2008;46(2):627–37.

Nelson CA, Saha S, Mead PS. Cat-scratch disease in the United States, 2005–2013. Emerg Infect Dis. 2016;22(10):1741–6.

BRUCELLOSIS

María Negrón, Rebekah Tiller, Grishma Kharod

INFECTIOUS AGENT: *Brucella* spp.	
ENDEMICITY	Worldwide
TRAVELER CATEGORIES AT GREATEST RISK FOR EXPOSURE & INFECTION	People who consume unpasteurized dairy products or who have contact with infected animals
PREVENTION METHODS	Avoid contact with infected animals Practice safe food habits and avoid unpasteurized dairy products Use personal protective equipment, as appropriate
DIAGNOSTIC SUPPORT	A clinical laboratory certified in high complexity testing; state health department; CDC's Bacterial Special Pathogens Branch (bspb@cdc.gov); or the CDC Emergency Operations Center (770-488-7100)

INFECTIOUS AGENT

Brucella spp., the causative agents for brucellosis, are facultative, intracellular, gram-negative coccobacilli. The main *Brucella* spp. known to cause human disease are *Brucella abortus* (including the livestock vaccine strain *Brucella abortus* RB51), *B. melitensis, B. suis,* and *B. canis.*

EPIDEMIOLOGY & TRANSMISSION

Over 500,000 new human cases of brucellosis—a bacterial zoonosis—are reported worldwide each year. This number is likely an underestimate, however, because cases are underreported and often misdiagnosed because clinical symptoms are nonspecific, physicians might lack awareness, and laboratory capacity for diagnosis is limited. *B. melitensis* is the most frequently reported cause of brucellosis worldwide, but the most widespread potential source of infection is *B. abortus.*

Human infections occur most frequently among travelers to, or people living in, areas where the disease is endemic in animals—primarily cattle, goats, and sheep—in Africa, Central and South America, Asia, eastern Europe, along the Mediterranean Basin, and the Middle East. In North America, *Brucella* spp. are endemic to the feral swine population and wildlife around the Greater Yellowstone Area.

Humans most commonly acquire *Brucella* through consumption of unpasteurized dairy products (e.g., raw milk, and butter, soft cheese, or ice cream made from raw milk) from infected animals. The bacteria can also enter the body via skin wounds, mucous membranes, or inhalation, so direct contact with infected animal tissues or fluids can be an exposure risk. Activities such as carcass dressing and assisting birthing animals can increase the risk for contact with infective tissues and fluids.

Travelers' brucellosis can be caused by *B. suis* or *B. canis* infection because certain travelers might have contact with animal populations infected with these *Brucella* species (e.g., *B. suis* in feral swine and caribou or reindeer, and *B. canis* in dogs). Consumption of undercooked meat from infected animals can lead to infection, but this exposure risk is less likely because bacterial loads are lower in muscle. Person-to-person transmission has been reported but is rare. Exposure to *Brucella* during pregnancy can increase the risk for miscarriage, so travelers who are or might be pregnant should take extra precautions.

CLINICAL PRESENTATION

The incubation period of brucellosis is usually 2–4 weeks (range 5 days–6 months). Initial clinical presentation is nonspecific and includes arthralgia, fatigue, fever, headache, malaise, myalgia, and night sweats. Focal infections are common and can affect most organs in the body. Osteoarticular involvement is the most common brucellosis complication, as is reproductive system involvement. Although rare, endocarditis can occur and is the principal cause of death among patients with brucellosis.

DIAGNOSIS

Blood culture is considered the diagnostic gold standard, but isolation rates can vary considerably (25%–80%) depending on stage of infection, previous use of antimicrobial drugs, type and volume of clinical specimen, and culture method used. Bacterial growth in culture can be observed within 3–5 days but might take longer; therefore, laboratories should hold cultures for ≥10 days before considering a sample negative.

To increase recovery of the organism, collect samples during a febrile episode and prior to starting antimicrobial drugs; when focal disease is suspected, collect samples for culture from the affected area (e.g., cerebrospinal fluid, joint aspirate). Inform the laboratory that brucellosis is suspected when submitting blood, bone marrow, or other clinical specimens for culture because the bacteria take longer to grow, and laboratory personnel require additional personal protective equipment when handling the clinical specimens and culture.

Serologic testing is the most common method for diagnosis. The serum agglutination test (SAT) is the standard method for serologic diagnosis and detects IgM, IgG, and IgA. The Bacterial Special Pathogens Branch at the Centers for Disease Control and Prevention (CDC) performs a modified version of the SAT, known as the *Brucella* microagglutination test (BMAT). In general, ELISA tests have good sensitivity and specificity and can detect IgM or IgG, and US commercial diagnostic laboratories have the capacity to perform these assays.

Because most *Brucella* serologic assays show variable levels of cross-reactivity with other gram-negative bacteria (e.g., *Escherichia coli* O:157, *Francisella tularensis, Yersinia enterocolitica*), consider the limitations of serologic testing for diagnosing brucellosis. In addition, *Brucella* antibodies can persist for >1 year despite successful antibiotic treatment. Finally, no validated serologic assays are available to detect antibodies produced against infections caused by *B. canis* and *B. abortus* RB51 strain in humans. If infection with either of these organisms is possible or suspected, perform a culture on a specimen taken prior to the start of antimicrobial drug therapy.

For diagnostic support and specimen submission guidance, contact the local, territorial, tribal, or state public health department. CDC's Bacterial Special Pathogens Branch (bspb@cdc.gov) can coordinate testing needs in conjunction with the public health department; CDC-specific guidance on specimen submission can be found at the CDC Test Directory (www.cdc.gov/laboratory/specimen-submission/list.html; enter *Brucella* in the search bar).

TREATMENT

A combined regimen of doxycycline (or oral tetracycline) and rifampin for ≥6 weeks is recommended for the treatment of uncomplicated infection. For complicated brucellosis (endocarditis, meningitis, osteomyelitis), consider adding an aminoglycoside in combination with doxycycline and extend the duration of therapy to 4–6 months. *B. abortus* RB51 is resistant to rifampin; modify treatment for brucellosis caused by this strain accordingly (e.g., doxycycline in combination with trimethoprim-sulfamethoxazole, unless contraindicated). Other antimicrobial agents have been used in various combinations; treatment should be guided by a clinician with expertise in infectious diseases. Incorrect or incomplete therapy, or late diagnosis, can result in relapse.

PREVENTION

Travelers should avoid unpasteurized dairy products, undercooked meat, and potentially contaminated meat products in countries where brucellosis is endemic. People who dress or butcher wild animals or who handle birthing products from animals potentially infected with *Brucella* spp. should wear appropriate protective equipment, including rubber gloves, goggles or face shields, and gowns. Inform clinical microbiology laboratories when submitting specimens from patients with suspected brucellosis to ensure proper biosafety precautions in the laboratory handling of specimens and specimen derivatives.

For questions on laboratory diagnostics, post-exposure guidance, or treatment, contact the local, territorial, tribal, or state public health department, or CDC's Bacterial Special Pathogens Branch (bspb@cdc.gov).

CDC website: www.cdc.gov/brucellosis

BIBLIOGRAPHY

Al Dahouk S, Nockler K. Implications of laboratory diagnosis on brucellosis therapy. Expert Rev Anti Infect Ther. 2011;9(7):833–45.

Ariza J, Bosilkovski M, Cascio A, Colmenero JD, Corbel MJ, Falagas ME, et al. Perspectives for the treatment of brucellosis in the 21st century: the Ioannina recommendations. PLoS Med. 2007;4(12):e317.

Brown SL, Klein GC, McKinney FT, Jones WL. Safranin O–stained antigen microagglutination test for detection of brucella antibodies. J Clin Microbiol. 1981;13:398–400.

Centers for Disease Control and Prevention. *Brucellosis reference guide: exposures, testing, and prevention.* Atlanta: The Centers; 2017. Available from: www.cdc.gov/brucellosis/pdf/brucellosi-reference-guide.pdf.

Corbel M; Food and Agricultural Organization of the United Nations, World Organisation for Animal Health, World Health Organization. Brucellosis in humans and animals. Geneva: The Organizations; 2006. Available from: www.who.int/publications/i/item/9789241547130.

Ghanem-Zoubi N, Eljay SP, Anis E, Paul M. Association between human brucellosis and adverse pregnancy outcome: a cross-sectional population-based study. Eur J Clin Microbiol Infect Dis. 2018;37(5):883–8.

Memish ZA, Balkhy HH. Brucellosis and international travel. J Travel Med. 2004;11(1):49–55.

Rhodes HM, Williams DN, Hansen GT. Invasive human brucellosis infection in travelers to and immigrants from the Horn of Africa related to the consumption of raw camel milk. Travel Med Infect Dis. 2016;14(3):255–60.

Roushan M, Baiaini M, Asnafi N, Saedi F. Outcomes of 19 pregnant women with brucellosis in Babol, northern Iran. Trans R Soc Trop Med Hyg. 2011;105(9):540–2.

Yousefi-Nooraie R, Mortaz-Hejri S, Mehrani M, Sadeghipour P. Antibiotics for treating human brucellosis. Cochrane Database Syst Rev. 2012;10:CD007179.

CAMPYLOBACTERIOSIS

Farrell Tobolowsky, Mark Laughlin, Rachael Aubert, Daniel Payne

INFECTIOUS AGENT: *Campylobacter* spp.	
ENDEMICITY	Worldwide
TRAVELER CATEGORIES AT GREATEST RISK FOR EXPOSURE & INFECTION	Children <5 years old Adults ≥65 years old Males People with immunodeficiencies
PREVENTION METHODS	Follow safe food and water precautions Practice good hand hygiene
DIAGNOSTIC SUPPORT	A clinical laboratory certified in moderate complexity testing

INFECTIOUS AGENT

Campylobacteriosis is caused by gram-negative, curved microaerophilic bacteria of the family *Campylobacteriacae*. Most infections are caused by *Campylobacter jejuni*; ≥18 other species, including *C. coli*, also cause human infections. *C. jejuni* and *C. coli* are carried normally in the intestinal tracts of many domestic and wild animals.

TRANSMISSION

The major modes of transmission include eating contaminated foods, especially undercooked chicken and foods contaminated by raw chicken, and consuming contaminated water or dairy products, most commonly unpasteurized milk. Transmission also occurs less commonly from contact with pets, particularly kittens and puppies, and farm animals (e.g., cows, poultry). Rarely, *Campylobacter* can be transmitted from person to person by the fecal–oral route. The infectious dose is small; <500 organisms can cause disease.

5

EPIDEMIOLOGY

Campylobacter is a leading cause of bacterial diarrheal disease worldwide and caused ≈96 million cases in 2010. In the United States, *Campylobacter* causes ≈1.5 million human illnesses every year. About 15% of illnesses are associated with international travel, and *Campylobacter* comprises a large proportion of travel-related enteric infections. All travelers are at risk for infection, but children <5 years of age, adults ≥65 years of age, males, and people with immunodeficiencies are at increased risk. Risk is greatest in US travelers to Africa, Asia, and South America, especially to areas where food handling practices and sanitation might not be adequate. The incidence of *Campylobacter* infection is greater in rural areas. Infection occurs year-round in low- and middle-income countries and exhibits late summer and fall seasonality in developed countries.

CLINICAL PRESENTATION

The incubation period is typically 2–4 days but can range from 1–10 days. Illness is characterized by diarrhea (frequently bloody), abdominal pain, fever, and occasionally nausea and vomiting. More severe illness can occur, characterized by dehydration, bloodstream infection, or symptoms mimicking acute appendicitis or ulcerative colitis. Postinfectious complications include irritable bowel syndrome (in 9%–13% of patients), reactive arthritis (2%–5%), and Guillain-Barré syndrome (GBS; 0.1%). *C. jejuni* is the most frequently observed bacterial infection preceding GBS, and ≈5%–41% of all GBS cases could be attributed to campylobacteriosis; symptoms usually begin 1–3 weeks after the onset of enteritis.

DIAGNOSIS

Campylobacteriosis diagnosis is traditionally based on isolation of the organism from stool specimens or rectal swabs by using selective media incubated under reduced oxygen tension at 42°C (107.6°F) for 72 hours. Direct detection in stool specimens using multi-analyte PCR panels has become common.

Collect stool specimens as early as possible after symptoms begin and before initiating antimicrobial drug treatment. Because the organism is fastidious, a delay in transporting the specimen to the laboratory will affect viability. If transport and processing are not possible within 2 hours of stool sample collection, place specimens in a transport medium, (e.g., Cary-Blair) according to standard guidelines. Laboratories might reject stool specimens without preservative that have been in transit for >2 hours. Campylobacter cannot be recovered from frozen specimens.

Culture and isolation of *Campylobacter* from the specimen are needed to subtype and test for antimicrobial susceptibility. Identification to the species level can be difficult using traditional biochemical methods; molecular methods, including PCR, 16S rRNA sequencing, or whole-genome sequencing often are required. Matrix-assisted laser desorption ionization time of flight (MALDI-TOF) mass spectroscopy provides a rapid, sensitive method for identifying *Campylobacter* species.

Culture-independent methods for direct detection of *Campylobacter* from stool specimens include both immunologic (antigen-based) and nucleic-acid amplification-based tests (NAATs). Several NAAT gastrointestinal panels are approved by the US Food and Drug Administration (FDA) to detect *Campylobacter* and a variety of other gastrointestinal pathogens. However, many of these panels detect only *Campylobacter* species, and reflex culture is required for further identification, subtyping, and antimicrobial susceptibility testing (AST). The Clinical and Laboratory Standards Institute (CLSI) provides methods and interpretive criteria for AST.

Broth microdilution or disk diffusion can be performed under microaerophilic conditions, and clinical interpretive criteria (also known as susceptibility breakpoints) are available for both methods for ciprofloxacin, erythromycin, and tetracycline. Broth microdilution breakpoints are also available for doxycycline. Azithromycin susceptibility or resistance can be predicted by erythromycin testing.

Sensitivity and specificity of stool antigen tests are variable; in settings of low prevalence, the positive predictive value is likely to be low. Therefore, laboratories should confirm positive results of stool antigen tests by culture. Campylobacteriosis is a nationally notifiable disease in the United States.

TREATMENT

Campylobacteriosis is generally self-limited in healthy people, lasting ≤1 week and requiring only fluids and supportive care. Antimicrobial drug therapy decreases the duration of symptoms and bacterial shedding if administered early during illness. Because campylobacteriosis generally cannot be distinguished from other causes of travelers' diarrhea without a diagnostic test, use of empiric antibiotics in travelers should follow the guidelines for travelers' diarrhea (see Sec. 2, Ch. 6, Travelers' Diarrhea).

Rates of antibiotic resistance, especially fluoroquinolone resistance, have risen sharply in the past 20 years, and high rates of resistance are now seen in many regions, especially in South America and Southeast Asia. Travel abroad is a risk factor for infection with antimicrobial-resistant *Campylobacter*. Suspect resistant infections in returning travelers with campylobacteriosis in whom empiric fluoroquinolone treatment has failed. Macrolides like azithromycin are the current drugs of choice when antimicrobial drug treatment is indicated. Intravenous antibiotics might rarely be required for severe infections or for highly resistant strains.

5

PREVENTION

No vaccine is available. Travelers can best prevent infection by adhering to standard food and water safety precautions (see Sec. 2, Ch. 8, Food & Water Precautions) and by washing hands thoroughly with soap and water after contact with animals or environments that might be contaminated with animal feces. Antibiotic prophylaxis is not recommended.

CDC website: www.cdc.gov/foodsafety/diseases/campylobacter

BIBLIOGRAPHY

Havelaar AH, Kirk MD, Torgerson PR, Gibb HJ, Hald T, Lake RJ, et al. World Health Organization global estimates and regional comparisons of the burden of foodborne disease in 2010. PLoS Med. 2015;12(12):e1001923.

Kaakoush NO, Castaño-Rodríguiz N, Mitchell HA, Man SM. Global epidemiology of *Campylobacter* infection. Clin Microbiol Rev. 2015;28(3):687–720.

Kendall ME, Crim S, Fullerton K, Han PV, Cronquist AB, Shiferaw B, et al. Travel-associated enteric infections diagnosed after return to the United States, Foodborne Diseases Active Surveillance Network (FoodNet), 2004–2009. Clin Infect Dis. 2012;54 Suppl_5:S480–7.

Nachamkin, I. Campylobacter and Arcobacter. In: Carroll KC, Pfaller M, Landry ML, McAdam AJ, Patel R, Richter SS, Warnock DW, editors. American Society of Microbiology manual of clinical microbiology, 12th edition. Washington, DC: ASM Press; 2019. pp. 1028–43.

Olson CK, Ethelberg S, van Pelt W, Tauxe RV. Chapter 9: epidemiology of *Campylobacter jejuni* infections in industrialized nations. In: Nachamkin I, Szymanski C, Blaser M, editors. Campylobacter, 3rd edition. Washington, DC: ASM Press; 2008. pp. 163–89.

Scallan Walter EJ, Crim SM, Bruce BB, Griffin PM. Incidence of *Campylobacter*-associated Guillain-Barre syndrome estimated from health insurance data. Foodborne Pathog Dis. 2020;17(1):23–8.

Tack DM, Marder EP, Griffin PM, Cieslak PR, Dunn J, Hurd S, et al. Preliminary incidence and trends of infections with pathogens transmitted commonly through food—Foodborne Diseases Active Surveillance Network, 10 US sites, 2015–2018. MMWR Morb Mortal Wkly Rep. 2014;63(15):328–32.

CHOLERA

Talia Pindyck, Bruce Gutelius, Eric Mintz

INFECTIOUS AGENT: Toxigenic *Vibrio cholerae* O1 or O139	
ENDEMICITY	Africa Americas (island of Hispaniola at very low levels) South and Southeast Asia
TRAVELER CATEGORIES AT GREATEST RISK FOR EXPOSURE & INFECTION	Humanitarian aid workers Refugees and internally displaced people Travelers going to endemic or outbreak areas
PREVENTION METHODS	Travelers who consistently observe safe food, water, sanitation, and hand hygiene precautions have virtually no risk of infection Cholera is a vaccine-preventable disease
DIAGNOSTIC SUPPORT	A clinical laboratory certified in moderate complexity testing; state health department

5

INFECTIOUS AGENT

Cholera is an acute bacterial intestinal infection caused by toxigenic *Vibrio cholerae* O-group 1 (O1) or O-group 139 (O139). Many other serogroups of *V. cholerae*, with or without the cholera toxin gene (including the nontoxigenic strains of the O1 and O139 serogroups), can cause a cholera-like illness. Only toxigenic strains of serogroups O1 and O139 have caused widespread epidemics and are reportable to the World Health Organization (WHO) as "cholera." Toxigenic strains of *V. cholerae* O1 are the source of an ongoing global pandemic that began in 1961, but the O139 serogroup is localized to a few areas in Asia.

V. cholerae O1 has 2 biotypes, classical and El Tor, and each biotype can be divided into distinct serotypes, Inaba Ogawa, and rarely, Hikojima. The symptoms of infection are indistinguishable, but more people infected with the El Tor biotype remain asymptomatic or have only a mild illness. Globally, most cholera cases are caused by O1 El Tor organisms. In recent years, an El Tor variant with characteristics of both classical and El Tor biotypes has emerged in Asia and spread to Africa and the Caribbean. This is the strain responsible for the epidemic on Hispaniola, the island shared by Haiti and the Dominican Republic; compared to older El Tor strains, this newer variant appears to be more virulent, causing a greater proportion of severe episodes of cholera with the potential for higher death rates.

TRANSMISSION

Toxigenic *V. cholerae* O1 and O139 are free-living bacterial organisms found in fresh and brackish water, often in association with copepods or other zooplankton, shellfish, and aquatic plants. Cholera infections are acquired most often from untreated drinking water in which toxigenic *V. cholerae* naturally occurs or has been introduced from the feces of an infected person. Other common vehicles include raw or undercooked food, especially fish and shellfish. Other foods, including produce, are less commonly implicated. Direct person-to-person transmission, including to health care workers during epidemics, has been reported.

When in countries affected by cholera, travelers who consistently observe recommendations regarding safe drinking water, food preparation and consumption, handwashing, and sanitation have virtually no risk of acquiring the disease.

EPIDEMIOLOGY

Cholera is endemic to ≈50 countries, primarily in South and Southeast Asia and Africa. During 2007–2017, the United States had 117 confirmed cholera cases among people who traveled internationally in the week before illness; ≈16% reported travel to India or Pakistan. Other reported destinations included other countries in Southeast Asia, East and West Africa, and the Caribbean. Sporadic cases in the United States associated with travel to or from cholera-affected countries in Asia and Africa continue to occur.

More than half (70/117, ≈60%) of US cases during 2007–2017 were linked to travel to Haiti, the Dominican Republic, or Cuba, the 3 Caribbean countries affected by a large cholera epidemic that began in Haiti in October 2010. Ninety-four percent (66/70) of case-patients reported travel to either Haiti or the Dominican Republic sometime during 2010–2017. The other case-patients had been to Cuba sometime during 2013–2015.

In 2018 and 2019, the most recent years for which data are available, no cholera cases in the United States were associated with travel to Haiti or the Dominican Republic, and those 2 countries reported far fewer cholera cases to WHO during these 2 years than in previous years. Although efforts were underway to eliminate cholera from Hispaniola, in October 2022, the Pan American Health Organization reported a resurgence of the disease in Haiti. Before 2022, the last confirmed case of cholera in Haiti was in 2019, and in the Dominican Republic in 2018.

Travelers to areas where cholera is endemic or where an active epidemic is occurring are at risk for cholera infection. Health care and response workers in cholera-affected areas (e.g., during an outbreak, after a disaster) also might be at increased risk for cholera. People who do not follow handwashing recommendations, and/or do not use latrines or other sanitation systems are at increased risk for infection. People who have low gastric acidity have a greater risk for infection, and they, along with those with blood type O, are at greater risk for developing severe disease if infected.

CLINICAL PRESENTATION

Cholera most commonly manifests as acute watery diarrhea in an afebrile person. The pathogen typically remains in the gastrointestinal tract and does not invade the bloodstream. Infection is often mild or asymptomatic, but it can be severe. Severe cholera (*cholera gravis*) occurs in ≈10% of cholera episodes and is characterized by profuse watery diarrhea, described as rice-water stools, often accompanied by nausea and vomiting that can rapidly lead to severe volume depletion.

Clinical findings include dry mucous membranes and loss of skin turgor, hypotension, tachycardia, and thirst. Additional symptoms, including muscle cramps, are secondary to the resulting electrolyte imbalances. Untreated cholera can cause rapid loss of body fluids, which can lead to severe dehydration, hypovolemic shock, and death within hours. The case-fatality ratio for untreated cholera can reach >50%, but with adequate and timely rehydration, the case-fatality ratio is <1%.

DIAGNOSIS

In the United States, cholera traditionally is confirmed by isolation and identification of toxigenic *V. cholerae* O1 recovered from a stool sample of a patient with acute, watery diarrhea. Before administering antimicrobial treatment, collect patient stool samples and preserve samples in Cary-Blair medium for transport at ambient temperature. Selective media (e.g., taurocholate-tellurite-gelatin agar, thiosulfate-citrate-bile salts agar) also can be used for pathogen isolation.

Reagents for serogrouping *V. cholerae* isolates are available in most state health department laboratories. Antigen-based rapid diagnostic tests (RDTs) do not yield an isolate for toxin detection, antimicrobial susceptibility testing, or subtyping. Reflex culture to recover an isolate should always be performed when a *V. cholerae* diagnosis is derived from an RDT, and clinicians should send the isolate to a public health laboratory for additional characterization.

Currently available commercial RDTs, which detect O1 and O139 antigens in human stool specimens using monoclonal antibodies, are useful for cholera outbreak detection and response, but should not be used to diagnose individual patients. Molecular methods (e.g., PCR, whole-genome sequencing) can detect *V. cholerae* and characterize its genetic profile and are increasingly used in public health laboratories. Cholera is a nationally notifiable disease in the United States, and all isolates obtained in the United States should be sent to the Centers for Disease Control and Prevention (CDC) via state health department laboratories for identification and virulence testing.

TREATMENT

Rehydration is the cornerstone of cholera treatment. Administer oral rehydration solution and, when necessary, intravenous fluids and electrolytes; timely administration in adequate volumes will reduce case-fatality ratios to <1%. Antibiotics will reduce fluid requirements and duration of illness and are indicated in conjunction with aggressive hydration for severe cases and for patients with moderate dehydration and ongoing fluid losses.

5

Whenever possible, antimicrobial susceptibility testing should inform treatment choices. In most countries, doxycycline is recommended as the first-line antibiotic treatment for children, adults, and pregnant people. Previously, tetracycline antibiotics (including doxycycline) were not recommended for children due to concern for dental discoloration, or pregnant people due to concern for teratogenic effects. A recent systematic review among young children and pregnant people receiving doxycycline did not demonstrate a safety risk.

Multidrug-resistant isolates are emerging, particularly in South Asia, with resistance to quinolones, trimethoprim-sulfamethoxazole, and tetracycline. The strain from Hispaniola is also multidrug resistant; as of 2013, however, tested isolates were still sensitive to doxycycline and tetracycline. Macrolides, including erythromycin and azithromycin, are alternative agents for multidrug-resistant isolates. Zinc supplementation reduces the severity and duration of cholera and other diarrheal diseases in children living in resource-limited areas.

PREVENTION

Food & Water

Travelers should follow safe food and water precautions and frequently wash hands (see Sec. 2, Ch. 8, Food & Water Precautions). Antibiotic chemoprophylaxis is not recommended.

Vaccine

No country or territory requires vaccination against cholera as a condition for entry. CVD 103-HgR, a live, attenuated, single-dose oral cholera vaccine (Vaxchora, PaxVax), is licensed in the United States. The vaccine was previously marketed under the names Orochol and Mutacol in other countries.

INDICATIONS

The Advisory Committee on Immunization Practices (ACIP) recommends CVD 103-HgR vaccine for both pediatric and adult travelers (2–64 years old) visiting areas of active cholera transmission. An area of active cholera transmission is defined as a province, state, or other administrative subdivision within a country with endemic or epidemic cholera caused by toxigenic *V. cholerae* O1. It includes areas that are prone to recurrence of cholera epidemics that have had cholera activity within the past year. Locations where rare sporadic cholera cases have been reported are not considered active cholera areas.

CDC provides a list of countries for which cholera vaccine can be considered for travelers (see "Who is at risk?") at https://wwwnc.cdc.gov/travel/diseases/cholera. Cholera activity can occur in certain parts of a country or in certain settings, however, and information about places with cholera activity might be incomplete because of variations in surveillance and reporting. The vaccine is not routinely recommended for most travelers from the United States because they do not visit areas with active cholera transmission. Clinicians and travelers can find additional country-specific information on CDC's Travelers' Health website at https://wwwnc.cdc.gov/travel/destinations/list.

EFFICACY

In clinical efficacy trials, adults aged 18–45 years who received Vaxchora were protected against severe diarrhea after oral *V. cholerae* O1 challenge at 10 days (vaccine efficacy 90%) and at 3 months (vaccine efficacy 80%) after vaccination. In adults aged 46–64 years, vibriocidal antibody seroconversion rates, the best available marker for protection against cholera, were comparable to the response seen in adults aged 18–45 years. Multicenter randomized clinical efficacy trials of CVD 103-HgR in children (published in 2020) demonstrated CVD 103-HgR induced serum vibriocidal antibody seroconversion on day 11 in >97% of recipients aged 2–17 years; efficacy was not assessed.

ADMINISTRATION

Prepare and administer Vaxchora in a health care setting equipped to dispose of medical waste. To prepare Vaxchora, reconstitute the buffer component in 100 milliliters (mL) of cold or room temperature, purified, non-carbonated, non-flavored bottled or spring bottled water. The package insert indicates that for children aged 2–5 years, half of the reconstituted buffer solution (50 mL) should be discarded before adding the active component (lyophilized *V. cholerae* CVD 103-HgR); after preparation, a single oral dose of Vaxchora for children aged 2–5 years is 50 mL. Patients should avoid eating or drinking for 60 minutes before and after taking Vaxchora vaccine. Administer Vaxchora as a single oral dose ≥10 days before potential cholera exposure.

BOOSTER DOSES

The safety and efficacy of revaccination with CVD 103-HgR have not been established.

SAFETY & ADVERSE REACTIONS

Serious adverse events were rare among recipients of Orochol and Mutacol, the previously marketed formulation of the CVD 103-HgR vaccine.

In clinical safety trials involving adults aged 18–45 years, headache, tiredness, and nausea, vomiting, and diarrhea were reported more commonly by CVD 103-HgR recipients than by placebo recipients within 7 days of vaccination. Among children and adolescents aged 2–17 years, adverse events more commonly reported by vaccine than by placebo recipients included abdominal pain, anorexia, headache, and tiredness. No vaccine-related serious adverse events were reported among participants aged 2–64 years.

Vaxchora is not currently licensed for use in children <2 years or adults >65 years of age. The safety and effectiveness of Vaxchora have not been established in pregnant or lactating people, or in immunocompromised people. No difference in adverse events were reported among HIV-positive recipients of an older formulation of the CVD 103-HgR vaccine and those who received placebo.

PRECAUTIONS & CONTRAINDICATIONS

Vaxchora is contraindicated in people with a history of severe allergic reaction to the ingredients of this or any other cholera vaccine. A study with the older formulation of CVD 103-HgR showed that concomitant use of chloroquine decreased the immune response to the vaccine; therefore, antimalarial prophylaxis with chloroquine should begin ≥10 days after administration of Vaxchora. Coadministration of mefloquine and proguanil with CVD 103-HgR did not diminish the vaccine's immunogenicity. Antimicrobial drugs might decrease the immune response to CVD 103-HgR, so clinicians should not administer the vaccine to patients who have received antibiotics in the previous 14 days.

Vaxchora might be shed in the stool for ≥7 days, and the vaccine strain could be transmitted to nonvaccinated close contacts. Clinicians and travelers should use caution when considering whether to use the vaccine in people with close contacts who are immunocompromised.

CDC website: www.cdc.gov/cholera

BIBLIOGRAPHY

Centers for Disease Control and Prevention. Cholera and Other *Vibrio* Illness Surveillance (COVIS) System. 2020. Available from: www.cdc.gov/vibrio/surveillance.html.

Chen WH, Cohen MB, Kirkpatrick BD, Brady RC, Galloway D, Gurwith M, et al. Single-dose live oral cholera vaccine CVD 103-HgR protects against human experimental infection with *Vibrio cholerae* O1 El Tor. Clin Infect Dis. 2016;62(11):1329–35.

Danzig L, editor. Vaxchora clinical data summary. Meeting of the Advisory Committee on Immunization Practices; February 24, 2016; Atlanta, GA.

Freedman DO. Re-born in the USA: another cholera vaccine for travelers. Travel Med Infect Dis. 2016; 14(4):295–6.

Harris JB, LaRocque RC, Qadri F, Ryan ET, Calderwood SB. Cholera. Lancet. 2012;379(9835):2466–76.

Kollaritsch H, Que JU, Kunz C, Wiedermann G, Herzog C, Cryz SJ, Jr. Safety and immunogenicity of live oral cholera and typhoid vaccines administered alone or in combination with antimalarial drugs, oral polio vaccine, or yellow fever vaccine. J Infect Dis. 1997;175(4):871–5.

Schilling KA, Cartwright EJ, Stamper J, Locke M, Esposito DH, Balaban V, et al. Diarrheal illness among US residents providing medical services in Haiti during the cholera epidemic, 2010–2011. J Travel Med. 2014;21(1):55–7.

Wong KK, Burdette E, Mahon BE, Mintz ED, Ryan ET, Reingold RL. Recommendations of the Advisory Committee on Immunization Practices for use of cholera vaccine. MMWR Morb Mortal Wkly Rep. 2017;66(18):482–5.

Wong KK, Mahon BE, Reingold A. CVD 103-HgR vaccine for travelers. Travel Med Infect Dis. 2016;14(6):632–3.

World Health Organization. Cholera 2019. Wkly Epidemiol Rec. 2020;37:441–8.

DIPHTHERIA

Anna Acosta, Sarah Bennett

5

INFECTIOUS AGENT: Toxigenic strains of *Corynebacterium diphtheriae* biotypes *mitis*, *gravis*, *intermedius*, or *belfanti*	
ENDEMICITY	The Americas (Haiti and the Dominican Republic) Asia and the South Pacific Eastern Europe Middle East
TRAVELER CATEGORIES AT GREATEST RISK FOR EXPOSURE & INFECTION	Travelers not current with diphtheria toxoid vaccine
PREVENTION METHODS	Diphtheria is a vaccine-preventable disease
DIAGNOSTIC SUPPORT	A clinical laboratory certified in high complexity testing; state health department; request Elek testing for toxin production by contacting CDC Emergency Operations Center (770-488-7100)

INFECTIOUS AGENT

Diphtheria is caused by toxigenic strains of *Corynebacterium diphtheriae* biotype *mitis*, *gravis*, *intermedius*, or *belfanti*. Toxigenic strains of *C. ulcerans* also cause rare cases of a diphtheria-like illness.

TRANSMISSION

Transmission occurs person-to-person through respiratory droplets or direct contact with secretions from cutaneous diphtheria lesions, and rarely, by fomites.

EPIDEMIOLOGY

Diphtheria is endemic to many regions around the world: Haiti and the Dominican Republic in the Americas; Asia and the South Pacific; Eastern Europe; and the Middle East. Since 2016, respiratory diphtheria outbreaks have occurred in Bangladesh, Burma (Myanmar), Haiti, Indonesia, South Africa, Ukraine, Venezuela, Vietnam, and Yemen. Cutaneous diphtheria is common in tropical countries. Respiratory and cutaneous diphtheria have been reported in travelers to countries with endemic disease. The last case of respiratory diphtheria in a US traveler was reported in 2003, but toxin-producing cutaneous *C. diphtheriae* was identified from 4 US residents who returned from travel between September 2015 and March 2018. Diphtheria can affect any age group, especially people who are not fully vaccinated with diphtheria toxoid vaccine.

CLINICAL PRESENTATION

The incubation period is 2–5 days (range 1–10 days). Affected anatomic sites include the mucous membranes of the upper respiratory tract (nose, pharynx, tonsils, larynx, and trachea [respiratory diphtheria]), skin (cutaneous diphtheria), or rarely, mucous membranes at other sites (eye, ear, vulva). Nasal diphtheria can be asymptomatic or mild, with a blood-tinged discharge.

Respiratory diphtheria has a gradual onset and is characterized by a mild fever (rarely >101°F [38.3°C]), sore throat and difficulty swallowing, malaise, loss of appetite, and if the larynx is involved, hoarseness. The hallmark of respiratory diphtheria is a pseudomembrane that appears within 2–3 days of illness onset, covers the mucous lining of the tonsils, pharynx, larynx, or nares, and that can extend into the trachea. The pseudomembrane is firm, fleshy, grey, and adherent; it typically will bleed after attempts to remove or dislodge it. Fatal airway obstruction can result if the pseudomembrane extends into the larynx or trachea or if a piece of it becomes dislodged. The case-fatality ratio is 5%–10%.

DIAGNOSIS

A presumptive diagnosis is usually based on clinical features. Diagnosis is confirmed by isolating *C. diphtheriae* from culture of nasal or throat swabs or pseudomembrane tissue and testing for toxin production by the Elek test. Laboratory capacity for diphtheria culture and Elek testing varies by country, and testing might be available through national reference or commercial laboratories. In the United States, the Centers for Disease Control and Prevention (CDC) has the only laboratory able to perform Elek testing. Diphtheria is a nationally notifiable disease in the United States, and clinicians can contact their state health department or the CDC Emergency Operations Center for more information.

TREATMENT

Patients with respiratory diphtheria require hospitalization to monitor response to treatment and manage complications. Equine diphtheria antitoxin (DAT) is the mainstay of treatment and can be administered without waiting for laboratory confirmation. In the United States, DAT is available to physicians under an investigational new drug protocol by contacting their state health department, followed by the CDC Emergency Operations Center at 770-488-7100.

In addition to DAT, treating physicians should prescribe an antibiotic (erythromycin or penicillin) to eliminate the causative organisms, stop toxin production, and reduce communicability. Patients will require supportive care, including airway and cardiac monitoring. In addition, close contacts of patients should receive antimicrobial prophylaxis with erythromycin or penicillin.

PREVENTION

All travelers should be up to date with diphtheria toxoid vaccine before departure. After a primary series and childhood and adolescent boosters, all adults should receive booster doses with a diphtheria toxoid–containing vaccine at 10-year intervals, given either as Td (tetanus-diphtheria) or Tdap (tetanus-diphtheria-acellular pertussis). This booster is particularly important for travelers who will live or work in countries where diphtheria is endemic.

CDC website: www.cdc.gov/diphtheria

BIBLIOGRAPHY

Centers for Disease Control and Prevention. Fatal respiratory diphtheria in a US traveler to Haiti—Pennsylvania, 2003. MMWR Morb Mortal Wkly Rep. 2004;52(53):1285–6.

Clarke KEN, MacNeil A, Hadler S, Scott C, Tiwari TSP, Cherian T. Global epidemiology of diphtheria, 2000–2017. Emerg Infect Dis. 2019;25(10):1834–42.

Griffith J, Bozio CH, Poel AJ, Fitzpatrick K, DeBolt DA, Cassiday P, et al. Imported toxin-producing cutaneous diphtheria—Minnesota, Washington, and New Mexico, 2015–2018. MMWR Morb Mortal Wkly Rep. 2019;68:281–4.

Havers FP, Moro PL, Hunter P, Hariri S, Bernstein H. Use of tetanus toxoid, reduced diphtheria toxoid, and acellular pertussis vaccines: updated recommendations of the Advisory Committee on Immunization Practices—United States, 2019. MMWR Morb Mortal Wkly Rep. 2020;69:77–83.

Liang JL, Tiwari T, Moro P, Messonnier ME, Reingold A, Sawyer M, et al. Prevention of pertussis, tetanus, and diphtheria with vaccines in the United States: recommendations of the Advisory Committee on Immunization Practices (ACIP). MMWR Recomm Rep. 2018;67(2):1–44.

Pan American Health Organization/World Health Organization. Epidemiological update: diphtheria. 17 November 2020. Washington, DC: The Organizations; 2020. Available from: https://iris.paho.org/handle/10665.2/53173.

World Health Organization. Diphtheria vaccine: WHO position paper—August 2017. Wkly Epidemiol Rec. 2017;92(31):417–36.

ESCHERICHIA COLI, DIARRHEAGENIC

Jennifer Collins, Danielle Tack, Talia Pindyck, Patricia Griffin

5

INFECTIOUS AGENT: *Escherichia coli* (diarrheagenic)	
ENDEMICITY	Worldwide
TRAVELER CATEGORIES AT GREATEST RISK FOR EXPOSURE & INFECTION	All travelers, especially those going to low- and middle-income countries
PREVENTION MEASURES	Follow safe food and water precautions
DIAGNOSTIC SUPPORT	A clinical laboratory certified in moderate complexity testing

INFECTIOUS AGENT

Escherichia coli are gram-negative bacteria that inhabit the gastrointestinal tract. Most types do not cause illness, but 5 pathotypes are associated with diarrhea: enterotoxigenic *E. coli* (ETEC), Shiga toxin–producing *E. coli* (STEC), enteropathogenic *E. coli* (EPEC), enteroaggregative *E. coli* (EAEC), and enteroinvasive *E. coli* (EIEC). In addition, diffusely adherent *E. coli* (DAEC) might also be associated with diarrhea. Pathotypes that are common causes of urinary tract infections, bloodstream infections, and meningitis are not covered here.

E. coli serotypes are determined by surface antigens (O and H), and specific serotypes tend to cluster within specific pathotypes. Pathotype determination typically is based on testing for virulence genes. Some *E. coli* have virulence genes of >1 pathotype; for example, the O104:H4 strain that caused a 2011 outbreak in Germany produced Shiga toxin and had adherence properties typical of EAEC.

STEC also are called verotoxigenic *E. coli* (VTEC), and the term enterohemorrhagic *E. coli* (EHEC) commonly is used to specify STEC strains capable of causing human illness, especially bloody diarrhea and hemolytic uremic syndrome (HUS).

TRANSMISSION

Diarrheagenic *E. coli* pathotypes can be passed in the feces of humans and other animals. Transmission occurs through the fecal–oral route, via consumption of contaminated food or water, and through person-to-person contact, contact with animals or their environment, and swimming in untreated water. Humans constitute the main reservoir for non-STEC pathotypes that cause diarrhea in humans. The intestinal tracts of animals, especially cattle and other ruminants, are the primary reservoirs of STEC.

EPIDEMIOLOGY

The 2010 World Health Organization (WHO) Global Burden of Foodborne Diseases report estimated ≈111 million illnesses and ≈63,000 deaths caused by diarrheagenic *E. coli* globally each year. Rates of infection vary by region, and certain types of diarrheagenic *E. coli* infections, mainly ETEC, are associated with travel to low- and middle-income countries. The incidence of travel-associated diarrhea caused by *E. coli* is likely underestimated because many travelers do not seek medical care or have stool testing performed, particularly if diarrhea is non-bloody, as commonly occurs with ETEC infection. Moreover, many clinical laboratories do not use methods that can detect diarrheagenic *E. coli* other than STEC in stool samples.

Risk for travelers' diarrhea can be divided into 3 levels, according to the destination country. Low-risk countries include Australia, Canada, Greenland, Japan, New Zealand, the United States, and countries in northern and western Europe. Intermediate-risk countries include Argentina, Brazil, Chile, Morocco, Portugal, South Africa, Thailand (in Bangkok, Chiang Mai, and Phuket; risk to travelers going to rural areas is likely greater), Uruguay, and most countries in the Caribbean, eastern Europe, and the Middle East. High-risk countries include Afghanistan, Burma (Myanmar), the Indian subcontinent, Indonesia, Iran, Malaysia, Mexico, Papua New Guinea, most countries in Africa, and countries in Central America and northern South America, including Bolivia and Paraguay.

STEC infections are most commonly reported in industrialized countries, and ≈85% of STEC infections among international travelers are caused by non-O157 serotypes. Additional information about travelers' diarrhea is available in Sec. 2, Ch. 6, Travelers' Diarrhea.

CLINICAL PRESENTATION

Diarrheagenic *E. coli* infections, other than STEC, have incubation periods ranging from 8 hours to 3 days. The median incubation period of STEC infection is 3–4 days, with a range of 1–10 days. Clinical manifestations of diarrheagenic *E. coli* vary by pathotype (see Table 5-02).

DIAGNOSIS

Diagnostic testing is not usually recommended for uncomplicated travelers' diarrhea unless treatment is indicated. Until recently, diarrheagenic *E. coli* other than STEC could not be distinguished from non-pathogenic *E. coli* in stool using routine tests in clinical laboratories. Commercial molecular tests have increasingly become available and can identify ETEC, EPEC, EAEC, and EIEC through detection of virulence genes.

Consider several caveats when interpreting results of such tests. The combination of virulence genes that confer pathogenicity has not been determined for all pathotypes, and *E. coli* sometimes have virulence genes from >1 pathotype due to transfer of mobile genetic elements. Some studies have identified some genes, including the *eae* gene used to diagnose EPEC, at a similar frequency in stools from healthy people as from those with acute diarrhea. Identification of 2 virulence genes in a specimen does not mean they are carried by the same organism. Finally, molecular tests detect genetic material, which does not always correspond to the presence of viable organisms.

Using PCR or whole-genome sequence analysis to facilitate recognition of specific *E. coli* pathotypes, state public health and Centers for Disease Control and Prevention laboratories can assist in outbreak investigations. When STEC infection is suspected, stool samples should be cultured for *E. coli* O157 and simultaneously tested for Shiga toxins or the genes that encode them. For more information, see www.cdc.gov/mmwr/preview/mmwrhtml/rr5812a1.htm. Send all presumptive *E. coli* O157 isolates and Shiga toxin–positive specimens to a public health laboratory for further characterization and for outbreak detection. Rapid, accurate diagnosis of STEC infection is important because early clinical management decisions can affect patient outcomes, and early detection can help prevent further transmission.

TREATMENT

Maintenance of hydration and electrolyte balance with oral rehydration is important, especially in patients with vomiting or profuse diarrhea. Travelers with mild non-bloody diarrhea can use

Table 5-02 Mechanism of pathogenesis & typical clinical syndrome of *Escherichia coli* pathotypes

PATHOTYPE	MECHANISM OF PATHOGENESIS	INCUBATION PERIOD	ILLNESS DURATION	TYPICAL CLINICAL SYNDROME
DAEC	Diffuse adherence to epithelial cells	Unknown	Unknown	Watery diarrhea but pathogenicity not conclusively demonstrated
EAEC	Small and large bowel adherence mediated via various adhesins and accessory proteins; enterotoxin and cytotoxin production	8–48 hours	3–14 days; persistent diarrhea (>14 days) has been reported	Watery diarrhea with mucous, occasionally bloody; can cause prolonged or persistent diarrhea in children
EIEC	Mucosal invasion and inflammation of large bowel	10–18 hours	4–7 days	Watery diarrhea that might progress to bloody diarrhea (dysentery-like syndrome); fever
EPEC	Small bowel adherence and epithelial cell effacement mediated by intimin	9–12 hours	12 days	Severe acute watery diarrhea that can be persistent; common cause of infant diarrhea in developing countries
ETEC	Small bowel adherence via various adhesins that confer host specificity; heat-stable or heat-labile enterotoxin production	10–72 hours	1–5 days	Acute watery diarrhea, occasionally severe; afebrile
STEC	Large bowel adherence mediated via intimin (or less commonly by other adhesins); Shiga toxin 1, Shiga toxin 2 production; Shiga toxin production is linked to induction of the bacteriophages carrying the Shiga toxin genes; some antibiotics induce these bacteriophages	1–10 days (usu. 3–4 days)	Typically, 5–7 days; persistent diarrhea (>14 days) has been reported	Watery diarrhea that progresses (often for STEC O157, less often for non-O157) to bloody diarrhea in 1–3 days; abdominal cramps and tenderness; fever is low-grade, if present; hemolytic uremic syndrome complicates ≈6% of diagnosed STEC O157 infections (15% among children aged <5 years) and 1% of non-O157 STEC infections

Abbreviations: DAEC, diffusely adherent *Escherichia coli*; EAEC, enteroaggregative *E. coli*; EIEC, enteroinvasive *E. coli*; EPEC, enteropathogenic *E. coli*; ETEC, enterotoxigenic *E. coli*; STEC, Shiga toxin–producing *E. coli*.

loperamide to decrease the frequency of loose stools. Travelers with moderate illness can consider self-treatment with an antibiotic, and those with bloody diarrhea or severe illness (that keeps them confined to their room) should generally receive antibiotic therapy. Travelers can use loperamide as an adjunctive therapy to antibiotics taken for moderate or severe travelers' diarrhea.

Azithromycin is preferred for bloody diarrhea or severe illness and is an option for moderate non-bloody diarrhea. Fluoroquinolones (e.g., ciprofloxacin) can be effective, but resistant strains are increasing in frequency, particularly in Asia; other agents are also preferred because fluoroquinolones have been associated with adverse effects, including tendinopathies, QT interval prolongation (a cardiac conduction abnormality), and *Clostridioides difficile* enterocolitis.

If treatment with azithromycin or a fluoroquinolone does not improve the condition within 24 hours, travelers should continue the antibiotic for no longer than 3 days. A 3-day course of rifaximin is effective for some non-bloody diarrheal illnesses. Administering certain antimicrobial agents to patients whose clinical syndrome suggests STEC infection could increase their risk of developing HUS (Table 5-02). Studies of children with STEC O157 infection have shown that early use of intravenous fluids (within the first 4 days of diarrhea onset) might decrease the risk of oligoanuric renal failure.

Antimicrobial-resistant *E. coli* are increasing worldwide. Carefully weigh the decision to use an antibiotic against the severity of illness; the possibility that the pathogen is resistant; and the risk for adverse reactions (e.g., HUS, rash, other manifestations of allergy), antibiotic-associated colitis, and vaginal yeast infection. Some studies suggest that loperamide combined with antibiotics can be used safely in many patients. Due to a potential risk for complications, including toxic megacolon and HUS, avoid treating bloody diarrhea or STEC infection solely with antimotility drugs.

PREVENTION

No vaccine is available for *E. coli* infection. Although bismuth subsalicylate and certain antimicrobial agents (e.g., fluoroquinolones, rifaximin) can prevent *E. coli* diarrhea, chemoprophylaxis is not recommended for most travelers. Furthermore, antimicrobial drug use can adversely affect the intestinal microbiota and increase susceptibility to gut infections.

5

Remind travelers of the importance of adhering to food and water precautions (see Sec. 2, Ch. 8, Food & Water Precautions), and instruct travelers about the importance of handwashing. Because soap and water might not be readily available, travelers should consider taking hand sanitizer with ≥60% alcohol with them when they travel.

CDC website: www.cdc.gov/ecoli

BIBLIOGRAPHY

Frank C, Werber D, Cramer JP, Askar M, Faber M, an der Heiden M, et al. Epidemic profile of Shiga-toxin–producing *Escherichia coli* O104: H4 outbreak in Germany. New Engl J Med. 2011;365(19):1771–80.

Guiral E, Gonçalves Quiles M, Muñoz L, Moreno-Morales J, Alejo-Cancho I, Salvador P, et al. Emergence of resistance to quinolones and β-lactam antibiotics in enteroaggregative and enterotoxigenic *Escherichia coli* causing traveler's diarrhea. Antimicrob Agents Chemother. 2019;63(2):e01745-18.

Havelaar AH, Kirk MD, Torgerson PR, Gibb HJ, Hald T, Lake RJ, et al. World Health Organization global estimates and regional comparisons of the burden of foodborne disease in 2010. PLoS Med. 2015;12(12):e1001923.

Kaper JB, Nataro JP, Mobley HL. Pathogenic *Escherichia coli*. Nat Rev Microbiol. 2004;2(2):123–40.

Kotloff KL, Nataro JP, Blackwelder WC, Nasrin D, Farag TH, Panchalingam S, et al. Burden and aetiology of diarrhoeal disease in infants and young children in developing countries (the Global Enteric Multicenter Study, GEMS): a prospective, case-control study. Lancet. 2013;382(9888):209–22.

Mintz ED. Enterotoxigenic *Escherichia coli*: outbreak surveillance and molecular testing. Clin Infect Dis. 2006;42(11):1518–20.

Mody RK, Griffin PM. Editorial commentary: increasing evidence that certain antibiotics should be avoided for Shiga toxin–producing *Escherichia coli* infections: more data needed. Clin Infect Dis. 2016;62(10):1259–61.

Riddle MS, Connor BA, Beeching NJ, DuPont HL, Hamer DH, Kozarsky P, et al. Guidelines for the prevention and treatment of travelers' diarrhea: a graded expert panel report. J Travel Med. 2017;24(suppl_1):S63–80.

Shane AL, Mody RK, Crump JA, Tarr PI, Steiner TS, Kotloff K, et al. 2017 Infectious Diseases Society of America clinical practice guidelines for the diagnosis and management of infectious diarrhea. Clin Infect Dis. 2017;65(12):e45–80.

HELICOBACTER PYLORI

Bradley Connor

INFECTIOUS AGENT: *Helicobacter pylori*	
ENDEMICITY	Worldwide
TRAVELER CATEGORIES AT GREATEST RISK FOR EXPOSURE & INFECTION	All travelers
PREVENTION METHODS	None
DIAGNOSTIC SUPPORT	A clinical laboratory certified in moderate complexity testing

5

INFECTIOUS AGENT

Helicobacter pylori is a small, curved, microaerophilic, gram-negative, rod-shaped bacterium.

TRANSMISSION

H. pylori is believed to be transmitted mainly by fecal–oral route, but also possibly by oral–oral.

EPIDEMIOLOGY

H. pylori is recognized as one of the most common chronic bacterial infections worldwide, and about two-thirds of the world's population is infected; it is more common in developing countries. Short-term travelers appear to be at low risk of acquiring *H. pylori* through travel, but expatriates and long-stay travelers could be at greater risk.

CLINICAL PRESENTATION

Although usually asymptomatic, *H. pylori* infection is the major cause of peptic ulcer disease and gastritis worldwide, which often present as gnawing or burning epigastric pain. Less commonly, symptoms include loss of appetite, nausea, or vomiting. Designated as a carcinogen by the World Health Organization, *H. pylori* infection is the strongest known risk factor for non-cardia gastric adenocarcinoma. Infected people have a 2–6-fold increased risk of developing gastric cancer and mucosal associated-lymphoid-type (MALT) lymphoma compared with their uninfected counterparts.

DIAGNOSIS

H. pylori diagnosis can be made through fecal antigen assay, urea breath test, rapid urease test, or histology of a biopsy specimen. A positive serology indicates present or past infection.

TREATMENT

Asymptomatic infections generally do not need to be treated. Determine treatment on an individual basis, and treat patients with active duodenal or gastric ulcers if they are infected. Standard treatment is bismuth quadruple therapy: proton pump inhibitor (PPI) or H2-blocker + bismuth + metronidazole + tetracycline. Clarithromycin triple therapy (PPI + clarithromycin + amoxicillin or metronidazole) is an option in regions where *H. pylori* clarithromycin resistance is known to be <15% and in patients with no previous history of macrolide exposure.

Recently, combination therapies using rifabutin have become available, especially for refractory cases. Longer treatment durations (14 days vs. 7 days) provide higher eradication success rates (see http://gi.org/guideline/treatment-of-helicobacter-pylori-infection).

PREVENTION

No specific recommendations.

BIBLIOGRAPHY

Chey WD, Leontiadis GI, Howden CW, Moss SF. ACG clinical guideline: treatment of *Helicobacter pylori* infection. Am J Gastroenterol. 2017;112(2):212–39.

Lindkvist P, Wadstrom T, Giesecke J. *Helicobacter pylori* infection and foreign travel. J Infect Dis. 1995;172(4):1135–6.

Potasman, I, Yitzhak A. *Helicobacter pylori* serostatus in backpackers following travel to tropical countries. Am J Trop Med Hyg. 1998;58(3):305–8.

Shah, SC, Iyer PG, Moss SF. AGA clinical practice update on the management of refractory *Helicobacter pylori* infection: expert review. Gastroenterology. 2021;160(5):1831–41.

LEGIONNAIRES' DISEASE & PONTIAC FEVER

William (Chris) Edens

5

INFECTIOUS AGENT: *Legionella* spp.	
ENDEMICITY	Worldwide
TRAVELER CATEGORIES AT GREATEST RISK FOR EXPOSURE & INFECTION	Travelers >50 years of age, current or former smokers, have chronic lung conditions, or are immunocompromised
PREVENTION METHODS	Travelers at increased risk for infection should avoid recognized high-risk exposures (e.g., hot tubs)
DIAGNOSTIC SUPPORT	A clinical laboratory certified in moderate or high complexity testing; state health department

INFECTIOUS AGENT

Gram-negative bacteria of the genus *Legionella* cause Legionnaires' disease and Pontiac fever. Most cases of Legionnaires' disease are caused by *Legionella pneumophila*, but all species of *Legionella* can cause disease.

TRANSMISSION

The most common route of transmission is by inhalation of aerosolized water containing the bacteria, although transmission can sometimes occur through aspiration of water containing the bacteria. A single episode of possible person-to-person transmission of Legionnaires' disease has been reported.

Legionella is ubiquitous in freshwater sources worldwide, but quantities of *Legionella* in these environments are insufficient to cause disease. In the built environment, *Legionella* can amplify in water systems, depending on the conditions. Factors associated with amplification include warm water temperatures of 77°F–108°F [25°C–42°C]); water stagnation; presence of scale, sediment, and biofilm in the pipes and fixtures; and absence of disinfectant.

To cause disease, *Legionella* spp. must be aerosolized and inhaled by a susceptible host. The most common sources of transmission include potable water (via showerheads and faucets), cooling towers, hot tubs, and decorative fountains.

EPIDEMIOLOGY

Legionella growth and transmission can occur anywhere in the world when the right conditions exist. The capacity to diagnose and report cases of Legionnaires' disease is better established, however, in industrialized settings. In the United States, the incidence of Legionnaires' disease is increasing; the number of reported Legionnaires' disease cases increased nearly 900% between 2000 and 2018.

Legionnaires' disease cases and outbreaks have been reported worldwide. Large outbreaks associated with cooling towers were reported in Spain in 2001 (449 confirmed cases) and Portugal in 2014 (377 cases). In 2015, a cooling tower in Bronx, New York, was associated with 138 cases of Legionnaires' disease. Travel-associated outbreaks have also been reported. In 2015, 114 cases (11 confirmed Legionnaires' disease, 29 suspected Legionnaires' disease, and 74 Pontiac fever cases) were identified among visitors to a hotel in Chicago, Illinois; and during 2016–2017, 51 confirmed cases of Legionnaires' disease were associated with travel to Dubai.

5

Despite the presence of *Legionella* spp. in many aquatic environments, the risk of developing Legionnaires' disease is low for most people. Travelers who are >50 years old, are current or former smokers, have chronic lung conditions, or are immunocompromised are at increased risk for infection when exposed to aerosolized water containing *Legionella* spp. Travel-associated Legionnaires' disease outbreaks can occur on cruise ships, in hotels, and at resorts. A common feature among these settings is the presence of a large, often complex, water system that can be challenging to maintain properly.

Approximately 10% of all reported cases of Legionnaires' disease in the United States occur in people who have traveled during the 10 days before symptom onset. Exposures among travelers can occur when a person is in or near a hot tub, showering in a hotel, standing near a decorative fountain, or touring in cities with buildings that have cooling towers. Patients with Legionnaires' disease often do not recall specific water exposures because exposure frequently occurs during normal activities.

CLINICAL PRESENTATION

Legionellosis is primarily composed of 2 clinically and epidemiologically distinct syndromes: Legionnaires' disease and Pontiac fever. Though rare, *Legionella* spp. have also been associated with disease outside of the lungs (extrapulmonary). Legionnaires' disease typically presents with severe pneumonia, which usually requires hospitalization and can be fatal in ≈10% of cases. Symptom onset occurs 2–10 days (rarely, ≤19 days) after exposure. In outbreak settings, <5% of people exposed to the source of the outbreak develop Legionnaires' disease. Nearly all cases of legionellosis in the United States are reported as Legionnaires' disease.

Pontiac fever is milder than Legionnaires' disease and presents with fever, headache, or muscle aches, but no signs of pneumonia. Pontiac fever can affect healthy people as well as those with underlying illnesses, and symptoms occur within 72 hours of exposure. Nearly all patients fully recover without antimicrobial drug therapy or hospitalization. Up to 95% of people exposed during outbreaks of Pontiac fever can develop symptoms of disease.

DIAGNOSIS

The preferred diagnostic tests for Legionnaires' disease are the *Legionella* urinary antigen test and culture of lower respiratory secretions (sputum, bronchoalveolar lavage) on media that supports growth of *Legionella* spp. The most common diagnostic test, the urinary antigen test, only detects *L. pneumophila* serogroup 1; this serogroup accounts for 80%–90% of cases.

Isolation of *Legionella* by culture is important to detect non–*L. pneumophila* serogroup 1 infections and is necessary to compare clinical to environmental isolates during an outbreak investigation. Diagnosis by PCR of lower respiratory secretions also is possible, but the number of commercially available tests is limited. Because of differences in the mechanisms of disease, *Legionella* spp. cannot be isolated in people who have Pontiac fever. Legionnaires' disease, Pontiac fever, and extrapulmonary legionellosis are nationally notifiable diseases in the United States.

TREATMENT

For travelers with suspected Legionnaires' disease, administer specific antimicrobial drug treatment promptly while diagnostic tests are being processed. Preferred antimicrobial agents include fluoroquinolones and macrolides. Patients with severe cases might have prolonged intensive care unit stays. Treating physicians should consult with an infectious disease specialist. Because Pontiac fever is a self-limited illness, antimicrobial drugs have no benefit, and treatment is focused on supportive care.

PREVENTION

No vaccine for Legionnaires' disease is available, and antibiotic prophylaxis is not effective. Water management programs for building water systems and devices at risk for *Legionella* growth and transmission can lower the potential for illnesses and outbreaks. Travelers at increased risk for infection, such as older people or people with immunocompromising conditions (e.g., cancer, diabetes), might choose to avoid high-risk exposures (e.g., hot tubs). If exposure cannot be avoided, travelers should seek medical attention promptly if they develop symptoms of Legionnaires' disease or Pontiac fever.

CDC website: www.cdc.gov/legionella

BIBLIOGRAPHY

Centers for Disease Control and Prevention. Surveillance for travel-associated Legionnaires' disease—United States, 2005–2006. MMWR Morb Mortal Wkly Rep. 2007;56(48):1261–3.

Centers for Disease Control and Prevention. Vital signs: deficiencies in environmental control identified in outbreaks of Legionnaires' disease—North America, 2000–2014. MMWR Morb Mortal Wkly Rep. 2016;65(22):576–84.

Chitasombat MN, Ratchatanawin N, Visessiri Y. Disseminated extrapulmonary *Legionella pneumophila* infection presenting with panniculitis: case report and literature review. BMC Infect Dis. 2018;18(1):467.

Dabrera G, Brandsema P, Lofdahl M, Naik F, Cameron R, et al. Increase in Legionnaires' disease cases associated with travel to Dubai among travelers from the United Kingdom, Sweden, and the Netherlands, October 2016 to end August 2017. Euro Surveill. 2017;22(38):1–4.

de Jong B, Payne Hallstrom L, Robesyn E, Ursut D, Zucs P, Eldsnet. Travel-associated Legionnaires' disease in Europe, 2010. Euro Surveill. 2013;18(23):1–8.

George F, Shivaji T, Pinto CS, Serra LAO, Valente J, Albuquerque MJ, et al. A large outbreak of Legionnaires' disease in an industrial town in Portugal [in Portuguese]. Rev Port Saude Publica. 2016;34(3):199–208.

Mouchtouri VA, Rudge JW. Legionnaires' disease in hotels and passenger ships: a systematic review of evidence, sources, and contributing factors. J Travel Med. 2015;22(5):325–37.

Smith S, Ritger K, Samala U, Black S, Okodua M, et al. (2015). Legionellosis outbreak associated with a hotel fountain. Open Forum Infect Dis. 2015;2(4):ofv164.

LEPTOSPIROSIS

Ilana Schafer, Renee Galloway, Robyn Stoddard

INFECTIOUS AGENT: *Leptospira* spp.	
ENDEMICITY	Worldwide, higher incidence in tropical areas
TRAVELER CATEGORIES AT GREATEST RISK FOR EXPOSURE & INFECTION	Adventure tourists, outdoor athletes, and others exposed to fresh water or mud Humanitarian aid workers, particularly at sites of hurricanes or floods Military personnel
PREVENTION METHODS	Avoid contact with animal urine and water or soil contaminated with animal urine Use personal protective equipment Use chemoprophylaxis
DIAGNOSTIC SUPPORT	A clinical laboratory certified in high complexity testing; state health department; or contact CDC's Bacterial Special Pathogens Branch (bspb@cdc.gov) for additional identification and genotyping, molecular detection, or serology.

INFECTIOUS AGENT

Leptospira spp., the causative agent of leptospirosis, are obligate aerobic, gram-negative spirochete bacteria.

TRANSMISSION

Leptospira are transmitted through abrasions or cuts in the skin, or through the conjunctiva and mucous membranes. Macerated skin resulting from prolonged water exposure is another suspected route of infection. Humans can be infected by direct contact with urine or reproductive fluids from infected animals, through contact with urine-contaminated freshwater sources or wet soil, or by consuming contaminated food or water. Infection rarely occurs through animal bites or human-to-human contact. Rodents are an important reservoir for *Leptospira*, but most mammals, including dogs, horses, cattle, and swine, and many wildlife species, can be infected and shed the bacteria in their urine.

EPIDEMIOLOGY

Leptospirosis has a worldwide distribution; incidence is greater in tropical climates, however. Regions with the highest estimated morbidity and mortality include parts of sub-Saharan Africa, parts of Latin America, and in the Caribbean, South and Southeast Asia, and Oceania. Travelers to endemic areas are at increased risk when participating in recreational freshwater activities (e.g., boating, swimming), particularly after heavy rainfall or flooding. Prolonged exposure to contaminated water and activities that involve head immersion or swallowing water increase the risk for infection.

Participating in activities involving mud (e.g., adventure races) also increases a traveler's risk for infection, as does working directly with animals in endemic areas, especially when exposed to their body fluids, and visiting or residing in areas with rodent infestation. Leptospirosis occurs most commonly in adult males. The estimated worldwide annual incidence is >1 million cases, including ≈59,000 deaths.

Outbreaks can occur after heavy rainfall or flooding in endemic areas, especially in urban areas of low- and middle-income countries, where housing conditions and sanitation are poor and rodent infestation is common. Outbreaks of leptospirosis have occurred after flooding in popular US travel destinations, including Florida, Hawaii, Puerto Rico, and the US Virgin Islands. Nearly half of the leptospirosis cases reported in the continental United States during 2014–2018 that had an identified geographic source of infection were associated with international travel. Most US cases are reported outside the continental United States in the domestic travel destinations of Hawaii and Puerto Rico.

CLINICAL PRESENTATION

The incubation period for leptospirosis is 2–30 days, but illness usually occurs 5–14 days after exposure. Most infections are thought to be asymptomatic, but clinical illness can present as a self-limiting acute febrile illness, estimated to occur in ≈90% of clinical infections, or as a severe, potentially fatal illness with multiorgan dysfunction in 5%–10% of patients. In patients who progress to severe disease, the illness can be biphasic, with a temporary decrease in fever between phases.

The acute, septicemic phase lasts ≈7 days and presents as an acute febrile illness with symptoms including headache, which can be severe and include photophobia and retro-orbital pain; chills; myalgias, characteristically involving the calves and lower back; conjunctival suffusion, characteristic of leptospirosis but not occurring in all cases; nausea; vomiting; diarrhea; abdominal pain; cough; and rarely, a skin rash.

The second or immune phase is characterized by antibody production and the presence of leptospires in the urine. In patients who progress to severe disease, clinical findings can include cardiac arrhythmias, hemodynamic collapse, hemorrhage, jaundice, liver failure, aseptic meningitis, pulmonary insufficiency, and renal failure. The classically described syndrome, Weil's disease, consists of renal and liver failure.

Among patients with severe disease, the case-fatality ratio is 5%–15%. Severe pulmonary hemorrhagic syndrome is a rare but severe form of leptospirosis that can have a case-fatality ratio >50%. Poor prognostic indicators include older age, development of altered mental status, respiratory insufficiency, or oliguria.

DIAGNOSIS

Submit a combination of samples for leptospirosis testing, including serum samples; whenever possible, obtain acute and convalescent sample pairs. During early disease, PCR analysis of whole blood (collected in the first week of illness) and urine (collected after the first week of illness) can be helpful. PCR analysis of cerebrospinal fluid (CSF) also can be helpful in diagnosing patients with signs of meningitis.

Diagnosis of leptospirosis is often based on serology; microscopic agglutination test (MAT) is the reference standard and can only be performed at certain reference laboratories. Various serologic screening tests are available at commercial laboratories, including ELISA and ImmunoDOT/DotBlot rapid diagnostic tests. The use of IgM-specific serologic screening tests is recommended, and positive screening tests should be confirmed with MAT.

Detection of the organism in acute whole blood using real-time PCR can provide a more timely diagnosis during the early, septicemic phase, and PCR also can be performed on CSF or convalescent urine. A positive PCR result is confirmatory for infection. Culture is insensitive, slow, and requires special media; it is therefore not recommended as the sole diagnostic method.

The Zoonoses and Select Agent Laboratory at the Centers for Disease Control and Prevention (CDC) performs MAT and PCR for diagnosis of leptospirosis as well as culture identification and genotyping of isolates. Clinicians can find information on diagnostic testing at CDC and sample submission instructions at www.cdc.gov/ncezid/dhcpp/bacterial_special/zoonoses_lab.html. Clinicians can consult on a suspected leptospirosis case by contacting CDC's Bacterial Special Pathogens Branch, by calling the CDC Emergency Operations Center (770-488-7100). Leptospirosis is a nationally notifiable disease, and the Council for State and Territorial Epidemiologists' case definition can be found at https://ndc.services.cdc.gov/case-definitions/leptospirosis-2013.

TREATMENT

If leptospirosis is suspected, initiate antimicrobial therapy as soon as possible, without waiting for diagnostic test results. Early treatment can be effective in decreasing the severity and duration of infection. For patients with mild symptoms, doxycycline is a drug of choice, unless contraindicated; alternative options include ampicillin, amoxicillin, or azithromycin. Intravenous penicillin is the drug of choice for patients with severe leptospirosis; ceftriaxone and cefotaxime are alternative antimicrobial agents. As with other spirochetal diseases, antibiotic treatment of patients with leptospirosis might cause a Jarisch-Herxheimer reaction; the reaction is rarely fatal. Patients with severe leptospirosis might require hospitalization and supportive therapy, including intravenous hydration and electrolyte supplementation, dialysis in cases of oliguric renal failure, and mechanical ventilation in cases of respiratory failure.

5

PREVENTION

The best way to prevent infection is to avoid exposure. Advise travelers to avoid exposure to potentially contaminated bodies of freshwater, flood waters, potentially infected animals or their body fluids, and areas with rodent infestation. Educate travelers who might be at increased risk for infection to consider taking additional preventive measures (e.g., wearing protective clothing, especially footwear), instructing them to cover cuts and abrasions with occlusive dressings, counseling them on boiling or chemically treating potentially contaminated drinking water, and providing chemoprophylaxis. Limited studies have shown that chemoprophylaxis with doxycycline (200 mg orally, weekly) begun 1–2 days before and continuing through the period of exposure, might be effective in preventing clinical disease in adults and could be considered for people at high risk and with short-term exposures. No human vaccine is available in the United States.

CDC website: www.cdc.gov/leptospirosis

BIBLIOGRAPHY

Brett-Major DM, Coldren R. Antibiotics for leptospirosis. Cochrane Database Syst Rev. 2012;(2):CD008264.

Brett-Major DM, Lipnick RJ. Antibiotic prophylaxis for leptospirosis. Cochrane Database Syst Rev. 2009;(3):CD007342.

Costa F, Hagan JE, Calcagno J, Kane M, Torgerson P, Martinez-Silveira MS, et al. Global morbidity and mortality of leptospirosis: a systematic review. PLoS Negl Trop Dis. 2015;9(9):e0003898.

Haake DA, Levett PN. Leptospira species (leptospirosis). In: Bennett JE, Dolin R, Blaser MJ, editors. Principles and practice of infectious diseases, 8th edition. Philadelphia: Saunders; 2015. pp. 2714–20.

Haake DA, Levett PN. Leptospirosis in humans. Curr Top Microbiol Immunol. 2015;387:65–97.

Jensenius M, Han PV, Schlagenhauf P, Schwartz E, Parola P, Castelli F, et al. Acute and potentially life-threatening tropical diseases in western travelers—a GeoSentinel multicenter study, 1996–2011. Am J Trop Med Hyg. 2013;88(2):397–404.

Lau C, Smythe L, Weinstein P. Leptospirosis: an emerging disease in travellers. Travel Med Infect Dis. 2010;8(1):33–9.

Marinova-Petkova A, Guendel I, Strysko JP, Ekpo LL, Galloway R, Yoder J, et al. First reported human cases of leptospirosis in the United States Virgin Islands in the aftermath of Hurricanes Irma and Maria, September–November 2017. Open Forum Infect Dis. 2019;6(7):ofz261.

Picardeau M, Bertherat E, Jancloes M, Skouloudis AN, Durski K, Hartskeerl RA. Rapid tests for diagnosis of leptospirosis: current tools and emerging technologies. Diagn Microbiol Infect Dis. 2014;78(1):1–8.

Sejvar J, Bancroft E, Winthrop K, Bettinger J, Bajani M, Bragg S, et al. Leptospirosis in "Eco-Challenge" athletes, Malaysian Borneo, 2000. Emerg Infect Dis. 2003;9(6):702–7.

5

LYME DISEASE

Paul Mead, David McCormick

INFECTIOUS AGENT: *Borrelia burgdorferi* sensu lato complex	
ENDEMICITY	North America, in the Northeast, mid-Atlantic, and upper Midwest of the United States Northern Asia (temperate forest regions) Europe
TRAVELER CATEGORIES AT GREATEST RISK FOR EXPOSURE & INFECTION	Adventure tourists Long-term travelers and expatriates
PREVENTION METHODS	Avoid tick bites
DIAGNOSTIC SUPPORT	A clinical laboratory certified in moderate complexity testing; Contact CDC's Division of Vector-Borne Diseases (970-221-6400; dvbid@cdc.gov)

INFECTIOUS AGENT

Lyme disease is caused by spirochetes belonging to the *Borrelia burgdorferi* sensu lato complex, including *B. afzelii*, *B. burgdorferi* sensu stricto, and *B. garinii*.

TRANSMISSION

Borrelia spirochetes are transmitted through the bite of infected *Ixodes* (blacklegged) ticks, typically immature (nymphal) ticks. Nymphal ticks are small, about the size of a poppy seed, and elude easy detection. Patients with Lyme disease might be unaware that they were ever bitten.

EPIDEMIOLOGY

Borrelia transmission has not been documented in the tropics. In Europe, Lyme disease is endemic from southern Scandinavia into the northern Mediterranean countries of Greece, Italy, and

Spain, and east from the British Isles into central Russia. Incidence is greatest in central and eastern European countries. In Asia, infected ticks range from western Russia through Mongolia, northeastern China, and into Japan; human infection appears to be uncommon in most of these areas, however. In North America, highly endemic areas include the northeastern and north-central United States.

Lyme disease is occasionally reported in travelers to the United States returning to their home countries. Consider Lyme disease in the differential diagnosis of patients with consistent symptoms and a history of camping, hiking, or outdoor activities. Some case reports describe Lyme disease in Australian and US travelers returning from Europe and endemic regions of the United States, but no data are available regarding the incidence of travel-acquired infection.

CLINICAL PRESENTATION

The incubation period of Lyme disease is typically 3–30 days. Approximately 80% of people infected with *B. burgdorferi* develop a characteristic rash, erythema migrans (EM), within 30 days of exposure. EM is a red, expanding rash, with or without central clearing, often accompanied by symptoms of fatigue, fever, headache, mild stiff neck, arthralgia, or myalgia.

Within days or weeks, infection can spread to other parts of the body, causing more serious neurologic conditions (meningitis, radiculopathy, and facial palsy) or cardiac abnormalities (myocarditis with atrioventricular heart block). Left untreated, infection can progress over several months to cause monoarticular or oligoarticular arthritis, peripheral neuropathy, or rarely, encephalopathy. These long-term sequelae can occur over variable periods of time, ranging from months to years.

Infection with European strains of *Borrelia* can result in manifestations rarely seen in the United States, specifically lymphocytoma, an acute blister-like lesion, and acrodermatitis chronica atrophicans, characterized by atrophic patches of bluish-red skin that develop over a period of years and typically involve the extremities.

DIAGNOSIS

In people with a history of recent travel to an endemic area (with or without a recollection of a tick bite) a diagnosis of Lyme disease can be made by identifying an EM rash. For patients with evidence of disseminated infection (cardiac, musculoskeletal, neurologic manifestations), serologic testing using commercial assays can aid in diagnosis. Lyme disease is nationally notifiable.

Serological tests used to diagnose domestically acquired Lyme disease might not reliably identify infections acquired internationally. Some laboratories offer testing for additional *Borrelia* species that cause Lyme disease in Europe but are not found in the United States. These tests are only appropriate for people with a history of travel outside the United States. For diagnostic support, contact the Centers for Disease Control and Prevention (CDC)'s Division of Vector-Borne Diseases (970-221-6400; dvbid@cdc.gov).

TREATMENT

Most patients can be treated with oral doxycycline, amoxicillin, or cefuroxime axetil; or with intravenous ceftriaxone (for details, see www.cdc.gov/lyme). Diagnosis and management of disseminated infection can be complicated and may require referral to an infectious disease specialist or rheumatologist.

PREVENTION

Advise patients to avoid tick habitats (e.g., wooded, brushy, or grassy areas); use an Environmental Protection Agency–registered insect repellent on exposed skin and clothing; and carefully check every day for attached ticks. Instruct patients to minimize areas of exposed skin by wearing long-sleeved shirts, long pants, and closed shoes, and to tuck in shirts and tuck pants into socks to help reduce risk for tick bites (see Sec. 4, Ch. 6, Mosquitoes, Ticks & Other Arthropods).

CDC website: www.cdc.gov/lyme

BIBLIOGRAPHY

Hu LT. Lyme disease. Ann Intern Med. 2016;165(9):677.

Lantos PM, Rumbaugh J, Bockenstedt LK, Falck-Ytter YT, Aguero-Rosenfeld ME, Auwaerter PG, et al. Clinical practice guidelines by the Infectious Diseases Society of America (IDSA), American Academy of Neurology (AAN), and American College of Rheumatology (ACR): 2020 guidelines for the prevention, diagnosis and treatment of Lyme disease. Clin Infect Dis. 2021;72(1):1–8.

Sanchez E, Vannier E, Wormser GP, Hu LT. Diagnosis, treatment, and prevention of Lyme disease, human granulocytic anaplasmosis, and babesiosis: a review. JAMA. 2016;315(16):1767–77.

Steere AC, Strle F, Wormser GP, Hu LT, Branda JA, Hovius JW, et al. Lyme borreliosis. Nat Rev Dis Primers. 2016;2:16090.

MELIOIDOSIS

Lindy Liu, Jay Gee, David Blaney

INFECTIOUS AGENT: *Burkholderia pseudomallei*	
ENDEMICITY	Tropical and subtropical regions worldwide Primarily Southeast Asia, South Asia, and Australia Some parts of Africa, the Americas, and Middle East
TRAVELER CATEGORIES AT GREATEST RISK FOR EXPOSURE & INFECTION	Adventure travelers and ecotourists Construction and resource extraction workers Military personnel Travelers who contact contaminated soil or water
PREVENTION METHODS	Avoid contaminated soil and water
DIAGNOSTIC SUPPORT	A clinical laboratory certified in high complexity testing; state health department; or contact CDC's Bacterial Special Pathogens Branch (bspb@cdc.gov) for additional support

INFECTIOUS AGENT

Burkholderia pseudomallei, a saprophytic gram-negative bacillus, is the causative agent of melioidosis. The bacteria are found in soil and water and are widely distributed in tropical and subtropical countries.

TRANSMISSION

B. pseudomallei can infect both animals and humans through damaged skin (e.g., open wounds, cuts, burns) or mucous membranes. Damaged skin coming in direct contact with contaminated soil or water is the most frequent route for natural infection. Ingestion and inhalation are two other routes of infection. The risk of spread from person-to-person is considered extremely low as there are few documented cases of transmission via this route.

EPIDEMIOLOGY

Melioidosis goes underreported or unrecognized in many tropical and subtropical areas; >165,000 cases are estimated to occur annually, mainly in Southeast Asia and in northern Australia. *B. pseudomallei* is endemic to Southeast Asia, Papua New Guinea, much of the Indian subcontinent, southern China, Hong Kong, and Taiwan. It is considered highly endemic to northeast Thailand, Malaysia, Singapore, and northern Australia.

B. pseudomallei has also been found in the Americas, including the Caribbean and the Gulf Coast of the United States (Mississippi).

Sporadic cases of disease have been reported among residents of or travelers to Aruba, British Virgin Islands, Colombia, Costa Rica, Ecuador, El Salvador, Guatemala, Guadeloupe, Guyana, Honduras, Martinique, Mexico, Panama, Peru, Puerto Rico, US Virgin Islands, and Venezuela. Clusters of melioidosis have been reported in northeastern Brazil. The true extent of distribution the bacteria remains unknown.

Among the average of 12 melioidosis cases reported annually to the Centers for Disease Control and Prevention (CDC), most occur in people with a history of recent travel to a region where *B. pseudomallei* is known to be endemic. Risk for infection is greatest for adventure travelers, construction and resource extraction workers, ecotourists, military personnel, and other people whose contact with contaminated soil or water might expose them to the bacteria. The bacteria can also be present in untreated water and raw or undercooked food. Infections have been reported in people who spent <1 week in an endemic area. Cases, especially those presenting as pneumonia, are often associated with periods of high rainfall (e.g., during typhoons or the monsoon season).

Even in regions where melioidosis is highly endemic (e.g., northern Australia, Thailand), most healthy people exposed to *B. pseudomallei* never develop melioidosis. People with certain conditions, however, are at greater risk for disease. Risk factors for developing melioidosis include diabetes, excessive alcohol use, chronic lung disease (e.g., chronic obstructive pulmonary disease or cystic fibrosis), chronic renal disease, thalassemia, and malignancy or other non-HIV–related immune suppression.

CLINICAL PRESENTATION

Incubation period is generally 1–21 days, with a median of 4 days; people who receive a high inoculum can become symptomatic within a few hours. Melioidosis also can remain latent for months or years before symptoms develop. It can present as a localized infection, pneumonia, bacteremia, or disseminated infection involving any organ, including the brain.

Symptoms are nonspecific and will vary depending on the route of infection. Symptoms can include abdominal discomfort; abscesses or ulcerations; chest pain, cough, and respiratory distress; disorientation, headache, and seizures; fever; localized pain and swelling; muscle or joint pain; and weight loss. Patients generally present with acute illness, but ≈9% present with ≥2 months of symptoms. Chronic melioidosis often mimics *Mycobacterium tuberculosis* infection clinically. Subclinical infection is also possible.

DIAGNOSIS

Prompt diagnosis and treatment are critical. Guided by clinical syndrome, collect specimens from all relevant infection sites for culture. Depending on the site(s) of suspected infection, recommended specimens for collection include blood, cerebrospinal fluid, pericardial fluid, peritoneal fluid, purulent exudate (from skin or internal abscesses), sputum, synovial fluid, and urine; throat and rectal swabs can also be collected. Culturing *B. pseudomallei* from any clinical specimen is diagnostic for melioidosis because the bacterium is not considered part of the natural microbiota. Alert clinical laboratory personnel in advance that specimen cultures may grow *B. pseudomallei* and to follow proper safety precautions.

Although an indirect hemagglutination assay (IHA) is widely used, no serologic test can confirm melioidosis. In the United States, the Laboratory Response Network (https://emergency.cdc.gov/lrn) can perform confirmatory testing on isolates. CDC laboratories can conduct confirmatory testing in addition to other complex tests (e.g., antimicrobial susceptibility testing, IHA, and genetic analysis by whole-genome sequencing). Submissions to CDC are handled through coordination with local or state public health labs; clinicians should consult local or state public health departments to arrange testing. Information and procedures for submitting specimens to CDC's Bacterial Special Pathogens Branch in the Division of High-Consequence Pathogens and Pathology are available at www.cdc.gov/ncezid/dhcpp/bacterial_special/zoonoses_lab.html.

TREATMENT

Treatment of melioidosis requires long-term antibiotic therapy (acute phase followed by eradication phase), and consultation with an infectious disease or tropical medicine specialist is strongly advised. Intravenous ceftazidime, or meropenem for severe cases with sepsis, is typically used for initial treatment, for a minimum of 14 days.

BOX 5-01 Melioidosis infection precautions: a checklist for travelers visiting areas where *Burkholderia pseudomallei* is endemic

- ☐ Avoid contact with soil or muddy water, particularly after heavy rains
- ☐ Protect open wounds, cuts, or burns. Use waterproof bandages to help keep damaged skin from contacting soil or water. Thoroughly wash any open wounds, cut, or burns that contact soil.
- ☐ For people with diabetes, foot care and preventing contamination of foot or other open wounds is important.
- ☐ Wear protective footwear and gloves when doing yard work, agricultural work.
- ☐ Wear waterproof boots during and after flooding or storms to prevent infection through the feet and lower legs.
- ☐ Avoid drinking untreated water and eating undercooked or raw foods.

5

Depending on response to therapy, clinicians can extend intravenous treatment for up to 8 weeks in severe cases. After initial treatment, provide 3–6 months of eradication treatment with oral trimethoprim-sulfamethoxazole (TMP-SMX) or amoxicillin-clavulanic acid (for patients unable to tolerate TMP-SMX). Relapses can occur, especially in patients who receive a shorter-than-recommended course of therapy.

PREVENTION

People who live in or who visit areas where *B. pseudomallei* is endemic—especially those individuals with underlying health conditions that place them at increased risk for developing melioidosis—should follow the precautions listed in Box 5-01.

CDC website: www.cdc.gov/melioidosis

BIBLIOGRAPHY

Benoit TJ, Blaney DD, Doker TJ, Gee JE, Elrod MG, Rolim DB, et al. A review of melioidosis cases in the Americas. Am J Trop Med Hyg. 2015;93(6):1134–9.

CDC Health Alert Network (HAN). HAN no. 470: Melioidosis locally endemic in areas of the Mississippi Gulf Coast after *Burkholderia pseudomallei* isolated in soil and water and linked to two cases—Mississippi, 2020 and 2022. Available from: https://emergency.cdc.gov/han/2022/han00470.asp.

Cheng JW, Hayden MK, Singh K, Heimler I, Gee JE, Proia L, et al. *Burkholderia pseudomallei* infection in US traveler returning from Mexico, 2014. Emerg Infect Dis. 2015;21(10):1884–5.

Currie BJ. Melioidosis: evolving concepts in epidemiology, pathogenesis, and treatment. Semin Respir Crit Care Med. 2015;36(1):111–25.

Currie BJ, Mayo M, Ward LM, Kaestli M, Meumann EM, Webb JR, et al. The Darwin prospective melioidosis study: a 30-year prospective, observational investigation. Lancet Infect Dis. 2021;21(12):1737–46.

Doker TJ, Sharp TM, Rivera-Garcia B, Perez-Padilla J, Benoit TJ, Ellis EM, et al. Contact investigation of melioidosis cases reveals regional endemicity in Puerto Rico. Clin Infect Dis. 2015;60(2):243–50.

Gee JE, Bower WA, Kunkel A, Petras J, Gettings J, Bye M, et al. Multistate outbreak of melioidosis associated with imported aromatherapy spray. N Engl J Med. 2022;386(9):861–8.

Limmathurotsakul D, Golding N, Dance DA, Messina JP, Pigott DM, Moyes CL, et al. Predicted global distribution of *Burkholderia pseudomallei* and burden of melioidosis. Nat Microbiol. 2016;1:15008.

Limmathurotsakul D, Kanoksil M, Wuthiekanun V, Kitphati R, deStavola B, Day NP, et al. Activities of daily living associated with acquisition of melioidosis in northeast Thailand: a matched case-control study. PLoS Negl Trop Dis. 2013;7(2):e2072.

Wiersinga WJ, Virk HS, Torres AG, Currie BJ, Peacock SJ, Dance DAB, et al. Melioidosis. Nat Rev Dis Primers. 2018;4:17107.

MENINGOCOCCAL DISEASE

Lucy McNamara, Amy Blain

INFECTIOUS AGENT: *Neisseria meningitidis*	
ENDEMICITY	Worldwide, but greatest incidence occurs in the meningitis belt of Africa (see Map 5-01)
TRAVELER CATEGORIES AT GREATEST RISK FOR EXPOSURE & INFECTION	Unvaccinated travelers to countries in the meningitis belt, particularly travelers having prolonged contact with local populations during an epidemic
PREVENTION METHODS	Meningococcal disease is vaccine-preventable
DIAGNOSTIC SUPPORT	A clinical laboratory certified in moderate complexity testing; state health department

INFECTIOUS AGENT

Neisseria meningitidis is a gram-negative diplococcus bacterium. Meningococci are classified into serogroups based on the composition of their capsular polysaccharide. The 6 major meningococcal serogroups associated with disease are A, B, C, W, X, and Y.

TRANSMISSION

Meningococci spread through respiratory secretions and require close contact for transmission. Both asymptomatic carriers and people with overt meningococcal disease can be sources of infection. Asymptomatic carriage is transient and typically affects ≈5%–10% of the population at any given time.

EPIDEMIOLOGY

N. meningitidis is found worldwide, but incidence is greatest in the "meningitis belt" of sub-Saharan Africa (Map 5-01). Meningococcal disease is hyperendemic in this region, and periodic epidemics during the dry season (December–June) reach an incidence of up to 1,000 cases per 100,000 population. By contrast, rates of disease in Australia, Europe, South America, and the United States range from 0.10–2.4 cases per 100,000 population per year.

Although meningococcal disease outbreaks can occur anywhere in the world, they are most common in the African meningitis belt, where large-scale epidemics occur every 5–12 years. Historically, outbreaks in the meningitis belt were primarily due to serogroup A. With the introduction of a monovalent serogroup A meningococcal conjugate vaccine (MenAfriVac) in the region starting in 2010, however, recent meningococcal outbreaks in the meningitis belt have primarily been caused by serogroups C and W; serogroup X outbreaks also have been reported.

Outside the meningitis belt, infants, adolescents, and adults >80 years of age have the highest rates of disease. In meningitis belt countries, high rates of disease are seen in people ≤30 years old; the highest rates are in children and adolescents aged 5–14 years.

Unvaccinated travelers visiting meningitis belt countries and having prolonged contact with local populations during an epidemic are at greatest risk for meningococcal disease. The Hajj pilgrimage to Saudi Arabia also has been associated with outbreaks of meningococcal disease among returning pilgrims and their contacts, including 4 cases in travelers from the United States during a large Hajj-associated outbreak in 2000.

CLINICAL PRESENTATION

Meningococcal disease generally occurs 1–10 days after exposure and presents as meningitis in ≈50% of cases in the United States. Meningococcal

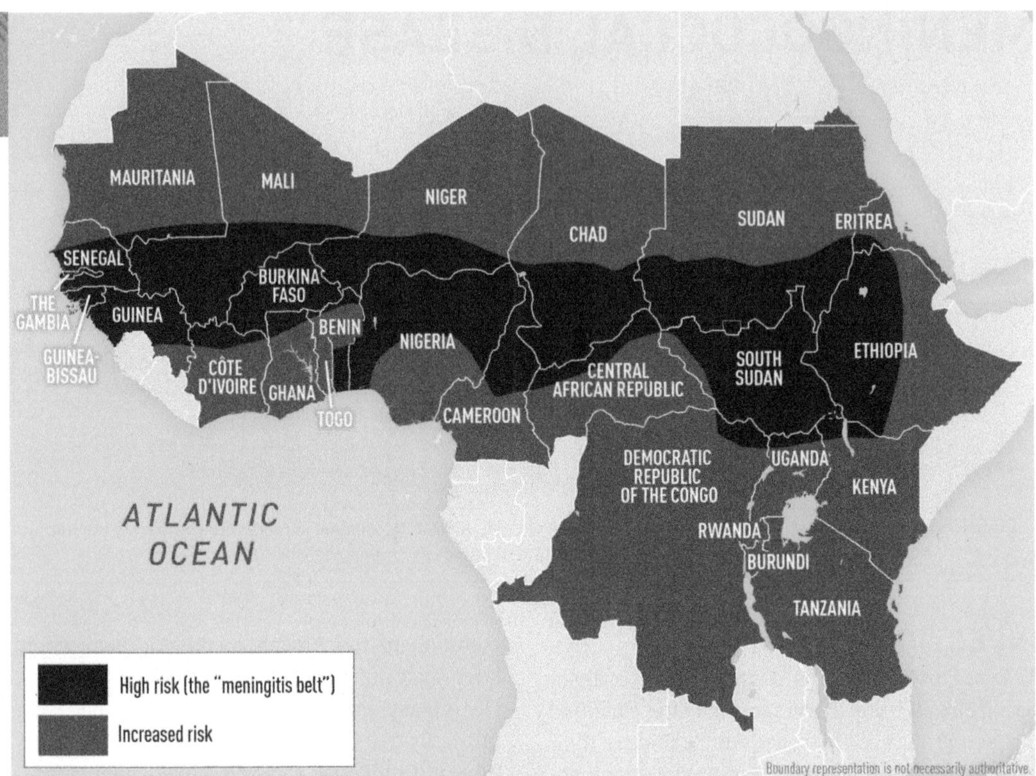

MAP 5-01 The meningitis belt & other areas at risk for meningococcal meningitis epidemics
Disease data source: World Health Organization. International Travel and Health. Geneva, Switzerland: 2015.

meningitis is characterized by sudden onset of headache, fever, and neck stiffness, sometimes accompanied by nausea, vomiting, photophobia, or altered mental status. Meningococcal disease progresses rapidly and has a case-fatality rate of 10%–15%, even with antimicrobial drug treatment. Without rapid treatment, fatality rates can be much higher.

Approximately 30% of people with meningococcal disease present with meningococcal sepsis, known as meningococcemia. Symptoms of meningococcemia can include abrupt onset of fever, chills, vomiting, diarrhea, and a petechial or purpuric rash, which can progress to purpura fulminans. Meningococcemia often involves hypotension, acute adrenal hemorrhage, and multiorgan failure. An additional 15% of meningococcal disease cases in the United States, primarily among adults >65 years of age, present as bacteremic pneumonia.

Other presentations (e.g., septic arthritis) also occur. Among infants and children aged <2 years, meningococcal disease can have nonspecific symptoms. Neck stiffness, usually seen in people with meningitis, might be absent in this age group.

DIAGNOSIS

Early diagnosis and treatment are critical. If bacterial meningitis is suspected, collect blood for culture right away and perform a lumbar puncture (LP) to collect cerebrospinal fluid (CSF) for microscopic examination and Gram stain. In general, diagnosis is made by isolating *N. meningitidis* from a normally sterile body site (e.g., blood, CSF) either by culture or by PCR detection of *N. meningitidis*–specific nucleic acid. State health departments can provide diagnostic and testing support if needed.

Signs and symptoms of meningococcal meningitis are like those of other causes of bacterial meningitis (e.g., *Haemophilus influenzae, Streptococcus pneumoniae*). Proper treatment and prophylaxis depend on correctly identifying the causative organism. Meningococcal disease is nationally notifiable in the United States; report cases to the state or local health department without delay.

TREATMENT

Meningococcal disease can be rapidly fatal and should always be viewed as a medical emergency. As soon as disease is suspected and blood cultures and CSF have been collected, deliver appropriate treatment; if the LP is to be delayed for any reason (e.g., imaging studies of the head prior to LP), administer antimicrobial drugs immediately after collecting blood cultures. Begin empiric antimicrobial drug treatment early and prior to receiving diagnostic test results.

Third-generation cephalosporins are recommended for empiric treatment. Although ampicillin or penicillin also can be used for treatment, determine meningococcal isolate susceptibility before switching to one of these antibiotics; recent reports indicate emerging penicillin resistance among meningococcal isolates in the United States. If a patient presents with suspected bacterial meningitis of uncertain etiology, some treatment algorithms recommend empiric use of dexamethasone in addition to an antimicrobial drug until a bacterial etiology is established; if meningococcal meningitis is confirmed or suspected, steroids can be discontinued.

PREVENTION

Vaccine

Five meningococcal vaccines (3 quadrivalent, 2 monovalent) are licensed and available in the United States. Travelers should receive vaccines 7–10 days before travel to enable time for protective antibody levels to develop. See Table 5-03 for more information about available meningococcal vaccines.

ROUTINE IMMUNIZATION

The Advisory Committee on Immunization Practices (ACIP) recommends routine administration of a quadrivalent meningococcal conjugate vaccine (MenACWY) for all people aged 11–18 years. Administer a single dose of vaccine to patients at age 11 or 12 years and a booster dose at age 16 years. Routine immunization with MenACWY is not recommended for other age groups in the United States, except for people at increased risk for meningococcal disease, including those with a persistent complement component deficiency (C3, C5-9, properdin, factor D, factor H); people taking a complement component inhibitor (e.g., eculizumab [Soliris] or ravulizumab [Ultomiris]); people who have functional or anatomic asplenia; or people with HIV. ACIP describes vaccine, product, number of doses, and booster dose recommendations, based on age and risk factors for each risk group, in Meningococcal Vaccination: Recommendations of the Advisory Committee on Immunization Practices, United States, 2020 (www.cdc.gov/mmwr/volumes/69/rr/rr6909a1.htm).

ACIP also recommends adolescents and young adults aged 16–23 years be vaccinated with a serogroup B meningococcal (MenB) vaccine series, based on shared clinical decision-making. A MenB vaccine series provides short-term protection against most strains of serogroup B meningococcus; 16–18 years is the optimal age for MenB vaccination. ACIP also recommends routine use of MenB vaccine for people aged ≥10 years who are at increased risk for meningococcal disease, including people who have persistent complement component deficiency and those with functional or anatomic asplenia. ACIP recommendations for use of MenB vaccines can be found in Meningococcal Vaccination: Recommendations of the Advisory Committee on Immunization Practices, United States, 2020 (www.cdc.gov/mmwr/volumes/69/rr/rr6909a1.htm).

IMMUNIZATION FOR TRAVELERS

QUADRIVALENT MENINGOCOCCAL CONJUGATE (MENACWY) VACCINES

ACIP recommends that travelers aged ≥2 months who visit or reside in parts of the meningitis belt of sub-Saharan Africa (see Map 5-01) during the dry season (December–June) receive vaccination with a MenACWY vaccine before travel. The Centers for Disease Control and Prevention (CDC) issues advisories for travelers to other countries when outbreaks of meningococcal disease are recognized; travelers should check the CDC Travelers' Health website (https://wwwnc.cdc.gov/travel/notices) before travel. There are 3 meningococcal vaccines licensed and available in

Table 5-03 Meningococcal vaccines licensed & available in the United States: recommendations for travelers to or residents of countries where meningococcal disease is hyperendemic or epidemic[1]

VACCINE	TRADE NAME (MANUFACTURER)	AGE AT VACCINE INITIATION	DOSE	SERIES
Meningococcal (serogroups A, C, W, and Y) oligosaccharide diphtheria CRM_{197} conjugate vaccine (MenACWY-CRM)	Menveo (GlaxoSmithKline)	2 months old	0.5 mL IM	4-dose series[2] DOSE 1: Infant is 2 months old DOSE 2: 2 months after DOSE 1 (infant is 4 months old) DOSE 3: 2 months after DOSE 2 (infant is 6 months old) DOSE 4: 6 months after DOSE 3 (infant is 12 months old)
		3–6 months old	0.5 mL IM	Multi-dose series[2] (number of doses depends on age at vaccine initiation) DOSE 1: Infant is between 3–6 months old SUBSEQUENT DOSES: After DOSE 1, give 1 dose every 8 weeks until the infant is ≥7 months old, then give 1 additional dose after the infant is ≥12 months old
		7–23 months old	0.5 mL IM	2-dose series[2] DOSE 1: Child is 7–23 months old DOSE 2: ≥12 weeks after DOSE 1 *and* the child is ≥12 months old
		≥2 years old	0.5 mL IM	1 dose[2,3]
Meningococcal (serogroups A, C, W, and Y) polysaccharide diphtheria toxoid conjugate vaccine (MenACWY-D)	Menactra (Sanofi Pasteur)	9–23 months old	0.5 mL IM	2-dose series[2] DOSE 1: Child is 9–23 months old DOSE 2: ≥12 weeks after DOSE 1[4]
		≥2 years old	0.5 mL IM	1 dose[2,3]

Meningococcal (serogroups A, C, W, and Y) polysaccharide tetanus toxoid conjugate vaccine (MenACWY-TT)	MenQuadfi (Sanofi Pasteur)	≥2 years old	0.5 mL IM	1 dose[2,3]
Meningococcal serogroup B vaccine (MenB-FHbp)[5]	Trumenba (Pfizer)	10–25 years old	0.5 mL IM	2-dose series[6,7,8] DOSE 1: Between 10–25 years old DOSE 2: 6 months after DOSE 1
Meningococcal serogroup B vaccine (MenB-4C)[5]	Bexsero (GlaxoSmithKline)	10–25 years old	0.5 mL IM	2-dose series[7,8] DOSE 1: Between 10–25 years old DOSE 2: ≥1 month after DOSE 1

Abbreviations: IM, intramuscular

[1]Source: TABLE 9. Recommended vaccination schedule and intervals for people who travel to or are residents of countries where meningococcal disease is hyperendemic or epidemic—Advisory Committee on Immunization Practices, United States, 2020 (www.cdc.gov/mmwr/volumes/69/rr/rr6909a1.htm#T9_down).

[2]For people at continued risk, revaccination (booster) with meningococcal conjugate vaccine (MenACWY-CRM, -D, or -TT) is recommended for the following age groups: <7 years old, a single dose 3 years after primary vaccination and every 5 years thereafter; ≥7 years old, a single dose 5 years after primary vaccination and every 5 years thereafter.

[3]A 2-dose primary series (DOSE 2 given 8–12 weeks after DOSE 1) is recommended for the following groups: people with HIV; people with anatomic or functional asplenia; people with persistent complement component deficiency (C3, C5-9, properdin, factor D, factor H); and people taking a complement component inhibitor (e.g., eculizumab [Soliris] or ravulizumab [Ultomiris]).

[4]Can be administered ≥8 weeks apart in travelers.

[5]MenB-FHbp and MenB-4C are not interchangeable; the same vaccine should be used for all doses, including booster doses.

[6]A 3-dose primary series (DOSE 2 given 1–2 months after DOSE 1; DOSE 3 given 6 months after DOSE 2) is recommended for the following groups: people with anatomic or functional asplenia; people with persistent complement component deficiency (C3, C5-9, properdin, factor D, factor H); people taking a complement component inhibitor (e.g., eculizumab [Soliris] or ravulizumab [Ultomiris]); microbiologists routinely exposed to *Neisseria meningitidis* isolates; and people at risk during a serogroup B meningococcal disease outbreak.

[7]A single booster dose of MenB vaccine is recommended for people at increased risk due to a serogroup B meningococcus outbreak if they completed the MenB primary series ≥1 year prior (≥6 months might also be considered by public health professionals). See: www.cdc.gov/meningococcal/downloads/meningococcal-outbreak-guidance.pdf.

[8]A booster dose of MenB vaccine is recommended 1 year after completion of the primary vaccination series and every 2–3 years thereafter for people who remain at increased risk of serogroup B meningococcal disease for any other reason.

the United States for children; the age at vaccine initiation and schedule differs for each. See Table 5-03 for more information about meningococcal vaccines for young children.

The Kingdom of Saudi Arabia (KSA) requires travelers >2 years of age making the Umrah or Hajj pilgrimage to provide documentation of quadrivalent vaccine ≥10 days and ≤3 years before arrival for polysaccharide vaccine (MPSV4, no longer available in the United States) and ≤5 years before arrival for conjugate vaccine (see www.moh.gov.sa/en/Hajj/HealthGuidelines/HealthGuidelinesDuringHajj/Pages/HealthRequirements.aspx). Travelers should confirm visa requirements with the KSA embassy. Although the KSA Ministry of Health advises against travel to Hajj for pregnant people or children, these groups should receive meningococcal vaccination according to licensed indications for their age if they travel.

5

International travelers at risk for meningococcal disease who were previously vaccinated with a quadrivalent vaccine should receive a booster dose. For children who completed the primary dose or series at <7 years of age, administer a booster dose of MenACWY after 3 years and repeat every 5 years thereafter for those who live in or travel to hyperendemic areas. For people who received the primary dose or series at ≥7 years of age, administer a booster dose after 5 years and every 5 years thereafter for people who live in or travel to a hyperendemic area.

MONOVALENT VACCINES (SEROGROUPS A, B & C)

In 2010, the Meningitis Vaccine Project introduced MenAfriVac, a monovalent serogroup A meningococcal conjugate vaccine, into meningitis belt countries through mass vaccination campaigns and the routine childhood immunization schedule. This vaccine is not licensed for use in the United States. US travelers going to live or work in the meningitis belt should receive a quadrivalent meningococcal conjugate vaccine (MenACWY) before leaving, to protect against 4 serogroups.

MenB vaccine is not recommended for people who live in or travel to meningitis belt countries, because serogroup B disease is extremely rare in this region. MenB vaccine is not routinely recommended for travelers to other regions of the world unless an outbreak of serogroup B disease has been reported.

In some countries outside the meningitis belt, meningococcal vaccination (e.g., monovalent conjugate C vaccine or MenB vaccine) might be recommended as part of the routine immunization program for infants. Clinicians can consider meningococcal vaccination for infants residing in these countries, according to the routine immunization recommendations of that country.

SAFETY & ADVERSE REACTIONS

Side effects after MenACWY vaccination include low-grade fevers and local reactions (e.g., injection-site pain, arm swelling, pain that limits movement of the injected arm). Symptoms are generally mild to moderate and resolve within 48–72 hours. Severe adverse events (e.g., high fever, chills, joint pain, rash, seizures) are rare (<5% of vaccinees).

Although no clinical trials of meningococcal vaccines have been conducted in people who are pregnant or lactating, post-licensure safety data have not identified any serious safety concerns to the mother or fetus. Pregnancy or lactation should not preclude vaccination with MenACWY if indicated.

PRECAUTIONS & CONTRAINDICATIONS

People with moderate or severe acute illness should defer vaccination until their condition improves. Vaccination is contraindicated for people who have had a severe allergic reaction to any component of the vaccines or to a prior dose of the vaccine. A severe allergic reaction to any diphtheria toxoid- or CRM_{197}-containing vaccine also is a contraindication for MenACWY-D and MenACWY-CRM; severe allergic reaction to any tetanus toxoid–containing vaccine is a contraindication for MenACWY-TT.

To avoid interference with the immune response to meningococcal vaccine, MenACWY-D should be given either before or at the same time as DTaP in children. MenACWY-D may be given at any time in relation to Tdap or Td.

All meningococcal vaccines are inactivated and can be given to people who are immunosuppressed.

POSTEXPOSURE PROPHYLAXIS

In the United States and most industrialized countries, antibiotic chemoprophylaxis is recommended for close contacts of a patient with invasive meningococcal disease to prevent secondary cases. Chemoprophylaxis ideally should be initiated within 24 hours after the index patient is identified; prophylaxis given >2 weeks after exposure has little value.

Antibiotics used for prophylaxis include ceftriaxone, ciprofloxacin, and rifampin. Ceftriaxone is recommended for pregnant people. CDC provides detailed information on meningococcal prophylaxis in the Manual for the Surveillance of Vaccine-Preventable Diseases (www.cdc.gov/vaccines/pubs/surv-manual/chpt08-mening.html).

CDC website: www.cdc.gov/meningococcal

BIBLIOGRAPHY

American Academy of Pediatrics. Meningococcal infections. In: Kimberlin DW, Brady MT, Jackson M, Long SS, editors. Red Book: 2015 report of the Committee on Infectious Diseases, 30th edition. Elk Grove Village (IL): American Academy of Pediatrics; 2015. pp. 547–58.

Centers for Disease Control and Prevention. Public health dispatch: Update: assessment of risk for meningococcal disease associated with the Hajj 2001. MMWR Morb Mortal Wkly Rep. 2001;50(12):221–2.

Folaranmi T, Rubin L, Martin SW, Patel M, MacNeil JR. Use of serogroup B meningococcal vaccines in persons aged >/=10 years at increased risk for serogroup B meningococcal disease: recommendations of the Advisory Committee on Immunization Practices, 2015. MMWR Morb Mortal Wkly Rep. 2015;64(22):608–12.

Halperin SA, Bettinger JA, Greenwood B, Harrison LH, Jelfs J, Ladhani SN, et al. The changing and dynamic epidemiology of meningococcal disease. Vaccine. 2012;30(Suppl 2):B26–36.

MacNeil JR, Rubin L, Folaranmi T, Ortega-Sanchez IR, Patel M, Martin SW. Use of serogroup B meningococcal vaccines in adolescents and young adults: recommendations of the Advisory Committee on Immunization Practices, 2015. MMWR Morb Mortal Wkly Rep. 2015;64(41):1171–6.

Mbaeyi SA, Bozio CH, Duffy J, Rubin LG, Hariri S, Stephens DS, et al. Meningococcal vaccination: recommendations of the Advisory Committee on Immunization Practices, United States, 2020. MMWR Recomm Rep. 2020;69(9):1–41.

McNamara LA, Potts C, Blain AE, Retchless AC, Reese N, Swint S, et al. Detection of ciprofloxacin-resistant, β-lactamase-producing *Neisseria meningitidis* serogroup Y isolates—United States, 2019–2020. MMWR Morb Mortal Wkly Rep. 2020;69(24):735–9.

Patton ME, Stephens D, Moore K, MacNeil JR. Updated recommendations for use of MenB-FHbp serogroup B meningococcal vaccine—Advisory Committee on Immunization Practices, 2016. MMWR Morb Mortal Wkly Rep. 2016;66(19);509–13.

Trotter CL, Lingani C, Fernandez K, Cooper LV, Bita A, Tevi-Benissan C, et al. Impact of MenAfriVac in nine countries of the African meningitis belt, 2010–2015: an analysis of surveillance data. Lancet Infect Dis. 2017;17(8):867–72.

World Health Organization. Epidemic meningitis control in countries of the African meningitis belt, 2016. Wkly Epidemiol Rec. 2017;92(13):145–54.

5

PERTUSSIS / WHOOPING COUGH

Tami Skoff, Anna Acosta

INFECTIOUS AGENT: *Bordetella pertussis*	
ENDEMICITY	Worldwide
TRAVELER CATEGORIES AT GREATEST RISK FOR EXPOSURE & INFECTION	Infants <1 year of age People who are pregnant People who have not been vaccinated against pertussis
PREVENTION METHODS	Pertussis is a vaccine-preventable disease
DIAGNOSTIC SUPPORT	A clinical laboratory certified in moderate complexity testing; state health department

INFECTIOUS AGENT

Pertussis is caused by *Bordetella pertussis*, a fastidious gram-negative coccobacillus.

TRANSMISSION

B. pertussis transmission occurs person-to-person via aerosolized respiratory droplets or by direct contact with respiratory secretions.

EPIDEMIOLOGY

Pertussis is endemic worldwide, even in areas with high vaccination rates. International travel, therefore, does not generally place US travelers at increased risk for infection, as compared to home. Travelers are, however, at increased risk if they come into close contact with infected people. Pertussis has resurged in many countries with successful vaccination programs, especially countries that have transitioned from whole-cell pertussis vaccine formulations to acellular pertussis preparations, including the United States. Although limited data are available on the global burden of pertussis, disease rates are presumed to be highest among young children in countries where vaccination coverage is low, primarily developing countries. In industrialized countries, reported pertussis incidence is highest among infants too young to be vaccinated.

Immunity conferred by childhood vaccination and natural disease wanes with time; therefore, adolescents and adults who have not received a tetanus-diphtheria-pertussis (Tdap) booster vaccination can become infected or reinfected with pertussis. Infants, especially those too young to be protected by a complete vaccination series, are at highest risk for severe illness and death from pertussis.

CLINICAL PRESENTATION

In classic pertussis disease, mild upper respiratory tract symptoms typically begin 7–10 days (range 5–21 days) after exposure (catarrhal stage), after which a cough develops and becomes paroxysmal (paroxysmal stage). Coughing paroxysms can vary in frequency and often are followed by vomiting. Fever is absent or minimal. The coughing paroxysms gradually resolve into milder and less frequent coughing, but paroxysms can recur with subsequent respiratory infections (convalescent stage). The clinical case definition for pertussis includes cough for ≥2 weeks with paroxysms, whoop, post-tussive vomiting, or apnea with or without cyanosis.

Infants aged <6 months can have atypical disease, with a short catarrhal stage, gagging, gasping, or apnea as early manifestations. Among infants aged <2 months, the case-fatality ratio is ≈1%. The illness can be milder, and the characteristic paroxysmal cough and whoop might be absent, in children, adolescents, and adults who were previously vaccinated.

DIAGNOSIS

Factors such as prior vaccination status, disease stage, antibiotic use, specimen collection and transport conditions, and use of nonstandardized tests can affect the sensitivity, specificity, and interpretation of available diagnostic tests for *B. pertussis*. Centers for Disease Control and Prevention (CDC) guidelines for laboratory confirmation of pertussis include culture and PCR when the above clinical case definition is met. Serology is not included as a confirmatory test in the current case definition for reporting purposes. Direct fluorescent antibody (DFA) testing is no longer recommended for diagnosing pertussis because of poor sensitivity and specificity. Testing for *B. pertussis* is widely available in commercial laboratories. Clinicians can consult Vaccine-Preventable Diseases Reference Centers for additional testing support if needed (www.aphl.org/programs/infectious_disease/Pages/VPD.aspx). Pertussis is a nationally notifiable disease

TREATMENT

Clinicians can treat pertussis in people aged ≥1 month with a macrolide antibiotic (azithromycin, clarithromycin, or erythromycin); for infants aged <1 month, azithromycin is preferred. Antimicrobial drug therapy with a macrolide antibiotic administered <3 weeks after cough onset can limit transmission to others.

PREVENTION

Vaccine

Travelers should be up to date on pertussis vaccinations before departure. Multiple pertussis vaccines are available in the United States for infants and children; 2 vaccines are available for adolescents and adults. A complete listing of licensed vaccines is available at www.fda.gov/BiologicsBloodVaccines/Vaccines/ApprovedProducts/ucm093833.htm.

INFANTS & CHILDREN

In the United States, all infants and children should receive 5 doses of acellular pertussis vaccine in combination with diphtheria and tetanus toxoids (DTaP) at ages 2, 4, 6, and 15–18 months, and at 4–6 years. Providers can use an accelerated schedule of doses to complete the DTaP series before travel, if needed.

Children aged 7–10 years who are not fully vaccinated against pertussis and for whom no contraindication to pertussis vaccine exists should receive a single dose of tetanus toxoid, reduced diphtheria toxoid, and acellular pertussis vaccine (Tdap) to provide protection against pertussis. If children need additional doses of tetanus and diphtheria toxoid–containing vaccines, administer them according to catch-up guidance, with Tdap preferred as the first dose (see www.cdc.gov/vaccines/schedules/hcp/imz/catchup.html).

ADOLESCENTS & ADULTS

Adolescents aged 11–18 years who have completed the recommended childhood DTaP vaccination series should receive a single dose of Tdap, preferably at age 11–12 years. Adults aged ≥19 years who have not previously received Tdap should receive a single dose of Tdap instead of tetanus and diphtheria toxoids (Td) vaccine for booster immunization against tetanus, diphtheria, and pertussis, regardless of the interval since their last tetanus or diphtheria toxoid–containing vaccine.

To ensure continued protection against tetanus and diphtheria, administer booster doses of either Td or Tdap every 10 years throughout a patient's life. Follow the catch-up schedule for Td/Tdap for adolescents and adults who have never been immunized against pertussis, tetanus, or diphtheria; who have not completed an immunization series; or whose immunity is uncertain.

PREGNANT PEOPLE

Even if vaccinated previously, a person should receive a dose of Tdap with each pregnancy. Although Tdap can be given at any time during pregnancy, to maximize the maternal antibody response and passive antibody transfer to the infant, optimal timing for Tdap administration is at 27–36 weeks' gestation, preferably during the earlier part of the period.

POSTEXPOSURE PROPHYLAXIS

Postexposure prophylaxis is recommended for all household contacts of cases and for people at high risk of developing severe disease (e.g., infants, people in the third trimester of their pregnancy, anyone who will have contact with a person at high risk of severe illness). The recommended agents and dosing regimens for prophylaxis are the same as for the treatment of pertussis.

CDC website: www.cdc.gov/pertussis

BIBLIOGRAPHY

Centers for Disease Control and Prevention. Pertussis (whooping cough) postexposure antimicrobial prophylaxis: Information for Health Professionals. Available from: www.cdc.gov/pertussis/pep.html.

Havers FP, Moro PL, Hunter P, Hariri S, Bernstein H. Use of tetanus toxoid, reduced diphtheria toxoid, and acellular pertussis vaccines: updated recommendations of the Advisory Committee on Immunization Practices—United States, 2019. MMWR Morb Mortal Wkly Rep. 2020;69:77–83.

Liang JL, Tiwari T, Moro P, Messonnier NE, Reingold A, Sawyer M, et al. Prevention of pertussis, tetanus, and diphtheria with vaccines in the United States: recommendations of the Advisory Committee on Immunization Practices (ACIP). MMWR Recomm Rep. 2018;67(2):1–44.

Skoff TH, Hadler S, Hariri S. The epidemiology of nationally reported pertussis in the United States, 2000–2016. Clin Infect Dis. 2019;68(10):1634–40.

Tiwari T, Murphy TV, Moran J. Recommended antimicrobial agents for the treatment and postexposure prophylaxis of pertussis: 2005 CDC Guidelines. MMWR Recomm Rep. 2005;54(RR-14):1–16.

Yeung KHT, Duclos P, Nelson EAS, Hutubessy RCW. An update of the global burden of pertussis in children younger than 5 years: a modelling study. Lancet Infect Dis. 2017;17(9):974–80.

PLAGUE

David McCormick, Paul Mead

INFECTIOUS AGENT: *Yersinia pestis*	
ENDEMICITY	Sub-Saharan Africa and Madagascar North America (Western United States) South America Central and Southeast Asia, and India
TRAVELER CATEGORIES AT GREATEST RISK FOR EXPOSURE & INFECTION	Adventure tourists Long-term travelers and expatriates
PREVENTION METHODS	Avoid insect bites Use postexposure prophylaxis
DIAGNOSTIC SUPPORT	A clinical laboratory certified in high complexity testing; state health department; or contact CDC's Division of Vector-Borne Diseases (970-221-6400; dvbid@cdc.gov)

INFECTIOUS AGENT

Yersinia pestis, the causative organism for plague, is a gram-negative coccobacillus.

TRANSMISSION

Y. pestis transmission usually occurs through the bite of infected rodent fleas. Less common exposures include handling infected animal tissues (e.g., among hunters and wildlife personnel); inhaling infectious droplets from cats or dogs with plague; and, rarely, contact with a patient who has pneumonic plague.

EPIDEMIOLOGY

Plague is endemic to rural areas in central and southern Africa, especially eastern Democratic Republic of the Congo, northwestern Uganda, and Madagascar; parts of the southwestern United States; the northeastern part of South America; central Asia; and the Indian subcontinent. The overall risk for travelers is low, and encountering *Y. pestis* while traveling is unlikely.

Although travelers' risk is negligible (no plague cases have been reported among travelers returning to the United States in >40 years), cases of plague can lead to societal disruptions that complicate travel. For example, during a plague outbreak in India in the 1980s, planes from India were temporarily prevented from landing in Europe, although none of the passengers had symptoms of plague. In 2017, schools in the Republic of Seychelles were closed and large public gatherings banned in response to a plague outbreak in neighboring Madagascar.

CLINICAL PRESENTATION

The incubation period is typically 1–6 days. Plague illness has 3 possible clinical presentations: bubonic (the most common), pneumonic, or septicemic. Clinical symptoms and signs of bubonic plague include rapid onset of fever and painful, swollen, and tender lymph nodes, usually axillary, cervical, or inguinal. Pharyngeal plague is rare and presents with fever, sore throat, and cervical lymphadenitis; in its early stages, it may be clinically indistinguishable from more common causes of pharyngitis. For pneumonic plague, signs and symptoms include high fever, overwhelming pneumonia, cough, bloody sputum, and chills. For septicemic plague, signs and symptoms include fever, prostration, and hemorrhagic or thrombotic phenomena, progressing to acral gangrene. Meningitis can also develop in up to 10% of patients with plague.

DIAGNOSIS

Y. pestis can be isolated from bubo aspirates, blood cultures, or sputum culture if pneumonic. State public health laboratories or Centers for Disease Control and Prevention (CDC) laboratories can confirm diagnosis by culture or serologic tests for the *Y. pestis* F1 antigen. Plague is a nationally notifiable disease. For diagnostic support, clinicians can contact CDC's Division of Vector-Borne Diseases (970-221-6400; dvbid@cdc.gov).

TREATMENT

Treatment for plague differs by clinical presentation and illness severity. Several different classes of antimicrobials effectively treat plague, but aminoglycosides and fluoroquinolones are considered first-line. Treating physicians can use doxycycline for bubonic or pharyngeal plague, but these should not be used for pneumonic or septicemic plague, or plague meningitis. If plague meningitis is suspected, use dual antibiotic therapy with chloramphenicol and a fluoroquinolone or aminoglycoside. For full treatment recommendations, see Antimicrobial Treatment and Prophylaxis of Plague: Recommendations for Naturally Acquired Infections and Bioterrorism Response (www.cdc.gov/mmwr/volumes/70/rr/rr7003a1.htm).

PREVENTION

Travelers can prevent plague by reducing contact with fleas and potentially infected rodents and other wildlife. Although a live attenuated vaccine has been in use in Russia since the 1930s, no plague vaccine is currently available for commercial use in the United States or western Europe. A killed whole-cell vaccine was available in the United States for people with occupational risk, but this vaccine was discontinued in 1999. Australia continued to use this vaccine until 2005. Newer vaccines using a recombinant F1 antigen are in development, but none are commercially available or currently approved for use by the US Food and Drug Administration. Oral antibiotics, including doxycycline, ciprofloxacin, and levofloxacin can be prescribed for postexposure prophylaxis.

CDC website: www.cdc.gov/plague

5

BIBLIOGRAPHY

Bertherat E. Plague around the world, 2010–2015. WHO Wkly Epidemiol Rec. 2016;91:89–104.

Butler T. Plague gives surprises in the first decade of the 21st century in the United States and worldwide. Am J Trop Med Hyg. 2013;89:788–93.

Nelson CA, Meaney-Delman D, Fleck-Derderian S, Cooley KM, Yu PA, Mead PS. Antimicrobial treatment and prophylaxis of plague: recommendations for naturally acquired infections and bioterrorism response. MMWR Recomm Rep. 2021;70(3):1–27.

Perry RD, Fetherston JD. *Yersinia pestis*—etiologic agent of plague. Clin Microbiol Rev. 1997;10(1):35–66.

PNEUMOCOCCAL DISEASE

Jennifer Loo Farrar

INFECTIOUS AGENT: *Streptococcus pneumoniae*	
ENDEMICITY	Worldwide
TRAVELER CATEGORIES AT GREATEST RISK FOR EXPOSURE & INFECTION	Very young children and older adults Travelers with chronic illnesses or immunosuppressed
PREVENTION METHODS	Pneumococcal disease is vaccine-preventable
DIAGNOSTIC SUPPORT	A clinical laboratory certified in moderate complexity testing; or call the CDC Emergency Operations Center (770-488-7100) and ask for the Respiratory Diseases Branch, *Streptococcus* Laboratory, or email pneumococcus@cdc.gov

INFECTIOUS AGENT

A gram-positive diplococcus *Streptococcus pneumoniae*, also called pneumococcus, causes pneumococcal disease.

TRANSMISSION

S. pneumoniae is transmitted person-to-person through close contact via respiratory droplets.

EPIDEMIOLOGY

S. pneumoniae is a major cause of bacterial meningitis and the most common bacterial cause of community-acquired pneumonia worldwide. Disease incidence is higher in low- and middle-income countries than in high-income countries. Pneumococcal meningitis outbreaks have occurred recently in countries in the meningitis belt of Africa (see Sec. 5, Part 1, Ch. 13, Meningococcal Disease). Infections from pneumococcus also have been reported in travelers attending mass gatherings (e.g., the Hajj pilgrimage, Olympic Games) due to crowded conditions and limited space. Risk for infection is greatest in very young children, older adults, and people with chronic illnesses or immune suppression.

5

CLINICAL PRESENTATION

The major clinical syndromes of pneumococcal disease are pneumonia, bacteremia, and meningitis. Pneumococcal pneumonia classically presents with sudden onset of fever and malaise, pleuritic chest pain, cough with purulent or blood-tinged sputum, or dyspnea. In older people, fever, shortness of breath, or altered mental status are possible initial symptoms.

Symptoms of pneumococcal meningitis include headache, lethargy, vomiting, irritability, fever, neck stiffness, and seizures. People with cochlear implants are at increased risk for pneumococcal meningitis. *S. pneumoniae* infection causes meningitis less frequently than it causes pneumonia.

DIAGNOSIS

S. pneumoniae infection is diagnosed by isolation of the organism from blood or other normally sterile body sites (e.g., pleural fluid, cerebrospinal fluid [CSF]). Tests are also available to detect pneumococcal antigen in body fluids (e.g., urine). The urinary antigen test is commercially available, simple to use, and has reasonable specificity to detect pneumococcal infection in adults, making it a useful addition for diagnostic evaluation.

Suspect pneumococcal pneumonia when a sputum specimen contains gram-positive diplococci, polymorphonuclear leukocytes, and few epithelial cells. Gram-positive diplococci on staining of CSF might indicate pneumococcal meningitis. High white blood cell counts should raise suspicion for bacterial infection.

TREATMENT

Therapy depends on the syndrome, and clinicians should treat patients presenting with community-acquired pneumonia empirically for pneumococcal infection. In 30% of severe cases, pneumococcal bacteria are resistant to ≥1 antimicrobial drug, although the level and type of resistance varies geographically. Studies show that pneumococcal macrolide resistance is widely variable, between 20%–90%. Pneumococcal resistance to fluoroquinolones is relatively low in the United States and Europe. Global prevalence of drug-resistant *S. pneumoniae* causing community-acquired pneumonia is currently unknown.

In outpatient settings, current clinical practice guidelines for pneumonia management recommend amoxicillin for children, and macrolides (e.g., azithromycin) or doxycycline for previously healthy adults. For adults with chronic or immunosuppressing conditions, a respiratory fluoroquinolone (e.g., moxifloxacin, levofloxacin) or a β-lactam plus a macrolide are recommended.

In inpatient settings, the initial treatment includes a broad-spectrum cephalosporin plus a macrolide or a respiratory fluoroquinolone alone. For some pneumococcal infections, consider adding vancomycin until antimicrobial susceptibility results are available. Use a broad-spectrum cephalosporin plus vancomycin to treat patients with presumptive pneumococcal meningitis by CSF staining until susceptibility results are available.

PREVENTION

The 13-valent pneumococcal conjugate vaccine (PCV13) provides protection against the 13 serotypes responsible for most severe illness. PCV13 has been part of the US infant immunization schedule since 2010, and Advisory Committee on Immunization Practices (ACIP) recommends

PCV13 for some adults aged ≥65 years and adults aged 19–64 with immunocompromising conditions.

ACIP recommends 23-valent pneumococcal polysaccharide vaccine (PPSV23) for all adults aged ≥65 years and people aged 2–64 years with underlying medical conditions. PCV13 and PPSV23 should not be coadministered. Intervals between administering PCV13 and PPSV23 differ by age and risk group (see www.cdc.gov/vaccines/vpd/pneumo/hcp/recommendations.html).

A 20-valent pneumococcal conjugate vaccine (PCV20) was licensed for use in adults in June 2021, and the 15-valent pneumococcal conjugate vaccine (PCV15) was licensed for use in adults in July 2021. On October 20, 2021, the ACIP approved recommendations to use PCV20 alone, or PCV15 in series with PPSV23, for all adults aged ≥65 years and for adults aged 19–64 years with underlying medical conditions who have not previously received a pneumococcal conjugate vaccine or whose vaccination history is unknown. Official guidance on use of these vaccines is being developed.

CDC website: www.cdc.gov/pneumococcal

BIBLIOGRAPHY

Aliberti S, Cook GS, Babu BL, Reyes LF, Rodriguez AH, Sanz F, et al. International prevalence and risk factors evaluation for drug-resistant *Streptococcus pneumoniae* pneumonia. J Infect. 2019;79(4):300–11.

Bradley JS, Byington CL, Shah SS, Alverson B, Carter ER, Harrison C, et al. The management of community-acquired pneumonia in infants and children older than 3 months of age: clinical practice guidelines by the Pediatric Infectious Diseases Society and the Infectious Diseases Society of America. Clin Infect Dis. 2011;53(7):e25–76.

Centers for Disease Control and Prevention. Pneumococcal vaccine recommendations 2020. Available from: www.cdc.gov/vaccines/vpd/pneumo/hcp/recommendations.html.

Cilloniz C, Garcia-Vidal C, Ceccato A, Torres A. Antimicrobial resistance among *Streptococcus pneumoniae*. In: Fong I, Shlaes D, Drlica K editors. Antimicrobial resistance in the 21st century. Emerging infectious diseases of the 21st century. Geneva: Springer Nature; 2018. pp. 13–38.

Metlay JP, Waterer GW, Long AC, Anzueto A, Brozek J, Crothers K, et al. Diagnosis and treatment of adults with community-acquired pneumonia. An official clinical practice guideline of the American Thoracic Society and Infectious Diseases Society of America. Amer J Resp and Crit Care Med. 2019;200(7):e45–67.

Wahl B, O'Brien KL, Greenbaum A, Majumder A, Liu L, Chu Y, et al. Burden of *Streptococcus pneumoniae* and *Haemophilus influenzae* type b disease in children in the era of conjugate vaccines: global, regional, and national estimates for 2000–15. Lancet Global Health. 2018;6:e744–57.

5

Q FEVER

Gilbert Kersh

INFECTIOUS AGENT: *Coxiella burnetii*	
ENDEMICITY	Worldwide, except New Zealand
TRAVELER CATEGORIES AT GREATEST RISK FOR EXPOSURE & INFECTION	Animal handlers, e.g., veterinarians, butchers, farmers, and farm workers People visiting rural areas and farms with livestock
PREVENTION METHODS	Avoid exposure to infected animals Follow safe food precautions and avoid unpasteurized dairy products Vaccine available in Australia, but not in the United States
DIAGNOSTIC SUPPORT	A clinical laboratory certified in high complexity testing; state health department; call the CDC Emergency Operations Center (770-488-7100) and ask for the Rickettsial Zoonoses Branch; or consult www.cdc.gov/qfever/public-health/index.html

INFECTIOUS AGENT

The causative agent of Q fever is the gram-negative intracellular bacterium *Coxiella burnetii*.

TRANSMISSION

C. burnetii is most commonly transmitted through inhalation of aerosols or dust contaminated with dried birth fluids or excreta from infected animals, usually cattle, goats, or sheep. *C. burnetii* is highly infectious and persists in the environment. Infections via ingestion of contaminated unpasteurized dairy products and human-to-human transmission via sexual contact have been reported, but rarely.

EPIDEMIOLOGY

C. burnetti has a worldwide distribution but is absent from New Zealand. *C. burnetti* prevalence is greatest in Africa and countries in the Middle East. Reported rates of human infection are higher in France and Australia than in the United States. The largest known Q fever outbreak reported to date involved ≈4,000 human cases during 2007–2010 in the Netherlands. Cases of Q fever in travelers are most often reported in people who visited rural areas or farms with cattle, goats, sheep, or other livestock. During 1990–2013, ≥250 travel-related cases of Q fever were reported in the literature.

Occupational exposure to infected animals, particularly during parturition, poses a high risk for infection among butchers, farmers, meat packers, veterinarians, and seasonal or migrant farm workers. Examples of travel-acquired Q fever include cases in soldiers deployed to rural areas, travelers with livestock contact and consumption of unpasteurized milk, and travelers obtaining treatments that involved the injection of fetal sheep cells. In a 2008 review of 708 returned travelers evaluated for fever, Q fever was diagnosed in 5 people (0.7%).

CLINICAL PRESENTATION

The incubation period is typically 2–3 weeks but can be shorter after exposure to large numbers of organisms. Estimates suggest that over half of acute infections are mild or asymptomatic. The most common clinical presentation of acute infection is a self-limiting febrile illness, with hepatitis or pneumonia associated with more severe acute infections. Chronic infections occur primarily in patients with preexisting cardiac valvulopathies, vascular abnormalities, or immunosuppression. Without proper treatment, infection during pregnancy poses a risk for adverse pregnancy outcomes. The most common manifestations of chronic disease are endocarditis and endovascular infections. Chronic infections might become apparent months or years after the initial exposure.

DIAGNOSIS

Serologic evidence of a 4-fold rise in phase II IgG by indirect fluorescent antibody test between paired acute and convalescent serum samples collected 3–4 weeks apart is the gold standard for diagnosis. Consider a single high serum phase II IgG titer (>1:64) in conjunction with clinical evidence of infection as indicative of probable acute Q fever. PCR testing of serum or whole blood is useful for confirmation of acute Q fever if samples are taken ≤14 days after symptom onset.

Chronic Q fever diagnosis requires a phase I IgG titer >1:512 and clinical evidence of persistent infection (e.g., endocarditis, infected vascular aneurysm, osteomyelitis). Identifying *C. burnetii* in whole blood, serum, or tissue samples by PCR, immunohistochemical staining, or isolation can be used to confirm chronic disease. Tests for direct detection of *C. burnetii* might not be widely available, but the Rickettsial Zoonoses Branch at the Centers for Disease Control and Prevention (CDC) can assist. Information about diagnostic testing is available at www.cdc.gov/qfever/public-health/index.html, or call the CDC Emergency Operations Center (770-488-7100) and ask to be directed to the Rickettsial Zoonoses Branch. Q fever is a nationally notifiable disease.

TREATMENT

Doxycycline is the most frequently used and most effective treatment for acute Q fever. For pregnant people, children aged <8 years with mild illness, and patients allergic to doxycycline, trimethoprim-sulfamethoxazole is an alternative treatment option. Treatment for acute Q fever is not recommended for asymptomatic people or for those whose symptoms have resolved. Chronic *C. burnetii* infections require long-term combination therapy, and the combination of doxycycline and hydroxychloroquine for ≥18 months provides the best treatment outcomes. Alternative treatments include trimethoprim-sulfamethoxazole and fluoroquinolones, but these are less effective. Treatment of Q fever also might involve surgery to remove infected tissue.

PREVENTION

To prevent Q fever, travelers should avoid areas where potentially infected animals are kept and avoid consumption of unpasteurized dairy products. A human vaccine for Q fever has been developed and used in Australia but is not available in the United States.

CDC website: www.cdc.gov/qfever

BIBLIOGRAPHY

Anderson A, Bijlmer H, Fournier PE, Graves S, Hartzell J, Kersh GJ, et al. Diagnosis and management of Q fever—United States, 2013: recommendations from CDC and the Q Fever Working Group. MMWR Recomm Rep. 2013;62(RR-03):1–30.

Delord M, Socolovschi C, Parola P. Rickettsioses and Q fever in travelers (2004–2013). Travel Med Infect Dis. 2014;12(5):443–58.

Million M, Thuny F, Richet H, Raoult D. Long-term outcome of Q fever endocarditis: a 26-year personal survey. Lancet Infect Dis. 2010;10(8):527–35.

Robyn MP, Newman AP, Amato M, Walawander M, Kothe C, Nerone JD, et al. Q fever outbreak among travelers to Germany who received live cell therapy—United States and Canada, 2014. MMWR Morb Mortal Wkly Rep. 2015;64(38):1071–3.

Roest HI, Tilburg JJ, van der Hoek W, Vellema P, van Zijderveld FG, Klaassen CH, et al. The Q fever epidemic in The Netherlands: history, onset, response and reflection. Epidemiol Infect. 2011;139(1):1–12.

RICKETTSIAL DISEASES

William Nicholson, Christopher Paddock

INFECTIOUS AGENTS: *Rickettsia, Orientia, Anaplasma, Ehrlichia, Neoehrlichia, Neorickettsia* spp.	
ENDEMICITY	Worldwide
TRAVELER CATEGORIES AT GREATEST RISK FOR EXPOSURE & INFECTION	People exposed to vector fleas, lice, mites, or ticks
PREVENTION METHODS	Avoid insect and arthropod bites
DIAGNOSTIC SUPPORT	A clinical laboratory certified in high complexity testing; state health department; or contact CDC's Rickettsial Zoonoses Branch (rzbepidiag@cdc.gov)

INFECTIOUS AGENTS

Rickettsial infections are caused by various bacteria within 6 genera of the order Rickettsiales: *Rickettsia, Orientia, Anaplasma, Ehrlichia, Neoehrlichia,* and *Neorickettsia* (Table 5-04). *Rickettsia* spp. are classically divided into the spotted fever group (SFG) and the typhus group, although more recently these have been classified into as many as 4 groups. *Orientia* spp. comprise the scrub typhus group, which has only recently expanded from the single species *O. tsutsugamushi.*

Rickettsial species (and diseases) that travelers are more likely to encounter outside the United

States include the SFG pathogens, *Rickettsia africae* (African tick-bite fever), *R. conorii* (Mediterranean spotted fever), *R. rickettsii* (Rocky Mountain spotted fever [RMSF], also known as Brazilian spotted fever); *R. typhi* (murine typhus); *Orientia tsutsugamushi* (scrub typhus); and *Anaplasma phagocytophilum* (anaplasmosis). Many other rickettsial agents cause human infections across the globe, but the true burden remains undetermined.

TRANSMISSION

Most rickettsial pathogens are transmitted directly to humans by infected arthropod vectors (i.e., fleas, lice, mites, or ticks) during feeding. Rickettsia also might be transmitted when a person inadvertently inoculates the arthropod bite wound (or other breaks in the skin) with rickettsial pathogens; this can happen by scratching skin contaminated with an arthropod's infectious fluids or feces, or by crushing the arthropod vector at the bite site. Inhaling bacteria or inoculating conjunctiva with infectious material also can initiate infection for some rickettsial pathogens.

5

Vectors that transmit each rickettsial species are listed in Table 5-04; some details are discussed here. Transmission of a few pathogens, particularly *Anaplasma* and *Ehrlichia* spp., through transfusion of infected blood products or by organ transplantation, is less common.

EPIDEMIOLOGY

Regardless of the length of travel (short- or long-term), all age groups are at risk for rickettsial infections during visits to endemic areas. Transmission risk increases with time spent participating in outdoor activities, particularly during seasons of peak feeding and lifecycle activity for the vector. In many parts of the world, however, rickettsial infections occur year-round. The most diagnosed rickettsial diseases in travelers are in the spotted fever or typhus groups; notably, rickettsial infections can also be caused by emerging and newly recognized species.

Spotted Fever Group

Tickborne spotted fever rickettsioses are the most frequently reported travel-associated rickettsial infections.

AFRICAN TICK-BITE FEVER

Travelers who go on safari—especially those traveling to national parks, game hunters, and ecotourists to sub-Saharan Africa—are at risk for African tick-bite fever caused by *R. africae*. *R. africae* is also endemic to several islands of the Caribbean West Indies, and imported cases have been described from this region.

R. africae remains the most frequently reported rickettsial infection acquired during travel. Commonly, cases of African tick-bite fever cluster among people traveling together, and diagnosis of the disease in 1 member of a family or tourist group can alert other similarly exposed people to seek care if they develop compatible signs and symptoms.

CAT FLEA RICKETTSIOSIS

R. felis, the cause of cat flea rickettsiosis, has been identified in various invertebrate hosts worldwide and has been reported as a major cause of febrile illness in some countries of Africa.

MEDITERRANEAN SPOTTED FEVER

Travel-associated cases of Mediterranean spotted fever (also known as Boutonneuse fever), caused by *R. conorii*, are less commonly reported but occur over a large geographic area, including but not limited to Africa, much of Europe, India, and the Middle East.

RICKETTSIALPOX

The causative agent of rickettsialpox, *R. akari*, is transmitted by house mouse mites, and circulates mainly in urban centers in the Balkan states, Korea, South Africa, Ukraine, and the United States. Outbreaks of rickettsialpox most often occur after contact with infected peridomestic rodents and their mites, especially during natural die-offs or exterminations of infected rodents that cause the mites to seek out new hosts, including humans. Urban rodents seem more often associated with human cases, but the agent has been identified in a few wild rodent populations.

ROCKY MOUNTAIN SPOTTED FEVER OR BRAZILIAN SPOTTED FEVER

RMSF (also known as Brazilian spotted fever and other local names) is caused by *R. rickettsii*. It occurs

Table 5-04 Rickettsial diseases in humans[1]

SPOTTED FEVER GROUP				
DISEASE	**RICKETTSIAL SPECIES**	**GEOGRAPHIC DISTRIBUTION**	**ANIMAL HOST(S)**	**VECTORS**
African tick-bite fever	*Rickettsia africae*	Sub-Saharan Africa; West Indies	Domestic and wild ruminants	Ticks
Aneruptive fever	*R. helvetica*	Asia; central and northern Europe	Rodents	Ticks
Astrakhan spotted fever	*R. conorii*, subsp. *caspiae* (proposed)	North Caspian region of Russia		Ticks
Cat flea rickettsiosis	*R. felis*	Africa; North and South America; Asia; Europe	Domestic cats, opossums, rodents	Fleas
Far Eastern spotted fever	*R. heilongjiangensis*	East Asia; northern China; far east Russia	Rodents	Ticks
Flinders Island spotted fever Thai tick typhus	*R. honei*, including strain "marmionii"	Australia; Thailand	Reptiles, rodents	Ticks
Indian tick typhus	*R. conorii*, subsp. *indica* (proposed)	South Asia		Ticks
Israeli tick typhus	*R. conorii*, subsp. *israelensis* (proposed)	Southern Europe; Middle East		Ticks
Japanese spotted fever	*R. japonica*	Japan	Rodents	Ticks
Lymphangitis-associated rickettsiosis	*R. sibirica mongolotimonae*	Africa; Asia (China); Europe (southern France, Portugal)	Rodents	Ticks
Maculatum infection	*R. parkeri*	North and South America	Rodents	Ticks
Mediterranean spotted fever (Boutonneuse fever)	*R. conorii*, subsp. *conorii* (proposed)	Africa; southern Europe; southern and western Asia (India)	Dogs, rodents	Ticks
Mediterranean spotted fever–like illness	*R. massiliae*	Central Africa (Mali); North America (USA); Europe (France, Greece, Portugal, Sicily, Spain, Switzerland)	Unknown (maybe dogs)	Ticks

(*continued*)

Table 5-04 Rickettsial diseases in humans (continued)

Mediterranean spotted fever–like illness	*R. monacensis*	North Africa; Europe	Lizards, possibly birds	Ticks
North Asian tick typhus Siberian tick typhus	*R. sibirica*	China; Mongolia; Russia	Rodents	Ticks
Queensland tick typhus	*R. australis*	Australia; Tasmania	Rodents	Ticks
Rickettsialpox	*R. akari*	Africa (South Africa); North and South America; Asia (Korea); southern and eastern Europe (Balkans, Turkey, Ukraine and former Soviet Union)	House mice, wild rodents	Mites
Rickettsiosis	*R. aeschlimannii*	South Africa; Morocco; Mediterranean littoral	Unknown	Ticks
Rocky Mountain spotted fever (RMSF; also known as Brazilian spotted fever; febre maculosa; São Paulo exanthematic typhus; Minas Gerais exanthematic typhus)	*R. rickettsii*	North, Central, and South America	Rodents	Ticks
Tickborne lymphadenopathy (TIBOLA) *Dermacentor*-borne necrosis and lymphadenopathy (DEBONEL)	*R. raoultii*	Asia; Europe	Unknown	Ticks
Tickborne lymphadenopathy (TIBOLA) *Dermacentor*-borne necrosis and lymphadenopathy (DEBONEL)	*R. slovaca*	Asia; southern and eastern Europe; recently found in a US tick colony (origin unknown)	European boar, lagomorphs, rodents	Ticks
TYPHUS GROUP				
DISEASE	**RICKETTSIAL SPECIES**	**GEOGRAPHIC DISTRIBUTION**	**ANIMAL HOST(S)**	**VECTORS**
Epidemic typhus Sylvatic typhus	*Rickettsia prowazekii*	Central Africa; North, Central and South America; Asia	Humans Flying squirrels	Human body louse Flying squirrel ectoparasites

Table 5-04 Rickettsial diseases in humans (continued)

Murine typhus	*R. typhi*	Temperate, tropical, and subtropical areas worldwide	Rodents	Fleas
SCRUB TYPHUS GROUP				
DISEASE	**RICKETTSIAL SPECIES**	**GEOGRAPHIC DISTRIBUTION**	**ANIMAL HOST(S)**	**VECTORS**
Scrub typhus	*Orientia tsutsugamushi*	Asia-Pacific region (north Australia, China, Indonesia, maritime Russia); Middle East (Afghanistan); possibly several countries in sub-Saharan Africa	Rodents	Trombiculid mites and chiggers
	O. chuto	United Arab Emirates (UAE)		
	O. chiloensis	Southern Chile		
ANAPLASMA GROUP				
DISEASE	**RICKETTSIAL SPECIES**	**GEOGRAPHIC DISTRIBUTION**	**ANIMAL HOST(S)**	**VECTORS**
Human anaplasmosis	*Anaplasma bovis*	USA	Unknown	Ticks
	A. capra	China	Goats, sheep	Ticks
	A. ovis	China; Cyprus; Greece	Sheep	Ticks
	A. phagocytophilum	Worldwide (primarily USA)	Deer, small mammals, rodents	Ticks
	A. platys	Argentina	Dogs	Ticks
EHRLICHIA GROUP				
DISEASE	**RICKETTSIAL SPECIES**	**GEOGRAPHIC DISTRIBUTION**	**ANIMAL HOST(S)**	**VECTORS**
Human ehrlichiosis	*Ehrlichia chaffeensis*	USA and possibly elsewhere worldwide	Deer; domestic and wild dogs; domestic ruminants; rodents	Ticks
	E. ewingii			

(*continued*)

5

Table 5-04 Rickettsial diseases in humans (continued)

	E. muris eauclairensis			
	E. muris muris			
	E. canis	Worldwide Human cases in Costa Rica, Venezuela	Dogs	Ticks
	E. ruminantium	South Africa	Domestic and wild ruminants	Ticks
NEOEHRLICHIA GROUP				
DISEASE	**RICKETTSIAL SPECIES**	**GEOGRAPHIC DISTRIBUTION**	**ANIMAL HOST(S)**	**VECTORS**
Human neoehrlichiosis	*Neoehrlichia mikurensis*	Asia; Europe	Rodents	Ticks
NEORICKETTSIA GROUP				
DISEASE	**RICKETTSIAL SPECIES**	**GEOGRAPHIC DISTRIBUTION**	**ANIMAL HOST(S)**	**VECTORS**
Sennetsu fever	*Neorickettsia sennetsu*	Japan; Malaysia; possibly other parts of Asia	Fish	Trematodes

[1]Highlighted rows indicate diseases described in more detail in the text.

throughout much of the Western Hemisphere, and cases are reported from Canada, Mexico, the United States, and many countries of Central and South America, including Argentina, Brazil, Colombia, Costa Rica, and Panama. Clusters of illness might be reported in families or in geographic areas. Contact with dogs in rural and urban settings, and outdoor activities (e.g., camping, fishing, hiking, hunting) increase the risk for infection.

Typhus Group

EPIDEMIC TYPHUS

Louseborne or epidemic typhus, caused by *R. prowazekii*, is rarely reported among tourists; more commonly, it occurs among people living in crowded conditions where body lice are prevalent (e.g., refugees housed in camps, incarcerated populations). Outbreaks often happen during the colder months. Travelers at greatest risk for epidemic typhus include people who provide medical or humanitarian aid to people living in refugee camps and those who visit impoverished areas affected by war, famine, or natural disasters. Active foci of epidemic typhus are in the Andes region of South America and some parts of Africa, including but not limited to Burundi, Ethiopia, and Rwanda.

Classical louseborne typhus has not occurred in the United States for approximately the past century; however, a zoonotic reservoir exists in the southern flying squirrel, and sporadic sylvatic epidemic typhus cases are reported when these animals invade people's homes or cabins.

MURINE TYPHUS

Murine typhus, caused by *R. typhi*, is distributed worldwide, particularly in and around port cities and coastal regions with large rodent populations. People are at risk for fleaborne rickettsioses when traveling in endemic regions and when they are exposed to flea-infested cats, dogs, and peridomestic animals, or enter or sleep in areas infested with rodents. Murine typhus has been reported among travelers returning from Africa, Asia, and the Mediterranean Basin. Most cases acquired in the United States are reported from California, Hawaii, and Texas.

Scrub Typhus Group

Scrub typhus can be transmitted by many species of trombiculid mites that live in high grass and brush. Scrub typhus is endemic to regions of east Asia (China, northern Japan), Southeast Asia (India, Indonesia, Sri Lanka), the Pacific (eastern Australia), and several parts of south-central Russia. Cases of disease also have been described from several unexpected regions, including the United Arab Emirates and southern Chile, and appear to be caused by newly recognized species of *Orientia*.

More people worldwide are at risk for scrub typhus than for any other rickettsial disease; >1 million cases occur annually, mostly in farmers or people with occupational exposure. Travel-acquired cases of scrub typhus occasionally are reported among people who visit rural regions of countries where *O. tsutsugamushi* is endemic, and exposure is often associated with participating in recreational activities (e.g., camping, hiking, rafting). Rare urban cases have been described.

Anaplasmosmis & Ehrlichiosis

Although anaplasmosis (caused predominately by *A. phagocytophilum*) and ehrlichiosis (caused predominately by *E. chaffeensis*, *E. ewingii*, and *E. muris euclairensis*) are tickborne infections commonly reported in the United States, pathogenic species can be found in many regions of the world. Infections with these and other *Anaplasma* and *Ehrlichia* spp. have been reported in Africa, South America, Asia, and Europe, and occasionally among travelers.

Neoehrlichia & Neorickettsia

Neoehrlichia mikurensis is a tickborne pathogen that occurs in many parts of Asia and Europe. It generally infects people who are older or who are immunocompromised. Sennetsu fever, caused by *N. sennetsu*, occurs in Japan, Malaysia, and parts of Southeast Asia. This disease can be contracted from eating raw fish infested with neorickettsiae-infected flukes.

CLINICAL PRESENTATION

Rickettsial diseases are difficult to diagnose, even by health care providers experienced with these diseases. The incubation period for most rickettsial diseases ranges from 5–10 days. Travelers can experience signs and symptoms during their trip or not until 1–2 weeks after returning home.

Most symptomatic rickettsial diseases cause moderate illness, but others, including RMSF (also called Brazilian spotted fever), epidemic typhus, scrub typhus, and Mediterranean spotted fever, can be life-threatening in some cases, particularly when treatment is delayed. Clinical presentations vary with the causative agent and patient. Common symptoms that typically develop within 1 week of infection include fever, headache, malaise, nausea, or vomiting. Many rickettsioses also are accompanied by a maculopapular, petechial, or vesicular rash, or sometimes an eschar (a dark necrotic scab) at the site of the tick or mite bite (see Sec. 11, Ch. 8, Dermatologic Conditions).

Spotted Fever Group

AFRICAN TICK-BITE FEVER

African tick-bite fever is typically milder than most other rickettsioses, but recovery is facilitated with antimicrobial treatment. Suspect this disease in patients presenting with fever, headache, myalgia, and ≥1 eschars after recent travel to sub-Saharan Africa or the Caribbean.

MEDITERRANEAN SPOTTED FEVER

Mediterranean spotted fever can be life-threatening, and clinicians should suspect it in patients with fever, rash, and an eschar after recent travel to northern Africa or the Mediterranean Basin.

ROCKY MOUNTAIN SPOTTED FEVER OR BRAZILIAN SPOTTED FEVER

RMSF is characterized by fever, headache, abdominal pain, and nausea, and can progress rapidly into a serious systemic disease. A maculopapular or petechial rash is commonly reported, but eschars are not. RMSF is the most severe of the spotted fever rickettsioses, and case fatality ratios of 20%–40% are seen among patients for whom antimicrobial drug treatment was delayed.

5

Typhus Group

MURINE TYPHUS

Patients with murine typhus usually present with a moderately severe but nonspecific febrile illness. Only about half of patients develop a maculopapular rash, typically on the trunk. Although generally less severe than diseases like RMSF or scrub typhus, patients with murine typhus can develop organ failure or other severe sequelae requiring hospital-based management. Death can occur.

Scrub Typhus

Clinicians should include scrub typhus in the differential diagnosis of patients with a fever, headache, myalgias, and eschar after recent travel to destinations where the disease is endemic. Cough, encephalitis, lymphadenopathy, and rash might be present, and multisystem organ failure can develop.

Anaplasmosis & Ehrlichiosis

Clinicians should consider anaplasmosis or ehrlichiosis in febrile patients with leukopenia and an appropriate exposure history. Rash might occur in some children with ehrlichiosis, but is not a feature of anaplasmosis. Other clinical signs are similar to those of other rickettsioses.

DIAGNOSIS

As noted above, rickettsial diseases are difficult to diagnose, even by experienced clinicians. Timely presumptive diagnosis and initiation of antibiotic therapy is almost always based on clinical recognition and epidemiologic context. Serologic testing provides retrospective confirmation and is most accurate when acute and convalescent phase serum samples are compared; a ≥4-fold rise in antibody titer between paired specimens is diagnostic in indirect immunofluorescence antibody assays. Because of cross-reactivity of antigens, some antibodies might react in group-targeted serologic tests and provide evidence of exposure to the group level.

PCR assays and immunohistochemical analyses can be helpful, but results are highly dependent on the type and timing of submitted specimens. If an eschar is present, a swab or biopsy sample of the lesion can be evaluated by PCR to provide a species-specific diagnosis. Similarly, biopsy specimens of rash lesions or whole blood specimens can be evaluated by PCR but are generally less sensitive than samples derived from an eschar.

If anaplasmosis or ehrlichiosis is suspected, PCR of a whole blood specimen provides the best diagnostic test. A buffy coat might provide presumptive evidence of infection if examined to identify characteristic inclusion bodies within leukocytes (called intraleukocytic morulae).

Spotted fever rickettsiosis, anaplasmosis, and ehrlichiosis are nationally notifiable diseases in the United States. Commercial laboratories offer testing for rickettsioses, scrub typhus, anaplasmosis, and ehrlichiosis. Some species-targeted serologic tests are not routinely available at commercial laboratories, however, and are available only through CDC's Rickettsial Zoonoses Branch (rzbepidiag@cdc.gov).

TREATMENT

Because some rickettsioses can progress rapidly to severe illness, clinicians should initiate therapy as soon as infection is suspected and not wait to receive confirmatory test results. Immediate empiric treatment with a tetracycline (most commonly, doxycycline) is recommended for patients of all ages. Almost no other broad-spectrum antibiotic provides effective treatment.

Rigorous reevaluation of earlier reports of doxycycline-resistant scrub typhus has revealed those reports to be incorrect. *Orientia* spp. are doxycycline sensitive. Limited clinical experience has shown that *A. phagocytophilum* and *R. africae* infections respond to treatment with rifampin, which can be an alternative for pregnant or doxycycline-intolerant patients. Chloramphenicol is the only recognized alternative treatment for diseases caused by *Orientia* and *Rickettsia* species, but oral formulations are not available in many areas; moreover, chloramphenicol use is associated with more deaths, particularly with *R. rickettsii* infection. Seek expert advice if considering treatment with an alternative antibiotic.

PREVENTION

No vaccine is available for preventing rickettsial infections. Antibiotic prophylaxis is not recommended for rickettsial diseases, and antimicrobial agents should not be given to asymptomatic people.

Instruct travelers going to rickettsia endemic areas to minimize their exposure to infectious arthropods (including fleas, lice, mites, ticks) and avoid animal reservoirs (particularly dogs and rats). Travelers can reduce risk for infection by properly using insect repellents on skin and clothing, conducting a self-examination after visits to vector-infested areas, and wearing protective clothing (see Sec. 4, Ch. 6, Mosquitoes, Ticks & Other Arthropods). These precautions are especially important for travelers with immune-compromising conditions, because they might be more susceptible to severe disease.

CDC websites: www.cdc.gov/rmsf/; www.cdc.gov/otherspottedfever/; www.cdc.gov/typhus/murine/; www.cdc.gov/anaplasmosis/; www.cdc.gov/ehrlichiosis/

BIBLIOGRAPHY

Biggs HM, Barton Behravesh C, Bradley KK, Dahlgren FS, Drexler NA, Dumler JS, et al. Diagnosis and management of tickborne rickettsial diseases: Rocky Mountain spotted fever and other spotted fever group rickettsioses, ehrlichiosis, and anaplasmosis—United States: A practical guide for health care and public health professionals. MMWR Recomm Rep. 2016;65:1–44.

Botelho-Nevers E, Socolovschi C, Raoult D, Parola P. Treatment of *Rickettsia* spp. infections: a review. Exp Rev Anti Infect Ther. 2012;10:1425–37.

Cherry CC, Denison AM, Kato CY, Thornton K, Paddock CD. Diagnosis of spotted fever group rickettsioses in U.S. travelers returning from Africa, 2007–2016. Am J Trop Med Hyg. 2018;99(1):136–42.

de Vries SG, van Eekeren LE, van der Linden H, Visser BJ, Grobusch MP, Wagenaar JFP, Goris MGA, Goorhuis A. Searching and finding the hidden treasure: a retrospective analysis of rickettsial disease among Dutch international travelers. Clin Infect Dis. 2021;72:1171–8.

Eldin C, Parola P. Update on tick-borne bacterial diseases in travelers. Curr Infect Dis Rep. 2018;20(7):17.

Paris DH, Neumayr A. Ticks and tick-borne infections in Asia: implications for travellers. Trav Med Infect Dis. 2018;26:3–4.

Rauch J, Eisermann P, Noack B, Mehlhoop U, Muntau B, Schäfer J, Tappe D. Typhus group rickettsiosis, Germany, 2010–2017. Emerg Infect Dis 2018;24:1213–20.

Silaghi C, Beck R, Oteo JA, Pfeffer M, Sprong H. Neoehrlichiosis: an emerging tick-borne zoonosis caused by *Candidatus Neoehrlichia mikurensis*. Exp Appl Acarol. 2016;68:279–97.

Strand A, Paddock CD, Rinehart AR, Condit ME, Marus JR, Gillani S, et al. African tick bite fever treated successfully with rifampin in a patient with doxycycline intolerance. Clin Infect Dis. 2017;65:1582–4.

Wangrangsimakul T, Phuklia W, Newton PN, Richards AL, Day NPJ. Scrub typhus and the misconception of doxycycline resistance. Clin Infect Dis. 2020;70:2444–9.

Weitzel T, Acosta-Jamett G, Martinez-Valdebenito C, Richards AL, Grobusch MP, Abarca K. Scrub typhus risk in travelers to southern Chile. Trav Med Infect Dis. 2019;29:78–9.

SALMONELLOSIS, NONTYPHOIDAL

Ian Plumb, Patricia (Patti) Fields, Beau Bruce

INFECTIOUS AGENT: Nontyphoidal *Salmonella* serotypes	
ENDEMICITY	Worldwide
TRAVELER CATEGORIES AT GREATEST RISK FOR EXPOSURE & INFECTION	Adventurous eaters Travelers who pet, touch, or handle animals
PREVENTION	Follow safe food and water precautions; avoid untreated water and undercooked or raw meat, eggs, dairy, and produce Practice good hand hygiene, especially after contact with animals or their environments
DIAGNOSTIC SUPPORT	A clinical laboratory certified in moderate complexity testing

INFECTIOUS AGENT

Salmonella are gram-negative, rod-shaped bacilli. More than 2,500 *Salmonella* serotypes have been described. *Salmonella* serotypes can be categorized as typhoidal, which cause typhoid and paratyphoid fever, and nontyphoidal serotypes, which cause other human illness, typically acute diarrhea. See the Sec. 5, Part 1, Ch. 24, Typhoid & Paratyphoid Fever, for illness caused by *Salmonella* serotypes Typhi, Paratyphi A, tartrate negative Paratyphi B, and Paratyphi C.

TRANSMISSION

Animal reservoirs include both domestic and wild animals, including food animals, amphibians, and reptiles. Human infection can result from direct contact with infected animals or their environments. Transmission usually occurs from eating contaminated foods (e.g., dairy, eggs, meat, raw produce); drinking contaminated water; or from contact with people who have a diarrheal illness. The risk for infection after exposure is increased by taking antibiotics or antacid medication.

EPIDEMIOLOGY

Nontyphoidal *Salmonella* is one of the leading bacterial causes of diarrhea, causing ≈150 million illnesses and ≈60,000 deaths globally each year. *Salmonella* infection is diagnosed in ≈5 per 1,000 travelers who return with diarrhea. Among travelers returning to the United States, the rate of confirmed infection per 100,000 air travelers is estimated to be 26 after travel to Africa; 6–9 after travel to the Caribbean, Central America, or Asia; and 2–3 after travel to South America, Europe, or Oceania.

CLINICAL PRESENTATION

Nontyphoidal *Salmonella* infection usually presents with an acute diarrheal illness. The incubation period of salmonellosis is typically 12–96 hours, but it can be ≥7 days. Illness manifests commonly with acute diarrhea, abdominal cramps, and fever, and usually resolves without treatment after 1–7 days.

Approximately 5% of people develop bacteremia or focal invasive infection (e.g., osteomyelitis, meningitis, endovascular infection, septic arthritis). Rates of invasive disease are generally higher among infants, older adults, and people who are immunocompromised, including those with HIV. People with atherosclerosis, hemoglobinopathies, or malignant neoplasms also have increased risk for extraintestinal infection. Infection with antibiotic-resistant organisms has been associated with a greater risk for bloodstream infection and hospitalization.

DIAGNOSIS

Culture provides confirmation of nontyphoidal *Salmonella* infection. Approximately 90% of isolates are obtained from routine stool culture; isolates also can be obtained from other sites of infection (e.g., abscesses, blood, cerebrospinal fluid, urine). Although clinical laboratories increasingly use culture-independent diagnostic tests to detect *Salmonella* infection, isolates are necessary for antimicrobial susceptibility testing and for characterization during public health investigations. Reflex bacterial culture is recommended, if possible, on the same specimen, for positive culture-independent specimens. Serologic testing is unreliable and not advised.

Salmonellosis is a nationally notifiable disease. Most states mandate that *Salmonella* isolates or clinical material be submitted to the local or state public health laboratory. Clinical laboratory staff should be aware of disease reporting and mandatory isolate submission regulations for their state; they can contact their local public health department with questions.

TREATMENT

Indications for Antibiotic Therapy

Most patients can be treated with supportive care alone, including oral rehydration therapy. Antibiotic therapy is not recommended for most patients with uncomplicated salmonellosis caused by nontyphoidal *Salmonella*; it does not shorten the duration of illness and can prolong bacterial shedding.

Consider antibiotic therapy for patients with suspected invasive disease (e.g., patients with severe diarrhea, high fever, manifestations of extraintestinal infection) and for patients at increased risk for invasive disease (e.g., infants, older adults, people who are immunocompromised, patients with known atherosclerosis). For these populations, treat infections empirically until susceptibility results are available.

Bacteremic patients generally require ≥7 days of antimicrobial drug therapy and an investigation for possible sites of infection. Longer therapy, specialist consultation, and surgical intervention might be required for extraintestinal infections. Immunocompromised patients are at risk for recurrent invasive disease and require therapy of longer duration.

Choice of Empiric Antimicrobial Drug Therapy

Salmonella resistance to older antimicrobial agents (ampicillin, chloramphenicol, and trimethoprim-sulfamethoxazole) has been recognized for many years; none of these should be considered first-line empiric agents in returning travelers (see Sec. 2, Ch. 6, Travelers' Diarrhea). Resistance to antimicrobial agents varies by *Salmonella* serotype and geographic region.

FLUOROQUINOLONES

Fluoroquinolones are considered first-line treatment in adult travelers. Resistance to fluoroquinolones among *Salmonella* strains has been rising globally, however; among travelers returning to the United States with a diagnosis of nontyphoidal salmonellosis during 2004–2014, decreased susceptibility to fluoroquinolones was present in 41% of isolates from travelers to Asia.

CEFTRIAXONE

Ceftriaxone can be used to treat children or adults with invasive disease. Although ceftriaxone resistance is rare, it has increasingly been detected among bloodstream isolates in sub-Saharan Africa. Azithromycin can be used for children and is an alternative agent for adults. Decreased susceptibility to azithromycin is rare, but has been documented in multiple settings globally. Clinical laboratories do not commonly test for resistance to azithromycin, however, because susceptibility breakpoints have not been established.

PREVENTION

No vaccine against nontyphoidal *Salmonella* infection is available. Travelers should follow preventive measures, such as eating food that is adequately cooked and drinking from safe sources (see Sec. 2, Ch. 8, Food & Water Precautions), and by frequently washing hands, especially after contact with animals or their environments. In general, travelers should avoid uncooked vegetables, but travelers can gain some protection by washing raw produce properly.

People with diarrheal illness should avoid preparing food for others. After their symptoms have resolved, people who had diarrheal illness should continue to practice safe food preparation and carefully wash hands regularly because they can shed bacteria for weeks afterward.

CDC website: www.cdc.gov/salmonella

BIBLIOGRAPHY

American Academy of Pediatrics. *Salmonella* infections. In: Kimberlin DW, Brady MT, Jackson MA, Long SS, editors. Red Book: 2018 report of the Committee on Infectious Diseases. Itasca (IL): American Academy of Pediatrics; 2018. pp. 711–18. Available from: https://redbook.solutions.aap.org/chapter.aspx?sectionid=247326914&bookid=2591.

Crump JA, Sjölund-Karlsson M, Gordon MA, Parry CM. Epidemiology, clinical presentation, laboratory diagnosis, antimicrobial resistance, and antimicrobial management of invasive salmonella infections. Clin Microbiol Rev. 2015;28(4):901–37.

Grass JE, Kim S, Huang JY, Morrison SM, McCullough AE, Bennett C, et al. Quinolone nonsusceptibility among enteric pathogens isolated from international travelers–Foodborne Diseases Active Surveillance Network (FoodNet) and National Antimicrobial Monitoring System (NARMS), 10 United States sites, 2004–2014. PLOS ONE; 2019;14(12):e0225800.

Pegues DA, Miller SI. Salmonella species. In: Bennett JE, Dolin R, Blaser MJ, editors. Mandell, Douglas, and Bennett's principles and practice of infectious diseases, 9th edition. Philadelphia: Elsevier Saunders; 2020. pp. 2725–36.

Shane AL, Mody RK, Crump JA, Tarr PI, Steiner TS, Kotloff K, et al. 2017 Infectious Diseases Society of America clinical practice guidelines for the diagnosis and management of infectious diarrhea. Clin Infect Dis; 2017;65(12):e45–e80.

5

SHIGELLOSIS

Amanda Garcia-Williams, Kayla Vanden Esschert, Naeemah Logan

INFECTIOUS AGENT: *Shigella* spp.	
ENDEMICITY	*Shigella flexneri* in low- and middle-income countries *S. sonnei* in high-income countries
TRAVELER CATEGORIES AT GREATEST RISK FOR EXPOSURE & INFECTION	Children Immigrants and refugees Mass gathering attendees Men who have sex with men Tourists Travelers visiting friends and relatives
PREVENTION METHODS	Practice good hand hygiene Follow safe food and water safety precautions Minimize fecal-oral exposures during sexual activity
DIAGNOSTIC SUPPORT	A clinical laboratory certified in moderate complexity testing; state health department

INFECTIOUS AGENT

Shigellosis is an acute infection of the intestine caused by bacteria in the genus *Shigella*. There are 4 species of *Shigella: S. dysenteriae, S. flexneri, S. boydii*, and *S. sonnei* (also referred to as group A, B, C, and D, respectively). Several distinct serotypes are recognized within the first 3 species.

TRANSMISSION

Shigella is transmitted via the fecal–oral route, through direct person-to-person contact, or indirectly through contaminated food, water, or fomites. Transmission directly from one person to another or via fomite is likely the most common mode of transmission in high resource settings; foodborne and waterborne transmission are additional important transmission routes in both high- and low-resource settings. Spread of *Shigella* through both direct and indirect sexual contact has been widely reported, primarily among men who have sex with men (MSM). Shigellosis is highly contagious; as few as 10 organisms can cause infection. Humans are the primary natural reservoir, although nonhuman primates also can be infected.

EPIDEMIOLOGY

Shigella spp. are endemic to temperate and tropical climates. Shigellosis is caused predominantly by *S. sonnei* in high-income countries, whereas *S. flexneri* is prevalent in low- and middle-income countries. Infections caused by *S. boydii* and *S. dysenteriae* are less common globally. *S. boydii* is mostly restricted to the Indian subcontinent, and *S. dysenteriae* accounts for most *Shigella* spp. isolated in sub-Saharan Africa and South Asia.

Worldwide, *Shigella* is estimated to cause 80–165 million cases of disease and 600,000 deaths annually, and most cases and deaths are among children. Among shigellosis cases worldwide, approximately 20–119 million illnesses and 6,900–30,000 deaths are attributed to foodborne transmission. Foodborne transmission has been reported among travelers in multiple outbreaks, and tourists became ill after eating contaminated foods in hotels and on airplanes and cruise ships. Common food vehicles include cold salads, vegetables, lettuce, and herbs; meat and dairy items and hot dishes also have been implicated.

Numerous outbreaks have also been attributed to waterborne transmission, in both treated and untreated recreational water, and through ingesting contaminated drinking water. Outbreaks of shigellosis tend to occur in settings where sanitation and hygiene practices are inadequate; common settings include schools and daycare centers, private residences, and restaurants. Other populations with reported outbreaks of shigellosis include MSM, people experiencing homelessness, and people in refugee camps.

Shigella spp. have been detected in stool samples of 5%–18% of patients with travelers' diarrhea, and studies in Australia and Canada found that 40%–50% of locally diagnosed shigellosis cases were associated with international travel. In the United States, ≈25% of sporadic cases of shigellosis are travel-associated, and *Shigella* spp. account for 13% of travel-associated enteric infections. In a study conducted among US travelers, most infections caused by *S. dysenteriae* (56%) and *S. boydii* (44%) were travel-associated, whereas infections caused by *S. flexneri* and *S. sonnei* were less often associated with travel (24% and 12%, respectively). In another study among US travelers, the risk for infection caused by *Shigella* spp. was greatest for people who had traveled to Africa, and then travelers to Central America, South America, and Asia. Infections caused by Shiga toxin–producing *S. flexneri* and *S. dysenteriae* have been reported repeatedly among travelers to Haiti and the Dominican Republic (Hispaniola).

Antimicrobial resistance is common in *Shigella*; resistant strains can be acquired during travel to areas of high endemicity. A systematic review of travel-associated *Shigella* infections from 139 countries showed that the percentage of antibiotic-resistant infections increased from 19% during 1990–1999, to 65% during 2000–2009. Moreover, most resistant *Shigella* spp. isolates originated from Asia (25%, excluding West Asia) and Central and South America (18%). The study also documented an increase in quinolone-resistant *Shigella* spp. from 30% during 1990–1999 to 53% during 2000–2009.

Likewise, in the United States, infection with quinolone-resistant *Shigella* spp. has been linked to international travel. Bowen et al. identified a large outbreak of ciprofloxacin-resistant shigellosis in San Francisco after international travel, primarily to the Dominican Republic, Haiti, and India. Similarly, Grass et al. analyzed *Shigella* infections using linked data collected during 2004–2014 from the Foodborne Diseases Active Surveillance Network (FoodNet) and National Antimicrobial Resistance Monitoring System (NARMS). The authors found that international travel was associated with a 6-fold higher odds of infection with quinolone-resistant *Shigella*.

Resistance to third- and fourth-generation cephalosporins is less common but has also been documented in the United States and is more common in South and East Asia. Additionally, reduced susceptibility to azithromycin and ciprofloxacin has been documented among MSM in several countries, including the United States. Finally, widespread and extensive resistance to former first-line agents, including ampicillin, cotrimoxazole, and nalidixic acid, exists.

CLINICAL PRESENTATION

Illness typically begins 1–2 days after exposure with symptoms lasting 5–7 days. Disease severity varies according to species. *S. dysenteriae* serotype 1 (Sd1) is the agent of epidemic dysentery and often causes severe illness, whereas *S. sonnei* commonly causes milder, nondysenteric diarrheal illness. *Shigella* of any species can cause severe illness among people with compromised immune systems.

Shigellosis is characterized by watery, bloody, or mucoid diarrhea, fever, and stomach cramps. Tenesmus is also a common symptom. Illness in immunocompetent people is usually mild and self-limited. Occasionally, patients experience intestinal or extraintestinal complications, including intestinal perforation, seizures (in young children), and invasive focal infections. Postinfectious manifestations, including reactive arthritis, and hemolytic-uremic syndrome (HUS), can occur weeks after infection. HUS is associated with Shiga toxin–producing *Shigella* strains, particularly Sd1.

DIAGNOSIS

To confirm the diagnosis of shigellosis, perform a stool culture. Conduct antimicrobial susceptibility testing for patients who might require antimicrobial treatment. Rapid PCR-based diagnostic tests for *Shigella* are now increasingly available in the United States. This method cannot determine whether viable *Shigella* organisms are present in stool, however, and does not yield an isolate for susceptibility testing or for public health investigation and control. As such, if *Shigella* is detected using a PCR assay, consider performing reflex culture and susceptibility testing.

If additional diagnostic support is required, consult a clinical laboratory first. Testing performed at the Centers for Disease Control and Prevention, if appropriate, should be arranged through the state or county public health department. Shigellosis is a nationally notifiable disease in the United States.

TREATMENT

Shigellosis usually resolves within 5–7 days with supportive care alone; antimicrobial treatment given early in the course of illness can, however, shorten the duration of symptoms and of carriage (asymptomatic shedding of the organism in the stool). Consider antimicrobial treatment for patients with severe disease or those with compromised immune systems. Antimicrobial treatment can also be considered for patients working in occupations where their risk of transmitting *Shigella* to others is high (e.g., childcare workers, food handlers, health care workers) or to limit transmission in outbreak settings.

Whenever possible, use antimicrobial susceptibility results to direct antibiotic therapy. If empiric therapy is indicated, current clinical guidelines recommend azithromycin, ciprofloxacin, or ceftriaxone as first-line options. Given widespread resistance to commonly used first- and second-line agents, review local resistance trends and pertinent sexual and travel history before initiating empiric therapy. In the United States, populations at increased risk for multidrug-resistant *Shigella* infections include international travelers, people experiencing homelessness, MSM, and people infected with HIV. Information on antimicrobial resistance among shigellosis cases in the United States is available at https://wwwn.cdc.gov/narmsnow. Additional discussion of symptomatic management can be found in Sec. 2, Ch. 6, Travelers' Diarrhea.

PREVENTION

No vaccines are available for *Shigella*. The best defense against shigellosis is thorough, frequent handwashing; strict adherence to standard food and water safety precautions (see Sec. 2, Ch. 8, Food & Water Precautions); and minimizing fecal–oral exposures during sexual activity by using barriers during sex, washing the genitals and anal area before and after sex, and washing sex toys after use. When soap and water are not available, travelers can use alcohol-based hand sanitizers. Sec. 2, Ch. 6, Travelers' Diarrhea, contains general recommendations to prevent diarrhea while traveling.

CDC website: www.cdc.gov/shigella

BIBLIOGRAPHY

American Academy of Pediatrics. *Shigella* infections. In: Kimberlin DW, Brady MT, Jackson MA, Long SS, editors. Red Book: 2018 report of the Committee on Infectious Diseases, 31st edition. Itasca (IL): American Academy of Pediatrics; 2018. pp. 723–7.

Bowen A, Hurd J, Hoover C, Khachadourian Y, Traphagen E, Harvey E, et al. Importation and domestic transmission of *Shigella sonnei* resistant to ciprofloxacin—United States, May 2014–February 2015. MMWR Morb Mortal Wkly Rep. 2015;64(12):318–20.

Centers for Disease Control and Prevention. Shigellosis outbreak associated with an unchlorinated fill-and-drain wading pool—Iowa, 2001. MMWR Morb Mortal Wkly Rep. 2001;50(37):797–800.

Grass JE, Kim S, Huang JY, Morrison SM, McCullough AE, Bennett C, et al. Quinolone nonsusceptibility among enteric pathogens isolated from international travelers—Foodborne Diseases Active Surveillance Network (FoodNet) and National Antimicrobial Monitoring System (NARMS), 10 United States sites, 2004–2014. PLoS One. 2019;14(12):e0225800.

Kendall ME, Crim S, Fullerton K, Han PV, Cronquist AB, Shiferaw B, et al. Travel-associated enteric infections diagnosed after return to the United States, Foodborne Diseases Active Surveillance Network (FoodNet), 2004–2009. Clin Infect Dis. 2012;54(Suppl 5):S480–7.

Kirk MD, Pires SM, Black RE, Caipo M, Crump JA, Devleesschauwer B, et al. World Health Organization estimates of the global and regional disease burden of 22 foodborne bacterial, protozoal, and viral diseases, 2010: a data synthesis. PLoS Med. 2015;12(12):e1001921.

Klontz KC, Singh N. Treatment of drug-resistant *Shigella* infections. Expert Rev Anti Infect Ther. 2015;13(1):69–80.

Kotloff KL, Riddle MS, Platts-Mills JA, Pavlinac P, Zaidi AK. Shigellosis. The Lancet. 2018;391(10122):801–12.

Puzari M, Sharma M, Chetia P. Emergence of antibiotic resistant *Shigella* species: A matter of concern. J Infect Public Health. 2018;11(4):451–4.

Williams PCM, Berkley JA. Guidelines for the treatment of dysentery (shigellosis): a systematic review of the evidence. Paediatr Int Child Health. 2018;38(suppl):S50–65.

TETANUS

Anna Minta, Fiona Havers, Rania Tohme

INFECTIOUS AGENT: *Clostridium tetani*	
ENDEMICITY	Worldwide
TRAVELER CATEGORIES AT GREATEST RISK FOR EXPOSURE & INFECTION	Humanitarian aid workers Pregnant travelers Travelers not current with tetanus toxoid–containing vaccine
PREVENTION METHODS	Tetanus is a vaccine-preventable disease Properly manage wounds (vaccination + tetanus immune globulin)
DIAGNOSTIC SUPPORT	No confirmatory laboratory tests are available for tetanus; consult CDC's Tetanus website, www.cdc.gov/tetanus/clinicians.html

INFECTIOUS AGENT

The causative agent of tetanus is *Clostridium tetani*, a spore-forming, anaerobic, gram-positive bacterium. Ubiquitous in the environment, spores of *C. tetani* germinate into toxin-producing bacteria when they enter the body under specific conditions.

TRANSMISSION

Tetanus is transmitted via direct contamination of open wounds and non-intact skin. Non-neonatal tetanus typically is acquired when spores enter certain wounds, including wounds contaminated with dirt, animal or human excreta or saliva, or necrotic tissue. Burns, crush injuries, and deep punctures are also at increased risk for tetanus infection. Even wounds without visible contamination can become infected with tetanus spores; tetanus transmission has been associated with abortion, dental infection, injection drug use, otitis media, pregnancy, and surgery. Neonatal tetanus is typically acquired when spores contaminate the umbilical cord due to unhygienic delivery practices. Direct person-to-person transmission does not occur.

EPIDEMIOLOGY

Tetanus is distributed worldwide. It is more common in rural and agricultural regions; areas where contact with soil or animal excreta is likely; warm and moist environments; and areas where immunization against tetanus is inadequate. Because the spores exist in the environment, tetanus cannot be eradicated. In 2020, over 11,750 tetanus cases across the globe were reported to the World Health Organization / United Nations Children's Fund, of which 2,230 occurred in neonates. Most tetanus cases were reported from countries in Africa and Southeast Asia.

Maternal and neonatal tetanus elimination, defined as <1 neonatal tetanus case per 1,000 live births per year in every district in a country, has not been achieved in Afghanistan, Angola, Central African Republic, Guinea, Mali, Nigeria, Pakistan, Papua New Guinea, Somalia, Sudan, South Sudan, or Yemen. Any traveler not up to date with tetanus vaccination is at risk of acquiring tetanus infection. Because hygienic obstetric care might not be available, travelers (especially pregnant travelers) going to countries that have not eliminated maternal and neonatal tetanus might be at increased risk for morbidity and mortality from tetanus infection; in addition, proper wound management and tetanus immune globulin (TIG) are less likely to be available in these settings.

Tetanus can affect any age group. The risk for injuries after natural disasters is high; therefore, humanitarian aid workers should be up to date on tetanus vaccination before travel. The number of US travelers who acquire tetanus infection abroad is unknown; surveillance might be limited because travelers with injuries are unlikely to seek care at a travel clinic when they return from their trip. Injuries are common among travelers, however, and any tetanus-prone wound is a risk, so ensure that all travelers are properly vaccinated.

CLINICAL PRESENTATION

The incubation period is on average 10 days (range 3–21 days). The duration of the incubation period is inversely related to the severity of symptoms, and shorter incubation periods are associated with injuries closer to the central nervous system. Tetanus is classified as generalized, localized, and cephalic. Generalized tetanus, which occurs in >80% of cases, is characterized by lockjaw, generalized spasms, risus sardonicus, and opisthotonus. Symptoms of localized tetanus include muscle spasms confined to the injury site. Cephalic tetanus is characterized by a head or face wound and flaccid cranial nerve palsies. Progression from localized and cephalic tetanus to generalized tetanus can occur. Neonatal tetanus occurs in newborns who have contaminated umbilical stumps and whose mothers are unimmunized or inadequately immunized. Neonatal tetanus can lead to long-term sequelae, including behavioral, intellectual, and neurologic abnormalities. Severe tetanus can lead to respiratory failure and death. Case-fatality ratios for generalized tetanus vary between 25% and 100% and can only be reduced to 10%–20% where modern intensive care is available. The case-fatality ratio is <1% for localized tetanus.

DIAGNOSIS

Diagnosis is based on clinical findings with epidemiologic support; no confirmatory laboratory tests are available. Tetanus is a nationally notifiable disease in the United States.

TREATMENT

The goals of treatment are to inactivate circulating toxin by immediately administering tetanus immune globulin (TIG); eliminate the bacteria with aggressive wound care and debridement to stop further toxin formation; provide supportive care; and provide antibiotic treatment for 7–10 days. Metronidazole is the most appropriate antibiotic; parenteral penicillin G is an alternative treatment. Patients with tetanus must be hospitalized in a quiet, dim room to minimize spasms. Additional supportive care measures include agents to control muscle spasm and autonomic dysfunction, and respiratory support. Patients should be vaccinated and receive TIG as described below. Additional information about diagnosis and treatment can be found at the Centers for Disease Control and Prevention (CDC) Tetanus website (www.cdc.gov/tetanus/clinicians.html).

PREVENTION

Vaccine

INDICATIONS FOR USE

Tetanus disease does not result in immunity. Vaccination is the only prevention against tetanus. Because immunity after vaccination wanes over time, lifelong vaccination with tetanus toxoid–containing vaccine (TTCV) is necessary to attain and sustain immunity against tetanus. All travelers should be up to date with vaccination before departure.

CHILDREN

DTaP (diphtheria-tetanus-acellular pertussis) and DT (diphtheria-tetanus) are indicated for children <7 years, while Tdap (tetanus-diphtheria-acellular pertussis) and Td (tetanus-diphtheria) are indicated for children ≥10 years. Infants and children should receive 5 doses of DTaP at 2, 4, 6, and 15–18 months, and at 4–6 years; adolescents should receive 1 dose of Tdap at 11–12 years of age. Children ≥7 years old can receive Tdap for catch-up vaccination.

ADULTS

Adults should receive TTCV booster doses every 10 years. Adults who have never received Tdap should receive Tdap; otherwise, clinicians can administer either Td or Tdap. Previously unvaccinated pregnant people should receive 2 doses of TTCV during their pregnancy. Pregnant people also should be properly vaccinated to prevent infant pertussis, irrespective of their vaccination history, by receiving Tdap during every pregnancy at 27–36 weeks' gestation, preferably earlier in this period. See the CDC Immunization Schedules website (www.cdc.gov/vaccines/schedules/index.html) for routine and catch-up vaccination schedules and minimum intervals between TTCV doses.

ADVERSE REACTIONS & SAFETY

TTCV are safe. The most common adverse reactions are fatigue, headache, and injection site pain.

CONTRAINDICATIONS & PRECAUTIONS

A severe allergic reaction (e.g., anaphylaxis) to a previous dose or a component of the vaccine is a contraindication for any TTCV (DTaP, DT, Tdap, or Td). For DTaP or Tdap, encephalopathy without an identifiable cause occurring within ≤7 days of a previous dose of DTP, DTaP, or Tdap is a contraindication to vaccine administration. Encephalopathy is a contraindication for the pertussis component of the vaccines; therefore, people with this contraindication should receive either DT in place of DTaP or Td in place of Tdap, to ensure protection against diphtheria and tetanus.

Precautions for all TTCV include Guillain-Barré syndrome ≤6 weeks after a previous dose of TTCV, history of Arthus-type hypersensitivity after a previous dose of tetanus or diphtheria toxoid–containing vaccine (in which case, vaccination should be deferred until ≥10 years after the last TTCV), and moderate or severe acute illness with or without fever.

Due to the pertussis component of these vaccines, an additional precaution for DTaP and Tdap is a progressive or neurologic disorder, in which case vaccination should be deferred. Please see Liang et al. (www.cdc.gov/mmwr/volumes/67/rr/rr6702a1.htm) for additional information about when TTCV can be given.

Table 5-05 Tetanus prophylaxis for wound management

HISTORY OF TTCV	CLEAN, MINOR WOUND		ALL OTHER WOUNDS[1]	
	TTCV[2]	TIG	TTCV[2]	TIG[3]
Unknown or <3 doses	Yes	No	Yes	Yes
≥3 doses	No[4]	No	No[5]	No

Abbreviations: TIG, tetanus immune globulin; TTCV, tetanus toxoid–containing vaccine.

Source: Table adapted from Liang et al. MMWR. 2018;67(2):1–44.

[1] *All other wounds* include, but are not limited to, wounds contaminated with dirt, feces, saliva, or soil; avulsions; puncture wounds; and wounds resulting from burns, crush injuries, frostbite, or missiles.
[2] Use age-appropriate TTCV: DTaP for children <7 years of age; Tdap or Td for children ≥7 years of age and adults; Tdap is preferred for people who have not already received Tdap. Do not use Tdap for people who are pregnant.
[3] People with severe immunodeficiency or HIV infection with contaminated wounds should receive TIG regardless of TTCV status.
[4] Yes, if ≥10 years have passed since last TTCV.
[5] Yes, if ≥5 years have passed since last TTCV.

Wound Management

Patients with wounds should be evaluated for risk for tetanus infection based on the type of wound and TTCV status, and clinicians should provide prophylaxis accordingly (see Table 5-05). Complete information on tetanus prophylaxis and the use of TIG when indicated for wound management is available from Liang et al. (www.cdc.gov/mmwr/volumes/67/rr/rr6702a1.htm).

CDC websites: www.cdc.gov/tetanus; www.cdc.gov/vaccines/pubs/pinkbook/tetanus.html

BIBLIOGRAPHY

Afshar M, Raju M, Ansell D, Bleck TP. Narrative review: tetanus—a health threat after natural disasters in developing countries. Ann Intern Med. 2011;154(5):329–35.

Centers for Disease Control and Prevention. National Notifiable Diseases Surveillance System, 2018 annual tables of infectious disease data. Available from: https://wonder.cdc.gov/nndss/static/2018/annual/2018-table2n.html.

Chen LH, Wilson ME, Davis X, Loutan L, Schwartz E, Keystone J, et al. Illness in long-term travelers visiting GeoSentinel clinics. Emerg Infect Dis. 2009;15(11):1773–82.

Havers FP, Moro PL, Hunter P, Hariri S, Bernstein H. Use of tetanus toxoid, reduced diphtheria toxoid, and acellular pertussis vaccines: updated recommendations of the Advisory Committee on Immunization Practices—United States, 2019. MMWR Morb Mortal Wkly Rep. 2020;69(3):77–83.

Liang JL, Tiwari T, Moro P, Messonnier NE, Reingold A, Sawyer M, et al. Prevention of pertussis, tetanus, and diphtheria with vaccines in the United States: recommendations of the Advisory Committee on Immunization Practices (ACIP). MMWR Morb Mortal Wkly Rep. 2018;67(2):1–44.

McInnes RJ, Williamson LM, Morrison A. Unintentional injury during foreign travel: a review. J Travel Med. 2002;9(6):297–307.

Roper M, Wassilak S, Scobie H, Ridpath A, Orenstein W. Tetanus toxoid. In: Plotkin S, Orenstein W, Offit P, Edwards K, editors. Vaccines, 7th edition. Philadelphia: Elsevier; 2018. pp. 1052–79.e18.

World Health Organization. Tetanus reported cases and incidence. Available from: https://immunizationdata.who.int/pages/incidence/ttetanus.html

TUBERCULOSIS

John Jereb

INFECTIOUS AGENT: *Mycobacterium tuberculosis* complex	
ENDEMICITY	Worldwide, but with wide variations by region and social context
TRAVELER CATEGORIES AT GREATEST RISK FOR EXPOSURE & INFECTION	Humanitarian aid workers and health care personnel working in high-prevalence settings (e.g., refugee camps; HIV clinics, and in-patient hospital wards) Immigrants and refugees
PREVENTION METHODS	Avoid high-risk social contexts Obtain pre- and posttravel testing and preventive treatment for new infections Get fit-tested and use respiratory protection (e.g., N95 respirators) in high-risk occupational settings Consider vaccination with bacillus Calmette-Guérin (no longer available in the United States)
DIAGNOSTIC SUPPORT	A clinical laboratory certified in moderate or high complexity testing; state or local health department; or consult with US TB Centers of Excellence for Training, Education, and Medical Consultation, www.cdc.gov/tb/education/tb_coe/default.htm

INFECTIOUS AGENT

Mycobacterium tuberculosis complex is a group of closely related rod-shaped, nonmotile, slow-growing, acid-fast bacteria, which includes *M. bovis* and *M. tuberculosis hominis*, the most common cause of human tuberculosis (TB), usually referred to as *M. tuberculosis*.

TRANSMISSION

TB transmission occurs when a patient with a contagious form of the infection coughs, spreading bacilli through the air. People can acquire bovine TB (caused by *M. bovis*) by consuming unpasteurized dairy products from infected cattle.

The risk for *M. tuberculosis* transmission on an airplane is low, but instances of in-flight TB transmission have occurred. The risk of transmission is dependent on the contagiousness of the person with TB, seating proximity, flight duration, and host factors. To prevent transmission, people with contagious TB should not travel by commercial airplanes or other commercial conveyances. Typically, only TB of the lung or airway is contagious in community contexts, and health department authorities determine whether TB is contagious based on a person's chest radiograph, sputum tests, symptoms, and treatment received. The World Health Organization (WHO) issued guidelines for notifying passengers potentially exposed to TB on airplanes. Passengers concerned about possible TB exposure should see their primary health care provider or visit their local health department clinic for evaluation.

Bovine TB is a risk for travelers who consume unpasteurized dairy products in countries (e.g., Mexico) where *M. bovis* in cattle is common. *M. bovis* risk in some African countries has been postulated, but human *M. bovis* statistics are unavailable for those countries.

EPIDEMIOLOGY

According to the World Health Organization, ≈10 million new TB cases and ≈1.2 million TB-related deaths occurred in 2019. TB occurs throughout the world, but the incidence varies (see Map 5-02). In some countries in sub-Saharan Africa and Asia,

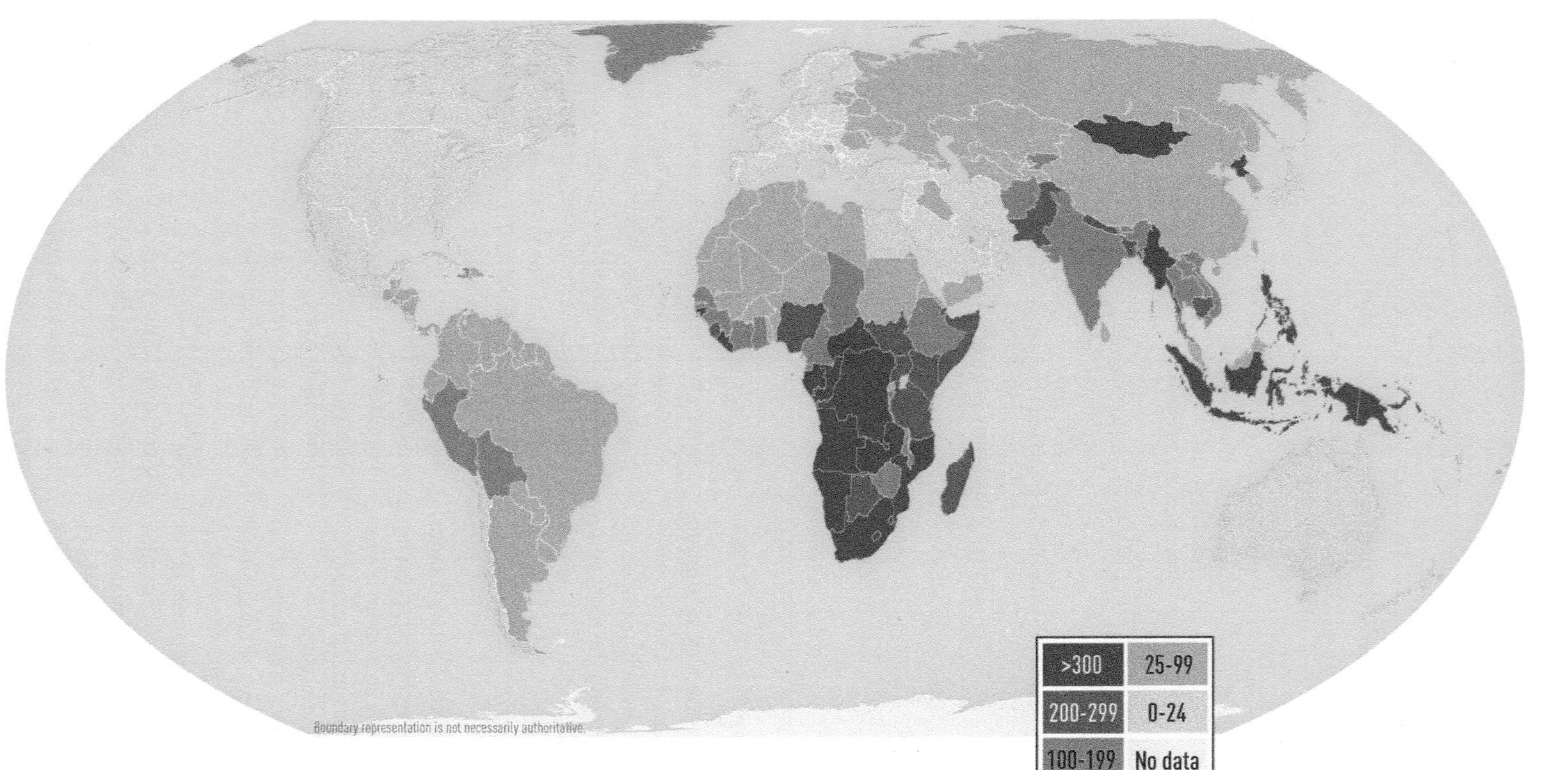

MAP 5-02 Estimated tuberculosis incidence rates per 100,000 population

Disease data sources: World Health Organization. Global tuberculosis report 2020 (https://apps.who.int/iris/bitstream/handle/10665/336069/9789240013131-eng.pdf); for French Guiana, *Tableau 5: Taux de déclaration de tuberculose maladie par Nouvelles régions (taux pour 100 000), France entière*, 2015–2020; Santé publique France; *La tuberculose: données* (Table 5: Tuberculosis disease reporting rate by New regions [rate per 100,000], Whole France, 2015–2020, Public Health France, Tuberculosis: data; www.santepubliquefrance.fr/maladies-et-traumatismes/maladies-et-infections-respiratoires/tuberculose/donnees/#tabs); for Taiwan, Statistics of Communicable Diseases and Surveillance Report 2019, Centers for Disease Control, Ministry of Health and Welfare, R.O.C. (Taiwan), November 2020 (www.cdc.gov.tw/En/File/Get/0nnMQjC37VAuhzVY3Vuq-A).

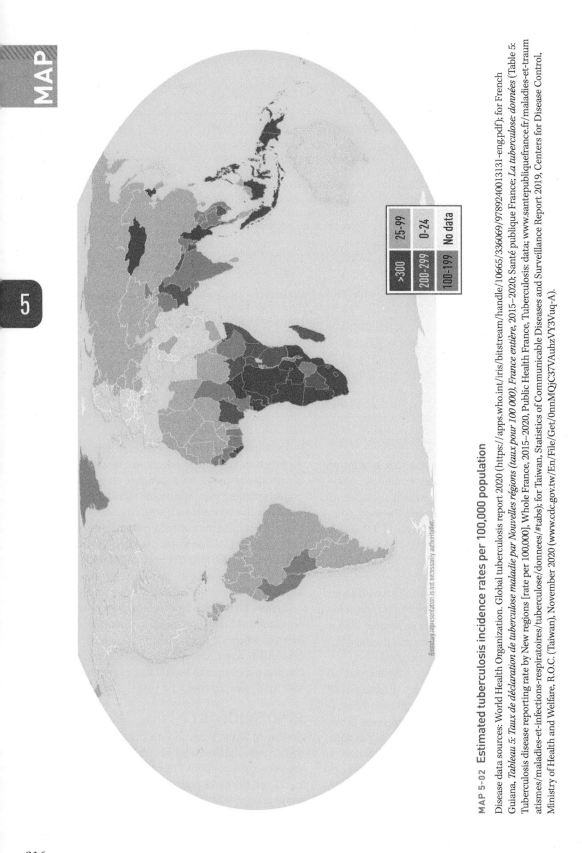

the annual incidence is several hundred per 100,000 population. In the United States, the annual incidence is <3 per 100,000 population, but immigrants from countries with a high TB burden and long-term residents of high-burden countries have a 10× greater incidence of TB than the US national average. Of note, US surveillance does not capture travel-related cases of TB.

Drug-resistant TB is an increasing concern. Multidrug-resistant (MDR) TB is resistant to at least the 2 most effective drugs, isoniazid and rifampin. MDR TB is less common than drug-susceptible TB, but globally ≈363,000 cases of MDR TB were diagnosed in 2019, and MDR TB accounts for >25% of TB cases in some countries (Table 5-06). MDR and higher-order resistance

Table 5-06 Estimated proportion of multidrug-resistant (MDR) tuberculosis (TB) cases in countries with high MDR TB burden, 2019

COUNTRY	% OF NEW TB CASES THAT ARE MDR	% OF RETREATMENT MDR TB CASES
Angola	2.5%	14%
Azerbaijan	11%	24%
Bangladesh	0.7%	11%
Belarus	38%	60%
China	7.1%	23%
DPR Korea	2.2%	16%
DR Congo	1.8%	11%
Ethiopia	0.7%	12%
India	2.8%	14%
Indonesia	2.4%	13%
Kazakhstan	27%	44%
Kenya	1.3%	4.6%
Kyrgyzstan	29%	60%
Mozambique	3.7%	13%
Myanmar	4.9%	18%
Nigeria	4.3%	14%
Pakistan	4.2%	7.3%
Papua New Guinea	3.4%	26%

(continued)

5

5

Table 5-06 Estimated proportion of multidrug-resistant (MDR) tuberculosis (TB) cases in countries with high MDR TB burden, 2019 (continued)

COUNTRY	% OF NEW TB CASES THAT ARE MDR	% OF RETREATMENT MDR TB CASES
Peru	6.3%	20%
Philippines	1.8%	28%
Republic of Moldova	33%	60%
Russian Federation	35%	71%
Somalia	8.7%	88%
South Africa	3.4%	7.1%
Tajikistan	29%	40%
Thailand	1.7%	10%
Ukraine	27%	43%
Uzbekistan	12%	22%
Vietnam	3.6%	17%
Zimbabwe	3.1%	14%

are of particular concern among HIV-infected or other immunocompromised people.

CLINICAL PRESENTATION

M. tuberculosis infection can be detected by a positive tuberculin skin test (TST) or interferon-γ release assay (IGRA) 8–10 weeks after exposure. Overall, only 5%–10% of otherwise healthy people who are infected progress to TB disease during their lifetimes. Progression to TB disease can take weeks to decades after initial infection. People with TB disease have symptoms or other manifestations of illness (e.g., an abnormal chest radiograph). For most people who become infected, *M. tuberculosis* remains in an inactive state (latent TB infection or LTBI) in which the infected person has no symptoms and cannot spread the infection to others.

TB disease can affect any organ, but affects the lungs in 70%–80% of cases. Typical TB symptoms include prolonged cough, fever, hemoptysis, night sweats, decreased appetite, and weight loss. The most common sites for TB outside the lungs (i.e., extrapulmonary TB) are the bladder, bones and joints, brain and meninges, genitalia, kidneys, lymph nodes, and pleura.

The risk for progression to disease is much higher in immunosuppressed people; for example, progression is 8%–10% per year in HIV-infected people not receiving antiretroviral therapy. People receiving tumor necrosis factor blockers to treat rheumatoid arthritis and other chronic inflammatory conditions also are at increased risk for disease progression.

DIAGNOSIS

Pretravel & Posttravel Testing

Before leaving the United States, travelers who anticipate possible prolonged exposure to TB (e.g., people who will care for patients, or who will work in health care facilities, prisons or jails, refugee camps, or homeless shelters) and those planning prolonged stays in TB-endemic countries should have a pretravel IGRA (e.g., QuantiFERON-TB Gold Plus, T-SPOT.*TB*, 2-step tuberculin skin test [TST]). For details, see the following chapter in this section, . . . *perspectives*: Testing Travelers for *Mycobacterium tuberculosis* Infection.

If the predeparture test is negative, repeat IGRA or single TST 8–10 weeks after the traveler returns. The predeparture test and follow-up test should be the same test type to facilitate interpretation of results. People with HIV infection or other immunocompromising conditions are more likely to have an impaired response to either a skin or a blood test; be sure to ask travelers about such underlying conditions.

Travelers who suspect they have been exposed to TB should inform their health care provider of the possible exposure and receive a medical evaluation. Because drug resistance is relatively common in some parts of the world, consult with experts in infectious diseases or pulmonary medicine regarding proper management and coordinate consultations with input from the public health department.

Diagnostic Testing Recommendations

The Centers for Disease Control and Prevention (CDC), the American Thoracic Society (ATS), and the Infectious Diseases Society of America (IDSA) jointly published diagnostic recommendations for both TB disease and LTBI. Collect sputum or other respiratory specimens for culture and smears for acid-fast bacilli (AFB) from people being examined for pulmonary TB.

Although diagnosis of TB disease can be made using clinical criteria in the absence of microbiologic confirmation, perform laboratory testing to confirm the diagnosis, guide treatment decisions, and provide bacterial DNA for molecular epidemiology. Molecular tests for mutations that confer drug resistance can be performed directly on specimens and can guide initial treatment while culture results are pending. Culture-based susceptibility testing is recommended for all patients with a positive culture result, to help determine the appropriate drug regimen.

CULTURE METHODS

Culture methods, with referral to a public health reference laboratory in some instances, are necessary to identify the *M. tuberculosis* complex species responsible for infection. Culture and identification of *M. tuberculosis* takes ≈2 weeks, even with rapid culture techniques.

MICROSCOPY

A preliminary diagnosis of TB can be made when AFB are seen by microscopy on a sputum smear or in other body tissues or fluids. Microscopy cannot distinguish *M. tuberculosis* from nontuberculous mycobacteria, however, which is particularly problematic in countries like the United States, where the prevalence of infections with nontuberculous mycobacteria is greater than that of TB.

NUCLEIC ACID AMPLIFICATION TESTS

Less sensitive than culture but more sensitive than AFB smear, nucleic acid amplification tests (NAAT) are specific for the *M. tuberculosis* complex. NAAT methods detect all members of the *M. tuberculosis* complex. Thus, a positive NAAT result can rapidly confirm a diagnosis and help guide initial treatment until culture results return.

The availability of NAAT methods and the policies for ordering these tests are locally determined, and clinicians should consult their state health department. Diagnosis of extrapulmonary TB disease can be confirmed with a NAAT positive for *M. tuberculosis* complex or a culture positive for *M. tuberculosis* from affected body tissues or fluids.

Diagnostic Support

TB disease is a nationally notifiable condition in the United States. LTBI is also notifiable in many jurisdictions. LTBI is diagnosed by a positive result from an IGRA or TST after further examinations (e.g., chest radiograph, symptom review) have excluded TB disease.

Expertise in the diagnosis of TB and its specialty laboratory services, or local referral for such expertise, is available from the health departments of cities, counties, and states. In most settings, contact tracing is managed by public health officials. General information and expert medical consultation also are available from the CDC-sponsored US TB Centers of

Excellence for Training, Education, and Medical Consultation (www.cdc.gov/tb/education/tb_coe/default.htm).

TREATMENT

Latent Tuberculosis Infection

People with LTBI can be treated, and treatments are effective at preventing progression to TB disease. Clinicians must exclude TB disease before starting LTBI treatment. In the United States, several regimens exist for the treatment of drug-susceptible LTBI, including 3 months of once-weekly isoniazid and rifapentine; 4 months of daily rifampin; 3 months of daily isoniazid and rifampin; and 6–9 months of daily isoniazid. Given the low completion rates of the 6- to 9-month isoniazid regimen, shorter duration regimens are preferred.

Choose a regimen for patients based on coexisting medical conditions, potential for drug interactions, and drug-susceptibility results of the presumed source of exposure, if known. For example, rifampin has interactions with oral contraceptives and certain antiretroviral medications taken by people with HIV/AIDS. Individuals at especially high risk for TB disease who might have difficulty adhering to treatment, or who are given an intermittent dosing regimen, might be candidates for directly observed therapy for LTBI.

Tuberculosis Disease

CDC/ATS/IDSA published guidelines for treating drug-susceptible TB disease with a multiple-drug regimen administered by directly observed therapy for 6–9 months. Usually, the regimen is isoniazid, rifampin, ethambutol, and pyrazinamide for 2 months, then isoniazid and rifampin for an additional 4 months. Drug-resistant TB is more difficult to treat, historically requiring 4–6 drugs for 18–24 months and best managed by an expert. In a randomized controlled trial, a newer 6-month all-oral regimen of bedaquiline, pretomanid, and linezolid was effective in treating highly drug-resistant TB or patients who could not tolerate other regimens. This and other new regimens are being used in the United States.

PREVENTION

Travelers should avoid exposure to people with TB disease in crowded and enclosed environments (e.g., health care facilities, prisons or jails, or homeless shelters). Advise travelers who will be caring for patients, or who will be working in health care facilities where people with TB are likely to be patients, to consult infection control or occupational health experts about baseline LTBI screening, procedures for obtaining personal respiratory protective devices (e.g., N95 respirators), and recommendations for respirator selection and training.

Based on WHO recommendations, bacillus Calmette-Guérin (BCG) vaccine is used once, at birth, in countries with higher TB burdens to reduce the severe consequences of TB in infants and children. BCG vaccine has low and variable efficacy in preventing TB in adults, however. Some experts advocate vaccinating health care providers likely to be exposed to drug-resistant TB in settings where infection control measures like those recommended in the United States are not fully implemented; US Food and Drug Administration–approved vaccine formulations of BCG are no longer available in the United States. All people, including those who have received BCG vaccination, must follow recommended TB infection control precautions to the greatest extent possible. IGRA is preferred over the TST for pretravel and posttravel testing in those vaccinated with BCG, because BCG might induce false-positive TST results. No BCG effects on IGRA results have been detected in multiple studies.

To prevent infections from *M. bovis* and other foodborne pathogens, travelers should avoid consuming unpasteurized dairy products.

CDC website: www.cdc.gov/tb

BIBLIOGRAPHY

Brown ML, Henderson SJ, Ferguson RW, Jung P. Revisiting tuberculosis risk in Peace Corps volunteers, 2006–13. J Travel Med. 2016;23(1):tav005.

Centers for Disease Control and Prevention. Availability of an assay for detecting *Mycobacterium tuberculosis*, including rifampin resistant strains, and considerations for its use—United States, 2013. MMWR Morb Mortal Wkly Rep. 2013;62(41):821–7.

Conradie F, Diacon AH, Ngubane N, Howell P, Everitt D, Crook AM, et al. Treatment of highly drug-resistant pulmonary tuberculosis. N Engl J Med. 2020;382(10):893–902.

Jensen PA, Lambert LA, Iademarco MF, Ridzon R. Guidelines for preventing the transmission of *Mycobacterium tuberculosis* in health-care settings, 2005. MMWR Recomm Rep. 2005;54(RR-17):1–141.

Lewinsohn DM, Leonard MK, LoBue PA, Cohn DL, Daley CL, Desmond E, et al. Official American Thoracic Society/Infectious Diseases Society of America/Centers for Disease Control and Prevention clinical practice guidelines: diagnosis of tuberculosis in adults and children. Clin Infect Dis. 2017;64(2):111–5.

Nahid P, Dorman SE, Alipanah N, Barry PM, Brozek JL, Cattamanchi A, et al. Official American Thoracic Society/Centers for Disease Control and Prevention/Infectious Diseases Society of America clinical practice guidelines: treatment of drug-susceptible tuberculosis. Clin Infect Dis. 2016;63(7):e147–95.

National Society of Tuberculosis Clinicians and National Tuberculosis Controllers Association. Testing and treatment of latent tuberculosis infection in the United States: clinical recommendations. Smyrna (GA): The Association; 2021. Available from www.tbcontrollers.org/resources/tb-infection/clinical-recommendations.

Seaworth BJ, Armitige LY, Aronson NE, Hoft DF, Fleenor ME, Gardner AF, et al. Multidrug resistant tuberculosis. Recommendations for reducing risk during travel for healthcare and humanitarian work. Ann Am Thorac Soc. 2014;11(3):286–95.

Sterling TR, Njie G, Zenner D, Cohn DL, Reves R, Ahmed A, et al. Guidelines for the treatment of latent tuberculosis infection: recommendations from the National Tuberculosis Controllers Association and CDC, 2020. MMWR Recomm Rep 2020;69(RR-1):1–11.

World Health Organization. Global tuberculosis report 2020. Geneva: The Organization; 2020. Available from: https://apps.who.int/iris/bitstream/handle/10665/336069/9789240013131-eng.pdf.

World Health Organization. Tuberculosis and air travel: guidelines for prevention and control, 3rd edition. Geneva: The Organization; 2008. Available from: www.who.int/publications/i/item/9789241547505.

TESTING TRAVELERS FOR *MYCOBACTERIUM TUBERCULOSIS* INFECTION

John Jereb

5

Screening for asymptomatic *Mycobacterium tuberculosis* infections should only be carried out for travelers at risk of acquiring tuberculosis (TB) at their destinations (see Sec. 5, Part 1, Ch. 22, Tuberculosis). Screening with a tuberculin skin test (TST) or interferon-γ release assay (IGRA) in very-low-risk travelers might produce false-positive test results, leading to unnecessary additional screening or treatment. IGRAs, which require a single blood draw, are approximately as specific as TST in people who have not been vaccinated with bacillus Calmette-Guérin (BCG) and are more specific in BCG-vaccinated populations. Moreover, TST is prone to boosting sensitivity in serial testing, necessitating a 2-step initial test for establishing a baseline, which is unneeded with IGRAs. Using screening tests in very-low-prevalence populations will probably produce more false positives than true positives.

Travelers at risk for TB infection include those going to live in a TB-endemic country or anyone intending to spend any length of time in routine contact with patients in health care facilities or populations living in congregate settings (e.g., homeless shelters, prisons, refugee camps). People at low risk for exposure to TB, which includes most travelers, do not need to be screened before or after travel.

For travelers who anticipate a long stay or contact with a high-risk population, perform pretravel screening by using an IGRA or, when IGRA is not available, 2-step TST screening. CDC guidelines recommend testing with an IGRA (as opposed to TST) for people aged ≥5 years in low-risk populations. The American Academy of Pediatrics guidelines recommend an IGRA for children ≥2 years old; some pediatric TB experts use IGRAs for all children. If an IGRA is used for pretravel testing and there is concern for a false positive in an otherwise low-risk traveler, a second test can be used, which confirms TB infection only if both tests are positive. If the IGRA result is negative, repeat the traveler's test 8–10 weeks after they return from their trip; however, data supporting a recommendation for regular serial testing for a long-term traveler are limited.

If TST is used for pretravel testing, use the 2-step TST for any traveler undergoing TST testing for the first time. The 2-step method is not needed for travelers who have already been tested and found to have a negative result within the previous 2 years. For the 2-step method, anyone whose baseline TST yields a negative result should be retested 1–3 weeks after the initial test; if the second test result is negative, the patient can be considered not infected. If the second test result is positive, the patient is classified as having skin test boosting, possibly because of previous *M. tuberculosis* infection.

The 2-step TST is recommended over single TST in this population because some people infected with *M. tuberculosis* years earlier (or who were sensitized by BCG or nontuberculous mycobacteria) exhibit waning delayed-type hypersensitivity to tuberculin. When skin tested years after infection, these people might have a negative initial TST result even though they had been sensitized previously. The first TST might stimulate the ability to react to subsequent tests, however, resulting in a "booster" reaction. When the test gets repeated at some future date, a positive result could be misinterpreted as a new *M. tuberculosis* infection (recent conversion) rather than a boosted reaction. For travelers who do not have enough time to complete a 2-step TST before departure, a single-step TST is an acceptable alternative, but an IGRA is preferred.

If the result of a pretravel test (either IGRA or 2-step TST) for *M. tuberculosis* infection is negative, a traveler should have a posttravel test with the same type of test used pretravel, 8–10 weeks after returning from their trip. People who have repeat TSTs should be tested with the same tuberculin purified protein derivative solution, because switching products can lead to different test results. The US Food and Drug Administration has approved 2 commercially available tuberculin solutions for skin testing: Aplisol (JHP Pharmaceuticals) and Tubersol (Sanofi Pasteur). During extended (>6 months) stays in, or repeated travel to, high-risk settings, travelers should have repeat testing every 6–12 months while traveling outside the United States and then 8–10 weeks after final return, all with the same type of test used pretravel.

In general, do not mix the types of tests used for a person. The discordance between TST and IGRA results is ≤15%; in most instances of discordance, the TST result is positive and the IGRA is negative. Multiple reasons for the discordance exist, and clinicians cannot be confident about the reason for discordance in any single person. If a clinician does decide to mix tests, going from TST to IGRA is better than the other way around, because the likelihood of a discordant result with the TST negative and the IGRA positive is much lower. Such discordant results might become unavoidable as more medical establishments switch from TSTs to IGRAs.

When testing travelers who were born or took up residence in TB-endemic areas, consider the greater background prevalence of infection in these places. In a study among 53,000 adults in Tennessee, the prevalence of a positive TST results among foreign-born participants was >11× that of US-born participants (34% vs. 3%). Confirming *M. tuberculosis* test status before travel would prevent the conclusion that a positive result after travel was due to recent infection.

5

BIBLIOGRAPHY

Hagmann SH, Han PV, Stauffer WM, Miller AO, Connor BA, Hale DC. Travel-associated disease among US residents visiting US GeoSentinel clinics after return from international travel. Fam Pract. 2014;31(6):678–87.

Lewinsohn DM, Leonard MK, LoBue PA, Cohn DL, Daley CL, Desmond E, et al. American Thoracic Society/Infectious Diseases Society/Centers for Disease Control and Prevention clinical practice guidelines: diagnosis of tuberculosis in adults and children. Clin Infect Dis. 2017;64(2):111–5.

US Preventive Services Task Force. Screening for latent TB infection in adults: US Preventive Services Task Force recommendation statement. JAMA. 2016:316(9):962–9.

. . . *perspectives* chapters supplement the clinical guidance in this book with additional content, context, and expert opinion. The views expressed do not necessarily represent the official position of the Centers for Disease Control and Prevention (CDC).

TYPHOID & PARATYPHOID FEVER

Michael Hughes, Grace Appiah, Louise Francois Watkins

TYPHOID FEVER

INFECTIOUS AGENT: *Salmonella enterica* serotype Typhi	
ENDEMICITY	Africa Latin America Asia (greatest risk for infection is in South Asia)
TRAVELER CATEGORIES AT GREATEST RISK FOR EXPOSURE & INFECTION	Travelers to low- and middle-income countries where typhoid and paratyphoid fever are endemic Travelers to mass gatherings Travelers visiting friends and relatives
PREVENTION METHODS	Follow safe food and water precautions Typhoid fever is a vaccine-preventable disease
DIAGNOSTIC SUPPORT	A clinical laboratory certified in moderate complexity testing; state health department

PARATYPHOID FEVER

INFECTIOUS AGENTS: *Salmonella enterica* serotypes Paratyphi A, B, C	
ENDEMICITY	Africa Latin America Asia (greatest risk for infection is in South Asia)
TRAVELER CATEGORIES AT GREATEST RISK FOR EXPOSURE & INFECTION	Travelers to low- and middle-income countries where typhoid and paratyphoid fever are endemic Travelers to mass gatherings Travelers visiting friends and relatives
PREVENTION METHODS	Follow safe food and water precautions
DIAGNOSTIC SUPPORT	A clinical laboratory certified in moderate complexity testing; state health department

INFECTIOUS AGENT

Salmonella enterica serotypes Typhi, Paratyphi A, Paratyphi B, and Paratyphi C cause potentially severe and occasionally life-threatening bacteremic illnesses referred to as typhoid fever (for Typhi serotype) and paratyphoid fever (for Paratyphi serotypes), and collectively as enteric fever. Paratyphi B strains are differentiated into 2 distinct pathotypes on the basis of their ability to ferment tartrate: the first pathotype, Paratyphi B, is unable to ferment tartrate and is associated with paratyphoid fever; the second pathotype, Paratyphi B var. L(+) tartrate(+), ferments tartrate and is associated with gastroenteritis typical of nontyphoidal salmonellosis. For more details on nontyphoidal salmonellosis, see the Sec. 5, Part 1, Ch. 19, Nontyphoidal Salmonellosis.

TRANSMISSION

Humans are the only source of the bacteria that cause enteric fever; no animal or environmental reservoirs have been identified. Typhoid and paratyphoid fever are acquired through consumption of water or food contaminated by feces of an acutely infected or convalescent person, or a person with chronic, asymptomatic carriage. Risk for infection is high in low- and middle-income countries with endemic disease and poor access to safe food and water, and poor sanitation. Sexual contact, particularly among men who have sex with men, has been documented as a rare route of transmission.

EPIDEMIOLOGY

An estimated 11–21 million cases of typhoid fever and 5 million cases of paratyphoid fever occur worldwide each year, causing an estimated 135,000–230,000 deaths. In the United States during 2016–2018, ≈400 culture-confirmed cases of typhoid fever and 50–100 cases of paratyphoid fever caused by Paratyphi A were reported each year; paratyphoid fever caused by Paratyphi B and Paratyphi C is rarely reported. Approximately 85% of typhoid fever and 92% of paratyphoid fever cases in the United States occur among international travelers; most are in travelers returning from South Asia, primarily Bangladesh, India, and Pakistan. Other high-risk regions for infection include Africa, Latin America, and Southeast Asia; lower-risk regions include East Asia and the Caribbean.

Travelers visiting friends and relatives are at increased risk because they might be less careful with food and water while abroad than other travelers and might not seek pretravel health consultation or typhoid vaccination (see Sec. 9, Ch. 9, Visiting Friends & Relatives: VFR Travel). Although the risk of acquiring illness increases with the duration of stay, travelers have acquired typhoid fever even during visits of <1 week to countries where the disease is highly endemic (e.g., Bangladesh, India, Pakistan).

CLINICAL PRESENTATION

The incubation period of both typhoid and paratyphoid infections is 6–30 days. The onset of illness is insidious, with gradually increasing fatigue and a fever that increases daily from low-grade to 102°F–104°F (38°C–40°C) by the third or fourth day of illness. Fever is commonly lowest in the morning, peaking in the late afternoon or evening. Anorexia, headache, and malaise are nearly universal, and abdominal pain, constipation, or diarrhea are common. Diarrhea and vomiting are more common in children than in adults. People also can have dry cough, fatigue, myalgias, and sore throat. Hepatosplenomegaly often can be detected. A transient, maculopapular rash of rose-colored spots can occasionally be seen on the trunk.

The clinical presentation is often confused with malaria. Suspect enteric fever in a person with a history of travel to an endemic area who is not responding to antimalarial medication. Untreated, the disease can last for a month, and reported case-fatality ratios are 10%–30%. By comparison, the case-fatality ratio in patients treated early is usually <1%. Serious complications of typhoid fever occur in 10%–15% of hospitalized patients, generally after 2–3 weeks of illness, and include life-threatening gastrointestinal hemorrhage, intestinal perforation, and encephalopathy. Paratyphoid fever appears to have a lower case-fatality ratio than typhoid fever; however, severe cases do occur.

DIAGNOSIS

Typhoid and paratyphoid fever are nationally notifiable diseases in the United States. Clinicians should report cases to their state or local health department. Identification of a domestically acquired case should prompt a public health investigation to prevent other cases.

Blood Culture

Patients with typhoid or paratyphoid fever typically have bacteremia; blood culture is therefore the preferred method of diagnosis. A single culture is positive in only ≈50% of cases, however. Multiple blood cultures increase the sensitivity and might be required to make the diagnosis. Depending on the blood culture system used, cultures might need to be held and observed for up to 7 days before reporting a negative result. Although bone marrow culture is more invasive (and therefore less commonly performed), it increases the sensitivity to ≈80% of cases and is relatively unaffected by previous or concurrent antibiotic use. Stool culture is not usually positive during the first week of illness and has less diagnostic sensitivity than blood culture. Urine culture has a lower diagnostic yield than stool culture.

Rapid Diagnostic Tests

Globally, several commercial rapid diagnostic tests for typhoid fever are available, but their sensitivity and specificity are not optimal. The Widal test measures elevated antibody titers; it is unreliable but widely used in developing countries because of its low cost. Serologic tests do not distinguish acute from past infection or vaccination and lack specificity; thus, blood culture remains the preferred method to diagnose acute infections.

5

Clinical Diagnosis

Poor sensitivity and specificity of rapid antibody tests and the time it takes to obtain a positive culture mean that the initial diagnosis must often be made clinically. Typhoid and paratyphoid fever are clinically indistinguishable. The combination of risk factors for infection and gradual onset of fever that increases in severity over several days should raise suspicion of enteric fever.

TREATMENT

Antibiotic therapy shortens the clinical course of enteric fever and reduces the risk for death. Treatment decisions are complicated by high rates of resistance to many antimicrobial agents, and antimicrobial treatment should be guided by susceptibility testing. A careful travel history can inform empiric treatment choices while awaiting culture results.

Multidrug-Resistant Infection

Established resistance to older antibiotics (e.g., ampicillin, chloramphenicol, trimethoprim-sulfamethoxazole) has led to these agents being recommended only as alternative antibiotics for infections with known susceptibility. Multidrug-resistant (MDR) Typhi with resistance to all 3 of these antibiotics has been present for decades. Regional estimates for MDR Typhi range from 9% in South Asia (2015–2018) to 35%–59% in parts of Africa (2010–2014).

Fluoroquinolones (e.g., ciprofloxacin) are still considered the treatment of choice for fluoroquinolone-susceptible infections in adults. Most Typhi and Paratyphi A infections in the United States are fluoroquinolone-nonsusceptible, however, and most (>90%) have occurred among travelers returning from South Asia. Fluoroquinolone-nonsusceptible infections have been associated with treatment failure or delayed clinical response. Therefore, azithromycin and ceftriaxone, antibiotics with historically low rates of resistance globally, are increasingly being used as empiric treatment for enteric fever.

Extensively Drug-Resistant Infection

In 2017, among all Typhi and Paratyphi A isolates tested by CDC's National Antimicrobial Resistance Monitoring System (NARMS), <1% were resistant to azithromycin or to ceftriaxone, based on resistance criteria for Typhi. Resistance to both agents is emerging, however. In 2016, an outbreak of extensively drug-resistant (XDR) typhoid fever began in Sindh Province, Pakistan. These XDR *Salmonella* Typhi isolates are typically resistant to ampicillin, ceftriaxone, chloramphenicol, ciprofloxacin, and trimethoprim-sulfamethoxazole, but susceptible to azithromycin and carbapenem antibiotics.

The first US cases of XDR typhoid fever associated with travel to Pakistan were diagnosed in 2018, and by early 2021 >70 XDR infections had been documented among residents of the United States, including 9 cases among patients who did not travel internationally in the 30 days before illness began (https://emergency.cdc.gov/han/2021/han00439.asp). Ceftriaxone resistance also has been identified in Typhi isolates from US travelers returning from Iraq. Additionally, resistance to azithromycin has been identified among Typhi and Paratyphi strains isolated from patients in Bangladesh, Cambodia, India, Nepal, Pakistan, Saudi Arabia, and the United States.

Empiric treatment should be guided by the patient's travel history. For patients with suspected typhoid fever who traveled to Iraq or Pakistan, or who did not travel internationally before their illness began, empirically treat uncomplicated illness with azithromycin, and treat complicated illness with a carbapenem. Ceftriaxone remains an appropriate empiric treatment option for travelers returning from most other countries. Once culture results are available, use susceptibility information to guide treatment. Case reports have suggested that patients with XDR Typhi infection who do not improve on a carbapenem alone might benefit from the addition of a second antibiotic (e.g., azithromycin). Updated information about antimicrobial resistance among isolates from US patients with enteric fever in the United States can be found at the NARMS website (www.cdc.gov/narmsnow).

Cases Unresponsive to Treatment

Patients treated with antimicrobial agents can continue to have fever for 3–5 days, but the maximum temperature generally decreases each day. Patients sometimes feel worse during the first few days after commencing antibiotic treatment. If fever in a person with typhoid or paratyphoid infection does not subside within 5 days of initiating antibiotic therapy, however, consider treatment with alternative antibiotics or begin looking for a persistent focus of infection (e.g., an abscess, or an infection in a bone, joint, or other extraintestinal site).

Relapse, Reinfection & Chronic Carriage

Relapse, reinfection, and chronic carriage also can occur. Relapse occurs in ≤10% of patients 1–3 weeks after clinical recovery, requiring further antibiotic treatment. An estimated 1%–4% of treated patients become asymptomatic chronic carriers (defined as people who excrete the organism in stool for ≥12 months); a prolonged antibiotic course is usually required to eradicate the organism.

PREVENTION

Food & Water Precautions

Safe food and water precautions and frequent handwashing, especially before meals, are important in preventing both typhoid and paratyphoid fever (see Sec. 2, Ch. 8, Food & Water Precautions). Although recommended by the Advisory Committee on Immunization Practices (ACIP), typhoid vaccines are not 100% effective, and a large bacterial inoculum can overwhelm vaccine-induced immunity. Therefore, vaccinated travelers should follow recommended food and water precautions to prevent enteric fever and other infections. No vaccines are available for paratyphoid fever; thus, food and water precautions are the only prevention methods.

Vaccines

INDICATIONS

The ACIP recommends typhoid vaccine for travelers going to areas where risk for exposure to Typhi is recognized. Destination-specific vaccine recommendations are available at the CDC Travelers' Health website (https://wwwnc.cdc.gov/travel). Two typhoid vaccines are licensed for use in the United States: Vi capsular polysaccharide vaccine (ViCPS) (Typhim Vi, manufactured by Sanofi Pasteur) for intramuscular use; and live attenuated vaccine (Vivotif, manufactured from the Ty21a strain of serotype Typhi by PaxVax) for oral use. Both vaccines are unconjugated, which means the polysaccharide antigens are not paired with a protein to elicit a strong response from the immune system. Because these vaccines protect 50%–80% of recipients, remind travelers that typhoid immunization is not 100% effective, and take the opportunity to reinforce safe food and water precautions. Neither vaccine is licensed to prevent paratyphoid fever, although limited data from efficacy trials suggest that the Ty21a vaccine might provide some cross-protection against Paratyphi B.

Newer, protein conjugated Vi vaccines have greater efficacy in children <2 years old and protect people for longer than Vi unconjugated polysaccharide vaccines. Three typhoid Vi conjugate vaccines (TCV) have been licensed in India: Peda Typh (manufactured by Biomed); Typbar-TCV (manufactured by Bharat Biotech); and Zyvac TCV (manufactured by Zydus Cadila). Typbar-TCV also is licensed in Cambodia, Nepal, and Nigeria. Although none of these vaccines are licensed or available in the United States, Tybar-TCV received prequalification from the World Health Organization in 2018. The vaccine is approved for use in people ≥6 months old. In a human challenge study, Typbar-TCV had ≈87% protective efficacy. Interim analysis from a large field study in Nepal has shown Typbar-TCV effectiveness of 81.6% in children after 15 months of follow-up.

ADMINISTRATION

For information on dosage, administration, and revaccination for the 2 typhoid vaccines licensed in the United States, see Table 5-07. The time required for primary vaccination differs, as do the lower age limits for each.

VI CAPSULAR POLYSACCHARIDE VACCINE

Primary vaccination with ViCPS consists of one 0.5-mL (25-µg) dose administered intramuscularly ≥2 weeks before travel. The vaccine is approved for use in people ≥2 years old. A dose is recommended every 2 years for those who remain at risk.

5

LIVE ATTENUATED TY21A VACCINE

Primary vaccination with Ty21a vaccine consists of 4 capsules, 1 taken every other day. The capsules should be kept refrigerated (not frozen), and all 4 doses must be taken to achieve maximum efficacy. Each capsule should be swallowed whole (not chewed) and taken with cool liquid no warmer than 98.6°F (37°C), approximately 1 hour before a meal and ≥2 hours after a previous meal. The manufacturer recommends avoiding alcohol consumption 1 hour before and 2 hours after administration, because alcohol can disintegrate the enteric coating.

Travelers should complete the Ty21a vaccine regimen ≥1 week before potential exposure. The approach for addressing a missed oral vaccine dose or taking a dose late is undefined. Some suggest that minor deviations in the dosing schedule (e.g., taking a dose 1 day late) might not alter vaccine efficacy; no studies have shown the effect of such deviations, however. If travelers do not complete 4 doses as directed, they might not achieve an optimal immune response. The vaccine is approved for use in people ≥6 years old. A booster dose is recommended every 5 years for those who remain at risk.

ADVERSE REACTIONS

Adverse reactions most often associated with ViCPS vaccine include headache, injection-site reactions, fever, and general discomfort. Adverse reactions to Ty21a vaccine are rare and mainly consist of abdominal discomfort, diarrhea, fever, headache, nausea, vomiting, and rash. Report adverse reactions to the Vaccine Adverse Event Reporting System at the website, https://vaers.hhs.gov/index.html, or by calling 800-822-7967.

Table 5-07 Typhoid fever vaccines

VACCINE	APPROVED AGES FOR USE	DOSE & ROUTE OF ADMINISTRATION	NUMBER OF DOSES	DOSING INTERVAL	REPEAT DOSES
Vi Capsular Polysaccharide Vaccine (ViCPS)—Typhim Vi					
Primary series	≥2 years	0.5 mL, IM injection	1	NA	NA
Booster	≥2 years	0.5 mL, IM injection	1	NA	Every 2 years
Live Attenuated Ty21a Vaccine—Vivotif[1]					
Primary series	≥6 years	1 capsule, orally every other day[2]	4	48 hours	NA
Booster	≥6 years	1 capsule, orally every other day[2]	4	48 hours	Every 5 years

Abbreviations: IM, intramuscular; NA, not applicable.

[1]Vaccine must be kept refrigerated at 35°F–46°F (2°C–8°C).

[2]Capsules should be taken with cool liquid, no warmer than 98.6°F (37°C)

PRECAUTIONS & CONTRAINDICATIONS

Neither the ViCPS nor the Ty21a vaccine should be given to people with an acute febrile illness; in addition, Ty21a is not recommended for use in people with acute gastroenteritis. Live vaccines, including Ty21a vaccine, should not be given to pregnant or immunocompromised people, including those with HIV. No information is available on the safety of the inactivated vaccine (ViCPS) in pregnancy; consider ViCPS for pregnant people when the benefits of vaccination outweigh potential risks (e.g., when the likelihood of exposure to Typhi is high).

The intramuscular vaccine (ViCPS) presents a theoretically safer alternative than the live, oral vaccine (Ty21a) for immunocompromised travelers. The Ty21a vaccine can be administered to household contacts of immunocompromised people; although vaccine organisms can be shed transiently in the stool of vaccine recipients, secondary transmission of vaccine organisms has not been documented. The only contraindication to vaccination with ViCPS vaccine is a history of severe local or systemic reactions after a previous dose.

Theoretical concerns have been raised about the immunogenicity of Ty21a vaccine in people concurrently receiving antimicrobial agents, live vaccines, or immune globulin. The growth of the live Ty21a strain is inhibited in vitro by various antimicrobial agents. The manufacturer advises that vaccination with the Ty21a vaccine should be delayed for >72 hours after the administration of any antimicrobial agent, and antibiotics should not be given to a patient ≤72 hours after the last dose of the Ty21a vaccine.

Ty21a vaccine can be administered simultaneously or at any interval before or after live virus vaccines (e.g., measles-mumps-rubella, oral polio, or yellow fever vaccines). Available data do not suggest that simultaneous administration of live virus vaccines decreases the immunogenicity of the Ty21a vaccine. If typhoid vaccination is warranted, it should not be delayed because of administration of viral vaccines. No data are available on coadministration of the Ty21a vaccine and the oral cholera vaccine (lyophilized CVD 103-HgR [Vaxchora]); taking the first Ty21a vaccine dose ≥8 hours after oral cholera vaccine might decrease potential interference between the vaccines. Simultaneous administration of the Ty21a vaccine and immune globulin does not appear to pose a problem.

CDC website: www.cdc.gov/typhoid-fever

5

BIBLIOGRAPHY

Browne AJ, Kashef Hamadani BH, Kumaran EAP, Rao P, Longbottom J, Harris E, et al. Drug-resistant enteric fever worldwide, 1990 to 2018: a systematic review and meta-analysis. BMC Med. 2020;18(1):1.

Crump JA. Progress in typhoid fever epidemiology. Clin Infect Dis. 2019;68(Suppl 1):S4–9.

Crump JA, Sjölund-Karlsson M, Gordon MA, Parry CM. Epidemiology, clinical presentation, laboratory diagnosis, antimicrobial resistance, and antimicrobial management of invasive *Salmonella* infections. Clin Microbiol Rev. 2015;28(4):90137.

Date KA, Bentsi-Enchill A, Marks F, Fox K. Typhoid fever vaccination strategies. Vaccine. 2015;33:C55–61.

Date KA, Newton AE, Medalla F, Blackstock A, Richardson L, McCullough A, et al. Changing patterns in enteric fever incidence and increasing antibiotic resistance of enteric fever isolates in the United States, 2008–2012. Clin Infect Dis. 2016;63(3):322–9.

Effa EE, Lassi ZS, Critchley JA, Garner P, Sinclair D, Olliaro P, Bhutta ZA. Fluoroquinolones for treating uncomplicated typhoid and paratyphoid fever (enteric fever). Cochrane Database Syst Rev. 2011(10):CD004530.

François Watkins LK, Winstead A, Appiah GD, Friedman CR, Medalla F, Hughes MJ, et al. Update on extensively drug-resistant *Salmonella* serotype Typhi infections among travelers to or from Pakistan and report of ceftriaxone-resistant *Salmonella* serotype Typhi infections among travelers to Iraq—United States, 2018–2019. MMWR Morb Mortal Wkly Rep. 2020;69(20):618–22.

Jackson BR, Iqbal S, Mahon B. Updated recommendations for the use of typhoid vaccine—Advisory Committee on Immunization Practices, United States, 2015. MMWR Morb Mortal Wkly Rep. 2015;64(11):305–8.

Klemm EJ, Shakoor S, Page AJ, Qamar FN, Judge K, Saeed DK, et al. Emergence of an extensively drug-resistant *Salmonella enterica* serovar Typhi clone harboring a promiscuous plasmid encoding resistance to fluoroquinolones and third-generation cephalosporins. mBio. 2018;9(1):e00105-18.

Lynch MF, Blanton EM, Bulens S, Polyak C, Vojdani J, Stevenson J, et al. Typhoid fever in the United States, 1999–2006. JAMA. 2009;302(8):859–65.

McAteer J, Derado G, Hughes M, Bhatnagar A, Medalla F, Chatham-Stephens K, et al. Typhoid fever in the US pediatric population, 1999–2015: opportunities for improvement. Clin Infect Dis. 2021;(73)11:e4581–9.

Stanaway JD, Reiner RC, Blacker BF, Goldberg EM, Khalil IA, Troeger CE, et al. The global burden of typhoid and paratyphoid fevers: a systematic analysis for the Global Burden of Disease Study 2017. Lancet Infect Dis. 2019;19(4):369–81.

Syed KA, Saluja T, Cho H, Hsiao A, Shaikh H, Wartel TA, et al. Review on the recent advances on typhoid vaccine development and challenges ahead. Clin Infect Dis. 202029;71(Suppl_2):S141–50.

YERSINIOSIS

Louise Francois Watkins, Cindy Friedman

5

INFECTIOUS AGENTS: *Yersinia enterocolitica* and *Y. pseudotuberculosis*	
ENDEMICITY	Northern, temperate regions: northern Europe (particularly Scandinavia), Canada, Japan
TRAVELER CATEGORIES AT GREATEST RISK FOR EXPOSURE & INFECTION	Adventurous eaters Children
PREVENTION METHODS	Follow safe food and water precautions Avoid unpasteurized dairy products, raw or undercooked pork products, and untreated water
DIAGNOSTIC SUPPORT	A clinical laboratory certified in moderate complexity testing; state health department

INFECTIOUS AGENT

Yersinia species are facultative anaerobic gram-negative coccobacilli. The most common species that cause yersiniosis are *Yersinia enterocolitica* (serogroups O:3, O:5,27, O:8, and O:9), but disease is also caused by *Y. pseudotuberculosis.* The term "yersinosis" does not include illness caused by *Yersinia pestis*, the causative agent of plague, which is discussed separately (see Sec. 5, Part 1, Ch. 15, Plague); discussion of *Yersinia* spp. in this chapter excludes *Y. pestis.*

TRANSMISSION

Transmission of *Yersinia* spp. can occur from consuming or handling contaminated food, commonly raw or undercooked pork products (e.g., chitterlings); consuming milk that was not pasteurized, inadequately pasteurized, or contaminated after pasteurization; or drinking untreated water. *Yersinia* spp. also can be transmitted by direct or indirect contact with animals through the fecal–oral route. Pigs are a major reservoir of pathogenic *Y. enterocolitica*, but a variety of other domestic (e.g., dogs), farm (e.g., cattle), and wild (e.g., deer) animals can harbor *Yersinia* spp. Transmission through blood product transfusions has been reported.

EPIDEMIOLOGY

Most yersiniosis cases are reported from northern Europe, particularly Scandinavia, and from Canada and Japan. Yersiniosis is not, however, a reportable condition in most countries (including the United States), and infections in countries without surveillance programs might be underrepresented. In the United States, *Y. enterocolitica* causes ≈92% of infections with known species information, accounting for approximately 117,000 illnesses, 640 hospitalizations, and 35 deaths every year.

In temperate climates, the risk for infection is increased during cooler months. Children are infected more often than adults. People with diseases that cause high iron levels (e.g., hemochromatosis, thalassemia), including those on iron chelation treatment, are at greater risk for infection and severe disease. The incidence among travelers to low- and middle-income countries is generally low, and most cases are believed to be due to foodborne transmission. A US study found that ≈6% of *Y. enterocolitica* infections were travel-associated.

CLINICAL PRESENTATION

The incubation period is 4–6 days (range 1–14 days), and symptom onset might be more gradual compared with infections caused by other enteric pathogens. Enterocolitis is the most common clinical presentation; symptoms typically include abdominal pain, diarrhea (which can be bloody and persist for several weeks), and fever. Sore throat also can occur, particularly in children. Mesenteric adenitis, which presents as pain mimicking appendicitis, has been well described. Necrotizing enterocolitis has been described in young infants. Reactive arthritis affecting the wrists, knees, and ankles can occur, usually 1 month after the initial diarrhea episode, resolving after 1–6 months. Erythema nodosum, manifesting as painful, raised red or purple lesions along the trunk and legs, can occur, and usually resolves spontaneously within 1 month.

DIAGNOSIS

Diagnosis is frequently made by isolating the organism from bile, blood, cerebrospinal fluid, mesenteric lymph nodes, peritoneal fluid, stool, a throat swab, or wounds. If yersiniosis is suspected, notify the clinical laboratory because cold enrichment, alkali treatment, or plating of a clinical specimen on CIN agar can be used to increase the likelihood of a positive culture. Several culture-independent diagnostic tests (CIDTs) are now available and have more than doubled the detection rate of *Yersinia* spp. in the United States. CIDT panels typically target only *Y. enterocolitica*, and the rarity of yersiniosis has precluded robust evaluation of the specificity and sensitivity of CIDT platforms through prospective studies. Culture is required to determine the species and for antimicrobial susceptibility testing. For questions about diagnostic testing beyond the capacity of the clinical laboratory, contact a local or state public health department. Public health officials can provide information and guidance on specimen submission, including submission to the Centers for Disease Control and Prevention (CDC) if appropriate.

5

TREATMENT

Most infections are self-limited. Antimicrobial drug therapy has not been shown to shorten the duration of uncomplicated enterocolitis or to alter the likelihood of postinfectious sequelae. Prescribe antibiotics for moderate to severe illness. *Y. enterocolitica* isolates are usually susceptible to aminoglycosides, third-generation cephalosporins, fluoroquinolones, tetracyclines, and trimethoprim-sulfamethoxazole and are typically resistant to first-generation cephalosporins and most penicillins.

PREVENTION

Travelers can reduce the risk for *Yersinia* spp. infection by avoiding consumption of unpasteurized milk products, raw or undercooked pork products, and untreated water (see Sec. 2, Ch. 8, Food & Water Precautions). Washing hands with soap and water before eating and preparing food, after contact with animals, and after handling raw meat helps reduce risk.

CDC website: www.cdc.gov/yersinia

BIBLIOGRAPHY

Chakraborty A, Komatsu K, Roberts M, Collins J, Beggs J, Turabelidze G, et al. The descriptive epidemiology of yersiniosis: a multistate study, 2005–2011. Public Health Rep. 2015;130(3):269–77.

Frydén A1, Bengtsson A, Foberg U, Svenungsson B, Castor B, Kärnell A, et al. Early antibiotic treatment of reactive arthritis associated with enteric infections: clinical and serological study. BMJ. 1990;301(6764):1299–302.

Kendall ME, Crim S, Fullerton K, Han PV, Cronquist AB, Shiferaw B, et al. Travel-associated enteric infections diagnosed after return to the United States, Foodborne Diseases Active Surveillance Network (FoodNet), 2004–2009. Clin Infect Dis. 2012;54 Suppl 5:S480–7.

Long C, Jones TF, Vugia DJ, Scheftel J, Strockbine N, Ryan P, et al. *Yersinia pseudotuberculosis* and *Y. enterocolitica* infections, FoodNet, 1996–2007. Emerg Infect Dis. 2010;16(3):566–7.

Mead PS. *Yersinia* species, including plague. In: Bennett JE, Dolin R, Blaser MJ, editors. Mandell, Douglas, and Bennett's principles and practice of infectious diseases, 8th edition. Philadelphia: Saunders Elsevier; 2015. pp. 2615–7.

Pai CH, Gillis F, Tuomanen E, Marks MI. Placebo-controlled double-blind evaluation of trimethoprim-sulfamethoxazole treatment of *Yersinia enterocolitica* gastroenteritis. J Pediatr. 1984;104(2):308–11.

Press N, Fyfe M, Bowie W, Kelly M. Clinical and microbiological follow-up of an outbreak of *Yersinia pseudotuberculosis* serotype Ib. Scand J Infect Dis. 2001;33(7):523–6.

Sato K, Ouchi K, Komazawa M. Ampicillin vs. placebo for *Yersinia pseudotuberculosis* infection in children. Pediatr Infect Dis J. 1988;7(10):686–9.

Tack DM, Marder EP, Griffin PM, Cieslak PR, Dunn J, Hurd S, et al. Preliminary incidence and trends of infections with pathogens transmitted commonly through food—Foodborne Diseases Active Surveillance Network, 10 U.S. Sites, 2015–2018. MMWR Morb Mortal Wkly Rep. 2018;68(16);369–73.

PART 2: VIRAL

5

Table 5-08 Vaccine-Preventable Diseases: Viral

VACCINE	TRADE NAME (MANUFACTURER)	DESCRIPTION[1] & ROUTE OF ADMINISTRATION	AGE LIMITS	DOSES	PRESCRIBING & BOOSTER INFORMATION, RECOMMENDATIONS & RESTRICTIONS
COVID-19	COMIRNATY (Pfizer-BioNTech)	mRNA, IM	www.fda.gov/emergency-preparedness-and-response/coronavirus-disease-2019-covid-19/comirnaty-and-pfizer-biontech-covid-19-vaccine www.cdc.gov/vaccines/hcp/acip-recs/vacc-specific/covid-19.html		
	SPIKEVAX (Moderna)	mRNA, IM	www.fda.gov/emergency-preparedness-and-response/coronavirus-disease-2019-covid-19/spikevax-and-moderna-covid-19-vaccine www.cdc.gov/vaccines/hcp/acip-recs/vacc-specific/covid-19.html		
	NOVAVAX (Novavax)	Recombinant, IM	www.fda.gov/emergency-preparedness-and-response/coronavirus-disease-2019-covid-19/novavax-covid-19-vaccine-adjuvanted www.cdc.gov/vaccines/hcp/acip-recs/vacc-specific/covid-19.html		
Dengue	DENGVAXIA (Sanofi Pasteur)	Live-attenuated, SC	9–16 y	3	*Restrictions apply* www.fda.gov/vaccines-blood-biologics/dengvaxia www.cdc.gov/vaccines/hcp/acip-recs/vacc-specific/dengue.html
Ebola Zaire	ERVEBO (Merck)	Live-attenuated, IM	≥18 y	1	*Restrictions apply* www.fda.gov/vaccines-blood-biologics/ervebo www.cdc.gov/vhf/ebola/clinicians/vaccine/index.html
Enterovirus-A71 (Hand, Foot & Mouth)	Available in China only				
Hepatitis A	HAVRIX (GlaxoSmithKline)	Inactivated, IM	**0.5 mL**		www.fda.gov/vaccines-blood-biologics/vaccines/havrix www.cdc.gov/vaccines/hcp/acip-recs/vacc-specific/hepa.html
			≥12 mo to <19 y	2	
			1.0 mL		
			≥19 y	2	

	VAQTA (Merck)	Inactivated, IM	**0.5 mL**		www.fda.gov/vaccines-blood-biologics/vaccines/vaqta www.cdc.gov/vaccines/hcp/acip-recs/vacc-specific/hepa.html
			≥12 mo to <19 y	2	
			1.0 mL		
			≥19 y	2	
Hepatitis A + Hepatitis B	TWINRIX (GlaxoSmithKline)	Inactivated HAV + Recombinant HBV, IM	**STANDARD DOSING**		www.fda.gov/vaccines-blood-biologics/vaccines/twinrix www.cdc.gov/vaccines/hcp/acip-recs/vacc-specific/hepa.html
			≥18 y	3	
			ACCELERATED DOSING		
			≥18 y	3 (+ booster)	
Hepatitis B	ENGERIX-B (GlaxoSmithKline)	Recombinant, IM	<20 y	3	www.fda.gov/vaccines-blood-biologics/vaccines/engerix-b www.cdc.gov/vaccines/hcp/acip-recs/vacc-specific/hepb.html
			≥20 y	3	
	HEPLISAV-B (Dynavax Technologies)	Recombinant, IM	≥18 y	2	www.fda.gov/vaccines-blood-biologics/vaccines/heplisav-b www.cdc.gov/vaccines/hcp/acip-recs/vacc-specific/hepb.html
	PREHEVBRIO (VBI Vaccines)	Recombinant, IM	≥18 y	3	www.fda.gov/vaccines-blood-biologics/prehevbrio www.cdc.gov/vaccines/hcp/acip-recs/vacc-specific/hepb.html
	RECOMBIVAX HB (Merck)	Recombinant, IM	**0.5 mL**		www.fda.gov/vaccines-blood-biologics/vaccines/recombivax-hb www.cdc.gov/vaccines/hcp/acip-recs/vacc-specific/hepb.html
			<20 y	3	
			1.0 mL		
			11–15 y	2	
			≥20 y	3	

(continued)

5

Table 5-08 Vaccine-Preventable Diseases: Viral (continued)

VACCINE	TRADE NAME (MANUFACTURER)	DESCRIPTION[1] & ROUTE OF ADMINISTRATION	AGE LIMITS	DOSES	PRESCRIBING & BOOSTER INFORMATION, RECOMMENDATIONS & RESTRICTIONS
Influenza	For the list of influenza vaccines licensed for use in the United States, see: www.fda.gov/vaccines-blood-biologics/vaccines/vaccines-licensed-use-united-states; www.cdc.gov/vaccines/hcp/acip-recs/vacc-specific/flu.html				
Japanese encephalitis	IXIARO (Valneva)	Inactivated, IM	**0.25 mL**		www.fda.gov/vaccines-blood-biologics/vaccines/ixiaro www.cdc.gov/vaccines/hcp/acip-recs/vacc-specific/je.html
			≥2 mo to <3 y	2	
			0.5 mL		
			≥3 y	2	
Mumps	M-M-R II (Merck)	Live-attenuated, SC	<12 mo	3	www.fda.gov/vaccines-blood-biologics/vaccines/measles-mumps-and-rubella-virus-vaccine-live www.cdc.gov/vaccines/hcp/acip-recs/vacc-specific/mmr.html
			≥12 mo	2	
	ProQuad (Merck)	Live-attenuated, SC	≥12 mo to <13 y	2	www.fda.gov/vaccines-blood-biologics/vaccines/proquad www.cdc.gov/vaccines/hcp/acip-recs/vacc-specific/mmrv.html
Polio	IPOL (Sanofi Pasteur)	Inactivated, IM or SC	**CHILDREN**		www.fda.gov/vaccines-blood-biologics/vaccines/ipol-poliovirus-vaccine-inactivated-monkey-kidney-cell www.cdc.gov/vaccines/hcp/acip-recs/vacc-specific/polio.html www.cdc.gov/polio/what-is-polio/travelers.html
			≥6 wks	3	
			ADULTS TRAVELING TO AREAS WITH INCREASED RISK OF POLIO		
			UNVACCINATED, PARTLY VACCINATED, VACCINATION STATUS UNKNOWN		
			≥18 y	3	
			COMPLETELY VACCINATED		
			≥18 y	1-time booster	

Rabies	IMOVAX (Sanofi Pasteur)	Inactivated (human diploid cell), IM	all ages	2–3	www.fda.gov/vaccines-blood-biologics/vaccines/imovax www.cdc.gov/vaccines/hcp/acip-recs/vacc-specific/rabies.html
	RabAvert (Novartis)	Inactivated (purified chick embryo cell), IM	all ages	2–3	www.fda.gov/vaccines-blood-biologics/vaccines/rabavert-rabies-vaccine www.cdc.gov/vaccines/hcp/acip-recs/vacc-specific/rabies.html
Rubella	M-M-R II (Merck)	Live-attenuated, SC	<12 mo	3	www.fda.gov/vaccines-blood-biologics/vaccines/measles-mumps-and-rubella-virus-vaccine-live www.cdc.gov/vaccines/hcp/acip-recs/vacc-specific/mmr.html
			≥12 mo	2	
	ProQuad (Merck)	Live-attenuated, SC	≥12 mo to <13 y	2	www.fda.gov/vaccines-blood-biologics/vaccines/proquad www.cdc.gov/vaccines/hcp/acip-recs/vacc-specific/mmrv.html
Rubeola / Measles	M-M-R II (Merck)	Live-attenuated, SC	<12 mo	3	www.fda.gov/vaccines-blood-biologics/vaccines/measles-mumps-and-rubella-virus-vaccine-live www.cdc.gov/vaccines/hcp/acip-recs/vacc-specific/mmr.html
			≥12 mo	2	
	ProQuad (Merck)	Live-attenuated, SC	≥12 mo to <13 y	2	www.fda.gov/vaccines-blood-biologics/vaccines/proquad www.cdc.gov/vaccines/hcp/acip-recs/vacc-specific/mmrv.html
Tick-borne encephalitis	TICOVAC (Pfizer)	Inactivated, IM	**0.25 mL**		www.fda.gov/vaccines-blood-biologics/ticovac
			≥1–15 y	3	
			0.5 mL		
			≥16 y	3	

(*continued*)

Table 5-08 Vaccine-Preventable Diseases: Viral (continued)

VACCINE	TRADE NAME (MANUFACTURER)	DESCRIPTION[1] & ROUTE OF ADMINISTRATION	AGE LIMITS	DOSES	PRESCRIBING & BOOSTER INFORMATION, RECOMMENDATIONS & RESTRICTIONS
Varicella / Chickenpox	VARIVAX (Merck)	Live-attenuated, SC	1–12 y	2	www.fda.gov/vaccines-blood-biologics/vaccines/varivax www.cdc.gov/vaccines/vpd/varicella/hcp/
			≥13 y	2	
	ProQuad (Merck)	Live-attenuated, SC	≥12 mo to <13 y	2	www.fda.gov/vaccines-blood-biologics/vaccines/proquad www.cdc.gov/vaccines/hcp/acip-recs/vacc-specific/mmrv.html
Variola / Smallpox + Monkeypox	ACAM2000 (Emergent BioSolutions)	Live-attenuated vaccinia virus, percutaneous via bifurcated needle	all ages	1	*Restrictions apply* www.fda.gov/vaccines-blood-biologics/vaccines/acam2000 www.cdc.gov/vaccines/hcp/acip-recs/vacc-specific/smallpox.html
	JYNNEOS (Bavarian Nordic)	Live-attenuated non-replicating vaccinia virus, SC	≥18 y	2	Restrictions apply www.fda.gov/vaccines-blood-biologics/jynneos www.cdc.gov/vaccines/hcp/acip-recs/vacc-specific/smallpox.html
Yellow Fever	YF-VAX (Sanofi Pasteur)	Live-attenuated, SC	≥9 mo	1	www.fda.gov/vaccines-blood-biologics/vaccines/yf-vax www.cdc.gov/vaccines/hcp/acip-recs/vacc-specific/yf.html

Abbreviations: IM, intramuscular; SC, subcutaneously

[1]For an overview and description of vaccine types, see: www.hhs.gov/immunization/basics/types/index.html

B VIRUS

Ludmila Perelygina

INFECTIOUS AGENT: B Virus (*Macacine Herpesvirus* 1)	
ENDEMICITY	North Africa Asia
TRAVELER CATEGORIES AT GREATEST RISK FOR EXPOSURE & INFECTION	Children Tourists, particularly adventure tourists Veterinarians and laboratory workers
PREVENTION METHODS	Avoid feeding or petting macaque monkeys
DIAGNOSTIC SUPPORT	National B Virus Resource Center (404-413-6560; http://biotech.gsu.edu/virology/contactUs.html; http://bvirus.org)

5

INFECTIOUS AGENT

B virus (*Macacine herpesvirus* 1) is an enveloped, double-stranded DNA virus in the family *Herpesviridae*, genus *Simplexvirus*. B virus is also commonly referred to as herpes B, monkey B virus, herpesvirus B, and herpesvirus simiae. B virus is commonly found among macaques, a genus of Old World monkeys.

TRANSMISSION

B virus is typically transmitted to humans through bites or scratches from an infected macaque, but also can occur through contact with body fluids or tissues of an infected macaque. A single case of human-to-human transmission has been documented, in which a woman became infected through direct contact with lesions on her infected spouse.

EPIDEMIOLOGY

Macaques are the natural reservoir for B virus. No other primates are known to carry B virus unless they become infected through contact with infected macaques. Although B virus infections in macaques are usually asymptomatic or cause only mild disease, ≈70% of untreated infections in humans are fatal.

Infections in humans are rare. Since B virus was identified in 1932, <50 cases of human infection have been documented. People at greatest risk for B virus infection are laboratory workers, veterinarians, and others who have close contact with macaques or macaque cell cultures. International travelers visiting temples and parks with exotic animal life often come in direct contact with free-roaming macaques, which often carry B virus. Children are more likely to be bitten than adults. Although transmission of B virus from macaques to humans in public settings has not been documented, the potential risk for transmission exists.

CLINICAL PRESENTATION

Disease onset typically occurs within 1 month of exposure, although the actual incubation period can be as short as 3–7 days. The first signs of disease typically include influenza-like symptoms (fever, headache, myalgia) and sometimes vesicular lesions near the exposure site. Localized neurologic symptoms (e.g., pain, numbness, itching) might occur near the wound site. Lymphadenitis, lymphangitis, nausea, vomiting, and abdominal pain also can occur.

Spread of the infection to the central nervous system (CNS) causes acute ascending encephalomyelitis. Most patients with CNS involvement die despite antiviral therapy and supportive care. People who survive usually suffer serious neurologic sequelae. Respiratory failure associated with ascending paralysis is the most common cause of death.

DIAGNOSIS

Before collecting clinical specimens for diagnostic testing, cleanse all wound sites thoroughly (see First Aid & Treatment, next). Obtaining specimens from wound sites before proper cleansing could force virus more deeply into exposed tissue.

In the United States, diagnostic testing of human specimens is performed only at the National B Virus Resource Center at Georgia State University (http://biotech.gsu.edu/virology). Detection of viral DNA by B virus PCR from clinical specimens is the standard for diagnosis.

5

Detection of B virus–specific antibodies in serum is also diagnostic. Collect and submit a baseline serum sample as close as possible to the time of injury, and again 14–21 days post-injury for serological testing to evaluate for B virus infection. Testing paired specimens is essential for a reliable diagnosis. Viral culture is generally unsuccessful because the virus is unlikely to remain viable during transit or after being frozen and thawed. For more information on specimen collection, storage, and shipment, see National B Virus Resource Center (http://biotech.gsu.edu/virology).

FIRST AID & TREATMENT

For suspected exposure, travelers should administer immediate first aid. Travelers should cleanse wounds by thoroughly washing and scrubbing the area with soap, concentrated detergent solution, povidone iodine, or chlorhexidine and water, then irrigate the area with running water for 15–20 minutes. For urine splashes to the eyes, travelers should perform repeated eye flushes for several minutes.

Antiviral therapy is recommended as postexposure prophylaxis in high-risk exposures (see www.cdc.gov/herpesbvirus/firstaid-treatment.html). When recommended, the drug of choice is valacyclovir, and an alternative is acyclovir. If B virus infection is diagnosed, initiate treatment with intravenous acyclovir or ganciclovir, depending on whether CNS symptoms are present.

PREVENTION

No vaccine is available for B virus. Laboratories should adhere to laboratory and animal facility protocols to reduce the risk for B virus transmission among workers. Visitors to parks and tourist destinations with free-roaming macaques should avoid feeding or petting the animals, and seek care for possible postexposure prophylaxis if a high-risk exposure occurs. Immediate cleaning of bite and scratch wounds is of utmost importance for disease prevention. Consider postexposure antiviral prophylaxis for high-risk exposures, including any deep bites, and scratches or other wounds to the head, neck, or torso. Contact a medical expert familiar with B virus infections at the earliest opportunity.

CDC website: www.cdc.gov/herpesbvirus/index.html

BIBLIOGRAPHY

Centers for Disease Control and Prevention. Notice to readers: occupational safety and health in the care and use of nonhuman primates. MMWR Morb Mortal Wkly Rep. 2003;52(38):920.

Cohen JI, Davenport DS, Stewart JA, Deitchman S, Hilliard JK, Chapman LE; B virus Working Group. Recommendations for prevention of and therapy for exposure to B virus (*Cercopithicine herpesvirus 1*). Clin Infect Dis. 2002;35(10):1191–203.

NASPHV; Centers for Disease Control and Prevention; Council of State and Territorial Epidemiologists; American Veterinary Medical Association. Compendium of measures to prevent disease associated with animals in public settings, 2009: National Association of State Public Health Veterinarians, Inc. (NASPHV). MMWR Recomm Rep. 2009;58(RR-05):1–15.

National Institute for Occupational Safety and Health (NIOSH). Hazard ID 5—*Cercopithicine herpesvirus 1* (B virus) infection resulting from ocular exposure; publication no. 99–100. Atlanta: The Institute; 1999.

Schmid DS, Chapman LE, Cohen JI. Herpes B virus infection (updated 2022 Mar 23). BMJ Best Practice. Available from: https://bestpractice.bmj.com/topics/en-gb/1608.

Wu AC, Rekant SI, Baca ER, Jenkins RM, Perelygina LM, Hilliard JK, et al. Notes from the field: monkey bite in a public park and possible exposure to herpes B virus—Thailand, 2018. MMWR Morb Mortal Wkly Rep. 2020;69(9):247–8.

CHIKUNGUNYA

J. Erin Staples, Susan Hills, Ann Powers

INFECTIOUS AGENT: Chikungunya virus	
ENDEMICITY	Tropical and subtropical regions worldwide
TRAVELER CATEGORIES AT GREATEST RISK FOR EXPOSURE & INFECTION	Adventure tourists Long-term travelers and expatriates Travelers visiting friends and relatives
PREVENTION METHODS	Avoid insect bites
DIAGNOSTIC SUPPORT	A clinical laboratory certified in high complexity testing; state health department; or contact CDC's Arboviral Diseases Branch (www.cdc.gov/ncezid/dvbd/specimensub/arboviral-shipping.html; 970-221-6400; dvbid@cdc.gov)

5

INFECTIOUS AGENT

Chikungunya virus is a single-stranded RNA virus that belongs to the family *Togaviridae*, genus *Alphavirus*.

TRANSMISSION

Chikungunya virus is transmitted to humans via the bite of an infected mosquito of the *Aedes* spp., predominantly *Aedes aegypti* and *Ae. albopictus*. Mosquitoes become infected when they feed on viremic nonhuman or human primates, both of which are likely the main amplifying reservoirs of the virus. Humans are typically viremic shortly before and in the first 2–6 days of illness.

Bloodborne transmission is possible; 1 case has been documented in a health care worker who sustained a needle stick after drawing blood from an infected patient. Furthermore, chikungunya virus has been identified in donated blood products undergoing screening, although no transfusion-associated cases have been identified to date. Cases also have been documented among laboratory personnel handling infected blood, through percutaneous punctures, and through aerosol exposure in the laboratory.

Maternal–fetal transmission has been documented during pregnancy; the greatest risk occurs in the perinatal period when the pregnant person is viremic at the time of delivery. Although chikungunya viral RNA was identified in the breast milk of 1 infected person, the breastfed infant had no symptoms or evidence of infection based on laboratory testing. Additionally, chikungunya viral RNA has been identified in semen, but no evidence of sexual transmission has been noted to date.

EPIDEMIOLOGY

Chikungunya virus occurs in tropical and subtropical regions. It often causes large outbreaks with high attack rates, affecting up to 75% of the population in areas where the virus is circulating. Outbreaks of chikungunya have occurred in Africa, the Americas, Asia, Europe, and islands in the Indian and Pacific Oceans. In late 2013, the first locally acquired cases of chikungunya were reported in the Americas on islands in the Caribbean. By the end of 2017, >2.6 million suspected cases of chikungunya had been reported in the Americas. Since then, the virus has continued to circulate and cause sporadic cases and periodic outbreaks in many areas of the world, including Africa, South America, and Asia.

Risk to travelers is greatest in areas experiencing ongoing chikungunya epidemics. Most epidemics occur during the tropical rainy season and abate during the dry season. Outbreaks in Africa have occurred after periods of drought, however, where open water containers near human habitats served as vector-breeding sites. Risk for infection exists primarily during the day, because the primary vector, *Ae. aegypti*, aggressively bites during daytime. *Ae. aegypti* mosquitoes bite indoors or outdoors near dwellings and lay their eggs in domestic containers that hold water, including buckets and flowerpots.

Both adults and children can become infected and be symptomatic with chikungunya. After the outbreaks in the Americas during 2014–2017, >4,000 chikungunya cases were reported among US travelers, and 13 locally acquired cases were reported in the continental United States. In addition, the US territories of American Samoa, US Virgin Islands, and Puerto Rico reported locally acquired cases during 2014–2015; Puerto Rico also has been reporting sporadic cases since 2016. During 2018–2020, 340 US traveler cases were reported, with noticeably fewer cases in 2020 due to decreases in international travel during the coronavirus disease 2019 (COVID-19) pandemic.

CLINICAL PRESENTATION

Approximately 3%–28% of people infected with chikungunya virus will remain asymptomatic. For people who develop symptomatic illness, the incubation period is typically 3–7 days (range 1–12 days). Disease is most often characterized by sudden onset of high fever (temperature typically >102°F [39°C]) and joint pains. Fevers typically last for ≤1 week; the fever can be biphasic. Joint symptoms are typically severe, can be debilitating, and usually involve multiple joints, typically bilateral and symmetric. Joint pain occurs most commonly in hands and feet but can affect more proximal joints. Other symptoms include conjunctivitis, headache, myalgia, nausea, vomiting, or a rash. The rash, which is typically maculopapular, occurs after onset of fever and involves the trunk and extremities but also can include the palms, soles, and face.

Abnormal laboratory findings can include elevated creatinine and liver function tests, lymphopenia, and thrombocytopenia. Rare but serious complications of the disease include hepatitis, myocarditis, neurologic disease (cranial nerve palsies, Guillain-Barré syndrome, meningoencephalitis, myelitis), ocular disease (uveitis, retinitis), acute renal disease, and severe bullous skin lesions. Groups identified as having increased risk for more severe disease include neonates exposed intrapartum, adults >65 years of age, and people with underlying medical conditions (e.g., diabetes, heart disease, hypertension).

Acute symptoms of chikungunya typically resolve in 7–10 days. Some patients will have a relapse of rheumatologic symptoms (e.g., polyarthralgia, polyarthritis, tenosynovitis, Raynaud syndrome) in the months after acute illness. Studies have reported variable proportions, ranging from 5% to 80%, of patients with persistent joint pains, and prolonged fatigue, for months or years after their illness. Fatalities associated with infection occur but are rare and are reported most commonly in older adults and those with comorbidities.

People who are pregnant have symptoms and outcomes similar to those of other people, and most infections that occur during pregnancy will not result in the virus being transmitted to the fetus. Intrapartum transmission can, however, result in neonatal complications, including hemorrhagic symptoms, myocardial disease, and neurologic disease. Rare spontaneous abortions after first-trimester maternal infection have been reported.

DIAGNOSIS

The differential diagnosis of chikungunya virus infection depends on clinical features (signs and symptoms) and when and where the person was suspected of being infected. Consider other infections and diseases in the differential diagnosis, including adenovirus, other alphaviruses (Barmah Forest, Mayaro, O'nyong-nyong, Ross River, and Sindbis), dengue, enterovirus, leptospirosis, malaria, measles, parvovirus, rubella, group A *Streptococcus*, typhus, Zika, and postinfectious arthritis and rheumatologic conditions.

Laboratory diagnosis is generally accomplished by testing serum to detect virus, viral nucleic acid, or virus-specific IgM and neutralizing antibodies. Because the virus develops high levels of viremia during the first week after symptom onset, chikungunya can often be diagnosed by performing viral culture or nucleic acid amplification on serum. Virus-specific IgM antibodies normally develop toward the end of the first week of illness but can remain detectable for months to years after infection. Rarely, serum IgM antibody testing can yield false-positive results due to cross-reacting antibodies against related alphaviruses (e.g., Mayaro virus, O'nyong-nyong virus). Plaque reduction neutralization tests (PRNT) can be used to confirm the infection and, if warranted, discriminate between cross-reacting antibodies.

Testing for chikungunya virus infection is performed at several state health department laboratories and commercial laboratories. Confirmatory testing for virus-specific neutralizing antibodies is available through the Centers for Disease Control and Prevention (CDC)'s Division of Vector-Borne Diseases (970-221-6400). Report suspected chikungunya cases to state or local health departments to facilitate diagnosis and mitigate the risk for local transmission. Because chikungunya is a nationally notifiable disease, state health departments should report laboratory-confirmed cases to CDC through ArboNET (https://wwwn.cdc.gov/arbonet), the national surveillance system for arboviral diseases.

TREATMENT

No specific antiviral treatment is available for chikungunya; a number of therapeutic options are being investigated, however. Treatment for symptoms include rest, fluids, and use of analgesics and antipyretics. Nonsteroidal anti-inflammatory drugs can be used to help with acute fever and pain. For patients who report travel to dengue-endemic areas, however, acetaminophen is the preferred first-line treatment for fever and joint pain to reduce the risk for hemorrhage until dengue can be ruled out. For patients with persistent joint pain, use of nonsteroidal anti-inflammatory drugs, corticosteroids, including topical preparations, and physical therapy might help lessen the symptoms.

PREVENTION

Currently, no vaccine or preventive drug is available; several candidate vaccines are in various stages of development. Travelers can best prevent infection by avoiding mosquito bites (see Sec. 4, Ch. 6, Mosquitoes, Ticks & Other Arthropods). Travelers at increased risk for more severe disease, including travelers with underlying medical conditions and people late in their pregnancy (because their fetuses are at increased risk), might consider avoiding travel to areas with ongoing chikungunya outbreaks. If travel is unavoidable, emphasize the importance of using protective measures against mosquito bites.

CDC website: www.cdc.gov/chikungunya

BIBLIOGRAPHY

Adams LE, Martin SW, Lindsey NP, Lehman JA, Rivera A, Kolsin J, et al. Epidemiology of dengue, chikungunya, and zika virus disease in U.S. states and territories, 2017. Am J Trop Med Hyg. 2019;101(4):884–90.

Brito Ferreira ML, Militão de Albuquerque MFP, de Brito CAA, de Oliveira França RF, Porto Moreira ÁJ, de Morais Machado MÍ, et al. Neurological disease in adults with Zika and chikungunya virus infection in northeast Brazil: a prospective observational study. Lancet Neurol. 2020;19(10):826–39.

Centers for Disease Control and Prevention. Chikungunya virus in the United States. Available from: www.cdc.gov/chikungunya/geo/united-states.html.

Guillot X, Ribera A, Gasque P. Chikungunya-induced arthritis in Reunion Island: a long-term observational follow-up study showing frequently persistent joint symptoms, some cases of persistent chikungunya immunoglobulin M positivity, and no anticyclic citrullinated peptide seroconversion after 13 years. J Infect Dis. 2020;222(10):1740–4.

Lindsey NP, Staples JE, Fischer M. Chikungunya virus disease among travelers—United States, 2014–2016. Am J Trop Med Hyg. 2018;98(1):192–7.

Pan American Health Organization. PLISA health information platform for the Americas: chikungunya. Available from: https://www3.paho.org/data/index.php/en/mnu-topics/chikv-en.html.

Pan American Health Organization and World Health Organization. Tool for the diagnosis and care of patients with suspected arboviral diseases. Washington, DC: The Organization; 2017. Available from: www.who.int/publications/i/item/tool-for-the-diagnosis-and-care-of-patients-with-suspected-arboviral-diseases.

Powers AM. Vaccine and therapeutic options to control chikungunya virus. Clin Microbiol Rev. 2017;31(1):e00104–16.

Simon F, Javelle E, Cabie A, Bouquillard E, Troisgros O, Gentile G, et al. French guidelines for the management of chikungunya (acute and persistent presentations); November 2014. Med Mal Infect. 2015;45(7):243–63.

COVID-19

The information included in this chapter was current as of August 2022. For the most recent information regarding coronavirus disease 2019 (COVID-19), see www.cdc.gov/coronavirus/2019-nCoV/index.html.

Sarah Anne Guagliardo, Cindy Friedman

5

INFECTIOUS AGENT: Severe acute respiratory syndrome coronavirus 2 (SARS-CoV-2)	
ENDEMICITY	Worldwide
TRAVELER CATEGORIES AT GREATEST RISK FOR EXPOSURE & INFECTION	All travelers
PREVENTION METHODS	Vaccination prevents hospitalization and deaths from COVID-19 Avoiding crowded, poorly ventilated spaces Hand hygiene Respiratory protection (wearing a well-fitting mask or respirator)
DIAGNOSTIC SUPPORT	A clinical laboratory certified in moderate complexity testing

INFECTIOUS AGENT

Severe acute respiratory syndrome coronavirus 2 (SARS-CoV-2), the cause of coronavirus disease 2019 (COVID-19), is a single-stranded, positive-sense RNA virus that belongs to the family *Coronaviridae*, genus *Betacoronavirus*.

TRANSMISSION

SARS-CoV-2 is primarily transmitted from person to person following close (≤6 ft, ≈2 m) exposure to respiratory fluids carrying infectious virus. When an infected person breathes, sings, talks, coughs, or sneezes, they release infectious aerosol particles (droplet nuclei) into the air. Exposure can occur when aerosol particles and small respiratory droplets are inhaled or contact exposed mucous membranes. Infection from contaminated surfaces or objects (fomites) is possible but is unlikely to contribute significantly to new infections.

Infection through inhalation is most likely to occur at closer distances (≤6 ft), but transmission over distances >6 ft by inhalation of very fine aerosolized, infectious particles (airborne transmission) has been documented. The risk of transmission is enhanced in poorly ventilated indoor spaces.

EPIDEMIOLOGY

The first cases of COVID-19 were reported in December 2019 in Wuhan, China, and since then, the virus has spread to all continents. International travel has played an ongoing role in the epidemiology of the pandemic, facilitating the initial global spread of the virus as well as each successive SARS-CoV-2 variant. From January 2020 to April 2022, there were 5 major epidemic waves in the United States; as of April 2022, the most recent 3 corresponded to the Alpha, Delta, and Omicron variants.

Mortality Rates

As of April 2022, there were an estimated 400 million cases and 6 million deaths reported worldwide. Case counts and deaths are likely an underestimate, since only a small proportion of infections are diagnosed and reported; in addition, self-testing options (for which positive results might go unreported) are now widely available. Estimates of the infection fatality rate (the mortality rate in infected individuals) among unvaccinated populations range from 0.15% to 1.7% Country-specific COVID-19 mortality rates can vary between destinations for multiple reasons, including differences in population-level immunity due to previous infection, vaccination rates, age distribution, prevalence of comorbidities, viral evolution, and access to health care. With the emergence of new variants, mortality rates may change.

Travel-Associated Risk

Reported travel-associated case counts and deaths also are likely an underestimate, and overall travel-related risk is difficult to ascertain. Investigating and identifying travel-associated cases of COVID-19 has unfortunately been hampered by a lack of complete passenger data for contact tracing, limited or incomplete reporting of contact tracing outcomes among exposed passengers, and difficulties in excluding non-travel–associated exposures. Tracking levels of transmission in countries globally is only one factor in determining travel-associated risk.

MODES OF TRANSPORTATION & TRANSMISSION RISK

Across all modes of transportation, not wearing a well-fitting mask or respirator (www.cdc.gov/coronavirus/2019-ncov/prevent-getting-sick/types-of-masks.htm]) within 6 ft of an infected person (e.g., sitting on a plane or train, sharing a cabin on a cruise) increases the risk for infection, underscoring the importance of prevention measures before and during travel.

AIR TRAVEL

Attack rates range from 0% to 8% on flights but can be as high as 60% in subsections of an aircraft, as was observed on a 10-hour flight in a business class cabin. The individuals affected in this outbreak were all seated within 6 feet of the index case; data regarding mask use were not available. The relationship between flight duration and attack rates is difficult to quantify due to other flight-specific variables (e.g., mask use among passengers and aircrew, passenger movement during the flight) that are not captured or difficult to measure. For more information about health concerns related to commercial air travel, see Sec. 8, Ch. 1, Air Travel.

CRUISE SHIP TRAVEL

Cruise ship travel facilitates the introduction and spread of respiratory viruses because of close indoor proximity and extensive social interactions between ever-changing cohorts of passengers from diverse geographic regions. Cruise ships were the source of many large COVID-19 outbreaks throughout the pandemic, with severe outcomes prior to COVID-19 vaccines.

In the earliest months of the pandemic (January–April 2020), attack rates on cruises were as high as 62%. Longer voyages were associated with more cases, and repeated outbreaks on the same ship (but different voyages) were common. Since then, the Centers for Disease Control and Prevention (CDC) has worked to develop guidance for the cruise ship industry to use to better manage risks associated with COVID-19 (www.cdc.gov/quarantine/cruise/index.html). See Sec. 8, Ch. 6, Cruise Ship Travel, for more details on health concerns related to cruises.

GROUND TRANSPORTATION

COVID-19 outbreaks on buses and trains have also been described. Attack rates on buses have been as high as 36%. On trains, attack rates among passengers within 3 rows of an index patient were lower, ranging from 0% to 10%, with an overall attack rate of <1%.

Sentinel Surveillance

In the context of declining global testing and reporting, determining country-level risk has become more challenging. Sentinel surveillance of international travelers may therefore be an important contribution to the global picture of disease burden and variant emergence. In September 2021, CDC launched a voluntary traveler-based SARS-CoV-2 genomic surveillance program to detect variants among travelers arriving at major US international airports. Through this program, CDC scientists detected Omicron subvariants BA.2 and BA.3 in the United States 7 and 45 days earlier, respectively, than any other US report.

CLINICAL PRESENTATION

SARS-CoV-2 infection can present with an array of clinical findings (www.cdc.gov/coronavirus/2019-ncov/symptoms-testing/symptoms.html), ranging from asymptomatic to severe (e.g., multiorgan involvement, respiratory failure, death). Most infections are mild, however; about 40% of people are asymptomatic. Among cases that do not result in severe disease or hospitalization, fatigue, headache, muscle aches, rhinitis, and sore throat are reported most often. Other reported symptoms and signs include fever, chills, cough, shortness of breath, loss of taste and smell, nausea, vomiting, and diarrhea.

There is evidence that clinical presentation and illness severity differ depending on the SARS-CoV-2 variant. For example, 34% of patients infected with the Delta variant experienced loss of taste and smell, as compared to 13% of patients infected with the Omicron variant. Omicron was also associated with proportionally less pneumonia and severe disease. For pre-Omicron variants, the median incubation period is 5 days with a range of 2–14 days after initial exposure; studies of the Omicron variant have estimated the incubation period to be 2–3 days.

Age and underlying medical conditions increase a person's risk for severe disease and death. The risk of severe disease and death increases significantly with age (≥50 years old), pregnancy, obesity, and with an increasing number of comorbidities (e.g., diabetes, hypertension, HIV infection). For a comprehensive list of risk factors, see www.cdc.gov/coronavirus/2019-ncov/hcp/clinical-care/underlyingconditions.html. See Sec. 3, Ch. 1, Immunocompromised Travelers, and Sec. 7, Ch. 1, Pregnant Travelers, for additional information about these populations.

Long COVID

People infected with SARS-CoV-2 can continue to experience symptoms ≥4 weeks after initial infection. Reported symptoms include shortness of breath, fatigue, headache, and difficulty thinking or concentrating. Commonly known as "long COVID," this condition goes by several other names, including post-COVID syndrome or condition, post-acute sequelae of COVID-19 (PASC), and chronic COVID Syndrome (CCS). For the most up-to-date definition of long COVID and an associated list of symptoms, see www.cdc.gov/coronavirus/2019-ncov/long-term-effects/index.html. Researchers are investigating risk factors and manifestations of long COVID.

In addition to the above, there is growing evidence of long-term cardiovascular consequences of the disease, including cerebrovascular disorders, dysrhythmias, heart failure, ischemic and non-ischemic heart disease, myocarditis, pericarditis, and thromboembolic disease.

DIAGNOSIS

Viral tests that detect current infection with SARS-CoV-2 are used for COVID-19 diagnosis, and include nucleic acid amplification tests (NAATs, e.g., reverse transcription PCR [RT-PCR]) and antigen tests. Tests that detect antibody to SARS-CoV-2 can be used to identify previous infection and might be useful for surveillance purposes, but are not typically used for diagnosis, except for multisystem inflammatory syndrome in children and adults (www.cdc.gov/coronavirus/2019-ncov/hcp/testing.html).

Nucleic Acid Amplification Testing

NAATs detect SARS-CoV-2 RNA and are highly sensitive and specific. The most common NAAT is the RT-PCR test. A positive RT-PCR provides evidence of current infection. Residual shedding of non-infectious viral RNA also can result in a positive test result, as demonstrated by reports of patients whose RT-PCR tests remain positive ≥3 months post-infection (www.cdc.gov/coronavirus/2019-ncov/hcp/testing-overview.html).

Acceptable specimens for SARS-CoV-2 RT-PCR tests include saliva and swab samples collected from the upper respiratory tract (e.g., nasopharynx, nasal mid-turbinate, anterior nasal, oropharynx). As new tests are developed, other specimen types might be identified as being suitable for testing. Each test should be performed as specified by the manufacturer and authorized or approved by the US Food and Drug Administration (FDA). NAAT results usually take 1–3 days, but some rapid tests available in the United States can be useful for travelers who need proof of a negative test for entry to international destinations; travelers should confirm with their air carrier and their destination in advance to ensure the acceptability of the test used.

Antigen Testing

Antigen tests detect the presence of viral proteins (antigens). In general, they are less sensitive than NAATs but are less expensive and can yield rapid results (≈15 minutes). Antigen tests can be used in a laboratory, at the point of care, or self-administered. For more information on antigen testing, see www.cdc.gov/coronavirus/2019-ncov/lab/resources/antigen-tests-guidelines.html.

TREATMENT

Before travel, encourage patients to have a health care contingency plan in place, should they test positive for COVID-19 while abroad; some countries require proof of travel insurance for COVID-19 (see Sec. 6, Ch. 1, Travel Insurance, Travel Health Insurance & Medical Evacuation Insurance). For mild disease, medications such as acetaminophen or ibuprofen can provide symptomatic relief. Patients also should rest and stay well hydrated.

For people at greater risk for progression to severe disease, the FDA has issued Emergency Use Authorization for several postexposure treatments, including antiviral medications and monoclonal antibodies. As of August 2022, preferred antiviral medications include oral nirmatrelvir + ritonavir (Paxlovid) and intravenous remdesivir. If neither of these drugs is available or clinically appropriate, alternative therapeutic options include prophylaxis with the oral antiviral molnupiravir or with monoclonal antibodies. For maximal efficacy, administer medications as soon as possible after diagnosis. Emergence of future variants might impact future treatment options.

The National Institutes of Health regularly updates COVID-19 treatment guidelines. See www.covid19treatmentguidelines.nih.gov/ for the most up-to-date information.

PREVENTION

During the initial months of the pandemic, global travel virtually halted, with many countries closing their borders to international travelers. Since then, travel has gradually returned to near prepandemic levels. In response to newly emerging variants of concern, many countries instituted measures (e.g., mask use, testing, isolation, quarantine, vaccination requirements) to slow travel-associated transmission. Several countries, including the United States, instituted travel bans, although evidence is limited that these are an effective prevention measure.

Inhalation of virus particles and deposition of virus on mucous membranes can be prevented by wearing a well-fitting mask or respirator and avoiding crowded indoor spaces with poor ventilation. Handwashing can help prevent transmission from contact with contaminated surfaces (fomite transmission). Used in combination, layered interventions (e.g., mask wearing, avoiding crowded indoor spaces with poor ventilation, testing, isolation, quarantine, vaccination) are measures that can reduce risk of transmission.

Coronavirus Disease 2019 Information by Destination

Because the situation continues to evolve, travelers and health care providers should review the travel restrictions, requirements, recommendations, and resources for all destination countries and the United States before departure. Knowing the most up-to-date information about COVID-19 by destination can help travelers and clinicians make informed decisions about travel based on COVID-19 levels, the travelers' risk for developing severe illness, and the health care capacity at the destination.

CDC's COVID-19 travel page (www.cdc.gov/coronavirus/2019-ncov/travelers/index.html)

BOX 5-02 Coronavirus disease 2019 (COVID-19) international travel preparation: a checklist for travelers

- ☐ Be up to date with your COVID-19 vaccines before international travel (www.cdc.gov/coronavirus/2019-ncov/vaccines/index.html; www.cdc.gov/coronavirus/2019-ncov/vaccines/stay-up-to-date.html)
- ☐ Learn about destination-specific entry requirements (e.g., vaccination; documentation of vaccination; predeparture and postarrival testing) and the return requirements for the end of your trip (https://travel.state.gov/content/travel/en/traveladvisories/COVID-19-Country-Specific-Information.html)
- ☐ CDC recommends wearing a well-fitting mask or respirator (www.cdc.gov/coronavirus/2019-ncov/travelers/masks-public-transportation.html)
- ☐ Practice mitigation measures (e.g., avoiding crowded, indoor spaces with poor ventilation; hand hygiene; cleaning and disinfection; www.cdc.gov/coronavirus/2019-ncov/global-covid-19/global-urban-areas.html)
- ☐ Learn about transportation-associated risk factors (e.g., avoid poorly ventilated, crowded trains, buses)
- ☐ Purchase travel health insurance (some countries require proof of travel insurance for COVID-19)
- ☐ Have plans ready in case you get sick or are exposed while abroad (e.g., know where you can be tested for COVID-19 at your destination or bring rapid test kits in your luggage; identify health care facilities that can manage severe illness at your destination; set aside additional resources for lodging needs in the event you need to quarantine and/or isolate)
- ☐ Know the international travel requirements and recommendations for the United States (www.cdc.gov/coronavirus/2019-ncov/travelers/international-travel/index.html)

5

provides guidance for travelers. Each country's ministry of health website is another source for information about COVID-19 levels at the destination as well as current entry requirements, including proof of vaccination.

Vaccination

As of August 2022, everyone ≥6 months old in the United States is eligible and recommended to receive COVID-19 vaccination (see www.cdc.gov/coronavirus/2019-ncov/vaccines/index.html, and Sec. 7, Ch. 4, Vaccine Recommendations for Infants & Children). At present, there are 4 vaccines authorized for use in the United States: 2 mRNA-based vaccines (Moderna, Pfizer-BioNTech), a DNA-based, adenovirus-vectored vaccine (Johnson & Johnson's Janssen), and a protein vaccine (Novavax). In most circumstances the 2 mRNA vaccines are preferred.

All eligible travelers should be up to date with their COVID-19 vaccines (www.cdc.gov/coronavirus/2019-ncov/vaccines/stay-up-to-date.html) before travel. Interim clinical considerations for the use of COVID-19 vaccines in the United States (www.cdc.gov/vaccines/covid-19/clinical-considerations/covid-19-vaccines-us.html) provide additional details regarding vaccine schedules, vaccine safety, and vaccination recommendations for people who are moderately to severely immunocompromised.

Testing

Conducting both a pretravel and posttravel test is estimated to reduce the risk of viral spread by up to 75%. Predeparture testing results in the greatest reduction of risk when a specimen is collected closest to the time of travel. Conducting a posttravel test 3–5 days after return can help prevent spread in the community. For the most up-to-date testing guidance for travelers, see www.cdc.gov/coronavirus/2019-ncov/travelers/international-travel/index.html, and www.cdc.gov/coronavirus/2019-ncov/travelers/travel-during-covid19.html.

Isolation

Isolation is the physical separation of a person with a confirmed or suspected infectious disease from people who are not infected. People who have symptoms or who test positive for COVID-19 should follow the latest CDC guidance regarding isolating themselves from others and the precautions to take after ending isolation (www.cdc.gov/coronavirus/2019-ncov/your-health/quarantine-isolation.html). If a person is symptomatic, they should avoid travel for 10 days after symptom onset; if asymptomatic, they should avoid travel for 10 days after the date the positive test was collected. Immunocompromised travelers (Sec. 3, Ch. 1, Immunocompromised Travelers) can be infectious for longer than 10 days and should consider longer isolation periods. For the most up-to-date information and guidance on isolation and travel, see www.cdc.gov/coronavirus/2019-ncov/travelers/index.html.

Quarantine

Quarantine is the physical separation from other people of a person who has had close contact with someone with confirmed or suspected infectious disease. A fundamental public health approach to disease containment, quarantine has been used throughout the COVID-19 pandemic (www.cdc.gov/coronavirus/2019-ncov/your-health/quarantine-isolation.html). For the most up-to-date information and guidance on quarantine and travel, see www.cdc.gov/coronavirus/2019-ncov/travelers/index.html.

Masks

Wearing a well-fitting mask or respirator that completely covers the nose and mouth reduces SARS-CoV-2 transmission. A properly fitted and appropriately worn respirator (e.g., N95 filtering facepiece respirator approved by the National Institute for Occupational Safety and Health) protects the wearer from inhaling airborne droplet nuclei. KN95s also offer a high level of protection. Well-fitting disposable surgical masks provide source control by helping reduce transmission from a person infected with SARS-CoV-2 to others within a shared space. Masks made from layered finely woven products afford some protection, with the least amount of protection being offered by loosely woven cloth products. For more details and updates on masking during travel, see www.cdc.gov/coronavirus/2019-ncov/travelers/face-masks-public-transportation.html.

CDC website: www.cdc.gov/coronavirus/2019-ncov/index.html

5

BIBLIOGRAPHY

Brooks JT, Butler JC. Effectiveness of mask wearing to control community spread of SARS-CoV-2. JAMA. 2021;325(10):998–9.

Guagliardo SAJ, Prasad PV, Rodriguez A, Fukunaga R, Novak RT, Ahart L, et al. Cruise ship travel in the era of coronavirus disease 2019 (COVID-19): a summary of outbreaks and a model of public health interventions. Clin Infect Dis. 2022;74(3):490–7.

Guan WJ, Ni ZY, Hu Y, Liang WH, Ou CQ, He JX, et al. Clinical characteristics of coronavirus disease 2019 in China. N Engl J Med. 2020 Apr 30;382:1708–20.

Hu M, Lin H, Wang J, Xu C, Tatem AJ, Meng B, et al. Risk of coronavirus disease 2019 transmission in train passengers: an epidemiological and modeling study. Clin Infect Dis. 2021;72(4):604.

Johansson MA, Quandelacy TM, Kada S, Prasad PV, Steele M, Brooks JT, et al. SARS-CoV-2 transmission from people without COVID-19 symptoms. JAMA Netw Open. 2021;4(1):e2035057.

Johansson MA, Wolford H, Paul P, Diaz PS, Chen TH, Brown CM, Cetron MS, Alvarado-Ramy F. Reducing travel-related SARS-CoV-2 transmission with layered mitigation measures: symptom monitoring, quarantine, and testing. BMC Medicine. 2021;19(1):94.

Johnson AG, Amin AB, Ali AR, Hoots B, et al. COVID-19 incidence and death rates among unvaccinated and fully vaccinated adults with and without booster doses during periods of Delta and Omicron variant emergence—25 U.S. jurisdictions, April 4–December 25, 2021. MMWR Morb Mortal Wkly Rep. 2022;71(4):132–8.

Khanh NC, Thai PQ, Quach HL, Thi NAH, Dinh PC, Duong TN, et al. Transmission of SARS-CoV 2 during long-haul flight. Emerg Infect Dis. 2020;26(11):2617.

Levin AT, Hanage WP, Owusu-Boaitey N, Cochran KB, Walsh SP, Meyerowitz-Katz G. Assessing the age specificity of infection fatality rates for COVID-19: systematic review, meta-analysis, and public policy implications. Euro J Epidemiol. 2020;35(12):1123–38.

Rosca EC, Heneghan C, Spencer EA, Brassey J, Plüddemann A, Onakpoya IJ, et al. Transmission of SARS-CoV-2 associated with aircraft travel: a systematic review. J Travel Med. 2021;28(7):taab133. doi: 10.1093/jtm/taab133.

Shen Y, Li C, Dong H, Wang Z, Martinez L, Sun L, et al. Community outbreak investigation of SARS-CoV-2 transmission among bus riders in eastern China. JAMA Intern Med. 2020;180(12):1665–71.

Wegrzyn RD, Appiah GD, Morfino R, Milford SR, Walker AT, Ernst ET, et al. Early detection of SARS-CoV-2 variants using traveler-based genomic surveillance at four US airports, September 2021–January 2022. Clin. Infect. Dis. 2022; ciac461.

DENGUE

Liliana Sánchez-González, Laura Adams, Gabriela Paz-Bailey

INFECTIOUS AGENT: Dengue virus 1, 2, 3, 4	
ENDEMICITY	Tropical and subtropical regions worldwide
TRAVELER CATEGORIES AT GREATEST RISK FOR EXPOSURE & INFECTION	All travelers, but increased risk for travelers on trips lasting >6 months
PREVENTION METHODS	Avoid insect bites Dengue is a vaccine-preventable disease (restrictions apply, see text for details)
DIAGNOSTIC SUPPORT	A clinical laboratory certified in high complexity testing; state health department; or CDC's Division of Vector-Borne Diseases, Dengue Branch (787-706-2399)

5

INFECTIOUS AGENT

Dengue, an acute febrile illness, is caused by infection with any of 4 related single-stranded RNA viruses of the genus *Flavivirus*, dengue virus 1, 2, 3, or 4 (DENV1–4). Infection with one DENV confers long-term immunity to that virus but conveys only short-lived protection against the other dengue viruses. The risk for severe dengue is greater during a second DENV infection; although severe dengue also can occur during the first, third, or fourth infection.

TRANSMISSION

Almost all DENV transmission occurs through the bite of infected *Aedes* species mosquitoes, primarily *Ae. aegypti* and *Ae. albopictus*. Because of the ≈7-day viremia in humans, bloodborne transmission is possible through exposure to infected blood, organs, or other tissues (e.g., bone marrow). In addition, perinatal DENV transmission occurs when the mother is infected near the time of birth; infection occurs via microtransfusions as the placenta detaches, or through mucosal contact with maternal blood during birth. No cases of congenital transmission have been documented, but it has been suggested. DENV can be transmitted through breast milk. DENV also has been detected in vaginal secretions and semen; sexual transmission has been reported but is considered rare.

EPIDEMIOLOGY

Dengue is endemic throughout the tropics and subtropics and occurs in >100 countries and destinations worldwide, including Puerto Rico, the US Virgin Islands, and US–affiliated Pacific Islands (Map 5-03, Map 5-04, and Map 5-05). The incidence of dengue among travelers to the tropics has increased in recent years, and dengue burden is expected to continue to grow in sub-Saharan Africa, Latin America, and Asia, with estimates of >50 million febrile illness cases per year.

More than 5,000 travel-related dengue cases were reported in the United States during 2010–2017, with an annual average of 626 cases; a total of 2,119 patients with travel-related dengue required hospitalization, and 18 died. The most frequently reported regions of travel among US cases were the Caribbean, Central America, and Asia. Sporadic outbreaks with local transmission have occurred in Florida, Hawaii, and Texas. Although the geographic distribution of dengue is similar to that of malaria, dengue is more of a risk in urban and residential areas than is malaria.

CLINICAL PRESENTATION

An estimated 40%–80% of DENV infections are asymptomatic. Symptomatic dengue most commonly presents as a mild to moderate, nonspecific, acute febrile illness; ≤5% of all dengue

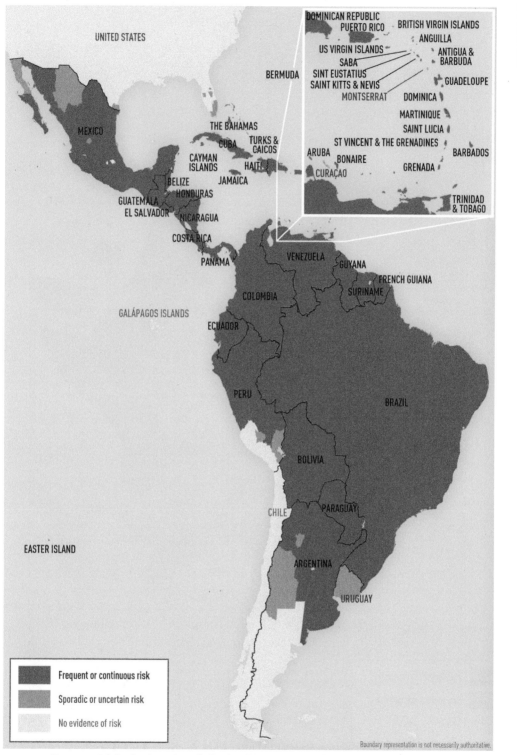

MAP 5-03 Dengue risk in the Americas & the Caribbean

Risk classification uses the methodology described in Jentes, et al. Evidence-based risk assessment and communication: a new global dengue-risk map for travellers and clinicians (www.ncbi.nlm.nih.gov/pmc/articles/PMC5345513/). *Frequent/continuous risk*: evidence of more than 10 dengue cases in at least 3 of the previous 10 years; *sporadic/uncertain risk*: evidence of at least 1 locally acquired dengue case during the last 10 years. Level of risk assigned to a destination reflects the highest risk level identified within that destination. Where data are available, subnational dengue risk levels are shown. Destination risk levels also are denoted using black (frequent/continuous risk) or gray (sporadic/uncertain risk) font for the place name.

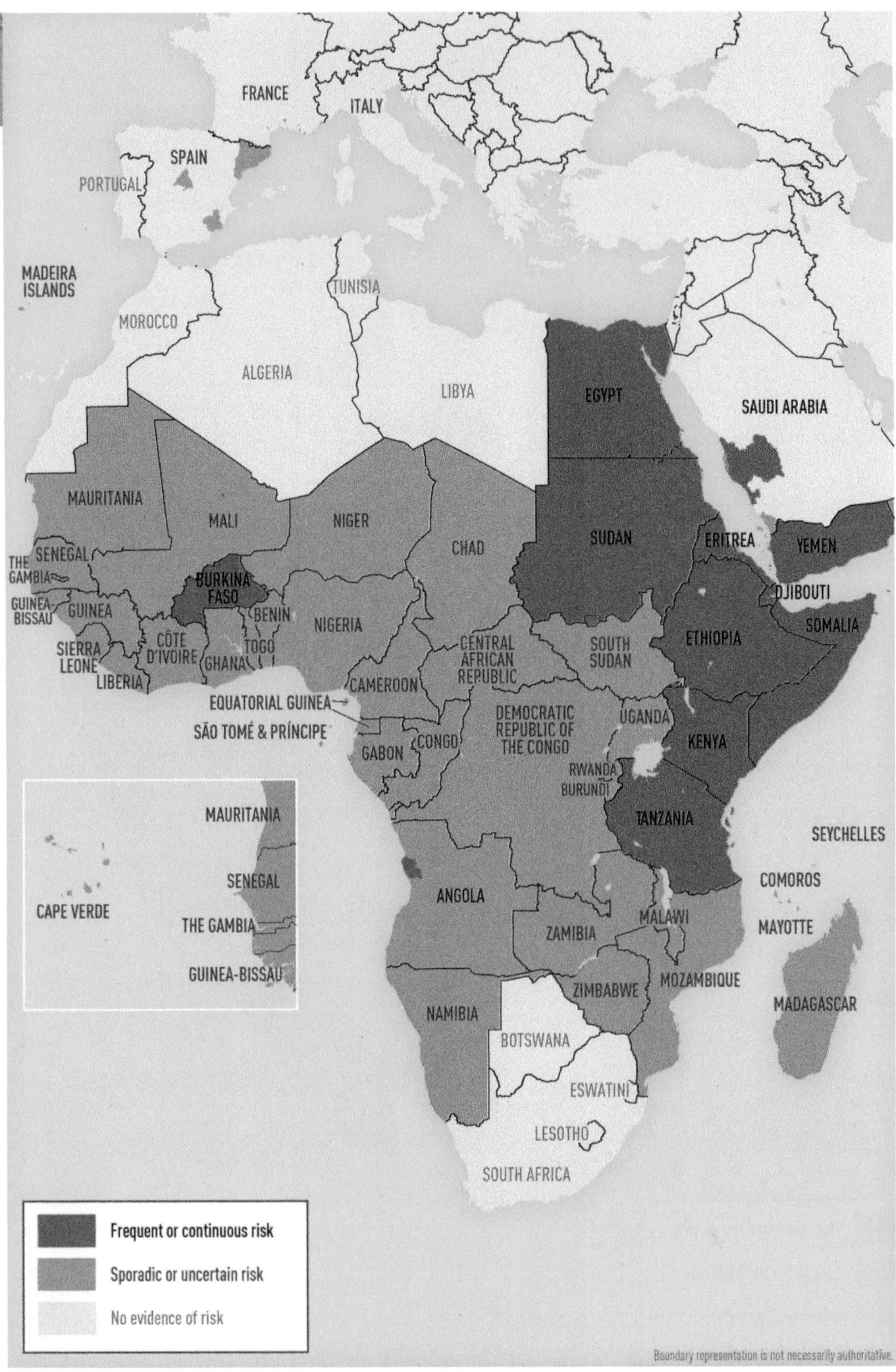

MAP 5-04 Dengue risk in Africa, Europe, & the Middle East

Risk classification uses the methodology described in Jentes, et al. Evidence-based risk assessment and communication: a new global dengue-risk map for travellers and clinicians (www.ncbi.nlm.nih.gov/pmc/articles/PMC5345513/). *Frequent/continuous risk*: evidence of more than 10 dengue cases in at least 3 of the previous 10 years; *sporadic/uncertain risk*: evidence of at least 1 locally acquired dengue case during the last 10 years. Level of risk assigned to a destination reflects the highest risk level identified within that destination. Where data are available, subnational dengue risk levels are shown. Destination risk levels also are denoted using black (frequent/continuous risk) or gray (sporadic/uncertain risk) font for the place name.

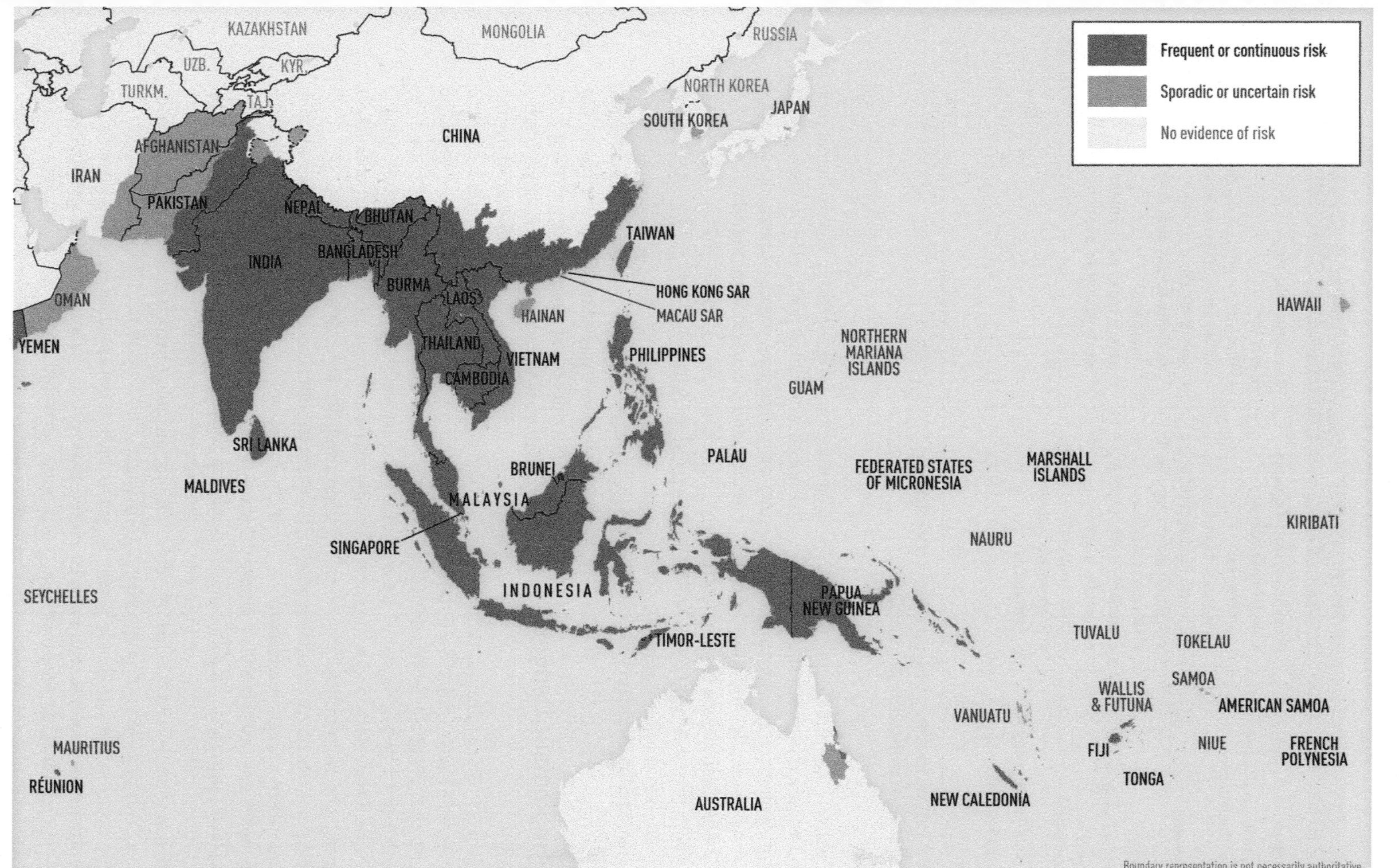

MAP 5-05 Dengue risk in Asia & Oceania

Risk classification uses the methodology described in Jentes, et al. Evidence-based risk assessment and communication: a new global dengue-risk map for travellers and clinicians (www.ncbi.nlm.nih.gov/pmc/articles/PMC5345513/). *Frequent/continuous risk*: evidence of more than 10 dengue cases in at least 3 of the previous 10 years; *sporadic/uncertain risk*: evidence of at least 1 locally acquired dengue case during the last 10 years. Level of risk assigned to a destination reflects the highest risk level identified within that destination. Where data are available, subnational dengue risk levels are shown. Destination risk levels also are denoted using black (frequent/continuous risk) or gray (sporadic/uncertain risk) font for the place name.

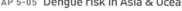

Table 5-09 Dengue Clinical Classification

DENGUE	DENGUE WITH WARNING SIGNS	SEVERE DENGUE
Probable Dengue Live in/travel to endemic area. **Fever** and 2 of the following criteria • Nausea/vomiting • Rash • Aches and pains • Tourniquet test positive • Leukopenia • Any warning sign **Laboratory-confirmed dengue** • Molecular techniques/ IgM or IgG seroconversion	Presence of warning signs • Abdominal pain or tenderness • Persistent vomiting • Clinical fluid accumulation (ascites, pleural effusion) • Mucosal bleeding • Lethargy, restlessness • Postural hypotension • Liver enlargement >2 cm • Progressive increase in hematocrit	One of the following manifestations • Shock or respiratory distress due to severe plasma leakage • Severe bleeding (based on evaluation by attending physician) • Severe organ involvement (such as liver or heart)

Source: Dengue: Guidelines for Patient Care in the Region of the Americas. Washington, DC: Pan-American Health Organization (2016).

5

patients develop severe, life-threatening disease. Early clinical findings are nonspecific but require a high index of suspicion; recognizing early signs of shock and promptly initiating intensive supportive therapy can reduce risk for death among patients with severe dengue by ≥20-fold. See Table 5-09 for information regarding the World Health Organization guidelines for classifying dengue.

Phases of Symptomatic Dengue

FEBRILE PHASE

Symptomatic dengue begins abruptly after an incubation period of 5–7 days (range 3–10 days) and has a 3-phase clinical course: febrile, critical, and convalescent. Fever typically lasts 2–7 days and can be biphasic. Other signs and symptoms include severe headache; retro-orbital pain; bone, joint, and muscle pain; macular or maculopapular rash; and minor hemorrhagic manifestations, including ecchymosis, epistaxis, bleeding gums, hematuria, petechiae, purpura, or a positive tourniquet test result. Some patients have an injected oropharynx and facial erythema in the first 24–48 hours after onset. Warning signs of progression to severe dengue occur in the late febrile phase around the time of defervescence (i.e., temperature <100.4°F [38°C]) and can include severe abdominal pain, difficulty breathing, extravascular fluid accumulation, progressive increase in hematocrit (hemoconcentration), postural hypotension, lethargy or restlessness, liver enlargement, mucosal bleeding, and persistent vomiting.

CRITICAL PHASE

The critical phase of dengue begins at defervescence and typically lasts 24–48 hours. Most patients improve clinically during this phase, but those with substantial plasma leak (resulting from marked increase in vascular permeability) progress to severe dengue. Patients with substantial plasma leak can develop ascites or pleural effusions, hemoconcentration, and hypoproteinemia. Physiologic compensatory mechanisms narrow the pulse pressure as diastolic blood pressure increases, initially maintaining adequate circulation; patients might appear well despite early signs of shock.

Once hypotension develops, however, systolic blood pressure rapidly declines, and irreversible shock and death can ensue despite resuscitation efforts. Especially in cases of prolonged shock, patients can develop severe hemorrhagic manifestations, including hematemesis, melena, or menorrhagia. Uncommon manifestations during this phase include encephalitis, hepatitis, myocarditis, and pancreatitis. Laboratory findings commonly include elevated aspartate aminotransferase and alanine aminotransferase, hyponatremia, leukopenia, lymphopenia, thrombocytopenia, and a normal erythrocyte sedimentation rate.

CONVALESCENT PHASE

As plasma leakage subsides, patients enter the convalescent phase and well-being improves; extravasated intravenous fluids and abdominal and pleural effusions are reabsorbed, hemodynamic status stabilizes (although bradycardia could manifest), and diuresis ensues. The patient's hematocrit stabilizes (or falls because of the dilutional effect of the reabsorbed fluid), and the white cell count usually starts to rise, after which the platelet count recovers. The convalescent phase rash might desquamate and be pruritic.

Dengue in Pregnancy

Data are limited on health outcomes of dengue in pregnancy and effects of maternal infection on the developing fetus. Perinatal transmission can occur, and peripartum maternal infection can increase the likelihood of symptomatic infection in the newborn. Signs and symptoms in perinatally infected neonates typically present during the first week of life and include ascites or pleural effusions, fever, hemorrhagic manifestations, hypotension, and thrombocytopenia. Placental transfer of maternal IgG against DENV from a previous maternal infection might increase risk for severe dengue among infants infected at 6–12 months of age when the protective effect of antibodies wanes.

DIAGNOSIS

Dengue is a nationally notifiable disease in the United States; report all suspected cases to the state or local health department. Consider dengue in the differential diagnosis of patients who develop onset of symptoms ≤2 weeks after returning from an endemic area. For patients presenting ≤7 days after fever onset, diagnostic testing should include a nucleic acid amplification test for DENV and IgM (Figure 5-01). For patients presenting >7 days after fever onset, IgM testing is recommended. In the United States, both IgM ELISA and real-time reverse transcription PCR (RT-PCR) are approved as in vitro diagnostic tests.

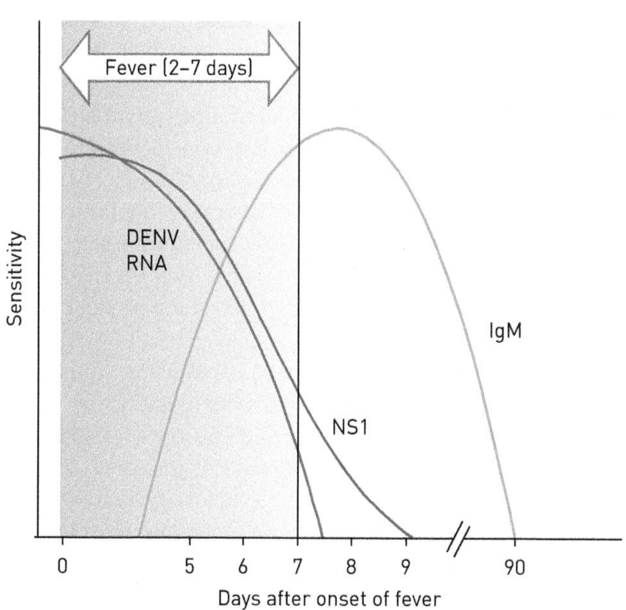

FIGURE 5-01 Relative sensitivity of detection of dengue virus nucleic acid, antigen, and IgM

Abbreviations: DENV, dengue virus; NS1, nonstructural protein 1

DENV RNA and NS1 are detectable during the first week of illness. DENV IgM is detectable starting ≈5 days after illness onset. Although most cases only have detectable DENV IgM for 14–20 days after illness onset, in some cases IgM might be detectable for up to 90 days. Routine testing of DENV IgG with a single sample is not useful in identifying patients with dengue.

Presence of virus by RT-PCR or DENV nonstructural protein 1 (NS1) antigen in a single diagnostic specimen is considered laboratory confirmation of dengue in patients with a compatible clinical and travel history. IgM in a single serum sample suggests a probable recent dengue infection. If a patient's travel history includes locations where other potentially cross-reactive flaviviruses circulate, perform both molecular and serologic diagnostic testing to detect DENV and other flaviviruses.

ELISA IgG in a single serum sample is not useful for routine diagnostic testing because IgG remains detectable for life after infection. In addition, people infected with or vaccinated against other flaviviruses (e.g., Japanese encephalitis, yellow fever) might produce cross-reactive flavivirus antibodies, yielding false-positive serologic dengue diagnostic test results.

Molecular and serologic DENV diagnostic testing are available from several commercial reference diagnostic laboratories, state public health laboratories, and the Centers for Disease Control and Prevention (CDC)'s Dengue Branch (www.cdc.gov/Dengue/clinicalLab/index.html). Clinicians can obtain consultation on dengue diagnostic testing from CDC at 787-706-2399 or by emailing dengue@cdc.gov.

TREATMENT

No specific antiviral agents exist for dengue. Depending on the clinical manifestations, patients might need only ambulatory care or might require hospitalization. Advise ambulatory patients to stay well hydrated and to avoid medications with anticoagulant properties, including aspirin (acetylsalicylic acid), aspirin-containing drugs, and other nonsteroidal anti-inflammatory drugs (e.g., ibuprofen). To control fever, advise patients to use acetaminophen and tepid sponge baths. Caution febrile patients to avoid mosquito bites to reduce risk for further community transmission.

Patients who develop severe dengue require hospitalization and close observation; monitoring in an intensive care unit might be required. Intravenous fluid therapy is the mainstay of treatment when plasma leakage is recognized. Prophylactic platelet transfusions in dengue patients are not beneficial and can contribute to fluid overload. Similarly, administration of corticosteroids has no demonstrated benefit and is potentially harmful. Avoid use of corticosteroids except in cases of autoimmune-related complications. CDC has additional dengue case management recommendations, available from www.cdc.gov/dengue/resources/DengueCheatSheet_ENG-P.pdf.

PREVENTION

In June 2021, the Advisory Committee on Immunization Practices (ACIP) recommended Dengvaxia for children aged 9–16 years with laboratory-confirmed previous dengue infection who are living in areas of the United States where dengue is endemic. These areas include the US territories of American Samoa, Puerto Rico, and the US Virgin Islands, and freely associated states including the Federated States of Micronesia, the Republic of Marshall Islands, and the Republic of Palau.

Dengvaxia is not approved for use in US travelers who are visiting but not living in areas where dengue is endemic. In people who have not already been infected with DENV, Dengvaxia can increase the risk for severe illness and hospitalization if the person gets dengue after vaccination. Serodiagnostic tests with acceptable performance (≥75% sensitivity and ≥98% specificity) recommended by health authorities are available to test people for evidence of previous dengue. Only people who test positive for previous DENV infection or who have other laboratory-confirmed evidence of a previous DENV infection are eligible for vaccination with Dengvaxia. Two other dengue vaccines are currently undergoing phase 3 clinical trials.

No specific medication is available to prevent dengue. Risk increases with duration of travel and disease incidence in the travel destination (e.g., during local epidemics or the rainy season). Travelers going to the tropics for any length of time should take steps to prevent mosquito bites by using the preventive measures listed below and in Sec. 4, Ch. 6, Mosquitoes, Ticks & Other Arthropods:

- Select accommodations with well-screened windows and doors or air conditioning, when possible. *Aedes* mosquitoes typically live indoors and often are found in dark, cool places (e.g., in closets, under beds, behind curtains, in bathrooms, on porches).

- Wear clothing that covers the arms and legs, especially during the early morning and late afternoon, when risk of being bitten by *Aedes* species mosquitoes is greatest.
- Use insect repellent.
- For longer-term travelers, empty and clean or cover any standing water that can be a mosquito-breeding site in the local residence (e.g., water storage tanks, flowerpots).

CDC website: www.cdc.gov/dengue

BIBLIOGRAPHY

Arragain L, Dupont-Rouzeyrol M, O'Connor O, Sigur N, Grangeon JP, Huguon E, et al. Vertical transmission of dengue virus in the peripartum period and viral kinetics in newborns and breast milk: new data. J Pediatric Infect Dis. 2017;6(4):324–31.

Blitvich BJ, Magalhaes T, Laredo-Tiscareño SV, Foy BD. Sexual transmission of arboviruses: a systematic review. Viruses. 2020;12(9):933.

Leder K, Torresi J, Libman MD, Cramer JP, Castelli F, Schlagenhauf P, et al. GeoSentinel surveillance of illness in returned travelers, 2007–2011. Ann Intern Med. 2013;158(6):456–68.

Rivera A, Adams LE, Sharp TM, Lehman JA, Waterman SH, Paz-Bailey G. Travel-associated and locally acquired dengue cases—United States, 2010–2017. MMWR Morb Mort Wkly Rep. 2020;69(6):149.

Schwartz E, Weld LH, Wilder-Smith A, von Sonnenburg F, Keystone JS, Kain KC, et al. Seasonality, annual trends, and characteristics of dengue among ill returned travelers, 1997–2006. Emerg Infect Dis. 2008;14(7):1081–8.

Sharp TM, Fischer M, Muñoz-Jordán JL, Paz-Bailey G, Staples JE, Gregory CJ, et al. Dengue and Zika virus diagnostic testing for patients with a clinically compatible illness and risk for infection with both viruses. MMWR Recomm Rep. 2019;68(1):1.

Simmons CP, Farrar JJ, van Vinh Chau N, Wills B. Dengue. N Engl J Med. 2012;366(15):1423–32.

Wilder-Smith A. Dengue infections in travellers. Paediatr Int Child Health. 2012;32(Suppl):28–32.

Wilder-Smith A, Ooi EE, Horstick O, Wills B. Dengue. Lancet. 2019;393(10169):350–63.

World Health Organization. Dengue guidelines for diagnosis, treatment, prevention and control: new edition. Geneva: The Organization; 2009. Available from: https://apps.who.int/iris/handle/10665/44188.

HAND, FOOT & MOUTH DISEASE

Eileen Yee

INFECTIOUS AGENT: Nonpolio enteroviruses	
ENDEMICITY	Worldwide, with outbreaks in the Asia-Pacific region
TRAVELERS CATEGORIES AT GREATEST RISK FOR EXPOSURE & INFECTION	Expatriates with children attending nursery school, daycare, elementary school Travelers with young children
PREVENTION METHODS	Practice hand hygiene Avoid close contact with infected people EV-A71 vaccine (licensed only in China)
DIAGNOSTIC SUPPORT	A clinical laboratory certified in moderate complexity testing; state health department; or CDC Polio and Picornavirus Laboratory (picornalab@cdc.gov)

INFECTIOUS AGENT

Hand, foot, and mouth disease (HFMD) is caused by nonpolio enteroviruses, a genus of the *Picornaviridae* family of nonenveloped RNA viruses (e.g., coxsackievirus A6, coxsackievirus A16, enterovirus A71). Enteroviruses that cause widespread outbreaks of HFMD worldwide can vary by type and region. In the Asia-Pacific region, enterovirus A71 (EV-A71) is the predominant etiologic agent, while in Europe and the United States, coxsackievirus viruses often are implicated in HFMD cases and outbreaks.

TRANSMISSION

Transmission occurs by direct person-to-person contact with the saliva, nose and throat secretions, vesicle fluid, or stool of an infected person and through contact with contaminated surfaces and objects (e.g., common diapering areas, shared toys, eating utensils).

EPIDEMIOLOGY

HFMD is a common infection among children worldwide and spreads quickly, causing large outbreaks that can lead to nursery, daycare, and school closures. Outbreaks often occur during summer and early fall in Australia and the United States, but seasonal patterns in the Asia-Pacific region can vary between climate zones. In the temperate climates, cases tend to peak during the early summer, whereas in tropical climates, including Hong Kong and Taiwan, outbreaks usually occur in late spring and fall.

Outbreaks also can happen sporadically throughout the year in other countries (e.g., Malaysia, Singapore, Thailand, Vietnam). Children <5 years old are most susceptible, but adults and adolescents also can become ill with HFMD. People traveling with young children should be aware of HFMD and any local outbreaks that might occur at their destinations and pay close attention to recommended preventive measures.

CLINICAL PRESENTATION

Incubation period is 3–6 days, and illness usually is self-limited, with recovery within 7–10 days. Patients usually present with fever and malaise; then sore throat and painful vesicles (herpangina) appear in the mouth, involving the buccal mucosa, tongue, or hard palate, and a peripheral rash, usually papulovesicular, appears on the hands (palms), feet (soles), or less often on the buttocks, genitals, elbows, and knees.

In rare cases, patients can develop brainstem encephalitis, aseptic meningitis, myocarditis, or pulmonary edema and can die from complications. Additionally, HFMD can have an atypical presentation, often in adults, beginning with a rash or lesion that enlarges and coalesces to form bullae; a thorough travel history or history of recent exposure to others with the infection is critical to making the diagnosis. Onychomadesis (shedding of the nails) and desquamation of the palms or soles can occur during convalescence.

DIAGNOSIS

Diagnosis is usually clinical, but confirmatory laboratory tests using reverse transcription PCR (RT-PCR) assays are available and performed for atypical or severe cases. Preferred samples for testing include vesicle fluid, throat or buccal swabs, or stool. Many commercial or reference laboratories can perform RT-PCR assays to detect enterovirus RNA.

The Centers for Disease Control and Prevention (CDC) Picornavirus Laboratory within the Division of Viral Diseases routinely performs qualitative pan-enterovirus molecular testing, after which the laboratory performs sequencing for enterovirus typing in consultation with state or local health departments in the United States. CDC can test nasopharyngeal or oropharyngeal swabs, nasal wash or aspirate samples, stool samples, rectal swabs, cerebrospinal fluid, serum, and tissue biopsy or autopsy specimens.

International laboratories seeking consultation can email the CDC laboratory, picornalab@cdc.gov. For information about specimen collection, storage, and shipping address, refer to CDC's Non-Polio Enterovirus website, www.cdc.gov/non-polio-enterovirus/lab-testing/index.html, and email the laboratory (picornalab@cdc.gov) prior to shipping.

TREATMENT

HFMD treatment mainly involves supportive care to treat symptoms of fever or pain caused by mouth sores, and to prevent dehydration, especially in young children.

PREVENTION

Travelers can prevent HFMD by avoiding close contact (e.g., hugging, kissing, sharing food utensils or drinking cups) with infected people. Travelers also should maintain good hand hygiene (see www.cdc.gov/handwashing), and clean and disinfect potentially contaminated surfaces and soiled items, including diapering and child potty areas, doorknobs, eating areas, and toys. People traveling with infants and young children and those affected by local school or daycare outbreaks especially should follow these precautions.

Travelers should use frequent handwashing with soap and water rather than hand sanitizers, because alcohol-based sanitizers might be less effective against nonenveloped enteroviruses. Travelers should choose a US Environmental Protection Agency–registered disinfecting product or a comparable product that kills nonenveloped viruses (e.g., norovirus). The public health response to large outbreaks of HFMD, particularly in Asia, includes isolation of cases, social distancing, and closures of schools and daycare centers.

Licensed EV-A71 vaccines to prevent severe HFMD have been approved in China since 2015. This vaccine might not provide cross-protection against other enterovirus serotypes, however. The US Food and Drug Administration has not approved any enterovirus vaccines for use in the United States.

5

CDC website: www.cdc.gov/hand-foot-mouth

BIBLIOGRAPHY

American Academy of Pediatrics. Enterovirus (nonpoliovirus). In: Kimberlin DW, Brady MT, Jackson MA, Long SS, editors. Red Book: 2018 report of the Committee on Infectious Diseases, 31st edition. Itasca (IL): American Academy of Pediatrics; 2018. pp. 331–4.

Chang Y-K, Chen K-H, Chen K-T. Hand, foot, and mouth disease and herpangina caused by EVA71 infections: a review of EVA71 molecular epidemiology, pathogenesis, and current vaccine development. Rev Inst Med Trop Sao Paulo. 2018;60:e70.

Koh WM, Bogich T, Seigel K, Jin J, Chong EY, Tan CY, et al. The epidemiology of hand, foot, and mouth disease in Asia: a systematic review and analysis. Pediatr Infect Dis J. 2016;35(10):e285–300.

Puenpa J, Wanlapakorn N, Vongpunsawad S, Poovorawan Y. The history of enterovirus A71 outbreaks and molecular epidemiology in the Asia-Pacific Region. J Biomed Sci. 2019;26(1):75.

World Health Organization. A guide to clinical management and public health response for hand, foot and mouth disease (HFMD). Geneva: The Organization; 2011. Available from: https://iris.wpro.who.int/bitstream/handle/10665.1/5521/9789290615255_eng.pdf.

World Health Organization. Hand, foot and mouth disease. Available from: www.who.int/westernpacific/emergencies/surveillance/archives/hand-foot-and-mouth-disease.

HENIPAVIRUS INFECTIONS

Trevor Shoemaker, Mary Joung Choi

INFECTIOUS AGENT: *Henipavirus* spp.	
ENDEMICITY	Southeast Asia, Bangladesh, India (Nipah virus) Australia (Hendra virus) China (Langya virus)
TRAVELER CATEGORIES AT GREATEST RISK FOR EXPOSURE & INFECTION	Travelers exposed to infected animals (e.g., bats, pigs) or their body fluids Travelers who eat foods (e.g., fallen fruit, palm sap) contaminated by body fluids of infected animals Health care workers treating infected patients
PREVENTION METHODS	Avoid bat roosting areas Avoid unprotected contact with blood, fluids, tissues of potentially infected animals (e.g., sick or dead bats, pigs) Follow safe food precautions: avoid cooking, eating, handling raw or undercooked meat or animal products; avoid eating fallen fruit, raw date palm sap Use standard barrier precautions and personal protective equipment in medical settings
DIAGNOSTIC SUPPORT	State health department; or call the CDC Emergency Operations Center at 770-488-7100.

INFECTIOUS AGENT

Enveloped, single-stranded RNA viruses in the genus *Henipavirus*, family Paramyxovirus can infect humans. Of the 6 identified *Henipavirus* species, Hendra virus and Nipah virus are highly virulent emerging pathogens that cause outbreaks in humans and are associated with high case-fatality ratios. In August 2022, a new *Henipavirus* species (Langya virus, LayV) was identified among febrile human cases in eastern China. Phylogenetic analysis of Langya shows it to be most closely related to Mojiang virus. Mojiang virus, along with two other *Henipavirus* species—Cedar virus and Ghanaian bat virus—are not known to cause human disease.

TRANSMISSION

Pteropid fruit bats (flying foxes) are *Henipavirus* reservoir hosts. Hendra virus is transmitted to humans through direct contact with infected horses or body fluids or tissues of infected horses; horses are infected through exposure to bat urine. Hendra virus is not transmitted person-to-person or directly from bats to humans.

Nipah virus is transmitted through contact with infected pigs or bats; consumption of date palm sap or fallen fruit contaminated with bat excretions is another route of exposure. Person-to-person transmission of Nipah virus has been reported through close contact with infected people, including respiratory droplets. Nipah transmission is facilitated by cultural and health care practices in which friends and family members care for ill patients.

Initial sampling of small wild mammals detected Langya virus predominantly in shrews (71 of 262 [26%] sampled) belonging to the species *Crocidura lasiura* and *Crocidura shantungensis*. More research is needed to definitively determine the natural animal reservoir(s), susceptible species, and routes of transmission to humans. Preliminary evidence is not suggestive of person-to-person transmission of Langya virus.

EPIDEMIOLOGY

To date, no *Henipavirus* infections have been reported among travelers. Hendra virus outbreaks in Australia are caused by exposure to sick or dead infected horses. Since 1994, Hendra virus has been reported nearly annually in the eastern states of Australia. Nipah virus outbreaks in humans were reported in 1999 in Malaysia and Singapore and are reported almost annually in Bangladesh and India, typically resulting from direct or indirect bat exposure, but also less commonly through person-to-person spread or exposure to sick or dead pigs. Pteropid bats can be found throughout the tropics and subtropics, however, and henipaviruses have been isolated from these animals in East Africa, Central and South America, Asia, and Oceania.

As of August 2022, researchers have identified a total of 35 non-fatal human cases of Langya virus infection. Further research is needed to determine the geographic distribution of this newly identified virus.

CLINICAL PRESENTATION

Incubation period is ≈5–16 days (and rarely ≤2 months). Both Hendra and Nipah virus infections can cause a severe influenza-like illness with dizziness, headache, fever, and myalgias. The disease can progress to severe encephalitis with confusion, abnormal reflexes, seizures, and coma; respiratory symptoms also might be present. Relapsing or late-onset encephalitis can occur months or years after acute illness. The case-fatality ratio of Hendra virus is 57%; among 7 known human cases, 4 were fatal. Case-fatality ratios for Nipah virus infection are 40%–70% but have been 100% in some human outbreaks.

Most of the 35 known cases of Langya virus infection have reported non-specific clinical symptoms (e.g., anorexia, cough, fatigue, fever, headache, myalgia, nausea, vomiting). No deaths due to Langya virus have yet been identified.

DIAGNOSIS

Laboratory diagnosis is made by using a combination of tests, including ELISA of serum or cerebrospinal fluid (CSF); reverse transcription PCR of serum, CSF, or throat swabs; and virus isolation from CSF or throat swabs. The Centers for Disease Control and Prevention (CDC) can test specimens from patients suspected to be infected with a *Henipavirus*. Prior to submitting specimens to CDC, contact the state or local health department to arrange a clinical consultation, or call the CDC Emergency Operations Center at 770-488-7100.

TREATMENT

No specific antiviral treatment is available for *Henipavirus* infections. Therapy consists of supportive care and management of complications. Ribavirin has shown in vitro effectiveness, but its clinical usefulness is unknown. A monoclonal serotherapy has been proposed for Hendra in Australia.

PREVENTION

Travelers should avoid contact with bats, sick horses and pigs, and their excretions. Travelers should not consume fallen fruit, raw date palm sap, or products made from raw sap. A Hendra virus vaccine for horses has been licensed in Australia and has potential future benefit to prevent *Henipavirus* infections in humans, but no licensed vaccines for humans currently are available.

CDC websites: www.cdc.gov/vhf/hendra/index.html; www.cdc.gov/vhf/nipah/index.html

BIBLIOGRAPHY

Ang BSP, Lim TCC, Wang L. Nipah virus infection. J Clin Microbiol. 2018;56(6):e01875–17.

Croser EL, Marsh GA. The changing face of the henipaviruses. Veterinary Microbiol. 2013;167(1–2):151–8.

Weatherman S, Feldmann H, de Wit E. Transmission of henipaviruses. Curr Opin Virol. 2018;28:7–11.

Zhang XA, Li H, Jiang FC, Zhu F, Zhang YF, Chen JJ, et al. A Zoonotic Henipavirus in Febrile Patients in China. N Engl J Med. 2022;387(5):470–2.

5

HEPATITIS A

Noele Nelson, Mark Weng

INFECTIOUS AGENT: Hepatitis A virus	
ENDEMICITY	High endemicity: parts of Africa and Asia Intermediate endemicity: parts of Asia; also, Central and South America, and eastern Europe Low endemicity: Western Europe, United States
TRAVELER CATEGORIES AT GREATEST RISK FOR EXPOSURE & INFECTION	Travelers not vaccinated against Hepatitis A Travelers going to areas with inadequate sanitation and limited access to clean water
PREVENTION METHODS	Follow safe food and water precautions Hepatitis A is a vaccine-preventable disease
DIAGNOSTIC SUPPORT	A clinical laboratory certified in moderate complexity testing; state health department; or for testing at CDC www.cdc.gov/laboratory/specimen-submission/list.html

5

INFECTIOUS AGENT

Hepatitis A virus (HAV) is a nonenveloped RNA virus classified as a picornavirus.

TRANSMISSION

HAV is transmitted through direct person-to-person contact (fecal–oral transmission) or through ingestion of contaminated food or water. HAV can survive in the environment for prolonged periods at low pH. Freezing does not inactivate the virus, and HAV can be transmitted through ice and frozen foods. Heat inactivation must occur at temperatures >185°F (>85°C) for 1 minute. HAV can be transmitted from raw or inadequately cooked foods contaminated during growing, processing, or distribution, and through contamination by an infected food handler. Recent large-scale outbreaks have been caused by common-source food exposures (e.g., frozen berries, fresh fruit and vegetables, seafood) and through person-to-person spread among people experiencing homelessness and people who use injection and non-injection drugs.

Infected people shed HAV in their feces. People are most infectious 1–2 weeks before the onset of clinical signs and symptoms of jaundice or elevation of liver enzymes, when virus concentration is greatest in the stool and blood. Viral excretion and the risk for transmission diminish rapidly after liver dysfunction or symptoms appear, which is concurrent with the appearance of circulating antibodies to HAV. Infants and children can shed virus for up to 6 months after infection.

EPIDEMIOLOGY

Hepatitis A is among the most common vaccine-preventable infections acquired during travel. Cases of travel-related hepatitis A can occur in travelers to developed and developing countries and who have standard tourist accommodations, eating behaviors, and itineraries. Risk is greatest for those who live in or visit rural areas, trek in backcountry areas, or frequently eat or drink in settings with poor sanitation. Common-source food exposures are increasingly recognized as a risk for hepatitis A, and sporadic outbreaks have been reported in Australia, Europe, North America, and other regions with low levels of endemic transmission. Multinational hepatitis A outbreaks among men who have sex with men (MSM) have been described, including, since 2016, among MSM who travel to areas in

European Union countries with ongoing HAV transmission among MSM.

Hepatitis A is common in areas with inadequate sanitation and limited access to clean water. In highly endemic areas (e.g., parts of Africa and Asia), a large proportion of adults in the population are infected as children, are immune to HAV, and epidemics are uncommon. In areas of intermediate endemicity (e.g., Central and South America, eastern Europe, parts of Asia), childhood transmission is less frequent, more adolescents and adults are susceptible to infection, and outbreaks are more likely. In areas of low endemicity (e.g., western Europe, the United States), infection is less common, but disease occurs among people in high-risk groups and as communitywide outbreaks. Determining HAV endemicity globally is complex, however, and limited data are available on subpopulation variation of HAV antibody seroprevalence within regions (Map 5-06).

In the United States, the most frequently identified risk factors for HAV infection vary from year to year. The Advisory Committee on Immunization Practices (ACIP) recommends routine hepatitis A vaccination for all children, and vaccination for adults at increased risk for HAV infection or at increased risk for severe disease from HAV infection.

CLINICAL PRESENTATION

The incubation period averages 28 days (range 15–50 days). Infection can range from mild illness lasting 1–2 weeks to severely disabling disease lasting several months. Clinical manifestations include abrupt onset of fever, malaise, anorexia, nausea, and abdominal discomfort, followed by jaundice within a few days. The likelihood of having symptoms with HAV infection is related to the age of the infected person. In children aged <6 years, most (70%) infections are asymptomatic; jaundice is uncommon in symptomatic young children. Among older children and adults, the illness usually lasts <2 months, but ≈10%–15% of infected people have prolonged or relapsing symptoms over 6–9 months.

Severe hepatic and extrahepatic complications, including fulminant hepatitis and liver failure, are rare but more common in older adults and people with underlying liver disease. Chronic infection does not occur. The overall case-fatality ratio varies according to the population affected.

DIAGNOSIS

Hepatitis A cannot be differentiated from other types of viral hepatitis based on clinical or epidemiologic features. Diagnosis requires a positive test for HAV IgM in serum, which is detectable 2 weeks before the onset of symptoms to ≈6 months after symptom onset.

Serologic total HAV IgG and IgM tests are available commercially. The combination of a positive total HAV result and a negative HAV IgM result indicates past infection or vaccination, and hence immunity. Presence of serum HAV IgM usually indicates current or recent infection and does not distinguish between immunity derived from infection versus vaccination. Hepatitis A is a nationally notifiable disease.

Information on how to obtain HAV diagnostic support from the Centers for Disease Control and Prevention (CDC), including contact information, which samples to send, and how to send them is available at www.cdc.gov/laboratory/specimen-submission/list.html. For research use and for outbreak investigations, select "Hepatitis A NAT and Genotyping." For testing regulated by Clinical Laboratory Improvement Amendments, select "Hepatitis A Serology."

TREATMENT

Provide supportive care.

PREVENTION

Travelers can prevent HAV through vaccination or immune globulin (IG), practicing food and water precautions, and maintaining standards of hygiene and sanitation.

Vaccine

Two single-antigen hepatitis A vaccines, Havrix (GlaxoSmithKline) and Vaqta (Merck), are approved for people ≥12 months of age in a 2-dose series. A combined hepatitis A and hepatitis B vaccine (Twinrix, GlaxoSmithKline) is approved for people ≥18 years of age in the United States (Table 5-10). The immunogenicity of the combination vaccine is equivalent to that of the single-antigen hepatitis A and hepatitis B vaccines when

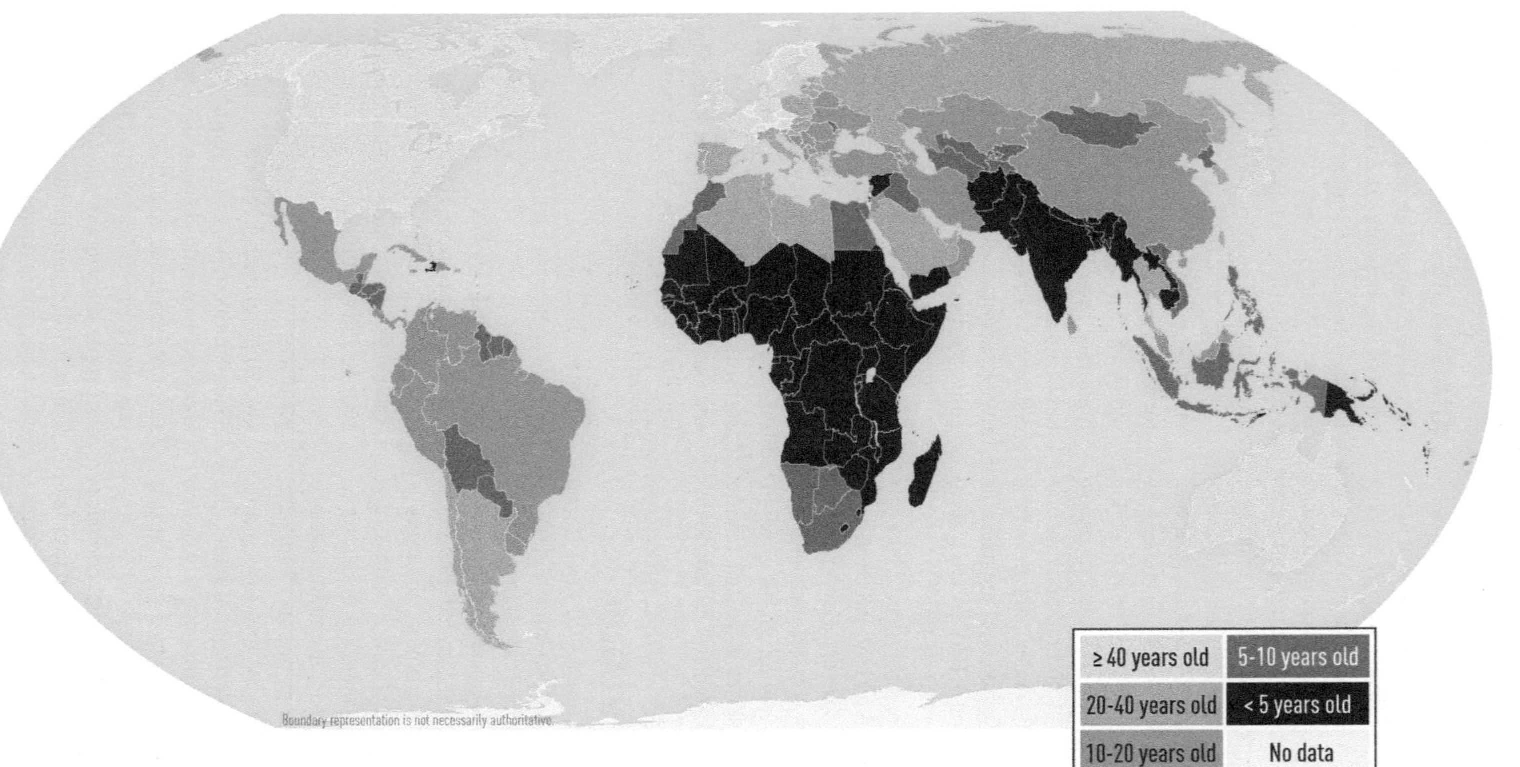

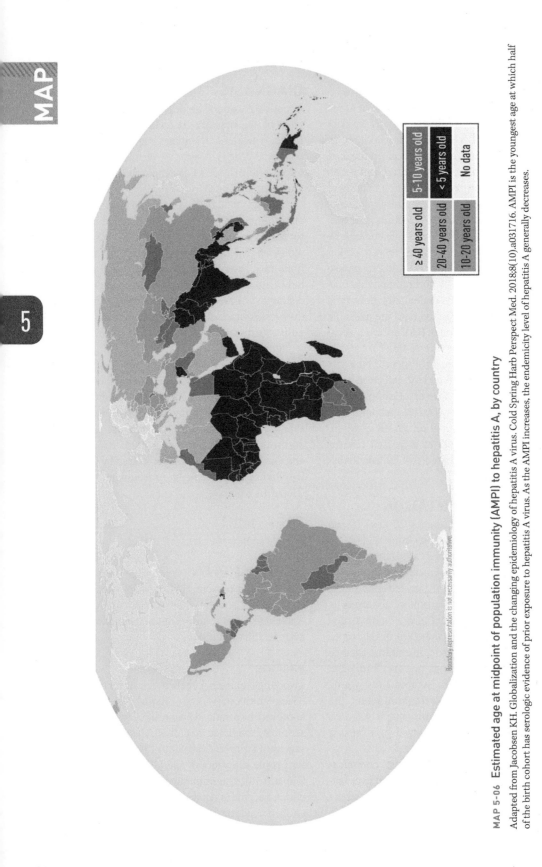

MAP 5-06 **Estimated age at midpoint of population immunity (AMPI) to hepatitis A, by country**

Adapted from Jacobsen KH. Globalization and the changing epidemiology of hepatitis A virus. Cold Spring Harb Perspect Med. 2018;8(10).a031716. AMPI is the youngest age at which half of the birth cohort has serologic evidence of prior exposure to hepatitis A virus. As the AMPI increases, the endemicity level of hepatitis A generally decreases.

Table 5-10 Vaccines used to prevent hepatitis A virus (HAV) infection

VACCINE	TRADE NAME (MANUFACTURER)	AGE IN YEARS	DOSE / ROUTE	SCHEDULE	BOOSTER
Hepatitis A vaccine, inactivated	Havrix (GlaxoSmithKline)	1–18	0.5 mL (720 ELU) IM	DOSE 1: 1–18 years old DOSE 2: 6–12 months after DOSE 1	None
		≥19	1 mL (1,440 ELU) IM	DOSE 1: ≥19 years old DOSE 2: 6–12 months after DOSE 1	None
Hepatitis A vaccine, inactivated	Vaqta (Merck)	1–18	0.5 mL (25 U) IM	DOSE 1: 1–18 years old DOSE 2: 6–18 months after DOSE 1	None
		≥19	1 mL (50 U) IM	DOSE 1: ≥19 years old DOSE 2: 6–18 months after DOSE 1	None
Combined hepatitis A and hepatitis B vaccine[1]	Twinrix (GlaxoSmithKline)	≥18	1 mL (720 ELU HAV + 20 µg HBsAg) IM	**STANDARD** DOSE 1: ≥18 years old DOSE 2: 1 month after DOSE 1 DOSE 3: 6 months after DOSE 1	None
		≥18	1 mL (720 ELU HAV + 20 µg HBsAg) IM	**ACCELERATED** DOSE 1: ≥18 years old DOSE 2: 7 days after DOSE 1 DOSE 3: 21–30 days after DOSE 1	12 months after DOSE 1

Abbreviations: ELU, ELISA units inactivated HAV; HBsAg, hepatitis B surface antigen; IM, intramuscular; U, units of HAV antigen

[1]Combined hepatitis A and hepatitis B vaccine (Twinrix) should not be used for postexposure prophylaxis.

tested after completion of the recommended schedule. Postvaccination testing for serologic response is not indicated for healthy people, but is recommended for people whose subsequent clinical management depends on knowledge of their immune status and people for whom revaccination might be indicated (e.g., people with HIV and other immunocompromised people).

INDICATIONS FOR USE

All susceptible people traveling for any purpose, frequency, or duration to countries with high or intermediate hepatitis A endemicity should be vaccinated or receive IG before departure. Furthermore, prevalence patterns of HAV infection vary among regions within a country; in some areas, limited data result in uncertainty in endemicity maps, especially in low- and middle-income countries. Countries with decreasing prevalence of HAV infection have growing numbers of susceptible people and are at risk for hepatitis A outbreaks. In recent years, large hepatitis A outbreaks have been reported in high-income countries among people exposed to imported HAV-contaminated food, among MSM, among people who use drugs, and among people experiencing

5

homelessness. Considering the complexity of interpreting hepatitis A risk maps and potential risk for foodborne hepatitis A in low-endemicity countries, some experts advise people traveling outside the United States to consider hepatitis A vaccination regardless of destination.

Vaccination is also recommended for unvaccinated household members and other people (e.g., regular babysitters) who anticipate close personal contact with an international adoptee from a high- or intermediate-endemicity country ≤60 days after the child's arrival in the United States. The first dose of the 2-dose hepatitis A vaccine series should be administered as soon as adoption is planned, ideally ≥2 weeks before the arrival of the child (see Sec. 7, Ch. 5, International Adoption).

5

ADMINISTRATION

All susceptible people (i.e., those unvaccinated or never infected) traveling to or working in countries with high or intermediate hepatitis A endemicity are at risk for HAV infection. Before departure, these travelers should be vaccinated, or receive IG if they are too young or have contraindications for hepatitis A vaccination. For travelers already partially vaccinated (i.e., did not receive a full series of hepatitis A-containing vaccine), administer a dose prior to travel according to the routine immunization schedule.

INFANTS YOUNGER THAN 6 MONTHS OLD

Infants aged <6 months and travelers allergic to a vaccine component, or who elect not to receive vaccine, should receive IG, which provides effective temporary protection against HAV infection. For travel duration ≤1 month, the manufacturer recommends 1 dose of IG at 0.1 mL/kg; for travel >1 month but ≤2 months, 1 dose of IG at 0.2 mL/kg is recommended. A 0.2 mL/kg dose of IG should be repeated every 2 months for the duration of travel if the traveler remains in a high-risk setting; but encourage hepatitis A vaccination if not contraindicated.

INFANTS 6–11 MONTHS OLD

Administer hepatitis A vaccine to infants aged 6–11 months traveling outside the United States when protection against hepatitis A is recommended. Although hepatitis A vaccine is considered safe and immunogenic in infants, hepatitis A vaccine doses administered before 12 months of age could result in a suboptimal immune response, particularly in infants with passively acquired maternal antibody. Therefore, hepatitis A vaccine doses administered at <12 months of age are not considered to provide long-term protection, and the 2-dose hepatitis A vaccine series should be initiated at age 12 months according to the routine immunization schedule.

ADULTS OVER 40 YEARS OLD

Adults aged >40 years, immunocompromised people, and people with chronic liver disease should receive a single dose of hepatitis A vaccine as soon as travel is considered. People planning travel in <2 weeks can receive IG (0.1 mL/kg) in addition to vaccine at a separate injection site (i.e., separate limbs) based on provider risk assessment, including considerations of the traveler's age, immune status, underlying conditions, risk for exposure, and availability of IG. The hepatitis A vaccine series should be completed according to the routine immunization schedule.

TWINRIX

An alternative accelerated 4-dose schedule is available for Twinrix; doses can be administered at 0, 7, and 21–30 days, then a dose at 12 months. For more details, refer to NP Nelson et al. in the bibliography of this chapter. Although vaccinating an immune traveler is not contraindicated and does not increase the risk for adverse effects, screening for total HAV antibodies before travel can be useful in some circumstances to determine susceptibility and avoid unnecessary vaccination.

SAFETY & ADVERSE REACTIONS

Based on passive surveillance, the most frequently reported adverse events after single-antigen hepatitis A vaccination were fever, injection site reactions, and rash. The most frequently reported adverse events after Twinrix vaccination were dizziness, fever, headache, and injection site reactions. These findings are similar to those for other inactivated vaccines routinely administered among similar age groups.

PRECAUTIONS & CONTRAINDICATIONS

Hepatitis A vaccines should not be administered to travelers with a history of hypersensitivity to any vaccine component, including neomycin. Twinrix should not be administered to people with a history of hypersensitivity to yeast. The tip caps of prefilled syringes of Havrix and Twinrix and the vial stopper, syringe plunger stopper, and tip caps of Vaqta might contain dry natural rubber, which can cause allergic reactions in latex-sensitive people. Because hepatitis A vaccine consists of inactivated virus, and hepatitis B vaccine consists of a recombinant protein, no special precautions are needed for vaccination of immunocompromised travelers with single-antigen vaccines or Twinrix. Check precautions and contraindications before administering IG.

PREGNANCY

The ACIP recommends vaccinating selected groups of pregnant people if they have not been vaccinated previously (see www.cdc.gov/vaccines/schedules/hcp/imz/adult-conditions.html). These include people (e.g., travelers) at increased risk for HAV infection during pregnancy as well as those at risk for having a severe outcome from HAV infection (e.g., those with chronic liver disease or HIV).

OTHER CONSIDERATIONS

The best approach is to administer hepatitis A vaccine according to the routine immunization schedule; however, an interrupted series does not need to be restarted. Over 90% of vaccinated people develop levels of antibodies to HAV that correlate with protection 1 month after the first dose of hepatitis A vaccines. Given their similar immunogenicity, a series that has been started with one brand of hepatitis A single-antigen vaccine can be completed with another brand of single-antigen vaccine. For children and adults who complete a primary series of hepatitis A-containing vaccine, booster doses of vaccine are not recommended. Measles-mumps-rubella and varicella vaccines should not be administered <6 months after IG administration.

POSTEXPOSURE PROPHYLAXIS

Travelers exposed to HAV who are asymptomatic and who have not received hepatitis A vaccine should receive 1 dose of single-antigen hepatitis A vaccine or IG (0.1 mL/kg) as soon as possible, ideally ≤2 weeks following exposure. The efficacy of IG or vaccine when administered >2 weeks after exposure has not been established.

Hepatitis A vaccines should be administered as postexposure prophylaxis (PEP) for all people aged ≥12 months who have been exposed to HAV ≤2 weeks and have not previously completed the hepatitis A vaccine series. In addition to hepatitis A vaccine, administer IG (0.1 mL/kg) to people who are immunocompromised or who have chronic liver disease, and to people aged >40 years, depending on the risk assessment, which should include consideration of the exposed person's age, immune status, underlying conditions, exposure type (risk of transmission), and availability of IG.

Administer PEP as soon as possible. If giving both hepatitis A vaccine and IG (0.1 mL/kg), administer both simultaneously in different anatomic sites (i.e., separate limbs). If only 1 product is available, administer it as soon as possible and have the exposed person return for the other product if it becomes available ≤2 weeks following exposure. When the dose of hepatitis A vaccine given postexposure is the first dose the exposed person has ever received, administer a second dose 6 months after the first for long-term immunity; however, the second dose is not necessary for PEP.

Infants <12 months of age and people who are allergic to a vaccine component or who elect not to receive vaccine should receive a single dose of IG (0.1 mL/kg) as soon as possible ≤2 weeks of exposure.

Do not use Twinrix for PEP. Twinrix contains half of the single-antigen hepatitis A adult dose, and no data are available on the efficacy of combination vaccine for prophylaxis after exposure to HAV.

CDC website: www.cdc.gov/hepatitis/HAV

BIBLIOGRAPHY

Centers for Disease Control and Prevention. Viral Hepatitis Surveillance 2019. Atlanta: U.S. Department of Health and Human Services; 2021.

Jacobsen KH. Globalization and the changing epidemiology of hepatitis A virus. Cold Spring Harb Perspect Med. 2018; 8(10):a031716.

Nelson NP. Updated dosing instructions for immune globulin (human) GamaSTAN S/D for hepatitis A virus prophylaxis. MMWR 2017;66(36):959–60.

Nelson NP, Weng MK, Hofmeister MG, Moore KL, Doshani M, Kamili S, et al. Prevention of hepatitis A virus infection in the United States: recommendations of the Advisory Committee on Immunization Practices, 2020. MMWR Recomm Rep. 2020;69(5):1–38.

HEPATITIS B

Aaron Harris

5

INFECTIOUS AGENT: Hepatitis B virus	
ENDEMICITY	Worldwide High prevalence in Africa and the Western Pacific
TRAVELER CATEGORIES AT GREATEST RISK FOR EXPOSURE & INFECTION	Expatriates Long-term development workers Medical tourists Missionaries and humanitarian aid workers Travelers not vaccinated against hepatitis B
PREVENTION METHODS	Ensure sterile medical and dental techniques Use safe injection practices Hepatitis B is a vaccine-preventable disease
DIAGNOSTIC SUPPORT	A clinical laboratory certified in moderate complexity testing; state health department; or contact CDC (www.cdc.gov/laboratory/specimen-submission/list.html). More information is available at www.cdc.gov/hepatitis/hbv/testingchronic.htm.

INFECTIOUS AGENT

Hepatitis B virus (HBV) is a small, circular, partially double-stranded DNA virus in the family *Hepadnaviridae*.

TRANSMISSION

HBV is transmitted by contact with contaminated blood, blood products, and other body fluids (e.g., semen). Travelers could be exposed to HBV through poor infection control during dental or medical procedures, receipt of blood products, injection drug use, tattooing or acupuncture, or unprotected sex.

EPIDEMIOLOGY

HBV is a leading cause of chronic hepatitis, liver cirrhosis, and hepatocellular carcinoma worldwide. In 2015, an estimated 257 million people globally were living with chronic HBV infection; that year, HBV caused an estimated 887,000 deaths. HBV infections are likely underestimated, however, because accurate data are lacking from many countries (Map 5-07).

Data demonstrating the specific risk to travelers are lacking; published reports of travelers acquiring hepatitis B are rare, however, and the risk for travelers who do not have high-risk

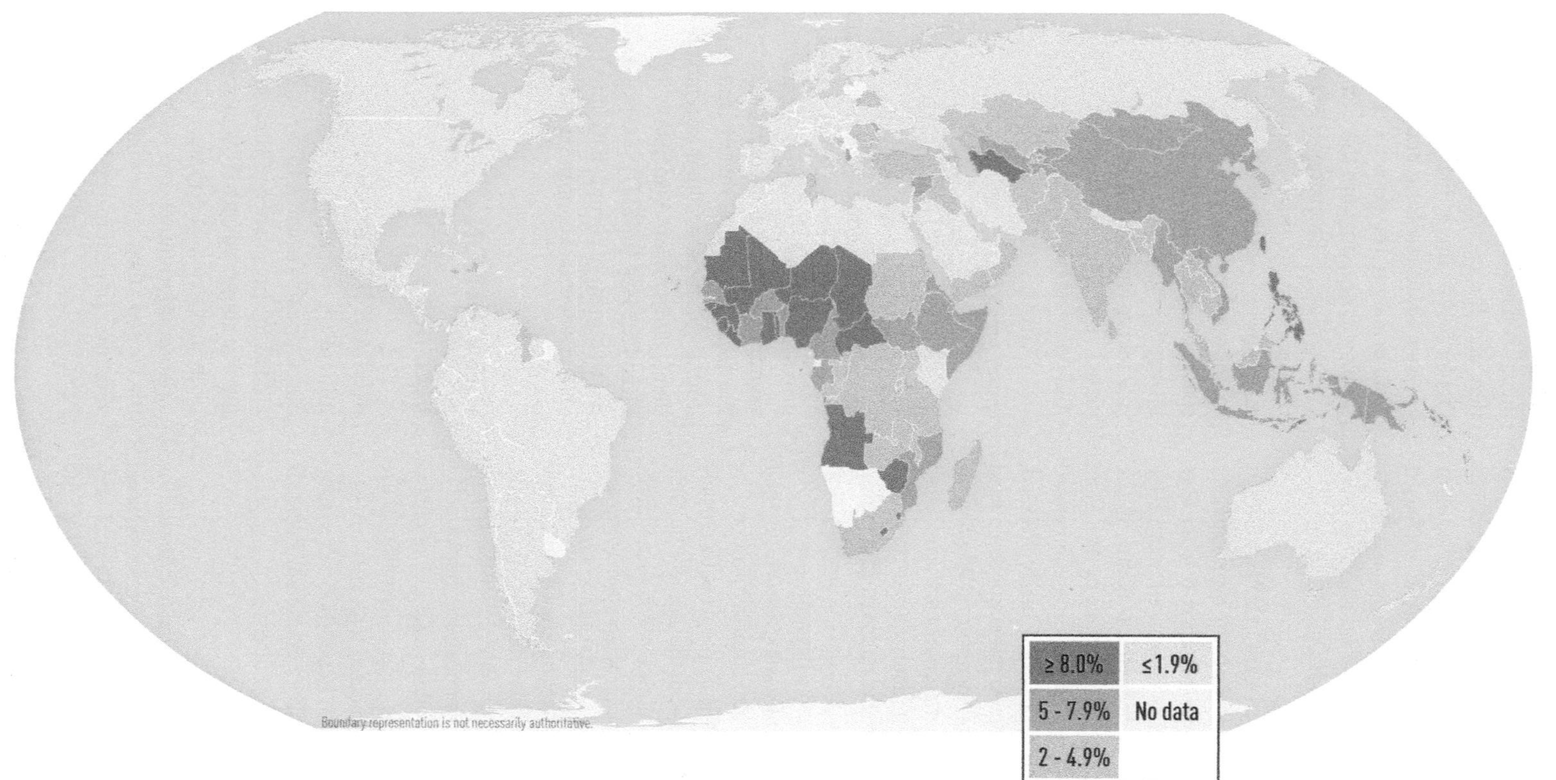

MAP 5-07 **Worldwide prevalence of hepatitis B virus infection**

Disease data source: 2021 estimates of hepatitis B virus disease burden. CDA Foundation Polaris Observatory. Available from: https://cdafound.org/polaris-countries-distribution/.

behaviors or exposures is low. The risk for HBV infection might be higher in countries where the prevalence of chronic HBV infection is ≥2% (e.g., in the western Pacific and African regions); expatriates, missionaries, and long-term development workers in those regions might be at increased risk for HBV infection. All travelers should be aware of how HBV is transmitted and take measures to minimize their exposures.

CLINICAL PRESENTATION

HBV infection primarily affects the liver. Typically, the incubation period for hepatitis B is 90 days (range 60–150 days). Newly acquired acute HBV infections only cause symptoms some of the time, and signs and symptoms vary by age. Most children <5 years of age and immunosuppressed adults are asymptomatic when newly infected, whereas 30%–50% of newly infected people aged ≥5 years have signs and symptoms. When present, typical signs and symptoms of acute infection include abdominal pain, anorexia, fatigue, fever, jaundice, joint pain, malaise, nausea and vomiting, light (clay-colored) stool, and dark urine. The overall case-fatality ratio of acute hepatitis B is ≈1%.

Some acute HBV infections resolve on their own, but some develop into chronic infection. The risk for acute hepatitis B to progress to chronic HBV infection depends on the age at the time of initial infection as follows: >90% of neonates and infants, 25%–50% of children aged 1–5 years, and <5% of older children and adults. Most people with chronic HBV infection are asymptomatic and have no evidence of liver disease. Fifteen percent to 40% of people with chronic HBV infection will, however, develop liver cirrhosis, hepatocellular carcinoma, or liver failure, and 25% of chronically infected people die prematurely from these complications. People infected with HBV are susceptible to infection with hepatitis D virus; coinfection increases the risk for fulminant hepatitis and rapidly progressive liver disease.

DIAGNOSIS

Hepatitis B is a nationally notifiable disease. The clinical diagnosis of acute HBV infection is based on signs or symptoms consistent with viral hepatitis and elevated hepatic transaminases and cannot be distinguished from other causes of acute hepatitis. Serologic markers specific for hepatitis B are necessary to diagnose HBV infection and for appropriate clinical management (Table 5-11). These markers can differentiate between acute, resolving, and chronic infection.

Information on how to obtain hepatitis B diagnostic support from the Centers for Disease Control and Prevention (CDC) Infectious Diseases Laboratories, including contact information, which samples to send, and how to send samples is available at www.cdc.gov/laboratory/specimen-submission/list.html. Select Hepatitis B Genotyping for research use only, and Hepatitis B Serology and Quantitative PCR if testing regulated by Clinical Laboratory Improvement Amendments is needed.

TREATMENT

No medications are available to treat acute HBV infection; treatment is supportive. Several antiviral medications are available for people with chronic HBV infection. People with chronic HBV infection should be under the care of a health professional and receive a thorough physical examination and laboratory testing to determine the need for antiviral therapy and ongoing monitoring for hepatocellular carcinoma and liver damage. American Association for the Study of Liver Diseases (AASLD) practice guidelines for the treatment of chronic HBV infection are available at www.aasld.org/publications/practice-guidelines-0.

PREVENTION

Vaccines

INDICATIONS FOR USE

Administer Hepatitis B vaccine to all unvaccinated people traveling to areas with intermediate to high prevalence of chronic HBV infection, namely, countries with HBV surface antigen positivity prevalence ≥2% (Map 5-07). Complete vaccination information and recommendations for the United States are available at www.cdc.gov/vaccines/hcp/acip-recs/vacc-specific/hepb.html.

Table 5-11 Interpretation of serologic test results for hepatitis B virus infection[1]

CLINICAL STATE	HBsAg	TOTAL ANTI-HBs	TOTAL ANTI-HBc	ACTION
Chronic infection	Positive	Negative	Positive	Link to hepatitis B-directed care[2]
Acute infection	Positive	Negative	Positive (HBc IgM)	Link to hepatitis B-directed care[2]
Resolved infection	Negative	Positive	Positive	Counseling, reassurance
Immune (immunization)	Negative	Positive[3]	Negative	Reassurance
Susceptible (never infected and no evidence of immunization)	Negative	Negative	Negative	Vaccinate
Isolated core antibody[4]	Negative	Negative	Positive	Depends on situation

Abbreviations: HBsAg, hepatitis B surface antigen; anti-HBc, antibody to hepatitis B core antigen; anti-HBs, antibody to hepatitis B surface antigen.

[1]Adapted from Abara WE, Qaseem A, Schillie S, McMahon BJ, Harris AM. Hepatitis B vaccination, screening, and linkage to care: best practice advice from the American College of Physicians and the Centers for Disease Control and Prevention. Ann Intern Med. 2017;167(11):794–804.

[2]Hepatitis B-directed care includes a physical examination and laboratory evaluation for liver transaminase, hepatitis B virus DNA, and hepatitis B e antigen.

[3]An anti-HBs titer of ≥10 mIU/mL correlates with protection only after a documented, complete hepatitis B vaccine series.

[4]If false-positive results are suspected, repeat testing. If results are from past infection or passive transfer to infants born to HBsAg-positive mother, no specific action is needed. If results could indicate occult hepatitis B virus infection, inform patient of risks from future chemotherapy, immunosuppression, or hepatitis C virus infection antiviral therapy, and consider checking hepatitis B virus DNA.

ADMINISTRATION

Several hepatitis B vaccines are available (Table 5-12). Hepatitis B vaccines are administered either as a 2-dose series at 0 and 1 month (Heplisav-B [Dynavax Technologies Corporation]), or as a 3-dose series at 0, 1, and 6 months (Engerix-B [GlaxoSmithKline], Recombivax HB [Merck], PreHevbrio [VBI], and the combined hepatitis A and hepatitis B vaccine, Twinrix [GlaxoSmithKline]). Heplisav-B is licensed for a 2-dose schedule for adults aged ≥18 years; the second dose should be given ≥1 month after the first dose.

Engerix B and Recombivax HB have also been licensed for use according to alternative vaccination schedules. Engerix-B can be administered using a 4-dose schedule, with the first 3 doses given within 2 months and a booster at 12 months (doses at 0, 1, 2, and 12 months). Recombivax HB can be given using a 2-dose schedule for children aged 11–15 years. Twinrix can be used on an accelerated 4-dose schedule (0, 7, and 21–30 days, with a booster at 12 months) to promote long-term immunity.

Always consult the prescribing information when administering alternative schedules and formulations. Whenever feasible, use the same manufacturer's vaccines to complete the patient's vaccine series; do not, however, defer vaccination when the manufacturer of previously administered doses is unknown or when the vaccine from the same manufacturer is unavailable. The 2-dose Heplisav-B vaccine series only applies when both doses in the series consist of Heplisav-B. Series consisting of a combination of 1 dose of Heplisav-B and a vaccine from a different manufacturer should adhere to the 3-dose schedule.

Table 5-12 Hepatitis B vaccines

VACCINE	TRADE NAME (MANUFACTURER)	AGE IN YEARS	DOSE & ROUTE	SCHEDULE	BOOSTER
Hepatitis B vaccine, recombinant with novel adjuvant (1018)	Heplisav-B (Dynavax Technologies)	≥18	0.5 mL (20 µg HBsAg and 3,000 µg of 1018) IM	DOSE 1: ≥18 years old DOSE 2: 1 month after DOSE 1	None
Hepatitis B vaccine, recombinant[1]	Engerix-B (GlaxoSmithKline)	0–19	0.5 mL (10 µg HBsAg) IM	**STANDARD** DOSE 1: 0–19 years old DOSE 2: 1 month after DOSE 1 DOSE 3: 6 months after DOSE 1	None
		0–10	0.5 mL (10 µg HBsAg) IM	**ACCELERATED** DOSE 1: 0–10 years old DOSE 2: 1 month after DOSE 1 DOSE 3: 2 months after DOSE 1	12 months after DOSE 1
		11–19	1 mL (20 µg HBsAg) IM	**ACCELERATED** DOSE 1: 11–19 years old DOSE 2: 1 month after DOSE 1 DOSE 3: 2 months after DOSE 1	12 months after DOSE 1
		≥20	1 mL (20 µg HBsAg) IM	**STANDARD** DOSE 1: ≥20 years old DOSE 2: 1 month after DOSE 1 DOSE 3: 6 months after DOSE 1	None
		≥20	1 mL (20 µg HBsAg) IM	**ACCELERATED** DOSE 1: ≥20 years old DOSE 2: 1 month after DOSE 1 DOSE 3: 2 months after DOSE 1	12 months after DOSE 1
Hepatitis B vaccine, recombinant[1]	Recombivax HB (Merck)	0–19	0.5 mL (5 µg HBsAg) IM	**STANDARD** DOSE 1: 0–19 years old DOSE 2: 1 month after DOSE 1 DOSE 3: 6 months after DOSE 1	None

Table 5-12 Hepatitis B vaccines (continued)

VACCINE	TRADE NAME (MANUFACTURER)	AGE IN YEARS	DOSE & ROUTE	SCHEDULE	BOOSTER
		11–15	1 mL (10 μg HBsAg) IM	**ADOLESCENT, ACCELERATED** DOSE 1: 11–15 years old DOSE 2: 4–6 months after DOSE 1	None
		≥20	1 mL (10 μg HBsAg) IM	**STANDARD** DOSE 1: ≥20 years old DOSE 2: 1 month after DOSE 1 DOSE 3: 6 months after DOSE 1	None
Hepatitis B vaccine, recombinant[1]	PreHevbrio (VBI)	≥18	1 mL (10 μg HBsAg) IM	DOSE 1: ≥18 years old DOSE 2: 1 month after DOSE 1 DOSE 3: 6 months after DOSE 1	None
Combined hepatitis A and B vaccine	Twinrix (GlaxoSmithKline)	≥18	1 mL (720 ELU HAV + 20 μg HBsAg) IM	**STANDARD** DOSE 1: ≥18 years old DOSE 2: 1 month after DOSE 1 DOSE 3: 6 months after DOSE 1	None
		≥18	1 mL (720 ELU HAV + 20 μg HBsAg) IM	**ACCELERATED** DOSE 1: ≥18 years old DOSE 2: 7 days after DOSE 1 DOSE 3: 21–30 days after DOSE 1	12 months after DOSE 1

Abbreviations: HBsAg, hepatitis B surface antigen; IM, intramuscular; ELU, ELISA units inactivated HAV; HAV, hepatitis A virus.

[1]Consult the prescribing information for differences in dosing for patients receiving hemodialysis, and other immunocompromised patients.

Protection from the standard vaccination series is robust, and >95% of healthy people achieve immunity after completion of the vaccination series. Serologic testing and booster vaccination are not recommended before travel for immunocompetent adults who have been previously vaccinated. Consider postvaccination serologic testing, however, for people whose subsequent clinical management depends on knowledge of their immune status, including health care personnel and public safety workers at risk for blood or body fluid exposure; those who require (or might require) outpatient hemodialysis; HIV-infected people; sex partners of HBsAg-positive people; and other immunocompromised people (e.g., hematopoietic stem-cell transplant recipients or people receiving chemotherapy).

SPECIAL SITUATIONS

The accelerated Twinrix vaccination schedule (0, 7, and 21–30 days, plus booster at 12 months) can be used for people traveling on short notice who face imminent HBV exposure or for emergency responders to disaster areas. Alternatively,

Heplisav-B can be used as a 2-dose series at 0 and 4 weeks to protect against hepatitis B alone. Ideally, vaccination with Heplisav-B should begin ≥1 month before travel so the full vaccine series can be completed before departure. When using vaccines other than Heplisav-B, begin vaccination ≥6 months before scheduled travel. Because some protection is provided by 1 or 2 doses, initiate the vaccine series, if indicated, even if the series cannot be completed before departure. Vaccines will not confer optimal protection, however, until after the series is completed; advise travelers to complete the vaccine series upon return.

SAFETY & ADVERSE REACTIONS

Safe hepatitis B vaccines are available for people of all ages, and serious adverse reactions are rare. The most common adverse reactions are soreness at the injection site (3%–29%) and low-grade fever (temperature >99.9°F [37.7°C]; 1%–6%). Hepatitis B vaccines should not be administered to people with a history of hypersensitivity to any vaccine component, including yeast. The vaccine contains a noninfectious recombinant protein (hepatitis B surface antigen) and an adjuvant (either 1018 [small synthetic immunostimulatory cytidine-phosphate-guanosine oligodeoxynucleotide motif for Heplisav-B] or aluminum [for Engerix-B, Recombivax HB, PreHevbrio, Twinrix]).

HBV infection affecting a pregnant person can result in serious disease for the mother and chronic infection for the newborn. Limited data indicate no apparent increased risk for adverse events to the mother (or the developing fetus) after maternal vaccination with Engerix-B, Recombivax HB, or Twinrix; no data are available on the use of Heplisav-B or PreHevbrio in pregnant or breastfeeding people. Until safety data are available for Heplisav-B and PreHevbrio, therefore, pregnant or breastfeeding people needing hepatitis B vaccination should receive Engerix-B, Recombivax HB, or Twinrix.

Personal Protective Measures

As part of the pretravel education process, educate all travelers about exposure risks for hepatitis B and other bloodborne pathogens, including activities or procedures that involve piercing the skin or mucosa; receiving blood products; contaminated equipment used during cosmetic (e.g., tattooing or piercing), dental, or medical procedures; injection drug use; and unprotected sexual activity. Caution travelers against providers who use inadequately sterilized or disinfected equipment, who reuse contaminated equipment, or who do not use safe injection practices (e.g., reusing disposable needles and syringes).

HBV and other bloodborne pathogens can be transmitted if medical equipment is not sterile or if personnel do not follow proper infection-control procedures. Travelers should consider the health risks when receiving dental or medical care overseas; US embassy country-specific websites might have information on medical concerns. Advise travelers to strongly consider health risks before obtaining a body piercing or a tattoo when traveling to destinations where adequate sterilization or disinfection procedures might not be available or practiced.

CDC website: www.cdc.gov/hepatitis/HBV

BIBLIOGRAPHY

Abara WE, Qaseem A, Schillie S, McMahon BJ, Harris AM. Hepatitis B vaccination, screening, and linkage to care: best practice advice from the American College of Physicians and the Centers for Disease Control and Prevention. Ann Intern Med. 2017;167(11):794–804.

CDA Foundation. Polaris observatory; 2019 [updated 2020 Mar 18]. Available from: https://cdafound.org/polaris.

Schillie S, Harris A, Link-Gelles R, Romero J, Ward J, Nelson N. Recommendations of the Advisory Committee on Immunization Practices for use of a hepatitis B vaccine with a novel adjuvant. MMWR Morb Mortal Wkly Rep. 2018;67(15);455–8.

Schillie S, Vellozzi C, Reingold A, Harris A, Haber P, Ward JW, et al. Prevention of hepatitis B virus infection in the United States: recommendations of the Advisory Committee on Immunization Practices. MMWR Recomm Rep 2018;67(RR-1):1–31.

Schweitzer A, Horn J, Mikolajczyk RT, Krause G, Ott JJ. Estimations of worldwide prevalence of chronic hepatitis B virus infection: a systematic review of data published between 1965 and 2013. Lancet. 2015;386(10003):1546–55.

Terrault NA, Lok ASF, McMahon BJ, Chang KM, Hwang JP, Jonas MM, et al. Update on prevention, diagnosis, and treatment of chronic hepatitis B: AASLD 2018 hepatitis B guidance. Hepatology. 2018;67(4):1560–99.

HEPATITIS C

Philip Spradling

INFECTIOUS AGENT: Hepatitis C virus	
ENDEMICITY	Worldwide Regions of high prevalence in Africa, central, southern, and eastern Asia, and eastern Europe
TRAVELER CATEGORIES AT GREATEST RISK FOR EXPOSURE & INFECTION	Medical tourists Travelers to destinations with poor infection-control practices who participate in activities with high injury potential
PREVENTION METHODS	Practice bloodborne pathogen precautions Use safe injection practices and syringe service programs
DIAGNOSTIC SUPPORT	A clinical laboratory certified in moderate complexity testing, state health department, or contact CDC's Division of Viral Hepatitis Diagnostic Reference Laboratory, www.cdc.gov/hepatitis/hcv/labtesting.htm

INFECTIOUS AGENT

Hepatitis C virus (HCV) is a spherical, enveloped, positive-strand RNA virus. Seven distinct HCV genotypes and 67 subtypes have been identified, the distribution of which vary geographically worldwide.

TRANSMISSION

HCV transmission is bloodborne and most often involves exposure to contaminated needles or syringes, or receipt of blood or blood products that have not been screened for HCV. Although infrequent, HCV can be transmitted through other procedures that involve blood exposure (e.g., tattooing, during sexual contact, perinatally from mother to child).

EPIDEMIOLOGY

Globally, an estimated 62 million people were living with HCV infection (chronically infected) in 2019. Although the quality of epidemiologic data and prevalence estimates vary widely across countries and within regions, the most recent global estimates from 2019 indicate that the viremic prevalence of HCV infection (prevalence of HCV RNA) is <1.0% in most developed countries, including the United States (Map 5-08). HCV prevalence is considerably higher in some countries in eastern Europe (3.1% in Ukraine, 2.9% in Russia, 2.9% in Moldova, 2.5% in Romania, 2.1% in Latvia) and certain countries in Africa (5.9% in Gabon, 3.6% in Burundi, 2.1% in Egypt), the Middle East (1.6% in Syria), and the South Caucasus and Central Asia (3.1% in Georgia, 3.0% in Uzbekistan, 2.7% in Tajikistan, 2.7% in Turkmenistan).

The most frequent mode of transmission in most high-, middle-, and low-income countries is sharing of drug preparation and drug-injection equipment. In countries where infection-control practices are poor, a predominant transmission mode is from unsafe injections and other health care exposures. Travelers' risk of contracting HCV infection is generally low, but they should exercise caution and avoid non-urgent dental or medical procedures, particularly in high-prevalence areas. Activities that can result in blood exposure include receiving blood transfusions that have not been screened for HCV; undergoing dental or medical procedures; participating in activities in which equipment has not been adequately sterilized or disinfected, or in which contaminated equipment is reused (e.g., acupuncture, injection drug use, shaving, and tattooing); and working in health care fields

5

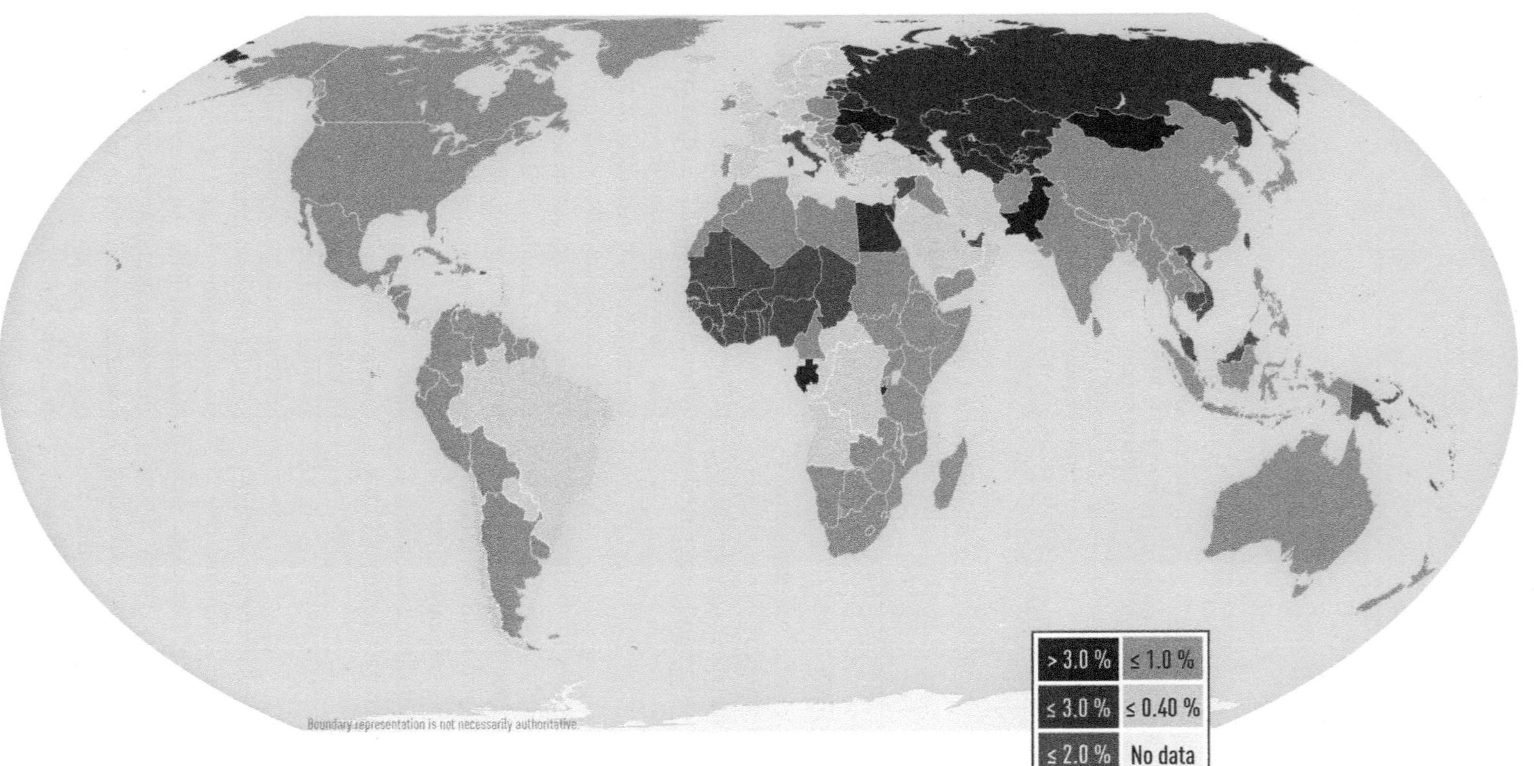

MAP 5-08 Worldwide prevalence of hepatitis C viremia, 2019

Disease data source: 2019 estimates of hepatitis C virus disease burden. CDA Foundation Polaris Observatory. Available from https://cdafound.org/polaris-countries-distribution/.

(dental, laboratory, or medical) that entail direct exposure to human blood.

CLINICAL PRESENTATION

HCV infection is a major cause of cirrhosis and liver cancer and is the leading reason for liver transplantation in the United States. Most (80%) people with acute HCV infection have no symptoms. When they occur, symptoms are indistinguishable from other forms of acute viral hepatitis and could include abdominal pain, anorexia and nausea, fatigue, jaundice, and dark urine. Among infected people, over half will remain chronically infected unless treated with antiviral medications. Cirrhosis develops in ≈10%–20% of people after 20–30 years of chronic infection, and progression is often clinically silent; evidence of liver disease might not occur until late in the course of the disease.

DIAGNOSIS

In the United States, hepatitis C is a nationally notifiable disease. Hepatitis C testing is required for diagnosis. Testing is not routinely performed in many countries, however, and most HCV-infected people are unaware of their infection. Two types of tests are available: IgG assays for HCV antibodies, and nucleic acid amplification tests to detect HCV RNA in blood (viremia). Both tests are commercially available in the United States and most countries. IgM assays, to detect early or acute infection, are not available. Because a positive HCV antibody test cannot discriminate between a previously infected person who resolved or cleared the infection and someone with current infection, be certain that HCV RNA testing follows a positive HCV antibody test to identify people with current (recent and chronic) HCV infection.

In 2020, CDC updated recommendations to include ≥1 hepatitis C screening test for all adults ≥18 years of age during a lifetime, and hepatitis C screening for all pregnant people during each pregnancy. Information on how to obtain hepatitis C diagnostic support from the Centers for Disease Control and Prevention (CDC), including contact information, which samples to send, and how to send samples is available at www.cdc.gov/hepatitis/hcv/hcvfaq.htm or by calling 800-CDC-INFO (800-232-4636).

TREATMENT

Since 2014, several new all-oral direct-acting antiviral agents have been approved for use to treat hepatitis C. These new regimens require only 8–12 weeks of treatment, have few side effects, and eliminate HCV infection in ≈95% of people who complete treatment, regardless of HCV genotype, prior treatment status, HIV co-infection, and the presence of cirrhosis. Treatment guidelines, which are updated frequently, can be found at www.hcvguidelines.org.

PREVENTION

No vaccine or postexposure prophylaxis is available to prevent HCV infection, nor does immune globulin provide protection. Travelers should check with their health care provider to understand the potential risk for infection and any precautions they should take. If seeking dental or medical care, travelers should be alert to the use of instruments, tools, and other equipment that has not been adequately sterilized or disinfected; reuse of contaminated equipment; and unsafe injection practices (e.g., reuse of disposable needles and syringes). People who travel to undergo dental, medical, or surgical procedures should be cognizant of potential HCV exposure (see Sec. 6, Ch. 4, Medical Tourism).

HCV and other bloodborne pathogens can be transmitted when medical instruments are not sterile or providers do not follow proper infection-control procedures (e.g., washing hands, using latex gloves, cleaning and disinfecting surfaces and instruments). In some parts of the world (e.g., parts of sub-Saharan Africa), blood donors might not be screened for HCV infection. Advise travelers to avoid body piercing, tattooing, being shaved by a barber, or having an elective dental or medical procedure in destinations where adequate sterilization or disinfection practices might not be used. Furthermore, instruct travelers to seek testing for HCV infection upon return if they received blood transfusions or sustained blood exposures for which they could not assess the risks, and to seek immediate medical care if they have signs or symptoms of acute hepatitis.

CDC website: www.cdc.gov/hepatitis/HCV

BIBLIOGRAPHY

American Association for Study of Liver Diseases (AASLD), Infectious Diseases Society of America (IDSA). Recommendations for testing, managing, and treating hepatitis C [Updated August 2020]. Available from: www.hcvguidelines.org.

CDA Foundation. Polaris observatory, 2020. Available from https://cdafound.org/polaris/.

Centers for Disease Control and Prevention. Testing for HCV infection: an update of guidance for clinicians and laboratorians. MMWR Morb Mortal Wkly Rep. 2013;62(18):362–5.

Messina JP, Humphreys I, Flaxman A, Brown A, Cooke GS, Pybus OG, et al. Global distribution and prevalence of hepatitis C virus genotypes. Hepatology. 2015;61(1):77–87.

Schillie S, Wester C, Osborne M, Wesolowski L, Ryerson AB. CDC recommendations for hepatitis C screening among adults—United States, 2020. MMWR Morb Mortal Recomm Rep. 2020;69(2):1–17.

Westbrook RH, Dusheiko G. Natural history of hepatitis C. J Hepatol. 2014;61(1 Suppl):S58–68.

HEPATITIS E

Eyasu Teshale

5

INFECTIOUS AGENT: Hepatitis E virus	
ENDEMICITY	Worldwide
TRAVELER CATEGORIES AT GREATEST RISK FOR EXPOSURE & INFECTION	Humanitarian aid workers Immigrants and refugees People who are pregnant Severely immunocompromised travelers Travelers to low- and middle-income countries
PREVENTION METHODS	Practice safe food and water precautions
DIAGNOSTIC SUPPORT	A clinical laboratory certified in high complexity testing; state health department; or contact CDC's Division of Viral Hepatitis Diagnostic Reference Laboratory, www.cdc.gov/hepatitis/hev/labtestingrequests.htm

INFECTIOUS AGENT

Hepatitis E is caused by hepatitis E virus (HEV), a spherical, nonenveloped, single-stranded, single-serotype, RNA virus belonging to the *Hepeviridae* family. Five HEV genotypes (HEV1–4 and HEV-7) are known to cause human disease. HEV-3 and HEV-4 cause hepatitis E in high-income countries, whereas HEV-1, HEV-2, HEV-4, and HEV-7 are associated with disease in low- and middle-income countries. Globally, HEV-1 is the most prevalent cause of hepatitis E. HEV is relatively stable in the environment but can be inactivated by chlorination or by heating to ≥70°C (≈160°F) for 5 minutes.

TRANSMISSION

HEV transmission routes vary by genotype distribution. HEV-1 and HEV-2 are transmitted primarily by the fecal–oral route, mainly through drinking contaminated water. Zoonotic foodborne transmission of HEV-3 is associated with eating uncooked or undercooked meat and offal (including liver), of boar, deer, and pig. Consumption of shellfish was implicated in an outbreak of hepatitis E on a cruise ship. HEV-7 infection has been associated with consumption of camel meat and milk.

Transfusion-related hepatitis E increasingly is reported in Europe. Rare, domestically acquired symptomatic disease has been observed in the United States, but its mode of transmission is generally unknown. Vertical transmission of HEV from people infected during pregnancy to their fetuses is common.

EPIDEMIOLOGY

Every year, ≈20 million HEV infections occur globally; ≈3.3 million cases are symptomatic hepatitis E, and ≈70,000 deaths occur. Large waterborne outbreaks have occurred in Africa, Central America, South and central Asia, and tropical East Asia. Many large outbreaks have occurred among refugees and in people living in camps for displaced persons. Sporadic illness is encountered in outbreak-prone areas, but also in regions not prone to outbreaks (e.g., North and South America, temperate East Asia [including China], Europe, the Middle East).

During hepatitis E outbreaks, clinical attack rates are highest among people aged 15–49 years. In areas endemic for HEV-1, infection in a pregnant person can progress to liver failure and death. Miscarriages and neonatal deaths are common complications of HEV infection during pregnancy. In areas where HEV-3 is prevalent, symptomatic disease occurs most frequently in adults aged >50 years. Among immunosuppressed people, particularly solid organ allograft recipients infected with HEV-3, hepatitis E can progress to chronic infection.

Due to the lack of systematic surveillance for hepatitis E, the incidence and characteristics of hepatitis E cases in the United States are unknown. Despite a lack of data on the risk for travel-associated HEV infections, US travelers are at greatest risk when they visit endemic countries and drink contaminated water. Most travel-associated hepatitis E cases have occurred among travelers returning from the Indian subcontinent. When traveling in countries where HEV-3 is found, eating raw or inadequately cooked boar, deer, or pig meat, or food products derived from any of these, can increase the risk for HEV infection.

CLINICAL PRESENTATION

The incubation period of HEV infection is 2–9 weeks (mean 6 weeks). The spectrum of illness ranges from asymptomatic to severe disease resulting in fulminant hepatitis and death. For most people, hepatitis E is a mild, self-limited disease. Infection with HEV-3 can progress to chronic infection, whereas infection with other genotypes results only in acute infection.

Signs and symptoms of acute hepatitis E include abdominal pain, anorexia, fever, jaundice, and lethargy, and are indistinguishable from other causes of viral hepatitis. Pregnant people with HEV-1 infection, especially those infected during the third trimester, might present with or progress to fulminant liver failure and death, and are at risk for spontaneous abortion and premature delivery. To date, no evidence shows severe outcomes associated with HEV-3 infection in people who are pregnant.

People with preexisting liver disease might have further hepatic decompensation with HEV superinfection. Recipients of solid organ transplants and people with severe immunosuppression tend to have asymptomatic acute HEV infection, but can develop chronic hepatitis E and progressive liver injury from HEV-3 infection.

DIAGNOSIS

Acute hepatitis E is diagnosed by detecting HEV IgM in serum. Detecting HEV RNA in serum or stool specimens further confirms the serologic diagnosis but seldom is required. Longer-term, serial detection of HEV RNA in serum or stool, regardless of the HEV antibody serostatus, suggests chronic HEV infection. No diagnostic test is approved by the US Food and Drug Administration (FDA) to detect HEV infection. Some commercial laboratories, however, perform both serologic and virologic tests upon request.

The Centers for Disease Control and Prevention (CDC), Division of Viral Hepatitis Diagnostic Reference Laboratory can provide diagnostic support for detecting HEV IgM and IgG in clinical samples by using commercially available kits, and offers a PCR assay for detection of HEV RNA in serum and stool samples. For information on sample handling and shipping to CDC's Division of Viral Hepatitis Diagnostic Reference Laboratory, see www.cdc.gov/hepatitis/hev/labtestingrequests.htm.

5

TREATMENT

Treatment for acute hepatitis E is supportive care. Oral ribavirin has been shown to be effective in the treatment of chronic hepatitis E.

PREVENTION

No FDA-approved vaccine or immune globulin is available to prevent HEV infection. Travelers should avoid drinking unboiled or unchlorinated water or any beverages containing unboiled water or ice. Travelers should eat only thoroughly cooked food, including seafood, meat, offal, and products derived from these.

CDC website: www.cdc.gov/hepatitis/HEV

BIBLIOGRAPHY

Ankcorn MJ, Tedder RS. Hepatitis E: the current state of play. Tranfus Med. 2017;27(2):84–95.

Kamar N, Izopet J, Tripon S, Bismuth M, Hillaire S, Dumortier J, et al. Ribavirin for chronic hepatitis E virus infection in transplant recipients. N Engl J Med. 2014;370(12):1111–20.

Nicolini LAP, Stoney RJ, Della Vecchia A, Grobusch M, Gautret P, Angelo KM, et al. Travel-related hepatitis E: a two-decade GeoSentinel analysis. J Travel Med. 2020;27(7):taaa132.

Riveiro-Barciela M, Minguez B, Girones R, Rodriguez-Frias F, Quer J, Buti M. Phylogenetic demonstration of hepatitis E infection transmitted by pork meat ingestion. J Clin Gastroenterol. 2015;49(2):165–8.

5

HUMAN IMMUNODEFICIENCY VIRUS / HIV

Robyn Neblett Fanfair, Katarzyna (Kate) Buchacz, Philip Peters

INFECTIOUS AGENT: Human immunodeficiency virus	
ENDEMICITY	Worldwide
TRAVELER CATEGORIES AT GREATEST RISK FOR EXPOSURE & INFECTION	Immigrants and refugees who come from environments with high rates of HIV in their cohorts or who have been abused Travelers who have cosmetic or medical procedures using contaminated needles, syringes, or other items Travelers who inject drugs using nonsterile equipment Travelers who have unprotected sex
PREVENTION METHODS	Avoid invasive procedures in locations where proper sterilization of instruments might not be used Avoid nonsterile injection use Practice safe sex Take preexposure prophylaxis (for some travelers)
DIAGNOSTIC SUPPORT	A clinical laboratory certified in moderate complexity testing; self-tests are also available

INFECTIOUS AGENT

HIV is an enveloped positive-strand RNA virus in the family *Retroviridae*.

TRANSMISSION

HIV is transmitted through sexual contact, needle or syringe sharing, unsafe medical injection or blood transfusion, and organ or tissue transplantation. It can also be transmitted from mother to child during pregnancy, at birth, and postpartum through breastfeeding.

EPIDEMIOLOGY

HIV infection occurs worldwide. In 2000, an estimated 37.7 million people were living with HIV infection globally (see www.unaids.org/en/topic/data). Sub-Saharan Africa is the most affected part of the world (25.4 million cases, or 67% of all people living with HIV infection); central Asia and eastern Europe have experienced the largest increases in new HIV infections (47% increase from 2010 to 2020). Although the reported adult HIV prevalence in many regions of the world is low, certain populations are disproportionately affected (e.g., sex workers, people who inject drugs, men who have sex with men, transgender people, and incarcerated people). People with HIV face an intersection of stigma, discrimination, violence, and criminalization that causes health inequities; international travelers should be aware of how their travel affects local communities, including people with HIV.

The risk for HIV infection is generally low for international travelers. Risk for HIV exposure and infection is determined less by a traveler's geographic destination and more by the behaviors in which they engage while traveling (e.g., sex without a condom, nonsterile injection drug use). Travelers who might undergo scheduled or emergency medical procedures should be aware that HIV can be transmitted by unsafe nonsterile medical injection practices (e.g., reusing needles, syringes, or single-dose medication vials). Unsafe medical practices might be greater in low-income countries where the blood supply and organs and tissues used for transplantation might not be screened properly for HIV.

CLINICAL PRESENTATION

As many as 90% of infected people will recall experiencing symptoms during the acute phase of HIV infection. Acute HIV infection can present as an infectious mononucleosis-like or influenza-like syndrome, but the clinical features are highly variable. Symptoms typically begin a median of 10 days after infection and can include arthralgias and myalgias, fatigue, fever, headache, lymphadenopathy, maculopapular rash, malaise, oral ulcers, pharyngitis, and weight loss. Although none of these symptoms are specific for acute HIV infection, certain features (e.g., oral ulcers), suggest the diagnosis.

DIAGNOSIS

HIV can be diagnosed with laboratory-based or point-of-care assays that detect HIV antibodies, HIV p24 antigen, or HIV-1 RNA. In the United States, the recommended laboratory-based screening test for HIV is a combination antigen/antibody assay that detects antibodies against HIV, and the p24 antigen. The combination antigen/antibody assay becomes reactive approximately 2–3 weeks after HIV infection. Estimates suggest that 99% of people will develop a reactive combination antigen/antibody result within 6 weeks of infection, but in rare cases, it can take up to 6 months to develop a reactive test result.

HIV self-tests also are available for retail purchase in the United States, including an HIV antibody test performed on oral fluid instead of blood. Although oral swab HIV tests have a lower sensitivity for detecting recent HIV infection, these can be an important testing method for people and their partners who would not otherwise get an HIV test (see Sec. 11, Ch. 2, Rapid Diagnostic Tests for Infectious Diseases). Acute HIV infection is characterized by markedly elevated HIV RNA levels; perform an HIV RNA viral load test if acute infection is suspected. Travelers with potential HIV exposures abroad, including those with symptoms consistent with acute HIV infection, should consider testing for HIV during travel or upon return to the United States. Travelers can find detailed information on HIV testing locations at https://gettested.cdc.gov.

TREATMENT

With timely diagnosis, prompt medical care, and daily antiretroviral therapy (ART), people with HIV can now live longer, healthier lives. Owing to the advances of ART, people with HIV who start

5

treatment can have close to the same life expectancy as people of the same age without HIV. Effective treatment also substantially reduces the risk of transmitting HIV to others. People with HIV who achieve and maintain an undetectable viral load by taking ART daily as prescribed cannot sexually transmit the virus to others (undetectable = untransmittable [U = U]).

Detailed information on specific treatments is available from the Department of Health and Human Services AIDSinfo website (www.aidsinfo.nih.gov). Travelers can contact HIVinfo toll free at 800-448-0440 (English or Spanish) or 888-480-3739 (TTY).

PREVENTION

5

Travelers can reduce their risk for HIV infection by avoiding sexual encounters with people whose HIV status is unknown, using condoms consistently and correctly with all partners who have HIV or whose HIV status is unknown, and using HIV prophylaxis when indicated. Travelers going abroad for medical procedures should try to ensure in advance that all blood or blood products at the facility have been screened for bloodborne pathogens (including HIV) and that all invasive medical equipment is sterilized between uses or is sterile and single use only (see Sec. 6, Ch. 2, Obtaining Health Care Abroad, and Sec. 6, Ch. 4, Medical Tourism). Travelers who inject drugs should avoid sharing needles or other injection equipment and use only sterile, single-use syringes and needles that are safely disposed of after every injection.

Preexposure Prophylaxis

Preexposure prophylaxis (PrEP) is a highly effective method to prevent HIV acquisition and is used by people without HIV who are at risk of being exposed to HIV. Two medications have been approved by the US Food and Drug Administration for use as PrEP; each consists of 2 drugs combined in a single oral tablet taken daily. F/TDF (brand name Truvada) combines 200 mg emtricitabine with 300 mg tenofovir disoproxil fumarate. F/TAF (brand name Descovy) combines 200 mg emtricitabine with 25 mg tenofovir alafenamide.

People already on PrEP should continue its use during international travel. Travel medicine providers can consider initiating PrEP for people who have a greater risk for HIV acquisition during international travel (see www.cdc.gov/hiv/pdf/risk/prep/cdc-hiv-prep-guidelines-2017.pdf). A comprehensive prevention plan includes not only prescribing (or considering prescribing) PrEP, but also reinforcing careful adherence to the PrEP regimen, educating travelers on the importance of consistent condom use to protect against HIV as well other sexually transmitted infections, and discussing other HIV prevention methods (see www.cdc.gov/hiv/clinicians/prevention/prep.html).

Travelers taking PrEP should carry proper documentation and be aware that some countries (see below for further information) deny entry to people with evidence of HIV infection, which PrEP medications might mistakenly indicate to customs officials. Free, expert PrEP advice is available to health care professionals through the National Clinician Consultation Center's PrEPline (855-448-7737; https://nccc.ucsf.edu/clinician-consultation/prep-pre-exposure-prophylaxis/).

Postexposure Prophylaxis

Postexposure prophylaxis (PEP) with antiretroviral medications is another method to prevent HIV infection (see www.cdc.gov/hiv/clinicians/prevention/pep.html). PEP is recommended as a prevention option after a single high-risk exposure to HIV during sex, through sharing needles or syringes, through a needlestick, or from a sexual assault. PEP must be started within 72 hours of a possible exposure. Travelers who will be working in medical settings (e.g., nurse volunteers drawing blood, medical missionaries performing surgeries) could have contact with HIV-infected or potentially infected biological materials.

Under certain conditions, a clinician can prescribe PEP medications for travelers to use in emergency situations. Free, expert PEP advice is available to health care professionals through the National Clinician Consultation Center's PEPline (888-448-4911; https://nccc.ucsf.edu/clinician-consultation/pep-post-exposure-prophylaxis/). See Sec. 9, Ch. 4, Health Care Workers, Including Public Health Researchers & Medical Laboratorians, for detailed advice regarding management of postexposure prophylaxis in occupational settings.

HIV TESTING REQUIREMENTS FOR US TRAVELERS ENTERING FOREIGN COUNTRIES

Advise international travelers that some countries screen incoming travelers for HIV (usually those with an extended stay) and might deny entry to people with evidence of HIV infection. People intending to visit a country for an extended stay should review that country's policies and requirements. This information is usually available from the consular officials of the individual nations. The US Department of State has compiled a list of entry, exit, and visa requirements by country, available at https://travel.state.gov/content/travel/en/international-travel/International-Travel-Country-Information-Pages.html.

CDC website: www.cdc.gov/hiv

BIBLIOGRAPHY

Brett-Major DM, Scott PT, Crowell TA, Polyak CS, Modjarrad K, Robb ML, et al. Are you PEPped and PrEPped for travel? Risk mitigation of HIV infection for travelers. Trop Dis Travel Med Vaccines. 2016;2:25.

Centers for Disease Control and Prevention. Preexposure prophylaxis for the prevention of HIV in the United States—2017 update: a clinical practice guideline. Atlanta: The Centers; 2018. Available from: www.cdc.gov/hiv/pdf/risk/prep/cdc-hiv-prep-guidelines-2017.pdf.

Centers for Disease Control and Prevention. Preexposure prophylaxis for the prevention of HIV in the United States—2017 update: clinical providers' supplement. Atlanta: The Centers; 2018. Available from: www.cdc.gov/hiv/pdf/risk/prep/cdc-hiv-prep-provider-supplement-2017.pdf

Centers for Disease Control and Prevention. HIV and COVID-19 Basics. Available from: www.cdc.gov/hiv/basics/covid-19.html.

Joint United Nations Programme on HIV/AIDS (UNAIDS). UNAIDS data 2020. Geneva: UNAIDS; 2020. Available from: www.unaids.org/sites/default/files/media_asset/UNAIDS_FactSheet_en.pdf.

Panel on Antiretroviral Guidelines for Adults and Adolescents. Guidelines for the use of antiretroviral agents in adults and adolescents with HIV. Washington, DC: Department of Health and Human Services; 2021. Available from https://clinicalinfo.hiv.gov/sites/default/files/guidelines/documents/AdultandAdolescentGL.pdf.

Patel P, Borkowf CB, Brooks JT, Lasry A, Lansky A, Mermin J. Estimating per-act HIV transmission risk: a systematic review. AIDS. 2014;28(10):1509–19.

World Health Organization. Coronavirus disease (COVID-19): COVID-19 vaccines and people living with HIV. Available from: www.who.int/news-room/q-a-detail/coronavirus-disease-(covid-19)-covid-19-vaccines-and-people-living-with-hiv.

INFLUENZA

Christine Szablewski, Michael Daugherty, Eduardo Azziz- Baumgartner

INFECTIOUS AGENT: Influenza virus	
ENDEMICITY	Worldwide
TRAVELER CATEGORIES AT GREATEST RISK FOR EXPOSURE & INFECTION	All travelers
PREVENTION METHODS	Influenza is a vaccine-preventable disease Practice hand hygiene Use appropriate personal protective equipment Use postexposure antiviral medication
DIAGNOSTIC SUPPORT	A clinical laboratory certified in moderate complexity testing; or contact CDC's Influenza Laboratory (404-639-2434)

INFECTIOUS AGENT

Influenza is caused by infection of the respiratory tract with influenza viruses, RNA viruses of the *Orthomyxovirus* genus. Influenza viruses are classified into 4 types: A, B, C, and D. Influenza A and B viruses commonly cause illness in humans and seasonal epidemics. Influenza A viruses are classified into subtypes based on the surface proteins hemagglutinin (HA) and neuraminidase (NA). Two influenza A virus subtypes, A(H1N1) and A(H3N2), and 2 influenza B virus lineages, B-Yamagata and B-Victoria, co-circulate in humans worldwide; the distribution of these viruses varies year to year and between geographic areas and time of year. Information about circulating seasonal viruses in various regions can be found on the Centers for Disease Control and Prevention (CDC) website (www.cdc.gov/flu/weekly) or World Health Organization website (www.who.int/teams/global-influenza-programme/surveillance-and-monitoring/influenza-updates/current-influenza-update).

5

Influenza type C infections generally cause mild illness and are not thought to cause human influenza epidemics. Influenza D viruses primarily affect cattle and are not known to infect or cause illness in people.

Novel influenza refers to viruses with a subtype different from seasonal influenza, and usually is caused by influenza A viruses that circulate among animals. Notably, avian influenza A(H5N1), A(H5N6), A(H7N9), and A(H9N2) viruses, and swine-origin variant viruses A(H1N1)v, A(H1N2)v, and A(H3N2)v have resulted in novel human influenza infections globally. An influenza virus that normally circulates in swine (but not people) but then is detected in a person is called a variant virus and is denoted with the letter *v*.

TRANSMISSION

Influenza viruses spread from person to person, primarily through respiratory droplets (e.g., when an infected person coughs or sneezes near a susceptible person). Transmission generally occurs via large particle droplets that require close proximity (≤6 feet) between the source and the recipient, but airborne transmission via small particle aerosols can occur within confined air spaces. Indirect transmission occurs when a person touches their face after touching a virus-contaminated surface (fomite).

The incubation period is usually 1–4 days after exposure. Most adults ill with influenza shed the virus in the upper respiratory tract and are infectious from the day before symptom onset to ≈5–7 days after symptom onset. Infectiousness is greatest within 3–4 days of illness onset and is correlated with fever. Children, immunocompromised people, and severely ill people might shed influenza virus for ≥10 days after symptom onset. Those who are asymptomatic can still shed the virus and infect others. Seasonal influenza viruses are rarely detected in blood or stool.

Influenza A virus transmission from animals to humans is rare but possible. Infected birds shed influenza virus in their droppings, mucus, and saliva, and transmission to humans can occur from direct contact with an animal (by touching an infected animal or by droplet spread) or contact with a sick animal's environment (by inhalation of airborne viruses or through fomite transmission). See CDC's Avian Influenza A Virus Infection in Humans website (www.cdc.gov/flu/avianflu/avian-in-humans.htm) for more details. Infected swine shed the virus in nasal secretions and can transmit viruses to humans in the same way seasonal influenza viruses spread among people. For more information, see CDC's website What People Who Raise Pigs Need to Know about Influenza (www.cdc.gov/flu/swineflu/people-raise-pigs-flu.htm).

EPIDEMIOLOGY

Seasonal Influenza

Influenza seasonality varies geographically. The risk for influenza exposure during travel depends on the time of year and destination. In temperate regions, influenza epidemics are more common during cooler months, October–March in the Northern Hemisphere and April–September in the Southern Hemisphere. In subtropical and tropical regions, seasonal influenza epidemics follow a similar pattern, but influenza illnesses can occur throughout the year. During the coronavirus disease 2019 pandemic in 2020 and 2021, there was a sharp decrease in global influenza activity. Although causality has not confirmed, the decrease has been attributed, in part, to community and personal implementation of nonpharmaceutical interventions to mitigate severe acute respiratory syndrome coronavirus 2 transmission.

CDC estimates that 9–45 million (symptomatic) illnesses, 4–21 million outpatient visits, 140,000–810,000 hospitalizations, and 12,000–61,000 deaths associated with influenza occur each year in the United States (see www.cdc.gov/flu/about/disease/burden.htm). Globally, annual influenza epidemics result in an estimated 3–5 million cases of severe illness and 290,000–650,000 respiratory deaths.

AT-RISK POPULATIONS

Certain groups are at increased risk for influenza complications (see Box 5-03 and www.cdc.gov/flu/highrisk/index.htm). The incidence of influenza illness is greatest among children, especially those aged 0–4 years, and adults aged 50–64 years. Rates of hospitalization (a marker of severe illness) and death due to influenza are typically higher among older adults (≥65 years old) followed by adults aged 50–64 years, children aged <2 years, and people of any age with underlying medical conditions that place them at increased risk for complications.

Zoonotic Influenza

Influenza A viruses circulate among animal populations and occasionally infect humans. The primary reservoirs for influenza A viruses are wild birds, like waterfowl, but influenza A viruses are also common in domestic poultry and swine populations. Influenza A viruses can infect other animal species (e.g., bats, cats, dogs, ferrets, horses, sea lions, seals).

In the United States, the last large outbreak of H5 lineage avian influenza virus in birds occurred in 2022. Although 34 different avian influenza subtypes have been reported globally since 2005, 94% of outbreaks reported in birds were caused by H5 lineage viruses. Since 2005, 23,754 outbreaks of H5 lineage avian influenza in animals have been reported from 97 countries (Map 5-09). Avian influenza virus outbreaks do not have to be reported to the World Organisation for Animal Health (OIE) if the virus is endemic in a country; avian influenza A(H5N1) was declared endemic in Indonesia in 2006 and in Egypt in 2008. Swine influenza is not reportable to OIE.

Novel Influenza A Viruses

Human infections with novel influenza A viruses are uncommon, but potentially could cause a pandemic if sustained human-to-human transmission occurs. Human infections with influenza A(H1N1)v, A(H1N2)v, and A(H3N2)v have been identified in the United States; the largest variant influenza outbreak occurred in 2012 and had a total of 309 infections and 1 death associated with an A(H3N2)v virus.

From 2011 through July 2021, 468 human infections with variant influenza viruses were identified in 24 US states. Most people identified with variant virus infections reported contact with swine preceding their illness, suggesting swine-to-human transmission. Limited cases of human-to-human transmission of variant viruses have also been reported. Seasonal human influenza viruses have infected swine, suggesting person-to-swine transmission. Agricultural fairs and swine farms are settings in which humans are exposed

BOX 5-03 Groups at increased risk for influenza complications

- Adults ≥65 years old
- Children <2 years old; although all children <5 years are considered at increased risk for serious influenza complications, the highest risk is for those <2
- Pregnant people and people ≤2 weeks post-partum
- People with certain medical conditions, including asthma, blood disorders, body mass index ≥40, chronic lung disease, endocrine disorders, heart disease, immunocompromise due to disease or medication, kidney disease, liver disorders, metabolic disorders, neurologic and neurodevelopment conditions, and history of stroke
- American Indians and Alaska Natives
- People living in nursing homes and other long-term care facilities

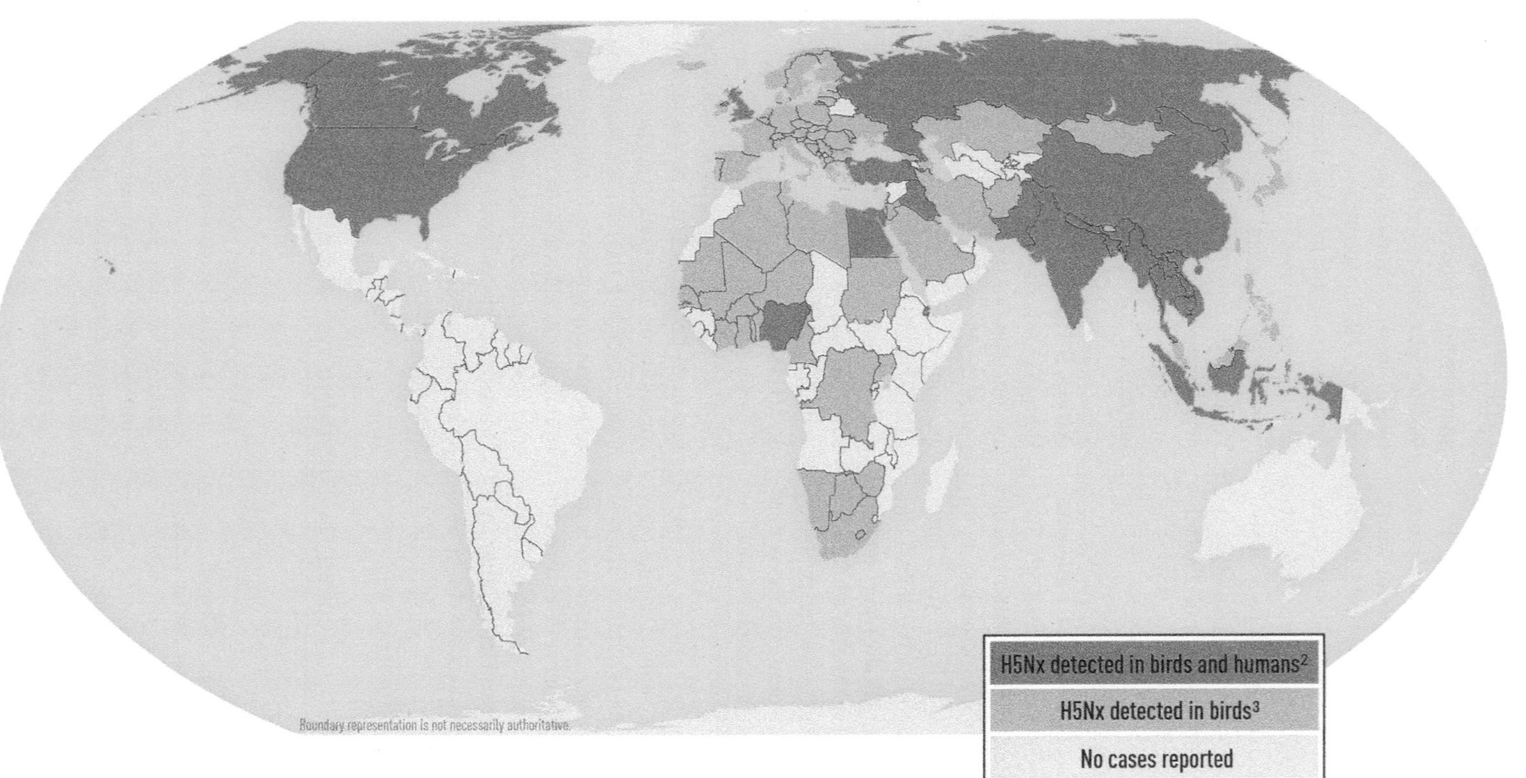

MAP 5-09 Global distribution of highly pathogenic avian influenza A (H5Nx) virus[1]

[1]Disease data source: Animal disease events. World Organisation for Animal Health, World Animal Health Information System (OIE-WAHIS). Available from: https://wahis.oie.int/#/events.

[2]H5Nx lineages include: H5N1, H5N6, and H5N8

[3]H5Nx lineages include: H5N1, H5N2, H5N3, H5N4, H5N5, H5N6, H5N8, H5N9, and H5Nx

to swine. Illnesses associated with variant virus infections are usually mild, with symptoms similar to those of seasonal influenza.

AVIAN INFLUENZA A(H5) LINEAGE VIRUSES

Avian influenza viruses do not commonly infect humans, but cases are reported globally each year (see www.cdc.gov/flu/avianflu/index.htm). During 2013–2020, 9 countries reported 281 human illnesses caused by avian influenza A(H5) lineage viruses, and a reported case-fatality ratio of ≈37% (Map 5-09). Most disease from A(H5) lineage viruses occurred after direct or close contact with sick or dead infected poultry. A(H5N1) and A(H5N6) viruses are widespread among poultry in some countries in Asia and the Middle East. Egypt and Indonesia account for 79% of A(H5N1) infections, and China accounts for 99% of A(H5N6) infections in humans globally. Instances of limited human-to-human A(H5N1) virus transmission have been reported. In February 2021, Russia reported 7 cases of human, asymptomatic infection with A(H5N8), the first report of influenza A(H5N8) infection in humans.

AVIAN INFLUENZA A(H7N9) VIRUS

Avian influenza A(H7N9) virus emerged in China in 2013; as of July 2021, it has caused 1,568 confirmed human infections. Most cases have been identified in mainland China, but several infections have been identified in Hong Kong Special Administrative Region (SAR), Macau SAR, Malaysia, and Taiwan, in travelers who reported exposure in mainland China. In 2014, Canada reported the first known imported influenza A(H7N9) virus infection in North America in a traveler returning from China. Most people with A(H7N9) infection were exposed to infected poultry or contaminated environments (e.g., live bird markets). The virus has been found in poultry and environmental samples collected in China. Most reported human A(H7N9) infections have been severe respiratory illnesses; the reported case-fatality ratio is 40%.

OTHER AVIAN INFLUENZA VIRUSES

Although uncommon, human infections with other avian influenza viruses, including A(H7N2), A(H7N3), and A(H9N2), have been reported globally in recent years, including 2 cases of A(H7N2) in humans exposed to infected cats in New York in 2016. And even though human infections with avian influenza viruses in the United States are rare, surveillance in domestic birds and people exposed to infected birds abides because of the low, but continued, risk for transmission to humans.

CLINICAL PRESENTATION

Physical Findings

Uncomplicated influenza illness, the most common presentation of seasonal influenza, is characterized by an abrupt onset of signs and symptoms that include nonproductive cough, fever, headache, malaise, muscle aches, rhinitis, sore throat, and vomiting, and, less commonly, rash. Illness without fever can occur, especially in older adults and infants. Children are more likely than adults to experience nausea, vomiting, or diarrhea when ill with influenza.

Physical findings are predominantly localized to the respiratory tract and include nasal discharge, pharyngeal inflammation without exudates, and occasionally rales on chest auscultation. Influenza illness typically resolves within 1 week for most previously healthy children and adults who do not receive antiviral medication, although cough and malaise can persist for >2 weeks, especially in older adults.

Humans infected with variant influenza viruses have a clinical presentation like seasonal influenza virus infections. Reported human infections with avian influenza A(H5N1) or A(H7N9) viruses often have severe pneumonia or respiratory failure and a high case-fatality ratio. These data might be skewed, however, because people with less severe illness often do not seek care for influenza or get tested for avian origin A(H5) or A(H7) viruses.

Complications

Complications of influenza virus infection include primary influenza viral pneumonia and secondary bacterial pneumonia; also, co-infections with other viral or bacterial pathogens, encephalopathy, exacerbation of underlying medical conditions (e.g., cardiac disease, pulmonary disease), Guillain-Barré syndrome (GBS), myocarditis, myositis, parotitis, seizures, and rarely, death.

DIAGNOSIS

Influenza can be difficult to distinguish from respiratory illnesses caused by other pathogens based on signs and symptoms alone. The positive predictive value of clinical signs and symptoms for influenza-like illness (fever with either cough or sore throat) for laboratory-confirmed influenza virus infection is 30%–88%, depending on host factors (e.g., age, community influenza activity levels).

Diagnostic Testing

Consider diagnostic testing for hospitalized patients with suspected influenza; patients for whom a diagnosis of influenza will inform clinical care decisions, including patients who do not improve on antiviral therapy and those with medical conditions that place them at increased risk for complications; and patients for whom results of influenza testing would affect infection control or management of close contacts, including other patients, such as in institutional outbreaks or other settings (e.g., cruise ships, tour groups).

For clinicians seeking laboratory confirmation of influenza, the Infectious Diseases Society of America recommends the use of rapid molecular assays in outpatients and nucleic acid amplification tests (e.g., reverse transcription PCR [RT-PCR]), in hospitalized patients. For suspected human infection with a novel influenza A virus of animal origin (e.g., avian influenza A virus, swine influenza A virus), contact the local and state health departments to perform RT-PCR for seasonal influenza viruses and novel influenza A viruses.

Other diagnostic tests available for influenza include antigen-based rapid influenza diagnostic tests, immunofluorescence assays, and viral culture (see www.cdc.gov/flu/professionals/diagnosis/overview-testing-methods.htm). Most patients with clinical illness consistent with uncomplicated influenza in communities where influenza viruses are circulating do not require diagnostic testing for empiric clinical management.

TEST SENSITIVITY

Nucleic acid assays are the most sensitive diagnostic assays. Thus, if infection with these viruses is suspected, contact the state health department in the United States or CDC outside the United States. Do not delay starting antiviral treatment while waiting for confirmatory laboratory testing results.

The sensitivity of antigen-based rapid influenza diagnostic tests varies but is substantially lower than RT-PCR or viral culture. Antigen-based rapid influenza diagnostic tests cannot distinguish between seasonal influenza A virus infections and animal-origin influenza A virus infections, and their sensitivity to detect these animal-origin influenza viruses can vary by test type and virus subtype. Therefore, a negative antigen-based rapid influenza diagnostic test result does not rule out influenza virus infection, and health care providers should not rely on a negative antigen-based rapid influenza diagnostic test result to make decisions about treatment.

TREATMENT

Antiviral Treatment

Early antiviral treatment (see Table 5-13) can shorten the duration of fever and other symptoms and reduce the risk for complications from influenza. Antiviral treatment is recommended as early as possible for any patient with confirmed or suspected influenza who is hospitalized; has severe, complicated, or progressive illness; or who is at increased risk for influenza-associated complications.

Treatment is most effective if it can be initiated ≤48 hours of symptom onset. For hospitalized patients, those with severe illness, or those at higher risk for complications, antiviral therapy might still be beneficial if started >48 hours after illness onset. Four antiviral agents are approved by the US Food and Drug Administration (FDA) for the treatment and prophylaxis of influenza (see www.cdc.gov/flu/professionals/antivirals/summary-clinicians.htm): oral oseltamivir, available as a generic (or as Tamiflu, Genentech); intravenous peramivir (Rapivab, BioCryst Pharmaceuticals); inhaled zanamivir (Relenza, GlaxoSmithKline); and oral baloxavir (Xofluza, Genentech).

Oseltamivir is the recommended treatment for people of all ages and is the preferred agent to treat patients with severe or complicated influenza illness who can tolerate oral medications. Peramivir is approved and recommended to treat patients aged ≥2 years and might be useful

Table 5-13 Treatment and prophylaxis for influenza A & B: approved and recommended antiviral medication dosing schedules

ANTIVIRAL	ROUTE	USE	PEDIATRIC DOSE	ADULT DOSE
Oseltamivir	Oral (PO)	Treatment[1]	**<1 year old**: 3 mg/kg PO, 2×/day ×5 days[2] **≥1 year old (weight-based dosing schedule):** ≤15 kg: 30 mg PO, 2×/day ×5 days >15–23 kg: 45 mg PO, 2×/day ×5 days >23–40 kg: 60 mg PO, 2×/day ×5 days >40 kg: 75 mg PO, 2×/day ×5 days	75 mg PO 2×/day ×5 days
		Prophylaxis[1]	**<3 months old:** unless the situation is judged critical, oseltamivir is not recommended due to limited data in this age group **≥3 months and <1-year old:** 3 mg/kg/dose PO 1×/day ×7 days[2] **≥1 year old (weight-based dosing schedule):** ≤15 kg: 30 mg PO, 1×/day ×7 days >15–23 kg: 45 mg PO, 1×/day ×7 days >23–40 kg: 60 mg PO, 1×/day ×7 days >40 kg: 75 mg PO, 1×/day ×7 days	75 mg PO 1×/day ×7 days
Peramivir	Intravenous (IV)	Treatment[3]	**2–12 years old:** 12-mg/kg dose (up to 600 mg maximum) by IV infusion over ≥15 minutes ×1	**≥13 years old**: 600 mg by IV infusion over ≥15 minutes ×1
		Prophylaxis[4]	Not recommended	Not approved
Zanamivir	Inhaled	Treatment[5]	**≥7 years old**: 10 mg (2 5-mg inhalations) 2×/day ×5 days	
		Prophylaxis	**≥5 years old**: 10 mg (two 5-mg inhalations) 1×/day ×7 days	
Baloxavir	Oral (PO)	Treatment[6]	**≥12 year old (weight-based dosing schedule):** 40 to <80 kg: 40 mg PO ×1 ≥80 kg: 80 mg PO ×1	
		Postexposure prophylaxis	**≥12 year old (weight-based dosing schedule):** 40 to <80 kg: 40 mg PO ×1 ≥80 kg: 80 mg PO ×1	

[1]Oseltamivir is approved by the US Food and Drug Administration (FDA) for the treatment of acute uncomplicated influenza ≤48 hours of illness onset. Although not part of the FDA-approved indications, use of oseltamivir to treat influenza in infants <14 days old, and for prophylaxis in infants 3 months to 1 year of age, is recommended by the Centers for Disease Control and Prevention (CDC) and the American Academy of Pediatrics (AAP).
[2]AAP provides alternative dosing guidelines for infants aged 9–11 months and for premature infants.
[3]Peramivir is FDA-approved and recommended for treatment of acute uncomplicated influenza ≤48 hours of illness onset. Daily dosing for a minimum of 5 days was used in clinical trials of hospitalized patients with influenza.
[4]No data for use of peramivir for influenza chemoprophylaxis are available.
[5]Zanamivir is FDA-approved and recommended for treatment of acute uncomplicated influenza ≤48 hours of illness onset.
[6]Baloxavir marboxil is FDA-approved and recommended for treatment of acute uncomplicated influenza ≤48 hours of illness onset.

in patients unable to tolerate or absorb oral antiviral therapy. Zanamivir is approved and recommended to treat patients aged ≥7 years and for prophylaxis in people aged ≥5 years. Inhaled zanamivir is not recommended for use in people with underlying chronic respiratory disease. Baloxavir is indicated to treat acute uncomplicated influenza in patients ≥12 years of age who have been symptomatic for ≤48 hours.

Two other FDA-approved influenza antiviral medications, amantadine and rimantadine, are not recommended for treatment or prophylaxis of influenza because of widespread viral resistance. Discuss antiviral treatment options with people at increased risk for complications of influenza before they travel to areas with influenza activity.

5

Postexposure Prophylaxis

To complement hand washing, face covering, and social distancing, antiviral drugs can be used for prophylaxis to prevent infection after close contact with a confirmed case. CDC does not, however, recommend routine use of antiviral medications for prophylaxis except as one of multiple interventions to control institutional influenza outbreaks. Initiate postexposure prophylaxis ≤48 hours of exposure, but never >48 hours, because of the risk of treating infection with a subtherapeutic dose. Alternatively, exposed people can monitor for symptoms and initiate antiviral treatment early after symptoms begin.

CDC recommendations for antiviral use for variant influenza virus infections are like those for seasonal influenza virus infection (see www.cdc.gov/flu/professionals/antivirals/index.htm). CDC recommends antiviral treatment for all suspected cases of human infection with avian influenza viruses (see www.cdc.gov/flu/avianflu/severe-potential.htm). Recommendations for postexposure prophylaxis of close contacts of confirmed human infections of avian influenza A(H5N1) and A(H7N9) viruses are available at www.cdc.gov/flu/avianflu/novel-av-chemoprophylaxis-guidance.htm.

Consider postexposure prophylaxis for anyone exposed to birds infected with influenza A(H5N1), A(H7N9), A(H5N2), and A(H5N8). The decision to initiate prophylaxis, however, should be based on clinical judgment, with consideration given to the type of exposure and whether the exposed person is at increased risk for complications from influenza. If antiviral prophylaxis is initiated for people exposed to avian influenza A viruses, CDC recommends twice daily treatment dosing for oseltamivir or zanamivir instead of once daily prophylaxis dosing (see www.cdc.gov/flu/avianflu/guidance-exposed-persons.htm).

PREVENTION

Vaccines

Vaccination is the most effective way to prevent influenza and its complications. In the United States, CDC recommends annual seasonal influenza vaccination for people aged ≥6 months. Several influenza vaccines are approved for use in the United States (see www.cdc.gov/flu/prevent/different-flu-vaccines.htm) and can be grouped into 3 categories: inactivated influenza vaccine (IIV) including cell-based, high-dose, and adjuvanted influenza vaccines; live attenuated influenza vaccine (LAIV); and recombinant influenza vaccine (RIV).

For updates and recommendations, refer to www.cdc.gov/flu/professionals/acip/summary/summary-recommendations.htm. For people for whom >1 type of vaccine is approved, clinicians can provide any category of vaccine. Children aged 6 months–8 years who have never received an influenza vaccine, or who have not previously received a lifetime total of ≥2 doses, require 2 doses of age-appropriate influenza vaccine given ≥4 weeks apart during their first season of vaccination to induce sufficient immune response.

Travelers—including people at increased risk for complications of influenza—who did not receive the current seasonal influenza vaccine and who are traveling to parts of the world where influenza activity is ongoing, should consider influenza vaccination ≥2 weeks before departure.

ADMINISTRATION

IIVs are administered by intramuscular injection and labeled for use in people aged ≥6 months, but specific age indications vary by manufacturer and product; follow label instructions. Cell-based inactivated vaccines are licensed for people aged

≥2 years. High-dose and adjuvanted IIV vaccines, which can elicit higher levels of antibodies than standard-dose vaccines, are available for people aged ≥65 years. LAIV is administered as a nasal spray and is labeled for use in people aged 2–49 years who do not have contraindications. RIV is labeled for use in people aged ≥18 years.

ADVERSE REACTIONS

INACTIVATED INFLUENZA VACCINE

The most frequent side effects of vaccination with IIV in adults are soreness and redness at the vaccination site. These local injection-site reactions are slightly more common with high-dose IIV. Reactions generally are mild and rarely interfere with the ability to conduct usual, daily activities. Fever, headache, malaise, myalgia, and other systemic symptoms sometimes occur after vaccination; symptoms might be more frequent in people with no previous exposure to the influenza virus antigens in the vaccine (e.g., young children) and are generally short-lived.

GBS is associated with influenza-like illness and was associated with the 1976 swine influenza vaccine, which had an increased risk of 1 additional case of GBS per 100,000 people vaccinated. None of the studies of influenza vaccines other than the 1976 influenza vaccine have demonstrated a risk for GBS of similar magnitude. The increased risk for GBS after seasonal influenza vaccines generally is small, ≈1–2 additional cases per 1 million people vaccinated, whereas the estimated risk for GBS after influenza is ≈17.2 cases per 1 million patients hospitalized with influenza.

LIVE ATTENUATED INFLUENZA VACCINE

The most frequent side effects of LAIV reported in healthy adults include minor upper respiratory symptoms, runny nose, and sore throat, which are generally well tolerated. Some children and adolescents have reported fever, myalgia, vomiting, and wheezing. These symptoms, particularly fever, are more often associated with the first administered LAIV dose and are self-limited.

Children aged 2–4 years who have a history of wheezing in the past year or who have a diagnosis of asthma should not receive LAIV. People 2–49 years of age who have conditions that increase their risk for severe influenza (e.g., immunocompromising conditions, pregnancy) should receive IIV or RIV, not LAIV. To decrease the risk of transmitting live virus to severely immunocompromised people, their caretakers also should not receive LAIV, or should avoid contact for 7 days after receiving LAIV.

COMPOSITION

Influenza vaccine composition can be trivalent, protecting against 3 different influenza viruses (2 influenza A subtypes and 1 influenza type B lineage), or quadrivalent, with protection against 4 different influenza viruses (2 influenza A subtypes and 2 influenza type B lineages). Quadrivalent vaccine includes a representative strain from antigenically distinct B-Yamagata and B-Victoria lineages. All influenza vaccines in the United States are quadrivalent vaccines.

5

COVERAGE

No information is available about the benefits of revaccinating people before summer travel who were vaccinated during the preceding fall, and revaccination is not recommended. People at increased risk for influenza complications should consult with their health care provider to discuss the risk for influenza or other travel-related diseases before traveling during the summer.

Seasonal influenza vaccines are not expected to provide protection against human infection with animal-origin novel influenza viruses, including influenza A(H5N1) and A(H7N9) viruses. No commercially available influenza vaccines are available to protect against avian or swine viruses.

PRECAUTIONS & CONTRAINDICATIONS

Influenza vaccine is contraindicated in people who have had a previous severe allergic reaction to influenza vaccine, regardless of which vaccine component was responsible for the reaction. Immediate hypersensitivity reactions (e.g., hives, angioedema, allergic asthma, or systemic anaphylaxis) rarely occur after influenza vaccination. These reactions likely result from hypersensitivity to vaccine components, one of which is residual egg protein. People with a history of egg allergy who have experienced only hives after exposure to eggs can receive any licensed and recommended influenza vaccine for their age and health status. Vaccine options are also available for people with a history of egg allergy with a history of severe reaction to egg, and are outlined at www.cdc.gov/flu/professionals/vaccination/vax-summary.htm#egg-allergy.

Personal Protective Measures

Measures that can help prevent influenza virus infection and other infections during travel include avoiding close contact with sick people and washing hands often with soap and water. In places where soap and a safe source of water are not available, CDC recommends using an alcohol-based hand sanitizer containing ≥60% alcohol. Face coverings are effective in preventing the spread of respiratory viruses, particularly among people in confined areas, and might have a role in the prevention of contagion during influenza epidemic periods. An ill person can help prevent the spread of illness to others by covering their nose and mouth with their elbow when coughing and sneezing and avoiding close contact with others. If symptomatic people cannot avoid contact with others, consider having them wear a mask when they are in close contact with others (see www.cdc.gov/flu/professionals/infectioncontrol/maskguidance.htm).

The best way to prevent infection with animal-origin influenza viruses, including A(H5N1) and A(H7N9), is to follow standard travel safety precautions, including using good hand hygiene, practicing food safety precautions, and avoiding contact with sources of exposure. Most human infections with animal-origin influenza viruses have occurred after direct or close contact with infected poultry or swine. In destinations where avian influenza virus outbreaks are occurring, travelers or those living abroad should avoid live animal markets and farms where animals are raised, avoid contact with sick or dead animals, avoid eating undercooked or raw animal products (including eggs), and avoid eating foods or drinking beverages that contain animal blood.

CDC website: www.cdc.gov/flu

BIBLIOGRAPHY

Centers for Disease Control and Prevention. Prevention and control of seasonal influenza with vaccines: recommendations of the Advisory Committee on Immunization Practices, United States, 2020–21 influenza season. MMWR Morb Mortal Wkly Rep. 2020;69(8):1–24.

Committee on Infectious Diseases. Recommendations for prevention and control of influenza in children, 2020–2021. Pediatrics. 2020;146(4):e2020024588.

Hirve S, Newman LP, Paget J, Azziz-Baumgartner E, Fitzner J, Bhat N, et al. Influenza seasonality in the tropics and subtropics–when to vaccinate? PLoS One. 2016;11(4):e0153003.

Iuliano AD, Roguski KM, Chang HH, Muscatello DJ, Palekar R, Tempia S, et al.; Global Seasonal Influenza-associated Mortality Collaborator Network. Estimates of global seasonal influenza-associated respiratory mortality: a modelling study. Lancet. 2018;391(10127):1285–300.

Lai S, Qin Y, Cowling BJ, Ren X, Wardrop NA, Gilbert M, et al. Global epidemiology of avian influenza A H5N1 virus infection in humans, 1997–2015: a systematic review of individual case data. Lancet Infect Dis. 2016;16(7):e108–18.

Merckx J, Wali R, Schiller I, Caya C, Gore GC, Chartrand C, et al. Diagnostic accuracy of novel and traditional rapid tests for influenza infection compared with reverse transcriptase polymerase chain reaction: a systematic review and meta-analysis. Ann Intern Med. 2017;167(6):394–409.

Olsen SJ, Azziz-Baumgartner E, Budd AP, Brammer L, Sullivan S, Pineda RF, et al. Decreased influenza activity during the COVID-19 pandemic-United States, Australia, Chile, and South Africa, 2020. MMWR Sept 18, 2020;69(37):1305–9.

Rolfes MA, Foppa IM, Garg S, Flannery B, Brammer L, Singleton JA. Annual estimates of the burden of seasonal influenza in the United States: a tool for strengthening influenza surveillance and preparedness. Influenza Other Respir Viruses. 2018;12(1):132–7.

Su S, Gu M, Liu D, Cui J, Gao GF, Zhou J, et al. Epidemiology, evolution, and pathogenesis of H7N9 influenza viruses in five epidemic waves since 2013 in China. Trends Microbiol. 2017;25(9):713–28.

Tsang TK, Lau LLH, Cauchemez S, Cowling BJ. Household transmission of influenza virus. Trends Microbiol. 2016;24(2):123–33.

Uyeki TM, Bernstein HH, Bradley JS, Englund JA, File TM, Fry AM, et al. Clinical practice guidelines by the Infectious Diseases Society of America: 2018 update on diagnosis, treatment, chemoprophylaxis, and institutional outbreak management of seasonal influenza. Clin Infect Dis. 2019;68(6):895–902.

JAPANESE ENCEPHALITIS

Susan Hills, Nicole Lindsey, Marc Fischer

INFECTIOUS AGENT: Japanese encephalitis (JE) virus	
ENDEMICITY	Asia and parts of the western Pacific
TRAVELER CATEGORIES AT GREATEST RISK FOR EXPOSURE & INFECTION	Adventure tourists Long-term travelers and expatriates
PREVENTION MEASURES	Avoid insect bites Japanese encephalitis is a vaccine-preventable disease
DIAGNOSTIC SUPPORT	State health department; or contact CDC's Division of Vector-Borne Diseases, Arboviral Diseases Branch (970-221-6400; www.cdc.gov/ncezid/dvbd/specimensub/arboviral-shipping.html)

INFECTIOUS AGENT

Japanese encephalitis (JE) virus is a single-stranded RNA virus that belongs to the genus *Flavivirus* and is closely related to dengue, West Nile, and Saint Louis encephalitis viruses.

TRANSMISSION

JE virus is transmitted to humans through the bite of an infected mosquito, primarily *Culex* species. The virus is maintained in an enzootic cycle between mosquitoes and amplifying vertebrate hosts, primarily wading birds and pigs. Humans are incidental or dead-end hosts because they usually do not develop a level or duration of viremia sufficient to infect mosquitoes.

EPIDEMIOLOGY

JE virus is the most common vaccine-preventable cause of encephalitis in Asia, occurring throughout most of Asia and parts of the western Pacific. Transmission principally occurs in rural agricultural areas, often associated with rice cultivation and flood irrigation. In some areas of Asia, these ecologic conditions can occur near, or occasionally within, urban centers. In temperate areas of Asia, transmission is seasonal, and human disease usually peaks in summer and fall. In the subtropics and tropics, seasonal transmission varies with monsoon rains and irrigation practices and might be prolonged or even occur year round.

In endemic countries, where adults have acquired immunity through natural infection, JE is primarily a disease of children. Travel-associated JE can occur among people of any age, however. For most travelers to Asia, the risk for JE is extremely low but varies based on destination, accommodations, activities, and duration and season of travel.

Before 1973, >300 cases of JE were reported among soldiers from the United States, the United Kingdom, Australia, and Russia. During 1973–2020, 88 JE cases among travelers or expatriates from nonendemic countries were published or reported to the Centers for Disease Control and Prevention (CDC). Since 1993, when a JE vaccine became available in the United States, only 13 JE cases among US travelers have been reported to CDC (1993–2020).

The overall incidence of JE among people from nonendemic countries traveling to Asia is estimated to be <1 case per 1 million travelers. However, expatriates and travelers who stay for prolonged periods in rural areas with active JE virus transmission might be at similar risk as the susceptible, pediatric resident population, which is 6–11 cases per 100,000 children per year. Travelers, even on brief trips, might be at increased risk if they have extensive outdoor or nighttime exposure in rural areas during periods of active transmission. Shorter-term (e.g., <1 month) travelers whose visits are restricted to major urban areas are at minimal risk for JE. In some endemic areas, few human cases occur among residents because of natural immunity among older people or vaccination, but JE virus is still maintained locally in an enzootic cycle between animals and mosquitoes. Therefore, susceptible visitors could be at risk for infection.

CLINICAL PRESENTATION

Most human infections with JE virus are asymptomatic; <1% of people infected with JE virus develop neurologic disease. Acute encephalitis is the most recognized clinical manifestation of JE virus infection. Milder forms of disease (e.g., aseptic meningitis, undifferentiated febrile illness) also can occur. The incubation period is 5–15 days. Illness usually begins with sudden onset of fever, headache, and vomiting. Mental status changes, focal neurologic deficits, generalized weakness, and movement disorders might develop over the next few days. The classical description of JE includes a parkinsonian syndrome with mask-like facies, tremor, cogwheel rigidity, and choreoathetoid movements. Acute flaccid paralysis, with clinical and pathological features like those of poliomyelitis, also has been associated with JE virus infection. Seizures are common, especially among children. The case-fatality rate is ≈20%–30%. Among survivors, 30%–50% have serious neurologic, cognitive, or psychiatric sequelae.

Common clinical laboratory findings include mild anemia, moderate leukocytosis, and hyponatremia. Cerebrospinal fluid (CSF) typically has a mild to moderate pleocytosis with a lymphocytic predominance, slightly elevated protein, and normal ratio of CSF to plasma glucose.

DIAGNOSIS

Suspect JE in a patient with evidence of a neurologic infection (e.g., encephalitis, meningitis, acute flaccid paralysis) who recently traveled to or resided in an endemic country in Asia or the western Pacific. Laboratory diagnosis of JE virus infection should be performed using a JE virus–specific IgM-capture ELISA on CSF or serum. JE virus–specific IgM can be measured in the CSF of most patients ≥4 days after symptom onset and in serum ≥7 days after symptom onset.

Plaque reduction neutralization tests can be performed to confirm the presence of JE virus–specific neutralizing antibodies and to discriminate between cross-reacting antibodies from closely related flaviviruses (e.g., dengue virus, West Nile virus). A ≥4-fold rise in JE virus–specific neutralizing antibodies between acute- and convalescent-phase serum specimens can be used to confirm recent infection. When interpreting laboratory results, clinicians must consider vaccination history, date of symptom onset, and information regarding other flaviviruses known to circulate in the geographic area that might cross-react in serologic assays.

Humans have low levels of transient viremia and usually have neutralizing antibodies by the time distinctive clinical symptoms are recognized. Virus isolation and nucleic acid amplification tests are insensitive in detecting JE virus or viral RNA in blood or CSF and should not be used for ruling out a diagnosis of JE. Contact the state or local health department or CDC's Arboviral Diseases Branch, Division of Vector-Borne Diseases (970-221-6400) for assistance with diagnostic testing. Instructions for submitting CSF and serum specimens to CDC for testing can be found at www.cdc.gov/ncezid/dvbd/specimensub/arboviral-shipping.html.

TREATMENT

No specific antiviral treatment for JE is available; therapy consists of supportive care and management of complications.

PREVENTION

Personal Protective Measures

Travelers can best prevent mosquito-borne diseases, including JE, by avoiding mosquito bites (see Sec. 4, Ch. 6, Mosquitoes, Ticks & Other Arthropods).

Vaccine

One JE vaccine is licensed and available in the United States, an inactivated Vero cell culture–derived vaccine, IXIARO, manufactured by Valneva Austria GmbH. IXIARO was approved in March 2009 for use in people aged ≥17 years, and in May 2013 for use in children aged 2 months through 16 years. Other inactivated and live attenuated JE vaccines are manufactured and used in other countries but are not licensed for use in the United States.

INDICATIONS FOR TRAVELERS

Based on each traveler's planned itinerary, assess the risks for mosquito exposure and JE virus infection and discuss ways to reduce these risks. Advise all travelers going to JE-endemic countries of the importance of personal protective measures to reduce the risk for mosquito bites. The decision whether to vaccinate should be individualized and include consideration of the risks related to the specific travel itinerary, likelihood of future travel to JE-endemic countries, the high rate of death and disability when JE occurs, availability of an effective vaccine, the possibility but low probability, of serious adverse events after immunization, and the traveler's personal perception and tolerance of risk.

Travel location, duration, activities, accommodations, and seasonal patterns of disease in the areas to be visited each influence risk for exposure. Interpret the data in Table 5-14 cautiously, because JE virus transmission activity varies within countries and from year to year, and surveillance data are often incomplete. Additional information on factors that increase risk is provided in Japanese encephalitis vaccine: Recommendations of the Advisory Committee on Immunization Practices (www.cdc.gov/mmwr/volumes/68/rr/rr6802a1.htm).

The Advisory Committee on Immunization Practices (ACIP) recommends JE vaccine for people moving to a JE-endemic country, longer-term (e.g., ≥1 month) travelers to JE-endemic areas, and frequent travelers to JE-endemic areas. Consider JE vaccine for shorter-term (e.g., <1 month) travelers with an increased risk for JE based on planned travel duration, season, location, activities, and accommodations. In addition, consider vaccination for travelers going to JE-endemic areas but who are uncertain of specific destinations, activities, or duration of travel.

ACIP does not recommend JE vaccine for travelers with very low risk itineraries (e.g., shorter-term travel limited to urban areas, travel that occurs outside a well-defined JE virus transmission season).

EFFICACY & IMMUNOGENICITY

No efficacy data are available for IXIARO. The vaccine was licensed in the United States based on its ability to induce JE virus–specific neutralizing antibodies as a surrogate for protection. In pivotal immunogenicity studies, 96% of adults and 100% of children developed protective neutralizing antibodies 28 days after receiving a primary immunization series of 2 doses administered 28 days apart. In a trial among adults aged ≥65 years, 65% were seroprotected at 42 days after the 2-dose primary series. An accelerated primary series of 2 doses administered 7 days apart was studied among adults aged 18–65 years and was noninferior to the conventional dosing schedule.

In a study where a booster dose was administered to adults at 15 months, 96% of subjects were still seroprotected ≈6 years later. In a study conducted among 150 children in a JE-endemic country who received a booster dose at 11 months, 100% were seroprotected at 24 months after the booster dose.

ADMINISTRATION

The primary vaccination dose and schedule for IXIARO varies by age (Table 5-15). To administer a 0.25-mL dose, expel and discard half of the volume from the 0.5-mL prefilled syringe by pushing the plunger stopper up to the edge of the red line on the syringe barrel before injection. For all age groups, the 2-dose series should be completed ≥1 week before travel.

BOOSTER DOSES

A booster dose (third dose) should be given at ≥1 year after completion of the primary IXIARO series if ongoing exposure or reexposure to JE virus is expected.

Limited data are available on the use of IXIARO as a booster dose after a primary series with the mouse brain–derived inactivated JE vaccine. Three studies have been conducted, 2 in US military personnel and the other at 2 travel clinics in Europe. Results showed that among adults who had previously received at

Table 5-14 Risk areas & transmission season for Japanese encephalitis (JE), by destination[1,2,3]

COUNTRY	RISK AREAS	TRANSMISSION SEASON	COMMENTS
AUSTRALIA	Outer Torres Strait Islands New South Wales Queensland South Australia Victoria	December–May All human cases reported February–April	Four cases previously reported from Outer Torres Strait Islands and 1 case from Tiwi Islands On Australian mainland, 1 case reported from Far North Queensland (1998) In 2022, cases reported in the states of New South Wales, South Australia, Victoria
BANGLADESH	Widespread	Year round Most cases reported July–November	Disease incidence is greatest in northwest Bangladesh
BHUTAN	Presumed widespread in non-mountainous areas	Unknown	Risk likely greatest in southern districts that share similar ecologic conditions with bordering JE-endemic states of India
BRUNEI DARUSSALAM	Presumed widespread	Unknown	Limited data, but outbreak reported in 2013 Proximity to Sarawak, Malaysia, suggests ongoing transmission likely
BURMA (MYANMAR)	Widespread	Year round Most cases reported May–September	Greatest risk in delta and lowland areas
CAMBODIA	Widespread	Year round Peak season May–October	Cases reported from most provinces, so transmission likely countrywide
CHINA	All provinces except Xinjiang and Qinghai	Peak season June–October	
INDIA	Andhra Pradesh, Arunachal Pradesh, Assam, Bihar, Goa, Haryana, Jharkhand, Karnataka, Kerala, Maharashtra, Manipur, Meghalaya, Nagaland, Odisha, Punjab, Tamil Nadu, Telangana, Tripura, Uttar Pradesh, Uttarakhand, West Bengal	Peak season May–November, especially in northern India Season can be extended or year round in some areas, especially in southern India	
INDONESIA	Widespread	Year round Peak season varies by island	Cases reported from many islands, including Bali, Java, Kalimantan, Nusa Tenggara, Papua, Sumatra Transmission likely on all islands Several cases reported among travelers to Bali in recent years

5

Table 5-14 Risk areas & transmission season for Japanese encephalitis (JE), by destination (continued)

COUNTRY	RISK AREAS	TRANSMISSION SEASON	COMMENTS
JAPAN	All islands	June–October	Rare sporadic cases reported from all islands except Hokkaido Enzootic transmission without reported human cases on Hokkaido
LAO PEOPLE'S DEMOCRATIC REPUBLIC	Widespread	Year round Peak season June–September	
MALAYSIA	Widespread	Year round Peak season in Sarawak, October–December	Much higher rates of disease reported from Sarawak than peninsular Malaysia
NEPAL	Southern lowlands (Terai), some hill and mountain districts	Peak season June–October	Highest rates of disease reported from southern lowlands (Terai) Vaccine not routinely recommended for those trekking in high-elevation areas
NORTH KOREA	Presumed widespread	Unknown Proximity to South Korea suggests peak transmission May–November	
PAKISTAN	Unknown	Unknown	Very limited data Previous case report and serosurvey data suggest transmission possible at least in Sindh Province
PAPUA NEW GUINEA	Widespread	Presumed year round	Sporadic cases reported from Western Province Serologic evidence of disease from Gulf and Southern Highland Provinces 1 case reported from near Port Moresby Transmission likely countrywide
PHILIPPINES	Widespread	Year round Peak season April–August	Human, animal, and mosquito studies indicate transmission in 32 provinces Transmission likely on all islands
RUSSIA	Primorsky Krai	June–September	Cases previously reported from Primorsky Krai Vaccine not routinely recommended
SINGAPORE	Presumed in focal areas	Year round	Very rare sporadic cases reported Vaccine not routinely recommended

(continued)

Table 5-14 Risk areas & transmission season for Japanese encephalitis (JE), by destination (continued)

COUNTRY	RISK AREAS	TRANSMISSION SEASON	COMMENTS
SOUTH KOREA	Widespread	May–November	
SRI LANKA	Widespread, except in mountainous areas	Year round Peak season November–February	
TAIWAN	Widespread	Peak season May–October	
THAILAND	Widespread	Year round Peak season May–October, especially northern Thailand	Highest rates of disease reported from Chiang Mai Valley Several traveler cases reported in recent years from resort and coastal areas of southern Thailand
TIMOR-LESTE	Presumed widespread	No data Proximity to West Timor suggests year-round transmission	
VIETNAM	Widespread	Year round Peak season May–October, especially northern Vietnam	

[1]When making decisions on vaccination, consider destination and transmission season information in association with travel duration and activities.

[2]Data are based on published and unpublished reports. Perform risk assessments cautiously; risk can vary within areas and from year to year, and surveillance data regarding human cases and JE virus transmission are often incomplete. In some endemic areas, human cases among residents are limited because of vaccination or natural immunity among older people. Because JE virus is maintained in an enzootic cycle between animals and mosquitoes, susceptible visitors to these areas still might be at risk for infection.

[3]Outbreaks previously occurred in the Western Pacific Islands of Guam (1947–1948) and Saipan (1990), but these are no longer considered risk areas and are not included in the table.

least a primary series of mouse brain–derived inactivated JE vaccine, a single dose of IXIARO provided good protection through 12–23 months.

SAFETY & ADVERSE REACTIONS

IXIARO was licensed in the United States based on safety evaluations in almost 5,000 adults. Since licensure, >1 million doses of IXIARO have been distributed in the United States without any identified safety concerns. Local symptoms of pain and tenderness were the most reported symptoms in a safety study among 1,993 adult participants who received 2 doses of IXIARO. Fatigue, headache, and myalgia were each reported at a rate of >10%. In children, fever was the most reported systemic reaction in studies. Serious adverse events are reported only rarely.

PRECAUTIONS & CONTRAINDICATIONS

A severe allergic reaction after a previous dose of IXIARO or any other JE vaccine, or to any component of IXIARO, is a contraindication to administration of IXIARO. IXIARO contains protamine sulfate, a compound known to cause hypersensitivity reactions in some people.

Table 5-15 Administration information for the inactivated Vero cell culture–derived Japanese encephalitis vaccine, IXIARO

AGE	DOSE	ROUTE	SCHEDULE	BOOSTER[1]
2 months–2 years	0.25 mL	IM	0, 28 days	≥1 year after primary series
3–17 years	0.5 mL	IM	0, 28 days	≥1 year after primary series
18–65 years	0.5 mL	IM	0, 7–28 days	≥1 year after primary series
>65 years	0.5 mL	IM	0, 28 days	≥1 year after primary series

Abbreviations: IM, intramuscular; mL, milliliter

[1]Administer a booster when potential for Japanese encephalitis virus exposure continues (e.g., repeated travel to endemic areas).

No studies of IXIARO in pregnant people have been conducted. Pregnancy is a precaution against the use of IXIARO, however, and in most instances, clinicians should defer vaccinating pregnant people. Further discussion (including the possibility of delaying travel) is merited before recommending vaccination to the pregnant person who must travel to areas where the risk for JE infection outweighs the theoretical risk from immunization.

CDC website: www.cdc.gov/japaneseencephalitis

BIBLIOGRAPHY

Deshpande BR, Rao SR, Jentes ES, Hills SL, Fischer M, Gershman MD, et al. Use of Japanese encephalitis vaccine in U.S. travel medicine practices in Global TravEpiNet. Am J Trop Med Hyg. 2014;91(4):694–8.

Dubischar KL, Kadlecek V, Sablan JB, Borja-Tabora CF, Gatchalian S, Eder-Lingelbach S, et al. Immunogenicity of the inactivated Japanese encephalitis virus vaccine Ixiaro in children from a Japanese encephalitis virus-endemic region. Pediatr Infect Dis J. 2017;36(9):898–904.

Dubischar KL, Kadlecek V, Sablan B Jr, Borja-Tabora CF, Gatchalian S, Eder-Lingelbach S, et al. Safety of the inactivated Japanese encephalitis virus vaccine Ixiaro in children: an open-label, randomized, active-controlled, phase 3 study. Pediatr Infect Dis J. 2017;36(9):889–97.

Hills SL, Fischer M, Biggerstaff BJ. Perceptions among the U.S. population of value of Japanese encephalitis (JE) vaccination for travel to JE-endemic countries. Vaccine. 2020;38(9):2117–21.

Hills SL, Walter EB, Atmar RL, Fischer M. Japanese encephalitis vaccine: recommendations of the Advisory Committee on Immunization Practices (ACIP). MMWR Recomm Rep. 2019;68:1–33.

Jelinek T, Burchard GD, Dieckmann S, Buhler S, Paulke-Korinek M, Nothdurft HD, et al. Short-term immunogenicity and safety of an accelerated preexposure prophylaxis regimen with Japanese encephalitis vaccine in combination with a rabies vaccine: a phase III, multicenter, observer-blind study. J Travel Med. 2015;22(4):225–31.

Jelinek T, Cromer MA, Cramer JP, Mills DJ, Lessans K, Gherardin AW, et al. Safety and immunogenicity of an inactivated Vero cell–derived Japanese encephalitis vaccine (Ixiaro, Jespect) in a pediatric population in JE non-endemic countries: an uncontrolled, open-label phase 3 study. Travel Med Infect Dis. 2018;22:18–24.

Paulke-Korinek M, Kollaritsch H, Kundi M, Zwazl I, Seidl-Friedrich C, Jelinek T. Persistence of antibodies six years after booster vaccination with inactivated vaccine against Japanese encephalitis. Vaccine. 2015;33(30):3600–4.

Rabe IB, Miller ER, Fischer M, Hills SL. Adverse events following vaccination with an inactivated, Vero cell culture-derived Japanese encephalitis vaccine in the United States, 2009–2012. Vaccine. 2015;33(5):708–12.

Ratnam I, Leder K, Black J, Biggs BA, Matchett E, Padiglione A, et al. Low risk of Japanese encephalitis in short-term Australian travelers to Asia. J Travel Med. 2013;20(3):206–8.

MIDDLE EAST RESPIRATORY SYNDROME / MERS

Claire Midgley, Marie Killerby, Aron Hall

INFECTIOUS AGENT: Middle East respiratory syndrome coronavirus (MERS-CoV)	
ENDEMICITY (IN CAMELS)	Arabian Peninsula Parts of North, West, and East Africa
TRAVELER CATEGORIES AT GREATEST RISK FOR EXPOSURE & INFECTION	Travelers in or near the Arabian Peninsula who have contact with camels or patients with known MERS infection, or who visit health care facilities
PREVENTION METHODS	Practice general hygiene measures, including regular hand washing, especially after contact with camels and people who are ill Immunocompromised people and those with underlying health conditions should avoid close contact with camels Follow safe food and water precautions and avoid drinking raw camel milk or camel urine, or eating improperly cooked meat, including camel meat
DIAGNOSTIC SUPPORT	Contact state or local health department

5

INFECTIOUS AGENT

Middle East respiratory syndrome coronavirus (MERS-CoV) is a single-stranded, positive-sense RNA virus that belongs to the family *Coronaviridae*, genus *Betacoronavirus*, which causes Middle East respiratory syndrome (MERS).

TRANSMISSION

MERS-CoV is a zoonotic virus known to transmit sporadically from the host reservoir, camels (specifically dromedaries [*Camelus dromedarius*]), to humans. Limited human-to-human transmission chains can subsequently occur, usually via close contact in health care or household settings.

Camel-to-Human Transmission

Transmission from camels to humans occurs via direct contact (e.g., grooming, petting), and possibly via indirect contact (e.g., contact with camel feces or camel products, being in settings where camels are present). Precise transmission mechanisms are unknown, but camel handlers with prolonged direct contact with live camels are thought to have the greatest risk for infection.

MERS-CoV has been detected in camels in North, West, and East Africa, and in or near the Arabian Peninsula, but most camel-to-human transmission has been reported within the Arabian Peninsula. Limited recent evidence suggests acute (RNA positive) infection among camel workers in parts of East Africa, and evidence for past (antibody positive) infection in camel workers in parts of North and East Africa. The extent of camel-to-human transmission on the African continent is not fully understood, however, and no current evidence of subsequent human-to-human transmission in Africa has been reported.

Person-to-Person Transmission

After camel-to-human transmission, MERS-CoV can be spread from person to person, resulting in outbreaks in households and in health care settings. MERS-CoV does not seem to pass easily between people and generally requires very close contact (e.g., in households, including sharing a bedroom with or caring for a person known to be infected with MERS-CoV, or when providing unprotected patient care in health care settings).

Large health care–related outbreaks have been documented, with transmission to other patients, visitors, and health care personnel; transmission has been reported in emergency departments, inpatient wards, and outpatient dialysis units. Superspreading events in health care facilities (generally, a single case linked to ≥5 subsequent cases) often have involved severely ill patients and have been associated with late recognition of people infected with MERS-CoV, crowding, delayed implementation of infection-control practices, and performance of aerosol-generating procedures prior to adopting airborne precautions.

Some evidence shows that symptomatic people, especially those with more severe illness, play a major role in human-to-human transmission, but little evidence supports transmission from asymptomatic people. Sustained community transmission of MERS-CoV has not been shown. A few MERS cases have been reported without camel, health care, or known MERS case exposure, indicating that MERS-CoV transmission pathways are not fully understood.

EPIDEMIOLOGY

First reported in September 2012, illnesses with onset as early as April 2012 were subsequently documented. To date, all MERS cases reported to the World Health Organization (WHO) have been linked to travel to, or residence in, countries in or near the Arabian Peninsula where risk of infection is ongoing, including Bahrain, Iran, Jordan, Kuwait, Lebanon, Oman, Qatar, Saudi Arabia, United Arab Emirates, or Yemen.

Cases among travelers to the Arabian Peninsula have been reported from North Africa, Asia, and Europe; subsequent transmission to travelers' contacts also has been documented. More than 1,300 people in the United States have been evaluated for MERS after travel to the Arabian Peninsula. To date, only 2 patients in the United States have tested positive for MERS-CoV infection; both were travelers who arrived from the Arabian Peninsula in May 2014, and no secondary transmission was identified for either case.

Most reported MERS cases have been linked to human-to-human transmission within health care facilities; people who have direct contact with camels or close contact with symptomatic MERS patients are at risk for MERS-CoV infection.

Camel-Associated Risk

While recent evidence has highlighted the potential for camel-to-human transmission within parts of North and East Africa, no subsequent human-to-human transmission has been reported after such exposures. The risk for MERS-CoV infection in North, West, or East Africa is thought to be minimal, but travelers to the region who have direct camel contact, including those who work with camels, could be at risk.

Health Care–Associated Risk

Health care personnel and others who visit or work in facilities experiencing known MERS-CoV transmission are at risk for exposure and infection. In addition, depending on their activities, travelers to, in, or near the Arabian Peninsula, including tourists, medical tourists, or business travelers, also could be at risk for infection. Close contacts of ill travelers who come from the Arabian Peninsula represent another group at potential risk for infection.

One of the largest health care–associated outbreaks (186 cases, 38 deaths), occurred in the Republic of Korea in 2015 because of delayed recognition of a single infected business traveler returning home from the Arabian Peninsula. Health care–associated transmission also has occurred in France and the United Kingdom from cases exported from the Arabian Peninsula. Rapid detection and isolation of patients with MERS seeking medical care is critical to preventing secondary transmission in health care facilities.

CLINICAL PRESENTATION

MERS is associated with a spectrum of illness that ranges from asymptomatic infection to mild upper respiratory tract illness to severe acute respiratory failure and multiple organ dysfunction. High mortality has been observed with MERS; ≈35% of confirmed cases have been fatal. For people who develop symptomatic illness, the incubation period is ≈2–14 days; median incubation period is slightly more than 5 days. Disease is most often characterized by cough, fever, and shortness of breath. Other nonspecific symptoms include abdominal pain, nausea, vomiting, and diarrhea; arthralgias and myalgias; chills; headache; and sore throat. Initial symptoms can progress to pneumonia. Chest radiographs have shown variable pulmonary involvement.

In addition to acute and often severe respiratory compromise, serious complications of MERS include acute renal injury and cardiovascular collapse. Abnormal laboratory findings can include elevated liver function tests, lymphopenia, and thrombocytopenia.

More severe illness and poorer outcomes have been observed in older adults, people who are immunocompromised, and people with underlying medical conditions (e.g., cardiovascular disease [including hypertension], diabetes mellitus, chronic kidney disease, chronic lung disease). Individuals with >1 underlying condition are at increased risk for poor outcomes.

DIAGNOSIS

Several diagnostic assays have been developed to detect acute infection with MERS coronavirus, including real-time reverse transcription PCR (rRT-PCR). These assays can reliably distinguish MERS coronavirus from other human coronaviruses, including severe acute respiratory syndrome coronavirus 2, the virus that causes coronavirus disease 2019 (COVID-19). Notably for MERS, specimens collected from the lower respiratory tract (e.g., bronchoalveolar lavage, endotracheal aspirates, sputum) are the priority for testing, although upper respiratory tract and serum specimens also can be used. To increase the likelihood of detecting MERS coronavirus, collect specimens from multiple sites and at multiple time points over the course of the illness.

In the United States, most state public health laboratories are approved to test for MERS-CoV using an rRT-PCR assay developed by the Centers for Disease Control and Prevention (CDC). Coordinate testing through state and local health departments, who will, in turn, contact CDC for additional diagnostic support as needed. For details on who should be evaluated as a person under investigation for MERS-CoV infection, see Box 5-04 and the CDC website, www.cdc.gov/coronavirus/mers/interim-guidance.html. Consult with public health

BOX 5-04 Patients in the United States who should be evaluated for Middle East respiratory syndrome coronavirus (MERS-CoV) infection

SEVERE ILLNESS: criteria for evaluation
Patient has fever and pneumonia or fever and acute respiratory distress syndrome, no alternative diagnosis, and ≥1 of the following epidemiologic risk factors

- Within 14 days before symptom onset, a history of travel from countries in or near the Arabian Peninsula

OR

- Within 14 days before symptom onset, history of close contact with a person who themselves developed fever and acute respiratory illness within 14 days of travel to countries in or near the Arabian Peninsula

OR

- Is a member of a cluster of patients with severe acute respiratory illness of unknown etiology

MILDER ILLNESS: criteria for evaluation
Patient has fever and symptoms of respiratory illness (e.g., cough and/or shortness of breath, not necessarily pneumonia), no alternative diagnosis, and ≥1 of the following epidemiologic risk factors

- Within 14 days of symptom onset, a history of being in a health care facility in a country or territory in or near the Arabian Peninsula where recent health care–associated cases of MERS have been identified

OR

- Within 14 days of symptom onset, a history of direct camel contact in or near the Arabian Peninsula

OR

- Within 14 days of symptom onset, a history of close contact with a person with confirmed MERS-CoV infection case while that person was ill departments for case-patients with equivocal clinical presentations or exposure histories (e.g., uncertain health care exposure).

Because the risk for MERS-CoV transmission from camels in North, West, and East Africa is not yet fully understood, consider MERS evaluation for travelers coming from these regions who develop severe respiratory illness (fever and pneumonia or acute respiratory distress syndrome) ≤14 days of direct camel contact.

TREATMENT

Treatment is currently limited to supportive care; no specific therapies for patients with MERS have yet been approved. As of April 2022, antiviral and monoclonal antibody therapies are in development or under investigation for potential use. In preclinical trials, some FDA-approved therapeutic options for adult patients with COVID-19 are also demonstrating efficacy against MERS-CoV.

PREVENTION

Although no vaccine or preventive drug has been approved for use in humans, several are under investigation. Because of the risk for nosocomial transmission resulting in sizeable hospital outbreaks, rapid detection and isolation of patients with MERS is critical. Standard, contact, and airborne infection-control precautions are recommended for hospitalized patients being evaluated for or diagnosed with MERS.

Travelers should practice general hygiene precautions (e.g., frequent handwashing; avoiding touching their eyes, noses, and mouths; avoiding contact with sick people). Additionally, WHO recommends as a general precaution that anyone visiting places where camels are present practice general hygiene measures, including regular handwashing before and after touching animals. In line with food hygiene practices, WHO recommends people avoid drinking raw camel milk or camel urine or eating meat (including camel meat) that has not been properly cooked. WHO also recommends that people at higher risk for severe MERS illness avoid close contact with camels.

CDC website: www.cdc.gov/coronavirus/mers

5

BIBLIOGRAPHY

Arabi YM, Arifi AA, Balkhy HH, Najm H, Aldawood AS, Ghabashi A, et al. Clinical course and outcomes of critically ill patients with Middle East respiratory syndrome coronavirus infection. Ann Intern Med. 2014;160(6):389–97.

Arabi YM, Asiri AY, Assiri AM, Balkhy HH, Al Bshabshe A, et al. Interferon beta-1b and lopinavir-ritonavir for Middle East respiratory syndrome, N Engl J Med. 2020;383(17):1645–56.

Arabi YM, Balkhy HH, Hayden FG, Bouchama A, Luke T, Baillie K, et al. Middle East respiratory syndrome. N Engl J Med. 2017;376(6):584–94.

Centers for Disease Control and Prevention. Interim infection prevention and control recommendations for hospitalized patients with Middle East respiratory syndrome coronavirus (MERS-CoV) [updated 2015 June]. Available from: www.cdc.gov/coronavirus/mers/infection-prevention-control.html.

De Wit E, Feldmann F, Cronon J, Jordan R, Okumua A, et al. Prophylactic and therapeutic remdesivir (GS-5734) treatment in the rhesus macaque model of MERS-CoV infection. Proc Natl Acad Sci USA. 2020;117(12):6771–76.

Dighe A, Jombart T, Van Kerkove MD, Ferguson N. A systematic review of MERS-CoV seroprevalence and RNA prevalence in dromedary camels: implications for animal vaccination. Epidemics. 2019;29:100350.

Killerby ME, Biggs HM, Midgley CM, Gerber SI, Watson JT. Middle East respiratory syndrome coronavirus transmission. Emerg Infect Dis. 2020;26(2):191–8.

Memish ZA, Zumla AI, Al-Hakeem RF, Al-Rabeeah AA, Stephens GM. Family cluster of Middle East respiratory syndrome coronavirus infections. N Engl J Med. 2013;368(26):2487–94.

Oboho IK, Tomczyk SM, Al-Asmari AM, Banjar AA, Al-Mugti H, Aloraini MS, et al. 2014 MERS-CoV outbreak in Jeddah—a link to health care facilities. N Engl J Med. 2015;372(9): 846–54.

World Health Organization. Middle East respiratory syndrome coronavirus (MERS-CoV)—Saudi Arabia (17 August 2021). Available from: www.who.int/emergencies/disease-outbreak-news/item/2021-DON333.

MUMPS

Mariel Marlow, Jessica Leung

INFECTIOUS AGENT: Mumps virus	
ENDEMICITY	Worldwide
TRAVELER CATEGORIES AT GREATEST RISK FOR EXPOSURE & INFECTION	All travelers, especially those not vaccinated against mumps
PREVENTION METHODS	Mumps is a vaccine-preventable disease
DIAGNOSTIC SUPPORT	A clinical laboratory certified in moderate complexity testing; or see CDC's Division of Viral Diseases (www.cdc.gov/mumps/lab/index.html)

INFECTIOUS AGENT

Mumps virus is an enveloped, single-stranded, negative-sense RNA virus of the family *Paramyxoviridae*, genus *Rubulavirus*.

TRANSMISSION

Transmission occurs by respiratory droplets or saliva from a person infected with mumps and usually requires close contact for spread. Transmission is most likely to occur 2 days before through 5 days after the onset of parotitis.

EPIDEMIOLOGY

Mumps is endemic throughout the world. On average >500,000 mumps cases are reported to the World Health Organization annually; global mumps incidence is challenging to estimate, however, because mumps is not a notifiable disease in many countries. As of 2018, mumps-containing vaccine is routinely used in 122 countries. Since the mid-2000s, large mumps outbreaks have been reported among populations with high 2-dose measles-mumps-rubella (MMR) vaccine coverage in countries with routine mumps immunization programs. Despite these outbreaks, mumps incidence is still much higher in countries that do not have routine mumps vaccination. The risk for potential exposure among travelers is unknown but could be high in many countries.

CLINICAL PRESENTATION

The average incubation period is 16–18 days (range 12–25 days). Mumps is an acute systemic illness that classically presents with parotitis (acute onset of unilateral or bilateral tender, self-limited swelling of the parotid) or other salivary gland swelling, usually lasting 5 days. Nonspecific prodromal symptoms of anorexia, low-grade fever, headache, malaise, and myalgias can occur several days before the onset of parotitis. Infections also can be asymptomatic or limited to nonspecific respiratory symptoms. Complications include aseptic meningitis, encephalitis, hearing loss, mastitis, oophoritis, orchitis, and pancreatitis, any of which can occur in the absence of parotitis. Fully vaccinated people can get mumps but are at much lower risk for mumps and mumps complications.

DIAGNOSIS

Mumps is usually clinically defined as acute parotitis or other salivary gland swelling or oophoritis or orchitis, without other apparent cause. Laboratory confirmation of mumps involves detecting mumps virus by real-time reverse transcription PCR (rRT-PCR) or virus isolation by culture. Laboratory confirmation of mumps can be challenging; therefore, mumps cases should not be ruled out by negative laboratory results.

Serologic testing for the presence of IgM antibodies in serum also can aid in the diagnosis of mumps but is not confirmatory. Mumps laboratory testing can be performed by commercial labs, most state and local public health laboratories, and the Centers for Disease Control and Prevention (CDC). For further information on laboratory testing, including optimal timing for specimen collection, see www.cdc.gov/mumps/lab/index.html. Mumps is a nationally notifiable disease.

TREATMENT

Supportive care is the mainstay of treatment for mumps.

PREVENTION

Before departure from the United States, travelers aged ≥12 months who do not have acceptable evidence of mumps immunity (as documented by 2 doses of a mumps virus–containing vaccine, laboratory evidence of immunity, laboratory confirmation of disease, or birth before 1957) should be vaccinated with 2 doses of MMR vaccine ≥28 days apart, or 1 dose of MMR if they previously received 1 MMR dose. Measles-mumps-rubella-varicella (MMRV) vaccine is licensed for children aged 12 months through 12 years and can be used if vaccination for measles, mumps, rubella, and varicella is indicated for this age group. There is no recommendation for infants aged <12 months to receive vaccination against mumps before international travel; the Advisory Committee on Immunization Practice (ACIP) recommends, however, that infants aged 6–11 months receive 1 dose of MMR vaccine before departure to protect against measles. There is no recommendation for a third dose of MMR vaccine for travelers to countries experiencing mumps outbreaks.

CDC website: www.cdc.gov/mumps

5

BIBLIOGRAPHY

Bankamp B, Hickman C, Icenogle JP, Rota PA. Successes and challenges for preventing measles, mumps and rubella by vaccination. Curr Opin Virol. 2019;34:110–6.

Centers for Disease Control and Prevention. Manual for the surveillance of vaccine-preventable diseases. Atlanta: The Centers; 2018. Available from: www.cdc.gov/vaccines/pubs/surv-manual/chpt09-mumps.pdf.

Centers for Disease Control and Prevention. Prevention of measles, rubella, congenital rubella syndrome, and mumps, 2013: summary recommendations of the Advisory Committee on Immunization Practices (ACIP). MMWR Recomm Rep. 2013;62(RR-04):1–34.

European Centre for Disease Prevention and Control. Mumps. In: ECDC. Annual epidemiological report for 2017. Stockholm: ECDC; 2020. Available from: www.ecdc.europa.eu/sites/default/files/documents/mumps-2017-aer.pdf.

World Health Organization. Mumps reported cases, 2018. Available from: http://apps.who.int/immunization_monitoring/globalsummary/timeseries/tsincidencemumps.html.

World Health Organization. The Immunological Basis for Immunization Series: module 16: Mumps; 2020. Available from: www.who.int/publications/i/item/9789241500661.

NOROVIRUS

Sara Mirza, Aron Hall

INFECTIOUS AGENT: Norovirus	
ENDEMICITY	Worldwide
TRAVELER CATEGORIES AT GREATEST RISK FOR EXPOSURE & INFECTION	All travelers
PREVENTION METHODS	Practice good hand hygiene with soap and water Carefully clean and disinfect surfaces and toilet areas contaminated with fecal material or vomit
DIAGNOSTIC SUPPORT	A clinical laboratory certified in moderate complexity testing; state health departments during outbreak investigations

5

INFECTIOUS AGENT

Norovirus infection is caused by nonenveloped, single-stranded RNA viruses of the genus *Norovirus*, which have also been referred to as Norwalk-like viruses, Norwalk viruses, and small round-structured viruses. Norovirus is a cause of viral gastroenteritis, sometimes referred to as stomach flu; however, norovirus has no biologic association with influenza or influenza viruses.

TRANSMISSION

Norovirus transmission occurs primarily through the fecal–oral route, either through direct person-to-person contact or indirectly via contaminated food or water. Norovirus also is spread through fomites and aerosols of vomitus.

EPIDEMIOLOGY

Norovirus outbreaks frequently occur in settings where people live in close quarters and can easily infect each other. Norovirus is a commonly reported cause of diarrhea among travelers in confined spaces (e.g., on cruise ships, and in camps, dormitories, hotels). Risk for infection is present anywhere food is prepared in an unsanitary manner and can be contaminated, or where drinking water is inadequately treated. Ready-to-eat cold foods (e.g., salads, sandwiches) are a particular risk. Raw shellfish, especially oysters, are a frequent source of infection because viral particles in contaminated water concentrate in the gut of these filter feeders. Contaminated ice has also been implicated in outbreaks.

Viral contamination of fomites can persist during and after outbreaks and be a source of infection. On cruise ships, for instance, environmental contamination has caused recurrent norovirus outbreaks on successive cruises with newly boarded passengers. Transmission of norovirus on airplanes has been reported during domestic and international flights and likely results from contamination of lavatories or from symptomatic passengers in the cabin.

Norovirus infections are common throughout the world. Globally, most children will have ≥1 infection by the time they are 5 years old. Norovirus infections can occur year round, but in temperate climates, activity peaks during the winter. Noroviruses are common in low-, middle-, and high-income countries. Globally, norovirus causes ≈18% of acute gastroenteritis cases and could be responsible for ≈200,000 deaths annually. In the United States, norovirus is the leading cause of medically attended gastroenteritis in young children and of outbreaks of gastroenteritis; norovirus causes ≈19–21 million illnesses a year and ≈50% of all foodborne disease outbreaks.

CLINICAL PRESENTATION

Infected people usually experience acute onset of vomiting and non-bloody diarrhea. The incubation period is 12–48 hours. Other symptoms include abdominal cramps, nausea, and sometimes a low-grade fever. Illness is generally self-limited, and most patients fully recover in 1–3 days. In some cases, especially among the very young or elderly, dehydration can occur and require medical attention.

DIAGNOSIS

Norovirus infection is generally diagnosed based on symptoms. Diagnostic testing is not widely performed to guide clinical management of individual patients, but laboratory testing is used to identify disease clusters during outbreak investigations.

PCR-based multipathogen diagnostic panels are increasingly available for clinical and research purposes. These panels have good sensitivity and specificity to detect norovirus. The most common diagnostic test used at state public health laboratories and at the Centers for Disease Control and Prevention (CDC) is real-time reverse-transcription quantitative PCR (RT-qPCR), which rapidly and reliably detects the virus in stool specimens. Several commercial enzyme immunoassays (EIAs) also are available to detect the virus in stool specimens, but the specificity and sensitivity of EIAs are relatively poor compared with RT-qPCR.

CDC recommends contacting local health departments for outbreak investigation and specimen testing. Whole stool specimens are preferred for testing; vomitus specimens might be acceptable. For more information on laboratory diagnostic testing and specimen collection, see www.cdc.gov/norovirus/lab-testing/index.html and www.cdc.gov/laboratory/specimen-submission/detail.html.

TREATMENT

Supportive care is the mainstay of norovirus treatment, especially oral or intravenous rehydration. Antidiarrheals and antiemetics are not recommended for the routine management of acute gastroenteritis in children. For adults, antiemetic, antimotility, and antisecretory agents can be useful adjuncts to rehydration. Antibiotics are not useful in treating patients with norovirus disease.

PREVENTION

No norovirus vaccine is currently available, but vaccine development is advancing. Noroviruses are common and highly contagious, but travelers can minimize their risk for infection by frequently and properly washing hands and avoiding possibly contaminated food and water. Washing hands with soap and water for ≥20 seconds is considered the most effective way to reduce norovirus contamination; alcohol-based hand sanitizers might be useful between handwashings, but should not be considered a substitute for soap and water.

In addition to handwashing, people traveling together can use measures to prevent transmission of noroviruses, including carefully cleaning up fecal material or vomit and disinfecting contaminated surfaces and toilet areas. Travelers should use products approved by the US Environmental Protection Agency for norovirus disinfection; alternatively, they can use a dilute bleach solution (5–25 tablespoons bleach per gallon of water). Travelers should wash soiled articles of clothing for the maximum available cycle length and machine dry clothing on high heat.

To help prevent the spread of noroviruses, consider isolation for ill people on cruise ships and in institutional settings, including hospitals, long-term care facilities, and schools.

CDC website: www.cdc.gov/norovirus

BIBLIOGRAPHY

Ahmed SM, Hall AJ, Robinson AE, Verhoef L, Premkumar P, Parashar UD, et al. Global prevalence of norovirus in cases of gastroenteritis: a systematic review and meta-analysis. Lancet Infect Dis. 2014;14(8):725–30.

Ajami NJ, Kavanagh OV, Ramani S, Crawford SE, Atmar RL, Jiang ZD, et al. Seroepidemiology of norovirus-associated travelers' diarrhea. J Travel Med. 2014;21(1):6–11.

Aliabadi N, Lopman BA, Parashar UD, Hall AJ. Progress toward norovirus vaccines: considerations for further development and implementation in potential target populations. Expert Rev Vaccines. 2015;14(9):1241–53.

Cardemil CV, Parashar UD, Hall AJ. Norovirus infection in older adults: epidemiology, risk factors, and opportunities for prevention and control. Infect Dis Clin North Am. 2017;31(4):839–70.

Hall AJ, Lopman BA, Payne DC, Patel MM, Gastañaduy PA, Vinje J, et al. Norovirus disease in the United States. Emerg Infect Dis. 2013;19(8):1198–205.

Hall AJ, Wikswo ME, Pringle K, Gould LH, Parashar UD. Vital signs: foodborne norovirus outbreaks—United States, 2009–2012. MMWR Morb Mortal Wkly Rep. 2014;63(22):491–5.

Kirk MD, Pires SM, Black RE, Caipo M, Crump JA, Devleesschauwer B, et al. World Health Organization estimates of the global and regional disease burden of 22 foodborne bacterial, protozoal, and viral diseases, 2010: a data synthesis. PLoS Med. 2015;12(12):e1001921.

Simons MP, Pike BL, Hulseberg CE, Prouty MG, Swierczewski BE. Norovirus: new developments and implications for travelers' diarrhea. Trop Dis Travel Med Vaccines. 2016;2:1.

POLIOMYELITIS

Concepción Estívariz, Janell Routh, Steven Wassilak

INFECTIOUS AGENT: Poliovirus (serotypes 1, 2, 3)	
ENDEMICITY	Type 1 wild poliovirus (WPV): endemic to Afghanistan and Pakistan only Circulating vaccine-derived poliovirus (cVDPV): countries in Africa and Asia (see www.polioeradication.org and https://wwwnc.cdc.gov/travel/notices)
TRAVELER CATEGORIES AT GREATEST RISK FOR EXPOSURE & INFECTION	Any unvaccinated or under-vaccinated traveler to countries with current or recent poliovirus circulation
PREVENTION METHODS	Polio is a vaccine-preventable disease
DIAGNOSTIC SUPPORT	CDC Emergency Operations Center (770-488-7100; ask to speak to the on-call polio subject matter expert) CDC's Polio and Picornavirus Laboratory (picornalab@cdc.gov) CDC's Poliovirus Laboratory Testing (www.cdc.gov/polio/what-is-polio/lab-testing/)

INFECTIOUS AGENT

Polioviruses (genus *Enterovirus*) are small, nonenveloped viruses with a single-stranded RNA genome. Polioviruses are rapidly inactivated by chlorine, formaldehyde, heat, and ultraviolet light. Poliovirus has 3 serotypes, 1, 2, and 3, that evoke minimal heterotypic immunity between them.

TRANSMISSION

Transmission occurs when the virus enters through the mouth and multiplies in the throat and gastrointestinal tract. Virus can be excreted in nasopharyngeal secretions for 1–2 weeks and in stool for 3–6 weeks, even in people who develop no symptoms after infection. Transmission occurs from person to person through the oral and fecal–oral routes.

EPIDEMIOLOGY

Before a vaccine was available, infection with wild poliovirus (WPV) was common worldwide and had seasonal peaks and epidemics in the summer and fall in temperate areas. The incidence of poliomyelitis (polio) in the United States declined rapidly after the licensure of inactivated poliovirus vaccine (IPV) in 1955 and live oral poliovirus vaccine (OPV) in the 1960s. The last cases of indigenously acquired polio in the United States occurred in 1979 and in the Americas in 1991.

Built on the success achieved in the Americas, the Global Polio Eradication Initiative (GPEI) began in 1988 and has made great progress in interrupting WPV transmission globally. Type 2 WPV was last isolated in 1999 and was declared eradicated in 2015; type 3 WPV was last detected in November 2012 and was declared eradicated in 2019. In 2021, type 1 WPV endemic circulation persisted in only 2 countries, Afghanistan and Pakistan. Despite achievements in eradicating WPV globally, polio-free countries with low vaccination coverage remain at risk for poliomyelitis outbreaks after importation of WPV. In February 2022, for example, a person in Malawi (onset of paralysis, November 2021) was identified with type 1 WPV, 18 months after Africa was certified free of indigenous WPV (in August 2020). The virus isolated from this patient was genetically linked to a type 1 WPV lineage last detected in Pakistan in 2019.

Countries that have low OPV coverage in routine immunization also are at risk of experiencing poliomyelitis cases and outbreaks caused by circulating vaccine-derived poliovirus (cVDPV). The live attenuated poliovirus strains contained in the Sabin OPV can circulate in areas with inadequate OPV coverage and revert to having wild-like characteristics. Rarely, OPV can cause paralytic poliomyelitis in vaccine recipients or their close contacts, known as vaccine-associated paralytic poliomyelitis (VAPP).

Because >90% of cVDPV cases detected between 2006 and 2014 were serotype 2, all OPV-using countries conducted a synchronized switch from trivalent OPV (tOPV, containing serotypes 1, 2, and 3) to bivalent OPV (bOPV, containing serotypes 1 and 3) in April 2016. Despite this effort, during 2019–2020, serotype 2 cVDPV caused 1,445 cases of poliomyelitis in 26 countries, whereas serotype 1 cVDPV caused 46 cases in 5 countries, and WPV caused 316 cases in 2 countries. In 2021, cVDPV serotypes 1 or 2 were isolated from 659 cases of poliomyelitis in 23 countries (data as of April 5, 2022).

Travelers to countries with current or recent WPV or cVDPV outbreaks can be at risk for exposure to poliovirus. The last documented case of WPV-associated paralysis in a US resident traveling abroad occurred in 1986 in a 29-year-old vaccinated adult who had been traveling in South and Southeast Asia. In 2005, an unvaccinated US adult traveling abroad acquired VAPP after contact with an infant recently vaccinated with OPV. Of special concern are people with underlying primary immunodeficiencies that prevent an adequate antibody response to viruses; they are at a greater risk for prolonged poliovirus infection and paralysis from WPV, cVDPV, or from exposure to people recently vaccinated with OPV.

For additional information on the status of polio eradication efforts, countries or areas with active WPV or VDPV circulation, and vaccine recommendations, consult the GPEI website (www.polioeradication.org) and the polio travel health notices on the Centers for Disease Control and Prevention (CDC)'s Travelers' Health website (https://wwwnc.cdc.gov/travel/notices).

CLINICAL PRESENTATION

Most poliovirus infections are asymptomatic; ≈25% cause minor illness with full recovery. Depending on poliovirus type, ≈1 in 200 to ≈1 in 2000 infections are associated with paralysis. Paralysis affects ≥1 limbs, and in severe cases can result in quadriplegia, respiratory failure, and rarely, death. Residual paralysis occurs in ≈2/3 cases, and for many people with residual deficits, and even for some who recover fully, worsening of weakness or paralysis can occur 20–30 years later, known as post-polio syndrome. Adults who develop paralysis usually have more severe disease and a worse prognosis than children.

DIAGNOSIS

Information on diagnostic testing for poliovirus is available from CDC's Polio Laboratory Testing website (www.cdc.gov/polio/what-is-polio/lab-testing) and Test Directory: Submitting Specimens to CDC (www.cdc.gov/laboratory/specimen-submission/list.html).

Poliovirus can be detected in clinical specimens (usually stool) obtained from an acutely ill patient. Shedding in fecal specimens can be intermittent and declines over time, but poliovirus can be detected for up to 60 days after onset of paralysis. During the first 3–10 days after paralysis onset, poliovirus also can be detected from oropharyngeal specimens, but stool specimens are the preferred source for diagnosis. Poliovirus rarely can be detected in the blood or cerebrospinal fluid; in most cases, blood antibody titers are not useful for diagnosis.

5

Poliovirus is detected by virus isolation in cultured cells. PCR testing of poliovirus isolates can identify the serotype and whether it is WPV, VDPV, or the vaccine (Sabin) strain. Genomic sequencing of poliovirus isolates can determine the geographic origin of WPV and the estimated time of circulation since the original OPV dose for VDPV.

Paralytic polio is designated an immediately notifiable, extremely urgent disease, which requires state and local health authorities to notify CDC within ≤4 hours of identification. Because of new safety requirements in handling polioviruses, CDC is the only laboratory in the United States permitted to test specimens from a suspected paralytic polio case. Notify CDC through the Emergency Operations Center (EOC, 770-488-7100) or through state health authorities. CDC's EOC will connect callers with polio subject matter experts who can provide consultation regarding the collection of clinical specimens and procedures.

TREATMENT

No licensed treatment exists for poliovirus infection, and only supportive care for symptoms is available. Two antiviral agents are undergoing clinical testing for the treatment of people with immunodeficiencies who are infected with and excreting VDPV.

PREVENTION

Vaccine

HEALTH PROTECTION RECOMMENDATIONS

Since 2000, IPV is the only polio vaccine available in the United States, but bivalent OPV is used in most low- and middle-income countries for routine immunization series and for global polio eradication activities. In response to cVDPV serotype 2 outbreaks, the population should be immunized with genetically stabilized novel OPV2, monovalent OPV2, or trivalent OPV when serotype co-circulation occurs, as in Afghanistan and Pakistan. For complete information on recommendations for poliomyelitis vaccination, consult the Advisory Committee on Immunization Practices (ACIP) website (www.cdc.gov/vaccines/hcp/acip-recs/vacc-specific/polio.html) and the March 2016 World Health Organization (WHO) position paper on poliovirus vaccines (https://cdn.who.int/media/docs/default-source/immunization/position_paper_documents/polio/who-pp-polio-mar2016-references.pdf?sfvrsn=f4e72554_2).

Before they go to areas where WPV or VDPV is circulating, ensure travelers have completed the recommended age-appropriate polio vaccine series (see Infants & Children, later in this chapter). Adults who have completed a primary series should receive a single lifetime IPV booster dose if traveling to those areas. CDC also recommends a single lifetime IPV booster dose for adult travelers going to some countries that border areas with WPV circulation based on evidence of historical cross-border transmission. These recommendations apply only to travelers going to bordering countries with a high risk for exposure to someone with imported WPV infection (e.g., people who will be working in health care settings, refugee camps, or other humanitarian aid settings).

Countries are considered to have WPV or VDPV circulation if they have evidence of poliovirus circulation during the previous 12 months, either endemic circulation of WPV, active WPV, or cVDPV outbreaks, or environmental isolation through sewage sampling. Because poliovirus circulation is dynamic, refer to CDC's Travelers' Health website destination pages for the most up-to-date polio vaccine recommendations by country (https://wwwnc.cdc.gov/travel/destinations/list).

COUNTRY REQUIREMENTS

In May 2014, the Director General of the WHO declared the international spread of poliovirus to be a public health emergency of international concern under the authority of the International Health Regulations (IHR). To prevent further spread of virus, WHO issued temporary polio vaccine recommendations for travelers staying >4 weeks and residents departing from countries with risk for poliovirus spread. The IHR emergency committee on polio meets every 3 months and updates the list of countries that must continue the temporary polio vaccine recommendations to reduce the risk for international spread of poliovirus. Updated IHR reports are available at www.who.int/news.

The polio vaccine must be received 4 weeks to 12 months before the date of departure from the polio-affected country. Be aware that long-term travelers and residents might be required to show proof of polio vaccination when departing from these countries, and document all polio vaccination administration on an International Certificate of Vaccination or Prophylaxis (ICVP). Country requirements might change, so check for updates on the CDC Travelers' Health website (https://wwwnc.cdc.gov/travel/notices) for a list of affected countries and guidance on meeting the vaccination requirements. For ordering information and instructions on how to fill out the ICVP, see https://wwwnc.cdc.gov/travel/page/icvp.

ADULTS

Before traveling to areas where WPV or VDPV is circulating, adults who are unvaccinated, incompletely vaccinated, or whose vaccination status is unknown should receive a series of 3 doses: 2 doses of IPV administered 4–8 weeks apart, and a third dose administered 6–12 months after the second dose. If 3 doses of IPV cannot be administered within the recommended intervals, alternative dosing schedules are available (see Table 5-16).

IMMUNOCOMPROMISED PEOPLE

IPV can be safely administered to immunocompromised travelers and their household contacts. Although a protective immune response cannot be ensured, IPV might confer some protection to people who are immunocompromised. Those with certain primary immunodeficiency diseases should not be given OPV and should avoid contact with children vaccinated with OPV overseas in the previous 6 weeks.

INFANTS & CHILDREN

In the United States, all infants and children should receive 4 doses of IPV, given at ages 2, 4, and 6–18 months, and 4–6 years. The final dose should be administered at ≥4 years of age, regardless of the number of previous doses, and should be given ≥6 months after the previous dose. A fourth dose in the routine IPV series is not necessary if the third dose was administered at ≥4 years of age and ≥6 months after the previous dose. If the routine series cannot be administered within the recommended intervals before protection is

Table 5-16 Alternative adult polio vaccine dosing schedules

TIME BEFORE TRAVEL	NUMBER OF DOSES[1]	INTERVAL BETWEEN DOSES
<4 weeks	1	Not Applicable
4–8 weeks	2	4 weeks
>8 weeks	3	4 weeks

[1]If <3 doses are administered, the remaining doses required to complete a 3-dose series should be administered when feasible—at the recommended intervals described in this chapter—if the person remains at risk for poliovirus exposure.

needed, CDC recommends the following alternative: give the first dose to infants at ≥6 weeks of age, give the second ≥4 weeks after dose 1, and the third dose ≥4 weeks after dose 2, then give the fourth dose ≥6 months after dose 3.

If the age-appropriate series is not completed before international travel, administer the remaining IPV doses to complete a full series when feasible, at the intervals recommended above. In addition, children completing the accelerated schedule should still receive a dose of IPV at ≥4 years of age, provided ≥6 months have passed since the last dose.

CHILDREN WHO RECEIVED POLIOVIRUS VACCINE OUTSIDE THE UNITED STATES

Vaccines administered outside the United States generally can be accepted as valid doses if the schedule is similar to that recommended in the United States. Vaccination against polio is also valid for children from countries that use an accelerated schedule. Only written, dated records are accepted as evidence of previous vaccination. Please see Guidance for Assessment of Poliovirus Vaccination Status and Vaccination of Children Who Have Received Poliovirus Vaccine Outside the United States (www.cdc.gov/mmwr/volumes/66/wr/mm6601a6.htm and its erratum, www.cdc.gov/mmwr/volumes/66/wr/mm6606a7.htm?s_cid=mm6606a7_w) for information on interpreting international poliovirus vaccination documentation.

Children with full vaccination status who received only bOPV in the primary series because they were born after April 2016, or who received a combination of tOPV and bOPV, should be revaccinated with a full IPV series to ensure protection against all 3 poliovirus types. If the child has documentation of receipt of an IPV dose, this can be considered the first dose in the US dosing schedule. In accordance with the age-appropriate US IPV schedule, vaccinate or revaccinate children <18 years old without adequate documentation of poliovirus vaccination.

International adoption from countries or areas where WPV or VDPV is actively circulating is a special situation. International adoptees might not have completed a primary polio vaccination series nor received a polio vaccine dose before departure. Thus, although the risk is small, they could be infected with WPV or VDPV and remain infectious upon entry into the United States, and potentially transmit to US household members and caregivers. As a measure of prudence, the polio vaccination status of all household members and caregivers of international adoptees from a country with active WPV or VDPV circulation should be assessed before the child enters the United States (see Sec. 7, Ch. 5, International Adoption). People who are unvaccinated, incompletely vaccinated, or whose vaccination status is unknown should be brought up to date.

PREGNANCY & BREASTFEEDING

If a pregnant person is unvaccinated or incompletely vaccinated and requires immediate protection against polio because of planned travel to a country or area where WPV or VDPV is actively circulating, IPV can be administered as recommended for adults. In addition, neither is breastfeeding a contraindication to receiving polio vaccine.

PRECAUTIONS & CONTRAINDICATIONS

IPV can be administered to people with diarrhea. Minor upper respiratory illnesses with or without fever, mild to moderate local reactions to a previous dose of IPV, current antimicrobial therapy, and the convalescent phase of acute illness are not contraindications to vaccination. IPV can be coadministered with other vaccines.

SAFETY & ADVERSE REACTIONS

Minor local reactions (pain and redness) can occur after IPV administration. Do not administer IPV to people who have experienced a severe allergic reaction (e.g., anaphylaxis) after a previous dose of the vaccine. Because IPV contains trace amounts of neomycin, polymyxin B, or streptomycin, hypersensitivity reactions can occur after IPV administration among people allergic to these antibiotics.

CDC website: www.cdc.gov/polio

BIBLIOGRAPHY

Bigouette JP, Wilkinson, AL, Tallis G, Burns CC, Wassalik SGF, Vertefeuille JF. Progress towards polio eradication—worldwide, January 2019–June 2021. MMWR Morb Mortal Wkly Rep. 2021;70(34):1129–35.

Burns CC, Diop OM, Sutter RW, Kew OM. Vaccine-derived polioviruses. J Infect Dis. 2014;210_Suppl 1:S283–93.

Centers for Disease Control and Prevention. Updated recommendations of the Advisory Committee on Immunization Practices (ACIP) regarding routine poliovirus vaccination. MMWR Morb Mortal Wkly Rep. 2009;58(30):829–30.

Macklin G, Diop OM, Humayun A, Shahmahmoodi S, El-Sayed ZA, Triki H, et al. Update on immunodeficiency-associated vaccine-derived polioviruses—worldwide, July 2018–December 2019. MMWR Morb Mortal Wkly Rep. 2020;69(28):913–7.

Marin M, Patel M, Oberste S, Pallansch MA. Guidance for assessment of poliovirus vaccination status and vaccination of children who have received poliovirus vaccine outside the United States. MMWR Morb Mortal Wkly Rep. 2017;66(01)23–5.

Sutter RW, Kew OM, Cochi SL, Aylward RB. Poliovirus vaccine—live. In: Plotkin SA, Orenstein WA, Offit PA, Edwards KM, editors. Vaccines, 7th edition. Philadelphia: Saunders Elsevier; 2017. pp. 866–917.

Vidor E, Plotkin SA. Poliovirus vaccine—inactivated. In: Plotkin SA, Orenstein WA, Offit PA, editors. Vaccines. 6th edition. Philadelphia: Saunders Elsevier; 2012. pp. 573–97.

Wallace GS, Seward JF, Pallansch MA. Interim CDC guidance for polio vaccination for travel to and from countries affected by wild poliovirus. MMWR Morb Mortal Wkly Rep. 2014;63(27):591–4.

Wilkinson AL, Diop OM, Jorba J, Gardner T, Snider CJ, Ahmed J. Surveillance to track progress toward polio eradication—worldwide, 2020–2021. MMWR Morb Mortal Wkly Rep 2022;71(15):538–44.

World Health Organization. Polio vaccines: WHO position paper—March 2016. Wkly Epidemiol Rec. 2016;91(12):145–68.

5

RABIES

Ryan Wallace, Brett Petersen, David Shlim

INFECTIOUS AGENT: Rabies virus	
ENDEMICITY	Worldwide, except Antarctica Some countries categorized as rabies virus–free are endemic for related viruses (e.g., Australian Bat Lyssavirus)
TRAVELER CATEGORIES AT GREATEST RISK FOR EXPOSURE & INFECTION	Primarily travelers with bat or dog contact (although a wide range of mammals can transmit virus)
PREVENTION METHODS	Avoid direct animal contact and animal bites If bitten, seek immediate medical attention and appropriate postexposure prophylaxis Rabies is a vaccine-preventable disease
DIAGNOSTIC SUPPORT	State health department; rabies@cdc.gov; or www.cdc.gov/rabies/specific_groups/hcp/ante_mortem.html

INFECTIOUS AGENTS

Rabies is a fatal, acute, progressive encephalomyelitis caused by neurotropic viruses in the family Rhabdoviridae, genus *Lyssavirus*. Numerous, diverse lyssavirus variants are found in various animal species throughout the world, all of which can cause fatal human rabies. Rabies virus is by far the most common *Lyssavirus* infection in humans. Tens of millions of potential human exposures and tens of thousands of deaths from rabies occur each year.

TRANSMISSION

The normal and most successful mode of rabies virus transmission is via the bite of a rabid animal. Rabies virus is neurotropic; it gains access to the nervous system through exposed peripheral nerve synapses in bite wounds. The virus travels from its point of entry along peripheral nerves to the central nervous system (CNS), where viral replication increases exponentially. Rabies virus then migrates from the CNS back to the peripheral nervous system (PNS) into, among other tissues, the salivary glands. Rabies virus secreted in saliva allows the transmission cycle to repeat. Viral shedding typically occurs just days prior to onset of clinical signs in infected animals and humans; early clinical signs can be nonspecific, however, and public health professionals should conduct a thorough risk assessment to determine if medical care is indicated.

Exposure of highly innervated tissues (e.g., those in the face and hands) can increase the risk for successful infection, and exposures occurring closer to the CNS (e.g., head, neck) can potentially shorten the incubation period. In addition to saliva, rabies virus can be found in CNS and PNS tissue, and in tears. Infection from non-bite exposures (e.g., organ transplantation from infected humans) has occurred, but human-to-human transmission generally does not occur otherwise.

All mammals are believed to be susceptible to rabies virus infection, but terrestrial mesocarnivores and bats are major rabies virus reservoirs. Dogs are the main reservoir in many low- and middle-income countries, and the epidemiology of the disease differs between regions and countries. All patients with mammal bites should be medically evaluated to ascertain if rabies postexposure prophylaxis is indicated.

Bat exposure anywhere in the world is a cause for concern and an indication to consider rabies postexposure prophylaxis.

EPIDEMIOLOGY

Lyssaviruses, the causative agent for rabies, have been found on all continents except Antarctica. Rabies virus is classified into 2 major genetic lineages: canine and New World bat. These 2 lineages can be further classified into rabies virus variants based on genetic differentiations and on the reservoir species in which they circulate. Regionally, different viral variants are adapted to various mammalian hosts and perpetuate in dogs and wildlife (e.g., bats, foxes, jackals, mongooses, raccoons, skunks).

Canine rabies remains enzootic in many areas of the world, including Africa, parts of Central and South America, and Asia. In addition to rabies virus, the *Lyssavirus* genus includes 14 other viruses that all cause rabies disease. Non–rabies *lyssaviruses* are found in Africa, Asia, Australia, and Europe; although non–rabies *lyssaviruses* have caused human deaths, these viruses contribute relatively little to the global rabies burden compared to rabies virus.

Timely and specific information about the global occurrence of rabies is often difficult to find. Surveillance levels vary, and reporting status can change suddenly because of disease reintroduction, emergence, or disruptions in surveillance operations. The rate of rabies exposures in travelers is an estimate, at best, and might range from 16–200 per 100,000 travelers.

CLINICAL PRESENTATION

After viral invasion of the PNS and then CNS, clinical illness in humans culminates in an acute, fatal encephalitis. After infection, the asymptomatic incubation period is variable, but signs and symptoms most commonly develop within several weeks to months after exposure.

Pain and paresthesia at the site of exposure are often the first symptoms of disease. The disease then progresses rapidly from a prodromal phase (fever and nonspecific, vague symptoms) to a neurologic phase characterized by anxiety, paralysis, paresis, and other signs of encephalitis. Swallowing muscle spasm can be stimulated by the sight, sound, or perception of water (hydrophobia). Delirium and convulsions can develop, followed soon thereafter by coma and death.

Approximately 80% of people with rabies will manifest with classic encephalitic disease in which fever, hydrophobia, hyperactivity, and spasms eventually progress to paralysis and coma; this progression corresponds to "furious" rabies in animals. Another 20% of people can present with paralytic rabies, in which paralysis often first involves the bitten extremity and then progresses as an ascending paralysis, ultimately leading to coma; this is the equivalent of paralytic or "dumb" rabies in animals. Once clinical signs appear, patients die quickly in the absence of intensive supportive care.

DIAGNOSIS

Diagnosis can be made in a patient with a compatible exposure history and a classic clinical presentation (Box 5-05). Clinical suspicion and prioritization of differential diagnoses can be complicated by variations in clinical presentation and a lack of exposure history, however. Because several weeks to months could have elapsed since exposure, and an accurate exposure history can be difficult to elicit, patients might not discuss potential rabies virus exposures with friends or family, and clinicians might not initially consider the possibility. As a result, rabies diagnosis in the United States is almost always missed at the first clinical encounter.

Definitive antemortem diagnosis requires use of specialized diagnostic methods on multiple specimens, including cerebrospinal fluid (CSF), saliva, serum, and skin biopsies taken from the nape of the neck. Because the probability of virus and antibody detection varies over the course of illness, sequential sample collection is indicated if initial testing is negative but clinical suspicion remains high. Finding rabies virus antigen or nucleic acid in any antemortem sample confirms the diagnosis.

A thorough review of all medical care provided to patients prior to sample collection is necessary to correctly interpret some diagnostic test results. Recent reports, for example, have described how human-derived products (e.g., intravenous immune globulin [IVIG]) administered to patients can be a passive source of high concentrations of donor-derived *Rabies lyssavirus*–neutralizing antibodies (RLNAs); in the absence of an accurate history of prior, recent IVIG administration, finding RLNAs in serum can incorrectly suggest a diagnosis of rabies. In unvaccinated encephalitic patients, however, the presence of rabies virus–neutralizing antibodies (particularly in CSF samples) confirms the diagnosis. For more information on diagnostic testing, see www.cdc.gov/rabies/specific_groups/hcp/ante_mortem.html.

Rabies is a nationally notifiable disease. The Centers for Disease Control and Prevention (CDC) is designated as the national rabies reference laboratory for the United States, along with the World Health Organization (WHO) Collaborating Center for Rabies and World Organisation for Animal Health (OIE) Rabies Reference Laboratory. In this capacity, CDC performs public health testing for domestic and international health agencies, for both human and animal rabies diagnoses. Clinicians submitting samples to CDC for rabies testing must first consult with program staff, obtain approval, and complete the requisite paperwork; step-by-step instructions are available from www.cdc.gov/rabies/resources/specimen-submission-guidelines.html.

5

BOX 5-05 World Health Organization, human rabies case definitions

CLINICAL CASE DEFINITION

A person presenting with an acute neurologic syndrome (encephalitis) dominated by forms of hyperactivity (furious rabies) or paralytic syndromes (paralytic rabies) progressing toward coma and death, usually by cardiac or respiratory failure, typically within 7–10 days after the first symptom if no intensive care is instituted.

Symptoms include any of the following: aerophobia, dysphagia, hydrophobia, nausea or vomiting, paresthesia or localized pain, localized weakness.

HUMAN RABIES: SUSPECTED

A case compatible with the clinical case definition.

HUMAN RABIES: PROBABLE

A suspected case plus a reliable history of contact with a suspected, probable, or confirmed rabid animal.

HUMAN RABIES: CONFIRMED

A suspected or probable case confirmed in the laboratory.

TREATMENT

No evidence-based "best practices" approach to treating rabies patients is available. Most cases are managed with symptomatic and palliative supportive care. Survival after the clinical phase of rabies virus infection is incredibly rare, but case reports continue to provide insight into potential therapeutic options, and experimental treatment regimens continue to be investigated. To date, early and robust production of rabies virus–neutralizing antibodies has been the primary factor associated with rare reports of survival. Rabies is still considered universally fatal for practical purposes; not getting bitten in the first place is therefore the most important prevention measure. For those who are (or who suspect they might have been) bitten by a rabid animal, urgently taking the other prevention measures described next is the only way to optimize survival.

5

PREVENTION

Travelers can best prevent rabies by learning about infection risks and the need to avoid bites from mammals, especially high-risk rabies reservoir species; consulting with travel health professionals to determine whether preexposure vaccination is recommended; knowing how to prevent rabies after a bite; and knowing how to obtain postexposure prophylaxis (PEP), which might involve urgent importation of rabies biologics or travel to somewhere PEP is available. Not seeking PEP or receiving inadequate care likely will result in death from rabies. See https://wwwnc.cdc.gov/travel/diseases/rabies for a list of pretravel rabies precautions.

Avoid Animal Bites

Avoiding bites is truly the best prevention measure for rabies. Although rabies can be completely prevented by appropriate postexposure care, obtaining that care and worrying about its effectiveness can be nerve-racking for patients. Warn travelers going to rabies-enzootic countries about the risks for rabies exposure. Counsel them to stay away from all free-roaming mammals, including puppies and kittens, and to avoid contact with bats and other wildlife.

Children are at greater risk for rabies exposure and subsequent illness because of their inquisitive nature and inability to read behavioral cues from dogs and other animals. The smaller a child's stature, the more likely they are to experience severe bites to high-risk areas (e.g., the head and face). Also contributing to the higher risk for children is their attraction to animals and the possibility that they might not report an exposure.

BATS & OTHER WILDLIFE

Besides rabies virus, other bat-associated pathogens include *Histoplasma* spp., coronaviruses, and viral hemorrhagic fever viruses (see Sec. 4, Ch. 7, Zoonotic Exposures: Bites, Stings, Scratches & Other Hazards). Educate travelers to avoid handling bats or other wildlife and to consider using personal protective equipment (PPE) before entering caves where bats are found. Many bats have tiny teeth, and the wounds they inflict might not be readily apparent. Warn travelers that any suspected or documented bite or wound from a bat should be grounds for seeking PEP.

DOGS

In many low- and middle-income countries, dogs stray freely in cities; encourage travelers to remain vigilant. Inadvertently approaching puppies when the mother is near, stepping on sleeping dogs, walking into dogs, or getting too close to dogs fighting or protecting food sources can provoke biting behavior.

Travelers bitten by a dog once are almost never bitten a second time, validating the observation that with proper awareness, bites can be avoided. Scanning for dogs on the street can become second nature for experienced travelers and expatriates. Knowledgeable travelers (even those never bitten) can travel for decades without ever having a dog bite.

NONHUMAN PRIMATES

Although nonhuman primates (NHPs) are rarely rabid, they are a common source of bites, mainly on the Indian subcontinent. In most instances, wild NHPs cannot be followed up for rabies assessments, and PEP is recommended for bite victims. Awareness of this risk and simple prevention are particularly effective: advise travelers not to approach or otherwise interact with NHPs or carry food while NHPs are near, especially those that have become habituated to tourists (see Sec. 4, Ch. 7, Zoonotic Exposures: Bites, Stings, Scratches & Other Hazards).

Preexposure Prophylaxis

Preexposure prophylaxis (PrEP) does not eliminate the need for additional medical attention after a rabies exposure, but it simplifies PEP (see Postexposure Prophylaxis later in this chapter). PrEP might also provide some protection when an exposure to rabies virus goes unrecognized, or PEP is otherwise delayed. Travelers who complete a recognized PrEP immunization series (see Revised Vaccine Schedule later in this chapter) or who receive full PEP are considered previously vaccinated and do not require routine boosters. Routine testing for rabies virus–neutralizing antibody is not recommended for international travelers who do not otherwise fall into the frequent or continuous risk categories (Table 5-17).

RECOMMENDED TRAVELER CATEGORIES

Recommendations for preexposure rabies vaccination can be made for certain international traveler categories based on multiple factors: the occurrence of animal rabies in the destination country; the availability of anti-rabies biologics; the traveler's intended activities, especially in remote areas; and the traveler's duration of stay. A decision to receive preexposure rabies immunization might also be based on the likelihood of repeat travel to at-risk destinations or long-term travel to a high-risk destination. Consider PrEP for animal handlers, field biologists, cavers, missionaries, veterinarians, and some laboratory workers. Table 5-17 provides criteria for PrEP. Regardless of whether PrEP is administered, encourage travelers to purchase medical evacuation insurance if they are going to areas where the risk for rabies is high (see Sec. 6, Ch. 1, Travel Insurance, Travel Health Insurance & Medical Evacuation Insurance).

REVISED VACCINE SCHEDULE

In the United States, PrEP previously consisted of a series of 3 intramuscular (deltoid) injections of human diploid cell rabies vaccine (HDCV) or purified chick embryo cell (PCEC) vaccine given on days 0, 7, and 21 or 28. Based on recent changes in WHO recommendations and the availability of empirical studies, the US Advisory Committee on Immunization Practices (ACIP) reviewed its own recommendations for PrEP and approved a 2-dose preexposure regimen, given on days 0 and 7 (Table 5-18).

The advantages of the revised schedule are that it is less expensive and easier to complete prior to travel. There are no data on how long this 2-dose series provides protection, however. Because of this uncertainty, travelers with a sustained risk for rabies exposure should either have a titer drawn or receive a third dose of vaccine within 3 years of the initial series. Travelers unlikely to visit an at-risk destination after 3 years require no further titers or boosters unless they have a subsequent exposure.

5

VACCINE SAFETY & ADVERSE REACTIONS

Advise travelers they might experience local reactions after vaccination (e.g., erythema, itching at the injection site, pain, swelling), or mild systemic reactions (e.g., abdominal pain, dizziness, headache, muscle aches, nausea). Approximately 6% of people receiving booster vaccinations with HDCV experience systemic hypersensitivity reactions characterized by malaise, pruritis, and urticaria. The likelihood of these reactions is less with PCEC vaccine.

Wound Management

If wounded by an animal, travelers should clean all animal bites and scratches with copious amounts of soap and water, povidone iodine, or other products with virucidal activity. Inform travelers that cleaning bite wounds immediately (or as soon as possible) substantially reduces the risk for rabies virus infection, especially when followed by timely administration of PEP. For unvaccinated patients, delay suturing any wounds for a few days. If suturing is necessary to control bleeding or for functional or cosmetic reasons, inject rabies immune globulin (RIG) into all exposed tissues before closing the wound. Use of local anesthetics is not contraindicated in wound management.

Table 5-17 Rabies preexposure prophylaxis recommendations—United States, 2022[1]

RISK CATEGORY	EXPOSURE TYPE[2]	TYPICAL POPULATION[2]	DISEASE BIOGEOGRAPHY[3]	RECOMMENDATIONS	
				PRIMARY PrEP VACCINE SERIES[4]	BOOSTERS[5]
CATEGORY 1 Elevated risk for unrecognized[6] and recognized[7] exposures, including unusual or high-risk exposures	Often high viral concentration exposures Could be recognized or unrecognized Could be unusual (e.g., aerosolized virus)	People working with live rabies virus in research or vaccine production facilities People performing testing for rabies in diagnostic laboratories	Laboratory	IM rabies vaccine DOSE 1: Day 0 DOSE 2: 7 days after DOSE 1	Check titers q6 months Provide booster for titers <0.5 IU/mL[8]
CATEGORY 2 Elevated risk for unrecognized[6] and recognized[7] exposures	Typically recognized Could be unrecognized Unusual exposures unlikely	People with frequent bat contact[9] People who perform animal necropsies	All geographic regions (domestic and international) where any rabies reservoir is present	IM rabies vaccine DOSE 1: Day 0 DOSE 2: 7 days after DOSE 1	Check titers q2 years Provide booster for titers <0.5 IU/mL[8]
CATEGORY 3 Elevated risk for recognized[7] exposures or sustained risk[10]	Exposure nearly always recognized Exposure risk exceeds that of the general population Duration of risk >3 years after primary 2-dose PrEP vaccine series	People who interact with animals that could be rabid[11] People whose occupational or recreational activities typically involve contact with animals[12] Selected travelers[13]	All domestic and international regions where any rabies reservoir is present International regions with rabies virus reservoirs, particularly where rabies virus is endemic in dog populations	IM rabies vaccine DOSE 1: Day 0 DOSE 2: 7 days after DOSE 1	One-time titer check during years 1–3 after the primary 2-dose PrEP vaccine series Provide booster for titers <0.5 IU/mL[8] **OR** Provide booster ≥21 days but <3 years after primary 2-dose PrEP vaccine series[14]

CATEGORY 4 Elevated risk for recognized[7] exposure, no sustained risk[10]	Exposure nearly always recognized Exposure risk exceeds that of the general population Duration of risk expected to be ≤3 years after primary 2-dose PrEP vaccine series	Same at-risk populations as CATEGORY 3 **BUT** Risk duration ≤3 years[15]	Same disease biogeography as CATEGORY 3	IM rabies vaccine DOSE 1: Day 0 DOSE 2: 7 days after DOSE 1	None
CATEGORY 5 Low risk for exposure	Exposure uncommon	Typical resident of the United States	Not applicable	None	None

Abbreviations: IM, intramuscular; IU, international units; PrEP, preexposure prophylaxis

[1]Source: Rao AK, Briggs D, Moore SM, et al. Use of a Modified Preexposure Prophylaxis Vaccination Schedule to Prevent Human Rabies: Recommendations of the Advisory Committee on Immunization Practices—United States, 2022. MMWR Morb Mortal Wkly Rep 2022;71:619–27 (www.cdc.gov/mmwr/volumes/71/wr/mm7118a2.htm).

[2]Exposure type and nature of work or travel are the most important variables to consider when determining a person's risk category. Perform risk categorization on a case-by-case basis; examples provided are intended as a guide only.

[3]Consult local or state health departments about local disease biogeography.

[4]Primary immunogenicity peaks 2–4 weeks after completing the recommended primary 2-dose PrEP vaccine series. People who are immunocompetent are expected to mount an appropriate response, and checking titers is not routinely recommended. Before people with altered immunity participate in high-risk activities, confirm a rabies antibody titer ≥0.5 IU/mL ≥1 week after booster vaccination (but ideally, 2–4 weeks after completing the recommended series). Individual facilities set their own rules regarding laboratory-confirmation of acceptable antibody titers for personnel.

[5]Need for boosters is based on long-term immunogenicity, the ability to mount an anamnestic response to rabies virus >3 years after completion of the primary 2-dose PrEP vaccine series.

[6]Unrecognized exposures: exposures that a person might not know occurred (e.g., a small scratch sustained during an inconspicuous breach in personal protective equipment might go unnoticed by a laboratorian testing neural tissue from rabid animals or by a field biologist conducting ecologic studies on bats).

[7]Recognized exposures: bites, scratches, splashes, etc., that are unusual for a person (e.g., bat contact) or painful (e.g., raccoon bite or scratch).

[8]Provide a booster dose of rabies vaccine when rabies antibody titers are <0.5 IU/mL. For people who are immunocompetent, checking antibody titers to verify booster response is not recommended. For people with altered immunity, verify antibody titers ≥1 week (ideally, 2–4 weeks) after each booster dose of vaccine administered.

[9]Includes people who: handle bats; have regular contact with bats; enter high-density bat environments (e.g., biologists who enter bat roosts or collect suspected rabies samples); perform animal necropsies (e.g., veterinary pathologists who frequently perform necropsies on mammals suspected to have had rabies). People for whom the frequency of handling rabies virus–infected tissues is low, or the procedures performed do not involve contact with neural tissue or opening of a suspected rabid animal's calvarium, could consider following the recommended immunization schedule for RISK CATEGORY 2 rather than RISK CATEGORY 1.

[10]Sustained risk: elevated risk for rabies virus exposure >3 years after the completion of the primary 2-dose PrEP vaccine series.

[11]Rabies virus is unlikely to persist outside a dead animal's body for an extended time due to virus inactivation by desiccation, ultraviolet irradiation, and other factors. Risk of transmission to people who handle animal products (e.g., hunters, taxidermists) is unknown but presumed to be low (RISK CATEGORY 5); direct skin contact with saliva and neural tissue of mammals should be avoided regardless of profession.

[12]Includes veterinarians, technicians, animal control officers, and their students/trainees; people who handle wildlife reservoir species (e.g., wildlife biologists, rehabilitators, trappers); spelunkers.

[13]PrEP considerations for travelers include: (1) Will the person be participating in occupational or recreational activities that increase their risk for exposure to potentially rabid animals (particularly dogs)? and (2) Will the person have difficulty getting prompt access to safe postexposure prophylaxis (PEP)? For example, will they be in rural areas or visiting destinations where PEP is not readily available (www.cdc.gov/rabies/resources/countries-risk.html).

[14]Unless the recipient has altered immunity, checking titers after recommended booster doses is not indicated.

[15]For example, short-term hands-on animal care volunteers, or infrequent travelers with no expected high-risk travel >3 years after their primary 2-dose PrEP vaccine series.

Table 5-18 Preexposure immunization for rabies[1]

VACCINE	DOSE (mL)	NUMBER OF DOSES	SCHEDULE (DAYS)[2]	ROUTE
HDCV, Imovax (Sanofi)	1.0	2	0 and 7	IM
PCEC, RabAvert (Novartis)	1.0	2	0 and 7	IM

Abbreviations: HDCV, human diploid cell vaccine; IM, intramuscular; PCEC, purified chick embryo cell

[1]People who are immunocompromised by disease or medications should postpone preexposure vaccinations and consider avoiding activities for which rabies preexposure prophylaxis is indicated during the period of expected immune compromise. If this is not possible, immunocompromised people at risk for rabies should have their antibody titers checked after vaccination.
[2]Every attempt should be made to adhere to recommended schedules; for most minor deviations (e.g., delays of a few days for individual doses), vaccination can be resumed as though the traveler were on schedule. Travelers with a sustained risk for rabies exposures should either have a titer drawn or receive a third dose of vaccine within 3 years of the initial series. Travelers unlikely to visit an at-risk destination after 3 years require no further titers or boosters unless they have an exposure.

5

Postexposure Prophylaxis

TRAVELERS WHO RECEIVED PREEXPOSURE PROPHYLAXIS

For previously vaccinated people, PEP consists of 2 doses of modern cell culture vaccine given 3 days apart (days 0 and 3), ideally initiated shortly after the exposure. The booster doses do not have to be the same brand as the one used for the original preexposure immunization series. RIG should not be administered to people who were previously vaccinated, because it can lead to a diminished immune response to vaccine and provides no benefit to the recipient.

TRAVELERS WHO DID NOT RECEIVE PREEXPOSURE PROPHYLAXIS

RABIES IMMUNE GLOBULIN + RABIES VACCINE

For unvaccinated people, PEP consists of RIG administration (20 IU/kg for human RIG [HRIG] or 40 IU/kg for equine RIG) and a series of 4 injections of rabies vaccine over 14 days; immunocompromised patients should receive 5 doses over a 1-month period (Table 5-19). After cleaning the wound, inject as much of the dose-appropriate volume of RIG (Table 5-19) as is anatomically feasible at wound sites. The intent is to put RIG anywhere saliva might have contaminated the wounded tissue.

Once initiated, rabies PEP should not be interrupted or discontinued because of local or mild systemic reactions to the vaccine. If an adverse event occurs with one of the vaccine types, consider switching to the alternative cell culture vaccine for the remainder of the series. Antihistamines or nonsteroidal anti-inflammatory medications taken before vaccination can help reduce mild adverse reactions in people with a history of such reactions.

RABIES IMMUNE GLOBULIN: AVAILABILITY & TIMING

HRIG is manufactured by plasmapheresis of blood from hyperimmunized volunteers. The total quantity of commercially produced HRIG falls short of worldwide demand, and it is not available in many low- and middle-income countries (www.cdc.gov/rabies/resources/countries-risk.html). Equine RIG, purified fractions of equine RIG, and rabies monoclonal antibody products might be available in some countries where HRIG is not. Such products are preferable to no RIG.

If access to RIG is delayed but modern cell culture vaccine is available, start the vaccine series as soon as possible, and add RIG to the regimen ≤7 days after the first dose of vaccine was administered. After day 7, RIG is unlikely to provide benefit, because antibodies from the patient's own vaccine-derived immune response should be present.

Because rabies virus can persist in tissue for a long time before invading a peripheral nerve, a previously unimmunized traveler who sustained a bite suspicious for rabies should receive full PEP, including RIG, even if a considerable length of time has passed since the initial exposure. If there is a scar, or the patient remembers where the bite

Table 5-19 Postexposure immunization for rabies[1]

IMMUNIZATION STATUS	PRODUCT	DOSE	NUMBER OF DOSES	SCHEDULE (DAYS)[2]	ROUTE
Not previously vaccinated[3]	RIG	20 IU/kg body weight	1	0	Infiltrate bite site (if possible) Give remainder IM
	Vaccine (HDCV or PCEC)	1.0 mL	4[4]	0, 3, 7, 14 (and 28 if immunocompromised)[5]	IM
Previously vaccinated[6,7]	Vaccine (HDCV or PCEC)	1.0 mL	2	0, 3	IM

Abbreviations: HDCV, human diploid cell vaccine; IM, intramuscular; PCEC, purified chick embryo cell; RIG, rabies immune globulin

[1]Begin all postexposure prophylaxis with immediate, thorough cleansing of all wounds with soap and water, povidone iodine, or other substances with virucidal activity.

[2]Every attempt should be made to adhere to recommended schedules; for most minor deviations (e.g., delays of a few days for individual doses), vaccination can be resumed as though the traveler were on schedule. When substantial deviations occur, assess immune status by serologic testing 7–14 days after the final dose is administered.

[3]For people not previously vaccinated against rabies, PEP consists of both RIG and a series of rabies vaccine injections.

[4]Immunocompromised patients should receive 5 vaccine doses. The first 4 vaccine doses are given on the same schedule as for an immunocompetent patient, and the fifth dose is given on day 28; patient follow-up should include monitoring antibody response. For more information, see Rupprecht et al., www.cdc.gov/mmwr/preview/mmwrhtml/rr5902a1.htm.

[5]The Centers for Disease Control and Prevention recommends 4 postexposure vaccine doses, on days 0, 3, 7, and 14, unless the patient is immunocompromised, in which case a fifth dose is given at day 28.

[6]Defined as preexposure immunization with HDCV or PCEC, prior postexposure prophylaxis with HDCV or PCEC, or prior vaccination with any other type of rabies vaccine and a documented history of positive rabies virus-neutralizing antibody response to that vaccination.

[7]RIG not recommended.

occurred, an appropriate amount of RIG should be injected in the area.

RABIES IMMUNE GLOBULIN: DILUTION

If the wound is small and on a distal extremity (e.g., a finger, toe), use clinical judgment to decide how much RIG to inject to avoid complications (e.g., ischemia) due to local distention of the digit or digits. Administer any remaining dose intramuscularly at a site distant from the site of vaccine administration. If wounds are extensive, do not exceed the dose-appropriate volume of RIG. If the indicated volume is inadequate to inject all wounds, dilute the RIG with dextrose 5% in water (D5W) to ensure sufficient volume to inject all wounds. Previous advice recommended normal saline as a diluent, but its use is incompatible with new formulations of HRIG. RIG dilution is particularly important in children whose body weight might be small in relation to the size and number of wounds.

RABIES IMMUNE GLOBULIN: SAFETY & ADVERSE EVENTS

The incidence of adverse events after the use of modern equine-derived RIG is low (0.8%–6.0%), and most reactions are minor. Because such products are not regulated by the US Food and Drug Administration, however, their use cannot be recommended unequivocally. In addition, unpurified anti-rabies serum of equine origin might still be used in some countries where neither human nor equine RIG is available.

CONTRAINDICATIONS & PRECAUTIONS

Pregnancy is not a contraindication to receiving PEP. In infants and children, the dose of HDCV or PCEC for PrEP or PEP is the same as that recommended for adults. The PEP RIG dose is based on body weight (Table 5-19).

Rabies vaccines were once manufactured from viruses grown in animal brains; some of these vaccines are still in use in low- and middle-income countries. Typically, travelers can identify brain-derived vaccines, also known as nerve tissue vaccines, if they are offered a daily large-volume injection (5 mL) for approximately 14–21 days. Because of variability in the potency in these preparations, which might limit their effectiveness, and the risk for severe adverse reactions, advise travelers to decline these vaccines and to travel to a location where acceptable vaccines and RIG are available.

VARIATIONS IN POSTEXPOSURE PROPHYLAXIS

Different PEP schedules, alternative routes of administration, and other rabies vaccines besides HDCV and PCEC might be used abroad. For example, commercially available purified Vero cell rabies vaccine is an acceptable alternative, if available. Other rabies vaccines or PEP regimens could require additional prophylaxis or confirmation of adequate rabies virus–neutralizing antibody titers. Encourage travelers to take photos of the rabies PEP products they receive and to be conscious of the vaccine storage conditions and corresponding administration schedule. This information is necessary for health care providers to determine whether additional vaccines or titers are indicated. Clinicians can obtain assistance managing complicated PEP scenarios from experienced travel medicine professionals, health departments, and CDC (rabies@cdc.gov).

Health care providers are justifiably concerned about getting everything right when trying to prevent a disease that is virtually 100% fatal, leading to overconcern about small variations in the administration of rabies vaccines. Modern-day cell culture rabies vaccines are highly immunogenic, however, and postexposure rabies vaccine schedules have been developed to provide the quickest onset of endogenous antibodies, which is why these vaccines are given on such a short schedule.

Make every effort to adhere to a recognized ACIP or WHO schedule. Variations of days to weeks are unlikely to diminish the immune response to vaccination but could delay the onset of protection. Numerous schedules and routes of administration have been recognized by international health authorities and have been shown to be highly effective at preventing rabies.

CDC website: www.cdc.gov/rabies

BIBLIOGRAPHY

Gautret P, Parola P. Rabies vaccination for international travelers. Vaccine. 2012;30(2):126–33.

Gautret P, Tantawichien T, Vu Hai V, Piyaphanee W. Determinants of pre-exposure rabies vaccination among foreign backpackers in Bangkok, Thailand. Vaccine. 2011;29(23):3931–4.

Malerczyk C, Detora L, Gniel D. Imported human rabies cases in Europe, the United States, and Japan, 1990 to 2010. J Travel Med. 2011;18(6):402–7.

Mills DJ, Lau CL, Weinstein P. Animal bites and rabies exposure in Australian travellers. Med J Aust. 2011;195(11-12):673–5.

Rupprecht CE, Briggs D, Brown CM, Franka R, Katz SL, Kerr HD, et al. Use of a reduced (4-dose) vaccine schedule for postexposure prophylaxis to prevent human rabies: recommendations of the Advisory Committee on Immunization Practices. MMWR Recomm Rep. 2010;59(RR-2):1–9.

Rupprecht CE, Gibbons RV. Clinical practice. Prophylaxis against rabies. N Engl J Med. 2004;351(25):2626–35.

Smith A, Petrovic M, Solomon T, Fooks A. Death from rabies in a UK traveller returning from India. Euro Surveill. 2005;10(30): E050728.5.

van Thiel PP, de Bie RM, Eftimov F, Tepaske R, Zaaijer HL, van Doornum GJ, et al. Fatal human rabies due to Duvenhage virus from a bat in Kenya: failure of treatment with coma-induction, ketamine, and antiviral drugs. PLoS Negl Trop Dis. 2009;3(7):e428.

Warrell MJ, Warrell DA. Rabies and other lyssavirus diseases. Lancet. 2004;363(9413):959–69.

World Health Organization. WHO expert consultation on rabies: third report. Geneva: The Organization; 2018. Available from: https://apps.who.int/iris/handle/10665/272364.

RABIES IMMUNIZATION

David Shlim

Prior to the coronavirus disease 2019 (COVID-19) pandemic, few topics in travel medicine prompted more concern and questions than the prevention of rabies in travelers. Rabies prevention presents unique issues for the travel medicine clinician, because it is the one infectious disease that can be prevented, either through a combination of pre- and postexposure immunizations or through postexposure treatment with rabies immune globulin (RIG) and vaccine. Prevention is possible because the time of the bite can almost always be recognized, and immunoprophylactic intervention can stop clinical disease from developing. The seeming complexity of the issues surrounding wound care, timing of administration, deviations from standard schedules, the cost of preexposure immunization, and the difficulty of finding vaccine and RIG while traveling can make the travel medicine practitioner's head spin.

The good news is that we have developed a method of preventing rabies encephalitis that is virtually 100% effective. The challenges that remain are the lack of availability of RIG in many areas of the world, the expense of both pre- and postexposure care, and the ongoing endemicity of rabies in street dogs in many areas. To keep the travel medicine approach to rabies prevention in perspective, 1–2 cases of rabies are reported in travelers per year, in contrast to >50,000 rabies deaths in resource-poor, low- and middle-income countries.

THE 2-DOSE PREEXPOSURE RABIES VACCINE SCHEDULE

World Health Organization Recommendations

In 2017—partly to address the lack of progress in decreasing rabies in the world—a World Health Organization (WHO) expert committee endorsed a 2-dose rabies preexposure immunization schedule in place of the previous 3-dose schedule. The committee was hoping to make preexposure immunization more affordable and convenient for local people, and more desirable and feasible for travelers. The seemingly sudden announcement spurred national health agencies to do their own research and decide whether to harmonize with WHO, or stick to their own recommendations. Conclusions so far have varied around the world.

WHO also endorsed the use of wound-only administration of RIG, in which an anatomically appropriate dose (not to exceed the weight-calculated amount) of RIG is injected around the wound, but where the remaining calculated dose is not administered intramuscularly. This idea was based on the thinking that RIG is most valuable at the site of the wound, and little additional RIG makes its way into the bloodstream. The further rationale behind this approach is that it leaves hard-to-obtain and expensive RIG available to treat more people. But measurable amounts of RIG are detected in the blood after its intramuscular administration, and whether this is critical to prevention of rabies encephalitis is not really known.

Advisory Committee on Immunization Practices Guidance

In the United States, the Advisory Committee on Immunization Practices (ACIP) convened a working group to evaluate similar questions to those considered by WHO. In 2021, ACIP voted to approve a 2-dose preexposure rabies immunization series, with the proviso that either a third dose be given within 3 years, or a serological

(continued)

RABIES IMMUNIZATION (CONTINUED)

test be performed to document seroconversion. Although the working group felt that "boostability" likely will extend beyond 3 years, there were no data yet available to support this.

In addition, and in contrast to WHO recommendations, ACIP elected to retain the current guidance of calculating RIG dose based on patient weight, administering an amount feasible around the wound and delivering the rest into muscle. This raises the question of whether Americans will receive the ACIP-recommended full RIG dose in countries that have adopted WHO's wound-only RIG administration guidance. This might be yet another reason for recommending preexposure prophylaxis.

5

After a high-risk exposure, travelers who received 2 (or 3) doses of rabies vaccine before travel need to receive 2 more doses of rabies vaccine, 3 days apart. Conversely, unimmunized travelers exposed to rabies and other lyssaviruses will require—according to US standards—a series of 4 or 5 doses of rabies vaccine intramuscularly over a 2- to 4-week period, and infiltration of RIG. Because human and equine RIG often are unavailable in low- and middle-income countries, preexposure rabies immunization can facilitate the traveler's access to adequate postexposure rabies prophylaxis.

In the United States, however, where a single dose of rabies vaccine can exceed $400, cost has been a deterrent to preexposure prophylaxis. Although the new ACIP guidelines have reduced the associated inconvenience of 3 pretravel clinic visits extending over several weeks to just 2 visits 7 days apart, the high price might influence a traveler's decision about whether to accept preexposure prophylaxis. Even when modern cell-culture rabies vaccine was first introduced in the early 1980s, at approximately $45 per dose, many people already considered the vaccine too expensive.

INTRADERMAL PREEXPOSURE RABIES IMMUNIZATION

Intradermal (ID) rabies immunization began almost as soon as the intramuscular (IM) human diploid cell vaccine (HDCV) was manufactured. By reconstituting the 1.0 mL of vaccine in the vial, practitioners could draw up approximately eight 0.1-mL doses. One problem was that the entire vial had to be used within a few hours of reconstituting, meaning that a provider had to either be working in a busy clinic or lining up groups of people (e.g., families) for rabies immunization all at the same time.

Early studies of the immune response to ID rabies vaccine, using HDCV and later, other rabies vaccines, were uniformly encouraging. Virtually 100% of vaccinees seroconverted. A 1982 statement by ACIP reviewed data on >1,500 vaccinees and declared, "It appears that, with this vaccine, the 0.1-mL ID regimen is an acceptable alternative to the currently approved 1.0-mL IM regimen for preexposure prophylaxis." ACIP called upon manufacturers to produce a product with appropriate packaging and labeling.

In 1986, the Mérieux Institute (now Sanofi Pasteur) received approval to market a 0.1-mL dose in an individual syringe. Sharing reconstituted vials of 1.0 mL between patients remained off-label. Although the new product solved the logistical problem of providing individual travelers with an ID dose, the cost of the prepackaged ID dose was still 75% of the full 1.0-mL IM dose.

ACIP continued to endorse the concept of ID preexposure rabies immunization in a 1999 statement on rabies prevention. Three lots of a prepackaged rabies ID vaccine were recalled in 2000, however, for having a potency that fell below the specification level before the expiration date. In 2001, the ID rabies vaccine was withdrawn from the market. Since then, authorities in the United States have not recommended sharing 1.0-mL vials for ID rabies immunization because the manufacturer has not applied to the US Food and Drug Administration for the appropriate packaging and labeling. This lack of endorsement of ID preexposure immunization has frustrated some travel medicine professionals.

With 2 decades more experience in using ID preexposure rabies immunization, the concept is now well accepted and routinely used in many parts of the world; ID administration remains off-label in the United States, however, due to the aforementioned packaging issues. Some clinics relying on preexposure ID dosing require vaccinated travelers to have a titer drawn after the series is completed to confirm seroconversion. This may save some money, but requires an additional clinic visit and even more time before travel.

POSTEXPOSURE PROPHYLAXIS

A wide variety of postexposure vaccine regimens are now used around the world, some of which use multisite intradermal vaccine doses. From the point of view of the traveler, perhaps the best strategy would be to try to use postexposure regimens that are approved in the traveler's home country, which could create the most confidence and make it easier to complete at home any regimens initiated abroad.

PREVENTION: THE BEST MEDICINE

I recently noticed that travelers are almost never bitten a second time in their entire lives, and experienced travelers and expatriates, including most travel medicine professionals, are never bitten at all. This led me to believe that it might be possible to educate travelers on how to avoid bites by making them better aware of animal behaviors and to keep their distance.

Perhaps greater emphasis on bite prevention should become a priority during the pretravel visit. As travel medicine professionals, we can analyze our own behaviors in avoiding bites and transmit that information to travelers. Avoiding bites altogether would be the best way to help reduce anxiety-ridden travel and urgent telephone calls to obtain postexposure immunization in resource-poor settings.

5

BIBLIOGRAPHY

Bernard KW, Fishbein DB, Miller KD, Parker RA, Waterman S, Sumner JW, et al. Pre-exposure rabies immunization with human diploid cell vaccine: decreased antibody responses in persons immunized in developing countries. Am J Trop Med Hyg. 1985 May;34(3):633–47.

Centers for Disease Control and Prevention. Recommendation of the Immunization Practices Advisory Committee supplementary statement on pre-exposure rabies prophylaxis by the intradermal route. MMWR Morb Mortal Wkly Rep. 1982;31(21):279–80, 85.

Mills DJ, Lau CL, Fearnley EJ, Weinstein P. The immunogenicity of a modified intradermal pre-exposure rabies vaccination schedule–a case series of 420 travelers. J Travel Med. 2011;18(5):327–32.

Muehlenbein MP, Angelo KM, Schlagenhauf P, Chen L, Grobusch MP, Gautret P, et al.; GeoSentinel Surveillance Network. Traveller exposures to animals: a GeoSentinel analysis. J Travel Med. 2020;27(7):taaa010.

Rao AK, Briggs D, Moore SM, et al. Use of a Modified Preexposure Prophylaxis Vaccination Schedule to Prevent Human Rabies: Recommendations of the Advisory Committee on Immunization Practices—United States, 2022. MMWR Morb Mortal Wkly Rep. 2022;71:619–27.

Soentjens P, Andries A, Aerssens A, Tsoumanis A, Ravinetto R, Heuninckx W, et al. Pre-exposure intradermal rabies vaccination: a non-inferiority trial in healthy adults on shortening the vaccination schedule from 28 to 7 days. Clin Infect Dis. 2019;68(4):607–14.

World Health Organization. Rabies vaccine and immunoglobulins: WHO position. Geneva: The Organization; 2018. Available from: http://apps.who.int/iris/bitstream/10665/259855/1/WHO-CDS-NTD-NZD-2018.04-eng.pdf?ua=1.

. . . *perspectives* chapters supplement the clinical guidance in this book with additional content, context, and expert opinion. The views expressed do not necessarily represent the official position of the Centers for Disease Control and Prevention (CDC).

RUBELLA

Michelle Morales, Tatiana Lanzieri, Susan Reef

INFECTIOUS AGENT: Rubella virus	
ENDEMICITY	Worldwide
TRAVELER CATEGORIES AT GREATEST RISK FOR EXPOSURE & INFECTION	Unvaccinated travelers
PREVENTION METHODS	Rubella is a vaccine-preventable disease
DIAGNOSTIC SUPPORT	A clinical laboratory certified in moderate complexity testing; state health department; or CDC Rubella Laboratory Testing (www.cdc.gov/rubella/lab/index.html)

INFECTIOUS AGENT

Rubella is a spherical, positive-sense, single-stranded RNA virus of the family *Matonaviridae*, genus *Rubivirus*.

TRANSMISSION

Rubella virus is transmitted through person-to-person contact or droplets shed from the respiratory secretions of infected people. People can shed virus from 7 days before the onset of the rash to ≈5–7 days after rash onset. Transmission from mother to fetus also can occur, with the highest risk for congenital rubella syndrome (CRS) if infection occurs in the first trimester. Infants with CRS can transmit virus for ≤1 year after they are born.

EPIDEMIOLOGY

In 2015, the World Health Organization Region of the Americas became the first in the world to be declared free of endemic rubella virus transmission. Rubella virus continues to circulate widely, however, especially in Africa, East Asia, and South Asia; ≈49,000 cases were reported worldwide in 2019, and ≈10,000 cases were reported in 2020. Globally, >100,000 infants are born each year with CRS; >80% are born in Africa and some countries in South and Southeast Asia. In the United States, endemic rubella virus transmission was interrupted in 2001 and elimination verified in 2004, but imported cases of rubella and CRS continue to occur. During 2016–2019, a median of 5 (range, 1–7) imported rubella cases were reported annually in the United States, and 8 CRS cases were reported during the same period.

CLINICAL PRESENTATION

The average incubation period is 14 days (range 12–23 days). Rubella usually presents with generalized lymphadenopathy, slight or no fever, and a mild, nonspecific, maculopapular, generalized rash that lasts up to 3 days. The rash usually starts on the face, becoming generalized within 24 hours. Appearance of the rash can sometimes be preceded by anorexia, mild conjunctivitis, low-grade fever, malaise, runny nose, and sore throat. Adolescents and adults, especially women, also can present with transient arthritis. Rare complications include encephalitis and thrombocytopenic purpura, but ≈25%–50% of infections are asymptomatic. Infection during early pregnancy can lead to miscarriage, fetal death, or an infant born with CRS, a constellation of birth defects.

DIAGNOSIS

Clinical diagnosis of rubella virus is unreliable and should not be considered in assessing immune status; ≤50% of all infections are subclinical or unapparent. Many rubella infections are not recognized because the rash resembles many other rash illnesses.

Diagnosis is based on serologic demonstration of specific rubella IgM or significant increase in rubella IgG in acute- and convalescent-phase specimens. Reverse transcription PCR (RT-PCR) can be used to detect virus infection; viral culture also is acceptable but is time consuming and expensive. Rubella is a nationally notifiable disease in the United States.

TREATMENT

Treatment of rubella involves supportive care. Counsel patients to isolate, and encourage household contacts to get tested and vaccinated.

PREVENTION

Unless contraindicated, vaccinate all travelers aged ≥12 months who do not have acceptable evidence of immunity to rubella (documented by ≥1 dose of rubella-containing vaccine on or after the first birthday, laboratory evidence of immunity, or birth before 1957) with measles-mumps-rubella (MMR) vaccine. Before departure from the United States, infants aged 6–11 months should receive 1 dose of MMR vaccine (for measles protection), and children aged ≥12 months and adults should receive 2 doses of MMR vaccine ≥28 days apart.

MMR vaccine is contraindicated during pregnancy. Advise pregnant people who do not have acceptable evidence of rubella immunity to avoid travel to countries where rubella is endemic or to areas with known rubella outbreaks, especially during the first 20 weeks of pregnancy. In addition, they should receive an MMR vaccination immediately postpartum. Ensure that all people of childbearing age and recent immigrants are up to date on immunization against rubella or have evidence of immunity to rubella, because these groups are at the greatest risk for maternal–fetal transmission of rubella virus, which can result in CRS.

CDC website: www.cdc.gov/rubella

5

BIBLIOGRAPHY

Centers for Disease Control and Prevention. National Notifiable Diseases Surveillance System, 2016–2019 annual tables of infectious disease data. Available from: www.cdc.gov/nndss/data-statistics/infectious-tables/index.html.

Grant GB, Desai S, Dumolard L, Kretsinger K, Reef SE. Progress toward rubella and congenital rubella syndrome control and elimination—worldwide, 2000–2018. MMWR Morb Mortal Wkly Rep. 2019;68(39):855–9.

Lanzieri T, Haber P, Icenogle JP, Patel M. Rubella. In: Rubella. In: Hall E, Wodi AP, Hamborsky J, Morelli V, Schillie S, editors. Epidemiology and prevention of vaccine-preventable diseases, 14th edition. Washington, DC: Public Health Foundation; 2021. pp. 301–14. Available from: www.cdc.gov/vaccines/pubs/pinkbook/rubella.html.

Reef SE, Plotkin SA. Rubella vaccines. In: Plotkin SA, Orenstein WA, Offit PA, Edwards KM, editors. Plotkin's vaccines, 7th edition. Philadelphia: Elsevier; 2018. pp. 970–1000.

Vynnycky E, Adams EJ, Cutts FT, Reef SE, Navar AM, Simons E, et al. Using seroprevalence and immunization coverage data to estimate the global burden of congenital rubella syndrome, 1996–2010: a systematic review. PLoS One. 2016;11(3):e0149160.

World Health Organization. Rubella vaccines: WHO position paper. Wkly Epidemiol Rec. 2020;95(27):306–24.

RUBEOLA / MEASLES

Paul Gastañaduy, James Goodson

INFECTIOUS AGENT: Measles virus	
ENDEMICITY	Worldwide
TRAVELER CATEGORIES AT GREATEST RISK FOR EXPOSURE & INFECTION	All travelers, especially unvaccinated travelers
PREVENTION METHODS	Rubeola is a vaccine-preventable disease
DIAGNOSTIC SUPPORT	A clinical laboratory certified in moderate complexity testing; state health department; or CDC Measles Virus Laboratory, www.cdc.gov/measles/lab-tools/measles-virus-lab.html

5

INFECTIOUS AGENT

Measles virus is a member of the genus *Morbillivirus* of the family *Paramyxoviridae.*

TRANSMISSION

Measles is transmitted from person to person via respiratory droplets and by the airborne route as aerosolized droplet nuclei. Infected people are usually contagious from 4 days before until 4 days after rash onset. Measles is among the most contagious viral diseases known; secondary attack rates are ≥90% among susceptible household and institutional contacts. Humans are the only natural host for sustaining measles virus transmission, which makes global eradication of measles feasible.

EPIDEMIOLOGY

Measles was declared eliminated (defined as the absence of endemic measles virus transmission in a defined geographic area for ≥12 months in the presence of a well-performing surveillance system) from the United States in 2000. Measles virus continues to be imported into the country from other parts of the world, however, and recent prolonged outbreaks in the United States resulting from measles virus importations highlight the challenges faced in maintaining measles elimination.

Given the large global measles burden and high communicability of the disease, travelers could be exposed to the virus in any country they visit where measles remains endemic or where large outbreaks are occurring. Most measles cases imported into the United States occur in unvaccinated US residents who become infected while traveling abroad, often to the World Health Organization (WHO)–defined Western Pacific and European regions. These travelers become symptomatic after returning to the United States and sometimes infect others in their communities, causing outbreaks.

Nearly 90% of imported measles cases are considered preventable by vaccination (i.e., the travelers lacked recommended age- and travel-appropriate vaccination). Furthermore, observational studies in travel clinics in the United States have shown that 59% of pediatric and 53% of adult travelers eligible for measles-mumps-rubella (MMR) vaccine at the time of pretravel consultation were not vaccinated at the visit, highlighting a missed opportunity to reduce the likelihood of measles introductions and subsequent spread. Encourage all eligible travelers to receive appropriate MMR vaccination. Outbreak investigations are costly and resource intensive, and infected people—in addition to productivity losses—can incur direct costs for the management of their illness, including treatment, quarantine, and caregiving.

CLINICAL PRESENTATION

The incubation period averages 11–12 days from exposure to onset of prodrome; rash usually appears ≈14 days after exposure. Symptoms include fever, with temperature ≤105°F (≤40.6°C); conjunctivitis; coryza (runny nose); cough; and small spots with white or bluish-white centers on an erythematous base appearing on the buccal mucosa (Koplik spots). A characteristic red, blotchy (maculopapular) rash appears 3–7 days after onset of prodromal symptoms. The rash begins on the face, becomes generalized, and lasts 4–7 days.

Common measles complications include diarrhea (8%), middle ear infection (7%–9%), and pneumonia (1%–6%). Encephalitis, which can result in permanent brain damage, occurs in ≈1 per 1,000–2,000 cases of measles. The risk for serious complications or death is highest for children aged ≤5 years, adults aged ≥20 years, and in populations with poor nutritional status or that lack access to health care.

Subacute sclerosing panencephalitis (SSPE) is a progressive neurologic disorder caused by measles virus that usually presents 5–10 years after recovery from the initial primary measles virus infection. SSPE manifests as mental and motor deterioration, which can progress to coma and death. SSPE occurs in ≈1 of every 5,000 reported measles cases; rates are higher among children <5 years of age.

DIAGNOSIS

Measles is a nationally notifiable disease. Laboratory criteria for diagnosis include a positive serologic test for measles-specific IgM, IgG seroconversion, or a significant rise in measles IgG level by any standard serologic assay; isolation of measles virus; or detection of measles virus RNA by reverse transcription PCR (RT-PCR) testing. The Centers for Disease Control and Prevention's Measles Virus Laboratory is the national reference laboratory; it provides serologic and molecular testing for measles and technical assistance to state public health laboratories for the collection and shipment of clinical samples for molecular diagnostics and genetic analysis. Detailed information on diagnostic support can be found at www.cdc.gov/measles/lab-tools/measles-virus-lab.html.

A clinical case of measles illness is characterized by generalized maculopapular rash lasting ≥3 days; temperature ≥101°F (38.3°C); and cough, coryza, or conjunctivitis. A confirmed case is one with an acute febrile rash illness with laboratory confirmation or direct epidemiologic linkage to a laboratory-confirmed case. In a laboratory-confirmed or epidemiologically linked case, the patient's temperature does not need to reach ≥101°F (38.3°C) and the rash does not need to last ≥3 days.

TREATMENT

Treatment is supportive. The WHO recommends vitamin A for all children with acute measles, regardless of their country of residence, to reduce the risk for complications. Administer vitamin A as follows: for infants <6 months old, give 50,000 IU, once a day for 2 days; for infants 6 months old and older, but younger than 12 months, give 100,000 IU once a day for 2 days; for children ≥12 months old give 200,000 IU once a day for 2 days. For children with clinical signs and symptoms of vitamin A deficiency, administer an additional (i.e., a third) age-specific dose of vitamin A 2–4 weeks following the first round of dosing.

PREVENTION

Measles has been preventable through vaccination since a vaccine was licensed in 1963. People who do not have evidence of measles immunity should be considered at risk for measles, particularly during international travel. Acceptable presumptive evidence of immunity to measles includes birth before 1957; laboratory confirmation of disease; laboratory evidence of immunity; or written documentation of age-appropriate vaccination with a licensed, live attenuated measles-containing vaccine[1], namely, MMR or measles-mumps-rubella-varicella (MMRV). For infants 6 months old and older, but younger than 12 months, this includes documented administration of 1 dose of MMR; for people aged ≥12 months, documentation should

[1] From 1963–1967, a formalin-inactivated measles vaccine was available in the United States and was administered to ≈600,000–900,000 people. It was discontinued when it became apparent that the immunity it produced was short-lived. Consider people who received this vaccine unvaccinated.

include 2 doses of MMR or MMRV (the first dose administered at age ≥12 months and the second dose administered no earlier than 28 days after the first dose). Verbal or self-reported history of vaccination is not considered valid presumptive evidence of immunity.

Vaccination

Measles vaccine contains live, attenuated measles virus, which in the United States is available only in combination formulations (e.g., MMR and MMRV vaccines). MMRV vaccine is licensed for children aged 12 months–12 years and can be used in place of MMR vaccine if vaccination for measles, mumps, rubella, and varicella is needed.

5

International travelers, including people traveling to high-income countries, who do not have presumptive evidence of measles immunity and who have no contraindications to MMR or MMRV, should receive MMR or MMRV before travel per the following schedule.

Infants (6 months old and older, but younger than 12 months): 1 MMR dose. Infants vaccinated before age 12 months must be revaccinated on or after the first birthday with 2 doses of MMR or MMRV separated by ≥28 days. MMRV is not licensed for children aged <12 months.

Children (aged ≥12 months): 2 doses of MMR or MMRV separated by ≥28 days.

Adults born in or after 1957: 2 doses of MMR separated by ≥28 days.

One dose of MMR is ≈85% effective when administered at age 9 months; MMR and MMRV are 93% effective when administered at age ≥1 year. Vaccine effectiveness of 2 doses is 97%.

ADVERSE REACTIONS

In rare circumstances, MMR vaccination has been associated with anaphylaxis (≈2–14 occurrences per million doses administered); febrile seizures (≈1 occurrence per 3,000–4,000 doses administered, but overall, the rate of febrile seizures after measles-containing vaccine is much lower than the rate with measles disease); thrombocytopenia (≈1 occurrence per 40,000 doses during the 6 weeks after immunization); or joint symptoms (arthralgia develops among ≈25% of nonimmune postpubertal females from the rubella component of the MMR vaccination, and ≈10% have acute arthritis-like signs and symptoms that generally persist for 1–21 days and rarely recur; chronic joint symptoms are rare, if they occur at all). No evidence supports a causal link between MMR vaccination and autism, type 1 diabetes mellitus, or inflammatory bowel disease.

CONTRAINDICATIONS

ALLERGY

People who experienced a severe allergic reaction (difficulty breathing, hives, hypotension, shock, swelling of the mouth or throat) following a prior dose of MMR or MMRV vaccine, or who had an anaphylactic reaction to topically or systemically administered neomycin, should not be vaccinated or revaccinated. People who are allergic to eggs can receive MMR or MMRV vaccine without prior routine skin testing or the use of special protocols.

IMMUNOSUPPRESSION

Enhanced replication of live vaccine viruses can occur in people who have immune deficiency disorders. Death related to vaccine-associated measles virus infection has been reported among severely immunocompromised people; thus, severely immunosuppressed people should not be vaccinated with MMR or MMRV vaccine. For a thorough discussion of recommendations for immunocompromised travelers, see Sec. 3, Ch. 1, Immunocompromised Travelers.

HIV

MMR vaccination is recommended for all people with HIV infection aged ≥12 months who do not have evidence of measles, mumps, and rubella immunity, and who do not have evidence of severe immunosuppression. The assessment of severe immunosuppression can be based on CD4 values (count or percentage); absence of severe immunosuppression is defined as CD4 ≥15% for ≥6 months for children aged ≤5 years, or CD4 ≥15% and CD4 count ≥200 cells/mL for ≥6 months for people aged >5 years.

LEUKEMIA

People with leukemia in remission and off chemotherapy, who were not immune to measles when diagnosed with leukemia, may receive MMR vaccine. At least 3 months should elapse after termination of chemotherapy before administering the first dose of vaccine.

STEROIDS & OTHER IMMUNOSUPPRESSIVE THERAPIES

Avoid vaccinating people who have received high-dose corticosteroid therapy (in general, considered to be ≥20 mg or 2 mg/kg body weight of prednisone, or its equivalent, daily for ≥14 days) with MMR or MMRV for ≥1 month after cessation of steroid therapy. Corticosteroid therapy usually is not a contraindication when administration is short-term (<14 days) or a low to moderate dose (<20 mg of prednisone or equivalent per day).

In general, withhold MMR or MMRV vaccine for ≥3 months after cessation of other immunosuppressive therapies and remission of the underlying disease. See Sec. 3, Ch. 1, Immunocompromised Travelers, for more details.

PREGNANCY

MMR vaccines should not be administered to pregnant people or people attempting to become pregnant. Because of the theoretical risk to the fetus, people should be counseled to avoid becoming pregnant for 28 days after receiving a live-virus (e.g., MMR) vaccine.

PRECAUTIONS

PERSONAL OR FAMILY HISTORY OF SEIZURES OF ANY ETIOLOGY

Compared with administration of separate MMR and varicella vaccines at the same visit, use of MMRV vaccine is associated with a higher risk for fever and febrile seizures 5–12 days after the first dose among children aged 12–23 months. Approximately 1 additional febrile seizure occurs for every 2,300–2,600 MMRV vaccine doses administered. Use of separate MMR and varicella vaccines avoids this increased risk for fever and febrile seizures.

THROMBOCYTOPENIA

The benefits of primary immunization are usually greater than the potential risks for vaccine-associated thrombocytopenia. Avoid giving subsequent doses of MMR or MMRV vaccine, however, if an episode of thrombocytopenia occurred ≤6 weeks after a previous dose of vaccine.

Postexposure Prophylaxis

Measles-containing vaccine or immune globulin (IG) can be effective as postexposure prophylaxis. MMR or MMRV administered ≤72 hours after initial exposure to measles virus might provide some protection. If the exposure does not result in infection, the vaccine should induce protection against subsequent measles virus infection.

When administered ≤6 days of exposure, IG can be used to confer temporary immunity in a susceptible person. If the exposure does not result in modified or typical measles, vaccination with MMR or MMRV is still necessary to provide long-lasting protection. Six months after receiving intramuscularly administered IG, or 8 months after receiving intravenously administered IG, administer MMR or MMRV vaccine, provided the patient is aged ≥12 months and the vaccine is not otherwise contraindicated.

CDC website: www.cdc.gov/measles

BIBLIOGRAPHY

Centers for Disease Control and Prevention. Prevention of measles, rubella, congenital rubella syndrome, and mumps, 2013: summary recommendations of the Advisory Committee on Immunization Practices (ACIP). MMWR Recomm Rep. 2013;62(RR-04):1–34.

Gastañaduy P, Redd S, Clemmons N, Lee AD, Hickman CJ, Rota PA, et al. Measles. In: Roush SW, Baldy LM, Kirkconnell Hall MA, editors. Manual for the surveillance of vaccine-preventable diseases. Atlanta: Centers for Disease Control and Prevention; 2019. Available from: www.cdc.gov/vaccines/pubs/surv-manual/chpt07-measles.html.

Hyle EP, Fields NF, Fiebelkorn AP, Taylor Walker A, Gastañaduy P, Rao SR, et al. The clinical impact and cost-effectiveness of measles-mumps-rubella vaccination to prevent measles importations among US international travelers. Clin Infect Dis. 2019;69(2):306–15.

Hyle EP, Rao SR, Bangs AC, Gastañaduy P, Parker Fiebelkorn A, Hagmann SHF, et al. Clinical practices for measles-mumps-rubella vaccination among US pediatric international travelers. JAMA Pediatr. 2020;174(2):e194515.

Hyle EP, Rao SR, Jentes ES, Parker Fiebelkorn A, Hagmann SHF, Taylor Walker A, et al. Missed opportunities for measles, mumps, rubella vaccination among departing U.S. adult travelers receiving pretravel health consultations. Ann Intern Med. 2017;167(2):77–84.

Lee AD, Clemmons NS, Patel M, Gastañaduy PA. International importations of measles virus into the United States during the post-elimination era, 2001–2016. J Infect Dis. 2019;219(10):1616–23.

National Notifiable Diseases Surveillance System. Measles (rubeola): 2013 case definition. Atlanta: CDC; 2013. Available from: https://ndc.services.cdc.gov/conditions/measles/.

Patel MK, Goodson JL, Alexander JP Jr., Kretsinger K, Sodha SV, Steulet C, et al. Progress toward regional measles elimination—Worldwide, 2000–2019. MMWR Morb Mortal Wkly Rep. 2020;69(45):1700–5.

Pike J, Leidner AJ, Gastañaduy PA. A review of measles outbreak cost estimates from the US in the post-elimination era (2004–2017): Estimates by perspective and cost type. Clin Infect Dis. 2020;1(6):1568–76.

World Health Organization. Measles vaccines: WHO position paper—April 2017. Wkly Epidemiol Rec. 2017;92(17):205–27.

5

SMALLPOX & OTHER ORTHOPOXVIRUS-ASSOCIATED INFECTIONS

The information included in this chapter was current as of August 2022. For the most recent information regarding monkeypox and the 2022 monkeypox outbreak, see www.cdc.gov/poxvirus/monkeypox/index.html.

Agam Rao, Andrea McCollum

SMALLPOX

INFECTIOUS AGENT: Variola virus	
ENDEMICITY	Eradicated worldwide Bioterrorism threat exists
TRAVELER CATEGORIES AT GREATEST RISK FOR EXPOSURE & INFECTION	None
PREVENTION METHODS	Smallpox is a vaccine-preventable disease (restrictions apply, see text below for details)
DIAGNOSTIC SUPPORT	CDC Poxvirus Inquiries (poxvirus@cdc.gov) CDC Emergency Operations Center (770-488-7100)

COWPOX, VACCINIA & SIMILAR ORTHOPOXVIRUSES

INFECTIOUS AGENTS: Cowpox virus, Vaccinia virus, Akhmeta virus	
ENDEMICITY	Cowpox virus: Europe and the Caucuses Vaccinia virus: the Americas (Argentina, Brazil, Colombia); Asia (Bangladesh, India) Akhmeta virus: Georgia
TRAVELER CATEGORIES AT GREATEST RISK FOR EXPOSURE & INFECTION	Travelers who come into direct contact with animals, specifically bovids
PREVENTION METHODS	Avoid agricultural bovids with signs of disease Wear appropriate personal protective equipment
DIAGNOSTIC SUPPORT	CDC Poxvirus Inquiries (poxvirus@cdc.gov) CDC Emergency Operations Center (770-488-7100)

MONKEYPOX

INFECTIOUS AGENT: Monkeypox virus	
ENDEMICITY	West and Central Africa, esp. Congo Basin, Nigeria
TRAVELER CATEGORIES AT GREATEST RISK FOR EXPOSURE & INFECTION	Travelers to monkeypox-endemic regions who have direct exposures to wild mammals, products derived from wild mammals, or monkeypox patients or their biological samples Travelers who have close skin-to-skin contact (including that which occurs during sex) with people infected with monkeypox virus
PREVENTION METHODS	Avoid sick or dead wild small mammals, tissues of wild mammals, and products made from wild mammals Avoid people with monkeypox Wear appropriate personal protective equipment Monkeypox is a vaccine-preventable disease (restrictions apply, see text below for details)
DIAGNOSTIC SUPPORT	CDC Poxvirus Inquiries (poxvirus@cdc.gov) CDC Emergency Operations Center (770-488-7100)

INFECTIOUS AGENT

Smallpox is caused by variola virus, genus *Orthopoxvirus*. Other members of this genus that can infect humans include cowpox virus, vaccinia virus, and monkeypox virus.

TRANSMISSION

Smallpox & Vaccinia

In 1980, the World Health Organization (WHO) officially declared smallpox eradicated; however, the threat of reemergence by intentional introduction (e.g., bioterrorism) persists. Before smallpox was eradicated, it spread from person to person principally through respiratory droplets. Contact with infectious skin lesions or scabs was a less common mode of transmission but sometimes occurred (e.g., when caregivers cared for patients or washed contaminated clothing). Rarely, smallpox spread through air in enclosed settings (airborne transmission).

Vaccinia virus is the live virus component of contemporary smallpox vaccines. One of these vaccines, ACAM2000, is a replication competent vaccinia virus; occasionally, infection occurs from touching the fluid or crust material from the inoculation lesion of someone recently vaccinated against smallpox, or from touching contaminated materials like sheets and towels. Human infections with vaccinia virus have occurred in Brazil, Colombia, and India after contact with agricultural animals, often bovids, infected with sylvatic vaccinia-like viruses.

Cowpox

Contrary to the disease name, wild rodents are considered the reservoirs for cowpox virus. Mammals (e.g., cats, cows, humans) are incidental hosts. Cowpox virus infection occurs after direct contact with infected animals including incidental hosts. Person-to-person transmission has not been observed.

Monkeypox

Small mammals, not monkeys, are the suspected reservoir for monkeypox virus. Historically, people at increased risk for transmission have had contact with infected wildlife or wildlife products, infected humans, or the bodily fluids or respiratory droplets from infected wildlife or people. Person-to-person spread of monkeypox virus can occur through exposure to respiratory secretions and through direct skin-to-skin contact with a lesion or lesions (including scabs). Contact with infectious materials (e.g., shared towels, bedding) is another, albeit less common, means of interpersonal spread. In 2022, a global, multinational monkeypox outbreak began; through August 2022, most cases had occurred among men who have sex with men and were predominately due to close skin-to-skin contact (including that which occurs during sex).

EPIDEMIOLOGY

Smallpox & Vaccinia

The last documented case of naturally occurring (endemic) smallpox was in 1977. A single confirmed case of smallpox today could be the result of an intentional act (bioterrorism) and would be considered a global public health emergency.

Infections with wild vaccinia-like viruses have been reported among cattle and buffalo herders in India and among dairy workers in southern Brazil and Colombia. Travelers touching affected bovines might acquire a localized, cutaneous infection. Immunosuppressed people or people with certain skin conditions are at an increased risk for developing systemic illness.

Cowpox

Human infections with cowpox virus and cowpox-like viruses have been reported in Europe and the Caucasus (e.g., cowpox and Akhmeta viruses in Georgia). Travelers having direct contact with infected bovines, felines, rodents (including pet rats), or captive exotic animals (e.g., zoo animals) can be at risk for cutaneous infection.

Monkeypox

Monkeypox is endemic to the tropical forested regions of West and Central Africa, notably the Congo Basin. Most cases are reported from the Democratic Republic of the Congo (DRC), where monkeypox was first recognized as a human disease in 1970. Travelers (including immigrants and refugees) leaving the DRC could be infected with monkeypox virus, but reports of disease imported from the DRC are rare.

In 2003, small mammals imported from Africa were the source of a human monkeypox outbreak in the United States. The infected, imported animals were housed with domestic prairie dogs being sold as pets. At least 37 people were infected.

Increases in human monkeypox cases across multiple African countries have occurred over the last few years in Cameroon, Central African Republic, Côte d'Ivoire, Gabon, Liberia, Nigeria, Republic of the Congo, and Sierra Leone. In many of these countries, decades had passed before new cases were detected. During 2018–2021, Nigeria was implicated as the country of origin for 8 cases of exported monkeypox in humans: 4 cases were diagnosed in people who traveled to the United Kingdom; 2 others traveled to the United States; 1 to Singapore; and 1 to Israel. In the United Kingdom, secondary cases occurred among family members of one of the patients and in a health care provider.

Most recently, a global monkeypox outbreak began in May 2022. On July 23, the WHO declared the outbreak a Public Health Emergency of International Concern, and on August 4, the United States declared the ongoing spread of the virus to be a public health emergency. As of August 2022, the outbreak had caused tens of thousands of cases in >90 countries, predominately among men who have sex with men; as previously noted, transmission has been associated with close skin-to-skin contact.

CLINICAL PRESENTATION

Table 5-20 summarizes key clinical characteristics of orthopoxvirus infections in humans. Immunocompromised patients or people with exfoliative skin conditions (e.g., atopic dermatitis or eczema) are at greater risk for severe illness or death. Ocular infections, although rare, have caused permanent corneal scarring. Poor pregnancy outcomes, including fetal death, have been observed when pregnant people have had variola or monkeypox virus infections.

Smallpox

Clinical signs and symptoms include acute onset of fever >101°F (38.3°C), head and body aches, malaise, and sometimes vomiting, then a characteristic, disseminated rash of firm, deep-seated vesicles or pustules in the same stage of development on

5

Table 5-20 Clinical characteristics of smallpox, cowpox, vaccinia (naturally occurring) and similar orthopoxviruses, and monkeypox

CLINICAL CHARACTERISTIC	SMALLPOX	COWPOX, VACCINIA, OR SIMILAR ORTHOPOXVIRUSES	MONKEYPOX	
			CLASSICAL	2022 OUTBREAK
INCUBATION PERIOD (DAYS)	7–19	2–4	4–17	Subject to change as the outbreak evolves
FEVER	Yes Febrile prodrome before lesions	Yes Often coincides with lesions	Yes Febrile prodrome before lesions	Not consistently reported
MALAISE	Yes	Yes	Yes	Not consistently reported
HEADACHE	Yes	Yes	Yes	Not consistently reported
LYMPHADENOPATHY	No	Yes	Yes	Not consistently reported
LESION DISTRIBUTION	Centrifugally disseminated Often present on palms/soles	Often localized to hands, face, and neck due to contact transmission	Centrifugally disseminated Present on the palms/soles	Often affecting anogenital region but also affecting face and extremities Sometimes present on palms/soles
LESION CHARACTERISTICS	Deep-seated, profound, well circumscribed, often with a central point of umbilication Rash progresses slowly from macule to papule to vesicle to pustule to crust, over 2–4 weeks			

each affected body site. Clinically, varicella is the most common rash illness likely to be confused with smallpox (see Sec. 5, Part 2, Ch. 24, Varicella / Chickenpox). Lesions on the palms or soles and a centrifugal distribution of lesions on the body, which are characteristic of smallpox, can sometimes help distinguish orthopoxvirus infection from varicella.

Cowpox & Vaccinia

Human infections with cowpox, cowpox-like viruses, vaccinia, and wild vaccinia-like viruses are most often self-limited, characterized by localized vesicular-pustular lesions, which in cowpox occasionally are ulcerative. Fever and other constitutional symptoms might occur briefly after lesions first appear. Lesions can be painful and persist for weeks.

5

Monkeypox

As with smallpox, a person infected with monkeypox virus classically experiences a febrile prodrome (characterized by high fever, malaise, headache, or back pain) followed by a widespread, characteristic, vesiculopustular rash that sometimes involves the palms and soles. Marked lymphadenopathy is common in classic presentations of monkeypox, distinguishing it from smallpox.

Cases associated with the worldwide outbreak that began in 2022 have exhibited a different clinical presentation than classic monkeypox. During the outbreak, rash lesions have been reported as being smaller and less diffusely spread; multiple lesions locally scattered over specific parts of the body or only a single lesion have been observed. In many cases, lesions have involved the anogenital area and caused pain and proctitis. The illness has been self-limited and most patients have not required hospitalization; some deaths have been reported, however.

DIAGNOSIS

PCR testing or virus isolation can confirm an orthopoxvirus infection. Do not send laboratory specimens to CDC without a prior consultation. Guidance on preparation and collection of specimens and other clinically relevant issues can be found at www.cdc.gov/poxvirus/monkeypox/clinicians/index.html and www.cdc.gov/smallpox/clinicians/index.html.

Monkeypox

During the 2022 monkeypox outbreak, public health laboratories and multiple commercial laboratories in the United States tested specimens prior to sending samples to CDC for additional characterization or specialized tests. CDC provides laboratory testing and consultation with monkeypox subject matter experts when requested.

Particularly during the 2022 outbreak, clinicians have confused monkeypox (in part due to its atypical presentation) with infections that can present similarly. Evaluate patients for these other infections as well as monkeypox. Moreover, co-infections with a sexually transmitted infection (e.g., syphilis) or with varicella have been known to occur. CDC is frequently updating its clinical guidance and management recommendations during the global monkeypox outbreak; see www.cdc.gov/poxvirus/monkeypox/clinicians/clinical-guidance.html for current information.

TREATMENT

Treatment of orthopoxvirus infections is mainly supportive care through hydration, nutritional supplementation, and prevention of secondary infections. To diminish the chances of spreading virus to other parts of the body or to other people, keep all pox lesions covered until the scab detaches; advise patients to avoid touching their eyes before proper hand washing. Managing orthopoxvirus infections in patients at high risk for severe outcomes (e.g., immunocompromised people, those with underlying skin conditions, those with eye involvement) can be challenging. Topical antivirals (e.g., trifluridine drops) have been used to treat ocular involvement. Tecovirimat (TPOXX), brincidofovir (Tembexa), and vaccinia immune globulin have been licensed by the US Food and Drug Administration to treat smallpox or vaccinia complications and are stocked in the US government's Strategic National Stockpile (SNS).

Monkeypox

During the 2022 global outbreak, health care providers have used Tecovirimat to treat patients with monkeypox. Anecdotally, use of this drug has been associated with shorter illness courses, although more evaluations are needed to better understand its role in treatment. Tecovirimat is available through a CDC–sponsored Investigational New Drug protocol for the treatment of monkeypox.

PREVENTION

To reduce the chances of contracting monkeypox and other orthopoxvirus infections, travelers should avoid contact with sick or dead animals, including wild animals, pets, and domestic ruminants (e.g., buffalo, cattle). They should also avoid direct contact with ill humans.

Two vaccines are licensed for the prevention of smallpox in the United States. People at occupational risk for orthopoxvirus infection (e.g., laboratorians who work with variola, monkeypox, or vaccinia viruses; military personnel who travel to regions in the world where variola virus could be encountered) are vaccinated for preexposure prophylaxis. The Advisory Committee on Immunization Practices only recommends preexposure prophylaxis for people at occupational risk for orthopoxvirus infection (e.g., because of health care delivery to a patient or laboratory work involving orthopoxviruses). Members of the US military might be required to receive the vaccine.

Monkeypox

Monkeypox is not considered a sexually transmitted infection, but it can be transmitted through close, sustained, physical contact, including sexual contact. Vaccinations might be recommended for people having direct or indirect exposure to a person with monkeypox; because of the evolving nature of the 2022 global outbreak, refer to the CDC website (www.cdc.gov/poxvirus/monkeypox/clinicians/vaccines/index.html) for the latest updates. Additional prevention strategies associated with safer sex, social gatherings, and monkeypox, can be found at www.cdc.gov/poxvirus/monkeypox/prevention/sexual-health.html.

CDC websites: www.cdc.gov/poxvirus/index.html; www.cdc.gov/smallpox/index.html

5

BIBLIOGRAPHY

Adler H, Gould S, Hine P, Snell LB, Wong W, Houlihan CF, et al. Clinical features and management of human monkeypox: a retrospective observational study in the UK. Lancet Infect Dis. 2022;22(8):1153–62.

Campe H, Zimmermann P, Glos K, Bayer M, Bergemann H, Dreweck C, et al. Cowpox virus transmission from pet rats to humans, Germany. Emerg Infect Dis. 2009;15(5):777–80.

Durski KN, McCollum AM, Nakazawa Y, Petersen BW, Reynolds MG, Briand S, et al. Emergence of monkeypox—West and Central Africa, 1970–2017. MMWR Morb Mortal Wkly Rep. 2018;67(10):306–10.

McCollum AM, Damon IK. Human monkeypox. Clin Infect Dis. 2014;58(2):260–7.

Petersen BW, Harms TJ, Reynolds MG, Harrison LH. Use of vaccinia virus smallpox vaccine in laboratory and health care personnel at risk for occupational exposure to orthopoxviruses—recommendations of the Advisory Committee on Immunization Practices (ACIP), 2015. MMWR Morb Mortal Wkly Rep. 2016;65(10):257–62.

Philpott D, Hughes CM, Alroy KA, Kerins JL, Pavlick J, Asbel L, et al. Epidemiologic and Clinical Characteristics of Monkeypox Cases—United States, May 17–July 22, 2022. MMWR Morb Mortal Wkly Rep. 2022;71(32):1018–22.

Trindade GS, Guedes MI, Drumond BP, Mota BE, Abrahao JS, Lobato ZI, et al. Zoonotic vaccinia virus: clinical and immunological characteristics in a naturally infected patient. Clin Infect Dis. 2009;48(3):e37–40.

TICK-BORNE ENCEPHALITIS

Susan Hills, Carolyn Gould, Caitlin Cossaboom

INFECTIOUS AGENT: Tick-borne encephalitis (TBE) virus	
ENDEMICITY	Western and northern Europe, extending to northern and eastern Asia
TRAVELER CATEGORIES AT GREATEST RISK FOR EXPOSURE & INFECTION	Adventurous eaters Expatriates living in endemic areas Travelers participating in outdoor activities in forested areas
PREVENTION METHODS	Avoid tick bites Practice safe food precautions and avoid unpasteurized dairy products Tick-borne encephalitis is a vaccine-preventable disease
DIAGNOSTIC SUPPORT	State health department; or contact CDC Arboviral Diseases Branch (www.cdc.gov/ncezid/dvbd/specimensub/arboviral-shipping.html; 970-221-6400; dvbid@cdc.gov)

INFECTIOUS AGENT

Tick-borne encephalitis (TBE) virus is a single-stranded RNA virus that belongs to the genus *Flavivirus*. TBE virus has 3 main subtypes: European, Far Eastern, and Siberian.

TRANSMISSION

TBE virus is transmitted to humans through the bite of an infected tick of the *Ixodes* species, primarily *I. ricinus* (European subtype) or *I. persulcatus* (Far Eastern and Siberian subtypes). Preferred habitats for these tick species include the edges of forests, areas with deciduous or coniferous trees, and low-growing dense brush and other vegetation. Ticks act as both the vector and virus reservoir, and small rodents are the primary amplifying host. People also can acquire TBE by ingesting unpasteurized dairy products (e.g., milk, cheese) from infected cows, goats, or sheep. Infrequently, TBE virus transmission has been reported through laboratory exposure and slaughtering viremic animals. Direct person-to-person spread of TBE virus occurs only rarely, through blood transfusion, solid organ transplantation, or breastfeeding.

EPIDEMIOLOGY

TBE is focally endemic in a geographic region spreading from western and northern Europe through to northern and eastern Asia. Approximately 5,000–10,000 TBE cases are reported from endemic countries each year, with large annual fluctuations. The number of human TBE cases reported from an area might not be a reliable predictor of a traveler's risk for infection because reporting of local cases depends on various factors, including the intensity of diagnosis and surveillance and the vaccine coverage in the population.

Russia, including Siberia, has the most reported cases. The highest disease incidence in recent years has been reported from the Baltic states (Estonia, Latvia, Lithuania), Czech Republic, and Slovenia. Other European countries with reported cases or known endemic areas include Austria, Belarus, Belgium, Bosnia, Bulgaria, Croatia, Denmark, Finland, France, Germany, Hungary, Italy, Liechtenstein, Moldova, Netherlands, Norway, Poland, Romania, Serbia, Slovakia, Sweden, Switzerland, Ukraine, and the United Kingdom. Asian countries with reported

TBE cases or virus activity include China, Japan, Kazakhstan, Kyrgyzstan, Mongolia, and South Korea.

Attack Rate Among Travelers

TBE virus transmission is highly variable by place and over time, and tick population density and infection rates in TBE virus–endemic areas are not consistent. The risk for TBE virus infection for an individual traveler is greatly affected by their planned itinerary and activities. Most infections result from tick bites acquired in forested areas while bicycling, birdwatching, camping, fishing, hiking, or collecting berries, flowers, or mushrooms. People with outdoor occupations, (e.g., farmers, forestry workers, military personnel training in forested areas) are also at increased risk. The risk is negligible for people who remain in urban or unforested areas and who do not consume unpasteurized dairy products.

During 2000–2020, 11 cases of TBE were reported among US civilian travelers. Of these, 10 (91%) cases occurred among males, and most (73%) were in people >19 years old. Destinations where infections likely were acquired included China, Russia, and several countries in Europe. During 2012–2020, an additional 9 TBE cases were reported among US military personnel or their dependents residing in Germany.

Travelers at risk for TBE virus infection might also be at risk for other tickborne diseases because the same ticks that transmit TBE virus also can transmit other pathogens, including *Borrelia burgdorferi* (the agent for Lyme disease), *Anaplasma phagocytophilum* (anaplasmosis), and *Babesia* spp. (babesiosis); simultaneous infection with multiple organisms has been described.

Seasonality & Geographic Range

Most TBE cases occur during April–November, with peaks in early and late summer when ticks are most active. Most cases occur in areas <2,500 ft (≈750 m) in elevation. During the past 30 years, the range of TBE virus transmission appears to have expanded to new geographic areas and to higher elevations; the virus has been found at ≥5,000 ft (≈1,500 m). These trends are likely due to a complex combination of changes in diagnostics and surveillance, changes in human activities, and other socioeconomic, ecologic, and climatic factors.

CLINICAL PRESENTATION

Most (≈2/3) infections are asymptomatic. The median incubation period for TBE is 8 days (range 2–28 days). Acute neuroinvasive disease is the most recognized clinical manifestation of TBE virus infection. Often, however, TBE presents with milder disease forms or a biphasic course.

Phases

The first phase of TBE is characterized by a nonspecific febrile illness sometimes accompanied by anorexia, headache, malaise, myalgia, and nausea, vomiting, or both. This phase usually lasts for several days and might be followed by an afebrile and relatively asymptomatic period. For patients who progress to more severe clinical illness, the second phase reflects central nervous system involvement, specifically aseptic meningitis, encephalitis, or meningoencephalomyelitis. Clinical findings can include altered mental status, ataxia, cognitive dysfunction, cranial nerve palsies, limb paresis, meningeal signs, rigidity, seizures, and tremors.

Sequelae

TBE disease severity increases with age; incidence and disease severity are greatest in people aged ≥50 years. Although TBE tends to be less severe in children, residual symptoms and neurologic deficits have been described. Clinical course and long-term outcome vary by TBE virus subtype, although some of the reported differences could be due to access to medical care, or testing or methodologic biases in published reports.

The European subtype is associated with milder disease, a case-fatality ratio of <2%, and neurologic sequelae in ≤30% of patients. The Far Eastern subtype is often associated with a more severe disease course, including a case-fatality ratio of 20%–40% among neurologic disease cases and higher rates of severe sequelae. The Siberian subtype has a case-fatality ratio of 6%–8%, with rare reports of cases with slow or chronic progression over months.

DIAGNOSIS

Suspect TBE in travelers who develop a nonspecific febrile illness that progresses to neuroinvasive disease ≤4 weeks after arriving from an endemic area. A history of tick bite might suggest TBE diagnosis; ≈30% of TBE patients do not recall a tick bite, however.

Serology

Serology is typically used for laboratory diagnosis. IgM-capture ELISA performed on serum or cerebrospinal fluid is almost always positive during the neuroinvasive phase of the illness. When interpreting results, consider the patient's vaccination history, date of symptom onset, and information about other flaviviruses known to circulate in the same geographic area that might cross-react with serologic assays.

5

Nucleic Acid Amplification Testing

During the first phase of the illness, TBE virus or viral RNA sometimes can be detected. By the time neurologic symptoms are recognized, however, the virus or viral RNA is usually undetectable. Therefore, virus isolation and reverse transcription PCR (RT-PCR) testing should not be used to rule out TBE diagnosis. No commercially available tests can diagnose TBE. Contact the state or local health department or the Centers for Disease Control and Prevention (CDC) Arboviral Diseases Branch, Division of Vector-Borne Diseases (970-221-6400), for assistance with diagnostic testing.

TREATMENT

No specific antiviral treatment is available for TBE. Therapy consists of supportive care and management of complications.

PREVENTION

Personal Protective Measures

Travelers should avoid consuming unpasteurized dairy products and use all measures to avoid tick bites (see Sec. 4, Ch. 6, Mosquitoes, Ticks & Other Arthropods).

Vaccine

In August 2021, the US Food and Drug Administration approved Pfizer's TICOVAC as the first TBE vaccine for use in the United States. Also marketed as FSME-IMMUN in Europe, TICOVAC is an inactivated, whole-virus vaccine with formulations for children (1–15 years) and adults (≥16 years). Five other TBE vaccines, not licensed for use in the United States, are available internationally.

INDICATIONS FOR USE

The risk for most US travelers visiting TBE-endemic areas is very low. Based on activities, destination, duration of travel, and season, some people who travel abroad are at increased risk for infection (Box 5-06). In February 2022, the Advisory Committee on Immunization Practices approved recommendations for vaccine use among people traveling or moving to a TBE-endemic area who will have extensive tick

BOX 5-06 Factors that increase the risk for tick-borne encephalitis (TBE) virus infection among travelers

Travel during the warmer spring and summer months when ticks are more active

Participating in recreational outdoor activities (e.g., camping, fishing, hiking, hunting) in or near tick habitats

Working in outdoor settings (e.g., farming, forestry work, field research) where there is an increased risk of contact with infected ticks

Longer stays in, or repeated travel to, endemic areas might increase a traveler's likelihood for exposure to TBE virus. The specific activities undertaken while in those areas, however, represent a more important risk for infection than time spent abroad.

BOX 5-07 Risk–benefit considerations for vaccination against tick-borne encephalitis (TBE)

RISK FOR TBE VIRUS EXPOSURE & INFECTION

Travelers most likely to be at greater risk for exposure and infection include both shorter-term (e.g., <1 month) travelers with daily or frequent exposure, and longer-term travelers with regular (e.g., a few times a month) exposure

Likelihood of exposure to TBE virus-infected ticks depends on activities and itinerary, including specific destination, rural vs. urban, season, duration

Future (additional) travel to TBE-endemic areas can also increase risk for exposure and infection

SEVERITY OF TBE DISEASE

Rare occurrence of TBE vs. potentially high morbidity and mortality

Increased risk for severe disease among certain populations (e.g., travelers ≥50 years old)

Individual perception and tolerance of risk for a potentially severe disease

VACCINE-ASSOCIATED RISKS

Availability of a vaccine with good long-term immunogenicity and safety profile

Possibility (but low probability) for serious adverse events from the vaccine

exposure based on planned outdoor activities and itinerary. In addition, consider TBE vaccine for people traveling or moving to a TBE-endemic area who might engage in outdoor activities in areas where ticks are likely to be found. Base a recommendation to vaccinate on an assessment of planned activities and itinerary, risk factors for a poorer medical outcome, and personal perception and tolerance of risk (Box 5-07).

ADMINISTRATION

Dose and primary vaccination schedule vary by age (Table 5-21). Each dose is administered intramuscularly.

SAFETY & ADVERSE REACTIONS

Although TICOVAC has only recently been licensed in the United States, the current vaccine formulation has been available internationally for >20 years, and >75 million doses have been administered with no serious safety concerns identified. Adverse events reported most commonly include tenderness and pain at the injection site in ≥10% of vaccine recipients. In children and adolescents, the most common systemic symptoms include fever, headache, and restlessness; in adults, headache, fatigue, and myalgia. Serious adverse events are reported only rarely.

Table 5-21 TICOVAC tick-borne encephalitis (TBE) vaccine administration schedule

AGE	DOSE	PRIMARY VACCINATION SCHEDULE	BOOSTER
1–15 years	0.25 mL	DOSE 1: Day 0 DOSE 2: 1–3 months after DOSE 1 DOSE 3: 5–12 months after DOSE 2	≥3 years after completion of primary immunization series if ongoing exposure or reexposure to TBE virus is expected
≥16 years	0.5 mL	DOSE 1: Day 0 DOSE 2: 14 days–3 months after DOSE 1 DOSE 3: 5–12 months after DOSE 2	≥3 years after completion of primary immunization series if ongoing exposure or reexposure to TBE virus is expected

CONTRAINDICTIONS & PRECAUTIONS

A severe allergic reaction to any component of TICOVAC is a contraindication to administration. Some individuals with altered immunocompetence might have reduced immune responses to TICOVAC, and immunocompromise and immunosuppression are precautions to vaccination. No studies have assessed the safety of TICOVAC in people who are pregnant or lactating.

CDC website: www.cdc.gov/tick-borne-encephalitis/index.html

BIBLIOGRAPHY

Centers for Disease Control and Prevention. Tick-borne encephalitis among US travelers to Europe and Asia—2000–2009. MMWR Morb Mortal Wkly Rep. 2010;59:335–8.

Hills SL, Broussard KR, Broyhill JC, Shastry LG, Cossaboom CM, White JL, et al. Tick-borne encephalitis among US travellers, 2010–20. J Travel Med. 2022;29(2):taab167.

Kunze U. Report of the 21st annual meeting of the International Scientific Working Group on Tick-Borne Encephalitis (ISW-TBE): TBE-record year 2018. Ticks Tick Borne Dis. 2020;11:101287.

Mancuso JD, Bazaco S, Stahlman S, Clausen SS, Cost AA. Tick-borne encephalitis surveillance in U.S. military service members and beneficiaries, 2006–2018. MSMR. 2019;26:4–10.

Ruzek D, Avšič Županc T, Borde J, Chrdle A, Eyer L, Karganova G, et al. Tick-borne encephalitis in Europe and Russia: Review of pathogenesis, clinical features, therapy, and vaccines. Antiviral Res. 2019;164:23–51.

Steffen R. Epidemiology of tick-borne encephalitis (TBE) in international travellers to Western/Central Europe and conclusions on vaccination recommendations. J Travel Med. 2016;23(4):taw018.

Suss J. Tick-borne encephalitis 2010: epidemiology, risk areas, and virus strains in Europe and Asia—an overview. Ticks Tick Borne Dis. 2011;2:2–15.

Taba P, Schmutzhard E, Forsberg P, Lutsar I, Ljostad U, Mygland A, et al. EAN consensus review on prevention, diagnosis, and management of tick-borne encephalitis. Eur J Neurol. 2017;24:1214-e61.

World Health Organization. Vaccines against tick-borne encephalitis: WHO position paper. Wkly Epidemiol Rec. 2011;86:241–56.

5

VARICELLA / CHICKENPOX

Mona Marin, Jessica Leung

INFECTIOUS AGENT: Varicella-zoster virus	
ENDEMICITY	Worldwide
TRAVELER CATEGORIES AT GREATEST RISK FOR EXPOSURE & INFECTION	Travelers without evidence of immunity
PREVENTION METHODS	Varicella is a vaccine-preventable disease
DIAGNOSTIC SUPPORT	A clinical laboratory certified in moderate complexity testing; state public health department; or CDC National VZV Laboratory, www.cdc.gov/chickenpox/lab-testing/collecting-specimens.html

INFECTIOUS AGENT

Varicella-zoster virus (VZV) is a member of the *Herpesviridae* family. Humans are the only VZV reservoir, and disease occurs only in humans. After primary infection as varicella (chickenpox), VZV remains latent in the sensory-nerve ganglia and can reactivate later, causing herpes zoster (shingles).

TRANSMISSION

VZV transmission occurs person to person, primarily via the respiratory route, by inhalation of aerosols from vesicular fluid of skin lesions of varicella or herpes zoster; VZV also can spread by direct contact with the vesicular fluid of skin lesions and possibly infected respiratory tract secretions. VZV enters the host through the upper respiratory tract or the conjunctiva. Varicella is a highly contagious viral disease with secondary attack ratios of ≈85% (range 61%–100%) in susceptible household contacts; contagiousness after community exposure is lower. Herpes zoster is ≈20% as infectious as varicella; in susceptible people, contact with herpes zoster rash causes varicella, not herpes zoster.

Virus communicability from patients with varicella begins ≈1–2 days before the onset of rash and ends when all lesions are crusted, typically 4–7 days after onset of rash in immunocompetent people; communicability might be longer in immunocompromised people. Vaccinated people who get chickenpox might develop lesions that do not crust. These people are considered contagious until no new lesions have appeared for 24 hours. Patients with herpes zoster are contagious while they have active, vesicular lesions (usually 7–10 days). In utero infection also can occur due to transplacental passage of the virus during maternal varicella infection.

EPIDEMIOLOGY

Varicella occurs worldwide. In temperate climates, varicella tends to be a childhood disease, with peak incidence among preschool and school-aged children; <5% of adults are susceptible to varicella. Disease typically occurs during late winter and early spring. In tropical climates, by contrast, infection tends to be more common later in childhood, with greater susceptibility among adults than in temperate climates, especially in less densely populated areas. The highest incidence of disease in tropical climates occurs during the driest, coolest months.

With the implementation of the childhood varicella vaccination program in the United States in 1996, substantial declines in disease incidence have occurred. Although still endemic, the risk for VZV exposure is now lower in the United States than in most other parts of the world. As of 2019, 18% of countries have introduced a routine varicella vaccination program, and an additional 6% have varicella vaccination programs for risk groups only.

Because varicella is endemic worldwide, all susceptible travelers are at risk for infection during travel. Additionally, exposure to herpes zoster poses a risk for varicella in susceptible travelers, although localized herpes zoster is much less contagious than varicella. Infants, adults, and immunocompromised people without evidence of immunity are at highest risk for severe varicella (see Box 5-08 for acceptable evidence of immunity).

CLINICAL PRESENTATION

Varicella is generally a mild disease in children, and most people recover without serious complications. The average incubation period is 14–16 days (range 10–21 days). Infection often is characterized by a short (1- or 2-day) prodromal period (fever, malaise), which might be absent in

BOX 5-08 Acceptable evidence of immunity to varicella

Birth in the United States before 1980 (not acceptable criterion for health care personnel, immunocompromised people, or pregnant people)

Documentation of age-appropriate vaccination
- Preschool-aged children (≥12 months through 3 years of age): 1 dose
- School-aged children (≥4 years of age), adolescents, and adults: 2 doses

Health care provider's diagnosis of varicella or verification of a history of varicella

Health care provider's diagnosis of herpes zoster or verification of a history of herpes zoster

Laboratory evidence of immunity or laboratory confirmation of disease children, and a generalized pruritic rash. The rash consists of crops of macules, papules, and vesicles (typically 250–500 lesions), which first appear on the chest, back, and face, then spread over the entire body in ≥3 successive waves and resolve by crusting. A characteristic of varicella is the presence of lesions in different stages of development at the same time.

Serious complications can occur, most commonly in infants, adults, and immunocompromised people. Complications include cerebellar ataxia, encephalitis, hemorrhagic conditions, pneumonia, and secondary bacterial infections of skin lesions, sometimes resulting in bacteremia or sepsis; rarely (≈1 in 40,000 varicella cases), these complications can cause death.

5

Modified varicella, also known as breakthrough varicella, can occur in vaccinated people. Breakthrough varicella is usually mild, with <50 lesions, low or no fever, and shorter duration for rash. The rash could be atypical in appearance, with fewer vesicles and predominance of maculopapular lesions. Breakthrough varicella is contagious, although less so than varicella in unvaccinated people.

DIAGNOSIS

Varicella is a nationally notifiable disease in the United States. Often based on an appropriate exposure history and the presence of a generalized maculopapulovesicular rash, the clinical diagnosis of varicella in the United States has become increasingly challenging because a growing number of cases now occur in vaccinated people in whom disease is mild and rash is atypical. Although not routinely performed, laboratory diagnosis is becoming increasingly useful. State public health and commercial laboratories can perform diagnostic tests for laboratory confirmation of varicella. See Collecting Specimens for Varicella-Zoster Virus (VZV) Testing (www.cdc.gov/chickenpox/lab-testing/collecting-specimens.html) for additional information on specimen collection and testing for varicella.

Nucleic Acid Amplification Testing

For laboratory confirmation, skin lesions are the preferred specimen source. Vesicular swabs or scrapings and scabs from crusted lesions can be used to identify varicella-zoster virus DNA by PCR testing (the preferred method because it is the most sensitive and specific) or direct fluorescent antibody. In the absence of vesicles or scabs, collect scrapings of maculopapular lesions for testing.

Serologic Testing

Serologic tests also can be used to confirm disease but are less reliable than PCR or direct fluorescent antibody methods for virus identification. A substantial rise in serum varicella IgG titers from acute- and convalescent-phase samples by any standard serologic assay can confirm a diagnosis retrospectively; these antibody tests might not be reliable in immunocompromised people. Additionally, in vaccinated people, baseline IgG levels might be high; thus, a 4-fold increase in convalescent serum samples might not be achieved. Of note, testing for varicella-zoster IgM by using commercial kits is not recommended, because available methods lack sensitivity and specificity; false-positive IgM results are common in the presence of high IgG levels. A positive IgM also does not distinguish between primary infection and reactivation.

TREATMENT

Treatment with antiviral medications is not recommended routinely for otherwise healthy children with varicella. Consider oral acyclovir treatment for people at increased risk for moderate to severe disease (e.g., people >12 years old); people with chronic cutaneous or pulmonary disorders; people who are receiving long-term salicylate therapy; people who are receiving short, intermittent, or aerosolized courses of corticosteroids; and possibly secondary cases among household contacts. Intravenous acyclovir is recommended for immunocompromised people, including patients being treated with high-dose corticosteroids for ≥2 weeks and people with virally mediated complications (e.g., pneumonia). Therapy initiated within 24 hours of illness onset maximizes efficacy. Do not use aspirin or aspirin-containing products to relieve fever from varicella; also avoid ibuprofen, if possible.

PREVENTION

Vaccine

INDICATIONS FOR USE

In the United States, all people, including those traveling or living abroad, should be assessed for varicella immunity; people who do not have evidence of immunity should receive age-appropriate vaccination if they do not have contraindications to vaccination. Vaccination against varicella is not a requirement for entry into any country, including the United States, but people who do not have evidence of immunity (Box 5-08) should be considered at risk for varicella during international travel.

ADMINISTRATION

Varicella vaccine contains live, attenuated VZV. Single-antigen varicella vaccine is licensed for people aged ≥12 months, and the combination measles-mumps-rubella-varicella (MMRV) vaccine is licensed only for children 1–12 years. CDC recommends varicella vaccine for all people aged ≥12 months without evidence of immunity to varicella who do not have contraindications to the vaccine. For children ≥12 months and <13 years, the recommendation is for 2 doses of vaccine administered ≥3 months apart. Typically, the first dose is given at 12–15 months of age and the second at 4–6 years of age. The second dose can be given before age 4, however, provided ≥3 months have passed since the first dose. For people aged ≥13 years, the recommendation is for 2 doses of vaccine administered ≥4 weeks apart. There is no recommendation for varicella vaccination for infants aged <12 months before international travel.

CONTRAINDICATIONS

Contraindications to vaccination include allergy to vaccine components, immunocompromising conditions or treatments, and pregnancy. When evidence of immunity is uncertain, a possible history of varicella is not a contraindication to varicella vaccination. Vaccine effectiveness is ≈80% after 1 dose and 92%–95% after 2 doses.

SAFETY & ADVERSE REACTIONS

The varicella vaccine is generally well tolerated. The most common adverse events after vaccination are self-limited injection-site reactions (e.g., pain, redness, swelling, soreness). Fever or a varicella-like rash, usually consisting of a few lesions at the injection site or generalized rash with a few lesions, are reported less frequently.

Compared with use of separate MMR and varicella vaccines at the same visit, use of the combination MMRV vaccine is associated with a higher risk for fever and febrile seizures, ≈1 additional febrile seizure for every 2,300–2,600 MMRV vaccine doses administered. Fever and febrile seizures typically occur 5–12 days after the first dose of MMRV; the greatest incidence occurs among children aged 12–23 months. Use of separate MMR and varicella vaccines helps avoid this risk. For detailed information regarding the varicella vaccine, visit CDC's website, Chickenpox (Varicella) Vaccination, www.cdc.gov/chickenpox/vaccination.html.

POSTEXPOSURE PROPHYLAXIS

Vaccine

CDC recommends administering postexposure varicella vaccine to unvaccinated healthy people aged ≥12 months without other evidence of immunity, to prevent or modify the disease. Administer the vaccine as soon as possible ≤5 days after exposure to rash, if the exposed person has no contraindications. Among children, protective efficacy was reported as ≥90% when vaccination occurred ≤3 days of exposure. Administration of a second postexposure dose is recommended for exposed people who previously received 1 dose, so their vaccinations are current and to best protect against future exposures.

Varicella-Zoster Immune Globulin

CDC recommends that people without evidence of immunity who have contraindications to vaccination and who are at risk for severe varicella and complications receive postexposure prophylaxis with varicella-zoster immune globulin. The varicella-zoster immune globulin product licensed in the United States is VariZIG.

People who should receive VariZIG after exposure include immunocompromised people, pregnant people without evidence of immunity, and some neonates and infants. VariZIG provides maximum benefit when administered as soon as possible after exposure, but might be effective if administered as late as 10 days after exposure. In the United States, VariZIG can be obtained from specialty distributors (see https://varizig.com).

If VariZIG is not available, consider administering a single dose (400 mg/kg) of intravenous immune globulin (IVIG) ≤10 days of exposure. In the absence of both VariZIG and IVIG, some experts recommend prophylaxis with acyclovir for people without evidence of immunity who have contraindications to varicella vaccination; the recommended dose is 80 mg/kg/day in 4 divided doses for 7 days, up to a maximum dose of 800 mg 4 times per day, beginning 7–10 days after exposure. Published data on the benefit of acyclovir as postexposure prophylaxis among immunocompromised people are limited.

CDC website: www.cdc.gov/chickenpox/

BIBLIOGRAPHY

American Academy of Pediatrics. Varicella-zoster infections. In: Kimberlin DW, Brady MT, Jackson MA, editors. Red Book: 2018 Report of the Committee on Infectious Diseases, 31st edition. Elk Grove Village (IL): American Academy of Pediatrics; 2018. pp. 869–82.

Centers for Disease Control and Prevention. Updated recommendations for use of VariZIG—United States, 2013. MMWR Morb Mortal Wkly Rep. 2013;62(28):574–6.

Leung J, Lopez AS, Mitchell T, Weinberg M, Lee D, Thieme M, et al. Seroprevalence of varicella-zoster virus in five US-bound refugee populations. J Immigrant Minority Health, 2015;17:310–3.

Lopez A, Leung J, Schmid S, Marin M. Varicella. In: Roush SW, Baldy LM, Kirkconnell Hall MA, editors. Manual for the surveillance of vaccine-preventable diseases. Atlanta: Centers for Disease Control and Prevention; 2018. Available from: www.cdc.gov/vaccines/pubs/surv-manual/chpt17-varicella.html.

Lopez AS, Zhang J, Marin M. Epidemiology of varicella during the 2-dose varicella vaccination program – United States, 2005–2014. MMWR Morb Mortal Wkly Rep. 2016;65:902–5.

Marin M, Broder KR, Temte JL, Snider DE, Seward JF. Use of combination measles, mumps, rubella, and varicella vaccine: recommendations of the Advisory Committee on Immunization Practices (ACIP). MMWR Recomm Rep. 2010;59(RR-3):1–12.

Marin M, Guris D, Chaves SS, Schmid S, Seward JF. Prevention of varicella: recommendations of the Advisory Committee on Immunization Practices (ACIP). MMWR Recomm Rep. 2007;56(RR-4):1–40.

VIRAL HEMORRHAGIC FEVERS

Trevor Shoemaker, Mary Joung Choi

ARENAVIRUSES

INFECTIOUS AGENT: Family *Arenaviridae*	
ENDEMICITY	Sub-Saharan Africa (Lassa, Lujo) South America (Chapare, Guanarito, Junin, Machupo, Sabia) United States (Lymphocytic choriomeningitis virus)
TRAVELER CATEGORIES AT GREATEST RISK FOR EXPOSURE & INFECTION	Travelers to rural areas or farmlands where rodent reservoir species are prevalent Health care workers treating infected patients
PREVENTION METHODS	Avoid areas where rodent reservoirs are present Use standard barrier precautions and personal protective equipment in medical settings
DIAGNOSTIC SUPPORT	Contact state or local health department

BUNYAVIRUSES

INFECTIOUS AGENT: Order *Bunyavirales*	
ENDEMICITY	Sub-Saharan Africa: Crimean-Congo hemorrhagic fever (CCHF, family *Nairoviridae*); Rift Valley fever (RVF, family *Phenuiviridae*) Eastern Europe through Central Asia: CCHF United States: Hantavirus (family *Hantaviridae*)
TRAVELER CATEGORIES AT GREATEST RISK FOR EXPOSURE & INFECTION	Travelers to areas with infected livestock, tick or mosquito vectors, or rodent reservoirs People handling infected raw meat or animal products Health care workers treating patients with CCHF People camping in rural areas or staying in homes infested with rodents or their excrement (hantavirus)
PREVENTION METHODS	Practice safe food precautions; avoid handling, cooking, or eating raw or undercooked meat or animal products Avoid unprotected contact with blood, fluids, or tissues of potentially infected animals; avoid touching sick or dead livestock Avoid mosquito and tick bites Use standard barrier precautions and personal protective equipment in medical settings (CCHF)
DIAGNOSTIC SUPPORT	Contact state or local health department

FILOVIRUSES

INFECTIOUS AGENT: Family *Filoviridae*	
ENDEMICITY	Sub-Saharan Africa Southeast Asia (Reston)
TRAVELER CATEGORIES AT GREATEST RISK FOR EXPOSURE & INFECTION	Travelers to areas where suspected bat reservoir species are prevalent Health care workers treating infected patients People in contact with sick or dead wildlife, or nonhuman primates
PREVENTION METHODS	Practice safe food precautions; avoid handling, cooking, or eating raw or undercooked meat or animal products Avoid touching sick or dead wildlife and nonhuman primates Avoid eating fruit found on the ground Use standard barrier precautions and personal protective equipment in medical settings Ebola is a vaccine-preventable disease (restrictions apply, see text below for details)
DIAGNOSTIC SUPPORT	Contact state or local health department

FLAVIVIRUSES

INFECTIOUS AGENT: Family *Flaviviridae*	
ENDEMICITY	Asia, Europe, former Soviet Union (Tick-borne encephalitis) Egypt, Saudi Arabia (Alkhurma) Southern India (Kyasanur Forest disease) Omsk and neighboring oblasts (Omsk)
TRAVELER CATEGORIES AT GREATEST RISK FOR EXPOSURE & INFECTION	People touching infected livestock or ticks (Alkhurma) Travelers to areas where rodent reservoirs and tick species are prevalent (Omsk) People with recreational or occupational exposure to rural or outdoor settings, or contact with infected ticks or animals (Tick-borne encephalitis, Kyasanur Forest disease, Omsk)
PREVENTION METHODS	Avoid unprotected contact with blood, fluids, or tissues of potentially infected animals (Alkhurma) Avoid tick bites
DIAGNOSTIC SUPPORT	Contact state or local health department

5

INFECTIOUS AGENTS

Viral hemorrhagic fever (VHF) diseases are caused by 3 families (*Arenaviridae*, *Filoviridae*, *Flaviviridae*) and 1 order (*Bunyavirales*) of enveloped RNA viruses. *Arenaviridae* (arenaviruses) include Chapare, Guanarito, Junin, Lassa, and Lujo viruses; lymphocytic choriomeningitis virus (LCMV); and Machupo and Sabia viruses. Viruses in the order *Bunyavirales* include the *Arenaviridae* family viruses, Crimean-Congo hemorrhagic fever (CCHF) virus (family *Nairoviridae*), hantaviruses (family *Hantaviridae*), and Rift Valley fever (RVF) virus (family *Phenuiviridae*). *Filoviridae* (filoviruses) include Ebola, Marburg, and Reston viruses. *Flaviviridae* (flaviviruses) include Alkhurma, Kyasanur Forest disease, Omsk hemorrhagic fever, dengue, and yellow fever viruses. For details on dengue and yellow fever, see the respective chapters in this section.

TRANSMISSION

Human-to-Human

Some VHF viruses (arenaviruses, CCHF virus, filoviruses) spread from person to person by direct contact with symptomatic patients, body fluids, or cadavers, or through inadequate infection control in a hospital setting. In the community, VHF viruses are generally transmitted through direct physical contact of unprotected skin or mucous membranes and the blood or other infectious body fluids of patients in the acute phase of disease or from patients who have died.

After recovery from acute Ebola virus disease (EVD) or Marburg virus disease (MVD), the virus or its RNA persists in some specific body fluids of convalescent patients. Ebola virus RNA has been detected in breast milk up to 21 days after the onset of the disease, and in vaginal secretions up to 33 days after onset. Ebola virus and Marburg virus have been cultured from ocular aqueous humor at 2 and 3 months after disease onset, respectively. Evidence suggests that Ebola and Marburg viruses can be sexually transmitted from a male survivor to his partner months after recovery. In pregnant people with EVD, in utero transmission of Ebola virus to the fetus can occur.

Zoonotic

ARTHROPOD VECTORS

Some bunyaviruses (RVF virus) and flaviviruses (dengue and yellow fever) can be transmitted by the bites of infected mosquitoes. Other bunyaviruses (CCHF virus) and flaviviruses (Alkhurma, Kyasanur Forest disease, and Omsk viruses) can be transmitted by the bites of infected ticks or by crushing infected ticks.

BATS
Bats are suspected reservoir species for filoviruses (Ebola and Marburg viruses) in the genus *Ebolavirus*; the natural reservoir for Marburg virus is the Egyptian fruit bat (*Rousettus aegyptiacus*).

LIVESTOCK
Some bunyaviruses (CCHF and RVF viruses) and flaviviruses (Alkhurma virus) can be transmitted during the slaughter of infected animals or from the consumption of raw meat or unpasteurized milk of an infected animal.

RODENTS & INSECTIVORES
Arenaviruses and some bunyaviruses (hantaviruses) can be transmitted by direct contact with infected animals or from inhalation of, or contact with, materials contaminated with rodent excreta.

EPIDEMIOLOGY
The viruses that cause VHF are distributed over much of the globe. Each virus is associated with ≥1 nonhuman host or vector species, restricting the virus and the initial contamination to the areas inhabited by these species. The diseases caused by these viruses are seen in people who live in or visit these areas. Humans are incidental hosts for these enzootic diseases; person-to-person transmission of some viruses can occur, however.

Arenaviral Diseases
Except Tacaribe virus—which was found in bats but has not been reported to cause disease in humans—arenaviruses are maintained in rodents and transmitted to humans. Most infections are mild, but some result in hemorrhagic fever with high death rates. Arenaviruses are categorized as Old World (Eastern Hemisphere) and New World (Western Hemisphere).

OLD WORLD ARENAVIRUSES
Old World arenaviruses (and the diseases they cause) include Lassa virus (Lassa fever), Lujo virus, and LCMV. In otherwise healthy people, LCMV infection can cause meningitis, encephalitis, and congenital fetal infection; in organ transplant recipients, it is reported to cause severe disease with multiple organ failure. Lassa fever occurs across rural West Africa, with hyperendemic areas in parts of Guinea, Liberia, Nigeria, and Sierra Leone. Lujo virus infection has been described in the Republic of South Africa during a health care–associated outbreak, and in Zambia.

NEW WORLD ARENAVIRUSES
New World arenaviruses (and the diseases they cause) include Chapare virus, Guanarito (Venezuelan hemorrhagic fever), Junin (Argentine hemorrhagic fever), Machupo (Bolivian hemorrhagic fever), and Sabia (Brazilian hemorrhagic fever).

RESERVOIR HOST SPECIES
Reservoir host species of arenaviruses include Old World rats and mice (family *Muridae*, subfamily *Murinae*) and New World rats and mice (family *Muridae*, subfamily *Sigmodontinae*). These rodent types are found worldwide, including Africa, the Americas, Asia, and Europe. Virus is transmitted through inhalation of rodent urine aerosols, ingestion of rodent-contaminated food, or by direct contact of broken skin or mucosa with rodent excreta.

Risk for Lassa virus infection is associated with peridomestic rodent exposure, where inappropriate food storage increases the risk for exposure. Several cases of Lassa fever have been confirmed in international travelers staying in traditional countryside dwellings. Health care–associated transmission and close family member infection with Lassa, Lujo, and Machupo viruses occurs through droplet spread and direct contact.

Bunyaviral Diseases
CRIMEAN-CONGO HEMORRHAGIC FEVER
CCHF is endemic to areas where ticks of the genus *Hyalomma* are found in Africa (including South Africa) and Eurasia (including the Balkans, the Middle East, Russia, and western China). CCHF is highly endemic to Afghanistan, Iran, Pakistan, and Turkey. In 2016, Spain reported its first identified human cases. *Hyalomma* ticks are primarily associated with livestock but will also bite humans.

Livestock and other tick hosts might develop CCHF viremia from tick bites but do not develop clinical disease. CCHF virus is transmitted to humans by infected ticks or by direct handling

5

and preparation of fresh carcasses of infected animals, usually domestic livestock. Human-to-human transmission can occur through droplets or direct contact.

HANTAVIRUS PULMONARY SYNDROME & HEMORRHAGIC FEVER WITH RENAL SYNDROME

Hantaviruses can cause hantavirus pulmonary syndrome (HPS) or hemorrhagic fever with renal syndrome (HFRS). Viruses that cause HPS are found in the Western Hemisphere (North, Central, and South America); those that cause HFRS occur worldwide. The viruses that cause both HPS and HFRS are transmitted to humans through contact with urine, feces, or saliva of infected rodents. Travelers staying in rodent-infested dwellings are at risk for HPS and HFRS. Human-to-human transmission of hantavirus has been reported only with Andes virus in Chile and Argentina. A reported case of imported Andes virus in the United States occurred in 2018 in a traveler returning from Chile and Argentina.

RIFT VALLEY FEVER

RVF primarily affects livestock, causing stillbirths and high mortality in neonatal cattle, goats, and sheep. In humans, RVF virus infection causes fever, hemorrhage, encephalitis, and retinitis. RVF virus is endemic to sub-Saharan Africa. Sporadic outbreaks have occurred in humans in Comoros, Egypt, Madagascar, Mali, Mauritania, Mayotte, Senegal, South Sudan, Sudan, and Uganda. Large epidemics occurred in Madagascar in 1990, and again in 2008; in Kenya, Somalia, and Tanzania during 1997–1998 and 2006–2007; in Saudi Arabia and Yemen in 2000; in Botswana, Mauritania, Namibia, and South Africa in 2010; and in Niger during 2016–2017. RVF virus is transmitted to livestock by mosquitoes; people more frequently become infected through direct contact with clinically affected animals or their body fluids, including through slaughter or consumption of infected animals.

Filoviral Diseases

People at greatest risk of EVD or MVD include family members, health care workers, or others who, without personal protective equipment (PPE), come into direct contact with infected patients or corpses. People who come into close contact or proximity to bats (e.g., those who visit caves or mines with bats) and people who handle infected primates or carcasses are also at risk. A postulated route of infection to humans (as well as to ground-dwelling animals) involves consumption of fallen or dropped fruit contaminated by the saliva or urine of infected, fruit-foraging bats. Additionally, the sexual partners of males who recently survived EVD or MVD might be at risk if they have had contact with virus-infected semen.

EBOLA VIRUS DISEASE

Countries where domestically acquired EVD cases have been reported and that should be considered areas where future epidemics could occur include Côte d'Ivoire, Democratic Republic of the Congo, Gabon, Guinea, Liberia, Republic of the Congo, Sierra Leone, South Sudan, and Uganda.

Prior to 2014, Ebola outbreaks typically had been limited in scope and geographic extent. In March of 2014, however, an outbreak of Ebola virus was detected in a rural area of Guinea near the borders with Liberia and Sierra Leone. By June 2014, cases were reported in all 3 countries and across many districts. Additional cases occurred in Italy, Mali, Nigeria, Senegal, Spain, the United Kingdom, and the United States, after infected people traveled from West Africa. The outbreak was the largest and most complex Ebola epidemic ever reported.

Since the 2014, Ebola outbreaks have been reported in the Democratic Republic of the Congo in 2017, 2018, 2020, and 2021, and in Guinea in 2021. Cases were also reported in Uganda in 2018–2019, and in 2022. Reston virus (in the genus *Ebolavirus*) is believed to be endemic to the Philippines but has not been shown to cause human disease.

MARBURG VIRUS DISEASE

Countries with confirmed human cases of MVD include Angola, Democratic Republic of the Congo, Guinea, Kenya, Uganda, and possibly Zimbabwe. Four cases occurred in travelers visiting caves harboring bats, including Kitum Cave in Kenya and Python Cave in Maramagambo Forest, Uganda. Miners in the Democratic Republic of the

Congo and Uganda have also acquired Marburg virus infection from working in underground mines harboring bats.

CLINICAL PRESENTATION

Signs and symptoms vary by disease, but in general, patients with VHF present with abrupt onset of fever, headache, myalgias, and prostration, followed by coagulopathy with a petechial rash or ecchymoses and sometimes overt bleeding in severe forms. Gastrointestinal symptoms (abdominal pain, diarrhea, vomiting) are commonly observed. Vascular endothelial damage leads to shock and pulmonary edema; liver injury is common.

Syndromic findings associated with specific *Arenaviridae* infections include pharyngitis, retrosternal pain, hearing loss in adults, and anasarca in newborns (Lassa); and spontaneous abortion and birth defects (Lassa fever, LCMV). Syndromic findings associated with specific *Bunyavirales* infections include ecchymoses and bruising (CCHF virus); renal failure (hantavirus, HFRS); and retinitis and partial blindness (RVF). Laboratory abnormalities include elevated liver enzymes, initial drop in leukocyte count, and thrombocytopenia. Because the incubation period can extend up to 21 days, patients might not develop illness until they return from travel; a thorough travel and exposure history is critical.

DIAGNOSIS

Immediately notify local health authorities of any suspected cases of VHF occurring in patients residing in the United States. For laboratory testing requests, notify your local or state health department. To notify the Centers for Disease Control and Prevention (CDC) directly about any patients requiring evacuation to the United States, contact the CDC Emergency Operations Center at 770-488-7100.

Appropriate PPE, including implementation of droplet and contact precautions, is indicated for any patients in whom a VHF is suspected. Airborne transmission of VHF viruses has not been documented in hospitals or households during any of the human outbreaks investigated to date. Certain procedures (e.g., bronchoscopy, endotracheal intubation) might, however, create mechanically generated aerosols that could be infectious. As such, airborne precautions are recommended for aerosol-generating procedures.

Postmortem samples of blood (collected by cardiac puncture) or skin collected within a few hours after death can be used for diagnosis. Whole blood or serum can be used for virologic testing by reverse transcription PCR (RT-PCR), antigen detection, or virus isolation, and to test for immunologic (IgM, IgG) evidence of infection. Skin biopsies fixed in formalin can be tested by immunohistochemistry, RT-PCR, and virus isolation. Consider collecting an oral swab from deceased patients when an alternative sample cannot be collected.

Special handling procedures are required when submitting blood and other body fluid specimens for diagnostic testing. Please contact the CDC Emergency Operations Center at 770-488-7100 for more information.

TREATMENT

The mainstay treatment for VHFs is early and aggressive supportive care directed at maintaining effective intravascular volume and correcting electrolyte imbalances. Convalescent-phase plasma is effective in treating Argentine hemorrhagic fever but is available only in Argentina. Ribavirin is effective if given early in the course of disease for treating Lassa fever and other Old World arenaviruses, New World arenaviruses, and potentially CCHF, but it is not approved for use by the US Food and Drug Administration (FDA) for these indications. Compassionate use intravenous ribavirin can be obtained from Bausch Health; initiate requests by contacting CDC's Viral Special Pathogens Branch (770-488-7100).

Two FDA-approved treatments are available for Ebola virus (species *Zaire ebolavirus*). Ebanga (single monoclonal antibody) and Inmazeb (triple monoclonal antibody cocktail) are both approved to treat acute EVD in adult and pediatric patients. In a randomized clinical control trial, Ebanga reduced mortality rates to 35%, and Inmazeb reduced rates to 33%. Both drugs particularly reduced deaths in patients with low viral loads; mortality rates in patients treated with Ebanga were 9.9% and were 11.2% in patients treated with Inmazeb.

Patients with EVD also might have concomitant malaria infection; consider empiric use of antimalarial therapy when rapid diagnostic testing is not immediately available. In general, avoid administering NSAIDs (e.g., diclofenac, ibuprofen) because of their antiplatelet activity.

PREVENTION

The risk of acquiring a VHF is very low for most international travelers. Travelers at increased risk for exposure include people who engage in animal research, and health care workers and others who do not have adequate PPE when caring for patients in communities where outbreaks are occurring. Prevention should focus on avoiding unprotected contact with sources of infection, including anyone suspected of having VHF, and host or vector species in endemic countries. Travelers should not visit locations where outbreaks are occurring. In addition, travelers should avoid contact with bats and rodents, and avoid blood or body fluids of livestock in RVF- or CCHF-endemic areas. To prevent vectorborne diseases, travelers should use insecticide-treated mosquito nets and use insect repellent (see Sec. 4, Ch. 6, Mosquitoes, Ticks & Other Arthropods).

For VHFs that can be transmitted person to person (EVD, MVD, Lassa Fever, CCHF), early identification and isolation of ill travelers, consistent implementation of basic infection-control measures and prompt notification of public health authorities are the keys to preventing secondary transmission. Early identification strategies include eliciting a travel history from all patients who present for care, and posting signs and placards asking patients with recent international travel to self-identify. Promptly isolate any patients with recent international travel who have symptoms consistent with a VHF by placing them in a private room or a separate enclosed area with a private bathroom or covered bedside commode. To minimize disease transmission risk, only essential health care providers wearing appropriate PPE should evaluate a patient and provide care. Prompt notification of the facility's infection-control program and state and local health departments is also key.

Vaccines

In February 2020, the Advisory Committee on Immunization Practices (ACIP) recommended ERVEBO for preexposure vaccination of adults aged ≥18 years in the United States at risk for Ebola exposure; groups meeting this definition include those responding to outbreaks of EVD due to Ebola virus (species *Zaire ebolavirus*). In November 2021, ACIP expanded its preexposure vaccination recommendations to include health care personnel at federally designated Ebola treatment centers in the United States, and laboratory workers or other staff at Biosafety Level 4 facilities in the United States that handle replication-competent Ebola virus (species *Zaire ebolavirus*).

Investigational vaccines exist for Argentine hemorrhagic fever and RVF, but neither is approved by FDA or commercially available in the United States.

CDC website: www.cdc.gov/vhf

BIBLIOGRAPHY

Bah EI, Lamah MC, Fletcher T, Jacob ST, Brett-Major DM, Sall AA, et al. Clinical presentation of patients with Ebola virus disease in Conakry, Guinea. N Engl J Med. 2015;372(1):40–7.

Centers for Disease Control and Prevention. Ebola (Ebola virus disease)—for clinicians—personal protective equipment (PPE). Available from www.cdc.gov/vhf/ebola/healthcare-us/ppe/index.html.

Choi MJ, Cossaboom CM, Whitesell AN, Dyal JW, Joyce A, Morgan RL, et al. Use of Ebola vaccine: recommendations of the Advisory Committee on Immunization Practices, United States, 2020. MMWR Recomm Rep. 2021;70(1):1–12.

Gunther S, Lenz O. Lassa virus. Crit Rev Clin Lab Sci. 2004;41(4):339–90.

Henao-Restrepo AM, Camacho A, Longini IM, Watson CH, Edmunds WJ, Egger M, et al. Efficacy and effectiveness of an rVSV-vectored vaccine in preventing Ebola virus disease: final results from the Guinea ring vaccination, open-label, cluster-randomised trial (Ebola Ça Suffit!). Lancet 2017;389:505–18.

Heyman P, Vaheri A, Lundkvist A, Avsic-Zupanc T. Hantavirus infections in Europe: from virus carriers to a major public-health problem. Expert Rev Anti Infect Ther. 2009;7(2):205–17.

Mulangu S, Dodd LE, Davey RT Jr, Tshiani Mbaya O, Proschan M, Mukadi D, et al; PALM Writing Group; PALM Consortium Study Team. A randomized, controlled trial of Ebola virus disease therapeutics. N Engl J Med 2019;381:2293–303.

Ozkurt Z, Kiki I, Erol S, Erdem F, Yilmaz N, Parlak M, et al. Crimean-Congo hemorrhagic fever in eastern Turkey: clinical features, risk factors and efficacy of ribavirin therapy. J Infect. 2006;52(3):207–15.

Regules JA, Beigel JH, Paolino KM, Voell J, Castellano AR, Munoz P, et al. A recombinant vesicular stomatitis virus Ebola vaccine—preliminary report. N Engl J Med. 2017;376(4):330–41.

Uyeki TM, Mehta AK, Davey RT Jr., Liddell AM, Wolf T, Vetter P, et al. Clinical management of Ebola virus disease in the United States and Europe. N Engl J Med. 2016;374(7):636–46.

World Health Organization. Clinical care for survivors of Ebola virus disease: interim guidance. Geneva: The Organization; 2016. Available from: https://apps.who.int/iris/handle/10665/204235.

YELLOW FEVER

Mark Gershman, J. Erin Staples

INFECTIOUS AGENT: Yellow fever virus	
ENDEMICITY	Sub-Saharan Africa Tropical South America
TRAVELER CATEGORIES AT GREATEST RISK FOR EXPOSURE & INFECTION	Unimmunized people visiting forested or savannah regions of endemic areas, or visiting destinations with ongoing yellow fever outbreaks
PREVENTION METHODS	Avoid insect bites Yellow fever is a vaccine-preventable disease
DIAGNOSTIC SUPPPORT	State health department; or contact CDC's Arboviral Diseases Branch (www.cdc.gov/ncezid/dvbd/specimensub/arboviral-shipping.html; 970-221-6400; dvbid@cdc.gov)

INFECTIOUS AGENT

Yellow fever (YF) virus is a single-stranded RNA virus that belongs to the genus *Flavivirus*.

TRANSMISSION

Vectorborne transmission of YF virus occurs via the bite of an infected mosquito, primarily *Aedes* or *Haemagogus* spp. Nonhuman primates and humans are the main reservoirs of the virus, and anthroponotic (human-to-vector-to-human) transmission occurs. YF virus has 3 transmission cycles: sylvatic (jungle), intermediate (savannah), and urban.

The sylvatic (jungle) cycle involves transmission of virus between nonhuman primates and mosquito species found in forest canopies. Virus is transmitted from monkeys to humans via mosquitoes when occupational or recreational activities encroach into the jungle. In Africa, an intermediate (savannah) cycle involves transmission of YF virus from tree hole–breeding *Aedes* spp. to humans in jungle border areas. YF virus can be transmitted from monkeys to humans or from human to human via these mosquitoes. The urban cycle involves transmission of virus between humans and peridomestic mosquitoes, primarily *Ae. aegypti*.

Humans infected with YF virus experience the highest levels of viremia shortly before onset of fever and for the first 3–5 days of illness, during which time they can transmit the virus to mosquitoes. Because of the high level of viremia, bloodborne transmission theoretically can occur via transfusion or needlesticks. One case of perinatal transmission of wild-type YF virus from a woman who developed symptoms of YF 3 days prior to delivery has been documented; the infant subsequently tested positive for YF viral RNA and died of fulminant YF on the 12th day of life.

EPIDEMIOLOGY

YF occurs in sub-Saharan Africa and tropical South America, where it is endemic and intermittently epidemic (see Table 5-22 and Table 5-23 for lists of countries with risk of YF virus transmission). Most YF disease in humans is due to sylvatic or intermediate transmission cycles. Urban YF occurs periodically in Africa and sporadically in the Americas. In areas of Africa with persistent circulation of YF virus, natural immunity accumulates with age; consequently, infants and children are at greatest risk for disease. In South America, YF occurs most frequently in unimmunized young people exposed to mosquito vectors through their work in forested areas.

RISK FOR TRAVELERS

A traveler's risk for acquiring YF is determined by their immunization status as well as destination-specific (e.g., local rate of virus transmission) and travel-associated (e.g., exposure duration, occupational and recreational activities, season) factors. Reported cases of human disease are the principal but crude indicator of disease risk. Case reports from a destination might be absent because of a low level of transmission, a high level of immunity in the population (e.g., due to vaccination), or failure of local surveillance systems to detect cases. Because "epidemiologic silence" does not mean absence of risk, travelers should not go into endemic areas without taking protective measures.

YF virus transmission in rural West Africa is seasonal; a period of elevated risk occurs at the end of the rainy season and the beginning of the dry season, usually July–October. In East Africa, YF virus transmission is generally less predictable because long periods (years) often pass between virus activity in this region; when YF

Table 5-22 Countries with risk for yellow fever (YF) virus transmission[1]

AFRICA		
Angola	Democratic Republic of the Congo	Mali[2]
Benin	Equatorial Guinea	Mauritania[2]
Burkina Faso	Ethiopia[2]	Niger[2]
Burundi	Gabon	Nigeria
Cameroon	The Gambia	Senegal
Central African Republic	Ghana	Sierra Leone
Chad[2]	Guinea	South Sudan
Congo, Republic of the	Guinea-Bissau	Sudan[2]
Côte d'Ivoire	Kenya[2]	Togo
	Liberia	Uganda
THE AMERICAS		
Argentina[2]	French Guiana	Peru[2]
Bolivia[2]	Guyana	Suriname
Brazil[2]	Panama[2]	Trinidad and Tobago[2]
Colombia[2]	Paraguay	Venezuela[2]
Ecuador[2]		

[1]Current as of November 2022. Defined by the World Health Organization (WHO) as countries or areas where YF "has been reported currently or in the past and vectors and animal reservoirs currently exist." See www.who.int/publications/m/item/countries-with-risk-of-yellow-fever-transmission-and-countries-requiring-yellow-fever-vaccination-(november-2022).
[2]These countries are not holoendemic (only a portion of the country has risk of YF virus + transmission). For details, see Map 5-10, Map 5-11, and YF vaccine recommendations (Sec. 2, Ch. 5, Yellow Fever Vaccine & Malaria Prevention Information, by Country).

Table 5-23 Countries with low potential for exposure to yellow fever (YF) virus[1]

AFRICA		
Eritrea[2] Rwanda	São Tomé and Príncipe Somalia[2]	Tanzania Zambia[2]

[1]The countries on this list have low potential for exposure to YF virus and are not included on the World Health Organization list of countries with risk for YF virus transmission (Table 5-22). Unless a country requires proof of YF vaccination from all arriving travelers (Table 5-25), or specifies otherwise, proof of YF vaccination should not be required for travelers arriving from the countries on this list.

[2]Classified as "low potential for exposure to YF virus" only in some areas; remaining areas are classified as having no risk of exposure to YF virus.

virus transmission occurs in East Africa, seasonality is similar to that in West Africa.

The risk for infection by sylvatic vectors in South America is greatest during the rainy season (January–May, with a peak incidence during February and March). *Ae. aegypti* can transmit YF virus episodically, however—even during the dry season—in both rural and densely settled urban areas.

During 1970–2015, 11 cases of YF were reported in people from the United States and Europe who traveled to West Africa (6 cases) or South America (5 cases); 8 (73%) died. Only 1 traveler had a documented history of YF vaccination; that traveler survived. Starting in 2016, the number of travel-associated YF cases increased substantially, primarily because of outbreaks in Angola and Brazil. During 2016–mid-2021, >37 travel-associated cases were reported in unvaccinated travelers who were residents of nonendemic areas or countries, including ≥15 European travelers and 1 American traveler to Peru.

The risk of acquiring YF during travel is difficult to predict because of variations in ecologic determinants of virus transmission. For a 2-week stay, the estimated risk for illness and for death due to YF for an unvaccinated traveler visiting an endemic area are as follows: for West Africa, risk for illness is 50 per 100,000 and risk for death is 10 per 100,000; for South America, risk for illness is 5 per 100,000 and risk for death is 1 per 100,000. These estimates are based on the risk to resident populations, often during peak transmission season, and might not accurately reflect the risk to travelers who have a different immunity profile, follow mosquito bite precautions, have less outdoor exposure, or who travel during off-peak periods. A traveler's risk for becoming infected is likely greater when outbreaks are occurring at their destination.

CLINICAL PRESENTATION

Most people infected with YF virus have minimal or no symptoms and are unlikely to seek medical attention. For those who develop symptomatic illness, the incubation period is typically 3–6 days. The initial illness is nonspecific: backache, chills, fever, headache, myalgia, nausea and vomiting, and prostration. Most improve after the initial presentation. After a brief remission of ≤48 hours, ≈12% of infected patients progress to a more serious form of the disease, characterized by hemorrhagic symptoms, jaundice, and eventually shock and multisystem organ failure. The case-fatality rate for severe cases is 30%–60%.

DIAGNOSIS

YF is a nationally notifiable disease. A preliminary diagnosis is based on clinical presentation and exposure details. Laboratory diagnosis is best performed by virus isolation or nucleic acid amplification tests (e.g., reverse transcription PCR [RT-PCR]) or by serologic assays. Perform virus isolation or nucleic acid amplification tests for YF virus or YF viral RNA early in the course of the illness. By the time more overt symptoms are recognized, the virus or viral RNA might no longer be detectable; thus, virus isolation and nucleic acid amplification testing should not be used to rule out a diagnosis of YF.

Serologic assays can be used to detect virus-specific IgM and IgG antibodies. Because of the possibility of cross-reactivity between antibodies against other flaviviruses, however, more specific antibody testing (e.g., a plaque reduction neutralization test) should be performed to confirm the infection. Contact your state or local health department or call the Centers for Disease Control and Prevention (CDC) Arboviral Diseases Branch at 970-221-6400 for assistance with diagnostic testing for YF virus infections.

TREATMENT

No specific medications are available to treat YF virus infections; treatment is directed at symptomatic relief or life-saving interventions. Fluids, rest, and use of analgesics and antipyretics might relieve symptoms of aching and fever. Avoid prescribing medications than can increase the risk for bleeding (e.g., aspirin or other nonsteroidal anti-inflammatory drugs). During the first few days of illness, protect infected people from further mosquito exposure by keeping them indoors or under a mosquito net, so they do not contribute to the transmission cycle.

PREVENTION

Personal Protective Measures

The best way to prevent mosquito-borne diseases, including YF, is to avoid mosquito bites (see Sec. 4, Ch. 6, Mosquitoes, Ticks & Other Arthropods).

Vaccine

YF is preventable by a relatively safe, effective vaccine. All YF vaccines currently manufactured are live attenuated viral vaccines. Only one YF vaccine (YF-VAX, Sanofi Pasteur) is licensed for use in the United States (Table 5-24). Periodically in the United States, shortages of YF-VAX have occurred due to production issues, including one that lasted from late 2015 until early 2021. To address this most recent shortage, Sanofi Pasteur collaborated with the CDC and the US Food and Drug Administration (FDA) to import and distribute Stamaril (a YF vaccine comparable to YF-VAX, manufactured at the company's facility in France) under an expanded-access investigational new drug protocol.

The different YF vaccine products, including those manufactured outside the United States, have no substantial differences in reactogenicity or immunogenicity. Consider people who receive YF vaccines licensed in other countries but not approved by the FDA to be protected against YF. For the most current information on YF vaccine availability, check the CDC Travelers' Health website at https://wwwnc.cdc.gov/travel.

INDICATIONS FOR USE

YF vaccine is recommended for people aged ≥9 months who are living in or traveling to areas with risk for YF virus transmission in Africa or South America. In addition, some countries require proof of YF vaccination for entry. For country-specific YF vaccination recommendations and requirements, see Sec. 2, Ch. 5, Yellow Fever Vaccine & Malaria Prevention Information, by Country.

Because of the risk for serious adverse events after YF vaccination, clinicians should only vaccinate people at risk for YF virus exposure or who require proof of vaccination to enter a country. To further minimize the risk for serious adverse events, carefully observe the contraindications and consider vaccination precautions before administering YF vaccine (Box 5-09). For

Table 5-24 Vaccine to prevent yellow fever (YF)

VACCINE	TRADE NAME (MANUFACTURER)	AGE	DOSE	ROUTE	SCHEDULE	BOOSTER
17D	YF-VAX (Sanofi Pasteur)	≥9 months[1]	0.5 mL[2]	Sub-cutaneous	1 dose	Not recommended for most people[3]

[1]Ages 6–8 months and ≥60 years are precautions, and age <6 months is a contraindication to receiving YF vaccine.

[2]YF-VAX is available in single-dose and multiple-dose (5-dose) vials.

[3]For further details regarding revaccination, see Prevention: Vaccine: Booster Doses, in this chapter.

BOX 5-09 Yellow fever vaccine contraindications & precautions

CONTRAINDICATIONS	PRECAUTIONS
Age <6 months Allergy to vaccine component[1] HIV infection (symptomatic) or CD4 T lymphocyte counts <200/mL (or <15% of total lymphocytes in children aged <6 years)[2,3] Primary immunodeficiencies Immunosuppressive and immunomodulatory therapies Malignant neoplasms Thymus disorder associated with abnormal immune cell function Transplantation	Age 6–8 months Age ≥60 years Breastfeeding HIV infection (asymptomatic) and CD4 T lymphocyte counts 200–499/mL (or 15%–24% of total lymphocytes in children aged <6 years)[2,3] Pregnancy

[1]If considering vaccination, desensitization can be performed under direct supervision of a physician experienced in the management of anaphylaxis.

[2]Symptoms of HIV are classified in Centers for Disease Control and Prevention. 1993 Revised classification system for HIV infection and expanded surveillance case definition for AIDS among adolescents and adults. MMWR Recomm Rep 1992;41(RR-17). Available from: www.cdc.gov/mmwr/preview/mmwrhtml/00018871.htm (see Table 1 Adults and Adolescents); and Panel on Antiretroviral Therapy and Medical Management of HIV-Infected Children. Guidelines for the use of antiretroviral agents in pediatric HIV infection 2010. pp. 20–2. Available from: www.hopkinsmedicine.org/som/faculty/appointments/_documents/_ppc_documents/portfolios/Hutton/Hutton-Portfolio-Samples/guidelines-for-the-use-of-antiretroviral-agents-in-pediatric-hiv-infection.pdf.

[3]In 2010, the Advisory Committee on Immunization Practices (ACIP) used this clinical classification of levels of immunosuppression among HIV-infected people to inform yellow fever vaccine recommendations (see Staples et al., Yellow fever vaccine: recommendations of the Advisory Committee on Immunization Practices). A revised surveillance case definition for HIV infection was published in 2014. To date, ACIP has not updated YF vaccine recommendations for people infected with HIV.

additional information, refer to the YF vaccine recommendations of the Advisory Committee on Immunization Practices (ACIP) at www.cdc.gov/vaccines/hcp/acip-recs/vacc-specific/yf.html.

ADMINISTRATION

For all eligible people, subcutaneously administer a single 0.5 mL injection of reconstituted vaccine, which is the standard dose.

COADMINISTRATION WITH OTHER VACCINES

INACTIVATED VACCINES

No evidence exists that inactivated vaccines interfere with the immune response to YF vaccine. Therefore, inactivated vaccines can be administered either simultaneously or at any time before or after YF vaccination.

LIVE ATTENUATED VIRAL VACCINES

ACIP recommends that YF vaccine be given at the same time as other live viral vaccines. If simultaneous administration is not possible, wait 30 days between vaccinations, because the immune response to a live viral vaccine could be impaired if it is administered within 30 days of another live viral vaccine. One study demonstrated that coadministration of YF vaccine and measles-mumps-rubella (MMR) vaccine decreased the seroconversion ratios to all antigens, except measles. Two more recent studies also showed a less robust antibody concentration in people who seroconverted after vaccine coadministration. These studies suggest that whenever possible, it is best to give YF and MMR vaccines 30 days apart. Of greater importance, however, is ensuring that travelers are vaccinated appropriately before travel; coadministration of YF and MMR vaccines is therefore acceptable.

No data are available on the immune response to nasally administered live attenuated influenza vaccine given simultaneously with YF vaccine.

LIVE BACTERIAL VACCINES

Data suggest that oral Ty21a typhoid vaccine (Vivotif), a live bacterial vaccine, can be administered simultaneously or at any interval before or after YF vaccine. No data are available on the immune response to live attenuated oral cholera vaccine (Vaxchora) administered simultaneously with YF vaccine.

FRACTIONAL DOSING

In recent years, several countries have extended vaccine supplies during large YF outbreaks by administering partial vaccine doses, usually 0.1 mL, a practice known as fractional dosing. Limited study data have demonstrated immunogenicity of fractional dosing is comparable to that of full-dose YF vaccination at 1 month and ≤1 year after subcutaneous administration; knowledge gaps regarding fractional dosing remain, however.

In the United States, FDA has not approved fractional dosing of YF vaccine. Furthermore, WHO notes that fractional dosing does not meet YF vaccination requirements under the International Health Regulations (IHR); proof of vaccination for international travel cannot be issued to a person who has received only a fractional dose.

BOOSTER DOSES

In 2014, the WHO Strategic Advisory Group of Experts on Immunization concluded that a single primary dose of YF vaccine provides sustained immunity and lifelong protection against YF disease and that revaccination (a booster dose) is not needed. In 2016, the IHR were officially amended to specify that a completed International Certificate of Vaccination or Prophylaxis (ICVP or "yellow card") is valid for the lifetime of the vaccinee, and countries cannot require proof of revaccination against YF as a condition of entry, even if the last vaccination was >10 years prior.

ACIP also has stated that a single dose of YF vaccine provides long-lasting protection and is adequate for most travelers. ACIP guidelines do differ slightly from those of WHO, however, by specifying that additional doses of YF vaccine are recommended for the following groups of travelers: people who were pregnant when they received their initial dose of vaccine (administer 1 additional dose before they are next at risk for YF); people who received a hematopoietic stem cell transplant after receiving a dose of YF vaccine (revaccinate before they are next at risk for YF as long as they are sufficiently immunocompetent); people infected with HIV when they received their last dose of YF vaccine (administer a dose every 10 years if they continue to be at risk for YF).

Consider administering a booster dose to travelers who received their last dose of YF vaccine ≥10 years previously if they will be going to higher-risk settings based on activities, duration of travel, location, and season. This consideration applies to travelers planning prolonged stays in endemic areas, those traveling to endemic areas (e.g., rural West Africa) during peak transmission season, or travelers visiting areas with ongoing outbreaks.

Although booster doses of YF vaccine are not recommended for most travelers, and despite the 2016 changes to the IHR, clinicians and travelers should nonetheless review the entry requirements for destination countries. For more information on country-specific recommendations and requirements, see Sec. 2, Ch. 5, Yellow Fever Vaccine & Malaria Prevention Information, by Country.

ADVERSE EVENTS

COMMON ADVERSE REACTIONS

Reactions to YF vaccine are generally mild; 10%–30% of vaccinees report mild systemic symptoms, including headache, low-grade fever, and myalgia, that begin within days after vaccination and last 5–10 days.

SERIOUS ADVERSE REACTIONS

HYPERSENSITIVITY REACTIONS

Immediate hypersensitivity reactions, characterized by bronchospasm, rash, or urticaria, are uncommon. Anaphylaxis after YF vaccine is reported to occur at a rate of 1.3 cases per 100,000 doses administered.

YELLOW FEVER VACCINE–ASSOCIATED NEUROLOGIC DISEASE

Yellow fever vaccine–associated neurologic disease (YEL-AND) represents a collection of clinical syndromes, including acute disseminated encephalomyelitis, Guillain-Barré syndrome, meningoencephalitis, and, rarely, cranial nerve palsies. Historically, YEL-AND was diagnosed primarily among infants as encephalitis, although more recent case reports have described various neurological syndromes among people of most age groups. YEL-AND is rarely fatal.

Almost all cases of YEL-AND reported globally occur in first-time vaccine recipients. The onset of illness for documented cases in the United States is 2–56 days after vaccination. The incidence of YEL-AND in the United States is 0.8 per 100,000 doses administered, but is greater (2.2 per 100,000 doses) in people aged ≥60 years.

YELLOW FEVER VACCINE–ASSOCIATED VISCEROTROPIC DISEASE

Yellow fever vaccine–associated viscerotropic disease (YEL-AVD) is a severe illness similar to wild-type YF disease, in which vaccine virus proliferates in multiple organs, often leading to multiorgan dysfunction or failure and occasionally death. Since 2001, >100 confirmed and suspected cases of YEL-AVD have been reported throughout the world.

YEL-AVD has been reported to occur only after the first dose of YF vaccine; no laboratory-confirmed YEL-AVD has been reported after booster doses. For YEL-AVD cases reported in the United States, the median time from YF vaccination until symptom onset is 4 days (range 1–18 days). The case-fatality ratio is ≈48% and the incidence is 0.3 cases per 100,000 doses of vaccine administered. The incidence of YEL-AVD is greater for people aged ≥60 years (1.2 per 100,000 doses) and greater still for people aged ≥70 years.

CONTRAINDICATIONS

Contraindications to receiving YF vaccine include age <6 months; various forms of altered immunity, including symptomatic HIV infection or HIV infection with severe immunosuppression; and hypersensitivity to vaccine components.

A person who has an absolute YF vaccine contraindication should not be vaccinated, because they have a condition that increases their risk for having a serious adverse event following vaccination. Encourage these people to consider alternative travel plans. If they cannot avoid travel to a YF-endemic area, provide them with a medical waiver (see below for details), emphasize the importance of strict adherence to protective measures against mosquito bites, and discuss risks associated with being unvaccinated.

AGE YOUNGER THAN 6 MONTHS

YF vaccine is contraindicated in infants aged <6 months because the rate of YEL-AND is high, 50–400 cases per 100,000 infants vaccinated. The mechanism of increased neurovirulence in infants is unknown, but could be due to the immaturity of the blood–brain barrier, an increased or more prolonged viremia, or immune system immaturity. Travel to YF-endemic countries for children aged <6 months should be postponed or avoided.

ALTERED IMMUNE STATUS

HIV INFECTION

YF vaccine is contraindicated in people with AIDS or other clinical manifestations of HIV infection, including those with CD4 T lymphocyte counts <200/mL, or <15% of total lymphocytes for children <6 years old. This contraindication is based on the potential increased risk for encephalitis in this population. See the section on Precautions (later in this chapter) for guidance regarding HIV-infected people who do not meet the above criteria.

THYMUS DISORDER

YF vaccine is contraindicated in people with a thymus disorder associated with abnormal immune cell function (e.g., myasthenia gravis, thymoma). There is no evidence of immune dysfunction or increased risk for YF vaccine–associated serious adverse events in people who have undergone incidental thymectomy or who have had indirect radiation therapy in the distant past; these people can be vaccinated.

OTHER IMMUNODEFICIENCIES

YF vaccine is contraindicated in people who are immunodeficient or immunosuppressed, whether due to an underlying (primary) disorder or medical treatment. Organ transplant recipients and patients with malignant neoplasms are among those for whom YF vaccine is contraindicated (see Sec. 3, Ch. 1, Immunocompromised Travelers).

IMMUNOSUPPRESSIVE & IMMUNOMODULATORY THERAPIES

YF vaccine is contraindicated in people whose immunologic response is either suppressed or modulated by current or recent radiation therapy or drugs. Drugs with known immunosuppressive or immunomodulatory properties (Table 3-04) include, but are not limited to, alkylating agents, antimetabolites, high-dose systemic corticosteroids, interleukin blocking agents (e.g., anakinra, tocilizumab), monoclonal antibodies targeting immune cells (e.g., alemtuzumab, rituximab), or tumor necrosis factor-α inhibitors (e.g., etanercept).

People receiving therapies such as those listed above are presumed to be at increased risk for YF vaccine–associated serious adverse events; administration of live attenuated vaccines is contraindicated in the package insert for most of these drugs (see Sec. 3, Ch. 1, Immunocompromised Travelers). Even among people who have discontinued immunosuppressive or immunomodulatory therapies, defer administration of live viral vaccines until their immune function has improved. Family members of people with altered immune status who themselves have no contraindications can receive YF vaccine.

HYPERSENSITIVITY

YF vaccine is contraindicated in people with a history of acute hypersensitivity reaction to a previous dose of the vaccine or to any of the vaccine components, including chicken proteins, eggs, egg products, or gelatin. If vaccination of a person with a questionable history of hypersensitivity to a vaccine component is considered essential, skin testing and, if indicated, desensitization should be performed by an experienced clinician according to instructions provided in the manufacturer's vaccine prescribing information (see www.fda.gov/media/76015/download).

PRECAUTIONS

A person with a precaution (relative contraindication) to YF vaccine has a condition that might increase their risk for having a serious adverse event following vaccination, or that could interfere with the ability of the vaccine to produce immunity. YF vaccination precautions include age 6–8 months, age ≥60 years, asymptomatic HIV infection with moderate immunosuppression, pregnancy, and breastfeeding.

Discussing the benefits and risks of YF vaccination with all patients—but particularly those with underlying precautions—is an essential part of the pretravel consultation. If travel to a YF risk area is unavoidable for a person with a vaccine precaution, the discussion about vaccination should balance the risk for YF virus exposure against the risk for having a serious post-vaccination adverse event.

Solicit information from the traveler about their risk tolerance level, and include this in the shared decision making about whether to administer YF vaccine. If the decision is made not to vaccinate the traveler, provide a medical waiver, emphasize the critical importance of adhering to insect bite precautions, and discuss risks associated with being unvaccinated. When no risk for YF exists in the itinerary, but international travel requirements are in effect in the traveler's destination(s), the vaccine risk outweighs the disease; avoiding vaccination and issuing a medical waiver to fulfill health regulations is reasonable, but this decision should be made in deliberation with the patient.

AGE 6–8 MONTHS

Two cases of YEL-AND have been reported in infants aged 6–8 months. By 9 months of age, risk for YEL-AND is believed to be substantially lower. ACIP recommends that, whenever possible, travel to YF-endemic countries for children aged 6–8 months should be postponed or avoided.

AGE ≥60 YEARS

The rate of reported serious adverse events after YF vaccination in people aged ≥60 years is 7.7 per 100,000 doses distributed, compared with 3.8 per 100,000 for all YF vaccine recipients. The risks for YEL-AND and YEL-AVD are increased in this age group. Because YEL-AVD has been reported exclusively, and YEL-AND almost exclusively, in primary vaccine recipients, carefully consider the risks and benefits of vaccinating older travelers against YF vaccine for the first time.

HIV INFECTION

Combined studies of >500 asymptomatic HIV-infected people classified as having moderate immune suppression, defined as CD4 T lymphocyte counts of 200–499/mL for people ≥6 years old (or 15%–24% of total lymphocytes for children aged <6 years) identified no serious adverse events after receipt of YF vaccine. HIV infection has, however, been associated with a reduced immunologic response to YF vaccine, and this diminished immune response has been correlated with HIV RNA levels and CD4 T cell counts.

If an asymptomatic HIV-infected person has no evidence of immune suppression based on CD4 counts (CD4 T lymphocyte counts ≥500/mL for people ≥6 years old or ≥25% of total lymphocytes for children aged <6 years), YF vaccine can be administered. Because YF vaccination might be less effective in eliciting an immune response in asymptomatic HIV-infected people, consider measuring their neutralizing antibody response to vaccination before travel. Contact your state health department or the CDC Arboviral Diseases Branch (970-221-6400) to discuss serologic testing.

PREGNANCY

Safety of YF vaccination during pregnancy has not been studied in any large prospective trials. In 2 observational studies of people vaccinated against YF during pregnancy, a slightly increased risk for minor congenital abnormalities (mainly pigmented nevi) was detected in one study, and a higher rate of spontaneous abortions was reported in the other. Neither finding was substantiated by subsequent studies.

If possible, pregnant people should avoid travel to YF risk areas. If travel is unavoidable and the risk for YF virus exposure is felt to outweigh the vaccination risk, recommending vaccination is appropriate. By contrast, if the vaccine risk is believed to outweigh the risk for YF virus exposure, suggest or offer a medical waiver to the traveler to fulfill health regulations.

The proportion of people vaccinated during pregnancy who develop a YF virus–specific IgG antibody response is variable depending on the study (39% or 98%) and might be correlated with the trimester when they received the vaccine. Because pregnancy can reduce immunologic responsiveness, consider serologic testing to document a protective immune response to the vaccine. Although no specific data are available, ACIP recommends that a person wait 4 weeks after receiving the YF vaccine before conceiving.

BREASTFEEDING

At least 3 YEL-AND cases have been reported in exclusively breastfed infants whose mothers were vaccinated with YF vaccine. All 3 infants were <1 month old at the time of exposure, and encephalitis was diagnosed in all 3 infants. Until specific research data are available, avoid vaccinating breastfeeding people against YF. When a person who is nursing cannot avoid or postpone travel to YF-endemic areas, however, recommend vaccination. Although no data are available to support the practice, some experts recommend that breastfeeding people should pump and discard their breast milk for ≥2 weeks after YF vaccination before resuming breastfeeding.

OTHER CONSIDERATIONS

No data are available regarding possible increased occurrence of adverse events or decreased vaccine efficacy after YF vaccine administration in people with other chronic medical conditions that can affect immune response (e.g., diabetes mellitus, liver disease [including hepatitis C virus infection], or renal disease). Limited data suggest that autoimmune disease, either by itself or in conjunction with other risk factors, including immunosuppressive medication, could increase the risk for YEL-AVD. Therefore, use caution if considering vaccination of such patients. Factors to consider when assessing a patient's general level of immune competence include clinical stability, comorbidities, complications, disease severity and duration, and which medications they are taking.

INTERNATIONAL CERTIFICATE OF VACCINATION OR PROPHYLAXIS

The IHR permit countries to require proof of YF vaccination documented on an ICVP (Figure 5-02) as a condition of entry for travelers arriving from certain countries, even if only in transit, to prevent YF virus importation and transmission in the destination country. Some countries require evidence

INTERNATIONAL CERTIFICATE OF VACCINATION OR PROPHYLAXIS
Certificat international de vaccination ou de prophylaxie

This is to certify that ① Jane Mary Doe (name - nom) ② 22 March 1960 (date of birth - né(e) le) F (sex - de sexe) United States (nationality - et de nationalité)
Nous certifions que

[passport number] (national identification document, if applicable - document d'identification national, le cas échéant) whose signature follows / dont la signature suit ③ Jane Mary Doe

has on the date indicated been vaccinated or received prophylaxis against / a été vacciné(e) ou a reçu une prophylaxie à la date indiquée ④ Yellow Fever (name of disease or condition - nom de la maladie ou de l'affection) in accordance with the International Health Regulations. / conformément au Règlement sanitaire international.

Vaccine or prophylaxis Vaccin ou agent prophylactique	Date	Signature and professional status of supervising clinician Signature et titre du professionel de santé responsable	Manufacturer and batch no. of vaccine or prophylaxis Fabricant du vaccin ou de l'agent prophylactique et numéro du lot	Certificate valid from: until: Certificat valable à partir du : jusqu'au :	Official stamp of the administering center Cachet officiel du centre habilité
④ Yellow Fever	⑤ 15 June 2018	⑥ John M. Smith, MD	[Batch (or lot) #]	⑦ 25 June 2018; life of person vaccinated	[⑧]

FIGURE 5-02 International Certificate of Vaccination or Prophylaxis (ICVP): instructions for completion[1,2]

[1]Clinics offering yellow fever vaccine can purchase ICVP (Form CDC 731; formerly PHS 731), from the US Government Publishing Office website
(http://bookstore.gpo.gov) or by phone (866-512-1800).
[2]Instructions for ICVP completion
(1) Print the traveler's name exactly as it appears in their passport.
(2, 5, 7) Enter all dates in the format shown: day (in numerals), month (spelled in letters), year. In the example above, the patient's date of birth is correctly entered as 22 March 1960.
(3) Space reserved for the patient's signature.
(4) For yellow fever (YF) vaccination, print "Yellow Fever" in both spaces. If the ICVP is used to document proof of another required vaccination or prophylaxis (following an amendment to the International Health Regulations or by recommendation of the World Health Organization), write the disease or condition name in this space. Other vaccinations may be listed on the other side of the ICVP booklet.
(5) Enter the date of vaccine administration, as shown.
(6) The health care provider should enter their handwritten signature, as shown. A signature stamp is not acceptable. For yellow fever vaccine, the health care provider signing the ICVP may be the stamp owner, or another health care provider authorized by the stamp holder to administer or supervise the administration of the vaccine.
(7) The ICVP is valid beginning 10 days after the date of primary YF vaccination. Add that date to this box along with the suggested wording "life of person vaccinated," as shown.
(8) Imprint the Uniform Stamp of the vaccinating center in this box.

of vaccination from all entering travelers, including those arriving directly from the United States (Table 5-25).

People with YF vaccine contraindications who must travel to destinations that require proof of vaccination should receive a medical waiver from a YF vaccine provider before their departure; see Medical Waivers (Exemptions) below. Travelers without proof of vaccination or a medical waiver arriving to destinations that require

Table 5-25 Countries that require proof of yellow fever (YF) vaccination from all arriving travelers[1]

AFRICA		
Angola Benin Burkina Faso Burundi Cameroon Central African Republic Congo, Republic of the	Côte d'Ivoire Democratic Republic of the Congo Gabon Ghana Guinea-Bissau Mali	Niger Sierra Leone South Sudan Togo Uganda
THE AMERICAS		
French Guiana		

[1]Current as of November 2022. Country requirements for YF vaccination are subject to change at any time; check with the destination country's embassy or consulate before departure.

5

this documentation for entry could be denied entry or face mandatory quarantine (up to 6 days) or vaccination on site.

ICVP Validation

Anyone who received YF vaccination after December 15, 2007, must provide proof of vaccination on the new ICVP. If the person received the vaccine before December 15, 2007, their original International Certificate of Vaccination against Yellow Fever (ICV) card is still valid as proof of vaccination. Vaccinees should receive a completed ICVP, signed by the vaccine provider and validated with the stamp of the center where the vaccine was given. Failure to secure validations can cause a traveler to be denied entry, quarantined, or possibly revaccinated at the point of entry to a country.

A properly completed ICVP is valid beginning 10 days after the date of primary vaccination. As of July 2016, the YF vaccine booster requirement was eliminated in the IHR, and a completed ICVP is considered valid for the lifetime of the vaccinee. Clinics offering YF vaccine can purchase ICVPs (Form CDC 731; formerly PHS 731) from the US Government Publishing Office website (http://bookstore.gpo.gov) or by phone (866-512-1800).

Designated Yellow Fever Vaccination Centers & Providers

The ICVP must bear the original signature of a YF vaccine provider, who can be a physician or other authorized licensed health care professional who supervises the administration of the vaccine. A signature stamp is not acceptable. YF vaccination must be given at a designated center that possesses an official "uniform stamp," which must be used to validate the ICVP. In the United States, state and territorial health departments are responsible for designating nonfederal YF vaccination centers and issuing uniform stamps to YF vaccine providers. Information about the location and hours of YF vaccination centers is available from the CDC Travelers' Health website (https://wwwnc.cdc.gov/travel/yellow-fever-vaccination-clinics/search).

Medical Waivers (Exemptions)

A YF vaccine provider issuing a medical waiver for YF vaccine should complete and sign the Medical Contraindications to Vaccination section of the ICVP (Figure 5-03). Reasons other than medical contraindications are not acceptable for exemption from vaccination. The YF vaccine provider should also provide the traveler with a signed and dated exemption letter on letterhead stationery,

MEDICAL CONTRAINDICATION TO VACCINATION
Contre-indication médicale à la vaccination

This is to certify that immunization against
Je soussigné(e) certifie que la vaccination contre

______________________________________ for
(Name of disease – Nom de la maladie) pour

______________________________________ is medically
(Name of traveler – Nom du voyageur) est médicalement

contraindicated because of the following conditions:
contre-indiquée pour les raisons suivantes:

____

____

____

____
(Signature and address of physician)
(Signature et adresse du médecin)

FIGURE 5-03 International Certificate of Vaccination or Prophylaxis (ICVP): Medical Contraindication to Vaccination section

clearly stating the contraindications to vaccination and bearing the imprint of the uniform stamp used by the YF vaccination center to validate the ICVP. Risks associated with not being vaccinated should be discussed, and the importance of strict adherence to mosquito bite prevention measures emphasized.

Medical waivers might not be accepted by the destination country. To improve the likelihood that a border official will grant a waiver holder entry to their intended destination, recommend that travelers contact the local embassy or consulate of the country or countries well in advance of travel to obtain specific and authoritative advice regarding waiver documentation requirements. All information provided should be kept with the completed Medical Contraindications to Vaccination and waiver letter.

VACCINE REQUIREMENTS VERSUS RECOMMENDATIONS

Country entry requirements for proof of YF vaccination under the IHR differ from CDC's recommendations. Countries are permitted to establish YF vaccine entry requirements to prevent the YF virus importation and transmission within their borders. Unless issued a medical waiver by a YF vaccine provider, travelers must comply with these requirements to enter the country.

Certain countries require vaccination from travelers arriving from all countries (Table 5-25); others require vaccination only for travelers above a certain age coming from countries with risk for YF virus transmission (see Sec. 2, Ch. 5, Yellow Fever Vaccine & Malaria Prevention Information, by Country). The WHO defines areas with risk for YF virus transmission as places where YF virus activity has been reported currently or in the past, and where vectors and animal reservoirs exist. Countries that contain areas with only low potential for YF virus exposure (Table 5-23) are not included on the official WHO list of countries with risk for YF virus transmission (Table 5-22). Unless a country requires proof of YF vaccination from all arriving travelers, proof

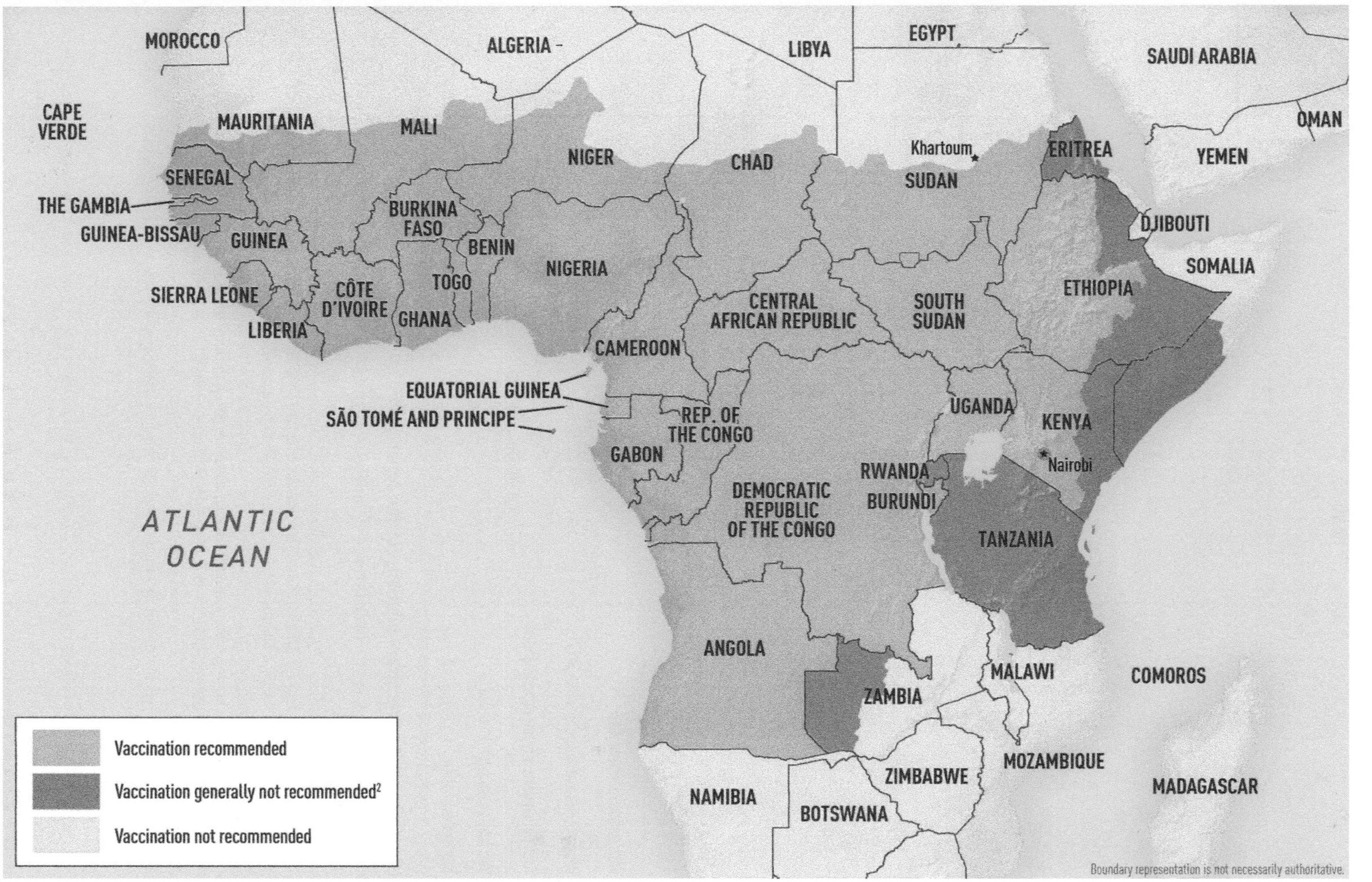

MAP 5-10 Yellow fever vaccine recommendations for Africa[1,2]

[1]Current as of November 2022. This map is an updated version of the 2010 map created by the Informal WHO Working Group on the Geographic Risk of Yellow Fever.

[2]Yellow fever (YF) vaccination is generally not recommended for travel to areas where the potential for YF virus exposure is low. Vaccination might be considered, however, for a small subset of travelers going to these areas who are at increased risk for exposure to YF virus due to prolonged travel, heavy exposure to mosquitoes, or inability to avoid mosquito bites. Factors to consider when deciding whether to vaccinate a traveler include destination-specific and travel-associated risks for YF virus infection; individual, underlying risk factors for having a serious YF vaccine-associated adverse event; and country entry requirements.

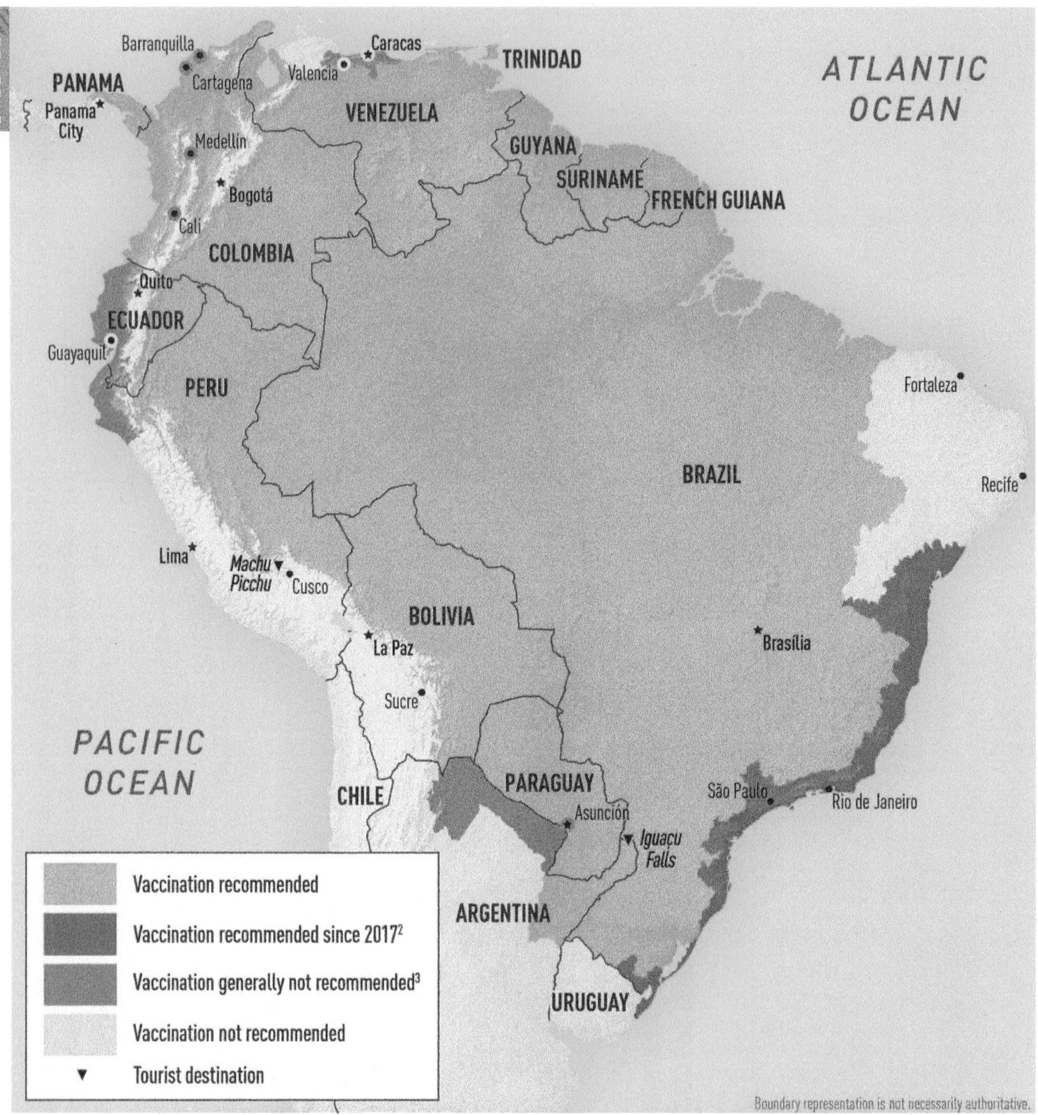

MAP 5-11 Yellow fever vaccine recommendations for the Americas[1,2,3]

[1]Current as of November 2022. This map is an updated version of the 2010 map created by the Informal WHO Working Group on the Geographic Risk of Yellow Fever.

[2]In 2017, the Centers for Disease Control and Prevention (CDC) expanded its yellow fever vaccine recommendations for travelers going to Brazil because of a large outbreak in multiple states in that country. For more information and updated recommendations, refer to the CDC Travelers' Health website (https://wwwnc.cdc.gov/travel).

[3]Yellow fever (YF) vaccination is generally not recommended for travel to areas where the potential for YF virus exposure is low. Vaccination might be considered, however, for a small subset of travelers going to these areas who are at increased risk for exposure to YF virus due to prolonged travel, heavy exposure to mosquitoes, or inability to avoid mosquito bites. Factors to consider when deciding whether to vaccinate a traveler include destination-specific and travel-associated risks for YF virus infection; individual, underlying risk factors for having a serious YF vaccine-associated adverse event; and country entry requirements.

of YF vaccination should not be required of travelers coming from countries identified as having low potential for YF virus exposure. Because country entry requirements are subject to change at any time, CDC encourages travelers and their health care providers to check with the relevant embassy or consulate before departure.

To make its recommendations for preventing travel-associated YF virus infections, CDC uses a destination-specific risk classification for YF virus transmission: endemic, transitional, low potential for exposure, and no risk. CDC recommends YF vaccination for travel to endemic or transitional areas (Map 5-10 and Map 5-11). Recommendations are subject to revision at any time because of changes in YF virus circulation; before departure, check the CDC Travelers' Health website destination pages for current vaccine information and relevant Travel Health Notices (https://wwwnc.cdc.gov/travel/notices).

CDC website: www.cdc.gov/yellowfever

BIBLIOGRAPHY

Gershman MD, Staples JE, Bentsi-Enchill AD, Breugelmans JG, Brito GS, Camacho LA, et al. Viscerotropic disease: case definition and guidelines for collection, analysis, and presentation of immunization safety data. Vaccine. 2012;30(33):5038–58.

Jentes ES, Poumerol G, Gershman MD, Hill DR, Lemarchand J, Lewis RF, et al. The revised global yellow fever risk map and recommendations for vaccination, 2010: consensus of the Informal WHO Working Group on Geographic Risk for Yellow Fever. Lancet Infect Dis. 2011;11(8):622–32.

Lindsey NP, Rabe IB, Miller ER, Fischer M, Staples JE. Adverse event reports following yellow fever vaccination, 2007–13. J Travel Med. 2016;23(5):taw045.

Monath TP, Cetron MS. Prevention of yellow fever in persons traveling to the tropics. Clin Infect Dis. 2002;34(10):1369–78.

Staples JE, Barrett ADT, Wilder-Smith A, Hombach J. Review of data and knowledge gaps regarding yellow fever vaccine-induced immunity and duration of protection. NPJ Vaccines. 2020;5(1):54.

Staples JE, Bocchini JA Jr, Rubin L, Fischer M. Yellow fever vaccine booster doses: recommendations of the Advisory Committee on Immunization Practices, 2015. MMWR Morb Mortal Wkly Rep. 20159;64(23):647–50.

Staples JE, Gershman M, Fischer M. Yellow fever vaccine: recommendations of the Advisory Committee on Immunization Practices (ACIP). MMWR Recomm Rep. 2010;59(RR-7):1–27.

Staples JE, Monath TP, Gershman MD, Barrett ADT. Yellow fever vaccine. In: Plotkin SA, Orenstein WA, Offit PA, editors. Vaccines, 7th edition. Philadelphia: Elsevier; 2018. pp. 1181–265.

World Health Organization. International health regulations, 2005. Geneva: The Organization; 2016. Available from: www.who.int/ihr/publications/9789241580496/en.

World Health Organization. Vaccines and vaccination against yellow fever. WHO position paper—June 2013. Wkly Epidemiol Rec. 2013;88(27):269–83.

ZIKA

Stacey Martin, J. Erin Staples

INFECTIOUS AGENT: Zika virus	
ENDEMICITY	Worldwide, periodic outbreaks in tropical and subtropical regions
TRAVELER CATEGORIES AT GREATEST RISK FOR EXPOSURE & INFECTION	Adventure tourists Long-term travelers and expatriates Travelers visiting friends and relatives
PREVENTION METHODS	Avoid insect bites Use condoms or abstain from sex if exposed (or possibly exposed)
DIAGNOSTIC SUPPORT	A clinical laboratory certified in high complexity testing; state health department; or contact CDC Arboviral Diseases Branch (www.cdc.gov/ncezid/dvbd/specimensub/arboviral-shipping.html; 970-221-6400; dvbid@cdc.gov)

5

INFECTIOUS AGENT

Zika virus is a single-stranded RNA virus of the *Flaviviridae* family, genus *Flavivirus.*

TRANSMISSION

Transmission occurs through the bite of an infected *Aedes* species mosquito. Intrauterine, perinatal, sexual, laboratory, and possible transfusion-associated transmission have been reported. Zika virus has been detected in breast milk, but the risk for transmission through breastfeeding is unknown.

EPIDEMIOLOGY

Zika virus occurs in tropical and subtropical regions. Since 2007, outbreaks of Zika virus disease have occurred throughout the Pacific Islands and in Southeast Asia. In 2015, Zika virus was identified in the Western Hemisphere, where large outbreaks occurred in Brazil. The virus then spread throughout much of the Americas, resulting in several hundred thousand cases. Since 2017, the number of reported Zika virus disease cases has declined worldwide, but occasional increases in cases have been noted from some countries. In 2020, only 4 Zika virus cases were reported in US international travelers. Current information on Zika virus transmission and travel guidance can be found at https://wwwnc.cdc.gov/travel/page/zika-travel-information.

CLINICAL PRESENTATION

Most Zika virus infections are either asymptomatic or result in mild clinical illness characterized by acute onset of fever, arthralgia, nonpurulent conjunctivitis, and maculopapular rash. Other symptoms can include edema, headache, lymphadenopathy, myalgia, retro-orbital pain, and vomiting. Severe disease requiring hospitalization and death are both uncommon. Guillain-Barré syndrome and rare reports of encephalopathy, meningoencephalitis, myelitis, uveitis, and severe thrombocytopenia have been associated with Zika virus infection, however. Vertical transmission of the virus leads to congenital Zika virus infection; sequelae include microcephaly with brain anomalies and other serious neurologic consequences, and fetal loss.

DIAGNOSIS

Consider Zika virus infection in patients with acute onset of fever, arthralgia, conjunctivitis, or maculopapular rash who, ≤2 weeks of illness onset, lived in or recently traveled to areas with ongoing Zika virus transmission or had sex with someone who lives in or traveled to those areas. Because Zika and dengue virus infections have similar clinical presentations, patients with suspected Zika virus infection also should be evaluated for possible dengue. Other considerations in the differential diagnosis include adenovirus, chikungunya, enterovirus, leptospirosis, malaria, measles, parvovirus, rickettsiosis, rubella, and group A streptococcal infections (see disease-specific chapters in this section).

Zika virus disease is a nationally notifiable condition. Report suspected cases of Zika virus infection to state or local health departments to facilitate diagnosis and mitigate the risk for local transmission in areas where *Aedes* species mosquitoes are active. State health departments should report laboratory-confirmed cases to the Centers for Disease Control and Prevention (CDC) according to the Council of State and Territorial Epidemiologists case definitions (https://ndc.services.cdc.gov).

Diagnostic Testing

Because Zika and dengue viruses share a similar global geographic distribution and cause infections that can be difficult to differentiate diagnostically, consider the global epidemiology of these 2 arboviruses when requesting testing and interpreting results. Zika virus testing guidance is updated as needed to address changes in the epidemiology. Current testing guidance is provided on the CDC website (www.cdc.gov/zika/hc-providers/testing-guidance.html). Some state health departments and many commercial laboratories perform Zika virus nucleic acid amplification testing (NAAT) and IgM testing. Confirmatory neutralizing antibody testing is available at CDC's Arboviral Diagnostic Reference Laboratory and selected health department laboratories.

NUCLEIC ACID AMPLIFICATION TESTING

NAAT is used to detect Zika viral RNA early in the course of infection and can be performed on amniotic fluid, whole blood, cerebrospinal fluid, semen, serum, tissues, and urine. Due to the temporal nature of Zika virus RNA in the body, a negative NAAT does not always exclude recent Zika virus infection. For this reason, Zika virus IgM antibody testing might be recommended in certain situations.

SEROLOGIC TESTING

Serum IgM antibody testing can detect Zika virus–specific IgM antibodies that typically develop toward the end of the first week of illness and can remain detectable for months to years after infection, making the determination of the timing of infection difficult. Serum IgM antibody testing can result in a false-positive result due to cross-reacting antibodies against related flaviviruses (e.g., dengue virus, yellow fever virus). Plaque reduction neutralization testing (PRNT) can be used to discriminate between cross-reacting antibodies in primary flavivirus infections, but neutralizing antibodies might still yield cross-reactive results in people who were previously infected with or vaccinated against a related flavivirus (secondary flavivirus infection).

TREATMENT

No specific antiviral treatment is available for Zika virus disease. Treatment is generally supportive and can include use of analgesics and antipyretics, fluids, and rest. Because aspirin and other nonsteroidal anti-inflammatory drugs (NSAIDs) can increase the risk for hemorrhage in patients with dengue, avoid use of these medications until dengue can be ruled out.

Protect people infected with Zika, chikungunya, or dengue virus from further mosquito exposure during the first week of illness to decrease the possibility of local transmission. Carefully evaluate pregnant people with laboratory evidence of Zika virus infection; closely manage these cases for possible adverse pregnancy outcomes. Guidance for the diagnosis, evaluation, and management of infants with possible congenital Zika virus infections is available at www.cdc.gov/pregnancy/zika/testing-follow-up/evaluation-testing.html.

PREVENTION

No vaccine or preventive drug is available for Zika virus. All travelers to areas with Zika virus transmission should take steps to avoid mosquito bites to prevent Zika virus and other vectorborne infections (see Sec. 4, Ch. 6, Mosquitoes, Ticks & Other Arthropods). Advise people with possible Zika virus exposure who want to reduce the risk for sexual transmission of Zika virus to an uninfected partner to follow current CDC recommendations (www.cdc.gov/zika/prevention/sexual-transmission-prevention.html). Although blood donations in the United States were previously screened for Zika virus RNA, the US Food and Drug Administration ceased this requirement in May 2021 because the virus no longer has sufficient incidence to affect the potential donor population.

Pregnancy

5

Pregnant people should not travel to areas with ongoing Zika outbreaks (https://wwwnc.cdc.gov/travel/page/zika-information). Before traveling to areas with current or past spread of Zika, pregnant people should discuss their travel plans with a health care provider. In deciding whether to travel, pregnant people should consider the destination, their reasons for traveling, and their ability to prevent mosquito bites. If used in accordance with the instructions on the product label, there are no restrictions on the use of insect repellents by people who are pregnant.

If a pregnant person or their partner travels to an area with current or past spread of Zika virus, advise the couple to use condoms or to abstain from sex for the entire pregnancy, even if the traveler does not have symptoms of Zika or feel sick. Couples trying to become pregnant who travel to areas with past or current Zika virus transmission should take steps to protect themselves from Zika and consider waiting to get pregnant according to the timeframes outlined in CDC guidance (www.cdc.gov/pregnancy/zika/women-and-their-partners.html).

Mothers are encouraged to breastfeed infants even after possible Zika virus exposure, because available evidence indicates the benefits of breastfeeding outweigh the theoretical risks associated with Zika virus infection transmission through breast milk.

CDC website: www.cdc.gov/zika

BIBLIOGRAPHY

Adebanjo T, Godfred-Cato S, Viens L, Fischer M, Staples JE, Kuhnert-Tallman W, et al. Update: interim guidance for the diagnosis, evaluation, and management of infants with possible congenital Zika virus infection—United States, October 2017. MMWR Morb Mortal Wkly Rep. 2017;66(41):1089–99.

Angelo KM, Stoney RJ, Brun-Cottan G, Leder K, Grobusch MP, Hochberg N, et al. Zika among international travellers presenting to GeoSentinel sites, 2012–2019: implications for clinical practice. J Travel Med. 2020;27(4): taaa061.

Gregory CJ, Oduyebo T, Brault AC, Brooks JT, Chung KW, Hills S, et al. Modes of transmission of Zika virus. J Infect Dis. 2017;216(10):S875–83.

Hills SL, Fischer M, Petersen LR. Epidemiology of Zika virus infection. J Infect Disease. 2017;216(10):S868–74.

Oduyebo T, Polen KD, Walke HT, Reagan-Steiner S, Lathrop E, Rabe IB, et al. Update: interim guidance for health care providers caring for pregnant women with possible Zika virus exposure—United States (including U.S. territories), July 2017. MMWR Morb Mortal Wkly Rep. 2017;66(29):781–93.

Sharp TM, Fischer M, Munoz-Jordan JL, Paz-Bailey G, Staples JE, Gregory CJ, et al. Dengue and Zika virus diagnostic testing for patients with a clinically compatible illness and risk for infection with both viruses. MMWR Recomm Rep. 2019;68(1):1–10.

Smoots AN, Olson SN, Cragan J, Delaney A, Roth NM, Gotfred-Cato NS, et al. Population-based surveillance of birth defects potentially related to Zika virus infection—22 States and U.S. territories, January 2016–June 2017. MMWR Morb Mortal Wkly Rep. 2020;69(3):67–71.

PART 3: PARASITIC

AMEBIASIS

Jennifer Cope, Ibne Ali

5

INFECTIOUS AGENT: *Entamoeba histolytica*	
ENDEMICITY	Worldwide, especially in tropical countries with poor sanitation
TRAVELER CATEGORIES AT GREATEST RISK FOR EXPOSURE & INFECTION	Humanitarian aid workers Immigrants and refugees Long-term travelers and expatriates
PREVENTION METHODS	Practice good hand hygiene Follow safe food and water safety precautions Minimize fecal–oral exposures during sexual activity
DIAGNOSTIC SUPPORT	Contact CDC's Free-Living and Intestinal Amebas (FLIA) Laboratory for confirmatory diagnostic testing (www.cdc.gov/laboratory/specimen-submission/detail.html?CDCTestCode=CDC-10478)

INFECTIOUS AGENT

The protozoan parasite *Entamoeba histolytica*, and possibly other *Entamoeba* spp., causes amebiasis.

TRANSMISSION

Transmission occurs through the fecal–oral route, either by eating or drinking fecally contaminated food or water or through person-to-person contact (e.g., diaper changing, sexual activity).

EPIDEMIOLOGY

Amebiasis is distributed worldwide, particularly in the tropics, most commonly in areas of poor sanitation. *E. histolytica* is a common diarrheal pathogen in returned travelers. Long-term travelers (duration >6 months) are much more likely than short-term travelers (duration <1 month) to develop *E. histolytica* infection. Recent immigrants and refugees from these areas also are at risk. Outbreaks among men who have sex with men have been reported. People at greater risk for severe disease are pregnant, immunocompromised, or receiving corticosteroids; severe disease has also been reported among people with diabetes and those who consume alcohol.

CLINICAL PRESENTATION

Most patients have a gradual illness onset days or weeks after infection. Symptoms include cramps, bloody or watery diarrhea, and weight loss, which might last several weeks. Occasionally, the parasite will spread to other organs (extraintestinal amebiasis), most commonly the liver. Amebic liver abscesses can be asymptomatic, but most patients present with right upper quadrant abdominal pain, fever, and weight loss, usually in the absence of diarrhea. Men are at greater risk of developing amebic liver abscess than are women for reasons not fully understood.

DIAGNOSIS

Microscopy does not distinguish between *E. histolytica* (known to be pathogenic), *E. bangladeshi*, *E. dispar*, and *E. moshkovskii*. Historically, *E. dispar* and *E. moshkovskii* have been considered nonpathogenic, but evidence is mounting that *E. moshkovskii* can cause illness; *E. bangladeshi* has only recently been identified, so its pathogenic potential is not well understood. ELISA or PCR are needed to confirm the diagnosis of *E. histolytica*. Additionally, serologic tests can help diagnose extraintestinal amebiasis.

5

The Free-Living and Intestinal Amebas (FLIA) laboratory of the Centers for Disease Control and Prevention (CDC) can make a specific diagnosis using a duplex real-time PCR capable of detecting and distinguishing *E. histolytica* and *E. dispar* in stool, liver aspirates, and tissue samples. More information about this testing and the CDC point of contact can be found at www.cdc.gov/laboratory/specimen-submission/detail.html; select test code CDC-10478 from the list.

The FLIA laboratory does not accept samples for routine screening purposes, and only accepts samples previously tested elsewhere but still requiring confirmatory testing. CDC requests that state public health officials assist clinical laboratories referring specimens for further testing, including providing information about testing, specimen submission forms, and shipping information.

TREATMENT

Treat patients with symptomatic intestinal infection and extraintestinal disease with metronidazole or tinidazole, then treat with iodoquinol or paromomycin. Also, treat asymptomatic patients infected with *E. histolytica* with iodoquinol or paromomycin, because they can infect others and because 4%–10% of asymptomatic patients develop disease within 1 year if untreated. In patients with large amebic liver abscesses (>5 cm in diameter), draining the abscess in addition to treating with metronidazole or tinidazole can aid in the early resolution of pain and tenderness.

PREVENTION

To reduce their risk for amebiasis, travelers should follow food and water precautions (see Sec. 2, Ch. 8, Food & Water Precautions), practice good hand hygiene, and avoid fecal exposure during sexual activity.

CDC website: www.cdc.gov/parasites/amebiasis

BIBLIOGRAPHY

Escolà-Vergé L, Arando M, Vall M, Rovira R, Espasa M, Sulleiro E, et al. Outbreak of intestinal amoebiasis among men who have sex with men, Barcelona (Spain), October 2017 and January 2017. Euro Surveill. 2017;22(30):30581.

Heredia RD, Fonseca JA, Lopez MC. *Entamoeba moshkovskii* perspectives of a new agent to be considered in the diagnosis of amebiasis. Acta Trop. 2012;123(3):139–45.

Kumar R, Ranjan A, Narayan R, Priyadarshi RN, Anand U, Shalimar. Evidence-based therapeutic dilemma in the management of uncomplicated amebic liver abscess: A systematic review and meta-analysis. Indian J Gastroenterol. 2019;38(6):498–508.

Lachish T, Wieder-Finesod A, Schwartz E. Amebic liver abscess in Israeli travelers: a retrospective study. Am J Trop Med Hyg. 2016;94(5):1015–9.

Shimokawa C, Kabir M, Taniuchi M, Mondal D, Kobayashi S, Ali IK, et al. *Entamoeba moshkovskii* is associated with diarrhea in infants and causes diarrhea and colitis in mice. J Infect Dis. 2012;206(5):744–51.

Shirley DT, Farr L, Watanabe K, Moonah S. A review of the global burden, new diagnostics, and current therapeutics for amebiasis. Open Forum Infect Dis. 2018;5(7):ofy161.

Shirley D, Moonah S. Fulminant amebic colitis after corticosteroid therapy: a systematic review. PLoS Negl Trop Dis. 2016;10(7):e0004879.

ANGIOSTRONGYLIASIS

Rebecca Chancey, Anne Straily

INFECTIOUS AGENT: *Angiostrongylus cantonensis*	
ENDEMICITY	Southeast Asia and the Pacific Basin Australia The Caribbean
TRAVELER CATEGORIES AT GREATEST RISK FOR EXPOSURE & INFECTION	All travelers, but especially adventurous eaters
PREVENTION METHODS	Follow safe food precautions Avoid fresh produce, which can contain infected slugs or snails Avoid raw and undercooked freshwater crabs, frogs, shrimp, and snails
DIAGNOSTIC SUPPORT	Contact CDC's Parasitic Diseases Branch, (www.cdc.gov/parasites; 404-718-4745; parasites@cdc.gov)

5

INFECTIOUS AGENT

Angiostrongylus cantonensis, rat lungworm, a nematode parasite, causes angiostrongyliasis.

TRANSMISSION

Various species of rats are the definitive hosts of rat lungworm. Parasites from rats only infect slugs and snails, which are the intermediate hosts. Infective larvae also have been found in paratenic (transport) hosts (e.g., freshwater crabs, frogs, shrimp), which become infected by consuming infected slugs and snails. Transmission to humans occurs by ingesting infected intermediate or paratenic hosts contaminating raw produce or vegetable juices.

EPIDEMIOLOGY

A. cantonensis is considered the most common infectious cause of eosinophilic meningitis in humans. Most described cases have occurred in Asia and the Pacific Basin (e.g., parts of Australia, mainland China, Taiwan, Thailand, Hawaii, and other Pacific Islands); cases have been reported in many areas of the world, however, including Central and South America, the Caribbean, and parts of the continental United States. A review of the published literature in 2018 identified ≥77 cases of neuroangiostrongyliasis among travelers. All travelers are at risk, but adventure travelers might have more risky eating behaviors, predisposing them to exposure.

CLINICAL PRESENTATION

Incubation period is typically 1–3 weeks but ranges from 1 day to >6 weeks. Common manifestations include body aches, headache, fatigue, photophobia, stiff neck, abnormal skin sensations (e.g., tingling or painful feelings), nausea, and vomiting. Low-grade fever is possible. Symptoms are usually self-limited but might persist for weeks or months. Severe cases can be associated with blindness, paralysis, or death.

DIAGNOSIS

Diagnosis is typically presumptive, based on clinical and epidemiologic criteria in people with otherwise unexplained eosinophilic meningitis. Request PCR testing of cerebrospinal fluid through the Centers for Disease Control and Prevention's DPDx laboratory (www.cdc.gov/dpdx; dpdx@cdc.gov), or the Parasitic Diseases Hotline for Healthcare Providers (404-718-4745;

parasites@cdc.gov). Immunodiagnostic tests have been developed in research settings but are not approved or licensed for clinical use in the United States.

TREATMENT

A. cantonensis larvae die spontaneously, and supportive care usually suffices, including analgesics for pain and corticosteroids to limit inflammation. No anti-helminthic drugs have been effective in treatment. Although albendazole has been combined with corticosteroids in some cases, concern remains that anti-helminthic drugs will exacerbate symptoms due to a systemic response to dying worms. Lumbar puncture is required for etiological diagnosis of eosinophilic meningitis and can be repeated if clinically indicated to reduce intracranial pressure.

5

PREVENTION

Travelers can reduce their risk for infection by following safe food and water precautions. In particular, travelers should avoid eating raw or undercooked slugs, snails, and other possible hosts; and avoid eating raw produce (e.g., lettuce) unless it has been thoroughly washed with clean water, which might provide some protection but might not fully eliminate the risk. If a catchment tank is used as a source of water, travelers should ensure that the tank is covered to prevent intrusion by slugs and snails (see Sec. 2, Ch. 9, Water Disinfection) and keep their drink containers covered. In addition, travelers should wear gloves if they handle slugs or snails, and thoroughly wash hands afterwards.

CDC website: www.cdc.gov/parasites/angiostrongylus

BIBLIOGRAPHY

Ansdell V, Wattanagoon Y. *Angiostrongylus cantonensis* in travelers: clinical manifestations, diagnosis, and treatment. Curr Opin Infect Dis. 2018;31(5):399–408.

Barratt J, Chan D, Sandaradura I, Malik R, Spielman D, Lee R, et al. *Angiostrongylus cantonensis*: a review of its distribution, molecular biology and clinical significance as a human pathogen. Parasitol. 2016;143(9):1087–118.

Eamsobhana P. Eosinophilic meningitis caused by *Angiostrongylus cantonensis*—a neglected disease with escalating importance. Trop Biomed. 2014;31(4):569–78.

Hochberg NS, Blackburn BG, Park SY, Sejvar JJ, Effler PV, Herwaldt BL. Eosinophilic meningitis attributable to *Angiostrongylus cantonensis* infection in Hawaii: clinical characteristics and potential exposures. Am J Trop Med Hyg. 2011;85(4):685–90.

Liu EW, Schwartz BS, Hysmith ND, DeVincenzo JP, Larson DT, Maves RC, et al. Rat lungworm infection associated with central nervous system disease—eight U.S. States, January 2011–January 2017. MMWR Morb Mortal Wkly Rep. 2018;67(30):825–8.

Qvarnstrom Y, Xayavong M, da Silva AC, Park SY, Whelen AC, Calimlim PS, et al. Real-time polymerase chain reaction detection of *Angiostrongylus cantonensis* DNA in cerebrospinal fluid from patients with eosinophilic meningitis. Am J Trop Med Hyg. 2016;94(1):176–81.

Rael RC, Peterson AC, Ghersi-Chavez B, Riegel C, Lesen AE, Blum MJ. Rat lungworm infection in rodents across post-Katrina New Orleans, Louisiana, USA. Emerg Infect Dis. 2018;24(12):2176–83.

Wang Q-P, Wu Z-D, Wei J, Owen RL, Lun Z-R. Human *Angiostrongylus cantonensis*: an update. Eur J Clin Microbiol Infect Dis. 2012;31(4):389–95.

CRYPTOSPORIDIOSIS

Michele Hlavsa, Dawn Roellig

INFECTIOUS AGENT: *Cryptosporidium* spp.	
ENDEMICITY	Worldwide
TRAVELER CATEGORIES AT GREATEST RISK FOR EXPOSURE & INFECTION	Children aged 1–4 years and their caregivers
PREVENTION	Follow safe food and water precautions Minimize fecal-oral exposures during sexual activity Practice good hand hygiene
DIAGNOSTIC SUPPORT	A clinical laboratory certified in moderate complexity testing; or contact CDC's Waterborne Disease Prevention Branch (healthywater@cdc.gov) for clinical and diagnostic questions (does not conduct cryptosporidiosis diagnostic testing)

5

INFECTIOUS AGENT

Among the many protozoan parasites in the genus *Cryptosporidium*, *Cryptosporidium hominis* and *C. parvum* cause >90% of human infections.

TRANSMISSION

Cryptosporidium is transmitted via the fecal–oral route. Its low infectious dose, prolonged survival in moist environments, protracted communicability, and extreme chlorine tolerance make *Cryptosporidium* ideally suited for transmission through contaminated drinking or recreational water (e.g., swimming pools). Transmission also can occur through contact with fecally contaminated surfaces, by eating contaminated food, or through contact with infected animals (particularly pre-weaned bovine calves) or people (e.g., when providing direct care, during oral–anal sex).

EPIDEMIOLOGY

Cryptosporidiosis is endemic worldwide; the highest rates are found in low- and middle-income countries. An estimated 823,000 cryptosporidiosis cases occur in the United States each year, of which 9.9% are thought be due to international travel. The highest US rates of reported cryptosporidiosis are in young children aged 1–4 years and in people aged 15–44 years, particularly females (likely caregivers changing diapers and helping with toileting). International travel is a risk factor for sporadic cryptosporidiosis in the United States (population attributable risk is 11%) and other high-income nations; few studies, however, have assessed the prevalence of cryptosporidiosis in travelers.

One report identified a 6% prevalence of *Cryptosporidium* infection in North American travelers to Mexico; among travelers to Cuernavaca or Guadalajara who experienced travelers' diarrhea, longer visits were associated with an increased risk for *Cryptosporidium* infection compared with bacterial diarrhea. Approximately 30% of patients with cryptosporidiosis in New York City reported international travel during their incubation period, particularly among those aged <20 years.

CLINICAL PRESENTATION

Symptoms—most commonly, frequent, non-bloody, watery diarrhea—begin ≤2 weeks (typically 5–7 days) after infection and are generally self-limited. Other symptoms include abdominal pain, flatulence and urgency, nausea, vomiting, and low-grade fever. In immunocompetent people, symptoms typically resolve within 2–3 weeks, although patients might experience a recurrence of symptoms after a brief period of recovery and before complete symptom resolution.

Clinical presentation in immunocompromised patients varies with the level of immunosuppression, ranging from no symptoms or transient disease to relapsing or chronic diarrhea or even cholera-like diarrhea, which can lead to dehydration and life-threatening wasting and malabsorption. Extraintestinal cryptosporidiosis in the biliary or respiratory tract, and rarely the pancreas, has been documented in children and immunocompromised people.

DIAGNOSIS

Routine testing for ova and parasites does not typically include *Cryptosporidium*; specifically request testing for this organism when *Cryptosporidium* infection is suspected. New molecular enteric panel assays generally include *Cryptosporidium* as a target pathogen. Because *Cryptosporidium* is intermittently excreted in the stool, collect multiple samples (i.e., collect specimens on 3 separate days) to increase test sensitivity.

Other diagnostic techniques include microscopy with direct fluorescent antibody (considered the gold standard), enzyme immunoassay kits, molecular assays, microscopy with modified acid-fast staining, and rapid immunochromatographic cartridge assays. Note that rapid immunochromatographic cartridge assays can generate false-positive results; consider confirmation with microscopy. The Centers for Disease Control and Prevention (CDC)'s Waterborne Disease Prevention Branch (healthywater@cdc.gov) can answer clinical and diagnostic questions but does not conduct cryptosporidiosis diagnostic testing. Health care professionals should contact their usual diagnostic laboratory for testing.

Infections caused by different *Cryptosporidium* species and subtypes can differ clinically. Most *Cryptosporidium* species, all with multiple subtypes, are indistinguishable by traditional diagnostic tests, however. To clarify cryptosporidiosis epidemiology and track infection sources, then, CDC coordinates CryptoNet (www.cdc.gov/parasites/crypto/cryptonet.html), which provides *Cryptosporidium* genotyping and subtyping services in collaboration with state public health agencies. CryptoNet recommends against using formalin to preserve stool for *Cryptosporidium* testing, because formalin impedes reliable genotyping and subtyping.

Cryptosporidiosis is a nationally notifiable disease in the United States.

TREATMENT

Most immunocompetent people recover from cryptosporidiosis without treatment; diarrhea can be managed by maintaining an adequate oral fluid intake. The US Food and Drug Administration has approved nitazoxanide as treatment for immunocompetent people aged ≥1 year with cryptosporidiosis (for details, see www.cdc.gov/parasites/crypto/treatment.html).

Nitazoxanide has not been shown to be effective in immunocompromised patients. Instead, reconstitution of the immune system can result in robust clinical improvement in the absence of specific treatment. Protease inhibitors might have anti-*Cryptosporidium* activity. All patients (immunocompromised and immunocompetent) might need rehydration and electrolyte replacement.

PREVENTION

Travelers can reduce their risk for cryptosporidiosis by carefully adhering to food and water precautions (see Sec. 2, Ch. 8, Food & Water Precautions) and using proper handwashing techniques (see www.cdc.gov/handwashing/when-how-handwashing.html and www.cdc.gov/parasites/crypto/gen_info/prevention-general-public.html). Alcohol-based hand sanitizers are not effective against this parasite.

Travelers can also decrease the risk for infection by filtering drinking water with an absolute 1-μm filter or heating drinking water to a rolling boil for 1 minute (see Sec. 2, Ch. 9, Water Disinfection, and www.cdc.gov/healthywater/drinking/travel/backcountry_water_treatment.html). *Cryptosporidium* oocysts are extremely tolerant of halogens (e.g., chlorine, iodine), so

CDC recommends filtering or boiling water in high-risk areas.

To protect themselves, swimmers should avoid ingesting recreational water. To protect others, people infected with cryptosporidiosis should not enter recreational water while ill with diarrhea, and for the first 2 weeks after symptoms have completely resolved, because of prolonged excretion of infectious oocysts.

Practicing safer sex (i.e., reducing contact with feces) can also decrease risk for infection.

CDC website: www.cdc.gov/parasites/crypto/index.html

BIBLIOGRAPHY

Adamu H, Petros B, Zhang G, Kassa H, Amer S, Ye J, et al. Distribution and clinical manifestations of *Cryptosporidium* species and subtypes in HIV/AIDS patients in Ethiopia. PLoS Negl Trop Dis. 2014;8(4):e2831.

Alleyne L, Fitzhenry R, Mergen KA, Espina N, Amorosos E, Cimini D, et al. Epidemiology of cryptosporidiosis, New York City, New York, USA, 1995–2018. Emerg Infect Dis. 2020;26(3):409–19.

Garcia LS, Arrowood M, Kokoskin E, Paltridge GP, Pillai DR, Procop GW, et al. Laboratory diagnosis of parasites from the gastrointestinal tract. Clin Microbiol Rev. 2017;31(1):e00025–17.

Kotloff KL, Nataro JP, Blackwelder WC, Nasrin D, Farag TH, Panchalingam S, et al. Burden and aetiology of diarrhoeal disease in infants and young children in developing countries (the Global Enteric Multicenter Study, GEMS): a prospective, case-control study. Lancet. 2013;382(9888):209–22.

Nair P, Mohamed JA, DuPont HL, Figueroa JF, Carlin LG, Jiang ZD, et al. Epidemiology of cryptosporidiosis in North American travelers to Mexico. Am J Trop Med Hyg. 2008;79(2):210–14.

Pantenburg B, Cabada MM, White AC Jr. Treatment of cryptosporidiosis. Expert Rev Anti Infect Ther. 2009;7(4):385–91.

Roy SL, DeLong SM, Stenzel SA, Shiferaw B, Roberts JM, Khalakdina A, et al. Risk factors for sporadic cryptosporidiosis among immunocompetent persons in the United States from 1999–2001. J Clin Microbiol. 2004;42(7):2944–51.

CUTANEOUS LARVA MIGRANS

Susan Montgomery, Mary Kamb

INFECTIOUS AGENT: *Ancylostoma* spp.	
ENDEMICITY	Worldwide
TRAVELER CATEGORIES AT GREATEST RISK FOR EXPOSURE & INFECTION	Travelers to tropical or subtropical regions who have unprotected skin contact with sand or soil
PREVENTION METHODS	Avoid direct skin contact with potentially contaminated sand or soil
DIAGNOSTIC SUPPORT	CDC's Parasitic Diseases Branch, (www.cdc.gov/parasites; 404-718-4745; parasites@cdc.gov) Parasitological diagnosis: DPDx (www.cdc.gov/DPDx)

INFECTIOUS AGENT

Larval stages of dog and cat hookworms (usually *Ancylostoma* spp.) can cause skin infections.

TRANSMISSION

Hookworm infections occur through direct skin contact with contaminated sand or soil.

EPIDEMIOLOGY

Zoonotic hookworms associated with cutaneous larva migrans (CLM)—also known as creeping eruption—have a worldwide distribution, but most cases are reported in travelers to Africa, South America, Asia, and the Caribbean. Beaches and sandboxes where free-roaming dogs and cats defecate are common sources of infection. Infection occurs in short-term and long-term travelers.

5

CLINICAL PRESENTATION

Creeping eruption usually appears 1–5 days after skin penetration, but the incubation period may be ≥1 month. Typically, a serpiginous, erythematous track appears in the skin and is associated with intense itching and mild swelling. Usual locations are the feet, lower legs, and buttocks, but any skin surface (e.g., trunk, upper extremities) that contacts contaminated soil can be affected (see Sec. 11, Ch. 8, Dermatologic Conditions).

DIAGNOSIS

CLM is diagnosed clinically based on a history of potential exposure and characteristic skin lesions. Biopsy is not recommended. Clinicians can obtain diagnostic assistance from the Centers for Disease Control and Prevention (CDC)'s Division of Parasitic Diseases and Malaria DPDx laboratory (www.cdc.gov/DPDx; dpdx@cdc.gov), or from the Parasitic Diseases Hotline for Healthcare Providers (404-718-4745; parasites@cdc.gov).

TREATMENT

CLM is self-limiting; migrating larvae usually die after 5–6 weeks. Albendazole is a very effective treatment. Ivermectin is effective but not approved by the US Food and Drug Administration for this indication. Symptomatic treatment can help relieve severe itching and reduce the chance of bacterial superinfection.

PREVENTION

Instruct travelers to reduce their contact with contaminated sand and soil by wearing shoes and protective clothing and using barriers (e.g., blankets, towels) when seated on the ground or sandy beaches, particularly in areas with free-roaming dogs and cats.

CDC website: www.cdc.gov/parasites/zoonotichookworm

BIBLIOGRAPHY

Caumes E. Treatment of cutaneous larva migrans. Clin Infect Dis. 2000;30(5):811–4.

Del Giudice P, Hakimi S, Vandenbos F, Magana C, Hubiche T. Autochthonous cutaneous larva migrans in France and Europe. Acta Derm Venereol. 2019;99(9):805–8.

Heukelbach J, Feldmeier H. Epidemiological and clinical characteristics of hookworm-related cutaneous larva migrans. Lancet Infect Dis. 2008;8(5):302–9.

Hochedez P, Caumes E. Hookworm-related cutaneous larva migrans. J Travel Med. 2007;14(5):326–33.

Lederman ER, Weld LH, Elyazar IR, von Sonnenburg F, Loutan L, Schwartz E, et al. Dermatologic conditions of the ill returned traveler: an analysis from the GeoSentinel Surveillance Network. Int J Infect Dis. 2008;12(6):593–602.

Vanhaecke C, Perignon A, Monsel G, Regnier S, Bricaire F, Caumes E. The efficacy of single dose ivermectin in the treatment of hookworm related cutaneous larva migrans varies depending on the clinical presentation. J Eur Acad Dermatol Venereol. 2014;28(5):655–7.

CYCLOSPORIASIS

Anne Straily, Rebecca Chancey

INFECTIOUS AGENT: *Cyclospora cayetanensis*	
ENDEMICITY	Tropical and subtropical regions
TRAVELER CATEGORIES AT GREATEST RISK FOR EXPOSURE & INFECTION	Any travelers to endemic regions who consume potentially contaminated fresh produce
PREVENTION METHODS	Follow safe food and water precautions
DIAGNOSTIC SUPPORT	A clinical laboratory certified in moderate complexity testing; or contact CDC's Parasitic Diseases Branch (www.cdc.gov/parasites; 404-718-4745; parasites@cdc.gov) Parasitological diagnosis: DPDx (www.cdc.gov/DPDx)

5

INFECTIOUS AGENT

Cyclospora cayetanensis, a coccidian protozoan parasite, causes cyclosporiasis.

TRANSMISSION

Transmission occurs through ingestion of infective *Cyclospora* oocysts, typically from contaminated food or water.

EPIDEMIOLOGY

Cyclosporiasis occurs in many countries around the world, but appears to be most common in tropical and subtropical regions. Outbreaks frequently are seasonal, but seasonality varies in different parts of the world. In Guatemala, detection rates increase during May–August. In Nepal, rates increase during the summer and rainy season (May–October). In Turkey, incidence rates are highest during July–November. No environmental conditions (e.g., temperature, rainfall) have yet been determined to be drivers for the seasonal variation in cyclosporiasis.

People typically become infected through the consumption of contaminated fresh produce or contaminated water. All travelers are at risk of infection, regardless of the purpose or length of their travel in an endemic area; even short-term travelers can become infected. Outbreaks in the United States and Canada typically occur during the spring and summer months; historically these have been linked to consumption of imported fresh produce. No commercially frozen or canned produce has yet been implicated as the source of an outbreak.

During 2011–2015, 415 cyclosporiasis cases were reported among US residents with a history of international travel during their incubation period. The most frequently reported destinations were in the Americas, including Mexico, the Caribbean, Central America, and South America; travel to Africa, Asia, and Europe was reported less frequently among identified case-patients.

CLINICAL PRESENTATION

The incubation period averages 1 week (range 2 days to ≥2 weeks). Symptom onset often is abrupt, but can be gradual; some people have an influenza-like prodrome. The most common symptom is watery diarrhea, which can be profuse. Other symptoms can include abdominal cramps, anorexia, bloating, body aches, low-grade fever, nausea, vomiting, and weight loss. If untreated, the illness can last for several weeks or months with a remitting–relapsing course.

DIAGNOSIS

Cyclosporiasis is diagnosed by detecting *Cyclospora* oocysts or DNA in stool specimens. Stool examinations for ova and parasites usually do not include methods for detecting *Cyclospora* unless testing for this parasite is specifically requested. Diagnostic assistance for *Cyclospora* and other parasitic diseases also is available from the Centers for Disease

Control and Prevention (www.cdc.gov/dpdx; 404-718-4745; parasites@cdc.gov). Cyclosporiasis is a nationally notifiable disease.

TREATMENT

Treatment includes trimethoprim-sulfamethoxazole; no highly effective alternatives have been identified. One case report documented resolution of symptoms after treatment with nitazoxanide in a patient with a sulfa allergy. Anecdotal data suggest that ciprofloxacin is ineffective.

PREVENTION

Travelers can reduce their risk for infection by following food and water precautions (see Sec. 2, Ch. 8, Food & Water Precautions), but using chlorine or iodine for water disinfection is unlikely to be effective because oocysts are extremely tolerant of halogens (see Sec. 2, Ch. 9, Water Disinfection).

CDC website: www.cdc.gov/parasites/cyclosporiasis

BIBLIOGRAPHY

Abanyie F, Harvey RR, Harris JR, Wiegand RE, Gaul L, Desvignes-Kendrick M, et al. 2013 multistate outbreaks of *Cyclospora cayetanensis* infections associated with fresh produce: focus on the Texas investigations. Epidemiol Infect. 2015;143(16):3451–8.

Cama VA, Mathison BA. Infections by intestinal coccidian and *Giardia duodenalis*. Clin Lab Med. 2015;35(2):423–44.

Casillas S, Hall R, Herwaldt BL. Cyclosporiasis surveillance—United States, 2011–2015. MMWR Surveill Summ. 2019;68(3):1–16.

Hall RL, Jones JL, Herwaldt BL. Surveillance for laboratory-confirmed sporadic cases of cyclosporiasis—United States, 1997–2008. MMWR Surveill Summ. 2011;60(2):1–11.

Herwaldt BL. *Cyclospora cayetanensis*: a review, focusing on the outbreaks of cyclosporiasis in the 1990s. Clin Infect Dis. 2000;31(4):1040–57.

Marques DFP, Alexander CL, Chalmers RM, Chiodini P, Elson R, Freedman J, et al. Cyclosporiasis in travelers returning to the United Kingdom from Mexico in summer 2017: lessons from the recent past to inform the future. Euro Surveill. 2017;22(32):30592.

Ortega YR, Sanchez R. Update on *Cyclospora cayetanensis*, a food-borne and waterborne parasite. Clin Microbiol Rev. 2010;23(1):218–34.

Zimmer SM, Schuetz AN, Franco-Paredes C. Efficacy of nitazoxanide for cyclosporiasis in patients with a sulfa allergy. Clin Infect Dis. 2007;44:466–7.

CYSTICERCOSIS

Paul Cantey, Sharon Roy

INFECTIOUS AGENT: *Taenia solium*	
ENDEMICITY	Worldwide Most prominent where sanitary conditions are poor, and pigs have access to human feces
TRAVELER CATEGORIES AT GREATEST RISK FOR EXPOSURE & INFECTION	Immigrants and refugees Long-term travelers Travelers visiting friends and relatives
PREVENTION METHODS	Follow safe food precautions Avoid eating food cooked by someone who does not practice good hand hygiene Practice good hand hygiene
DIAGNOSTIC SUPPORT	Serologic testing: CDC's Parasitic Diseases Branch (www.cdc.gov/parasites; 404-718-4745; parasites@cdc.gov)

INFECTIOUS AGENT

Cysticercosis is caused by *Taenia solium*, a cestode parasite.

TRANSMISSION

Transmission occurs through ingestion of eggs excreted by a human carrier of the adult *T. solium* tapeworm via fecally contaminated food or through close contact with the carrier. Autoinfection is also possible. Larval cysts of *T. solium* infect brain, muscle, or other tissues. Eating undercooked pork containing cysticerci results in tapeworm infection (taeniasis), not human cysticercosis.

EPIDEMIOLOGY

Cysticercosis occurs globally and is common where sanitary conditions are poor and where pigs have access to human feces. Endemic areas include Latin America, sub-Saharan Africa, East Asia, and India. Cysticercosis is uncommon in travelers, but is more likely in long-term travelers, in immigrants and refugees from endemic regions, and in people who visit friends and relatives in endemic areas.

CLINICAL PRESENTATION

The latent period for cysticercosis ranges from months to decades. Symptoms depend on the number, location, and stage of cysts. The most important clinical manifestations are caused by cysts in the brain, where cysts can be parenchymal or extraparenchymal (ventricular, subarachnoid). The most common presentations are seizures and increased intracranial pressure. Other presentations include encephalitis, symptoms of space-occupying lesions (e.g., seizures), and hydrocephalus. Cysticercosis should be considered in any adult with new-onset seizures who comes from an endemic area or has had potential exposure to a tapeworm carrier.

DIAGNOSIS

Neuroimaging studies (e.g., CT, MRI) are required, and confirmatory serologic testing is often needed. Visualization of a scolex on neuroimaging is diagnostic. The most specific serologic test is the enzyme-linked immunotransfer blot (EITB), but results can be negative in ≥30% of patients with a single parenchymal lesion. The sensitivity of the test is also reduced in patients with only calcified lesions. The EITB is available through the Parasitic Diseases Branch at the Centers for Disease Control and Prevention (CDC). Instructions on how to submit a serum specimen for testing at CDC can be found at www.cdc.gov/laboratory/specimen-submission/index.html.

TREATMENT

Control of symptoms is the cornerstone of cysticercosis therapy. Anticonvulsants, corticosteroids, or both might be indicated. Urgently manage increased intracranial pressure, if present. Antiparasitic treatment (albendazole, praziquantel) is not indicated for all presentations of neurocysticercosis; carefully consider the risks and benefits before starting treatment and consider expert consultation. Recommendations vary depending on whether the lesion is parenchymal or extraparenchymal; viable, enhancing, or calcified; has associated perilesional edema; and by location and number of lesions. For some intraventricular lesions, surgical intervention could be the treatment of choice.

In complicated cases, the priority is neurologic management (e.g., corticosteroids, mannitol), neurosurgery, or both. In 2018, the Infectious Diseases Society of America and the American Society of Tropical Medicine and Hygiene published guidelines for the clinical management of neurocysticercosis, which are available at https://doi.org/10.1093/cid/cix1084. Clinicians can contact CDC Parasitic Diseases Inquiries at 404-718-4745 or parasites@cdc.gov to obtain more information about diagnosis and treatment.

PREVENTION

To reduce the risk for infection, travelers should follow food and water precautions (see Sec. 2, Ch. 8, Food & Water Precautions) and practice good hand hygiene to reduce the risk for possible autoinfection.

CDC website: www.cdc.gov/parasites/cysticercosis

BIBLIOGRAPHY

Del Brutto OH. Neurocysticercosis among international travelers to disease-endemic areas. J Travel Med. 2012;19(2):112–17.

Garcia HH, Gonzales I, Lescano AG, Bustos JA, Pretell EJ, Saavedra H, et al. Enhanced steroid dosing reduces seizures during antiparasitic treatment for cysticercosis and early after. Epilepsia. 2014;55(9):1452–9.

Garcia HH, Gonzales I, Lescano AG, Bustos JA, Zimic M, Escalante D, et al. Efficacy of combined antiparasitic therapy with praziquantel and albendazole for neurocysticercosis: a double-blind, randomized controlled trial. Lancet Infect Dis. 2014;14(8):687–95.

White AC, Coyle CM, Rajshekhar V, Singh G, Hauser WA, Mohanty A, et al. Diagnosis and treatment of neurocysticercosis: 2017 clinical practice guidelines by the Infectious Diseases Society of America (IDSA) and the American Society of Tropical Medicine and Hygiene (ASTMH). Clin Infect Dis. 2018;66(8):e49–75.

ECHINOCOCCOSIS

Paul Cantey, Rebecca Chancey, Sharon Roy

5

INFECTIOUS AGENTS: *Echinococcus multilocularis* (alveolar echinococcosis) *Echinococcus granulosus* (cystic echinococcosis)	
ENDEMICITY	Alveolar echinococcosis: primarily in northern latitudes of North America, Asia, and Europe where canids ingest the rodent intermediate host Cystic echinococcosis: worldwide where canids ingest the organs of livestock
TRAVELER CATEGORIES AT GREATEST RISK FOR EXPOSURE & INFECTION	Immigrants and refugees Long-term travelers
PREVENTION METHODS	Avoid canids in affected areas Avoid drinking untreated water Avoid eating food cooked by someone who does not use good hand hygiene Practice good hand hygiene
DIAGNOSTIC SUPPORT	Serologic testing: CDC's Parasitic Diseases Branch (www.cdc.gov/parasites; 404-718-4745; parasites@cdc.gov) Parasitological diagnosis: DPDx (www.cdc.gov/DPDx)

INFECTIOUS AGENTS

Echinococcosis is caused by cestode parasites of the genus *Echinococcus*, including *E. multilocularis*, *E. granulosus*, and others.

TRANSMISSION

Humans become infected through ingestion of *Echinococcus* eggs shed in the feces of infected definitive hosts, including foxes and other canids for *E. multilocularis*, or dogs and other canids for *E. granulosus*. Ingestion can occur through hand-to-mouth transfer of eggs or by consuming fecally contaminated food, water, or soil.

EPIDEMIOLOGY

The 2 main forms of echinococcosis in humans are alveolar echinococcosis (AE), caused by *E. multilocularis*, and cystic echinococcosis (CE), caused by *E. granulosus* and other species. Rarer forms, referred to as neotropical echinococcosis

(NE), are caused by *E. vogeli* and *E. oligarthrus*. AE occurs in the northern hemisphere, in parts of North America and Eurasia. CE occurs in parts of Africa, the Americas (including South America [foci within Peru]), Australia, and Eurasia, including in pastoral and rangeland areas, where transmission often is maintained by dog-sheep-dog cycles. NE occurs in rural settlements near tropical forests in Central and South America. Although indigenous human cases of AE and CE have been reported in the United States, most US cases of echinococcosis have been imported.

CLINICAL PRESENTATION

People with AE and CE could remain asymptomatic for years. The nature and severity of the clinical manifestations depend in part on the location, size, and other characteristics of the lesions that develop and the associated complications. AE usually affects the liver; direct extension to and destruction of contiguous tissues can occur, as can metastatic lesions. In CE, lesions are cystic (referred to as hydatid cysts) and most commonly develop in the liver; the next most common site is the lungs, but cysts can develop in other organ systems. NE is rare; the polycystic form can be clinically similar to AE.

DIAGNOSIS

A presumptive diagnosis can be based on a combination of the person's exposure history and imaging studies (e.g., an ultrasound or CT scan). Lesions might be found incidentally in asymptomatic people. Serologic testing also can be helpful and is available through the Parasitic Diseases Branch at the Centers for Disease Control and Prevention (CDC). Instructions on how to submit a serum specimen for testing can be found at www.cdc.gov/laboratory/specimen-submission/index.html. For assistance with parasitological diagnosis, submit a request to the Division of Parasitic Diseases and Malaria DPDx (www.cdc.gov/dpdx/dxassistance.html).

TREATMENT

For AE, treatment strategies include complete surgical removal of infected tissue (if resectable) and long-term benzimidazole therapy; untreated AE progresses and ultimately leads to death. For CE, the World Health Organization has developed an image-based staging system that facilitates selecting among potential case-management strategies, including observation without treatment, percutaneous approaches, surgical resection, and drug treatment. Treatment of NE might involve surgical treatment or benzimidazole therapy; the role of percutaneous treatment is unclear. Clinicians can consult CDC to obtain more information about diagnosis and treatment (CDC Parasitic Diseases Inquiries: 404-718-4745 or parasites@cdc.gov).

PREVENTION

To reduce the risk for echinococcosis, travelers should avoid contact with dogs and wild canids in endemic areas; should not drink untreated water from canals, lakes, rivers, or streams; and should follow food and water precautions (see Sec. 2, Ch. 8, Food & Water Precautions). In addition, travelers should practice good hand hygiene after handling dogs and during food preparation in affected areas.

CDC website: www.cdc.gov/parasites/echinococcosis

BIBLIOGRAPHY

Brunetti E, Kern P, Vuitton DA; Writing Panel for the WHO-IWGE. Expert consensus for the diagnosis and treatment of cystic and alveolar echinococcosis in humans. Acta Trop. 2010;114(1):1–16.

Deplazes P, Rinaldi L, Alvarez Rojas CA, Torgerson PR, Harandi MF, Romig T, et al. Global distribution of alveolar and cystic echinococcosis. Adv Parasitol. 2017;95:315–493.

Kern P, Menezes da Silva A, Akhan O, Müllhaupt B, Vizcaychipi KA, Budke C, et al. The echinococcoses: diagnosis, clinical management and burden of disease. Adv Parasitol. 2017;96:259–369.

Mandal S, Mandal MD. Human cystic echinococcosis: epidemiologic, zoonotic, clinical, diagnostic and therapeutic aspects. Asian Pac J Trop Med. 2012;5(4):253–60.

Stojkovic M, Rosenberger K, Kauczor HU, Junghanss T, Hosch W. Diagnosing and staging of cystic echinococcosis: how do CT and MRI perform in comparison to ultrasound? PLoS Negl Trop Dis. 2012;6(10):e1880.

ENTEROBIASIS / PINWORM

Rebecca Chancey, Mary Kamb

INFECTIOUS AGENT: *Enterobius vermicularis*	
ENDEMICITY	Worldwide
TRAVELER CATEGORIES AT GREATEST RISK FOR EXPOSURE & INFECTION	Children People who take care of infected children
PREVENTION METHODS	Avoid handling contaminated bed linen and clothing Practice good hand hygiene, especially after using the toilet or changing diapers and before handling food
DIAGNOSTIC SUPPORT	Parasitological diagnosis: DPDx (www.cdc.gov/DPDx)

INFECTIOUS AGENT

Enterobiasis is caused by the intestinal nematode (roundworm) *Enterobius vermicularis.*

TRANSMISSION

People become infected, usually unknowingly, by ingesting infective pinworm eggs. Person-to-person transmission of infective pinworm eggs occurs through the fecal–oral route (including self-inoculation) by contaminated hands or eating contaminated food (rarely), or indirectly by handling bedding, clothing, or other articles contaminated by eggs. Because of their small size, pinworm eggs can become airborne, suggesting inhalation from air and dust could be another transmission route.

EPIDEMIOLOGY

Pinworm is endemic worldwide and commonly clusters within families. Infections are typically in preschool- and school-age children, people who care for young children, and people who are institutionalized. Based on limited data, travelers could be exposed in crowded conditions with infected people or through contaminated bedding.

CLINICAL PRESENTATION

The incubation period is usually 1–2 months; successive reinfections might be needed before symptoms appear. The most common symptom is perianal itching, which can be severe, causing sleep disturbances and irritability. Secondary infection of irritated skin also can occur. Adult worms can migrate from the anal area to the urethra, vagina, vulva, or other sites. Appendicitis and enuresis are reported as possible associated conditions.

DIAGNOSIS

Adult worms might be visible near the anus 2–3 hours after the infected person is asleep. Visual inspection of undergarments or bedding also might reveal pinworms. For microscopic identification, pinworm eggs can be collected by touching transparent tape to the affected person's anal area immediately after awakening and before washing, ideally on 3 consecutive mornings. Eggs also might be found in samples taken from under fingernails before handwashing. Examining stool samples is not recommended because pinworm eggs are sparse. Diagnostic assistance is available through the Centers for Disease Control and Prevention (CDC)'s DPDx laboratory in the Division of Parasitic Diseases and Malaria (www.cdc.gov/DPDx).

TREATMENT

Drugs of choice are albendazole, pyrantel pamoate, or mebendazole given as a single, initial dose, followed by a second dose of the same drug 2 weeks later to eliminate possible reinfection. Pyrantel pamoate is available without prescription in the United States. Mebendazole is available in the United States only through compounding pharmacies. Simultaneous treatment of all household members is warranted if >1 person is infected, or infection recurs. Offer treatment to exposed sexual partners.

PREVENTION

Careful hand hygiene is the most effective prevention method. During treatment, change bed linens and underclothing of infected children first thing in the morning. Advise patients and families to collect linens and clothing carefully to avoid contaminating the environment (e.g., not shaking out the clothing or linens), and then laundering promptly in hot (>40° C) water and drying in a hot dryer to kill any eggs that might be present. To prevent transmission or reinfection, counsel infected people to bathe (shower or stand-up baths) in the morning and change underwear daily and bed clothes frequently, including after treatment and preferably after bathing. Infected people should also practice personal hygiene measures, including washing hands with soap and water before eating or preparing food, keeping fingernails short, avoiding scratching the perianal region, and avoiding nail biting.

CDC website: www.cdc.gov/parasites/pinworm

BIBLIOGRAPHY

American Academy of Pediatrics. Pinworm infection (*Enterobius vermicularis*). In: Kimberlin DW, editor. Red Book: 2018 Report of the Committee on Infectious Disease, 31st edition. Itasca (IL): American Academy of Pediatrics; 2018. pp. 634–5.

American Public Health Association. Enterobiasis. In: Heyman DL, editor. Control of communicable diseases manual, 20th edition. Washington, DC: American Public Health Association; 2014. pp. 187–8.

Kang WH, Jee SC. *Enterobius vermicularis* (pinworm) infection. N Engl J Med. 2019;381(1):e1.

Kucik CJ, Martin GL, Sortor BV. Common intestinal parasites. Am Fam Physician. 2004;69(5):1161–9.

Wendt S, Trawinski H, Schubert S, Rodloff AC, Mössner J, Lübbert C. The diagnosis and treatment of pinworm infection. Dtsch Arztebl Int. 2019;116(13):213–9.

5

FILARIASIS, LYMPHATIC

Mary Kamb, Sharon Roy

INFECTIOUS AGENTS: *Wuchereria bancrofti*, *Brugia malayi*, and *B. timori*	
ENDEMICITY	Africa: Sub-Saharan Africa and Egypt Americas: Northeastern coast of Brazil; parts of Guyana, Haiti, and the Dominican Republic Asia and the Pacific: southern and southeast Asia; southwestern Pacific Islands
TRAVELER CATEGORIES AT GREATEST RISK FOR EXPOSURE & INFECTION	Immigrants and refugees from endemic areas Long-term travelers
PREVENTION METHODS	Avoid insect bites
DIAGNOSTIC SUPPORT	Serologic testing: National Institutes of Health Laboratory of Parasitic Diseases (301-496-5398) or CDC's Parasitic Disease Branch (www.cdc.gov/parasites; 404-718-4745; parasites@cdc.gov)

INFECTIOUS AGENT

Lymphatic filariasis is caused by 3 species of filarial nematodes, *Wuchereria bancrofti, Brugia malayi*, and *B. timori*.

TRANSMISSION

Infective larvae can be transmitted by both day- and night-biting mosquitoes; vectors include species from several genera, including *Aedes, Anopheles, Coquillettidia, Culex*, and *Mansonia*. Transmission occurs in rural, urban, and semiurban settings.

EPIDEMIOLOGY

Once widespread in Africa and Asia, and swaths of Latin America and the Pacific, sustained elimination efforts based on mass drug administration have greatly reduced the global prevalence of parasites that cause lymphatic filariasis. Currently, infections occur in parts of Africa (Egypt, sub-Saharan Africa); Asia (southeast Asia, the Indian subcontinent); and some southwestern Pacific Islands. In the Americas, focal distribution has been reported on the northeastern coast of Brazil, in Guyana, and on the island of Hispaniola (Dominican Republic, Haiti). Most infections in the United States occur in immigrants and refugees.

Because multiple exposures (bites from infected mosquitoes) over time are usually required for infection, travelers are at low risk for this disease. Infections have, however, been documented in long-term travelers (usually people living many months–years in endemic countries) and in visitors to areas with highly efficient mosquito vectors (e.g., *Aedes* in the Pacific) with as little as 1 month of exposure.

CLINICAL PRESENTATION

Infective filarial larvae grow into adult worms that inhabit the human lymphatic and subcutaneous tissues. Infections can be asymptomatic (subclinical) or associated with acute and chronic clinical manifestations involving moderate to severe lymphedema of the arm, breast, leg, penis, or scrotum. In people with lymphedema, episodes of acute secondary infections can involve painful swelling of an affected limb, fever, or chills; repeated episodes can hasten the progression of lymphedema to its advanced stage, known as elephantiasis.

Tropical pulmonary eosinophilia (TPE) syndrome is a potentially serious, progressive lung disease characterized by fever and nocturnal cough, wheezing, or both, which results from immune hyper-responsiveness to microfilariae in the pulmonary capillaries. Most cases of TPE have been reported in long-term residents from Asia, often men aged 20–40 years.

DIAGNOSIS

In symptomatic people with plausible exposure based on epidemiology, diagnosis can be made by microscopic detection of characteristic microfilariae on a thick blood film made from an appropriately timed sample collection. Microfilariae are usually not detected in patients with TPE.

Filarial antibody tests that detect elevated IgG and IgG4 can be useful, especially when microfilariae are not detected. Serologic assays are available through the National Institutes of Health (301-496-5398) or Centers for Disease Control and Prevention (CDC; www.cdc.gov/dpdx; 404-718-4745; parasites@cdc.gov). PCR tests exist in some research settings but are not yet commercially available. Ultrasound and lymphoscintigraphy can be used to detect presence of motile adult worms in lymphatic vessels, known as filarial dance sign.

TREATMENT

Diethylcarbamazine (DEC) is the drug of choice for lymphatic filariasis, regardless of the causative parasite species. Although no longer approved for use in the United States by the US Food and Drug Administration and not commercially available, DEC can be obtained under an investigational new drug protocol from the CDC Drug Service (M–F, 8 a.m.–4:30 p.m. Eastern, 404-639-3670; after hours/weekends/holidays, 770-488-7100; drugservice@cdc.gov).

Before initiating DEC treatment for lymphatic filariasis, first rule out co-infection with *Onchocerca volvulus* in at-risk patients (see Sec. 5, Part 3, Ch. 17, Onchocerciasis / River Blindness). DEC use is contraindicated in patients with *O. volvulus* infection due to the potential for causing a severe allergic response (Mazzotti reaction) that especially affects the eyes and skin. In addition, DEC must be used with extreme caution in patients with loiasis (*Loa loa* infection) due to possible life-threatening side effects in people with high circulating microfilariae loads.

People with lymphedema and hydrocele can benefit from lymphedema management and, in the case of hydrocele, surgical repair. Evidence suggests that a 4–8-week course of doxycycline (200 mg daily) can both sterilize adult worms and improve lymphatic pathologic features.

PREVENTION

No vaccines or drugs to prevent infection are available. Travelers should avoid mosquito bites (see Sec. 4, Ch. 6, Mosquitoes, Ticks & Other Arthropods).

CDC website: www.cdc.gov/parasites/lymphaticfilariasis

BIBLIOGRAPHY

Debrah AY, Mand S, Specht S, Marfo-Debrekyei Y, Batsa L, Pfarr K, et al. Doxycycline reduces plasma VEGF-C/sVEGFR-3 and improves pathology in lymphatic filariasis. PLoS Pathogens. 2006;2(9):e92.

Eberhard ML, Lammie PJ. Laboratory diagnosis of filariasis. Clin Lab Med. 1991;11(4):977–1010.

Hoerauf A, Pfarr K, Mand S, Bebrah AY, Specht S. Filariasis in Africa—treatment challenges and prospects. Clin Microbiol Infect. 2011;17(7):977–85.

Jones RT. Non-endemic cases of lymphatic filariasis. Trop Med Int Health. 2014;19(11):1377–83.

Lipner EM, Law MA, Barnett E, Keystone JS, von Sonnenburg F, Loutan L, et al. Filariasis in travelers presenting to the GeoSentinel Surveillance Network. PLoS Negl Trop Dis. 2007;1(3):e88.

Ryan ET, Hill DR, Solomon T, Magill AJ. Hunter's Tropical medicine and emerging infectious diseases, 9th edition. New York: Elsevier; 2012.

World Health Organization. Global programme to eliminate lymphatic filariasis: progress report, 2016. Wkly Epidemiol Rec. 2017;92(40):594–607.

5

FLUKES, LIVER

Sharon Roy, Paul Cantey

INFECTIOUS AGENTS: *Clonorchis*, *Fasciola* spp., and *Opisthorchis* spp.	
ENDEMICITY	*Clonorchis*: primarily East Asia *Fasciola* spp.: Worldwide *Opisthorchis* spp.: Regional
TRAVELER CATEGORIES AT GREATEST RISK FOR EXPOSURE & INFECTION	All travelers Expatriates and long-term travelers living in endemic areas
PREVENTION METHODS	Follow safe food and water precautions Avoid eating raw or undercooked crab, crayfish, or fish in areas where flukes are endemic Avoid eating watercress or other greens that might have been washed with water contaminated with fluke larvae
DIAGNOSTIC SUPPORT	A clinical laboratory certified in moderate complexity testing; or for serologic testing for *Fasciola* spp., contact CDC's Parasitic Diseases Branch (www.cdc.gov/parasites; 404-718-4745; parasites@cdc.gov) For *Clonorchis* and *Opisthorchis* spp. ova and parasite testing, contact Parasitological diagnosis DPDx (www.cdc.gov/DPDx)

INFECTIOUS AGENTS

Liver flukes are trematode flatworms, including *Clonorchis sinensis*; *Fasciola hepatica* and *F. gigantica*; *Opisthorchis felineus* and *O. viverrini*.

TRANSMISSION

Reservoir hosts for *Clonorchis* and *Opisthorchis* spp. are cats, dogs, and other fish-eating mammals, and human infection generally occurs by ingestion of raw or undercooked (e.g., pickled, salted, or smoked) freshwater fish. *Fasciola* spp. cause liver disease in cattle and sheep (definitive hosts) but can be transmitted to humans who consume watercress or other aquatic, freshwater plants contaminated with infective metacercariae, or who drink contaminated water.

5

EPIDEMIOLOGY

C. sinensis is found mainly in eastern Asia, including China, Korea, eastern Russia, Taiwan, and northern Vietnam; it was previously endemic in Japan, although the last human case there was reported in 1991. *F. hepatica* has worldwide distribution, especially in areas where cattle or sheep are raised. *F. gigantica* has a more limited distribution in parts of Africa and Asia. *O. felineus* is found mainly in eastern Europe and through central Asia to Siberia, including the Baltic countries, Belarus, Italy, Germany, Greece, Kazakhstan, Moldova, Poland, Romania, Russia, and the Ukraine. *O. viverrini* is found mainly in Burma (Myanmar), northeastern Cambodia, Laos, Thailand, and central and southern Vietnam.

Worldwide, men are more commonly infected with *Clonorchis* and *Opisthorchis* spp. than women; slightly more women are infected with *Fasciola* spp. than men. For fascioliasis, prevalence is greater during childhood and decreases somewhat in adulthood. For clonorchiasis and opisthorchiasis, prevalence increases during childhood, reaching a maximum prevalence at middle age, with a slight decrease in prevalence in older age.

Travelers to liver fluke–endemic areas can become infected by ingesting contaminated foods. The risk for infection increases with increasing exposure (i.e., ingestion of infective metacercariae on raw and inadequately washed plants), which is greater for people residing for long periods in known endemic areas (e.g., expatriates, immigrants, long-term travelers, refugees).

CLINICAL PRESENTATION

Clonorchiasis & Opisthorchiasis

Clonorchiasis and opisthorchiasis symptoms are related to worm burden and involve both the gallbladder and liver. Most low-intensity infections are asymptomatic or show only mild symptoms. Patients with high-intensity infections might show nonspecific signs and symptoms, which can include diarrhea, eosinophilia, fatigue, fever, nausea, and indigestion. They also could have abdominal pain, particularly in the right upper quadrant; intermittent colicky pain associated with worms obstructing the gallbladder; jaundice; and an enlarged or tender liver.

Generally, patients infected with *O. felineus* are more symptomatic in the acute phase than those infected with *O. viverrini* or *Clonorchis* spp. Chronic infections, at about 30 days post-infection, can result in various complications, including cholelithiasis, cholangitis, and cholecystitis. Liver abscesses and pancreatitis also have been linked to chronic clonorchiasis, as has developmental delay in children with high-intensity infections. Chronic *Clonorchis* and *Opisthorcis viverrini* from protracted episodes of reinfection over time are associated with the development of cholangiocarcinoma (CCA). Multiple nonparasitic risk factors for CCA exist, however, and liver fluke infections are very rarely associated with cases of CCA in the United States.

Fascioliasis

The acute phase of fascioliasis (also known as the migratory, invasive, or hepatic phase) can last up to 3–4 months. Although most infected people have low-intensity infections and are asymptomatic during the acute phase, ≈17.5% of patients with high-intensity infections can experience clinical manifestations, including abdominal pain and other gastrointestinal symptoms, marked eosinophilia, fever, respiratory symptoms (e.g., cough), and urticaria.

The chronic (biliary) phase begins 6 months after infection when immature worms (larval flukes) reach the bile ducts, mature into adult worms (which can live ≥10 years), and start to produce eggs. The clinical manifestations, if any, during the chronic phase reflect biliary tract disease (e.g., biliary tract obstruction, cholangitis, cholecystitis) or pancreatitis.

DIAGNOSIS

The primary mode of diagnosis of fascioliasis and liver flukes is detection of eggs in stool, or in duodenal or biliary aspirates. Distinguishing *Fasciola* eggs from those of *Fasciolopsis buski* can be difficult. *Fasciolopsis buski* is an intestinal fluke that requires a different treatment than *Fasciola*. In fascioliasis, egg production does not occur until ≥3–4 months after exposure; thus, serologic testing can be useful for fascioliasis diagnosis during the acute phase because parasite antibodies might be detectable in 2–4 weeks. Serology also can be useful during the chronic phase if egg production is intermittent or low.

Serologic testing for fascioliasis is available through the Centers for Disease Control and Prevention (CDC). Instructions for submitting specimens for testing at CDC can be found at www.cdc.gov/laboratory/specimen-submission/index.html; see the test directory for specific instructions on how to request *Fasciola* serology. Further information about diagnosis and management of the different liver flukes is available at www.cdc.gov/parasites, by emailing parasites@cdc.gov, or by calling 404-718-4745. No serologic tests are available in the United States for clonorchiasis or opisthorciasis. Imaging studies (e.g., CT, MRI, ultrasonography) of the hepatobiliary tract, can be helpful for the diagnosis of liver flukes of all species.

TREATMENT

First-line treatment of fascioliasis is with triclabendazole, approved for use in the United States by the Food and Drug Administration in 2019. Health care providers should contact the AllCare Plus Pharmacy at 888-774-7327 to order triclabendazole. AllCare will need the patient's name, address, telephone number, date of birth, weight, and clinical information; the pharmacy will arrange for free shipping of the drug to the patient. Nitazoxanide therapy might be helpful in some patients with fascioliasis.

First-line treatment for clonorchiasis and opisthorchiasis is praziquantel. Albendazole is an alternative drug for treatment of *Clonorchis* or *Opisthorchis*. In patients with biliary tract obstruction due to liver flukes of any of the species, removal of adult flukes (e.g., via endoscopic retrograde cholangiopancreatography) might be indicated.

PREVENTION

Travelers can prevent *Fasciola* infection by avoiding ingestion of uncooked, aquatic freshwater plants, including watercress, especially from endemic grazing areas. These include plants used in local dishes, appetizers, beverages, condiments, and juices. Additionally, travelers should avoid drinking water from untreated natural sources, particularly those frequented by livestock. Infection with other liver flukes can be prevented by avoiding ingestion of raw or undercooked, pickled, salted, or smoked freshwater fish in endemic areas (See Sec. 2, Ch. 8, Food & Water Precautions).

CDC website: www.cdc.gov/parasites/fasciola; www.cdc.gov/parasites/opisthorchis; www.cdc.gov/parasites/clonorchis

BIBLIOGRAPHY

Ashrafi K, Bargues MD, O'Neill S, Mas-Coma S. Fascioliasis: a worldwide parasitic disease of importance in travel medicine. Travel Med Infect Dis. 2014;12(6 Pt A):636–49.

Fürst T, Keiser J, Utzinger J. Global burden of human food-borne trematodiasis: a systematic review and meta-analysis. Lancet Infect Dis. 2012;12(3):210–21.

Keiser J, Utzinger J. Food-borne trematodiasis. Clin Micro Rev. 2009;22(3):466–83.

Mas-Coma S, Bargues MD, Valero MA. Human fascioliasis infection sources, their diversity, incidence factors, analytical methods and prevention measures. Parasitology. 2018; 145(13):1665–99.

Mas-Coma S, Valero MA, Bargues MD. Fascioliasis. In: Toledo R, Fried B, editors. Digenetic trematodes. Advances in experimental medicine and biology. 2019;1154:71–103.

Qian MB, Utzinger J, Keiser J, Zhou XN. Clonorchiasis. Lancet. 2016;387(10020):800–10.

Rowan SE, Levi ME, Youngwerth JM, Brauer B, Everson GT, Johnson SC. The variable presentations and broadening geographic distribution of hepatic fascioliasis. Clin Gastroenterol Hepatol. 2012;10(6):598–602.

FLUKES, LUNG

Susan Montgomery

INFECTIOUS AGENT: *Paragonimus* spp.	
ENDEMICITY	Africa The Americas East Asia (China, Japan, Korea) Southeast Asia
TRAVELER CATEGORIES AT GREATEST RISK FOR EXPOSURE & INFECTION	Adventurous eaters
PREVENTION METHODS	Practice safe food precautions Avoid raw or undercooked freshwater crab or crawfish
DIAGNOSTIC SUPPORT	A clinical laboratory certified in moderate complexity testing; or contact CDC's Parasitic Diseases Branch (www.cdc.gov/parasites; 404-718-4745; parasites@cdc.gov) Parasitological diagnosis: DPDx (www.cdc.gov/DPDx)

5

INFECTIOUS AGENTS

Paragonimiasis is caused by helminth parasites in the genus *Paragonimus*, especially *Paragonimus westermani*.

TRANSMISSION

Lung fluke infections are transmitted by eating raw or undercooked, pickled, or salted freshwater crab or crawfish infected with the immature form of the parasite. Ingested larval stages of the parasite are released when the infected crustacean is digested and then migrates from the intestines to other parts of the body. Most end up in the lungs, where they develop into adults and produce eggs. Human infections can persist for 20 years.

EPIDEMIOLOGY

Human disease is caused by ≥15 species of *Paragonimus*, which vary by geographic area and definitive host. *Paragonimus* species are found in western Africa, the Americas, and Asia. *P. westermani*, the most common cause of human disease, occurs predominantly in eastern and southern Asia.

CLINICAL PRESENTATION

Patients with *Paragonimus* infection can present with an acute syndrome within 2 days to 2 weeks after ingestion. Infections of longer duration can present with signs and symptoms like tuberculosis, with shortness of breath, cough, and hemoptysis. Extrapulmonary infections can occur and cause serious disease when the central nervous system is involved. Infections are usually associated with eosinophilia, especially during the larval migration stage.

DIAGNOSIS

Refer travelers to an infectious disease specialist if there is clinical suspicion of a lung fluke infection. Diagnosis is usually made by identifying eggs in stool or sputum. Serologic testing for *P. westermani*–specific antibodies can be helpful, especially for diagnosis of extrapulmonary infection; depending on the serologic assay, this testing can detect infections with other *Paragonimus* species because of differing levels of cross-reactivity among species.

Clinicians can obtain diagnostic assistance and confirmatory testing from the Centers for Disease Control and Prevention (CDC)'s Division of Parasitic Diseases and Malaria

DPDx laboratory (dpdx@cdc.gov), and from the Parasitic Diseases Hotline for Healthcare Providers (404-718-4745; parasites@cdc.gov).

TREATMENT

Treatment is with praziquantel; triclabendazole is an alternative.

PREVENTION

Travelers should avoid eating raw or undercooked freshwater crab or crawfish.

CDC website: www.cdc.gov/parasites/paragonimus/

BIBLIOGRAPHY

Fischer PU, Weil GJ. North American paragonimiasis: epidemiology and diagnostic strategies. Exp Rev Anti-Infect Ther. 2015;13(6):779–86.

World Health Organization. Foodborne parasitic infections: Paragonimiasis (Lung fluke). Available from: www.who.int/publications/i/item/WHO-UCN-NTD-VVE-2021.5

Xia Y, Ju Y, Chen J, You C. Hemorrhagic stroke and cerebral paragonimiasis. Stroke. 2014;45(11):3420–2.

5

GIARDIASIS

Katharine Benedict, Dawn Roellig

INFECTIOUS AGENT: *Giardia duodenalis*	
ENDEMICITY	Worldwide
TRAVELER CATEGORIES AT GREATEST RISK FOR EXPOSURE & INFECTION	Adventure tourists Children Humanitarian aid workers Immigrants and refugees Long-term travelers and expatriates
PREVENTION METHODS	Follow safe food and water safety precautions Minimize fecal–oral exposures during sexual activity Practice good hand hygiene
DIAGNOSTIC SUPPORT	A clinical laboratory certified in moderate complexity testing

INFECTIOUS AGENT

Giardiasis is an illness caused by the anaerobic protozoan parasite *Giardia duodenalis* (formerly known as *G. lamblia* or *G. intestinalis*).

TRANSMISSION

Giardia is transmitted via the fecal–oral route. Its low infectious dose, protracted communicability, and moderate chlorine tolerance make *Giardia* ideally suited for transmission through drinking and recreational water. Transmission also occurs through contact with feces (e.g., when providing direct patient care or during sexual activity), eating contaminated food, or contact with fecally contaminated surfaces.

EPIDEMIOLOGY

Giardia is endemic worldwide, including in the United States. Based on GeoSentinel Global Surveillance Network data from 2000–2012, *Giardia*-related acute diarrhea was a top 10 diagnosis in ill US travelers returning from destinations in Africa (North Africa and sub-Saharan Africa), the Americas (the Caribbean, Central America, and South America), Asia (South-Central Asia), Eastern Europe, and the Middle East. The risk for infection increases with duration of travel and travel within areas that have poor sanitation. Backpackers or campers who drink untreated water from lakes or rivers are also more likely to be infected. *Giardia* is commonly identified in routine screening of refugees and internationally adopted children, although many are asymptomatic.

CLINICAL PRESENTATION

Many infected people are asymptomatic; if symptoms develop, they typically develop 1–2 weeks after exposure and generally resolve within 2–4 weeks. Symptoms include abdominal cramps, anorexia, bloating, diarrhea (often with foul-smelling, greasy stools), flatulence, and nausea. Patients usually present with a history of gradual onset of 2–5 loose stools per day and increasing fatigue. Sometimes upper gastrointestinal symptoms are prominent. Weight loss can occur over time. Fever and vomiting are uncommon. Reactive arthritis, irritable bowel syndrome, and other chronic symptoms sometimes occur after infection with *Giardia* (see Sec. 11, Ch. 7, Persistent Diarrhea in Returned Travelers). In children, severe giardiasis can cause development delay, failure to thrive, malnutrition, and stunted growth.

DIAGNOSIS

Giardia cysts or trophozoites are not seen consistently in the stools of infected patients. Diagnostic sensitivity can be increased by examining ≤3 stool specimens over several days. New molecular enteric panel assays generally include *Giardia* as a target pathogen. Diagnostic techniques include microscopy with direct fluorescent antibody testing (considered the gold standard), microscopy with trichrome staining, enzyme immunoassay kits, rapid immunochromatographic cartridge assays, and molecular assays. Only molecular testing (e.g., DNA sequencing) can identify the genotypes and subtypes of *Giardia*. Retesting is recommended only if symptoms persist after treatment.

Health care professionals seeking laboratory support should consult their usual diagnostic laboratory with questions about appropriate testing. If testing beyond the capacity of the diagnostic laboratory is warranted, the diagnostic laboratory should reach out to public health officials (state or county as appropriate) for information and guidance on specimen submission, including submission to the Centers for Disease Control and Prevention (CDC), if appropriate.

TREATMENT

Effective treatments include metronidazole, tinidazole, and nitazoxanide. Alternative treatments include furozolidone, paromomycin, and quinacrine. Because a definitive diagnosis is difficult, empiric treatment can be used in patients with the appropriate history and typical symptoms.

PREVENTION

Travelers should follow safe water precautions, use appropriate sanitation, and practice good handwashing to avoid giardiasis. Travelers also should avoid drinking water and recreational water that could be contaminated. If the safety of drinking water is in doubt (e.g., during travel to a location with poor sanitation or lack of water treatment systems), travelers should follow recommended safe water precautions, including drinking commercially bottled water from an unopened factory-sealed container, or treating the water to make it safe for drinking. For more details, see Sec. 2, Ch. 8, Food & Water Precautions, and Sec. 2, Ch. 9, Water Disinfection.

Instruct travelers to avoid swallowing or drinking untreated water (even small amounts) from lakes, the ocean, ponds, rivers, springs, streams, or shallow wells. Travelers also should avoid swallowing water when swimming or recreating in hot tubs, interactive fountains, and swimming pools.

Travelers should wash hands frequently with soap and clean, running water for ≥20 seconds, rubbing hands together to make a lather, and making certain to lather backs of hands and between fingers and to scrub under nails. Travelers should especially wash hands before, during, and after preparing food; before eating; before and after caring for someone who is sick; after using the toilet, changing diapers, or cleaning a child who has used the toilet; and after touching an animal, animal waste, or animal environments.

In addition, travelers should prevent contact and contamination with feces during sex by using a barrier during oral–anal sex, and washing hands immediately after handling a condom used during anal sex and after touching the anus or rectal area of sexual partner(s).

In the United States, giardiasis is a nationally notifiable disease. State health departments should report outbreaks of giardiasis affecting multiple people to the CDC. Clinicians should inform local, state, and federal health authorities about cases of giardiasis so that appropriate public health responses can be taken to help control the spread of this disease.

CDC websites: www.cdc.gov/parasites/giardia; www.cdc.gov/healthywater/surveillance/nndss.html

BIBLIOGRAPHY

Abramowicz M, editor. Drugs for parasitic infections. New Rochelle (NY): The Medical Letter; 2013.

Adam EA, Yoder JS, Gould LH, Hlavsa MC, Gargano JW. Giardiasis outbreaks in the United States, 1971–2011. Epidemiol Infect. 2016;144(13):2790–801.

Escobedo AA, Lalle M, Hrastnik NI, Rodriguez-Morales AJ, Castro-Sanchez E, Cimerman S, et al. Combination therapy in the management of giardiasis: what laboratory and clinical studies tell us, so far. Acta Trop. 2016;162:196–205.

Halliez, MC, Buret AG. Extra-intestinal and long term consequences of *Giardia duodenalis* infections. World J Gastroenterol. 2013;19(47):8974–85.

Reses HE, Gargano JW, Liang JL, Cronquist A, Smith K, Collier SA, et al. Risk factors for sporadic *Giardia* infection in the USA: a case-control study in Colorado and Minnesota. Epidemiol Infect. 2018;146(9):1071–8.

Soares R, Tasca T. Giardiasis: an update review on sensitivity and specificity of methods for laboratorial diagnosis. J Microbiol Methods. 2016;129:98–102.

Swirski AL, Pearl DL, Peregrine AS, Pintar K. A comparison of exposure to risk factors for giardiasis in non-travellers, domestic travellers and international travellers in a Canadian community, 2006–2012. Epidemiol Infect. 2016;144(5):980–99.

5

HELMINTHS, SOIL-TRANSMITTED

Mary Kamb, Sharon Roy

INFECTIOUS AGENTS: *Ascaris lumbricoides* (roundworm) *Ancylostoma duodenale* and *Necator americanus* (hookworm) *Trichuris trichiura* (whipworm)	
ENDEMICITY	Worldwide
TRAVELER CATEGORIES AT GREATEST RISK FOR EXPOSURE & INFECTION	All travelers Immigrants and refugees from endemic countries
PREVENTION METHODS	Avoid contact with contaminated soil Follow safe food and water precautions Practice good hand hygiene Wear shoes
DIAGNOSTIC SUPPORT	A clinical laboratory certified in moderate complexity testing; or for clinical consultation, contact CDC's Parasitic Diseases Branch (www.cdc.gov/parasites; 404-718-4745; parasites@cdc.gov) Parasitological diagnosis: DPDx (www.cdc.gov/DPDx)

INFECTIOUS AGENTS

Ascaris lumbricoides (*Ascaris* or roundworm), *Ancylostoma duodenale* (hookworm), *Necator americanus* (hookworm), and *Trichuris trichiura* (whipworm) are helminths (parasitic worms) that infect the intestine. Due to the role of contaminated soil in their transmission, this group of nematode worms are known as soil-transmitted helminths (STH). *Strongyloides stercoralis* (threadworm) is sometimes included in the STH (see Sec. 5, Part 3, Ch. 21, Strongyloidiasis).

TRANSMISSION

STH are transmitted through ingestion of the tiny, infectious eggs of *Ascaris*, whipworm, and some hookworm, and through skin transmission for hookworm. People of all ages can become infected. Adult female worms produce thousands of eggs daily that are passed in feces and, if conditions allow, deposited in soil. Once in soil, infective larvae of *Ascaris* and whipworms develop in the fertile eggs and, if ingested by a human host, hatch and develop into adult worms over several months. Hookworm eggs are not infective—the eggs hatch and release larvae that must mature in soil before they become infective. Hookworm infection usually occurs when larvae penetrate the skin of people walking barefoot on contaminated soil; *Ancylostoma duodenale* also can be transmitted when larvae are ingested. Occasionally, human infection with *Ascaris suum* (pig roundworm) can occur due to ingestion of infectious eggs shed in pig feces.

EPIDEMIOLOGY

Globally, ≈2 billion people are infected with ≥1 STH, which together account for most parasitic disease burden worldwide. STH have widespread global distribution and are endemic in countries with tropical or subtropical climates and where sanitation is poor, human feces are used as fertilizer ("night soil"), or water supplies are contaminated. Although all travelers to endemic countries have some risk for STH infection, risk increases for long-term travelers and expatriates going to countries with poor general sanitation. Travelers can minimize risk by taking preventive measures.

Historically, STH infections were common in people living in US states where warm, moist climate and lack of sanitation enabled transmission; current prevalence of infection in those areas is unknown. Most reported infections in the United States are among immigrant and refugee populations. Since the introduction of predeparture treatment, stool testing for STH is unnecessary for most refugees. Because *Ascaris*, whipworm, and hookworm do not multiply in hosts (as opposed to threadworm), reinfection occurs only as a result of additional exposure to the infective-stage larvae.

CLINICAL PRESENTATION

Most STH infections are asymptomatic, especially when few worms are present. With *Ascaris*, pulmonary symptoms (Löffler syndrome) associated with marked eosinophilia and fever occur in a few patients when larvae pass through the lungs. Heavy roundworm infection also can cause intestinal discomfort, impaired nutritional status, and obstruction. Hookworm infection can lead to anemia due to blood loss and chronic protein deficiency, particularly in children. Whipworm infection can cause chronic abdominal pain, blood loss, diarrhea, dysentery, and rectal prolapse. Travelers rarely develop these more severe manifestations, however, which generally are associated with high worm burdens in indigenous populations.

DIAGNOSIS

Diagnosis is through detection of characteristic eggs using standard microscopy to examine fresh stool specimens. Stool concentration methods (e.g., Kato-Katz, McMaster, or FLOTAC techniques) can improve diagnostic yield. Collecting and testing 3 stool specimens on 3 separate days also improves detection because of variable shedding.

In returning travelers, parasitic eggs might not appear in stool for several months after exposure or symptom onset, because after infection female worms do not produce eggs for ≥40 days for *Ascaris* and ≥70 days for whipworm or hookworm. Serology to detect STH antibodies is not available in the United States. PCR testing is more sensitive and specific than microscopy, but tests are generally still unavailable commercially.

Co-infection with ≥1 STH or other parasitic worms common in some endemic areas can make diagnosis challenging. Request assistance with parasitological diagnosis through DPDx (www.cdc.gov/DPDx). Clinical consultations are available through the Parasitic Diseases Branch of the Centers for Disease Control and Prevention (www.cdc.gov/parasites; 404-718-4745; parasites@cdc.gov).

TREATMENT

Treatment of intestinal ascariasis consists of anthelminthic therapy, which effectively reduces morbidity but does not prevent reinfection. The drugs used most often to treat hookworm and *Ascaris* are albendazole and mebendazole, and for whipworm a combination of albendazole plus ivermectin. These drugs are safe for children but should be avoided or used with caution in pregnant or lactating people.

PREVENTION

No vaccines or drugs are available to prevent STH infection. Travelers can minimize infection risk by using preventive measures aimed at reducing ingestion or exposure to soil contaminated with human feces. Preventive measures include careful hand hygiene; washing, peeling, and cooking raw vegetables and fruit; and boiling or treating water (see Sec. 2, Ch. 8, Food & Water Precautions, and Sec. 2, Ch. 9, Water Disinfection). To avoid hookworm infection, travelers should avoid walking barefoot in areas where hookworm is common or where soil might be contaminated by human feces.

CDC website: www.cdc.gov/parasites/sth

5

BIBLIOGRAPHY

Bethony J, Brooker S, Albonico M, Geiger SM, Loukas A, Diemert D, et al. Soil-transmitted helminth infections: ascariasis, trichuriasis, and hookworm. Lancet. 2006;367(9521):1521–32.

Brooker S, Bundy DAP. Soil-transmitted helminths (geohelminths). In: Cook GC, Zumla A, editors. Manson's tropical diseases, 22nd edition. London: Saunders; 2009. pp. 1515–48.

Brooker S, Clements AC, Bundy DA. Global epidemiology, ecology and control of soil-transmitted helminth infections. Adv Parasitol. 2006;62:221–61.

Jourdan PM, Lamberton PHL, Fenwich A, Addis DG. Soil transmitted helminth infections. Lancet. 2018;391(10117):252–65.

LEISHMANIASIS, CUTANEOUS

Mary Kamb, Sharon Roy, Paul Cantey

INFECTIOUS AGENTS: >20 *Leishmania* spp.	
ENDEMICITY	Eastern Hemisphere: Africa, Asia, southern Europe, Middle East Western Hemisphere: Central and South America
TRAVELER CATEGORIES AT GREATEST RISK FOR EXPOSURE & INFECTION	Any traveler or migrant exposed to the vector
PREVENTION METHODS	Avoid insect bites
DIAGNOSTIC SUPPORT	A clinical laboratory certified in high complexity testing; or for tissue diagnostic techniques, contact CDC's Parasitic Diseases Branch (www.cdc.gov/parasites; 404-718-4745; parasites@cdc.gov) Parasitological diagnosis: DPDx (www.cdc.gov/DPDx)

INFECTIOUS AGENT

Leishmaniasis is caused by obligate intracellular protozoan parasites; >20 *Leishmania* species cause cutaneous leishmaniasis (CL). Leishmaniasis has different forms, including visceral leishmaniasis (the most severe form), but CL is the most common form. An aggressive form of CL, mucosal leishmaniasis (ML), affects mucosal areas.

TRANSMISSION

Leishmania parasites that cause CL are transmitted through the bites of infected female phlebotomine sand flies. CL also can occur after accidental occupational (laboratory) exposures to *Leishmania* parasites. Transmission risk is greatest from dusk to dawn because sand flies typically feed (bite) at night and during twilight hours. Although sand flies are less active during the hottest part of the day, they can bite if they are disturbed, for instance when people brush against tree trunks or other sites where sand flies are resting. Vector activity might easily be overlooked because sand flies are small and silent, and their bites can go unnoticed. Travelers with potentially increased risk for CL include adventure travelers, bird watchers, construction workers, ecotourists, military personnel, missionaries, Peace Corps volunteers, and people doing research or humanitarian work outdoors at night or twilight. Even short-term travelers in leishmaniasis-endemic areas have developed CL, however. Immigrants and refugees from endemic areas also might present with CL.

EPIDEMIOLOGY

As of 2017, CL was reported to be endemic in 87 countries on 6 continents, with an estimated annual prevalence of 4.13 million, including 700,000 new cases globally. The ecologic settings for leishmaniasis transmission range from rainforests to arid regions.

In the Eastern Hemisphere, CL is found in Africa, particularly the tropical region and North Africa; Asia, particularly central and southwest Asia; southern Europe, including southern France, Greece, Italy, Portugal, Spain, and the Mediterranean islands; and some countries of the Middle East. In the Western Hemisphere, CL is found in parts of Mexico, all countries of Central America, and most of South America. Endemic transmission in the United States has been identified in Texas, especially among people living in areas bordering northeastern Mexico, and in neighboring Oklahoma. CL is not found in Canada, Chile, or Uruguay.

GeoSentinel Surveillance from 1997–2017 indicated that among patients examined at specialized travel or tropical medicine clinics on 6 continents, including North America, and who had laboratory-confirmed diagnoses, common source countries for travel-associated CL were Bolivia; countries in the Amazon Basin, including Brazil, Colombia, Ecuador, and Peru; Costa Rica; El Salvador; and Israel. Among immigrants, common source countries were Afghanistan and Syria. Cases of CL in US service personnel have reflected military activities (e.g., in Afghanistan and Iraq). CL is usually more common in rural than urban areas but is found in some peri-urban and urban areas (e.g., in Kabul, Afghanistan).

CLINICAL PRESENTATION

CL can present with a broad variety of dermatologic manifestations ranging from small and localized skin lesions to large nodules or plaques covering multiple body surfaces; ≈10% of infections are asymptomatic. The clinical spectrum can mimic other skin conditions (e.g., leprosy, squamous cell cancer, fungal or other skin infections).

CL is characterized by skin lesions, which can be closed or open sores, that typically develop on exposed areas of the skin within several weeks or months after infection. In some people, however, the sores first appear months or years later, often in the context of trauma (e.g., skin wounds, surgery). The sores can change in appearance and size over time. Sores typically progress from small, erythematous papules or nodular plaques to open sores with a raised border and central crater (ulcer), which can be covered with crust or scales. Lesions usually are painless but can be painful if superinfected with bacteria. Satellite lesions, regional lymphadenopathy, and nodular lymphangitis can occur. Even without treatment, most sores eventually heal; they can last for months or years, however, and typically result in scarring.

Mucosal Leishmaniasis

Some *Leishmania* species in Central and South America are a potential concern because parasites might spread from the skin to the mucosal surfaces of the nose or mouth and cause sores in these areas. ML might not be apparent until years after the original skin sores appear to have healed. Although ML is uncommon, it has occurred in travelers and expatriates, including in people whose cases of CL were not treated or were treated inadequately. The initial clinical manifestations typically involve the nose, with bleeding, chronic stuffiness, and inflamed mucosa or sores; less often the mouth or larynx are involved, manifesting as a brassy cough or hoarseness.

In advanced cases, ulcerative destruction of the mouth, nose, larynx, and pharynx (e.g., perforation of the nasal septum, or laryngeal or tracheal damage) can occur. Thus, any patient with CL caused by a *Viannia* subgenus from the Western Hemisphere, regardless of symptoms, should undergo a careful examination of mucosal surfaces, including the vocal cords and oronasal pharynx, along with biopsy of any abnormal-appearing tissue, to avoid missing ML cases. Although most commonly associated with species of *Leishmania* found in the Western Hemisphere, ML has been documented on rare occasions with species of *Leishmania* found in various countries of the Eastern Hemisphere.

DIAGNOSIS

Consider CL in people with chronic, nonhealing skin lesions who have been in areas where leishmaniasis is found. Clinical signs and symptoms are not sufficiently specific to differentiate CL from other conditions. Obtain an explicit travel history, including, if possible, questioning fellow travelers about similar lesions. Obtain information about duration and progression of symptoms, whether the lesions are painful, prior treatment, and current medications (e.g., immunosuppressive agents); photographs are helpful to assess lesions over time. Conduct a careful physical examination including evaluation of skin, lymph nodes, and mucosal surfaces; referral to a specialist able to conduct an endoscopic laryngeal examination might be warranted if ML is suspected.

Laboratory confirmation of the diagnosis is achieved by detecting *Leishmania* parasites or DNA in infected tissue through light-microscopic examination of stained specimens, culture techniques, or molecular methods (e.g., PCR); conducting all 3 tests maximizes diagnostic yield. The Centers for Disease Control and Prevention (CDC) can assist in all aspects of the diagnostic evaluation. Because different *Leishmania* species have different management implications, species identification through molecular testing is important, particularly if >1 species is endemic to areas where the patient traveled.

Serologic testing generally is not useful for CL because the assays are insensitive and cannot distinguish between active and past infection. For consultative services, including collection and packaging of samples for molecular testing, contact CDC Parasitic Diseases Inquiries (404-718-4745; parasites@cdc.gov) or see www.cdc.gov/dpdx.

TREATMENT

The primary goal of treatment is to prevent morbidity. Individualize decisions about whether and how to treat CL, including whether to use a systemic (oral or parenteral) medication rather than a local or topical approach. Treat all cases of ML with systemic therapy. Clinicians can consult with CDC staff about the relative merits of various approaches to treat CL and ML (see the Diagnosis section for contact information). The response to a particular regimen can vary not only among *Leishmania* species but also for the same species in different geographic regions.

The oral agent miltefosine is approved by the US Food and Drug Administration (FDA) to treat CL caused by 3 Western Hemisphere species of the *Viannia* subgenus: *Leishmania* (*V.*) *braziliensis*, *L.* (*V.*) *guyanensis*, and *L.* (*V.*) *panamensis*, as well as for ML caused by *L.* (*V.*) *braziliensis*, in adults and adolescents ≥12 years old who weigh ≥30 kg and are not pregnant or breastfeeding during therapy or for 5 months after treatment. Various parenteral options, including liposomal amphotericin B, are commercially available, although not FDA-approved to treat CL or ML. The pentavalent antimonial compound sodium stibogluconate

5

(Pentostam) is no longer available through the CDC Drug Service.

PREVENTION

No vaccines or drugs to prevent infection are available. Travelers can reduce the risk for CL by using personal protective measures to avoid sand fly contact and sand fly bites (see Sec. 4, Ch. 6, Mosquitoes, Ticks & Other Arthropods). Advise travelers to avoid outdoor activities, to the extent possible, especially from dusk to dawn when sand flies are the most active; wear protective clothing and apply insect repellent to exposed skin and under the edges of clothing (e.g., shirt sleeves, pant legs) according to the manufacturer's instructions; and sleep in air-conditioned or well-screened areas. Spraying sleeping quarters with insecticide might provide some protection, and fans or ventilators might inhibit the movement of sand flies, which are weak fliers.

Sand flies are small (≈2–3 mm, <1/8 inch) and can pass through the holes in ordinary mosquito nets. Although fine mesh nets are available, these can be uncomfortable in hot climates. The effectiveness of mosquito nets can be enhanced by treating with a pyrethroid-containing (i.e., permethrin) insecticide. The same treatment can be applied to bed sheets and clothing, curtains, and window screens.

CDC website: www.cdc.gov/parasites/leishmaniasis

5

BIBLIOGRAPHY

Aronson N, Herwaldt BL, Libman M, Pearson R, Lopez-Velez R, Weina P, et al. Diagnosis and treatment of leishmaniasis: clinical practice guidelines by the Infectious Diseases Society of America (IDSA) and the American Society of Tropical Medicine and Hygiene (ASTMH). Clin Infect Dis. 2016;63(12):e202–64.

Blum J, Buffet P, Visser L, Harms G, Bailey MS, Caumes E, et al. LeishMan recommendations for treatment of cutaneous and mucosal leishmaniasis in travelers, 2014. J Travel Med. 2014;21(2):116–29.

Blum J, Lockwood DN, Visser L, Harms G, Bailey MS, Caumes E, et al. Local or systemic treatment for New World cutaneous leishmaniasis? Re-evaluating the evidence for the risk of mucosal leishmaniasis. Int Health. 2012;4(3):153–63.

Boggild AK, Caumes E, Grobusch MP, Schwartz E, Hynes NA, Libman M, et al. Cutaneous and mucocutaneous leishmaniasis in travellers and migrants: a 20-year GeoSentinel Surveillance Network analysis. J Travel Med. 2019; 26(8):taz055.

GBD 2017 Disease and Injury Incidence and Prevalence Collaborators. Global, regional, and national incidence, prevalence, and years lived with disability for 354 diseases and injuries for 195 countries and territories, 1990–2017: a systematic analysis for the Global Burden of Disease Study 2017. Lancet. 2018;392(10159):1789–858.

Hodiamont CJ, Kager PA, Bart A, de Vries HJC, van Thiel PPAM, Leenstra T, et al. Species-directed therapy for leishmaniasis in returning travelers: a comprehensive guide. PLoS Negl Trop Dis. 2014;8(5):e2832.

Karimkhani C, Wanga V, Coffeng LE, Naghavi P, Dellavalle RP, Naghavi M. Global burden of cutaneous leishmaniasis: a cross-sectional analysis from the Global Burden of Disease Study 2013. Lancet Infect Dis. 2016;16(5):584–91.

Kipp EJ, de Almeida M, Marcet PL, Bradbury RS, Benedict TK, Lin W, et al. An atypical case of autochthonous cutaneous leishmaniasis associated with naturally infected phlebotomine sand flies in Texas, United States. Am J Trop Med Hyg. 2020;103(4):1496–501.

Pan American Health Organization. Leishmaniasis in the Americas: treatment recommendations. Washington, DC: The Organization; 2018.

World Health Organization. Global leishmaniasis update, 2006–2015: a turning point in leishmaniasis surveillance. Wkly Epidemiol Rec. 2017;92(38):557–65.

LEISHMANIASIS, VISCERAL

Rebecca Chancey, Sharon Roy, Paul Cantey

INFECTIOUS AGENTS: *Leishmania* spp.	
ENDEMICITY	Eastern Hemisphere: East Africa, southwest Asia, southern Europe, Middle East Western Hemisphere: Brazil, Latin America
TRAVELER CATEGORIES AT GREATEST RISK FOR EXPOSURE & INFECTION	Adventure tourists Humanitarian aid workers Immigrants and refugees Long-term travelers and expatriates
PREVENTION METHODS	Avoid insect bites Avoid outdoor activities when sand flies are most active (especially from dusk to dawn)
DIAGNOSTIC SUPPORT	A clinical laboratory certified in high complexity testing; or for clinical consultation, CDC's Parasitic Diseases Branch (www.cdc.gov/parasites; 404-718-4745; parasites@cdc.gov) Parasitological diagnosis: DPDx (www.cdc.gov/DPDx)

5

INFECTIOUS AGENTS

Visceral leishmaniasis (VL) is caused by obligate intracellular protozoan parasites, primarily *Leishmania infantum* (considered synonymous with *L. chagasi*) and *L. donovani*. Leishmaniasis has several different forms. VL affects some of the internal organs of the body (e.g., bone marrow, liver, spleen).

TRANSMISSION

The parasites that cause VL are transmitted through the bite of infected female phlebotomine sand flies. Congenital transmission and parenteral transmission through blood transfusions and needle sharing have been reported.

EPIDEMIOLOGY

Leishmaniasis is a parasitic disease found in parts of the tropics, subtropics, and southern Europe. VL is usually more common in rural than urban areas, but it is found in some peri-urban areas (e.g., in northeastern Brazil). In the Eastern Hemisphere, VL is found in Africa, particularly East Africa; parts of Asia, particularly the Indian subcontinent and central and southwest Asia; southern Europe; and the Middle East. In the Western Hemisphere, most cases occur in Brazil; some cases occur in scattered foci elsewhere in Latin America. Overall, VL is found in focal areas of >70 countries; most (>90%) cases occur on the Indian subcontinent, in Bangladesh, India, and Nepal; countries in East Africa, including Ethiopia, Kenya, Somalia, South Sudan, and Sudan; and in Brazil. More information is available at https://apps.who.int/gho/data/node.main.NTDLEISHVNUM?lang=en.

The geographic distribution of VL cases evaluated in the United States and other countries reflects travel and immigration patterns. Although uncommon in most US travelers and expatriates, VL can occur in travelers returning from visits to endemic regions in European countries (e.g., France, Greece, Italy, Macedonia, and Spain) and among military personnel returning from the Middle East. Cases have been documented in short-term travelers to the Camino de Santiago in northern Spain and endemic areas of southern France, and in longer-term travelers (e.g., expatriates, deployed soldiers) to the Mediterranean region and Middle East.

CLINICAL PRESENTATION

Among symptomatic people, the incubation period typically ranges from weeks to months. Illness onset can be abrupt or gradual. Stereotypical clinical manifestations of VL include fever, hepatosplenomegaly (especially splenomegaly), night sweats, and weight loss; lymphadenopathy can occur. Laboratory findings characteristic of VL include pancytopenia (anemia, leukopenia, thrombocytopenia), high total protein, low albumin, and hypergammaglobulinemia. If untreated, severe (advanced) cases of VL typically are fatal. Latent infection can clinically manifest years to decades after exposure in people who become immunocompromised through HIV infection, biologic immunomodulatory therapy, or immunosuppressive therapy.

5

DIAGNOSIS

Consider VL in the differential diagnosis of people with a relevant travel history even in the distant past, and a persistent, unexplained febrile illness, especially if accompanied by other suggestive manifestations (e.g., pancytopenia or splenomegaly). Hemophagocytic lymphohistiocytosis (HLH) could be a complication and should prompt clinicians to consider VL in patients with the appropriate travel history.

Laboratory confirmation of the diagnosis is achieved by detecting *Leishmania* parasites or DNA in infected blood, bone marrow, liver, or lymph nodes through light-microscopic examination of stained specimens, molecular methods, or tissue culture techniques. Serologic testing can provide supportive evidence for the diagnosis.

The Centers for Disease Control and Prevention (CDC) can assist in all aspects of the diagnostic evaluation, including species identification. Information on specimen collection and diagnosis of leishmaniasis is available at www.cdc.gov/parasites/leishmaniasis/resources/pdf/cdc_diagnosis_guide_leishmaniasis_2016.pdf. For consultative services, contact CDC Parasitic Diseases Inquiries (404-718-4745; parasites@cdc.gov), or see www.cdc.gov/dpdx.

TREATMENT

Refer people with VL to an infectious disease or tropical medicine specialist who can help direct care and provide individualized treatment. CDC staff can discuss the relative merits of various approaches (see the Diagnosis section of this chapter for contact information). Risk for relapse and treatment failure is greater in patients with HIV, but also might occur rarely in immunocompetent patients.

Liposomal amphotericin B (AmBisome) is approved by the US Food and Drug Administration (FDA) to treat VL and is generally the drug of choice for US patients. The oral agent miltefosine is approved by the FDA to treat VL in patients infected with *L. donovani* who are ≥12 years old, who weigh ≥30 kg, and who are not pregnant or breastfeeding during therapy or for 5 months after treatment; the drug is available in the United States via www.profounda.com. Pentavalent antimonials (e.g., meglumine antimoniate, sodium stibogluoconate [Pentostam]) are used in endemic areas, except for India, where developing resistance is a concern. Pentavalent antimonial drugs are currently not FDA approved and not available for use in the United States; Pentostam is no longer available through the CDC Drug Service.

PREVENTION

No vaccines or drugs to prevent infection are available. Preventive measures are aimed at reducing contact with sand flies and avoiding sand fly bites (see Sec. 4, Ch. 6, Mosquitoes, Ticks & Other Arthropods, and Sec. 5, Part 3, Ch. 14, Cutaneous Leishmaniasis). Preventive measures include minimizing outdoor activities, to the extent possible, especially from dusk to dawn when sand flies generally are most active; wearing protective clothing; applying insect repellent to exposed skin; using bed nets treated with a pyrethroid-containing insecticide; and spraying dwellings with residual-action insecticides.

CDC website: www.cdc.gov/parasites/leishmaniasis

BIBLIOGRAPHY

Aronson N, Herwaldt BL, Libman M, Pearson R, Lopez-Velez R, Weina P, et al. Diagnosis and treatment of leishmaniasis: clinical practice guidelines by the Infectious Diseases Society of America (IDSA) and the American Society of Tropical Medicine and Hygiene (ASTMH). Clin Infect Dis. 2016;63(12):e202–64.

Fletcher K, Issa R, Lockwood DN. Visceral leishmaniasis and immunocompromise as a risk factor for the development of visceral leishmaniasis: a changing pattern at the hospital for tropical diseases, London. PLoS One. 2015;10(4):e0121418.

Haque L, Villanueva M, Russo A, Yuan Y, Lee E-J, Topal J, et al. A rare case of visceral leishmaniasis in an immunocompetent traveler returning to the United States from Europe. PLoS Negl Trop Dis. 2018;12(10):e0006727.

van Griensven J, Carrillo E, Lopez-Velez R, Lynen L, Moreno J. Leishmaniasis in immunosuppressed individuals. Clin Microbiol Infect. 2014;20(4):286–99.

van Griensven J, Diro E. Visceral leishmaniasis. Infect Dis Clin N Am. 2012;26(2):309–22.

Watkins ER, Shamasunder S, Cascino T, White KL, Katrak S, Bern C, et al. Visceral leishmaniasis–associated hemophagocytic lymphohistiocytosis in a traveler returning from a pilgrimage to the Camino de Santiago. J Travel Med. 2014;21(6):429–32.

World Health Organization. Control of the leishmaniases. Geneva: World Health Organization; 2010. Available from: http://apps.who.int/iris/bitstream/10665/44412/1/WHO_TRS_949_eng.pdf.

World Health Organization. Global leishmaniasis update, 2006–2015: a turning point in leishmaniasis surveillance. Wkly Epidemiol Rec. 2017;92(38):557–65.

MALARIA

Kathrine Tan, Francisca Abanyie

INFECTIOUS AGENT: *Plasmodium* spp.	
ENDEMICITY	Multiple countries in Africa, the Americas, and Asia
TRAVELER CATEGORIES AT GREATEST RISK FOR EXPOSURE & INFECTION	Children Long-term travelers and expatriates Pregnant travelers Tourists, business travelers, and missionaries Travelers visiting friends and relatives in areas with malaria
PREVENTION METHODS	Avoid insect bites Use malaria chemoprophylaxis
DIAGNOSTIC SUPPORT	A clinical laboratory certified in moderate complexity testing; state health department; or contact CDC's Malaria Hotline: ▪ 770-488-7788 (M–F 9 a.m.–5 p.m. Eastern) ▪ 770-488-7100 (after hours) Parasitological diagnosis: DPDx (www.cdc.gov/DPDx)

INFECTIOUS AGENT

Malaria in humans is caused by protozoan parasites of the genus *Plasmodium*, including *Plasmodium falciparum*, *P. malariae*, *P. ovale*, and *P. vivax*. In addition, zoonotic forms have been documented as causes of human infections and some deaths, especially *P. knowlesi*, a parasite of Old World (Eastern Hemisphere) monkeys, in Southeast Asia.

TRANSMISSION

Plasmodium species are transmitted by the bite of an infective female *Anopheles* mosquito.

Occasionally, transmission occurs by blood transfusion, needle sharing, nosocomially, organ transplantation, or vertically from mother to fetus. Malaria transmission occurs in large areas of Africa, Latin America, and parts of the Caribbean, Eastern Europe, the South Pacific, and in Asia including South Asia, Southeast Asia, and the Middle East (Map 5-12, Map 5-13, and Map 5-14).

EPIDEMIOLOGY

Malaria is a major international public health problem. According to the World Health Organization (WHO) World Malaria Report 2019, >90 countries reported ≈228 million infections and ≈405,000 deaths in 2018. Travelers going to malaria-endemic countries are at risk of contracting the disease, and almost all the ≈2,000 cases of malaria that occur each year in the United States are imported.

5

The risk of acquiring malaria differs substantially from traveler to traveler and from region to region, even within a single country. This variability is a function of the intensity of transmission within the various regions and the itinerary, duration, season, and type of travel. Risk also varies by travelers' adherence to mosquito precautions and prophylaxis recommendations. In 2016, 2,078 cases of malaria (including 7 deaths) were diagnosed in the United States and its territories and were reported to the Centers for Disease Control and Prevention (CDC). Of cases for which country of acquisition was known, 85% were acquired in Africa, 9% in Asia, 5% in the Caribbean and the Americas, and 1% in Oceania or the Eastern Mediterranean. Of US residents with malaria who reported a reason for travel, 69% were visiting friends and relatives.

Information about malaria transmission in specific countries is derived from various sources, including WHO (see Sec. 2, Ch. 5, Yellow Fever Vaccine & Malaria Prevention Information, by Country). The information presented here was accurate at the time of publication; the risk for malaria can change rapidly and from year to year, however, because of changes in local weather conditions, mosquito vector density, and prevalence of infection. Updated information can be found on the CDC website at www.cdc.gov/malaria.

CLINICAL PRESENTATION

Malaria is characterized by fever and influenza-like symptoms, including chills, headache, myalgias, and malaise; symptoms can occur intermittently. In severe disease, acute kidney injury, acute respiratory distress syndrome, mental confusion, seizures, coma, and death can occur. Malaria symptoms can develop as early as 7 days after being bitten by an infectious mosquito in a malaria-endemic area and as late as several months or more after exposure. Suspected or confirmed malaria, especially *P. falciparum*, is a medical emergency requiring urgent intervention, because clinical deterioration can occur rapidly and unpredictably. See Box 5-10 for frequently asked clinical questions.

DIAGNOSIS

Travelers with symptoms of malaria should seek medical evaluation as soon as possible, even if still traveling. Consider malaria in any patient with a febrile illness who has recently returned from a malaria-endemic country. Diagnostic assistance is available from state public health laboratories or CDC (www.cdc.gov/dpdx/dxassistance.html). The CDC malaria laboratory can assist in speciating malaria by blood smear microscopy, or confirm species by PCR testing. The CDC laboratory also can assess malaria parasites for mutations that confer resistance to medications. Serologic testing, used in certain situations (e.g., case investigations), can also be done by CDC laboratories (www.cdc.gov/dpdx/dxassistance.html).

In the United States, malaria is a notifiable disease. Health care providers must report cases of malaria diagnosed via microscopy or PCR in the United States and its territories to local or state health departments. More information on reporting malaria can be found at www.cdc.gov/malaria/report.html.

Blood Smear Microscopy

Blood smear microscopy remains the most important method for malaria diagnosis. Microscopy can provide immediate information about the presence of parasites, allow quantification of the density of the infection, and allow determination of the species of the malaria parasite—all of which are necessary for providing

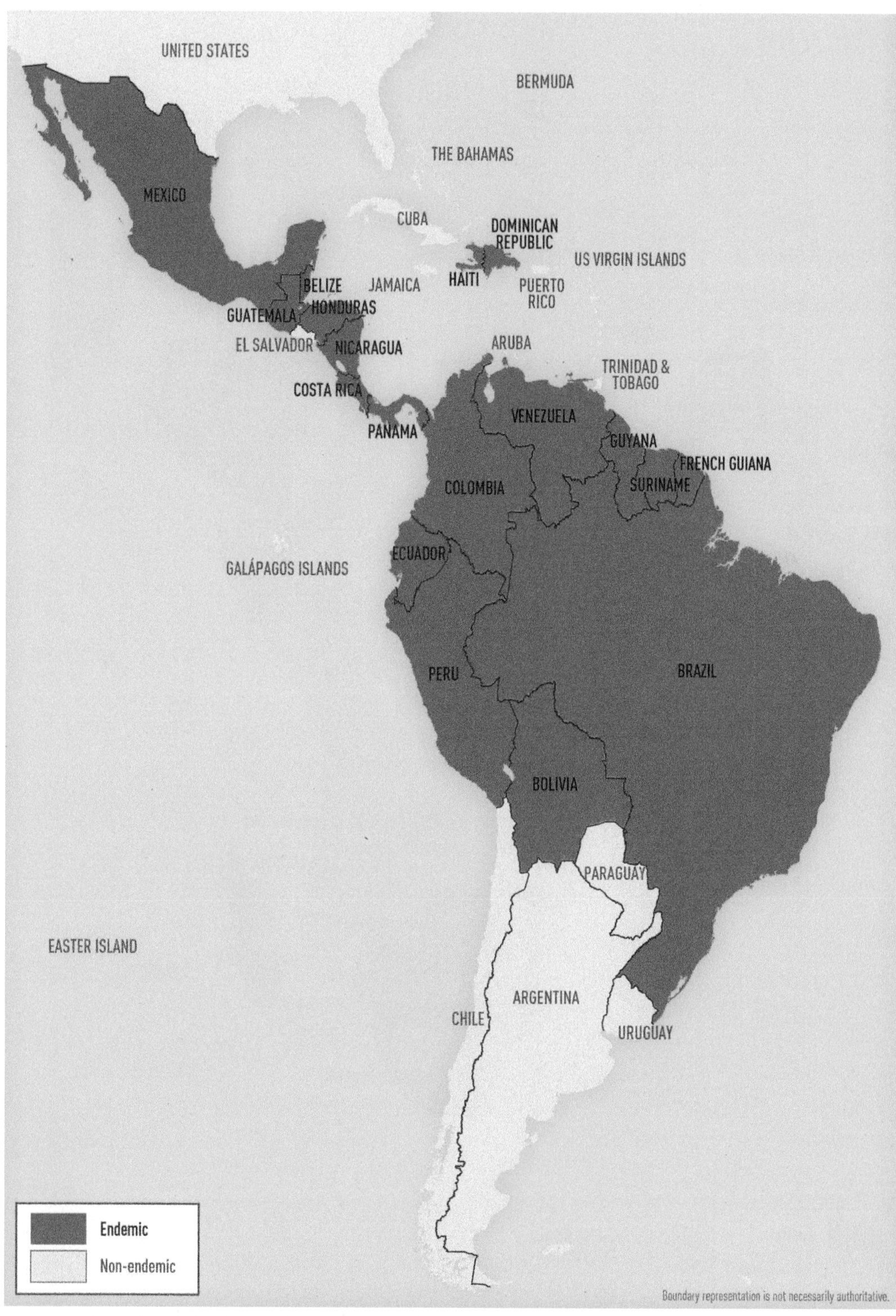

MAP 5-12 **Malaria-endemic destinations in the Americas & the Caribbean**

Malaria-endemic destinations are labeled using black font; destinations not endemic for malaria are labeled using gray font. Countries with areas endemic for malaria are shaded completely even if transmission occurs only in a small part of the country. For more specific within-country malaria transmission information, see Section 2, Yellow Fever Vaccine & Malaria Prevention Information, by Country.

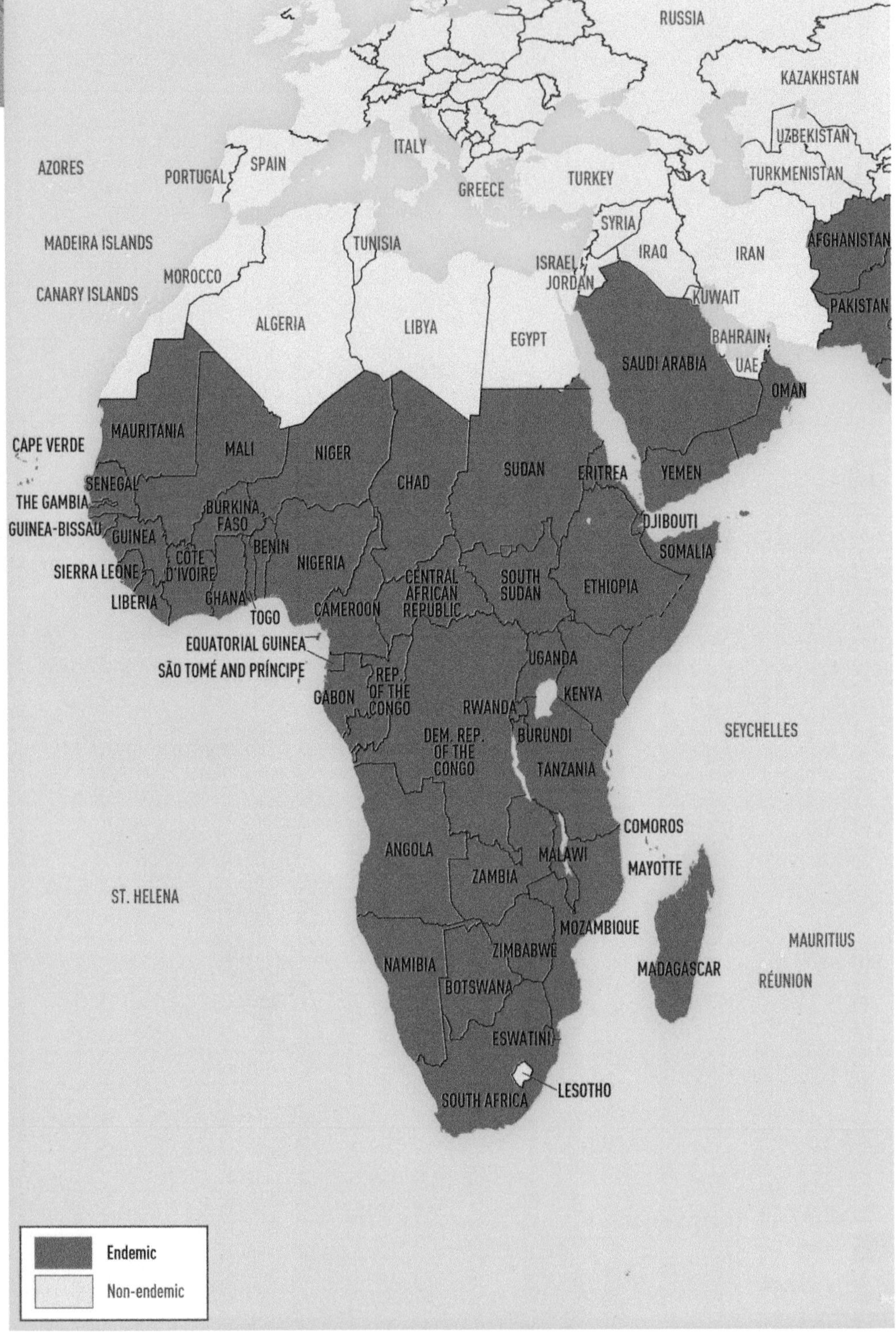

MAP 5-13 Malaria-endemic destinations in Africa & the Middle East

Malaria-endemic destinations are labeled using black font; destinations not endemic for malaria are labeled using gray font. Countries with areas endemic for malaria are shaded completely even if transmission occurs only in a small part of the country. For more specific within-country malaria transmission information, see Section 2, Yellow Fever Vaccine & Malaria Prevention Information, by Country.

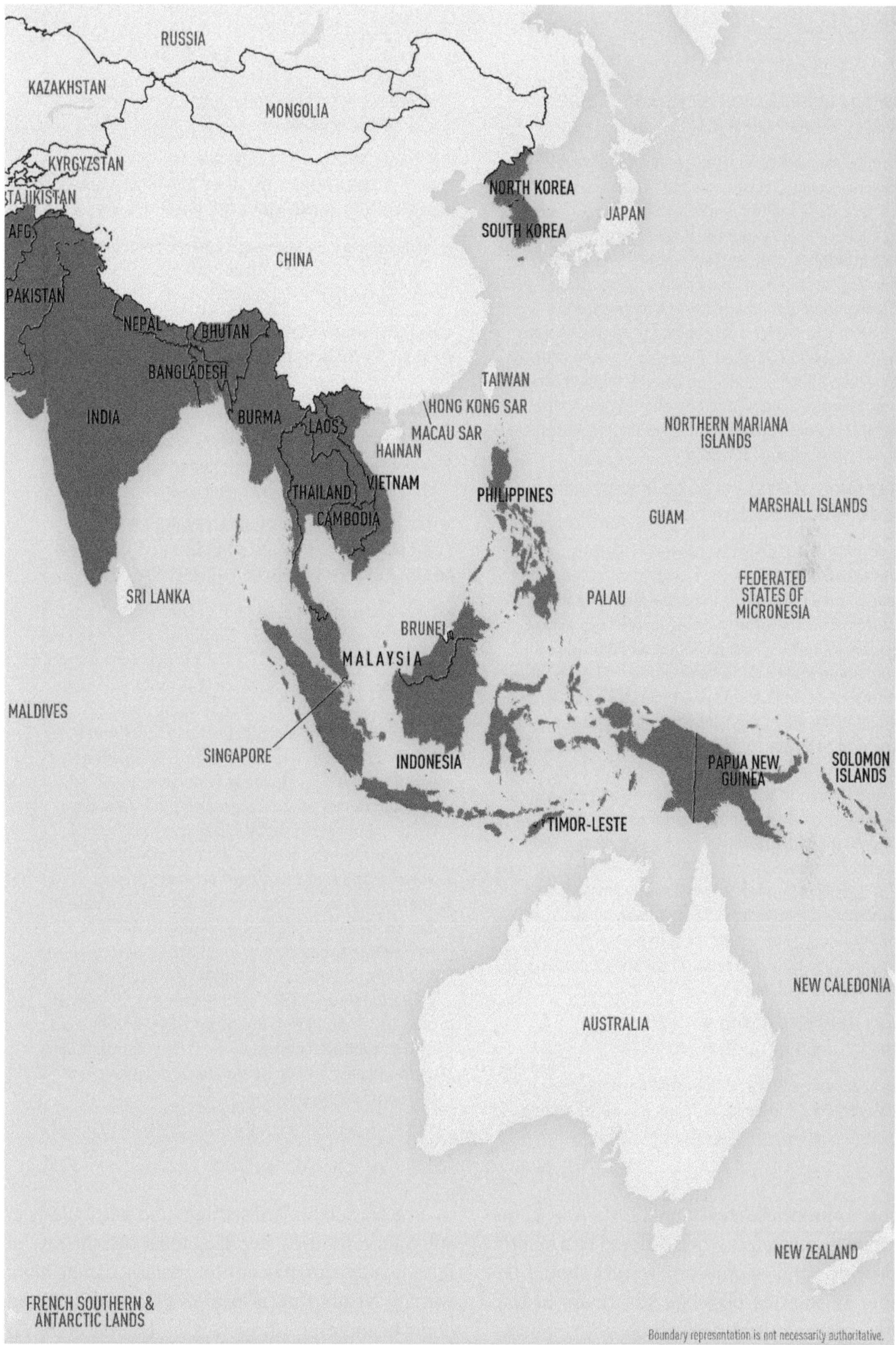

MAP 5-14 Malaria-endemic destinations in Asia & Oceania

Malaria-endemic destinations are labeled using black font; destinations not endemic for malaria are labeled using gray font. Countries with areas endemic for malaria are shaded completely even if transmission occurs only in a small part of the country. For more specific within-country malaria transmission information, see Section 2, Yellow Fever Vaccine & Malaria Prevention Information, by Country.

BOX 5-10 Frequently asked clinical questions

HOW DO I ADDRESS CONCERNS ABOUT SIDE EFFECTS FROM PROPHYLAXIS?

- Prophylaxis can be started earlier if the traveler has concerns about tolerating a particular medication. For example, mefloquine can be started 3–4 weeks in advance to allow potential adverse events to occur before travel. If unacceptable side effects develop, the clinician has time to change the medication before the traveler's departure.
- The drugs used for antimalarial prophylaxis are generally well tolerated. Side effects can occur, however. Minor side effects usually do not require stopping the drug. Clinicians should determine if symptoms are related to the medicine and make a medication change if needed.

WHAT SHOULD A TRAVELER DO IF THEY MISS A DOSE OF PROPHYLAXIS?

- Compared with drugs with short half-lives, which are taken daily, drugs with longer half-lives, which are taken weekly, offer the advantage of a wider margin of error if the traveler is late with a dose.
- For a weekly drug, prophylactic blood levels can remain adequate if the dose is only 1–2 days late. If this is the case, the traveler can take a dose as soon as possible, then resume weekly doses on the originally scheduled day. If the traveler is >2 days late, blood levels might not be adequate. The traveler should take a dose as soon as possible. The weekly doses should resume at this new day of the week (the next dose is 1 week later, then weekly thereafter).
- For a daily drug, if the traveler is 1–2 days late, protective blood levels are less likely to be maintained. The traveler should take a dose as soon as possible and resume the daily schedule at the new time of day.

WHAT HAPPENS IF TOO HIGH A DOSE OF PROPHYLAXIS IS TAKEN?

- Overdose of antimalarial drugs, particularly chloroquine, can be fatal. Medications should be stored in childproof containers out of reach of infants and children.

ISN'T MALARIA A TREATABLE DISEASE? WHY NOT CARRY A TREATMENT DOSE OF ANTIMALARIALS INSTEAD OF TAKING MALARIA PROPHYLAXIS?

- Malaria could be fatal even when treated, which is why prevention is always preferable to treating infections after they occur.

WHAT SHOULD BE DONE IF FEVER DEVELOPS WHILE TRAVELING IN A MALARIA-ENDEMIC AREA?

- Malaria and other potentially life-threatening infections acquired during travel could be fatal if treatment is delayed. Travelers should promptly seek medical help and continue to take malaria prophylaxis while in the malaria-endemic area.

WHAT SHOULD BE DONE IF A TRAVELER WHO TOOK MALARIA PROPHYLAXIS DEVELOPS FEVER AFTER RETURNING FROM THEIR TRIP?

- Malaria prophylaxis, while highly effective, is not 100% effective. Travelers should be advised to seek medical care immediately if fever develops, report their travel history, get tested for malaria, and get treated promptly if infection is confirmed.
- Malaria smear or a rapid diagnostic test must be performed, and results obtained immediately (within a few hours). These tests should not be sent out to reference laboratories that take days to weeks to return results. Empiric treatment with antimalarial drugs is not recommended because the malaria smear provides critical information for appropriate treatment. If a patient has an illness suggestive of severe malaria and a compatible travel history in an area where malaria transmission occurs, and malaria testing is not immediately available, start treatment as soon as possible, even before the diagnosis is established. CDC recommendations for malaria treatment can be found at www.cdc.gov/malaria/diagnosis_treatment/treatment.html.

the most appropriate treatment. Tests should be performed immediately when ordered by a health care provider, and microscopy results should be available as soon as possible, ≤24 hours of the patient's presentation. Assistance with speciation of malaria on smears is available from state health departments or CDC (www.cdc.gov/dpdx/dxassistance.html).

In resource-limited settings, and particularly in sub-Saharan Africa, overdiagnosis and the rate of false-positive microscopy for malaria can be high; warn travelers that a local diagnosis of malaria could be incorrect. In such cases, acutely ill travelers should seek the best available medical services and continue their prophylaxis regimen until they have a definitive diagnosis.

Rapid Diagnostic Testing

Rapid diagnostic tests (RDTs) for malaria detect antigens derived from malaria parasites. Malaria RDTs are immunochromatographic tests that most often use a dipstick or cassette format and provide results in 2–15 minutes. RDTs offer a useful alternative to microscopy in situations where reliable microscopic diagnosis is not immediately available. Although RDTs can detect malaria antigens within minutes, they have several limitations. RDTs cannot distinguish between all *Plasmodium* species that affect humans, they might be less sensitive than expert microscopy or PCR for diagnosis, they cannot quantify parasitemia, and an RDT-positive test result might persist for days or weeks after an infection has been treated and cleared. Thus, RDTs are not useful for assessing response to therapy. Furthermore, in some areas, mutations are increasingly being observed in malaria parasites, resulting in an absence of the malaria antigen usually detected by many RDTs, including the only RDT used in the United States. The absence of this parasite antigen in peripheral blood can lead to false-negative RDT test results.

Both positive and negative RDT results must always be confirmed by microscopy. Microscopy confirmation of the RDT result should occur as soon as possible, because the information on the presence, density, and parasite species is critical for optimal management of malaria. The US Food and Drug Administration (FDA) has approved an RDT (the BinaxNOW Malaria test) for hospital and commercial laboratory use; the test is not approved for use by clinicians or patients. Laboratories that do not provide in-house, on-the-spot microscopy services should maintain a stock of malaria RDTs so that they will be able to perform immediate malaria diagnostic testing when needed.

PCR Testing

PCR tests also are available to detect malaria parasites. These tests are more sensitive than routine microscopy, but results are not usually available as quickly as microscopy results, thus limiting the utility of PCR for acute diagnosis and initial clinical management. Use of PCR testing is encouraged to confirm the species of malaria parasite and detect mixed infections.

TREATMENT

Malaria can be treated effectively if treatment begins early in the disease; delaying therapy, however, can have serious or even fatal consequences. Specific treatment options depend on the species of malaria, the severity of infection, the likelihood of drug resistance (based on where the infection was acquired), the patient's age, and whether the patient is pregnant or breastfeeding.

Detailed CDC recommendations for malaria treatment can be found at www.cdc.gov/malaria/diagnosis_treatment/treatment.html. For assistance with the diagnosis or treatment of malaria, call the CDC Malaria Hotline (770-488-7788 or toll-free at 855-856-4713) from 9 a.m. to 5 p.m. Eastern Time. After hours, on weekends, or on holidays, call the CDC Emergency Operations Center at 770-488-7100 and ask the operator to contact the subject matter expert on call for the Malaria Branch. In addition, consult a clinician specializing in travel or tropical medicine or infectious diseases.

Travelers who decline to take prophylaxis, who choose a suboptimal drug regimen (e.g., chloroquine in an area with chloroquine-resistant *P. falciparum*), or who require a less-than-optimal drug regimen for medical reasons are at increased risk for acquiring malaria and then needing prompt treatment while abroad. Medications not used in the United States to treat malaria (e.g., halofantrine, sulfadoxine-pyrimethamine) are widely available abroad. CDC does not recommend halofantrine for treatment because of documented adverse cardiac events, including deaths. These adverse events have occurred in people with and without preexisting cardiac problems, and both in the presence and absence of other antimalarial drugs. Sulfadoxine-pyrimethamine is not recommended because of widespread drug-resistant *Plasmodium*.

Reliable Supply of Malaria Treatment

Some travelers who take effective prophylaxis but who will be in remote areas might decide, in consultation with their travel health provider, to also carry a reliable supply of a full course of an approved malaria treatment regimen. In the event a traveler carrying a reliable supply is diagnosed with malaria, they will have immediate access to an approved treatment.

CDC recommends that the reliable supply be acquired in the United States, so clinicians can consider the traveler's other medical conditions or medications when selecting an antimalarial drug and to avoid the possibility of travelers obtaining counterfeit drugs in the local pharmacy or market, or depleting local resources. In rare instances when access to medical care is not available and the traveler develops a febrile illness consistent with malaria, the reliable supply medication can be self-administered presumptively. Advise travelers that self-treatment of a possible malarial infection is only a temporary measure, and that prompt medical evaluation is imperative.

Two malaria treatment regimens available in the United States can be prescribed as a reliable supply for self-treatment: atovaquone-proguanil and artemether-lumefantrine. To treat malaria, CDC recommends against using the same (or related) drug that has been taken for prophylaxis. For example, atovaquone-proguanil can be used as a reliable supply medication by travelers who are not taking atovaquone-proguanil for prophylaxis. See Table 5-26 for dosing recommendations.

PREVENTION

Malaria prevention consists of a combination of mosquito avoidance measures and chemoprophylaxis. Prevention measures must address all malaria species in the travel area and apply to both short-term and long-term travelers. Although highly efficacious, interventions are not 100% effective, so all febrile persons returning from malaria-endemic areas should be tested for malaria even if they took chemoprophylaxis.

Table 5-26 Reliable supply regimens for malaria treatment[1]

DRUG	ADULT DOSE	PEDIATRIC DOSE	COMMENTS
ATOVAQUONE-PROGUANIL[2] Adult tablets: ▪ Atovaquone 250 mg ▪ Proguanil 100 mg Pediatric tablets: ▪ Atovaquone 62.5 mg ▪ Proguanil 25 mg	4 adult tablets taken orally (as a single daily dose) for 3 consecutive days	Weight-based daily dose taken orally (as a single daily dose) for 3 consecutive days 5–8 kg: 2 pediatric tablets 9–10 kg: 3 pediatric tablets 11–20 kg: 1 adult tablet 21–30 kg: 2 adult tablets 31–40 kg: 3 adult tablets >41 kg: 4 adult tablets	Contraindicated in people with severe renal impairment (creatinine clearance <30 mL/min). Not recommended for people taking atovaquone-proguanil prophylaxis. Not recommended for children weighing <5 kg, or people who are pregnant or breastfeeding infants weighing <5 kg.
ARTEMETHER-LUMEFANTRINE[2] One tablet ▪ Artemether 20 mg ▪ Lumefantrine 120 mg	Weight-based treatment schedule for both adult and pediatric patients. Patients should take an initial dose, followed by a second dose 8 hours later, then 1 dose twice a day for the next 2 days (total of 6 oral doses over 3 days). 5 kg to <15 kg: 1 tablet per dose 15 kg to <25 kg: 2 tablets per dose 25 kg to <35 kg: 3 tablets per dose ≥35 kg: 4 tablets per dose		Not recommended for people taking mefloquine prophylaxis. Not recommended for children weighing <5 kg, or people breastfeeding infants weighing <5 kg.

[1]A reliable supply is a complete course of an approved malaria treatment regimen obtained in the United States before travel. A reliable supply is not counterfeit or substandard; will not interact adversely with the patient's other medicines, including malaria chemoprophylaxis; will not deplete local resources in the destination country.
[2]If used for presumptive self-treatment, patients should seek medical care as soon as possible.

Preventing malaria involves striking a balance between effectiveness and safety: ensuring that all people at risk for infection use the recommended prevention measures, and preventing rare occurrences of adverse effects. Conduct an individual risk assessment for every traveler by collecting a detailed travel itinerary, including countries, specific areas to be visited in those countries (e.g., cities, rural areas, both), types of accommodation, season, and style of travel. Modify the risk assessment depending on traveler characteristics (e.g., pregnancy, underlying health conditions) and malaria characteristics at the destination (e.g., intensity of transmission, local parasite resistance to drugs). Depending on the level of risk, it might be appropriate to recommend no specific interventions, mosquito avoidance measures only, or mosquito avoidance measures plus chemoprophylaxis.

Several factors increase a traveler's risk for malaria. Travel, even for short periods of time, to areas with intense malaria transmission can result in infection. Malaria transmission is not distributed homogeneously throughout a country, so review the exact itinerary to determine if travel will occur in highly endemic areas. In countries where malaria is seasonal, travel during peak transmission season also increases risk. Travelers going to rural areas or staying in accommodations without screens or air conditioning also will be at greater risk. The greatest risk for malaria is associated with first- and second-generation immigrants living in nonendemic countries who return to their countries of origin to visit friends and relatives (VFRs). VFR travelers might perceive themselves to be at no risk because they grew up in a malaria-endemic country and consider themselves immune to the disease. Tolerance acquired through continuous exposure to malaria is quickly lost, however; consider VFRs to have the same risk as other nonimmune travelers (see Sec. 9, Ch. 9, Visiting Friends & Relatives: VFR Travel). Also remind travelers that they could become infected even if they had malaria before, and they still need to take preventive measures.

Mosquito Avoidance Measures

Because of the nocturnal feeding habits of *Anopheles* mosquitoes, malaria transmission occurs primarily between dusk and dawn. Travelers can reduce contact with mosquitoes by remaining in enclosed air-conditioned rooms or well-screened areas, sleeping under mosquito nets (preferably insecticide-treated), using an effective insecticide spray or mosquito coils in living and sleeping areas during evening and nighttime hours, and wearing clothes that cover most of the body.

All travelers should use an effective mosquito repellent, such as those that contain DEET (see Sec. 4, Ch. 6, Mosquitoes, Ticks & Other Arthropods). Repellents should be applied to exposed parts of the skin. If travelers are also wearing sunscreen, they should apply sunscreen first and insect repellent second. In addition to using a topical insect repellent, a permethrin-containing product can be applied to mosquito nets and clothing for additional protection against mosquitoes. Mosquito repellant–impregnated clothing also is available.

Chemoprophylaxis

CHOOSING A DRUG TO PREVENT MALARIA

All recommended primary prophylaxis regimens involve taking a medicine before, during, and after travel to an area with malaria. Beginning the drug before travel allows the antimalarial agent to be in the blood before the traveler is exposed to malaria parasites. In choosing a prophylaxis regimen before travel, the traveler and the travel health provider should consider several factors, including the presence of antimalarial drug resistance in the area of travel, length of travel, the patient's other medical conditions, allergy history, other medications prescribed or already being taken (to assess possible drug interactions), potential side effects, and the cost of the antimalarial. Long-term travelers, defined as people who travel for ≥6 months, have additional considerations (see Box 5-11). Table 5-27 lists some of the benefits and limitations of medicines used for malaria prophylaxis; additional information about choosing a malaria prophylaxis regimen can be found at www.cdc.gov/malaria/travelers/drugs.html.

Recommendations for drugs to prevent malaria by country of travel can be found in Sec. 2, Ch. 5, Yellow Fever Vaccine & Malaria Prevention Information, by Country. Recommended drugs for each country are listed in alphabetical order

BOX 5-11 Malaria prevention & prophylaxis considerations for the long-term traveler (travel >6 months)

CONSIDERATIONS

Malaria prevention measures are the same for both short- and long-term travelers.

Longer stays mean longer duration of exposure and increased risk of acquiring malaria.

Travelers' attention to mosquito avoidance can wane over time.

Travelers might not adhere to a lengthy course of malaria prophylaxis due to forgetfulness, fear of side effects, and the possible declining sense of risk and need over time.

Travelers might move between highly endemic or low endemic areas within a country or region.

Travelers might have a decreased sense of risk and concern about malaria after engaging in local conversations and lore, particularly regarding malaria immunity over time.

Travelers who become ill with malaria in countries with limited access and quality of health care might not receive appropriate or effective treatment.

ADDITIONAL ADVICE FOR LONG-TERM TRAVELERS

Travelers should not count on being able to obtain safe, reliable malaria prophylaxis medication abroad; strongly advise that before leaving the United States they purchase enough medication to last them for the entire duration of their travel to malaria-endemic areas.

Emphasize continued adherence to and safety of malaria prophylaxis drugs.

Develop a plan for seeking immediate care when ill with fever, including where to get promptly tested and treated for malaria.

Advise travelers to purchase travel insurance, including contingencies for medical evacuation.

Consider having a reliable supply of a treatment dose of antimalarial drugs available in case malaria is diagnosed while traveling.

and have comparable efficacy in that country. When >1 drug is recommended, Table 5-27 can help with the decision-making process. No antimalarial drug is 100% protective; therefore, travelers must combine prophylaxis with mosquito avoidance and personal protective measures (e.g., insect repellent, long sleeves, long pants, sleeping in a mosquito-free setting, using an insecticide-treated mosquito net).

MEDICATIONS USED FOR PROPHYLAXIS

ATOVAQUONE-PROGUANIL

Atovaquone-proguanil (Malarone) is a fixed combination of the drugs atovaquone and proguanil. Prophylaxis should begin 1–2 days before travel to malaria-endemic areas; the medication should then be taken daily, at the same time each day, while in the malaria-endemic areas, and daily for 7 days after leaving the endemic areas (see Table 5-28 for recommended dosages). Atovaquone-proguanil is well tolerated, and side effects are rare. The most common adverse effects reported in people using atovaquone-proguanil for prophylaxis or treatment are abdominal pain, nausea, vomiting, and headache.

Atovaquone-proguanil is not recommended for prophylaxis in children weighing <5 kg (11 lb), pregnant people, people breastfeeding infants <5 kg, or patients with severe renal impairment (creatinine clearance <30 mL/min). Proguanil can increase the effect of warfarin, so travelers might need international normalized ratio monitoring or adjustment of warfarin dosage. No data are available, however, regarding the clinical impact of taking atovaquone-proguanil and warfarin at the same time.

CHLOROQUINE & HYDROXYCHLOROQUINE

Chloroquine phosphate or hydroxychloroquine sulfate (Plaquenil) can be used to prevent malaria only in destinations where chloroquine-resistant *Plasmodium* spp. are not active (see Sec. 2, Ch. 5, Yellow Fever Vaccine & Malaria Prevention Information, by Country). Prophylaxis should begin 1–2 weeks before travel to malaria-endemic areas. Travelers should continue taking the drug once a week, on the same day of the week, during travel in malaria-endemic areas, and for 4 weeks after they leave endemic areas (see Table 5-28 for recommended dosages).

Table 5-27 Malaria chemoprophylaxis: prescribing considerations

DRUG	REASONS TO CONSIDER USING THIS DRUG	REASONS TO CONSIDER AVOIDING THIS DRUG
ATOVAQUONE-PROGUANIL	Good for last-minute travelers because the drug is started 1–2 days before travel. Some people prefer to take a daily medicine. Good choice for shorter trips because the traveler takes the medicine for only 7 days after leaving malaria-endemic area, rather than for 4 weeks. Well tolerated and side effects uncommon. Pediatric tablets are available and might be more convenient.	Cannot be used by people who are pregnant or who are breastfeeding a child that weighs <5 kg. Cannot be taken by people with severe renal impairment. Tends to be more expensive than some of the other options, especially for long trips. Some people (including children) would rather not take medicine every day.
CHLOROQUINE	Some people would rather take medicine weekly. Good choice for long trips because it is taken only weekly. Some people are already taking hydroxychloroquine chronically for rheumatologic conditions; in those instances, they might not have to take an additional medicine. Can be used in all trimesters of pregnancy.	Cannot be used in areas with chloroquine or mefloquine resistance. Can exacerbate psoriasis. Some people would rather not take a weekly medication. For short trips, some people would rather not take medication for another 4 weeks after leaving malaria-endemic areas. Not a good choice for last-minute travelers, because drug needs to be started 1–2 weeks before travel.
DOXYCYCLINE	Some people prefer to take a daily medicine. Good for last-minute travelers because the drug is started 1–2 days before travel. Tends to be the least expensive antimalarial drug. People already taking doxycycline chronically to prevent acne do not have to take an additional medicine. Doxycycline also can prevent other infections (e.g., rickettsial infections, leptospirosis); thus, might be preferred by people planning to camp, hike, and swim in fresh water where risk is high	Cannot be used by people who are pregnant or who are breastfeeding a child, or by children aged <8 years. Some people would rather not take medicine every day. For short trips, some people would rather not take medication for another 4 weeks after leaving malaria-endemic areas. People prone to getting vaginal yeast infections when taking antibiotics might prefer taking a different medicine. People might want to avoid the increased risk of sun sensitivity. Some people are concerned about the potential of getting an upset stomach from doxycycline.

(*continued*)

Table 5-27 Malaria chemoprophylaxis: prescribing considerations (continued)

DRUG	REASONS TO CONSIDER USING THIS DRUG	REASONS TO CONSIDER AVOIDING THIS DRUG
MEFLOQUINE	Some people would rather take medicine weekly. Good choice for long trips because it is taken only weekly. Can be used in all trimesters of pregnancy and during breastfeeding.	Cannot be used in areas with mefloquine-resistant *Plasmodium* spp. Cannot be used in patients with certain psychiatric conditions; some travelers without psychiatric conditions would prefer not taking a medication with known neuropsychiatric side effects. Cannot be used in patients with a seizure disorder. Not recommended for people with cardiac conduction abnormalities. Not a good choice for last-minute travelers because drug needs to be started ≥2 weeks before travel. Some people would rather not take a weekly medication. For short trips, some people would rather not take medication for another 4 weeks after leaving malaria-endemic areas.
PRIMAQUINE	One of the most effective drugs for prevention of *P. vivax*; thus, a good choice for travel to places with >90% *P. vivax*. Good choice for shorter trips because the traveler takes the medicine for 7 days after leaving a malaria-endemic area, rather than for 4 weeks. Good for last-minute travelers because the drug is started 1–2 days before travel. Some people prefer to take a daily medicine.	Cannot be used in patients with G6PD deficiency. Cannot be used in patients who have not been tested for G6PD deficiency. Costs and delays associated with getting a quantitative G6PD test might prohibit testing; however, the test only has to be done once. After a normal G6PD level is verified and documented, the test does not have to be repeated the next time primaquine or tafenoquine is considered. Cannot be used by people who are pregnant. Cannot be used by people who are breastfeeding unless the infant has also been tested for G6PD deficiency. Some people (including children) would rather not take medicine every day. Some people are concerned about the potential of getting an upset stomach from primaquine.
TAFENOQUINE	One of the most effective drugs for prevention of *P. vivax* malaria but also prevents *P. falciparum*. Good choice for shorter trips because the traveler takes the medicine once, 1 week after leaving malaria-endemic area, rather than for 4 weeks. Good for last-minute travelers because the drug is started 3 days before travel.	Cannot be used in people with G6PD deficiency. Cannot be used in patients who have not been tested for G6PD deficiency. Costs and delays associated with getting a quantitative G6PD test might prohibit testing; however, the test only has to be done once. After a normal G6PD level is verified and documented, the test does not have to be repeated the next time tafenoquine or primaquine is considered. Cannot be used by children. Cannot be used by people who are pregnant. Cannot be used by people who are breastfeeding unless the infant has also been tested for G6PD deficiency. Not recommended for patients with psychotic disorders.

Abbreviations: G6PD, glucose-6-phosphate-dehydrogenase

Reported side effects of chloroquine and hydroxychloroquine include blurred vision, dizziness, gastrointestinal disturbance, headache, insomnia, and pruritus, but generally, these effects do not require travelers to discontinue the drug. High doses of chloroquine (e.g., those used to treat rheumatoid arthritis) have been associated with retinopathy; this serious side effect appears to be extremely unlikely when chloroquine is used for routine weekly malaria prophylaxis. Chloroquine and related compounds reportedly can exacerbate psoriasis. People who experience uncomfortable side effects after taking chloroquine might tolerate the drug better by taking it with meals. As an alternative, a traveler experiencing side effects might better tolerate the related compound, hydroxychloroquine sulfate.

DOXYCYCLINE

Doxycycline prophylaxis should begin 1–2 days before travel to malaria-endemic areas. Doxycycline should then be taken once a day, at the same time each day, during travel in malaria-endemic areas and daily for 4 weeks after the traveler leaves endemic areas. Insufficient data exist on the antimalarial prophylactic efficacy of related compounds (e.g., minocycline, commonly prescribed for the treatment of acne). People on a long-term regimen of minocycline who need malaria prophylaxis should stop taking minocycline 1–2 days before travel and start doxycycline instead. Minocycline can be restarted after the full course of doxycycline is completed (see Table 5-28 for recommended dosages).

Doxycycline can cause photosensitivity, usually manifested as an exaggerated sunburn reaction. The risk for such a reaction can be minimized by avoiding prolonged, direct exposure to the sun and by using sunscreen (see Sec. 4, Ch. 1, Sun Exposure). In addition, doxycycline use is associated with an increased frequency of vaginal yeast infections.

Gastrointestinal side effects (nausea, vomiting) can be minimized by taking the drug with a meal or by specifically prescribing doxycycline monohydrate or the enteric-coated doxycycline hyclate, rather than the generic doxycycline hyclate, which is often less expensive. To reduce the risk for esophagitis, advise travelers to swallow the medicine with sufficient fluids and to avoid taking doxycycline shortly before going to bed.

Doxycycline is contraindicated in people with an allergy to tetracyclines, in pregnant people, and in infants and children aged <8 years. Vaccination with the oral typhoid vaccine Ty21a should be completed ≥24 hours before taking a dose of doxycycline.

MEFLOQUINE

Mefloquine prophylaxis should begin ≥2 weeks before travel to malaria-endemic areas. Travelers should continue taking the drug weekly, on the same day each week, during travel in malaria-endemic areas and for 4 weeks after leaving endemic areas (see Table 5-28 for recommended dosages).

At prophylactic doses, mefloquine has been associated with rare but serious adverse reactions (e.g., psychosis, seizures); these reactions are more frequent with the higher doses used for treatment. Other side effects reported in prophylaxis studies include abnormal dreams, anxiety disorder, depression, dizziness, gastrointestinal disturbance, headache, insomnia, and visual disturbances. Other neuropsychiatric disorders occasionally reported include aggressive behavior, agitation or restlessness, confusion, encephalopathy, forgetfulness, hallucinations, mood changes, panic attacks, paranoia, and sensory and motor neuropathies (e.g., ataxia, paresthesia, tremors). On occasion, psychiatric symptoms have been reported to continue long after mefloquine has been stopped. FDA also includes a boxed warning about rare reports of persistent dizziness after mefloquine use.

Mefloquine is contraindicated for travelers with a known hypersensitivity to the drug or related compounds (e.g., quinidine, quinine) and in people with active depression, a recent history of depression, generalized anxiety disorder, psychosis, schizophrenia and other major psychiatric disorders, or seizures. Mefloquine should be avoided in people with psychiatric disturbances or a history of depression.

A review of available data suggests that mefloquine can be used safely in people concurrently taking beta-blockers if they have no underlying arrhythmia. Mefloquine is not recommended for

Table 5-28 Malaria chemoprophylaxis: dosing information

DRUG	INDICATIONS	ADULT DOSE	PEDIATRIC DOSE	DOSING/CONTRAINDICATIONS/ PRECAUTIONS
ATOVAQUONE-PROGUANIL	Prophylaxis in all malaria-endemic areas	Adult tablets: • Atovaquone 250 mg • Proguanil 100 mg 1 adult tablet taken orally, 1×/day	Pediatric tablets: • Atovaquone 62.5 mg • Proguanil 25 mg Weight-based daily dosing schedule (taken orally, 1×/day) 5 kg to <8 kg: 1/2 pediatric tablet 8 kg to <10 kg: 3/4 pediatric tablet 10 kg to <20 kg: 1 pediatric tablet 20 kg to <30 kg: 2 pediatric tablets 30 kg to <40 kg: 3 pediatric tablets ≥40 kg: 1 adult tablet	Begin taking 1–2 days before travel to malaria-endemic areas. Take 1×/day, at the same time each day, while in malaria-endemic areas. Continue taking 1×/day for an additional 7 days after leaving endemic areas. Contraindicated in people with severe renal impairment (creatinine clearance <30 mL/min). Take with food or a milky drink. Not recommended for children weighing <5 kg, or people who are pregnant or breastfeeding infants weighing <5 kg. A pharmacist might need to prepare and dispense partial tablet doses in individual capsules, as described in the text.
CHLOROQUINE	Prophylaxis only in areas with chloroquine-sensitive malaria	300 mg base (500 mg salt) taken orally, once a week	5 mg/kg base (8.3 mg/kg salt), up to a maximum dose of 300 mg base (500 mg salt), taken orally, 1×/week	Begin taking 1–2 weeks before travel to malaria-endemic areas. Take 1×/week, on the same day each week, while in malaria-endemic areas. Continue taking 1×/week for another 4 weeks after leaving endemic areas. Can exacerbate psoriasis.
DOXYCYCLINE	Prophylaxis in all malaria-endemic areas	100 mg taken orally, 1×/day	≥8 years of age: 2.2 mg/kg, up to a maximum dose of 100 mg, taken orally, 1×/day	Begin taking 1–2 days before travel to malaria-endemic areas. Take 1×/day, at the same time each day, while in malaria-endemic areas. Continue taking 1×/day for another 4 weeks after leaving endemic areas. Contraindicated in children aged <8 years and in people who are pregnant.

Table 5-28 Malaria chemoprophylaxis: dosing information (continued)

DRUG	INDICATIONS	ADULT DOSE	PEDIATRIC DOSE	DOSING/CONTRAINDICATIONS/ PRECAUTIONS
HYDROXY-CHLOROQUINE	An alternative to chloroquine for prophylaxis only in areas with chloroquine-sensitive malaria	310 mg base (400 mg salt) taken orally, 1×/ week	5 mg/kg base (6.5 mg/kg salt), up to a maximum dose of 310 mg base (400 mg salt), taken orally, 1×/week	Begin taking 1–2 weeks before travel to malaria-endemic areas. Take 1×/week, on the same day each week, while in malaria-endemic areas. Continue taking 1×/week for another 4 weeks after leaving endemic areas.
MEFLOQUINE	Prophylaxis in areas with mefloquine-sensitive malaria	228 mg base (250 mg salt) taken orally, 1×/week	Weight-based weekly dosing schedule (taken orally, 1×/week) ≤9 kg: 4.6 mg/ kg base (5 mg/ kg salt) >9–19 kg: 1/4 tablet >19–30 kg: 1/2 tablet >30–45 kg: 3/4 tablet >45 kg: 1 tablet	Begin taking ≥2 weeks before travel to malaria-endemic areas. Take 1×/week, on the same day each week, while in malaria-endemic areas. Continue taking 1×/ week for another 4 weeks after leaving endemic areas. Contraindicated in people allergic to mefloquine or related compounds (quinidine, quinine) and in people with active depression, a recent history of depression, generalized anxiety disorder, psychosis, schizophrenia, other major psychiatric disorders, or seizures. Use with caution in people with psychiatric disturbances or a previous history of depression. Not recommended for people with cardiac conduction abnormalities.

(continued)

5

Table 5-28 Malaria chemoprophylaxis: dosing information (continued)

DRUG	INDICATIONS	ADULT DOSE	PEDIATRIC DOSE	DOSING/CONTRAINDICATIONS/ PRECAUTIONS
PRIMAQUINE[1]	Prophylaxis for short-duration travel to areas with principally *P. vivax*. Terminal prophylaxis (presumptive antirelapse therapy) to decrease the risk for relapses of *P. vivax* and *P. ovale*.	30 mg base (52.6 mg salt) taken orally, 1×/day. Same dose used for both primary and terminal prophylaxis; duration of therapy differs.	0.5 mg/kg base (0.8 mg/kg salt), up to maximum dose of 30 mg base (52.6 mg salt), taken orally, 1×/day Same dose for used both primary and terminal prophylaxis; duration of therapy differs.	Begin taking 1–2 days before travel to malaria-endemic areas. Take 1×/day, at the same time each day, while in malaria-endemic areas. Continue taking 1×/day for an additional 7 days after leaving endemic areas. Terminal prophylaxis indicated for people with prolonged exposure to *P. ovale*, *P. vivax*, or both. Take daily for 14 days after departure from the malaria-endemic area. Contraindicated in people with G6PD deficiency. Also contraindicated during pregnancy and breastfeeding unless the breastfed infant has a documented normal G6PD level.
TAFENOQUINE[1]	Prophylaxis in all malaria-endemic areas	200 mg orally	Not indicated for use in children	Begin taking 3 days before travel to malaria-endemic areas. Take 1×/week, on the same day each week, while in malaria-endemic areas. Take 1 additional dose 1 week after leaving endemic areas. Contraindicated in people with G6PD deficiency. Also contraindicated during pregnancy and breastfeeding unless the breastfed infant has a documented normal G6PD level.

Abbreviations: G6PD, glucose-6-phosphate-dehydrogenase

[1]Before prescribing primaquine or tafenoquine to any patient, document a normal G6PD level using a quantitative test.

5

people with cardiac conduction abnormalities, however. Any traveler receiving a prescription for mefloquine must also receive a copy of the FDA medication guide, which can be found at www.accessdata.fda.gov/drugsatfda_docs/label/2008/019591s023lbl.pdf.

PRIMAQUINE

> Primaquine can cause potentially life-threatening hemolysis in people with glucose-6-phosphate-dehydrogenase (G6PD) deficiency. Rule out G6PD deficiency with a quantitative laboratory test before prescribing primaquine to patients.

Primaquine phosphate has 2 distinct uses for malaria prevention in people with normal G6PD levels: primary prophylaxis in areas with primarily *P. vivax*, and terminal prophylaxis for travelers who have had prolonged exposure in malaria-endemic areas. Among people with normal G6PD levels taking primaquine, the most common adverse event is gastrointestinal upset; this occurs most commonly if the drug is taken on an empty stomach, and can be minimized or eliminated if it is taken with food.

PRIMARY PROPHYLAXIS

When taken for primary prophylaxis, primaquine should be taken 1–2 days before travel to malaria-endemic areas, daily (at the same time each day) while in the malaria-endemic area, and daily for 7 days after leaving the area (see Table 5-28 for recommended dosages).

TERMINAL PROPHYLAXIS

In addition to primary prophylaxis, terminal prophylaxis (also known as presumptive antirelapse therapy) generally is indicated for long-term travelers (e.g., military personnel, missionaries, Peace Corps volunteers) with prolonged exposure to *P. ovale* or *P. vivax* malaria. Terminal prophylaxis involves taking primaquine toward the end of the exposure period (or immediately thereafter) for the presumptive purpose of eliminating hypnozoites (dormant liver stages) of *P. ovale* or *P. vivax*, thereby preventing relapses or delayed-onset clinical presentations of malaria. Because most malaria-endemic areas of the world (except the Caribbean) have ≥1 species of relapsing malaria, travelers to these areas have some risk for acquiring either *P. ovale* or *P. vivax*, although the actual risk for an individual traveler is difficult to define.

When indicated, travelers should take primaquine for 14 days after leaving a malaria-endemic area, concurrently with their primary prophylaxis medication. If chloroquine, doxycycline, or mefloquine are used for primary prophylaxis, prescribe primaquine for travelers to take during the last 2 weeks of postexposure prophylaxis. When atovaquone-proguanil is used for primary prophylaxis, travelers can take primaquine during the final 7 days of atovaquone-proguanil, and then for an additional 7 days. If concurrent administration of primary and terminal prophylaxis is not feasible, instruct travelers to take primaquine after completing their primary prophylaxis medication. Primary prophylaxis with primaquine or with tafenoquine (see the following section) obviates the need for terminal prophylaxis.

5

TAFENOQUINE

> Tafenoquine can cause potentially life-threatening hemolysis in people with G6PD deficiency. Rule out G6PD deficiency with a quantitative laboratory test before prescribing tafenoquine to patients.

PRIMARY PROPHYLAXIS

Tafenoquine (Arakoda 100 mg tablets) can be used to prevent malaria in adults (see Table 5-28 for recommended dosages). Travelers should take a daily loading dose of tafenoquine for 3 days before leaving for a malaria-endemic area; starting 7 days after the loading dose is complete, they should take a weekly maintenance dose while in the malaria-endemic area; then take a final dose in the week after leaving the malaria-endemic area. Doses should be taken on the same day each week.

Tafenoquine is contraindicated in pregnant people and during breastfeeding. Avoid prescribing tafenoquine for people with a history of psychotic disorder; rare psychiatric adverse events have been observed in people with a history of psychotic disorder using higher doses of tafenoquine. The most common adverse events reported with use of tafenoquine are dizziness, gastrointestinal disturbances, headache, and clinically insignificant decreases in hemoglobin. Tafenoquine should be taken with food.

TERMINAL PROPHYLAXIS

As of 2020, CDC no longer recommends tafenoquine for terminal prophylaxis of *P. ovale* or *P. vivax* malaria.

PROPHYLAXIS FOR INFANTS, CHILDREN & ADOLESCENTS

All children traveling to malaria-endemic areas should use recommended prevention measures, which often include taking an antimalarial drug. In the United States, antimalarial drugs are not available in liquid formulation and can taste bitter. Calculate pediatric doses carefully according to the patient's body weight, but never exceed the adult dose. Pharmacists can pulverize tablets and prepare gelatin capsules for each measured dose. If a child is unable to swallow capsules or tablets, parents should prepare the child's medication dose by breaking open the gelatin capsule or crushing the pill and mixing the drug with a small amount of something sweet (e.g., condensed milk, chocolate syrup, chocolate spread) to ensure the entire dose is delivered to the child. Giving the dose on a full stomach can minimize stomach upset and vomiting.

Atovaquone-proguanil can be used as prophylaxis for infants and children weighing ≥5 kg (11 lb); prophylactic dosing for children weighing <11 kg (24 lb) constitutes off-label use in the United States. Chloroquine and mefloquine are options for infants and children of all ages and weights, depending on drug resistance at the destination. Doxycycline can be used for children aged ≥8 years. Primaquine can be used for children who are not G6PD-deficient and who are traveling to areas with principally *P. vivax*. Pediatric dosing regimens are included in Table 5-28.

PROPHYLAXIS DURING PREGNANCY

Malaria infection can be more severe in pregnant than in nonpregnant people. Malaria increases the risk for adverse pregnancy outcomes, including premature birth, spontaneous abortion, and stillbirth; thus, because no prophylaxis regimen is completely effective, advise people who are pregnant or likely to become pregnant to avoid travel to areas with malaria transmission if possible (see Sec. 7, Ch. 1, Pregnant Travelers). If travel to a malaria-endemic area cannot be deferred, an effective prophylaxis regimen and mosquito avoidance measures are essential.

Pregnant people traveling to areas where chloroquine-resistant *P. falciparum* has not been reported can take chloroquine prophylaxis. Chloroquine has not been found to have harmful effects on the fetus when used in the recommended doses for malaria prophylaxis; therefore, pregnancy is not a contraindication for malaria prophylaxis with chloroquine or hydroxychloroquine.

For travel to areas with known chloroquine-resistant *Plasmodium*, mefloquine is the only medication recommended for malaria prophylaxis during pregnancy. Studies of mefloquine use during pregnancy have found no indication of adverse effects on the fetus.

Atovaquone-proguanil is not recommended for use during pregnancy because of limited availability of data on its safety, and because other options are available. If other antimalarial drug options are not feasible, however, clinicians and patients should weigh the options, risks, and benefits of using atovaquone-proguanil to make the best decision for the patient. Doxycycline is contraindicated for malaria prophylaxis during pregnancy because of the risk for adverse effects seen with tetracycline, a related drug, on the fetus. These adverse effects include discoloration and dysplasia of the teeth and inhibition of bone growth. Neither primaquine nor tafenoquine should be used during pregnancy; both drugs can be passed transplacentally to a G6PD-deficient fetus and cause hemolytic anemia in utero.

People planning to become pregnant can use the same medications recommended for use during pregnancy (chloroquine or mefloquine, depending on the area of travel). CDC does not make recommendations about delaying pregnancy after the use of malaria prophylaxis medicines. If the traveler or their health care provider wishes to decrease the amount of antimalarial drug in the body before conception, however, Table 5-29 provides information on the half-lives of the recommended malaria prophylaxis

Table 5-29 Malaria chemoprophylaxis: half-lives

DRUG	HALF-LIFE
Atovaquone	2–3 days
Chloroquine	1–2 months
Doxycycline	15–24 hours
Hydroxychloroquine	1–2 months
Mefloquine	2–4 weeks
Primaquine	4–7 hours
Proguanil	12–25 hours
Tafenoquine	14–28 days

medicines. After 2 half-lives, ≈25% of the drug remains in the body, ≈6% remains after 4 half-lives, and ≈2% remains after 6 half-lives.

PROPHYLAXIS DURING BREASTFEEDING

The quantities of antimalarial drugs excreted in the breast milk of lactating people are insufficient to provide adequate protection to nursing infants. Therefore, infants who require prophylaxis should receive the recommended dosages of antimalarial drugs listed in Table 5-28. Because chloroquine and mefloquine can be prescribed safely to infants, infants also can be safely exposed to the small amounts excreted in breast milk. Data about the use of doxycycline in lactating people are very limited; most experts, however, consider the theoretical possibility of adverse events to the infant to be remote.

Although no information is available on the amount of primaquine or tafenoquine that enters human breast milk, test both the person breastfeeding and the infant for G6PD deficiency before initiating chemoprophylaxis with either one of these drugs. Because data are not yet available on the safety of atovaquone-proguanil prophylaxis in infants weighing <5 kg (11 lb), CDC does not recommend this drug to prevent malaria in people who are breastfeeding infants weighing <5 kg. Atovaquone-proguanil can, however, be used to treat people who are breastfeeding infants of any weight when the potential benefit outweighs the potential risk to the infant (e.g., treating a breastfeeding person who has acquired *P. falciparum* malaria in an area of multidrug-resistant strains and who cannot tolerate other treatment options).

TRAVEL TO AREAS WITH CHLOROQUINE-RESISTANT MALARIA

Chloroquine-resistant *P. falciparum* is found in all parts of the world except the Caribbean and countries west of the Panama Canal. Although chloroquine-resistant *P. falciparum* predominates in Africa, it is found in combination with chloroquine-sensitive *P. vivax* malaria in South America and Asia. Chloroquine-resistant *P. vivax* has been confirmed only in Papua New Guinea and Indonesia. For destinations with known chloroquine-resistant *Plasmodium* spp., in addition to mosquito avoidance measures, prescribe atovaquone-proguanil, doxycycline, mefloquine, or tafenoquine as prophylaxis.

TRAVEL TO AREAS WITH CHLOROQUINE-SENSITIVE MALARIA

Areas with chloroquine-sensitive *Plasmodium* spp. include many Latin American countries where malaria predominantly is caused by *P. vivax*. Chloroquine-sensitive *P. falciparum* is present in the Caribbean and Central American countries west of the Panama Canal. For destinations with known chloroquine-sensitive *Plasmodium* spp., in addition to mosquito avoidance measures, the many effective prophylaxis options include chloroquine, atovaquone-proguanil, doxycycline, mefloquine, and tafenoquine. In countries where *P. vivax* predominates, primaquine is also an option.

TRAVEL TO AREAS WITH MEFLOQUINE-RESISTANT MALARIA

Mefloquine-resistant *P. falciparum* has been confirmed in Southeast Asia on the borders of Thailand with Burma (Myanmar) and Cambodia, in the western provinces of Cambodia, in the eastern states of Burma on the border between Burma

Table 5-30 Malaria chemoprophylaxis: changing medications due to side effects

DRUG BEING STOPPED	DRUG BEING STARTED	DIRECTIONS FOR USE & COMMENTS
ATOVAQUONE-PROGUANIL	CHLOROQUINE	Not recommended
	DOXYCYCLINE	Begin taking doxycycline; continue taking 1×/day, at the same time each day, while in malaria-endemic areas. Take 1×/day for another 4 weeks after leaving the endemic area.
	MEFLOQUINE	Not recommended
	PRIMAQUINE	This switch would be unlikely because primaquine is recommended as primary prophylaxis for people with normal G6PD activity traveling to areas with mainly *Plasmodium vivax*. Should that be the case, begin taking primaquine. Continue taking 1×/day, at the same time each day, while in malaria-endemic areas. Take 1×/day for an additional 7 days after leaving the endemic area.
	TAFENOQUINE	Not recommended
CHLOROQUINE	ATOVAQUONE-PROGUANIL	If the switch occurs ≥3 weeks before departure from a malaria-endemic area, take atovaquone-proguanil 1×/day, at the same time each day. Continue taking 1×/day for an additional 7 days after leaving the area. If the switch occurs <3 weeks before departure from a malaria-endemic area, take atovaquone-proguanil 1×/day, at the same time each day, for 4 weeks after the switch. If the switch occurs after departure from a malaria-endemic area, take atovaquone-proguanil 1×/day, at the same time each day, for 4 weeks after leaving the area.
	DOXYCYCLINE	Begin taking doxycycline. Continue taking 1×/day, at the same time each day, while in malaria-endemic areas. Take 1×/day for another 4 weeks after leaving the area.
	MEFLOQUINE	Not recommended
	PRIMAQUINE	Primaquine is recommended as primary prophylaxis for people with normal G6PD activity traveling to areas with mainly *P. vivax*. Should that be the case, begin taking primaquine. Continue taking 1×/day, at the same time each day, while in malaria-endemic areas. Take 1×/day for an additional 7 days after leaving the area.
	TAFENOQUINE	For people with normal G6PD activity, begin taking tafenoquine as soon as possible after taking the last dose of chloroquine in a malaria-endemic area. Start by taking tafenoquine 1×/day for 3 days, then 1×/week while still in the area. Take 1 final dose during the week after leaving the endemic area.

Table 5-30 Malaria chemoprophylaxis: changing medications due to side effects (continued)

DRUG BEING STOPPED	DRUG BEING STARTED	DIRECTIONS FOR USE & COMMENTS
DOXYCYCLINE	ATOVAQUONE-PROGUANIL	If the switch occurs ≥3 weeks before departure from a malaria-endemic area, take atovaquone-proguanil 1×/day, at the same time each day. Continue taking 1×/day for an additional 7 days after leaving the endemic area. If the switch occurs <3 weeks before departure from a malaria-endemic area, take atovaquone-proguanil 1×/day, at the same time each day, for 4 weeks after the switch. If the switch occurs following departure from a malaria-endemic area, take atovaquone-proguanil 1×/day, at the same time each day, for 4 weeks after leaving the endemic area.
	CHLOROQUINE	Not recommended
	MEFLOQUINE	Not recommended
	PRIMAQUINE	This switch would be unlikely because primaquine is recommended as primary prophylaxis for people with normal G6PD activity traveling to areas with mainly *P. vivax*. Should that be the case, begin taking primaquine. Continue taking 1×/day, at the same time each day, while in malaria-endemic areas. Take 1×/day for an additional 7 days after leaving the endemic area.
	TAFENOQUINE	Not recommended
MEFLOQUINE	ATOVAQUONE-PROGUANIL	If the switch occurs ≥3 weeks before departure from a malaria-endemic area, take atovaquone-proguanil 1×/day, at the same time each day. Continue taking 1×/day for an additional 7 days after leaving the endemic area. If the switch occurs <3 weeks before departure from a malaria-endemic area, take atovaquone-proguanil 1×/day, at the same time each day, for 4 weeks after the switch. If the switch occurs after departure from a malaria-endemic area, take atovaquone-proguanil 1×/day, at the same time each day, for 4 weeks after leaving the endemic area.
	CHLOROQUINE	Not recommended
	DOXYCYCLINE	Begin taking doxycycline. Continue taking 1×/day, at the same time each day, while in malaria-endemic areas. Take 1×/day for another 4 weeks after leaving the endemic area.
	PRIMAQUINE	This switch would be unlikely because primaquine is recommended as primary prophylaxis for people with normal G6PD activity traveling to areas with mainly *P. vivax*. Should that be the case, begin taking primaquine. Continue taking 1×/day, at the same time each day, while in malaria-endemic areas. Take 1×/day for an additional 7 days after leaving the endemic area.

(continued)

5

Table 5-30 Malaria chemoprophylaxis: changing medications due to side effects (continued)

DRUG BEING STOPPED	DRUG BEING STARTED	DIRECTIONS FOR USE & COMMENTS
	TAFENOQUINE	For people with normal G6PD activity, begin taking tafenoquine as soon as possible after taking the last dose of mefloquine in a malaria-endemic area. Start by taking tafenoquine 1×/day for 3 days, then 1×/week while still in the endemic area. Take 1 final dose during the week after leaving the endemic area.
PRIMAQUINE	ATOVAQUONE-PROGUANIL	Begin taking atovaquone-proguanil. Continue taking 1×/day, at the same time each day, while in malaria-endemic areas. Take 1×/day for an additional 7 days after leaving the endemic area.
	CHLOROQUINE	Not recommended
	DOXYCYCLINE	Begin taking doxycycline. Continue taking 1×/day, at the same time each day, while in malaria-endemic areas. Take 1×/day for another 4 weeks after leaving the endemic area.
	MEFLOQUINE	Not recommended
	TAFENOQUINE	Not recommended
TAFENOQUINE	ATOVAQUONE-PROGUANIL	Begin taking atovaquone-proguanil. Continue taking 1x/day, at the same time each day, while in malaria-endemic areas. Take 1x/day for an additional 7 days after leaving the endemic area.
	CHLOROQUINE	Not recommended
	DOXYCYCLINE	Begin taking doxycycline. Continue taking 1×/day, at the same time each day, while in malaria-endemic areas. Take 1×/day for another 4 weeks after leaving the endemic area.
	MEFLOQUINE	Not recommended
	PRIMAQUINE	Not recommended

Abbreviations: G6PD, glucose-6-phosphate-dehydrogenase

and China, along the borders of Burma and Laos, and in southern Vietnam. For destinations with known mefloquine-resistant *Plasmodium* spp., in addition to mosquito avoidance measures, prophylaxis options are atovaquone-proguanil, doxycycline, and tafenoquine.

TRAVEL TO AREAS WITH LIMITED MALARIA TRANSMISSION

For destinations where malaria cases occur sporadically and risk for infection to travelers is considered low, CDC recommends that travelers use mosquito avoidance measures only, and no chemoprophylaxis (see Sec. 2, Ch. 5, Yellow Fever Vaccine & Malaria Prevention Information, by Country).

CHANGING MEDICATIONS AS A RESULT OF SIDE EFFECTS DURING PROPHYLAXIS

Medications recommended for malaria prophylaxis have different modes of action that affect the parasites at different stages of the life cycle. Thus, if the medication needs to be changed because of side effects before a full course has been completed, some special considerations exist (see Table 5-30).

Table 5-31 US Food and Drug Administration recommendations for deferring blood donation in people returning from malaria-endemic areas

GROUP	BLOOD DONATION DEFERRAL
Travelers to malaria-endemic areas	Not permitted to donate blood for 1 year after travel.
Former residents of malaria-endemic areas	Not permitted to donate blood for 3 years after departing. If they return to a malaria-endemic area within that 3-year period, they are deferred for an additional 3 years.
People diagnosed with malaria	Not permitted to donate blood for 3 years after treatment.

OBTAINING MEDICATIONS OVERSEAS

Medications recommended for malaria prophylaxis might be available at overseas destinations. Combinations of these medications and additional drugs that are not recommended might be commonly prescribed and used in other countries, however. Strongly discourage travelers from obtaining prophylaxis medications while abroad. The quality of these products is not known; products might be produced under substandard manufacturing practices, be counterfeit, contain contaminants, not be protective, or be dangerous. Additional information on medications obtained while traveling can be found in Sec. 6, Ch. 3, . . . *perspectives*: Avoiding Poorly Regulated Medicines & Medical Products During Travel, and on the FDA website, www.fda.gov/Drugs/ResourcesForYou/Consumers/BuyingUsingMedicineSafely/BuyingMedicinefromOutsidetheUnitedStates/default.htm.

BLOOD DONATION AFTER TRAVEL TO MALARIA-ENDEMIC AREAS

People who have been in an area where malaria transmission occurs should defer donating blood after returning from the malaria-endemic area to prevent transmission of malaria through blood transfusion (see Table 5-31).

Risk assessments can differ between travel health providers and blood banks. A travel health provider advising a traveler going to a country with relatively low malaria transmission for a short period of time and engaging in low-risk behaviors might suggest the traveler use only mosquito bite precautions and no prophylaxis. Upon the traveler's return, however, a blood bank might still choose to defer blood donations from that traveler for 1 year because of travel to an area where transmission occurs.

CDC website: www.cdc.gov/malaria

BIBLIOGRAPHY

Andrejko KL, Mayer RC, Kovacs S, Slutsker E, Bartlett E, Tan KR, Gutman JR. The safety of atovaquone-proguanil for the prevention and treatment of malaria in pregnancy: a systematic review. Travel Med Infect Dis. 2019;27:20–6.

Angelo KM, Libman M, Caumes E, Hamer DH, Kain KC, Leder K, et al. Malaria after international travel: a GeoSentinel analysis, 2003–2016. Malar J. 2017;16(1):293.

Boggild AK, Parise ME, Lewis LS, Kain KC. Atovaquone-proguanil: report from the CDC expert meeting on malaria chemoprophylaxis (II). Am J Trop Med Hyg. 2007;76(2):208–23.

Davlantes EA, Tan KR, Arguin PM. Quantifying malaria risk in travelers: a quixotic pursuit. J Travel Med. 2017;24(6):tax066.

Hill DR, Baird JK, Parise ME, Lewis LS, Ryan ET, Magill AJ. Primaquine: report from CDC expert meeting on malaria chemoprophylaxis I. Am J Trop Med Hyg. 2006;75(3):402–15.

Hwang J, Cullen KA, Kachur SP, Arguin PM, Baird JK. Severe morbidity and mortality risk from malaria in the United States, 1985–2011. Open Forum Infect Dis. 2014;1(1):ofu034.

Lupi E, Hatz C, Schlagenhauf P. The efficacy of repellents against *Aedes, Anopheles, Culex* and *Ixodes* spp.—a literature review. Travel Med Infect Dis. 2013;11(6):374–411.

Mace KE, Arguin PM, Lucchi NW, Tan KR. Malaria surveillance—United States, 2016. MMWR Surveill Summ 2019;68(SS-5):1–35.

Novitt-Moreno A, Ransom J, Dow, G, Smith B, Read LT, Toovey S. Tafenoquine for malaria prophylaxis in adults: an integrated safety analysis. Travel Med Infect Dis. 2017;17:19–27.

Tan KR, Magill AJ, Parise ME, Arguin PM. Doxycycline for malaria chemoprophylaxis and treatment: report from the CDC expert meeting on malaria chemoprophylaxis. Am J Trop Med Hyg. 2011;84(4):517–31.

ONCHOCERCIASIS / RIVER BLINDNESS

Paul Cantey, Sharon Roy

5

INFECTIOUS AGENT: *Onchocerca volvulus*	
ENDEMICITY	Sub-Saharan Africa Foci in South America and Yemen
TRAVELER CATEGORIES AT GREATEST RISK FOR EXPOSURE & INFECTION	Immigrants and refugees Long-term travelers and expatriates Travelers visiting friends and relatives
PREVENTION METHODS	Avoid blackfly habitats Avoid insect bites
DIAGNOSTIC SUPPORT	Serologic testing: National Institutes of Health Laboratory of Parasitic Diseases (301-496-5398) or CDC's Parasitic Diseases Branch (www.cdc.gov/parasites; 404-718-4745; parasites@cdc.gov) Parasitological diagnosis: DPDx (www.cdc.gov/DPDx)

INFECTIOUS AGENT

Onchocerca volvulus, a filarial nematode, causes onchocerciasis, also known as river blindness.

TRANSMISSION

Transmission occurs through female blackfly (genus *Simulium*) bites. *Simulium* vectors typically bite during the day and breed near rapidly flowing rivers and streams.

EPIDEMIOLOGY

Onchocerciasis is endemic to much of sub-Saharan Africa. Small endemic foci also are present in the Arabian Peninsula (Yemen) and in the Americas (Brazil and Venezuela). Foci center around blackfly breeding sites, located near rapidly flowing water. Most transmission occurs in rural areas, but some transmission occurs in semi-urban and urban areas. Infections diagnosed in the United States are most commonly in immigrants, people visiting friends and relatives in endemic areas, long-term travelers to endemic areas, and expatriates. Although rare, infection can occur in short-term (< 1 month) travelers, particularly to areas with intense exposure. The incidence of infections identified outside endemic areas might be declining due to successful implementation of ivermectin mass drug administration in many endemic areas.

CLINICAL PRESENTATION

Clinical signs and symptoms include highly pruritic, papular dermatitis; subcutaneous nodules; lymphadenitis; and ocular lesions, which can progress to vision loss and blindness. Symptoms begin after patent infections are established, which can take 18 months. Symptoms in travelers are primarily dermatologic, typically acute erythematous papular rash and pruritus, sometimes just edema, occurring years after departure from endemic areas. Signs of chronic skin changes are rare in travelers. Subcutaneous nodules and chronic skin changes (e.g., depigmentation, lichenification, hyperpigmented flat-topped papules), are more common in endemic populations. Peripheral eosinophilia is often present in symptomatic travelers and migrants.

DIAGNOSIS

The standard method of diagnosis is examination of a skin snip biopsy to determine the presence of microfilariae. The diagnosis also can be made by identifying adult worms in histologic sections of excised nodules or characteristic eye lesions. Serologic testing is most useful for detecting infection when microfilariae are not identifiable. Determination of serum filarial antibody is available through the National Institutes of Health (301-496-5398) or the Centers for Disease Control and Prevention (CDC). Instructions on how to submit a serum specimen to CDC for testing can be found at www.cdc.gov/laboratory/specimen-submission/index.html. Assistance with parasitological diagnosis can be obtained through DPDx (www.cdc.gov/DPDx). General assistance with the diagnosis or treatment of onchocerciasis can be obtained by contacting CDC's Parasitic Diseases Branch (parasites@cdc.gov; 404-718-4745).

TREATMENT

Ivermectin is the drug of choice to relieve symptoms. Patients might require repeated annual or semiannual doses to control symptoms, because the drug kills the microfilariae but not the adult worms. Some experts recommend treating patients with 1 dose of ivermectin, then 6 weeks of doxycycline to kill *Wolbachia*, an endosymbiotic rickettsia-like bacterium that appears to be required for the survival of the *O. volvulus* adult worm and for embryogenesis. Individuals at risk for co-infection with *Loa loa* should have blood evaluated to assess for the presence of *Loa loa* microfilariae. If co-infected, enlist the aid of a tropical medicine expert for management due to the risk of *Loa loa*–related fatal post-treatment reactions associated with ivermectin.

Diethylcarbamazine is contraindicated as a treatment for onchocerciasis because it leads to microfilarial death and, in some cases, systemic reactions associated with an increased risk for causing blindness in some patients with eye disease.

PREVENTION

Travelers should avoid blackfly habitats (e.g., fast-flowing rivers and streams) and use protective measures against biting insects (see Sec. 4, Ch. 6, Mosquitoes, Ticks & Other Arthropods).

CDC website: www.cdc.gov/parasites/onchocerciasis

BIBLIOGRAPHY

Hoerauf A, Pfarr K, Mand S, Bebrah AY, Specht S. Filariasis in Africa—treatment challenges and prospects. Clin Microbiol Infect. 2011;17(7):977–85.

Klion AD. Filarial infections in travelers and immigrants. Curr Infect Dis Rep. 2008;10(1):50–7.

Lipner EM, Law MA, Barnett E, Keystone JS, von Sonnenburg F, Loutan L, et al. Filariasis in travelers presenting to the GeoSentinel Surveillance Network. PLoS Negl Trop Dis. 2007;1(3):e88.

McCarthy JS, Ottesen EA, Nutman TB. Onchocerciasis in endemic and nonendemic populations: differences in clinical presentation and immunologic findings. J Infect Dis. 1994;170(3):736–41.

Murdoch ME, Hay RJ, Mackenzie CD, Williams JF, Ghalib HW, Cousens S, Abiose A, Jones BR. A clinical classification and grading system of the cutaneous changes in onchocerciasis. Brit J Derm. 1993;129(3):260–9.

Showler AJ, Nutman TB. Imported onchocerciasis in migrants and travelers. Curr Opin Infect Dis. 2018;31(5):393–8.

Tielsch JM, Beeche A. Impact of ivermectin on illness and disability associated with onchocerciasis. Trop Med Int Health. 2004;9(4):A45–56.

World Health Organization Department of Control of Neglected Tropical Diseases. Onchocerciasis—guidelines for stopping mass drug administration and verifying elimination of human onchocerciasis—criteria and procedures annexes. Geneva: The Organization; 2016. Available from: www.who.int/publications/i/item/9789241510011.

SARCOCYSTOSIS

Douglas Esposito

5

INFECTIOUS AGENT: *Sarcocystis* spp.	
ENDEMICITY	Intestinal disease endemic worldwide Muscular disease endemic in tropical and subtropical Southeast Asia; especially, Malaysia
TRAVELER CATEGORIES AT GREATEST RISK FOR EXPOSURE & INFECTION	Adventurous eaters
PREVENTION METHODS	Follow safe food and water precautions Avoid undercooked or raw beef and pork
DIAGNOSTIC SUPPORT	CDC's Parasitic Diseases Branch (www.cdc.gov/parasites; 404-718-4745; parasites@cdc.gov) Parasitological diagnosis: DPDx (www.cdc.gov/DPDx)

INFECTIOUS AGENT

Intracellular coccidian protozoan parasites in the genus *Sarcocystis* cause sarcosystosis.

TRANSMISSION

Intestinal Sarcocystosis

Humans are the natural definitive host for *Sarcocystis heydorni*, *S. hominis*, and *S. suihominis*, acquired by eating undercooked sarcocyst-containing beef or pork.

Muscular Sarcocystosis

Dead-end intermediate host infection with *S. nesbitti* and possibly other species can occur in humans who ingest food, water, or soil contaminated with the feces from a reptilian sporocyst-shedding definitive host, likely snakes.

EPIDEMIOLOGY

Human intestinal sarcocystosis occurs worldwide, but the prevalence is poorly defined and can vary regionally. Recent outbreaks of symptomatic muscular sarcocystosis among tourists in Malaysia suggest that intermediate-host infection could be a public health concern. Most reported cases have been acquired in the tropics and subtropics, particularly in Southeast Asia; only a few cases have been reported among US travelers and military personnel.

CLINICAL PRESENTATION

Most people with intestinal sarcocystosis are asymptomatic or experience mild gastroenteritis, but severe illness has been described. Differences in symptoms and illness severity and duration might reflect the number and species of the sarcocysts ingested. The disease is thought to be self-limited in immunocompetent hosts.

Intermediate-host infection can range from asymptomatic to severe and debilitating disease. In people who develop symptoms, onset occurs in the first 2 weeks after infection, and symptoms typically resolve in weeks to months.

Some patients can remain symptomatic for years, however. The most common symptoms are arthralgia, cough, fatigue, fever, headache, and myalgias. Less frequent symptoms include diarrhea, nausea, vomiting; lymphadenopathy; rash; wheezing; and symptoms reflecting cardiac involvement (e.g., palpitations). Fever and muscle pain can be relapsing and occur in 2 distinct phases: early (beginning during the second week after infection) and late (beginning during the sixth week after infection). Early-phase disease might reflect a generalized vasculitis, and late-phase disease can coincide with the onset of a diffuse focal myositis.

DIAGNOSIS

Consider intestinal sarcocystosis in patients with gastroenteritis and a history of eating raw or undercooked meat. Oocysts or sporocysts in stool can be confirmed by light or fluorescence microscopy; PCR testing is not widely available, and no serologic assays have been validated for use in humans.

Include muscular sarcocystosis in the differential diagnosis of people presenting with myalgia, with or without fever, and a history of travel to a tropical or subtropical region, especially Malaysia. Diagnosis during the early phase of infection is difficult, however, because of the lack of specificity of symptoms and clinical and laboratory findings. In the absence of an alternative diagnosis, consider serial investigations for evidence of myositis and eosinophilia. In people with myositis, exclude trichinellosis as a possible cause. Confirmation of muscular sarcocystosis requires biopsy and histologic observation of sarcocysts in muscle. Diagnostic assistance is available through the Centers for Disease Control and Prevention (www.cdc.gov/dpdx; dpdx@cdc.gov).

TREATMENT

No proven treatments are available for sarcocystosis. Trimethoprim-sulfamethoxazole might act against schizonts in the early phase of muscular sarcocystosis, but data are scant. Glucocorticoids and nonsteroidal anti-inflammatory medications can improve the symptoms associated with myositis.

5

PREVENTION

Intestinal sarcocystosis can be prevented by thoroughly cooking or freezing meat, which kills the infective bradyzoites. Travelers can reduce the risk for muscular sarcocystosis by following standard food and water precautions (see Sec. 2, Ch. 8, Food & Water Precautions).

CDC website: www.cdc.gov/parasites/sarcocystosis/index.html

BIBLIOGRAPHY

Arness MK, Brown JD, Dubey JP, Neafie RC, Granstrom DE. An outbreak of acute eosinophilic myositis attributed to human *Sarcocystis* parasitism. Am J Trop Med Hyg. 1999;61(4):548–53.

Esposito DH, Stich A, Epelboin L, Malvy D, Han PV, Bottieau E, et al. Acute muscular sarcocystosis: an international investigation among ill travelers returning from Tioman Island, Malaysia, 2011–2012. Clin Infect Dis. 2014;59(10):1401–10.

Fayer R, Esposito DH, Dubey JP. Human infections with *Sarcocystis* species. Clin Microbiol Rev. 2015;28(2):295–311.

Slesak G, Schafer J, Langeheinecke A, Tappe D. Prolonged clinical course of muscular sarcocystosis and effectiveness of cotrimoxazole among travelers to Tioman Island, Malaysia, 2011–2014. Clin Infect Dis. 2015;60(2):329.

SCABIES

Diana Martin

INFECTIOUS AGENT: *Sarcoptes scabiei* var. *hominis*	
ENDEMICITY	Worldwide
TRAVELER CATEGORIES AT GREATEST RISK FOR EXPOSURE & INFECTION	Long-term travelers Refugees and asylum seekers Study-abroad students
PREVENTION METHODS	Avoid contact with infected people
DIAGNOSTIC SUPPORT	CDC's Parasitic Diseases Branch (www.cdc.gov/parasites; 404-718-4745; parasites@cdc.gov)

5

INFECTIOUS AGENT

Scabies is caused by the human itch mite, *Sarcoptes scabiei* var. *hominis*.

TRANSMISSION

Direct transmission of conventional scabies occurs after prolonged skin-to-skin contact with a person infested with the mite. Indirect transmission of conventional scabies through contact with contaminated objects is rare. Animals are not a source of scabies.

Crusted scabies, by contrast, is more contagious than conventional scabies. Although <20 mites typically are found on a host with conventional scabies, a person with crusted scabies, formerly called Norwegian scabies, can harbor thousands of mites in just a small area of skin. The large number of mites present in crusted scabies greatly increases the chances that a person with crusted scabies will pass mites to others by both direct and indirect routes of transmission.

EPIDEMIOLOGY

Scabies occurs worldwide and is transmitted most easily in settings where skin-to-skin contact is common. Scabies also can be associated with sexual activity due to prolonged skin-to-skin contact. Scabies accounted for 1.5% of dermatologic complaints and <0.5% of all complaints in returning travelers presenting at GeoSentinel clinics. Scabies is more common in travelers with longer travel (>8 weeks) than in those who travel for shorter periods. Scabies is more common in tourists or volunteers than in business travelers or travelers visiting friends or family. Scabies is common in refugees and asylum seekers.

Crusted scabies most commonly occurs among debilitated, disabled, elderly, or immunosuppressed people, often in institutional settings. No reports of crusted scabies in travelers returning to the United States have been published.

CLINICAL PRESENTATION

The most common signs and symptoms of scabies are intense itching (pruritus), especially at night, and a papular itchy rash. The itching and rash each can affect much of the body or be limited to common sites (e.g., armpits, elbows, wrists, webbing between the fingers, nipples, the beltline or waist, penis, buttocks). The rash also can include small vesicles and scales.

Burrows, caused by the female scabies mite tunneling just beneath the surface of the skin, are sometimes seen. Burrows appear as tiny raised and crooked (serpiginous) grayish-white or skin-colored lines on the skin surface. Because infected people often only have a total of 10–15 mites, these burrows can be difficult to find; they are often in the webbing between the fingers, in the skin folds on the wrist, elbow, or knee, and on the breast, penis, or shoulder blades. In infants and very young children (but not usually in older children or adults), the head, face, neck, palms, and soles often are involved.

Symptoms occur 2–6 weeks after an initial infestation. For people who previously had scabies, symptoms appear much sooner, typically 1–4 days after exposure. Conventional scabies is characterized by intense itching, particularly at night, and by a papular or papulovesicular erythematous rash. Characteristic features of crusted scabies include widespread crusting and scales containing large numbers of mites; itching might be less prominent than in conventional scabies.

DIAGNOSIS

Scabies is diagnosed clinically. Telltale signs include burrows, typically found in skin folds and intertriginous areas in a patient with itching, and the characteristic rash. Although finding mites, mite eggs, or scybala (mite feces) under the microscope can confirm the diagnosis of scabies, microscopic identification of mites is far less sensitive than clinical diagnosis. Clinically, crusted scabies often is mistaken for psoriasis, but can be accurately diagnosed by using skin scrapings because of the high number of mites in the sores. The Centers for Disease Control and Prevention (CDC) Parasitic Diseases Branch provides consultations to health care providers at parasites@cdc.gov or 404-718-4745.

TREATMENT

Recommended treatments for conventional scabies include permethrin (5%) cream, which is approved by the US Food and Drug Administration (FDA), and ivermectin, which is not FDA-approved for scabies, but is indicated for scabies in the World Health Organization essential medicines list. Permethrin cream should be applied over the body from the neck down, left on for 8–12 hours or overnight, then washed off; patients will need a second application 1 week later. Treat household members and close contacts along with the index case. Oral ivermectin is reported to be safe and effective to treat conventional scabies at a single dose of 200 μg/kg, repeated after 1–2 weeks. Oral ivermectin should not be used in children weighing <15 kg or in pregnant people.

Treat crusted scabies more aggressively by using a combination of permethrin and ivermectin. Daily full-body application of permethrin for 7 days and ≤7 doses of oral ivermectin might be required. Details of the treatment regimen are found at the CDC's Parasitic Diseases Branch website (www.cdc.gov/parasites/scabies/health_professionals/meds.html). No over-the-counter treatments are available for scabies.

PREVENTION

Avoidance is the best way to prevent scabies; no chemoprophylaxis is known. Prolonged skin-to-skin contact with people with conventional scabies and even brief skin-to-skin contact with people with crusted scabies are the primary routes of transmission. Travelers should avoid sharing or handling clothing or bed linens used by an infected person, especially if the person has crusted scabies.

CDC website: www.cdc.gov/parasites/scabies

BIBLIOGRAPHY

Bouvresse S, Chosidow O. Scabies in healthcare settings. Curr Opin Infect Dis. 2010;23(2):111–8.

Chen LH, Wilson ME, Davis X, Loutan L, Schwartz E, Keystone J, et al.; GeoSentinel Surveillance Network. Illness in long-term travelers visiting GeoSentinel clinics. Emerg Infect Dis. 2009;15(11):1773–82.

Currie BJ, McCarthy JS. Permethrin and ivermectin for scabies. N Engl J Med. 2010;362(8):717–25.

Davis JS, McGloughlin S, Tong SY, Walton SF, Currie BJ. A novel clinical grading scale to guide the management of crusted scabies. PLoS Negl Trop Dis. 2013;7(9):e2387.

Lederman ER, Weld LH, Elyazar IR, von Sonnenburg F, Loutan L, Schwartz E, et al. Dermatologic conditions of the ill returned traveler: an analysis from the GeoSentinel Surveillance Network. Int J Infect Dis. 2008;12(6):593.

Warkowski JA, Bolan GA. Sexually transmitted diseases treatment guidelines, 2015. MMWR Morb Mortal Wkly Rep. 2015;64(RR-03):1–137.

SCHISTOSOMIASIS

Susan Montgomery, W. Evan Secor

INFECTIOUS AGENT: *Schistosoma* spp.	
ENDEMICITY	Mostly sub-Saharan Africa, Southeast Asia, China
TRAVELER CATEGORIES AT GREATEST RISK FOR EXPOSURE & INFECTION	Adventure travelers and ecotourists Immigrants and refugees from endemic areas Travelers who bathe, swim, or wade in contaminated freshwater
PREVENTION METHODS	Avoid bathing, swimming, wading, or other contact with freshwater in disease-endemic countries
DIAGNOSTIC SUPPORT	A clinical laboratory certified in moderate complexity testing; or contact CDC's Parasitic Diseases Branch (www.cdc.gov/parasites; 404-718-4745; parasites@cdc.gov) Parasitological diagnosis: DPDx (www.cdc.gov/DPDx)

5

INFECTIOUS AGENT

Schistosomiasis (also known as bilharzia and snail fever) is caused by helminth parasites of the genus *Schistosoma*. Other helminth infections are discussed in Sec. 5, Part 3, Ch. 13, Soil-Transmitted Helminths.

TRANSMISSION

Waterborne transmission occurs when larval cercariae, found in contaminated bodies of freshwater, penetrate the skin. Bathing, swimming, or wading in contaminated freshwater can result in infection; people of all ages are at risk. Human schistosomiasis is not acquired by contact with brackish or saltwater (oceans or seas). Schistosomiasis distribution is very focal and determined by the presence of competent snail intermediate hosts, inadequate sanitation, and infected humans. The specific snail intermediate hosts can be difficult to identify, and laboratory testing is the only way to determine whether snails are infected with human schistosome species.

EPIDEMIOLOGY

An estimated 85% of the world's cases of schistosomiasis are in Africa, where prevalence rates can exceed 50% in local populations. *Schistosoma mansoni* and *S. haematobium* are distributed throughout Africa. Only *S. haematobium* is found in areas of the Middle East, and only *S. mansoni* in parts of Brazil, Suriname, and Venezuela. In the Caribbean, risk is very low, but *S. mansoni* is found Guadeloupe, Martinique, and Saint Lucia, and previously in the Dominican Republic. *S. japonicum* is found in parts of China, in Indonesia, and in the Philippines. Although schistosomiasis had been eliminated in Europe for decades, transmission of *S. haematobium* was reported in Corsica in 2014, where cases were identified among travelers who had bathed in the Cavu River. Two other species can infect humans: *S. mekongi*, found in Cambodia and Laos, and *S. intercalatum*, found in parts of Central and West Africa. These 2 species are rarely reported causes of human infection.

Many but not all countries endemic for schistosomiasis have established control programs. Countries where development has led to widespread improvements in sanitation and water safety, especially where successful schistosomiasis control programs have been implemented, likely have eliminated this disease. No international guidelines currently exist for verification of elimination, however.

Travelers and expatriates potentially at increased risk for infection include adventure travelers and ecotourists, missionaries, Peace Corps volunteers, and soldiers. Outbreaks of schistosomiasis have occurred among adventure travelers on river trips in Africa. The geographic distribution of schistosomiasis acquired by travelers reflects travel and immigration patterns.

Most travel-associated cases of schistosomiasis are acquired in sub-Saharan Africa. Some African transmission sites frequently visited by travelers include rivers and water sources in the Banfora region (Burkina Faso) and areas populated by the Dogon people (Mali), Lake Malawi, Lake Tanganyika, Lake Victoria, the Nile River, the Omo River (Ethiopia), and the Zambezi River. As travel to more remote areas increases, travelers should remember that most freshwater surface water sources in Africa are potentially contaminated and can be sources of infection. Travelers should view with skepticism any local claim that a body of freshwater is free from schistosomiasis.

CLINICAL PRESENTATION

The incubation period is typically 14–84 days for acute schistosomiasis, and chronic asymptomatic infection can persist for years. Penetration of cercariae can cause a rash that develops within hours or up to a week after contaminated water exposure. Acute schistosomiasis (Katayama syndrome) is characterized by diarrhea, fever, headache, myalgia, and respiratory symptoms. Eosinophilia often is present; painful hepatomegaly or splenomegaly also can occur.

Clinical manifestations of chronic schistosomiasis are the result of host immune responses to schistosome eggs. Eggs secreted by adult worm pairs living in the bloodstream become lodged in the capillaries of organs and cause granulomatous reactions. *S. japonicum* and *S. mansoni* eggs most commonly lodge in the blood vessels of the liver or intestine and can cause blood in the stool, constipation, and diarrhea. Chronic inflammation can lead to bowel wall ulceration, hyperplasia, polyposis, and, with heavy infections, to periportal liver fibrosis and splenomegaly.

S. haematobium eggs typically lodge in the urinary tract and can cause dysuria and hematuria. Calcifications in the bladder might appear late in the disease. *S. haematobium* infection can cause genital symptoms and has been associated with increased risk for bladder cancer. As with acute schistosomiasis, eosinophilia might be present during chronic infection with any species.

Rarely, central nervous system manifestations of schistosomiasis develop; these are thought to result from aberrant migration of adult worms or eggs depositing in the spinal cord or brain. Signs and symptoms are related to ectopic granulomas in the central nervous system and can present as transverse myelitis.

DIAGNOSIS

Diagnosis is made by microscopic identification of parasite eggs in stool (*S. japonicum* or *S. mansoni*) or urine (*S. haematobium*). Serologic tests are useful to diagnose light infections, because egg shedding might not be consistent in travelers and in others who have not had schistosomiasis previously. Antibody tests do not distinguish between past and current infection but are useful for identifying infection in asymptomatic people who might have been exposed during travel and could benefit from treatment. Clinicians can obtain diagnostic assistance and confirmatory testing from the Centers for Disease Control and Prevention (CDC)'s Division of Parasitic Diseases and Malaria DPDx laboratory (www.cdc.gov/DPDx; dpdx@cdc.gov), and from the Parasitic Diseases Hotline for Healthcare Providers (404-718-4745; parasites@cdc.gov).

TREATMENT

Schistosomiasis is uncommon in the United States; clinicians unfamiliar with management of the condition should consult an infectious disease or tropical medicine specialist for assistance with diagnosis and treatment. Praziquantel is used to treat schistosomiasis. Praziquantel is most effective against adult forms of the parasite and requires a host immune response to the adult worm to be fully effective. Although a single course of treatment is usually curative, in lightly infected patients the immune response can be less robust and repeat treatment might be needed after 2–4 weeks to increase effectiveness.

PREVENTION

No vaccine or drugs are available to prevent infection. Travelers can prevent schistosomiasis by avoiding bathing, swimming, wading, or other contact with freshwater in disease-endemic countries. Untreated piped water coming directly from freshwater sources could contain cercariae; travelers should use fine-mesh filters, heat bathing water to 122°F (50°C) for 5 minutes, or allow water to stand for ≥24 hours before exposure to help prevent infection (see Sec. 2, Ch. 9, Water Disinfection).

Swimming in adequately chlorinated swimming pools is safe, even in disease-endemic countries, although confirming adequate levels of chlorination is difficult. Vigorous towel-drying after accidental exposure to water has been suggested as a method of removing cercariae before they can penetrate, but this should not generally be recommended as a preventive measure. Topical applications of insect repellents (e.g., DEET) can block penetrating cercariae, but the effect depends on the repellent formulation, could be short-lived, and does not provide adequate coverage to prevent infection reliably.

CDC website: www.cdc.gov/parasites/schistosomiasis

BIBLIOGRAPHY

5

Berry A, Mone H, Iriart X, Mouahid G, Aboo O, Boissier J, et al. Schistosomiasis haematobium, Corsica, France. Emerg Infect Dis. 2014;20(9):1595–7.

Campa P, Develoux M, Belkadi G, Magne D, Lame C, Carayon MJ, et al. Chronic *Schistosoma mekongi* in a traveler—case report and review of the literature. J Travel Med. 2014;21(5):361–3.

Clerinx J, van Gompel A. Schistosomiasis in travellers and migrants. Travel Med Infect Dis. 2011;9(1):6–24.

Colley DG, Bustinduy A, Secor WE, King CH. Human schistosomiasis. Lancet. 2014;383(9936):2253–64.

Lingscheid T, Kurth F, Clerinx J, Marocco S, Trevino B, Schunk M, et al. Schistosomiasis in European travelers and migrants: analysis of 14 years TropNet surveillance data. Am J Trop Med Hyg. 2017;97(2):567–74.

Ross AG, Vickers D, Olds GR, Shah SM, McManus DP. Katayama syndrome. Lancet Infect Dis. 2007;7(3):218–24.

World Health Organization Expert Committee. Prevention and control of schistosomiasis and soil-transmitted helminthiasis. World Health Organ Tech Rep Ser. 2002;912:1–57.

STRONGYLOIDIASIS

Susan Montgomery, Rebecca Chancey, Mary Kamb

INFECTIOUS AGENT: *Strongyloides stercoralis*	
ENDEMICITY	Worldwide in tropical and subtropical climates
TRAVELER CATEGORIES AT GREATEST RISK FOR EXPOSURE & INFECTION	Immigrants and refugees Immunocompromised travelers Long-term travelers and expatriates Military personnel on long deployments to endemic areas
PREVENTION METHODS	Avoid contact with fecal matter or sewage Wear shoes when walking on soil
DIAGNOSTIC SUPPORT	A clinical laboratory certified in moderate complexity testing; or contact CDC's Parasitic Diseases Branch (www.cdc.gov/parasites; 404-718-4745; parasites@cdc.gov) Parasitological diagnosis: DPDx (www.cdc.gov/DPDx)

INFECTIOUS AGENT

Strongyloidiasis is caused by an intestinal nematode, *Strongyloides stercoralis*.

TRANSMISSION

Transmission occurs when filariform larva, found in contaminated soil, penetrate human skin. Person-to-person transmission is rare but has been documented. Autoinfection can occur, leading to persistent infection if untreated.

EPIDEMIOLOGY

Strongyloidiasis is endemic to the tropics and subtropics; it has limited foci elsewhere, including Appalachia and the southeastern United States. Estimates of global prevalence range from 30–100 million. Most documented infections in the United States occur in immigrants, refugees, and military veterans living in *Strongyloides*-endemic areas for long periods. Risk for short-term travelers is low, but infections can occur.

CLINICAL PRESENTATION

Most acute and chronic infections are asymptomatic or have minimal symptoms. In acute infections, a localized, pruritic, erythematous papular rash can develop at the site of skin penetration, followed by pulmonary symptoms (a Löffler-like pneumonitis; for more details, see Sec. 5, Part 3, Ch. 13, Soil-Transmitted Helminths), abdominal pain, diarrhea, and eosinophilia. In chronic infections, migrating larvae in the skin can occasionally cause larva currens, a serpiginous urticarial rash on the perineum or upper thighs.

Immunocompromised people, especially those receiving systemic corticosteroids, those infected with human T cell lymphotropic virus type 1, and those with hematologic malignancies or who have had hematopoietic stem cell or organ transplants are at risk for hyperinfection or disseminated disease, characterized by abdominal pain, diffuse pulmonary infiltrates, and septicemia or meningitis from enteric bacteria. Untreated hyperinfection and disseminated strongyloidiasis are associated with high mortality rates.

DIAGNOSIS

Suspect strongyloidiasis in symptomatic patients who have a history of skin contact (i.e., bare feet) with soil in tropical or subtropical regions. Laboratory diagnosis usually involves blood and stool testing. Although common in intestinal strongyloidiasis, peripheral blood eosinophilia is often absent in hyperinfection and disseminated strongyloidiasis.

Rhabditiform larvae can be visualized on microscopic examination of stool, either directly or by culture on agar plates. Repeated stool examinations or examination of duodenal contents might be necessary. Hyperinfection and disseminated strongyloidiasis are diagnosed by examining cerebrospinal fluid, sputum, stool, and other body fluids and tissues, which typically contain high numbers of filariform larva.

Serologic testing is available through commercial laboratories; diagnostic assistance is available from the Centers for Disease Control and Prevention (CDC)'s Division of Parasitic Diseases and Malaria DPDx laboratory (www.cdc.gov/DPDx; dpdx@cdc.gov), and the Parasitic Diseases Hotline for Healthcare Providers (404-718-4745; parasites@cdc.gov).

TREATMENT

The treatment of choice for acute, chronic, and disseminated disease or hyperinfection is ivermectin. The alternative is albendazole, but it is associated with lower cure rates. Because of the potential for relapse, patients with hyperinfection, disseminated disease, or co-infection with human T cell lymphotropic virus 1 might need prolonged or repeated treatment.

PREVENTION

No vaccines or drugs are available to prevent infection. To protect against *Strongyloides* infection, travelers should wear shoes when walking in areas where humans might have defecated. Perform serologic testing for patients at risk for *Strongyloides* infection who will be placed on corticosteroids or other immunosuppressive drug regimens, or who will undergo procedures that involve immunosuppression (e.g., transplantation). If indicated, treat these patients for strongyloidiasis before initiating immunosuppressive therapy. Consider empiric treatment in people deemed at risk of strongyloidiasis who require immediate immunosuppression.

CDC website: www.cdc.gov/parasites/strongyloides

BIBLIOGRAPHY

Henriquez-Camacho C, Gotuzzo E, Echevarria J, White Jr AC, Terashima A, Samalvides F, et al. Ivermectin versus albendazole or thiabendazole for *Strongyloides stercoralis* infection. Cochrane Database Sys Rev. 2016(1):CD007745.

Keiser PB, Nutman TB. *Strongyloides stercoralis* in the immunocompromised population. Clin Microbiol Rev. 2004;17(1):208–17.

Krolewiecki A, Nutman TB. Strongyloidiasis: a neglected tropical disease. Infect Dis Clin North Am. 2019;33(1):135–51.

Nutman TB. Human infection with *Strongyloides stercoralis* and other related *Strongyloides* species. Parasitology. 2017;144(3):263–73.

Puthiyakunnon S, Boddu S, Li Y, Zhou X, Wang C, Li J, et al. Strongyloidiasis—an insight into its global prevalence and management. PLoS Negl Trop Dis. 2014;8(8):e3018.

Requena-Mendez A, Buonfrate D, Gomez-Junyent J, Zammarchi L, Bisoffi A, Munoz J. Evidence-based guidelines for screening and management of strongyloidiasis in non-endemic countries. Am J Trop Med Hyg. 2017;97(3):645–52.

Seybolt LM, Christiansen D, Barnett ED. Diagnostic evaluation of newly arrived asymptomatic refugees with eosinophilia. Clin Infect Dis. 2006;42(3):363–7.

5

TAENIASIS

Susan Montgomery, Sharon Roy

INFECTIOUS AGENTS: *Taenia* spp.	
ENDEMICITY	Africa Latin America South and Southeast Asia
TRAVELER CATEGORIES AT GREATEST RISK FOR EXPOSURE & INFECTION	Adventurous eaters Immigrants and refugees from endemic areas
PREVENTION METHODS	Follow safe food precautions Avoid raw or undercooked beef and pork
DIAGNOSTIC SUPPORT	A clinical laboratory certified in moderate complexity testing; or contact CDC's Parasitic Diseases Branch (www.cdc.gov/parasites; 404-718-4745; parasites@cdc.gov) Parasitological diagnosis: DPDx (www.cdc.gov/DPDx)

INFECTIOUS AGENTS

Taenia spp., including *T. asiatica*, *T. saginata* (beef tapeworm), and *T. solium* (pork tapeworm), cause human taeniasis.

TRANSMISSION

Transmission occurs through eating raw or undercooked contaminated beef (*T. saginata*) or pork (*T. asiatica*, *T. solium*).

EPIDEMIOLOGY

Taeniasis prevalence is greatest in Africa, Latin America, and South and Southeast Asia. Taeniasis has been reported at lower rates in Eastern Europe and the Iberian Peninsula (Portugal and Spain). Tapeworm infections are unusual in travelers.

CLINICAL PRESENTATION

The incubation period is 8–16 weeks for *T. asiatica*, 10–14 weeks for *T. saginata*, and 8–10 weeks for *T. solium*. Symptoms can include abdominal discomfort, anorexia, diarrhea, insomnia, nausea, nervousness, perianal pruritus, weakness, and weight loss. Symptoms are less likely for *T. solium* infection than for *T. saginata* infection.

DIAGNOSIS

Diagnosis is made by detecting eggs, proglottids (segments), or tapeworm antigens in the feces or on anal swabs. Differential diagnosis of *Taenia* spp. is based on morphology of the scolex and gravid proglottids. Clinicians can obtain diagnostic assistance and confirmatory testing from the Centers for Disease Control and Prevention's Division of Parasitic Diseases and Malaria DPDx laboratory (www.cdc.gov/DPDx; dpdx@cdc.gov) and from the Parasitic Diseases Hotline for Healthcare Providers (404-718-4745; parasites@cdc.gov).

TREATMENT

Praziquantel is the drug of choice for taeniasis, except for symptomatic neurocysticercosis (see Sec. 5, Part 3, Ch. 6, Cysticercosis). Niclosamide is an alternative but is not as widely available.

PREVENTION

Travelers should practice safe food precautions and especially avoid eating raw or undercooked meat.

CDC website: www.cdc.gov/parasites/taeniasis

BIBLIOGRAPHY

Cantey PT, Coyle CM, Sorvillo FJ, Wilkins PP, Starr MC, Nash TE. Neglected parasitic infections in the United States: cysticercosis. Am J Trop Med Hyg. 2014;90(5):805–9.

Eom KS, Rim HJ, Jeon HK. *Taenia asiatica*: historical overview of taeniasis and cysticercosis with molecular characterization. Adv Parasitol. 2020;108:133–73.

Wittner M, White ACJ, Tanowitz HB. Taenia and other tapeworm infections. In: Guerrant RL, Walker DH, Weller PF, editors. Tropical infectious diseases: principles, pathogens and practice, 3rd edition. Philadelphia: Saunders Elsevier; 2011. pp. 839–47.

Zammarchi L, Bonati M, Strohmeyer M, Albonico M, Requena-Mendez A, Bisoffi Z, et al. Screening, diagnosis and management of human cysticercosis and *Taenia solium* taeniasis: technical recommendations by the COHEMI project study group. Trop Med Int Health. 2017;22(7):881–94.

TOXOPLASMOSIS

Anne Straily, Susan Montgomery

INFECTIOUS AGENT: *Toxoplasma gondii*	
ENDEMICITY	Worldwide
TRAVELER CATEGORIES AT GREATEST RISK FOR EXPOSURE & INFECTION	All travelers Risk for congenital transmission when primary infection occurs during pregnancy
PREVENTION METHODS	Follow safe food and water precautions Pregnant people should avoid contact with cat feces
DIAGNOSTIC SUPPORT	A clinical laboratory certified in moderate complexity testing; or contact Sutter Health Palo Alto Medical Foundation Toxoplasma Serology Laboratory (www.pamf.org/serology)

INFECTIOUS AGENT

Toxoplasma gondii, an intracellular coccidian protozoan parasite, causes toxoplasmosis.

TRANSMISSION

T. gondii transmission occurs through ingestion of food, soil, or water contaminated with cat feces; ingestion of undercooked meat or shellfish; congenital transmission from a person infected during or shortly before pregnancy; and contaminated blood transfusions or organ transplantation.

EPIDEMIOLOGY

T. gondii is endemic throughout most of the world. Risk for infection is greater in developing and tropical countries, especially when people eat undercooked meat or shellfish, drink untreated water, or have extensive soil exposure. Congenital transmission also can occur if a person is infected shortly before becoming pregnant or during pregnancy.

CLINICAL PRESENTATION

Incubation period is 5–23 days. Symptoms can include influenza-like symptoms or a mononucleosis syndrome with prolonged fever, elevated liver enzymes, lymphadenopathy, lymphocytosis, and weakness. Rarely, chorioretinitis or disseminated disease can occur in immunocompetent people. In severely immunocompromised people, severe and even fatal encephalitis, pneumonitis, and other systemic illnesses can occur, most often from reactivation of a previous infection. Infants with congenital toxoplasmosis often are asymptomatic, but eye disease, neurologic disease, or other systemic symptoms can occur, and cognitive deficits, learning disabilities, or visual impairments could develop later in life.

DIAGNOSIS

Serologic tests for *T. gondii* antibodies are available at commercial diagnostic laboratories; because of the inherent difficulty in diagnosing acute toxoplasmosis, however, physicians are advised to seek confirmatory testing through the reference laboratory at Sutter Health Palo Alto Medical Foundation Toxoplasma Serology Laboratory (www.pamf.org/serology). Eye disease is diagnosed by ocular examination. Diagnosis of toxoplasmic encephalitis in immunocompromised people, most often seen in people with AIDS who are not receiving appropriate prophylaxis, can be based on typical clinical course and identification of ≥1 mass lesion by CT or MRI. Biopsy might be needed to make a definitive diagnosis.

TREATMENT

Treatment is reserved for acutely infected immunocompromised or pregnant people and people with severe disease. The recommended treatment regimen includes pyrimethamine, sulfadiazine, and leucovorin (folinic acid). Alternative treatment regimens include pyrimethamine with atovaquone, azithromycin, or clindamycin, but these have not been studied extensively. For the acutely infected pregnant person, recommended treatment depends on the timing of infection during gestation; seek consultation with an infectious disease specialist before initiating therapy in these patients.

PREVENTION

Travelers should adhere to safe food and water precautions (see Sec. 2, Ch. 8, Food & Water Precautions). In addition, travelers should avoid direct contact with sand or soil that could be contaminated with cat feces; if caring for a cat, change the litter box daily. Immunocompromised or pregnant people should avoid changing cat litter, if possible, and should not adopt or handle stray cats. Travelers should wash hands with soap and water after gardening, after contact with sand or soil, and after changing cat litter.

CDC website: www.cdc.gov/parasites/toxoplasmosis

BIBLIOGRAPHY

Anand R, Jones CW, Ricks JH, Sofarelli TA, Hale DC. Acute primary toxoplasmosis in travelers returning from endemic countries. J Travel Med. 2012;19(1):57–60.

Maldonado YA, Read JS; AAP Committee on Infectious Diseases. Diagnosis, treatment, and prevention of congenital toxoplasmosis in the United States. Pediatrics. 2017;139(2):e20163860.

Montoya JG, Liesenfeld O. Toxoplasmosis. Lancet. 2004;363(9425):1965–76.

Panel on Opportunistic Infections in HIV-Infected Adults and Adolescents. Guidelines for the prevention and treatment of opportunistic infections in HIV-infected adults and adolescents: recommendations from the Centers for Disease Control and Prevention, the National Institutes of Health, and the HIV Medicine Association of the Infectious Diseases Society of America; 2021. Available from: https://clinicalinfo.hiv.gov/sites/default/files/guidelines/documents/Adult_OI.pdf

Sepulveda-Arias JC, Gomez-Marin JE, Bobic B, Naranjo-Galvis CA, Djurkovic-Djakovic O. Toxoplasmosis as a travel risk. Travel Med Infect Dis. 2014;12(6 Pt A):592–601.

TRYPANOSOMIASIS, AFRICAN

Sharon Roy, Rebecca Chancey, Paul Cantey, Anne Straily

INFECTIOUS AGENTS: *Trypanosoma brucei rhodesiense* and *T. brucei gambiense*	
ENDEMICITY	Sub-Saharan Africa
TRAVELER CATEGORIES AT GREATEST RISK FOR EXPOSURE & INFECTION	Adventure tourists Humanitarian aid workers Immigrants and refugees Long-term travelers and expatriates Travelers visiting friends and relatives
PREVENTION METHODS	Avoid insect bites
DIAGNOSTIC SUPPORT	Contact CDC's Parasitic Diseases Branch for assistance with serologic testing for *T. b. gambiense* (www.cdc.gov/parasites; 404-718-4745; parasites@cdc.gov) Parasitological diagnosis: DPDx (www.cdc.gov/DPDx)

INFECTIOUS AGENTS

Trypanosomiasis is caused by 2 subspecies of the protozoan parasite *Trypanosoma brucei* (*T. brucei rhodesiense* and *T. brucei gambiense*).

TRANSMISSION

Trypanosomiasis is transmitted by the bite of an infected tsetse fly (*Glossina* spp.). Bloodborne, congenital, sexual, and transfusion or transplantation transmission are rare.

EPIDEMIOLOGY

African trypanosomiasis is endemic to rural sub-Saharan Africa. *T. brucei rhodesiense* is reported from eastern and southeastern Africa, mainly Malawi, Tanzania, Uganda, Zambia, and Zimbabwe. *T. brucei gambiense* is reported from central and west Africa, particularly in parts of the Democratic Republic of the Congo, as well as Angola, Cameroon, Central African Republic, Chad, Congo, Côte d'Ivoire, Equatorial Guinea, Gabon, Guinea, South Sudan, (northern) Uganda, and other countries. World Health Organization (WHO) maps and tables of African trypanosomiasis cases, by country, are available at www.who.int/data/gho/data/themes/topics/human-african-trypanosomiasis.

In 2018, WHO received 4,977 reports of sleeping sickness cases from African countries; *T. brucei gambiense* accounted for 98% of cases. Many cases, however, are likely not recognized or reported; exported cases also have been reported in expatriates, immigrants, refugees to countries outside of Africa, and tourists. Cases imported into the United States are rare; most cases in international travelers are due to *T. brucei rhodesiense*, typically acquired during visits to national parks or game reserves.

Tsetse flies inhabit rural areas, including forests and savannah areas, and areas of thick vegetation along rivers and waterholes, depending on the fly species. Travelers to urban areas are at minimal risk, although transmission has been observed in some urban settings in the past. Tsetse flies bite during the day, and <1% are infected. Risk for infection in travelers increases with the number of fly bites, which does not always correlate with duration of travel. People most likely to be exposed to African trypanosomiasis infection are hunters and villagers with infected cattle herds. Tourists and other people working in or visiting game parks are at risk for contracting African trypanosomiasis if they spend long periods in rural areas where the disease is present.

5

CLINICAL PRESENTATION

T. brucei rhodesiense

Clinical manifestations generally appear within 1–3 weeks after the infective bite and can include a chancre at the bite site that appears within a few days of the bite; high fever; headache; myalgia; skin rash; thrombocytopenia; and less commonly, cardiac dysfunction, renal failure, or splenomegaly. Central nervous system (CNS) involvement can occur within a few weeks of the exposure and results in sleep cycle disturbance, mental deterioration, and, if left untreated, death within months.

T. brucei gambiense

Clinical manifestations of *T. brucei gambiense* generally appear months to years after exposure, but the incubation period can be <1 month. Signs and symptoms are nonspecific and can include arthralgia, facial edema, intermittent fever, headache, lymphadenopathy, malaise, myalgia, pruritus, and weight loss. CNS involvement occurs after several months to years of infection and is characterized by daytime somnolence and nighttime sleep disturbance, headache, and other neurologic manifestations (e.g., behavioral changes, mood disorders, focal deficits). In residents of endemic areas, the clinical course of disease caused by *T. brucei gambiense* generally progresses more slowly (estimated average total duration of 3 years) than that caused by *T. brucei rhodesiense*, but if not treated, both forms of African trypanosomiasis typically are fatal.

DIAGNOSIS

Tsetse fly bites are characteristically painful, and a chancre can develop at the bite location. No serologic tests for *Trypanosoma brucei* are available in the United States. Diagnosis of *T. brucei rhodesiense* is made by microscopic identification of parasites in specimens of blood, chancre fluid, or tissue; cerebrospinal fluid (CSF); bone marrow aspirates; or lymph node aspirates. The level of parasitemia is lower in *T. brucei gambiense* than *T. brucei rhodesiense* infections. Microscopic identification generally requires serial examinations of samples concentrated by techniques such as centrifugation followed by buffy coat examination, microhematocrit centrifugation, or mini-anion exchange centrifugation.

Serologic testing for *T. brucei gambiense*, available outside of the United States, can assist in diagnosis; the Centers for Disease Control and Prevention (CDC) can provide contact information. All patients diagnosed with African trypanosomiasis must have their CSF examined on a wet preparation to look for motile trypomastigotes and white blood cells (WBC) to determine whether the CNS is involved; the choice of treatment drugs depends on the disease stage. Patients with ≤5 WBC/mL and no trypomastigotes in CSF are in the first stage, and those with >5 WBC/mL or trypomastigotes in CSF are in the second stage.

Diagnostic assistance is available from CDC's Division of Parasitic Diseases and Malaria DPDx laboratory (www.cdc.gov/DPDx; dpdx@cdc.gov), and from the Parasitic Diseases Hotline for Healthcare Providers (404-718-4745; parasites@cdc.gov).

TREATMENT

Treat people diagnosed with African trypanosomiasis with a drug course specific to the type of infection (*T. brucei rhodesiense* or *T. brucei gambiense*) and disease stage (i.e., presence or absence of CNS involvement). Pentamidine, the recommended treatment for first-stage *T. brucei gambiense* infection, is available in the United States. Nifurtimox was approved by the US Food and Drug Administration in August 2020 and is commercially available. Other drugs used to treat African trypanosomiasis (e.g., eflornithine [used in combination with nifurtimox], melarsoprol, suramin) are not commercially available in the United States but can be obtained from CDC. Physicians can consult with CDC staff to obtain otherwise unavailable treatment drugs (parasites@cdc.gov, 404-718-4745, or www.cdc.gov/parasites/sleepingsickness/health_professionals/index.html).

No test of cure is available for African trypanosomiasis. After treatment, closely follow patients for 24 months and monitor for relapse. Recurrence of symptoms will require examination of body fluids, including CSF, to detect the presence of trypanosomes.

PREVENTION

No vaccines or prophylactic drugs against African trypanosomiasis are available. To reduce the risk for infection, travelers should minimize contact with tsetse flies by wearing long-sleeved shirts and long pants made of medium-weight fabric in neutral colors. Tsetse flies are attracted to bright or dark colors, especially blue and black, and can bite through lightweight clothing. Travelers should inspect vehicles before entering, because the flies are attracted to the motion and dust from moving vehicles. Travelers should avoid bushes, because tsetse flies are less active during the hottest part of the day but will bite if disturbed. Although permethrin-impregnated clothing and insect repellent have not proven to be particularly effective against tsetse flies, travelers should use DEET repellent to prevent other insect bites that can cause illness (see Sec. 4, Ch. 6, Mosquitoes, Ticks & Other Arthropods).

CDC website: www.cdc.gov/parasites/sleepingsickness

5

BIBLIOGRAPHY

Büscher P, Cecchi G, Jamonneau V, Priotto G. Human African trypanosomiasis. Lancet. 2017;390(10110):2397–409.

Franco JR, Simarro PP, Diarra A, Jannin JG. Epidemiology of human African trypanosomiasis. Clin Epidemiol. 2014;6:257–75.

Kennedy PGE. Clinical features, diagnosis, and treatment of human African trypanosomiasis (sleeping sickness). Lancet Neurol. 2013;12(2):186–94.

Neuberger A, Meltzer E, Leshem E, Dickstein Y, Stienlauf S, Schwartz E. The changing epidemiology of human African trypanosomiasis among patients from nonendemic countries—1902–2012. PLoS One. 2014;9:e88647.

Simarro PP, Diarra A, Ruiz Postigo JA, Franco JR, Jannin JG. The human African trypanosomiasis control and surveillance programme of the World Health Organization 2000–2009: the way forward. PLoS Negl Trop Dis. 2011;5(2):e1007.

Simarro PP, Franco JR, Cecchi G, Paone M, Diarra A, Ruiz Postigo JA, Jannin JG. Human African trypanosomiasis in non-endemic countries (2000–2010). J Travel Med. 2012;19:44–53.

World Health Organization. Control and surveillance of human African trypanosomiasis. World Health Organ Tech Rep Ser. 2013;984:1–237.

TRYPANOSOMIASIS, AMERICAN / CHAGAS DISEASE

Susan Montgomery, Sharon Roy, Christine Dubray

INFECTIOUS AGENT: *Trypanosoma cruzi*	
ENDEMICITY	Parts of Mexico, and Central and South America
TRAVELER CATEGORIES AT GREATEST RISK FOR EXPOSURE & INFECTION	Immigrants and refugees from endemic areas Long-term travelers to endemic areas
PREVENTION METHODS	Avoid contact with triatomines (reduviid bugs) Avoid sleeping in thatch, mud, or adobe housing in endemic areas
DIAGNOSTIC SUPPORT	A clinical laboratory certified in high complexity testing; or contact CDC's Parasitic Diseases Branch (www.cdc.gov/parasites; 404-718-4745; parasites@cdc.gov) Parasitological diagnosis: DPDx (www.cdc.gov/DPDx)

5

INFECTIOUS AGENT

Chagas disease is caused by the protozoan parasite *Trypanosoma cruzi*.

TRANSMISSION

Human infection occurs when *T. cruzi* in the feces of an infected triatomine insect (reduviid bug) enters the body. Entry portals include breaks in the skin (e.g., at the site of a reduviid bug bite), through the eyes by touching or rubbing with contaminated fingers, and through the gastrointestinal tract by consuming contaminated food or beverages. *T. cruzi* also can be transmitted through blood transfusions, organ transplantation, and vertically, from mother to infant.

EPIDEMIOLOGY

T. cruzi is endemic to many parts of Mexico and Central and South America; rare locally acquired Chagas disease cases have been reported in the southern United States. No vectorborne transmission has been documented in the Caribbean islands. In the United States, Chagas disease is primarily a disease of immigrants from endemic areas of Latin America. The risk to travelers is extremely low, but travelers could be at risk if they stay in poor-quality housing or consume contaminated food or beverages in endemic areas.

CLINICAL PRESENTATION

Acute illness typically develops ≥1 week and ≤60 days after exposure. A chagoma (indurated local swelling) might develop at the site of parasite entry (e.g., Romaña's sign, edema of the eyelid and ocular tissues). Most infected people never develop symptoms, but remain infected throughout their lives. Approximately 20%–30% of infected people develop chronic manifestations after a prolonged asymptomatic period. Chronic Chagas disease usually affects the heart; clinical signs include conduction system abnormalities, ventricular arrhythmias, and, in late-stage disease, congestive cardiomyopathy. Chronic gastrointestinal problems (e.g., megaesophagus, megacolon) are less common. and can develop with or without cardiac manifestations. Reactivation disease can occur in immunocompromised patients.

DIAGNOSIS

During the acute phase, parasites can be detected in fresh preparations of buffy coat or stained peripheral blood specimens; PCR testing also can help detect acute infection. After the acute phase, diagnosis requires ≥2 serologic tests to detect *T. cruzi*–specific antibodies, most commonly ELISA, immunoblot, and immunofluorescent antibody test.

PCR is not a useful diagnostic test for chronic-phase infections because parasites cannot be detected in the peripheral blood during this phase. Clinicians can obtain diagnostic assistance and confirmatory testing from the Centers for Disease Control and Prevention (CDC)'s Division of Parasitic Diseases and Malaria DPDx laboratory (www.cdc.gov/DPDx; dpdx@cdc.gov), and from the Parasitic Diseases Hotline for Healthcare Providers (404-718-4745; parasites@cdc.gov).

TREATMENT

Antitrypanosomal drug treatment is always recommended for acute, early congenital, and reactivated *T. cruzi* infection, and for chronic *T. cruzi* infection in children <18 years old. In adults with chronic infection, treatment is usually recommended.

The 2 drugs used to treat Chagas disease are benznidazole and nifurtimox. Benznidazole is approved by the US Food and Drug Administration (FDA) for use in children 2–12 years old and is commercially available. Nifurtimox is approved by the FDA for treatment of children from birth to <18 years old who weigh at least 2.5 kg. The drug was approved in August 2020 and became commercially available later that year. Side effects are common with both drugs, and tend to be more frequent and more severe with increasing age. Contact CDC (parasites@cdc.gov; 404-718-4745) for assistance with clinical management (see www.cdc.gov/parasites/chagas/health_professionals/tx.html for more information).

PREVENTION

To avoid Chagas disease, travelers should follow insect bite precautions (see Sec. 4, Ch. 6, Mosquitoes, Ticks & Other Arthropods) and food and water precautions (see Sec. 2, Ch. 8, Food & Water Precautions). Travelers also should avoid sleeping in adobe, mud, or thatch housing in endemic areas, and use insecticides in and around such homes. Insecticide-treated bed nets are helpful. Screening blood and organs for Chagas disease prevents transmission via transfusion or transplantation. Screening of pregnant people coming from endemic areas and early detection and treatment of mother-to-baby (congenital) cases also will help reduce disease burden.

CDC website: www.cdc.gov/parasites/chagas

BIBLIOGRAPHY

Bern C. Antitrypanosomal therapy for chronic Chagas' disease. N Engl J Med. 2011;364(26):2527–34.

Bern C, Messenger LA, Whitman JD, Maguire JH. Chagas disease in the United States: a public health approach. Clin Microbiol Rev. 2019;33(1):e00023-19.

Bern C, Montgomery SP, Herwaldt BL, Rassi A Jr, Marin-Neto JA, Dantas RO, et al. Evaluation and treatment of Chagas disease in the United States: a systematic review. JAMA. 2007;298(18):2171–81.

Carter YL, Juliano JJ, Montgomery SP, Qvarnstrom Y. Acute Chagas disease in a returning traveler. Am J Trop Med Hyg. 2012;87(6):1038–40.

Edwards MS, Stimpert KK, Montgomery SP. Addressing the challenges of Chagas disease: an emerging health concern in the United States. Infect Dis Clin Pract. 2017;25(3):118–25.

Rassi A Jr, Rassi A, Marin-Neto JA. Chagas disease. Lancet. 2010;375(9723):1388–402.

PART 4: FUNGAL

COCCIDIOIDOMYCOSIS / VALLEY FEVER

Mitsuru Toda, Kaitlin Benedict, Tom Chiller

5

INFECTIOUS AGENTS: *Coccidioides immitis* and *C. posadasii*	
ENDEMICITY	The Americas (Central and South America, northern Mexico, and the United States, specifically Arizona and Southern California)
TRAVELER CATEGORIES AT GREATEST RISK FOR EXPOSURE & INFECTION	Adventure tourists Humanitarian aid workers Long-term travelers and expatriates Study abroad students Travelers visiting friends and relatives
PREVENTION METHODS	Limit exposure to outdoor dust in endemic areas Use personal protective equipment (e.g., N95 respirator) when working outdoors in endemic areas Preventive antifungal medication
DIAGNOSTIC SUPPORT	A clinical laboratory certified in moderate complexity testing; or contact CDC's Mycotic Diseases Branch Reference Laboratory Team (404-639-2569)

INFECTIOUS AGENTS

Valley fever (coccidioidomycosis) is caused by the fungi *Coccidioides immitis* and *C. posadasii.*

TRANSMISSION

Transmission occurs through inhalation of fungal conidia from the environment. Transmission from person to person does not occur.

EPIDEMIOLOGY

Coccidioides is endemic to the western United States, particularly Arizona and Southern California, and parts of Mexico and Central and South America. Travelers, including adventure tourists, expatriates, humanitarian aid workers, long-term travelers, and travelers visiting friends and relatives (VFRs) are at increased risk if they participate in activities that expose them to soil disruption and outdoor dust. Participating in activities like community housebuilding projects, gardening, four-wheeling, and horseback riding can put people at risk. Coccidioidomycosis outbreaks have been associated with activities such as archaeological excavation, construction, and military training exercises.

CLINICAL PRESENTATION

The incubation period is 7–21 days. About 40% of infected people develop symptomatic infections, ranging from primary pulmonary illness to severe disseminated disease. The most common symptoms of primary pulmonary coccidioidomycosis are cough and persistent fatigue, with only about half of patients reporting fever. Other symptoms include shortness of breath, headache, joint pain, muscle aches, night sweats, and rash. Symptoms can be indistinguishable from bacterial pneumonia. Coccidioidomycosis infections are often self-limited, typically resolving in a few weeks to months, but also can be severe, requiring hospitalization. An estimated 5%–10% of people develop serious or chronic lung disease (e.g., bronchiectasis, cavitary pneumonia, pulmonary fibrosis). About 1% of illnesses result in meningitis, which can require lifelong antifungal therapy; dissemination to bones, joints, and skin also can occur.

People ≥65 years of age, people with diabetes, people who smoke, and people with high inoculum exposure are at increased risk of developing severe pulmonary complications. Those with depressed cellular immune function (e.g., people with HIV, organ transplant recipients) and people who are pregnant are at increased risk for developing disseminated disease. Epidemiological data suggest that the risk for severe illness is increased among people of African American, Filipino, and Pacific Island descent, but further study is needed to understand the reasons for this association.

DIAGNOSIS

Coccidioidomycosis is a nationally notifiable disease in the United States. The most common methods to diagnose coccidioidomycosis are culture, histopathology, molecular techniques, and serology. Isolation of *Coccidioides* from fungal culture of respiratory specimens or tissue provides a definitive diagnosis. Microscopy of sputum or tissue can identify *Coccidioides* spherules but has low sensitivity. Molecular techniques include DNA probe for confirmation of cultures, as well as PCR for direct detection from clinical specimens, which became commercially available in early 2018. EIA is a sensitive serologic method to detect IgM and IgG antibodies. Immunodiffusion and complement fixation can also detect antibodies and are often used to confirm diagnosis. Lateral flow assays to detect any antibodies in serum became commercially available in 2018.

TREATMENT

Expert opinions differ on the proper management of patients with uncomplicated primary pulmonary disease in the absence of risk factors for severe or disseminated disease. Some experts recommend no therapy, since most illnesses are self-limited, whereas others advise treatment to reduce the intensity or duration of symptoms. Treatment with antifungal agents has not been proven to prevent dissemination. People at high risk for dissemination should receive antifungal therapy, as should people with clinical manifestations of severe acute pulmonary disease, chronic pulmonary disease, or disseminated disease. Depending on the clinical situation, a variety of antifungal agents can be used, including amphotericin B and fluconazole (or itraconazole).

PREVENTION

To reduce risk for coccidioidomycosis, travelers should limit exposure to outdoor dust in endemic areas, or wear an N95 respirator if they cannot avoid dusty areas while in this environment. During dust storms, travelers should stay inside and close windows. Travelers to known endemic areas also should avoid activities that require close contact with dirt or dust, including digging, gardening, and yard work. Air filtration measures can be used indoors. Preventive antifungal medication (fluconazole or itraconazole) can be taken in certain circumstances if recommended by a health care provider.

CDC websites: www.cdc.gov/fungal/diseases/coccidioidomycosis; www.cdc.gov/niosh/topics/valleyfever/; www.cdc.gov/fungal/diseases/coccidioidomycosis/factsheets/be-aware-of-valley-fever.html

BIBLIOGRAPHY

Diaz, JH. Travel-related risk factors for coccidioidomycosis. J Travel Med. 2018;25(1):tay027.

Galgiani JN, Ampel NM, Blair JE, Catanzaro A, Geertsma F, Hoover SE, et al. 2016 Infectious Diseases Society of America (IDSA) clinical practice guideline for the treatment of coccidioidomycosis. Clin Infect Dis. 2016;63(6):e112–46.

Freedman M, Jackson BR, McCotter O, Benedict K. Coccidioidomycosis outbreaks, United States and worldwide, 1940–2015. Emerg Infect Dis. 2018;24(3):417–23.

Rosenstein NE, Emery KW, Werner SB, Kao A, Johnson R, Rogers D, et al. Risk factors for severe pulmonary and disseminated coccidioidomycosis: Kern County, California, 1995–1996. Clin Infect Dis. 2001;32(5):708–15.

Toda M, Gonzalez FJ, Fonseca-Ford M, Franklin F, Huntington-Frazier M, Gutelius B, et al. Notes from the field: multistate coccidioidomycosis outbreak in U.S. residents returning from community service trips to Baja California, Mexico—July–August 2018. MMWR Morb Mortal Wkly Rep 2019;68(14):332–3.

HISTOPLASMOSIS

Jeremy Gold, Diego Caceres, Brendan Jackson, Kaitlin Benedict

5

INFECTIOUS AGENT: *Histoplasma capsulatum*	
ENDEMICITY	Worldwide
TRAVELER CATEGORIES AT GREATEST RISK FOR EXPOSURE & INFECTION	Adventure tourists Humanitarian aid workers Immigrants and refugees Long-term travelers and expatriates Study-abroad students Travelers visiting friends and relatives
PREVENTION METHODS	Avoid exposure to soil contaminated with bird droppings or bat guano Chemoprophylaxis might be appropriate in rare circumstances for immunocompromised people
DIAGNOSTIC SUPPORT	A clinical laboratory certified in moderate complexity testing; or contact CDC's Mycotic Diseases Branch Reference Laboratory Team (404-639-2569)

INFECTIOUS AGENT

Histoplasmosis is caused by *Histoplasma capsulatum*, a thermal-dimorphic fungus that grows as a mold in the environment and as a yeast in animal and human hosts.

TRANSMISSION

Histoplasmosis is transmitted through inhalation of spores (conidia) from the environment, often soil contaminated with bat guano or bird droppings, but is not transmitted from person to person.

EPIDEMIOLOGY

Knowledge of global histoplasmosis epidemiology is incomplete, and cases in travelers are likely underreported to public health authorities. Travelers, including adventure tourists, humanitarian aid workers, long-term travelers and expatriates, study-abroad students, and people visiting friends and relatives could be at increased risk for histoplasmosis if they engage in activities involving soil disruption (e.g., caving, construction, demolition, excavation, farming, gardening), particularly in areas where bats and birds roost. Histoplasmosis also occurs in immigrants from endemic regions who become immunocompromised.

CLINICAL PRESENTATION

Incubation period is typically 3–17 days for acute disease. About 90% of infections are asymptomatic or result in a mild influenza-like illness. Acute pulmonary histoplasmosis often involves body aches, chest pain, chills, cough, fatigue, fever, and headache. Most people spontaneously recover several weeks after symptom onset, but fatigue might persist longer. High-dose exposure can lead to severe disease. Dissemination, especially to the central nervous system and gastrointestinal tract, can occur in immunocompromised people. Histoplasmosis might be misdiagnosed as other illnesses, particularly as tuberculosis in people who travel from regions where both pathogens are endemic.

DIAGNOSIS

Several methods to diagnose histoplasmosis are available. Although culture and histopathologic identification remain the gold standards, a combination of antigen and antibody testing could be more useful in diagnosing travel-associated histoplasmosis. Rapid *Histoplasma* antigen testing by enzyme immunoassays, reagents for immunodiffusion, and complement fixation are commercially available as in vitro diagnostic kits. In immunocompetent patients, antigen testing is most useful when performed within 2 weeks of a high-dose exposure. Antibody testing of specimens collected during the acute and convalescent phases of illness can improve diagnostic yield; obtaining serial antigen and antibody titers can aid in monitoring response to treatment.

The Centers for Disease Control and Prevention (CDC)'s Mycotic Diseases Branch reference laboratory supports histoplasmosis diagnosis and outbreak investigations. Laboratory support includes immunodiagnostics by antibody and antigen testing, and molecular testing. To obtain diagnostic support from CDC, contact the Mycotic Diseases Branch reference laboratory team (404-639-2569).

TREATMENT

Treatment is not usually indicated for immunocompetent people with acute, localized pulmonary infection. People with more extensive disease or persistent symptoms lasting >1 month generally can be treated with an azole drug (e.g., itraconazole) for mild to moderate illness, or amphotericin B for severe infection. Patients with acute respiratory distress might benefit from steroids as well as antifungal treatment.

PREVENTION

People at increased risk for severe disease should avoid high-risk areas (e.g., bat-inhabited caves, hollow trees). No vaccine for histoplasmosis is available. Chemoprophylaxis with itraconazole is recommended for certain people living with HIV, and might be appropriate in specific circumstances for other immunosuppressed people.

CDC website: www.cdc.gov/fungal/diseases/histoplasmosis

BIBLIOGRAPHY

Adenis AA, Valdes A, Cropet C, McCotter OZ, Derado G, Couppie P, et al. (2018). Burden of HIV-associated histoplasmosis compared with tuberculosis in Latin America: a modelling study. Lancet Infect Dis. 2018;18(10):1150–9.

Armstrong PA, Beard JD, Bonilla L, Arboleda N, Lindsley MD, Chae S-R, et al. Outbreak of severe histoplasmosis among tunnel workers—Dominican Republic, 2015. Clin Infect Dis. 2018;66(10):1550–7.

Azar MM, Hage CA. Laboratory diagnostics for histoplasmosis. J Clin Microbiol. 2017;55(6):1612–20.

Bahr NC, Antinori S, Wheat LJ, Sarosi GA. Histoplasmosis infections worldwide: thinking outside of the Ohio River valley. Curr Trop Med Rep. 2015;2(2):70–80.

Centers for Disease Control and Prevention. Outbreak of histoplasmosis among travelers returning from El Salvador—Pennsylvania and Virginia, 2008. MMWR Morb Mortal Wkly Rep. 2018;57(50):1349–53.

Cottle LE, Gkrania-Klotsas E, Williams HJ, Brindle HE, Carmichael AJ, et al. A multinational outbreak of histoplasmosis following a biology field trip in the Ugandan rainforest. J Travel Med. 2013;20(2):83–7.

Kauffman CA. Histoplasmosis: a clinical and laboratory update. Clin Microbiol Rev. 2007;20(1):115–32.

Staffolani S, Buonfrate D, Angheben A, Gobbi F, Giorli G, Guerriero M, et al. Acute histoplasmosis in immunocompetent travelers: a systematic review of literature. BMC Infect Dis. 2018;18(1):673.

Wheat LJ, Freifeld AG, Kleiman MB, Baddley JW, McKinsey DS, Loyd JE, et al. Clinical practice guidelines for the management of patients with histoplasmosis: 2007 update by the Infectious Diseases Society of America. Clin Infect Dis. 2007;45(7):807–25.

Health Care Abroad

TRAVEL INSURANCE, TRAVEL HEALTH INSURANCE & MEDICAL EVACUATION INSURANCE

Rhett Stoney

Severe illness or injury abroad could cause a financial burden to travelers. Regardless of whether they have a domestic health insurance plan, travelers can substantially reduce their out-of-pocket costs for medical care received abroad by purchasing specialized insurance policies in advance of their trip. Three types of policies—travel insurance, travel health insurance, and medical evacuation insurance—each provide different types of coverage in the event of an illness or injury. Such policies might be particularly beneficial to travelers with preexisting medical conditions. Besides protection against costs, the insurance might also help travelers obtain medical care abroad.

Basic accident or travel health insurance might be necessary for travelers with certain itineraries. For example, although cruise lines employ health care staff, the cost for medical treatment delivered onboard a ship might not be included in the price of a passenger's ticket; thus, travelers on cruise ships might want to consider investing in specialized insurance policies.

DOMESTIC HEALTH INSURANCE & OVERSEAS TRAVEL

Some US health insurance carriers cover medical emergencies that occur when policyholders travel internationally. Encourage travelers to contact their insurer before traveling to learn what medical services, if any, their policies cover. Box 6-01 includes suggested questions travelers should ask their insurance company.

CDC Yellow Book 2024. Jeffrey Nemhauser, Oxford University Press.
DOI: 10.1093/oso/9780197570944.003.0006

BOX 6-01 Supplemental travel health insurance: suggested questions to ask before purchasing a policy

COVERAGE REQUIREMENTS

Do I need preauthorization before receiving treatment, hospital admission, or other medical services?

Do I need a second opinion before I can receive emergency treatment?

What are company policies regarding coverage of care received "out of network"?

Does the company provide policyholders access to a 24/7/365 physician-backed support center?

POTENTIAL EXCLUSIONS

Does this policy include or exclude coverage for treatment of injuries sustained while participating in high-risk activities (e.g., skydiving, scuba diving, mountain climbing)?

Does this policy include or exclude coverage for mental health (psychiatric) emergencies?

PREEXISTING MEDICAL CONDITIONS

Does this policy cover exacerbations of preexisting medical conditions?

Does this policy cover complications of pregnancy or neonatal intensive care?

PAYING FOR HEALTH SERVICES RECEIVED ABROAD

During the pretravel consultation, discuss insurance options and suggest that all travelers consider purchasing supplemental medical insurance coverage (see Box 6-02 for a discussion checklist), particularly if they are going to remote destinations or places lacking high-quality medical facilities. Strongly encourage supplemental medical insurance coverage for travelers planning extended international travel, those with underlying health conditions, and those participating in high-risk activities (e.g., scuba diving, mountain climbing) abroad. In addition to covering costs of treatment or medical evacuation, travel health insurers can assist the international traveler by organizing and coordinating care and by keeping relatives informed in the event of a medical emergency, which is especially important when the traveler is severely ill or injured and requires medical evacuation.

Nationalized health care services at a given destination do not necessarily cover health care costs of nonresidents. Even with a supplemental travel health insurance policy in force, receiving medical care abroad usually requires a cash or credit card payment at the point of service, which can result in expenditures of thousands of dollars. US citizens paying for health care abroad should obtain copies of all charges and receipts and, if necessary, contact a US consular officer, who can assist the traveler with transferring funds from the United States.

The US Department of State might be able to offer limited emergency medical assistance loans to US citizens who experience a medical emergency abroad but have no means to pay at point of service and cannot arrange for a transfer of funds from the United States. Travelers must repay these loans, but the funds might be available for temporarily destitute US citizens and their qualified dependents. Once a loan is issued, the Department of State will limit the traveler's US passport and, in most cases, will not issue a new passport until the loan is paid in full. US citizens should contact the nearest US embassy or consulate, or the US Department of State, Office of Overseas Citizens Services, at 888-407-4747 (or from abroad, +1-202-501-4444), for information about assistance options and eligibility requirements.

TRAVEL INSURANCE

Travel insurance protects the traveler's financial investment in a trip, including lost baggage and trip cancellation. Travelers who become ill before departing are more likely to avoid or postpone travel if they know their financial investment in the trip is protected. Depending on the policy, travel insurance might not cover medical expenses abroad, so travelers need to carefully research the coverage offered to determine their need for additional travel health and medical evacuation insurance.

BOX 6-02 Supplemental travel health insurance: discussion checklist

TRAVEL MEDICINE PROFESSIONAL RESPONSIBILITIES

- ☐ Determine travelers' health profile, including underlying medical conditions.
- ☐ Identify potential medical needs abroad, including health risks based on itinerary and destination, duration of travel, method of transportation (air-, land-, or water-based), lodgings or accommodations, and planned activities.
- ☐ Instruct travelers to review domestic health policies to identify gaps in coverage for identified potential medical needs.
- ☐ Discuss the differences between the 3 types of supplemental insurance (travel, travel health, and medical evacuation), and explain how to choose supplemental policies that cover potential medical needs abroad.
- ☐ Remind travelers of the steps to take should they require medical care abroad:
    - Travelers should be prepared to pay out of pocket at the time services are rendered, in some instances even before care is received, and then provide insurers with copies of bills and invoices to initiate reimbursement afterward.
    - Travelers should plan for potential emergencies in advance by identifying health care providers at the destination who see international travelers.

TRAVELER RESPONSIBILITIES

Before travel

- ☐ Review domestic health insurance policies to determine what medical services are or are not covered overseas.
- ☐ Purchase supplemental travel health insurance coverage based on potential medical needs and health risks.
- ☐ Identify medical service providers at destination (for a directory of English-speaking health care providers, see International Association for Medical Assistance to Travelers [www.iamat.org]).
- ☐ Check with the insurance company to confirm they reimburse for out-of-pocket payments made to healthcare providers abroad. In most cases, health care providers abroad do not accept payment from insurance carriers, and travelers must pay up front (with cash or credit card) for all services received.

During travel

- ☐ Carry insurance policy identity cards (including supplemental travel health insurance) and insurance claim forms while traveling.
- ☐ Have contact information of medical providers at destination(s).
- ☐ Keep copies of all charges and receipts for medical care received.

After travel

- ☐ Promptly seek medical attention upon return to the United States and at the first sign of any unexpected complications from care received internationally.
- ☐ Bring copies of all summary records, charges, and receipts for medical care received abroad.
- ☐ Give the US health care provider the following details: dates of travel, dates medical care received, contact information for the facility and all international health care providers seen.

SUPPLEMENTAL TRAVEL HEALTH & MEDICAL EVACUATION INSURANCE

Travel health insurance and medical evacuation insurance are 2 types of short-term supplemental policies that cover health care costs incurred while abroad. Each is relatively inexpensive. Many commercial companies offer travel health insurance; travelers can purchase such policies separately or together with medical evacuation insurance. Some recommended features to consider when purchasing supplemental travel health and medical evacuation insurance include whether the insurer arranges with hospitals to guarantee direct payment; provides assistance via a 24-hour physician-backed support center, which is critical for medical evacuation insurance; offers emergency medical transport to facilities in the home country (repatriation) or to facilities equivalent to those in the home country; and covers high-risk activities (e.g., scuba diving).

Although travel health insurance covers some international health care costs, the quality of care might be inadequate and medical evacuation (sometimes referred to as "medevac") from a resource-poor area to a hospital delivering definitive care might be necessary. The total cost of medevac varies by location, ranging from $25,000 for transport within North America to ≥$250,000 for more distant and remote locations. Costs increase when the patient being evacuated is critically ill or needs complex infection control measures. In such cases, medevac insurance covers the cost of transportation, including transportation to another country if necessary.

Some medical evacuation companies have more extensive experience working in some parts of the world than others; travelers should ask about a company's resources in each region of travel, especially if planning trips to hard-to-reach locations in a region. Even if travelers select their insurance provider carefully, unexpected delays in care can still arise, especially in remote destinations. Thus, if the health risks are too high, a traveler might want to postpone or cancel their international trip.

FINDING AN INSURANCE PROVIDER

Several organizations provide information about purchasing travel health and medical evacuation insurance, including the US Department of State (https://travel.state.gov/content/travel/en/international-travel/before-you-go/your-health-abroad/insurance-providers-overseas.html); International Association for Medical Assistance to Travelers (www.iamat.org); US Travel Insurance Association (www.ustia.org); and the American Association of Retired Persons (www.aarp.org), among others. The Centers for Disease Control and Prevention does not endorse any provider or medical insurance company.

TRAVELERS WITH UNDERLYING MEDICAL CONDITIONS

Travelers with underlying medical conditions should discuss any concerns with the insurer before departure. In a study of international travelers with travel health insurance claims, insurance companies fully paid only 2/3 of claims, and the main reasons for coverage refusal were preexisting illness and poor documentation of expenses incurred.

Beyond purchasing supplemental travel health insurance coverage, encourage travelers with medical conditions to take additional steps before departure. To facilitate ease of access to health records when overseas, travelers should store copies of their health records with a medical assistance company. Instruct travelers to obtain letters from their health care providers listing all medical conditions and current medications, including generic drug names, written in the local language if possible. Travelers should pack medications in the original packaging in carry-on luggage during transport. To facilitate ease of entry through customs, travelers should check with the destination country's embassy before departure to ensure that none of the medications they are bringing are considered illegal in that region. Anyone with a known heart condition should carry a copy (paper or electronic) of their most recent electrocardiogram.

MEDICARE BENEFICIARIES

Medicare beneficiaries are no different from other travelers; they need to examine their coverage carefully and supplement it with additional travel health insurance, as required. Except in limited circumstances, the Social Security Medicare program does not provide coverage for medical costs incurred outside the United States, nor does it cover medical evacuation. Medicare beneficiaries can purchase supplemental Medigap plans to fill gaps, including for travel coverage. Medigap plans C, D, F, G, M, and N cover some emergency care received outside the United States. After meeting the yearly $250 deductible, this benefit pays 80% of the cost of emergency care during the first 60 days of international travel. The coverage has a $50,000 lifetime maximum. International travelers can find more information on Medicare and Medigap options at www.medicare.gov/supplements-other-insurance/medigap-travel.

BIBLIOGRAPHY

American Association of Retired Persons. Overview of Medicare supplemental insurance 2010. Available from: www.aarp.org/health/medicare-insurance/info-10-2008/overview_medicare_supplemental_insurance.html.

Centers for Medicare and Medicaid Services. Medigap & travel. Available from: www.medicare.gov/supplements-other-insurance/medigap-travel.

Flaherty G, De Freitas S. A heart for travel: travel health considerations for patients with heart disease and cardiac devices. Ir Med J. 2016;109(10):486.

Leggat PA, Carne J, Kedjarune U. Travel insurance and health. J Travel Med. 1999;6(4):243–8.

Leggat PA, Leggat FW. Travel insurance claims made by travelers from Australia. J Travel Med. 2002;9(2):59–65.

Teichman PG, Donchin Y, Kot RJ. International aeromedical evacuation. N Engl J Med. 2007;356(3):262–70.

US Department of State. Emergency financial assistance for U.S. citizens abroad. Available from: https://travel.state.gov/content/travel/en/international-travel/emergencies/emergency-financial-assistance.html.

US Department of State. Insurance providers for overseas coverage. Available from: https://travel.state.gov/content/travel/en/international-travel/before-you-go/your-health-abroad/insurance-providers-overseas.html.

OBTAINING HEALTH CARE ABROAD

Stefan Hagmann

While abroad, travelers might seek medical care ranging from treatment for self-limited minor ailments, to care for chronic conditions, to sophisticated medical management of major illnesses or injuries. Insurance plans might not cover emergency health care, and travelers should check with their insurance carriers before departure to confirm the limits of their coverage and to identify any additional coverage requirements. For example, travel health insurance alone does not usually pay for the cost of an emergency medical evacuation or itinerary alterations needed to receive medical care during travel. Travelers can buy specific policies to cover these expenses, but should understand that such policies often do not cover expenses related to preexisting conditions.

Supplemental medical insurance plans purchased prior to traveling often furnish access to preselected local providers in many countries through a 24-hour emergency hotline; some even provide medical assistance via a nurse- or physician-backed support center (see Sec. 6, Ch. 1, Travel Insurance, Travel Health Insurance & Medical Evacuation Insurance, for more details). Travelers should be prepared to pay out of pocket when services are rendered and, in some instances, even before care is received, then provide insurers with copies of bills and invoices to initiate reimbursement afterward.

Travelers also should be aware (in advance) of destinations on their itinerary where coronavirus disease 2019 (COVID-19) vaccine coverage of the local population is low (https://ourworldindata.org/covid-vaccinations), or where case rates and hospitalizations are high (https://ourworldindata.org/covid-hospitalizations). Availability of health care resources in such places could be strained, and treatment options (for severe COVID-19 and other conditions) could be limited. Destination-specific COVID-19 travel recommendations are available at https://travel.state.gov/content/travel/en/traveladvisories/COVID-19-Country-Specific-Information.html.

6

LOCATING HEALTH CARE FACILITIES & PROVIDERS ABROAD

The level and availability of medical care around the world varies by country and even within countries. During pretravel preparation, travelers should consider how they will access health care during their trip should a medical problem or emergency arise (Box 6-03). Encourage travelers likely to need health care to research thoroughly and identify potential health care providers and facilities at their destination. For example, people who require regular dialysis treatments need to arrange appointments in advance at a site with appropriate equipment. Pregnant travelers should know the names and locations of reliable obstetric medical centers. Travelers should be aware that more choices are generally available in urban areas than in rural or remote locations.

Travelers, particularly those with preexisting or complicated medical issues, should know and ideally have documented in a doctor's letter the names

BOX 6-03 Obtaining health care abroad: a checklist for travelers

- ☐ Identify quality health care providers and facilities at destination, prior to traveling.
- ☐ Carry a provider letter that lists all active medical problems, current medications, and allergies. If possible, download travel health mobile applications to input medical records, medications, and other health information (e.g., electrocardiogram) so these are accessible if needed.
- ☐ Pack an adequate supply of medication in original, labeled containers, and know how to get additional safe and effective medications while abroad.
- ☐ Request documentation of any medical care received abroad, including medications, and share with health care providers delivering subsequent care while traveling and at home.
- ☐ If a blood transfusion is required while traveling, make every effort to ensure that the blood has been screened for transmissible diseases, including HIV.

6

of their conditions, any allergies, their blood type, and current medications, including generic names. If possible, this list should be in the local language of the travel destination. Travelers also should carry copies of prescriptions, including for glasses and contact lenses, and wear medical identification jewelry (e.g., a MedicAlert bracelet), as appropriate. Travelers should check with the foreign embassy of the countries they plan to visit to ensure current medications are permitted. Many mobile phone applications enable travelers to download their medical records, medications, electrocardiogram, and other information so that they can access these when needed. Remind travelers to request documentation of any medical care received during travel, including a list of medications received. Travelers can then share this information with any health care providers seen subsequently in the event they require ongoing care.

Box 6-04 includes a list of suggested resources international travelers can use to help identify health care providers and facilities around the world. The Centers for Disease Control and Prevention does not endorse any provider or medical insurance company, and accreditation does not necessarily ensure a good outcome.

BOX 6-04 Finding a health care provider overseas

The nearest US embassy or consulate (www.usembassy.gov) can help travelers locate medical services and notify friends, family, or employer of an emergency. Emergency consular services are available 24 hours a day, 7 days a week, overseas and in Washington, DC (888-407-4747 or 202-501-4444).

The US Department of State maintains a list of travel medical and evacuation insurance providers on their website, https://travel.state.gov/content/travel/en/international-travel/before-you-go/your-health-abroad/insurance-providers-overseas.html.

The International Society of Travel Medicine (www.istm.org) maintains a directory of health care professionals with expertise in travel medicine in more than 80 countries.

The International Association for Medical Assistance to Travelers (www.iamat.org/doctors_clinics.cfm) maintains a list of physicians, hospitals, and clinics that have agreed to provide care to members. Membership is free, although donations are suggested.

Travel agencies, hotels, and credit card companies (especially those with special benefits) also might provide information.

The following travel medicine websites, organized by country, provide access to clinicians:

AUSTRALIA: Travel Medicine Alliance (www.travelmedicine.com.au)

CANADA: Health Canada (www.phac-aspc.gc.ca and https://travel.gc.ca)

CHINA: International Travel Healthcare Association (www.itha.org.cn/)

GREAT BRITAIN: National Travel Health Network & Centre (www.nathnac.org) and British Global & Travel Health Association (www.bgtha.org)

SOUTH AFRICA: South African Society of Travel Medicine (www.sastm.org.za)

AVOIDING TRAVEL WHEN ILL

Advise travelers to self-evaluate before leaving home and to avoid or postpone travel if acutely ill with fever or other signs or symptoms of a communicable disease. Traveling while ill increases the chances that a person will have to interact with an unfamiliar and potentially inadequately equipped health care system and that they could transmit their illness to travel partners and/or other passengers. Moreover, travelers should be aware that airlines can request that they complete a brief health questionnaire and that local health authorities might conduct body temperature checks anywhere in the airport, including the waiting area and during boarding; passengers who fail such screenings might be prohibited from boarding their flight. Because people often are reluctant to postpone or cancel travel, trip cancellation insurance can protect some (or all) of their investment and increase compliance with the recommendation not to travel when ill.

DRUGS & OTHER PHARMACEUTICALS

The quality of drugs and medical products acquired abroad might not meet the same regulated standards established by the US Food and Drug Administration. Worse yet, drugs or medical products could be counterfeit and contain no active ingredients or could contain harmful ingredients (for more information, see the following chapter in this section, . . . *perspectives*: Avoiding Poorly Regulated Medicines & Medical Products During Travel). Travelers whose original supply of medication is used up, lost, stolen, or damaged should take steps to ensure that the replacement medicines they buy are safe and effective.

To minimize risks associated with substandard drugs and pharmaceuticals, travelers should bring enough medicine for the entire time they are away, and include an additional supply in case of trip delays. Travelers should carry all medications in the original labeled containers in their carry-on luggage, not in checked baggage; this also applies to travelers who might require an epinephrine autoinjector (Epi-Pen) to treat known severe, potentially life-threatening allergies. For Epi-Pens, travelers should carry a letter from the prescribing physician explaining their allergies and a copy of the written prescription.

Travelers who need injections while abroad should insist that health care providers use new needles and syringes. Travelers who know they require injections can bring their own supplies, but also should bring a letter from their provider attesting to the need for this equipment.

BLOOD SAFETY

A medical emergency abroad (e.g., a motor vehicle accident, other trauma) could require a lifesaving transfusion of whole blood or blood components (e.g., platelets, fresh frozen plasma). Not all countries accurately, reliably, and systematically screen blood donations for infectious agents, putting recipients at risk for transfusion-related diseases. Consequently, all travelers should consider receiving hepatitis B virus immunization before travel (see Sec. 2, Ch. 3, Vaccination & Immunoprophylaxis—General Principles, and Sec. 5, Part 2, Ch. 8, Hepatitis B). Hepatitis B vaccination is especially important for travelers who frequently visit or have long-term stays in low- and middle-income countries, travelers who have underlying medical conditions that increase their risk of requiring blood products while traveling, and travelers whose activities (e.g., adventure travel) put them at increased risk for serious injury.

Ensuring the safety of the blood supply can be difficult, but travelers can take a few measures to increase their chances of a safe blood transfusion. For instance, the traveler or a companion, if the traveler is incapacitated, can ask about blood supply screening practices for transfusion-transmissible infections, including HIV. Because obtaining information on the safety of the blood supply can be difficult at the point of service, travelers with known medical conditions that might require transfusions can identify medical services at their destination before travel to increase their chances of obtaining higher-quality care. Travelers also can register with agencies (e.g., the Blood Care Foundation [www.bloodcare.org.uk/blood-transfusionsabroad.html]) that attempt to deliver reliable blood products rapidly to members at international locations.

BIBLIOGRAPHY

Kolars JC. Rules of the road: a consumer's guide for travelers seeking health care in foreign lands. J Travel Med. 2002;9(4):198–201.

US Department of State, Bureau of Consular Affairs. Your health abroad. Available from: www.travel.state.gov/content/travel/en/international-travel/before-you-go/your-health-abroad.

World Health Organization. Blood safety and availability. Available from: www.who.int/news-room/fact-sheets/detail/blood-safety-and-availability.

World Health Organization. Substandard and falsified medical products. Available from: www.who.int/news-room/fact-sheets/detail/substandard-and-falsified-medical-products.

World Health Organization. Technical considerations for implementing a risk-based approach to international travel in the context of COVID-19: Interim guidance, 2 July 2021. Available from: www.who.int/publications/i/item/WHO-2019-nCoV-Risk-based-international-travel-2021.1.

6

AVOIDING POORLY REGULATED MEDICINES & MEDICAL PRODUCTS DURING TRAVEL

Michael Green

In many low- and middle-income countries, national drug regulatory authorities lack the capacity to monitor and enforce drug quality standards effectively and to keep poor-quality products, including drugs, vaccines, and medical devices, off the market. Consequently, substandard and fake medicines are a public health concern in these locations. Many poor-quality products also are trafficked by pharmacy websites that misrepresent themselves as reputable or located in countries with mature regulatory systems. Even high-income countries are not immune to the problem, because counterfeiters become adept at thwarting the efforts of more advanced regulatory systems.

Poor regulatory oversight breeds poor-quality medicines, whether they are counterfeit, falsified, substandard, or degraded (Box 6-05). A report from the World Health Organization identified that 10% of medical products circulating in low- and middle-income countries are either substandard or falsified. Another study found that 9%–41% of tested drugs failed quality specifications. In specific regions in Africa, Latin America, and Asia, the chance of purchasing a counterfeit drug can be >30%.

Because counterfeit drugs are not made by legitimate manufacturers and are produced under unlawful circumstances, improper or toxic ingredients in these products can cause serious harm. For example, the active pharmaceutical ingredient could be absent, present in small quantities, or replaced with a less effective compound. In addition, the wrong inactive ingredients (excipients) can contribute to poor drug dissolution, bioavailability, and toxicity. As a result, a patient might not respond to treatment or could have adverse reactions to unknown substituted or toxic ingredients.

Vaccines and other products (e.g., condoms, disinfectants, insecticide-treated mosquito nets, masks, water purification devices) also could have quality problems or be counterfeit. Vaccine integrity typically depends on a temperature-controlled supply chain, and, unlike medicines with stated amounts of active ingredients, the potency of vaccines is difficult to monitor and therefore easy to counterfeit. As expected, criminal networks have exploited the coronavirus disease 2019 (COVID-19) pandemic by producing fake vaccines. An international alert issued by INTERPOL resulted in confiscation of thousands of fake

BOX 6-05 Definitions of poorly regulated medical products

IMITATIONS

Counterfeit: A counterfeit product bears the unauthorized representation of a registered trademark on a product identical or similar to one for which the trademark is registered.

Falsified: A falsified product falsely represents the product's identity, source, or both.

AUTHENTICS

Substandard: A substandard product fails to meet national specifications cited in an accepted pharmacopeia or in the manufacturer's approved dossier.

Degraded: A degraded product has undergone chemical or physical changes due to incorrect storage conditions.

(continued)

AVOIDING POORLY REGULATED MEDICINES & MEDICAL PRODUCTS DURING TRAVEL (CONTINUED)

vaccines in China and in South Africa. INTERPOL's Secretary General described the number of seized vaccines as being "the tip of the iceberg."

AVOIDING COUNTERFEIT DRUGS WHEN TRAVELING

The best way to avoid counterfeit drugs is to reduce the need to purchase medications abroad. Instruct travelers to purchase anticipated amounts of medications for chronic conditions (e.g., arthritis, diabetes, hypertension), medications for travelers' diarrhea, and prophylactic medications for infectious diseases (e.g., malaria) before traveling. Advise travelers to avoid buying drugs online, because the source of the medication often cannot be verified. Travelers should also be aware that other health-related items obtained abroad (e.g., medical devices, insect repellents, mosquito nets) also could be counterfeit, falsified, or substandard.

In preparation for international travel, travelers should obtain all medicines and other health-related items needed for the trip. Prescriptions written in the United States usually cannot be filled overseas, and although many US prescription medications are available for over-the-counter purchase in foreign countries, some might not be available at all. Because checked baggage can get lost, travelers should pack medications and first aid items in a carry-on bag, and bring extra medicine in case of travel delays. Travelers should carry medicines in their original containers; for prescription drugs, the patient's name and dose regimen should appear on the container. Travelers also should bring the "patient prescription information" sheet, which provides information on common generic and brand names, use, side effects, precautions, and drug interactions. Travelers should check with the embassies of their destination countries for prohibited drugs; many countries have restrictions on medicines, including over-the-counter medications, entering their borders.

If travelers run out of and require additional medications, they should take steps to ensure the medicines they buy are safe (see Box 6-06

BOX 6-06 Purchasing medicines overseas: a good practices checklist for international travelers

- ☐ Obtain medicines from a legitimate pharmacy; the local US embassy or consulate might be able to help locate legitimate local pharmacies. Do not buy from open markets, street vendors, or suspicious-looking pharmacies; request a receipt when making the purchase.
- ☐ Do not buy medicines priced substantially lower than the typical price. Although generic medications are usually less expensive, many counterfeit brand names are sold at prices substantially lower than normal.
- ☐ Make sure the medicines are in their original packages or containers. If you receive medicines as loose tablets or capsules supplied in a plastic bag or envelope, ask the pharmacist to show you the container from which the medicine was dispensed. Record the brand, batch number, and expiration date. Sometimes a wary consumer will prompt the seller into supplying quality medicine rather than a counterfeit or substandard medicine.
- ☐ Be familiar with your medications. The size, shape, color, and taste of counterfeit medicines might be different from the authentic product. Discoloration, splits, cracks, spots, and stickiness of tablets or capsules are indications of possible counterfeit. These defects also could indicate improper storage. Keep examples of authentic medications to compare if you purchase the same brand.
- ☐ Be familiar with the packaging. Different color inks, poor-quality printing or packaging materials, and misspelled words are clues to counterfeit drugs. Keep an example of packaging for comparison and observe the expiration date.

Table 6-01 Online resources for travelers purchasing medicines & medical products overseas

ORGANIZATION / SOURCE	RESOURCE	AVAILABLE FROM
Drugs.com	Pill Identifier	www.drugs.com/pill_identification.html
International Society of Travel Medicine	Database on International Regulations on Importation of Medicines for Personal Use	www.istm.org/files/Documents/Groups/PPG/2nd%20Edition%20Carrying%20Medicines%20Database.pdf
Transportation Security Administration	Disabilities and Medical Conditions	www.tsa.gov/travel/special-procedures
US Centers for Disease Control and Prevention	Counterfeit Medicines	https://wwwnc.cdc.gov/travel/page/counterfeit-medicine
US Customs and Border Protection	Prohibited and Restricted Items (see Medication)	www.cbp.gov/travel/us-citizens/know-before-you-go/prohibited-and-restricted-items
US Food and Drug Administration	Drug Safety and Availability	www.fda.gov/drugs/drug-safety-and-availability
US Pharmacopeia	Medicines Quality Database (MQDB)	www.usp.org/global-public-health/medicines-quality-database
World Health Organization	Substandard and falsified medical products	www.who.int/news-room/fact-sheets/detail/substandard-and-falsified-medical-products

for a traveler checklist of good practices, and Table 6-01 for a list of online resources). One way to ensure medication safety is by comparing distinguishing features of the packaging, especially when authentic packaging is unavailable or if the traveler is not familiar with the brand. For example, the batch and lot numbers, manufacturing date, and expiration date printed on the outside of the box should match what is on the insert or blister pack.

BIBLIOGRAPHY

INTERPOL. Fake COVID vaccine distribution network dismantled after INTERPOL alert, 3 March 2021. Available from: www.interpol.int/News-and-Events/News/2021/Fake-COVID-vaccine-distribution-network-dismantled-after-INTERPOL-alert.

Institute of Medicine. Countering the problem of falsified and substandard drugs. Washington, DC: The National Academics Press; 2013.

Nayyar GML, Bremen JG, Herrington JE. The global pandemic of falsified medicines: laboratory and field innovations and policy perspectives. Am J Trop Med Hyg. 2015;92(6 suppl):2–7.

World Health Organization. Full list of WHO Medical Products Alerts. Available from: www.who.int/teams/regulation-prequalification/incidents-and-SF/full-list-of-who-medical-product-alerts.

World Health Organization. Medicines: counterfeit medicines [fact sheet no. 275]. Geneva: World Health Organization; 2018. Available from: www.who.int/news-room/fact-sheets/detail/substandard-and-falsified-medical-products.

. . . *perspectives* chapters supplement the clinical guidance in this book with additional content, context, and expert opinion. The views expressed do not necessarily represent the official position of the Centers for Disease Control and Prevention (CDC).

6

MEDICAL TOURISM

Matthew Crist, Grace Appiah, Laura Leidel, Rhett Stoney

Medical tourism is the term commonly used to describe international travel for the purpose of receiving medical care. Medical tourists pursue medical care abroad for a variety of reasons, including decreased cost, recommendations from friends or family, the opportunity to combine medical care with a vacation destination, a preference to receive care from a culturally similar provider, or a desire to receive a procedure or therapy not available in their country of residence.

Medical tourism is a worldwide, multibillion-dollar market that continues to grow with the rising globalization of health care. Surveillance data indicate that millions of US residents travel internationally for medical care each year. Medical tourism destinations for US residents include Argentina, Brazil, Canada, Colombia, Costa Rica, Cuba, the Dominican Republic, Ecuador, Germany, India, Malaysia, Mexico, Nicaragua, Peru, Singapore, and Thailand. Categories of procedures that US medical tourists pursue include cancer treatment, dental care, fertility treatments, organ and tissue transplantation, and various forms of surgery, including bariatric, cosmetic, and non-cosmetic (e.g., orthopedic).

Most medical tourists pay for their care at time of service and often rely on private companies or medical concierge services to identify foreign health care facilities. Some US health insurance companies and large employers have alliances with health care facilities outside the United States to control costs.

CATEGORIES OF MEDICAL TOURISM

Cosmetic Tourism

Cosmetic tourism, or travel abroad for aesthetic surgery, has become increasingly popular. The American Society of Plastic Surgeons (ASPS) reports that most cosmetic surgery patients are women 40–54 years old. The most common procedures sought by cosmetic tourists include abdominoplasty, breast augmentation, eyelid surgery, liposuction, and rhinoplasty. Popular destinations often are marketed to prospective medical tourists as low cost, all-inclusive cosmetic surgery vacations for elective procedures not typically covered by insurance. Complications, including infections and surgical revisions for unsatisfactory results, can compound initial costs.

Non-Cosmetic Medical Tourism

CANCER TREATMENT

Oncology, or cancer treatment, tourism often is pursued by people looking for alternative treatment options, better access to care, second opinions, or a combination of these. Oncology tourists are a vulnerable patient population because the fear caused by a cancer diagnosis can lead them to try potentially risky treatments or procedures. Often, the treatments or procedures used abroad have no established benefit, placing the oncology tourist at risk for harm due to complications (e.g., bleeding, infection) or by forgoing or delaying approved therapies in the United States.

DENTAL CARE

Dental care is the most common form of medical tourism among US residents, in part due to the rising cost of dental care in the United States; a substantial proportion of people in the United States do not have dental insurance or are underinsured. Dentists in destination countries might not be subject to the same licensure oversight as their US counterparts, however. In addition, practitioners abroad might not adhere to standard infection-control practices used in the United States, placing dental tourists at a potential risk for infection due to bloodborne or waterborne pathogens.

FERTILITY TREATMENTS

Fertility tourists are people who seek reproductive treatments in another country. Some do so to avoid associated barriers in their home country, including high costs, long waiting lists, and restrictive policies. Others believe they will receive higher quality care abroad. People traveling to other countries for fertility treatments often are in search of assisted reproductive technologies (e.g., artificial insemination by a donor, in vitro fertilization). Fertility tourists should be aware, however, that practices can vary in their level of clinical expertise, hygiene, and technique.

PHYSICIAN-ASSISTED SUICIDE

The practice of a physician facilitating a patient's desire to end their own life by providing either the information or the means (e.g., medications) for suicide is illegal in most countries. Some people consider physician-assisted suicide (PAS) tourism, also known as suicide travel or suicide tourism, as a possible option. Most PAS tourists have been diagnosed with a terminal illness or suffer from painful or debilitating medical conditions. PAS is legal in Belgium, Canada, Luxembourg, the Netherlands, Switzerland, and New Zealand, making these the destinations selected by PAS travelers.

REHAB TOURISM FOR SUBSTANCE USE DISORDERS

Rehab tourism involves travel to another country for substance use disorder treatment and rehabilitation care. Travelers exploring this option might be seeking a greater range of treatment options at less expense than what is available domestically (see Sec. 3, Ch. 5, Substance Use & Substance Use Disorders, and Box 3-10 for pros and cons of rehab tourism).

TRANSPLANT PROCEDURES

Transplant tourism refers to travel for receiving an organ, tissue, or stem cell transplant from an unrelated human donor. The practice can be motivated by reduced cost abroad or an effort to reduce the waiting time for organs. Xenotransplantation refers to receiving other biomaterial (e.g., cells, tissues) from nonhuman species, and xenotransplantation regulations vary from country to country. Many procedures involving injection of human or nonhuman cells have no scientific evidence to support a therapeutic benefit, and adverse events have been reported.

Depending on the location, organ or tissue donors might not be screened as thoroughly as they are in the United States; furthermore, organs and other tissues might be obtained using unethical means. In 2009, the World Health Organization released the revised Guiding Principles on Human Cell, Tissue, and Organ Transplantation, emphasizing that cells, tissues, and organs should be donated freely, in the absence of any form of financial incentive.

Studies have shown that transplant tourists can be at risk of receiving care that varies from practice standards in the United States. For instance, patients might receive fewer immunosuppressive drugs, increasing their risk for rejection, or they might not receive antimicrobial prophylaxis, increasing their risk for infection. Traveling after a procedure poses an additional risk for infection in someone who is immunocompromised.

THE PRETRAVEL CONSULTATION

Ideally, medical tourists will consult a travel medicine specialist for travel advice tailored to their specific health needs 4–6 weeks before travel. During the pretravel consultation, make certain travelers are up to date on all routine vaccinations, that they receive additional vaccines based on destination, and especially encourage hepatitis B virus immunization for unvaccinated travelers (see Sec. 2, Ch. 3, Vaccination & Immunoprophylaxis—General Principles, and Sec. 5, Part 2, Ch. 8, Hepatitis B). Counsel medical tourists that participating in typical vacation activities (e.g., consuming alcohol, participating in strenuous activity or exercise, sunbathing, swimming, taking long tours) during the postoperative period can delay or impede healing.

Advise medical tourists to also meet with their primary care provider to discuss their plan to seek medical care outside the United States, to address any concerns they or their provider might have, to ensure current medical conditions are well controlled, and to ensure they have a sufficient supply of all regular medications to last the duration of their trip. In addition, medical tourists should be aware of instances in which US medical professionals have elected not to treat medical tourists presenting with complications resulting from recent surgery, treatment, or procedures received abroad. Thus, encourage medical tourists to work with their primary care provider to identify physicians in their home communities who are willing and available to provide follow-up or emergency care upon their return.

Remind medical tourists to request copies of their overseas medical records in English and to provide this information to any health care providers they see subsequently for follow-up. Encourage medical tourists to disclose their entire travel history, medical history, and information about all surgeries or medical treatments received during their trip.

RISKS & COMPLICATIONS

All medical and surgical procedures carry some risk, and complications can occur regardless of where treatment is received. Advise medical tourists not to delay seeking medical care if they suspect any complication during travel or after returning home. Obtaining immediate care can lead to earlier diagnosis and treatment and a better outcome.

Infection

Among medical tourists, the most common complications are infection related. Inadequate infection-control practices place people at increased risk for bloodborne infections, including hepatitis B, hepatitis C, and HIV; bloodstream infections; donor-derived infections; and wound infections. Moreover, the risk of acquiring antibiotic-resistant infections might be greater in certain countries or regions; some highly resistant bacterial (e.g., carbapenem-resistant *Enterobacterales* [CRE]) and fungal (e.g., *Candida auris*) pathogens appear to be more common in some countries where US residents travel for medical tourism (see Sec. 11, Ch. 5, Antimicrobial Resistance).

Several infectious disease outbreaks have been documented among medical tourists, including CRE infections in patients undergoing invasive medical procedures in Mexico, surgical site infections caused by nontuberculous mycobacteria in patients who underwent cosmetic surgery in the Dominican Republic, and Q fever in patients who received fetal sheep cell injections in Germany.

Noninfectious Complications

Medical tourists have the same risks for noninfectious complications as patients receiving medical care in the United States. Noninfectious complications include blood clots, contour abnormalities after cosmetic surgery, and surgical wound dehiscence.

Travel-Associated Risks

Traveling during the post-operative or post-procedure recovery period or when being treated for a medical condition could pose additional risks for patients. Air travel and surgery independently increase the risk for blood clots, including deep vein thrombosis and pulmonary emboli (see Sec. 8, Ch. 3, Deep Vein Thrombosis & Pulmonary Embolism). Travel after surgery further increases the risk of developing blood clots because travel can require medical tourists to remain seated for long periods while in a hypercoagulable state.

Commercial aircraft cabin pressures are roughly equivalent to the outside air pressure at 6,000–8,000 feet above sea level. Medical tourists should not fly for 10 days after chest or abdominal surgery to avoid risks associated with changes in atmospheric pressure. ASPS recommends that patients undergoing laser treatments or cosmetic procedures to the face, eyelids, or nose, wait 7–10 days after the procedure before flying. The Aerospace Medical Association published medical guidelines for air travel that provide useful information on the risks for travel with certain medical conditions (see www.asma.org/asma/media/asma/Travel-Publications/paxguidelines.pdf).

RISK MITIGATION

Professional organizations have developed guidance, including template questions, that medical tourists can use when discussing what to expect with the facility providing the care, with the group facilitating the trip, and with their own domestic health care provider. For instance, the American Medical Association developed guiding principles on medical tourism for employers, insurance companies, and other entities that facilitate or incentivize medical care outside the United States (Box 6-07). The American College of Surgeons (ACS) issued a similar statement on medical and surgical tourism, with the additional recommendation

BOX 6-07 American Medical Association's guiding principles on medical tourism[1]

Employers, insurance companies, and other entities that facilitate or incentivize medical care outside the United States should adhere to the following principles:

- Receiving medical care outside the United States must be voluntary.
- Financial incentives to travel outside the United States for medical care should not inappropriately limit the diagnostic and therapeutic alternatives that are offered to patients or restrict treatment or referral options.
- Patients should only be referred for medical care to institutions that have been accredited by recognized international accrediting bodies (e.g., the Joint Commission International or the International Society for Quality in Health Care).
- Prior to travel, local follow-up care should be coordinated, and financing should be arranged to ensure continuity of care when patients return from medical care outside the United States.
- Coverage for travel outside the United States for medical care should include the costs of necessary follow-up care upon return to the United States.
- Patients should be informed of their rights and legal recourse before agreeing to travel outside the United States for medical care.
- Access to physician licensing and outcome data, as well as facility accreditation and outcomes data, should be arranged for patients seeking medical care outside the United States.
- The transfer of patient medical records to and from facilities outside the United States should be consistent with Health Insurance Portability and Accountability Action (HIPAA) guidelines.
- Patients choosing to travel outside the United States for medical care should be provided with information about the potential risks of combining surgical procedures with long flights and vacation activities.

[1]American Medical Association (AMA). New AMA Guidelines on Medical Tourism. Chicago: AMA; 2008. Available from: www.medretreat.com/templates/UserFiles/Documents/Whitepapers/AMAGuidelines.pdf.

6

that travelers obtain a complete set of medical records before returning home to ensure that details of their care are available to providers in the United States, which can facilitate continuity of care and proper follow-up, if needed.

Reviewing the Risks

Multiple resources are available for providers and medical tourists assessing medical tourism–related risks (see Table 6-02). When reviewing the risks associated with seeking health care abroad, encourage medical tourists to consider several factors besides the procedure; these include the destination, the facility or facilities where the procedure and recovery will take place, and the treating provider.

Make patients aware that medical tourism websites marketing directly to travelers might not include (or make available) comprehensive details on the accreditations, certifications, or qualifications of advertised facilities or providers. Local standards for facility accreditation and provider certification vary, and might not be the same as those in the United States; some facilities and providers abroad might lack accreditation or certification. In some locations, tracking patient outcome data or maintaining formal medical record privacy or security policies are not standard practices.

Medical tourists also should be aware that the drugs and medical products and devices used in other countries might not be subject to the same regulatory scrutiny and oversight as in the United States. In addition, some drugs could be counterfeit or otherwise ineffective because the medication expired, is contaminated, or was improperly stored (for more details, see the previous chapter in this section, . . . *perspectives*: Avoiding Poorly Regulated Medicines & Medical Products During Travel).

Checking Credentials

ACS recommends that medical tourists use internationally accredited facilities and seek care from providers certified in their specialties through a process equivalent to that established by the

Table 6-02 Online medical tourism resources

ORGANIZATION / SOURCE	RESOURCE	AVAILABLE FROM
Accreditation Association for Ambulatory Health Care	Accredited health care organization search tool	https://eweb.aaahc.org/eweb/dynamicpage.aspx?site=aaahc_site&webcode=find_orgs
Aerospace Medical Association	Medical Guidelines for Airline Passengers (2002)	www.asma.org/asma/media/asma/Travel-Publications/paxguidelines.pdf
The Aesthetic Society	Find a Plastic Surgeon search tool	www.surgery.org/consumers/find-a-plastic-surgeon
	Guidelines for patients seeking cosmetic procedures abroad	www.surgery.org/consumers/consumer-resources/consumer-tips/guidelines-for-patients-seeking-cosmetic-procedures-abroad
American Academy of Orthopaedic Surgeons	Bulletin (July 2007)	https://aaos.org/aaosnow/2007/jul/cover/cover1/
	Bulletin (February 2008)	https://aaos.org/aaosnow/2008/feb/managing/managing7/
American College of Surgeons	Statement on Medical and Surgical Tourism	www.facs.org/about-acs/statements/65-surgical-tourism
	Find a Surgeon search tool	www.facs.org/search/find-a-surgeon
American Medical Association	Ethics: Medical Tourism	www.ama-assn.org/delivering-care/ethics/medical-tourism
	Guidelines on Medical Tourism	www.medretreat.com/templates/UserFiles/Documents/Whitepapers/AMAGuidelines.pdf
American Society of Plastic Surgeons	ASPS Cautions Plastic Surgery Patients to Approach Holiday Medical Tourism with Vigilance (November 2012)	www.plasticsurgery.org/news/press-releases/asps-cautions-plastic-surgery-patients-to-approach-holiday-medical-tourism-with-vigilance
	Medical Tourism for Cosmetic Surgery High Risk of Complications, High Costs for Treatment (June 2017)	www.plasticsurgery.org/news/press-releases/medical-tourism-for-cosmetic-surgery-high-risk-of-complications-high-costs-for-treatment
	Plastic Surgery Abroad Can Lead to Severe Complications after Returning to the US (March 2018)	www.plasticsurgery.org/news/press-releases/plastic-surgery-abroad-can-lead-to-severe-complications-after-returning-to-the-us
	Medical Tourism Can Put Patients in Legal Limbo (September 2018)	www.plasticsurgery.org/news/press-releases/medical-tourism-can-put-patients-in-legal-limbo

Table 6-02 **Online medical tourism resources (continued)**

ORGANIZATION / SOURCE	RESOURCE	AVAILABLE FROM
	Briefing Paper: Cosmetic Surgery Tourism	www.plasticsurgery.org/news/briefing-papers/briefing-paper-cosmetic-surgery-tourism
	Plastic Surgeon match tool	https://find.plasticsurgery.org
International Society for Aesthetic Plastic Surgery	Find-a-surgeon search tool	www.isaps.org/member-directory/
Joint Commission International	Accredited facilities outside of the United States	www.jointcommissioninternational.org/JCI-Accredited-Organizations/
US Department of State	Your Health Abroad	https://travel.state.gov/content/travel/en/international-travel/before-you-go/your-health-abroad.html
World Health Organization	Guiding principles on human cell, tissue and organ transplantation	www.who.int/transplantation/Guiding_PrinciplesTransplantation_WHA63.22en.pdf

member boards of the American Board of Medical Specialties. Advise medical tourists to do as much advance research as possible on the facility and health care provider they are considering using. Also, inform medical tourists that accreditation does not guarantee a good outcome.

FACILITIES

Accrediting organizations (e.g., The Joint Commission International, Accreditation Association for Ambulatory Health Care) maintain listings of accredited facilities outside of the United States. Encourage prospective medical tourists to review these sources before committing to having a procedure or receiving medical care abroad.

PROVIDERS

ACS, ASPS, the American Society for Aesthetic Plastic Surgery, and the International Society of Aesthetic Plastic Surgery all accredit physicians abroad. Medical tourists should check the credentials of health care providers with search tools provided by relevant professional organizations.

Travel Health Insurance

Before travel, medical tourists should check their domestic health insurance plan carefully to understand what services, if any, are covered outside the United States. Additionally, travelers might need to purchase supplemental medical insurance coverage, including medical evacuation insurance; this is particularly important for travelers going to remote destinations or places lacking medical facilities that meet the standards found in high-income countries (see Sec. 6, Ch. 1, Travel Insurance, Travel Health Insurance & Medical Evacuation Insurance). Medical tourists also should be aware that if complications develop, they might not have the same legal recourse as they would if they received their care in the United States.

Planning for Follow-Up Care

Medical tourists and their domestic physicians should plan for follow-up care. Patients and clinicians should establish what care will be provided abroad, and what the patient will need upon return. Medical tourists should make sure they understand what services are included as part of the cost for their procedures; some overseas facilities and providers charge substantial fees for follow-up care in addition to the base cost. Travelers also should know whether follow-up care is scheduled to occur at the same facility as the procedure.

ADDITIONAL GUIDANCE FOR US HEALTH CARE PROVIDERS

Health care facilities in the United States should have systems in place to assess patients at admission to determine whether they have received medical care in other countries. Clinicians should obtain an explicit travel history from patients, including any medical care received abroad. Patients who have had an overnight stay in a health care facility outside the United States within 6 months of presentation should be screened for CRE. Admission screening is available free of charge through the Antibiotic Resistance Laboratory Network (www.cdc.gov/drugresistance/solutions-initiative/ar-lab-network.html).

Notify state and local public health as soon as medical tourism–associated infections are identified. Returning patients often present to hospitals close to their home, and communication with public health authorities can help facilitate outbreak recognition. Health care facilities should follow all disease reporting requirements for their jurisdiction. Health care facilities also should report suspected or confirmed cases of unusual antibiotic resistance (e.g., carbapenem-resistant organisms, *C. auris*) to public health authorities to facilitate testing and infection-control measures to prevent further transmission. In addition to notifying the state or local health department, contact the Centers for Disease Control and Prevention at medicaltourism@cdc.gov to report complications related to medical tourism.

6

BIBLIOGRAPHY

Adabi K, Stern C, Weichman K, Garfein ES, Pothula A, Draper L, et al. Population health implications of medical tourism. Plast Reconstr Surg. 2017;140(1):66–74.

Al-Shamsi, H, Al-Hajelli, M, Alrawi, S. Chasing the cure around the globe: medical tourism for cancer care from developing countries. J Glob Onc. 2018;4:1–3.

Kracalik I, Ham C, Smith AR, Vowles M, Kauber K, Zambrano M, et al. (2019). Notes from the field: Verona integron-encoded metallo-β-lactamase–producing carbapenem-resistant *Pseudomonas aeruginosa* infections in U.S. residents associated with invasive medical procedures in Mexico, 2015–2018. MMWR Morb Mortal Wkly Rep. 2019;68(20):463–4.

Pavli A, Maltezou HC. Infectious complications related to medical tourism. J Travel Med. 2021;28(1):taaa210.

Pereira RT, Malone CM, Flaherty GT. Aesthetic journeys: a review of cosmetic surgery tourism. J Travel Med. 2018;25(1):tay042.

Robyn MP, Newman AP, Amato M, Walawander M, Kothe C, Nerone JD, et al. Q fever outbreak among travelers to Germany who received live cell therapy—United States and Canada, 2014. MMWR Morb Mortal Wkly Rep. 2015;64(38):1071–3.

Salama M, Isachenko V, Isachenko E, Rahimi G, Mallmann P, Westphal LM, et al. Cross border reproductive care (CBRC): a growing global phenomenon with multidimensional implications (a systematic and critical review). J Assist Reprod Genet. 2018;35(7):1277–88.

Schnabel D, Esposito DH, Gaines J, Ridpath A, Barry MA, Feldman KA, et al. Multistate US outbreak of rapidly growing mycobacterial infections associated with medical tourism to the Dominican Republic, 2013–2014. Emerg Infect Dis. 2016;22(8):1340–7.

Stoney RJ, Kozarsky PE, Walker AT, Gaines JL. Population-based surveillance of medical tourism among US residents from 11 states and territories: findings from the Behavioral Risk Factor Surveillance System. Infect Control Hosp Epidemiol. 2022;43(7):870–5.

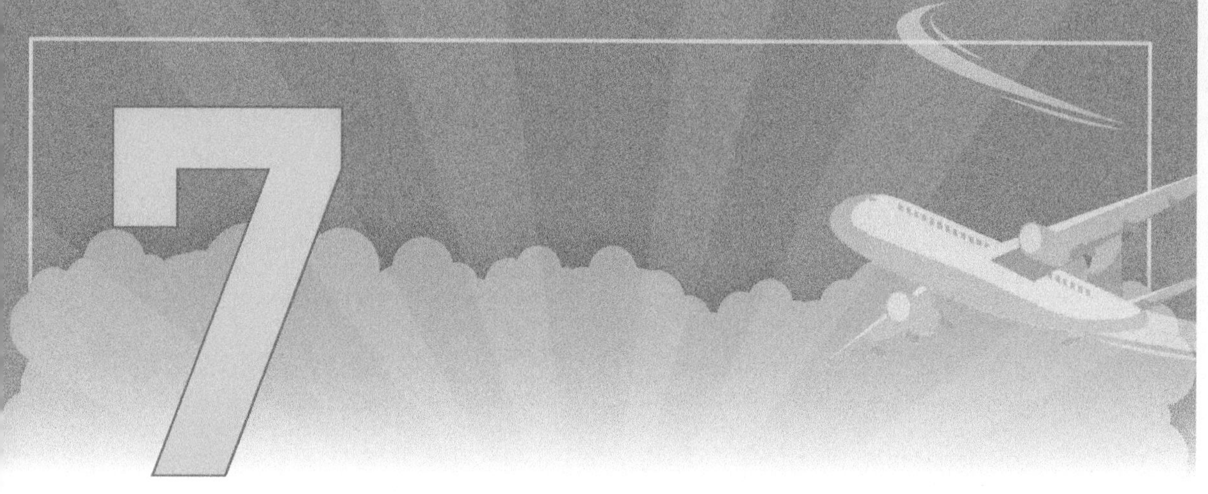

Family Travel

PREGNANT TRAVELERS

Romeo Galang, I. Dale Carroll, Titilope Oduyebo

Pregnancy can cause physiologic changes that require special consideration during travel. With careful preparation, however, most pregnant people can travel safely.

PRETRAVEL CONSULTATION

The pretravel consultation and evaluation of pregnant travelers (Box 7-01) should begin with a careful medical and obstetric history, specifically assessing gestational age and the presence of factors and conditions that increase risk for adverse pregnancy outcomes. A visit with an obstetric health care provider also should be a part of the pretravel assessment to ensure routine prenatal care and identify any potential problems. Instruct pregnant travelers to carry with them a copy of their prenatal records and physician's contact information.

Review the pregnant person's travel itinerary, including accommodations, activities, and destinations, to guide pretravel health advice. Discourage pregnant travelers from undertaking unaccustomed vigorous activity. Swimming and snorkeling during pregnancy generally are safe, but falls during waterskiing have been reported to inject water into the birth canal. Most experts advise against scuba diving for pregnant people because of risk for fetal gas embolism during decompression (see Sec. 4, Ch. 4, Scuba Diving: Decompression Illness & Other Dive-Related Injuries). Riding animals, bicycles, or motorcycles presents risks for abdominal trauma.

Educate pregnant people on how to avoid travel-associated risks, manage minor pregnancy discomforts, and recognize more serious complications. Advise pregnant people to seek urgent medical attention if they experience contractions or premature labor; symptoms of deep vein thrombosis (e.g., unusual leg swelling and pain in the calf or thigh) or pulmonary embolism (e.g., unusual shortness of breath); dehydration, diarrhea, or vomiting; severe pelvic or abdominal pain; symptoms of preeclampsia (e.g., severe headaches, nausea and vomiting, unusual

CDC Yellow Book 2024. Jeffrey Nemhauser, Oxford University Press. © Oxford University Press 2023.
DOI: 10.1093/oso/9780197570944.003.0007

BOX 7-01 Pretravel consultation for pregnant travelers: a checklist for health care providers

- ☐ Review vaccination history (e.g., COVID-19, hepatitis A, hepatitis B, measles, pertussis, rubella, varicella, tetanus) and update vaccinations as needed (see text for contraindications during pregnancy)
- ☐ Policies and paperwork
  - ○ Discuss supplemental travel insurance, travel health insurance, and medical evacuation insurance; research specific coverage information and limitations for pregnancy-related health issues
  - ○ Advise travelers to check airline and cruise line policies for pregnant travelers
  - ○ Provide letter confirming due date and fitness to travel
  - ○ Provide copy of medical records
- ☐ Prepare for obstetric care at destination
  - ○ Advise traveler to check medical insurance coverage
  - ○ Advise traveler to arrange for obstetric care at destination, as needed
- ☐ Review signs and symptoms requiring immediate care, including
  - ○ Bleeding
  - ○ Contractions or preterm labor
  - ○ Deep vein thrombosis or pulmonary embolism symptoms, which include unusual swelling of leg with pain in calf or thigh, unusual shortness of breath
  - ○ Pelvic or abdominal pain
  - ○ Preeclampsia symptoms (e.g., unusual swelling, severe headaches, nausea and vomiting, vision changes)
  - ○ Rupture of membranes
  - ○ Vomiting, diarrhea, dehydration

swelling, vision changes); prelabor rupture of the membranes; or vaginal bleeding.

7

Contraindications to Travel During Pregnancy

Absolute contraindications are conditions for which the potential harm of travel during pregnancy always outweighs the benefits of travel to the pregnant person or fetus. Relative contraindications are conditions for which travel should be avoided if the potential harm from travel outweighs its benefits (Box 7-02).

Although travel is rarely contraindicated during a normal pregnancy, pregnancies that require frequent antenatal monitoring or close medical supervision might warrant a recommendation that travel be delayed. Educate pregnant travelers that the risk of obstetric complications is greatest in the first and third trimesters of pregnancy.

Planning for Emergency Care

Obstetric emergencies are often sudden and life-threatening. Advise all pregnant travelers (but especially those in their third trimester or otherwise at high risk) to identify, in advance, international medical facilities at their destination(s) capable of managing complications of pregnancy, delivery (including by caesarean section), and neonatal problems. Counsel against travel to

BOX 7-02 Contraindications to travel during pregnancy

ABSOLUTE CONTRAINDICATIONS	RELATIVE CONTRAINDICATIONS
Abruptio placentae	Abnormal presentation
Active labor	Fetal growth restriction
Incompetent cervix	History of infertility
Premature labor	History of miscarriage or ectopic pregnancy
Premature rupture of membranes	Maternal age <15 or >35 years
Suspected ectopic pregnancy	Multiple gestation
Threatened abortion / vaginal bleeding	Placenta previa or other placental abnormality
Toxemia, past or present	

areas where obstetric care might be less than the standard at home.

Many health insurance policies do not cover the cost of medical treatment for pregnancy or neonatal complications that occur overseas. Pregnant people should strongly consider purchasing supplemental travel health insurance to cover pregnancy-related problems and care of the neonate, as needed. In addition, pregnant travelers should consider medical evacuation insurance coverage in case of pregnancy-related complications (see Sec. 6, Ch. 1, Travel Insurance, Travel Health Insurance & Medical Evacuation Insurance).

Medications

Over-the-counter drugs and nondrug remedies can help a pregnant person travel more comfortably. For instance, pregnant people can safely use a mild bulk laxative for constipation. In addition, several simple available remedies are effective in relieving the symptoms of morning sickness. Nonprescription remedies include ginger, available as a powder that can be mixed with food or drinks (e.g., tea), and as candy (e.g., lollipops). Similarly, pyridoxine (vitamin B6) is effective in reducing symptoms of morning sickness and is available in tablet form, as well as lozenges and lollipops. Antihistamines (e.g., dimenhydrinate, meclizine) often are used in pregnancy for morning sickness and motion sickness and appear to have a good safety record.

Carefully consider appropriate pain management and use of analgesics during pregnancy. Acetaminophen remains the nonopioid analgesic of choice during pregnancy. Although low-dose aspirin has been demonstrated to be relatively safe during pregnancy for certain clinical indications, it should be used cautiously. Aspirin can increase the incidence of abruption, and other anti-inflammatory agents can cause premature closure of the ductus arteriosus.

Various systems are used to classify drugs with respect to their safety in pregnancy (see www.fda.gov/consumers/free-publications-women/medicine-and-pregnancy). Refer to specific data about the effects of a given drug during pregnancy rather than depending on a classification. Counsel patients to help them make a balanced decision on the use of medications during pregnancy.

Vaccinations

In the best possible scenario, people should be up to date on routine vaccinations before becoming pregnant. The most effective way of protecting the infant against many diseases is to vaccinate the pregnant person. A summary of current Advisory Committee on Immunization Practices (ACIP) guidelines for vaccinating pregnant people is available at www.cdc.gov/vaccines/pregnancy/hcp/guidelines.html.

CORONAVIRUS DISEASE 2019

Pregnant people are more likely to become more severely ill from coronavirus disease 2019 (COVID-19) than people who are not pregnant. Having COVID-19 during pregnancy increases a person's risk of complications that can affect their pregnancy. For these reasons, the Centers for Disease Control and Prevention (CDC) recommends that people who are pregnant, trying to get pregnant, or who might become pregnant in the future get vaccinated against COVID-19 (www.cdc.gov/coronavirus/2019-ncov/vaccines/recommendations/pregnancy.html). As of August 2022, the COVID-19 vaccines authorized or approved for use in the United States are nonreplicating vaccines that do not cause infection in the pregnant person or the fetus. Pregnant people may choose to receive any of the COVID-19 vaccines authorized or approved for use in the United States; the ACIP does not state a preference.

COVID-19 vaccination can be safely provided before pregnancy or during any trimester of pregnancy. Available vaccines are highly effective in preventing severe COVID-19, hospitalizations, and deaths; data have shown that the benefits of vaccination during pregnancy, to both the pregnant person and their fetus, outweigh any potential risks. Pregnant people might want to speak with their health care provider before making a decision about receiving COVID-19 vaccine (www.acog.org/covid-19/covid-19-vaccines-and-pregnancy-conversation-guide-for-clinicians), but a consultation is not required before vaccination. Side effects from COVID-19 vaccination in pregnant people are like those expected among nonpregnant people. Pregnant people can take acetaminophen if they experience fever or other post-vaccination symptoms.

INFLUENZA

The ACIP recommends that all people who are or who will become pregnant during the influenza season have an annual influenza vaccine using inactivated virus. Influenza vaccines can be administered during any trimester.

HEPATITIS

The safety of hepatitis A vaccination during pregnancy has not been determined; because hepatitis A vaccine is produced from inactivated virus, though, the risk to the developing fetus is expected to be low. Weigh the risk associated with vaccination against the risk for infection in pregnant people who could be at increased risk for exposure to hepatitis A virus. According to the ACIP, pregnant people traveling internationally are at risk of hepatitis A virus infection; ACIP recommends vaccination during pregnancy for nonimmune international travelers (www.cdc.gov/mmwr/volumes/69/rr/rr6905a1.htm).

7

Limited data suggest that developing fetuses are not at risk for adverse events resulting from vaccination of pregnant people with hepatitis B vaccine (for details, see Sec. 5, Part 2, Ch. 8, Hepatitis B). ACIP recommends vaccinating pregnant people identified as being at risk for hepatitis B virus infection during pregnancy; risk factors include >1 sex partner during the previous 6 months, being evaluated or treated for a sexually transmitted infection, recent or current injection drug use, or having a HBsAg-positive sex partner. In November 2021, ACIP recommended vaccination of all adults 19–59 years old.

JAPANESE ENCEPHALITIS

Data are insufficient to make specific recommendations for use of Japanese encephalitis vaccine in pregnant people (see Sec. 5, Part 2, Ch. 13, Japanese Encephalitis).

LIVE-VIRUS VACCINES

Most live-virus vaccines, including live attenuated influenza, measles-mumps-rubella, live typhoid (Ty21a), and varicella, are contraindicated during pregnancy. Postexposure prophylaxis of a nonimmune pregnant person exposed to measles can be provided by administering measles immune globulin (IG) within 6 days of exposure; for varicella exposures, varicella-zoster IG can be given within 10 days. Advise people planning to become pregnant to wait ≥4 weeks after receiving a live-virus vaccine before conceiving.

YELLOW FEVER

Yellow fever vaccine is the exception to the rule about live-virus vaccines being contraindicated during pregnancy. ACIP considers pregnancy a precaution (i.e., a relative contraindication) for yellow fever vaccine. If travel is unavoidable, and the risk for yellow fever virus exposure outweighs the vaccination risk, it is appropriate to recommend vaccination. If the risks for vaccination outweigh the risks for yellow fever virus exposure, consider providing a medical waiver to the pregnant traveler to fulfill health regulations. Because pregnancy might affect immune responses to vaccination, consider performing serologic testing to document an immune response to yellow fever vaccine. Furthermore, if a person was pregnant (regardless of trimester) when they received their initial dose of yellow fever vaccine, they should receive 1 additional dose before they are next at risk for yellow fever virus exposure (see Sec. 5, Part 2, Ch. 26, Yellow Fever).

MENINGOCOCCAL

According to the ACIP, pregnant (and lactating) people should receive quadrivalent meningococcal vaccine, if indicated (www.cdc.gov/mmwr/volumes/69/rr/rr6909a1.htm). Meningococcal vaccine might be indicated for international travelers, depending on risk for infection at the destination (see Sec. 5, Part 1, Ch. 13, Meningococcal Disease).

POLIO

No adverse events linked to inactivated polio vaccine (IPV) have been documented among pregnant people or their fetuses. Vaccination of pregnant people should be avoided, however, because of theoretical concerns. IPV can be administered in accordance with the recommended immunization schedule for adults if a pregnant person is at increased risk for infection and requires immediate protection against polio (see Sec. 5, Part 2, Ch. 17, Poliomyelitis).

RABIES

Administer rabies postexposure prophylaxis with rabies immune globulin and vaccine after any moderate- or high-risk exposure to rabies; consider preexposure vaccine for travelers who have a substantial risk for exposure (see Sec. 5, Part 2, Ch. 18, Rabies).

TETANUS-DIPHTHERIA-PERTUSSIS

Tetanus, diphtheria, and acellular pertussis vaccine (Tdap) should be given during each pregnancy irrespective of a person's history of receiving the vaccine previously. To maximize maternal antibody response and passive antibody transfer to the infant, optimal timing for Tdap administration is between 27 and 36 weeks' gestation (earlier during this time frame is preferred), but it may be given at any time during pregnancy.

Malaria Prophylaxis

Malaria, caused by *Plasmodium* spp. parasites transmitted by mosquitoes, can be much more serious in pregnant than in nonpregnant people and is associated with high risks of illness and death for both mother and fetus. Malaria in pregnancy can be characterized by heavy parasitemia, severe anemia, and profound hypoglycemia, and can be complicated by cerebral malaria and acute respiratory distress syndrome. Placental sequestration of parasites might result in fetal loss due to abruption, premature labor, or miscarriage. An infant born to an infected mother is apt to be of low birth weight, and, although rare, congenital malaria is possible.

Because no prophylactic regimen provides complete protection, pregnant people should avoid or delay travel to malaria-endemic areas. If travel is unavoidable, the pregnant person should take precautions to avoid mosquito bites and use an effective prophylactic regimen.

Chloroquine is the drug of choice for pregnant travelers going to destinations with chloroquine-sensitive *Plasmodium* spp., and mefloquine is the drug of choice for pregnant travelers going to destinations with chloroquine-resistant *Plasmodium* spp. Doxycycline is contraindicated because of teratogenic effects on the fetus after the fourth month of pregnancy. Primaquine is contraindicated in pregnancy because the infant cannot be tested for glucose-6-phosphate dehydrogenase deficiency, putting the infant at risk for hemolytic anemia. Atovaquone-proguanil is not recommended because of lack of available safety data. A list of the available antimalarial drugs and their uses and contraindications during pregnancy can be found in Sec. 5, Part 3, Ch. 16, Malaria.

Travel Health Kits

In addition to the recommended travel health kit items for all travelers (see Sec. 2, Ch. 10, Travel Health Kits), pregnant travelers should pack antacids, antiemetic drugs, graduated compression stockings, hemorrhoid cream, medication for vaginitis or yeast infection, prenatal vitamins, and prescription medications. Encourage pregnant travelers to consider packing a blood pressure monitor if travel will limit access to a health center where blood pressure monitoring is available.

INFECTIOUS DISEASE CONCERNS

Respiratory and urinary infections and vaginitis are more likely to occur and to be more severe during pregnancy. Pregnant people who develop travelers' diarrhea or other gastrointestinal infections might be more vulnerable to dehydration than nonpregnant travelers. Stress the need for strict hand hygiene and food and water precautions (see Sec. 2, Ch. 8, Food & Water Precautions). Drinking bottled or boiled water is preferable to chemically treated or filtered water. Pregnant people should not consume water purified by iodine-containing compounds because of potential effects on the fetal thyroid (see Sec. 2, Ch. 9, Water Disinfection).

Coronavirus Disease 2019

As mentioned previously, pregnant people are at increased risk for severe COVID-19–associated illness (e.g., requiring invasive ventilation or extracorporeal membrane oxygenation) and death compared with people who are not pregnant (see www.cdc.gov/coronavirus/2019-ncov/need-extra-precautions/pregnant-people.html).

Underlying medical conditions (e.g., chronic kidney disease, diabetes, obesity) and other factors (e.g., age, occupation) can further increase a pregnant person's risk for developing severe illness. Additionally, pregnant people with COVID-19 are at greater risk for preterm birth and other adverse outcomes.

Pregnant people, recently pregnant people, and those who live with or visit them should take steps to protect themselves from getting COVID-19. CDC recommends that people (including those who are pregnant) not travel internationally until they are up to date with their COVID-19 vaccines (www.cdc.gov/coronavirus/2019-ncov/vaccines/stay-up-to-date.html). Additional information for international travelers is available at www.cdc.gov/coronavirus/2019-ncov/travelers/international-travel/index.html.

Hepatitis

Hepatitis A and hepatitis E are both spread by the fecal–oral route (see Sec. 5, Part 2, Ch. 7, Hepatitis A, and Sec. 5, Part 2, Ch. 10, Hepatitis E). Hepatitis A has been reported to increase the risk for placental abruption and premature delivery. Hepatitis E is more likely to cause severe disease during pregnancy and could result in a case-fatality rate of 15%–30%; when acquired during the third trimester, hepatitis E is also associated with fetal complications and fetal death.

7

Listeriosis & Toxoplasmosis

Listeriosis and toxoplasmosis (see Sec. 5, Part 3, Ch. 23, Toxoplasmosis) are foodborne illnesses of particular concern during pregnancy because the infection can cross the placenta and cause spontaneous abortion, stillbirth, or congenital or neonatal infection. Warn pregnant travelers to avoid unpasteurized cheeses and uncooked or undercooked meat products. Risk for fetal infection increases with gestational age, but severity of infection is decreased.

Other Parasitic Infections & Diseases

Parasitic infections and diseases can be a concern, particularly for pregnant people visiting friends and relatives in low- and middle-income countries. In general, intestinal helminths rarely cause enough illness to warrant treatment during pregnancy. Most, in fact, can be addressed safely with symptomatic treatment until the pregnancy is over. On the other hand, protozoan intestinal infections (e.g., *Cryptosporidium*, *Entamoeba histolytica*, *Giardia*) often do require treatment. These parasites can cause acute gastroenteritis, severe dehydration, and chronic malabsorption resulting in fetal growth restriction. *E. histolytica* can cause invasive disease, including amebic liver abscess and colitis. Pregnant people also should avoid bathing, swimming, or wading in freshwater lakes, rivers, and streams that can harbor the parasitic worms (schistosomes) that cause schistosomiasis (see Sec. 5, Part 3, Ch. 20, Schistosomiasis).

Travelers' Diarrhea

The treatment of choice for travelers' diarrhea is prompt and vigorous oral hydration; azithromycin or a third-generation cephalosporin may, however, be given to pregnant people if clinically indicated. Avoid use of bismuth subsalicylate because of the potential impact of salicylates on the fetus. In addition, fluoroquinolones are contraindicated in pregnancy due to toxicity to developing cartilage, as noted in experimental animal studies.

Vectorborne Infections

Pregnant people should avoid mosquito bites when traveling in areas where vectorborne diseases are endemic. Preventive measures include use of Environmental Protection Agency–registered insect repellants (see www.epa.gov/insect-repellents), protective clothing, and mosquito nets (see Sec. 4, Ch. 6, Mosquitoes, Ticks & Other Arthropods). For details on yellow fever vaccine and malaria prophylaxis during pregnancy, see above.

ZIKA

Zika virus is spread primarily through the bite of an infected *Aedes* mosquito (*Ae. aegypti* and *Ae. albopictus*) but can also be sexually transmitted. The illness associated with Zika can be asymptomatic or mild; some patients report acute onset of conjunctivitis, fever, joint pain, and rash that last for several days to a week after infection.

Birth defects caused by Zika virus infection during pregnancy include brain, eye, and neurodevelopmental abnormalities. Because of the risk for birth defects, CDC recommends pregnant people avoid travel to areas with a Zika outbreak, and, for the duration of the pregnancy, to avoid sex or use condoms with anyone who has traveled to a risk area.

Advise pregnant people considering travel to areas with Zika to carefully assess the risks of Zika infection during pregnancy; provide information about prevention strategies, signs and symptoms, and the limitations of Zika testing. Pregnant people should strictly follow steps to prevent mosquito bites and sexual transmission. Additional information, including the most current list of countries and territories where Zika is active, is available at https://wwwnc.cdc.gov/travel/page/zika-information. Guidance for pregnant people can be found on the CDC Zika website, www.cdc.gov/pregnancy/zika/index.html.

ENVIRONMENTAL HEALTH CONCERNS

Pregnant people should be aware of specific current environmental issues in their international destinations (e.g., natural disasters, special events or gatherings, travel warnings). More information can be found at the CDC Travelers' Health website (https://wwwnc.cdc.gov/travel/notices) and on the destination pages of the US Department of State website (https://travel.state.gov/content/travel/en/international-travel/International-Travel-Country-Information-Pages.html).

Air Quality

Air pollution causes more health problems during pregnancy because ciliary clearance of the bronchial tree is slowed, and mucus is more abundant. For more details on traveling to destinations where air quality is poor, see Sec. 4, Ch. 3, Air Quality & Ionizing Radiation.

Extremes of Temperature

Body temperature regulation is not as efficient during pregnancy, and temperature extremes can create more physiological stress on the pregnant person (see Sec. 4, Ch. 2, Extremes of Temperature). In addition, increases in core temperature (e.g., heat exhaustion, heat stroke), might harm the fetus. The vasodilatory effect of a hot environment and dehydration might cause fainting. For these reasons, then, encourage pregnant travelers to seek air-conditioned accommodations and restrict their level of activity in hot environments. If heat exposure is unavoidable, the duration should be as short as possible to prevent an increase in core body temperature. Pregnant travelers should take measures to avoid dehydration and hyperthermia.

High Elevation Travel

Pregnant people should avoid activities at high elevation unless they have trained for and are accustomed to such activities; those not acclimated to high elevation might experience breathlessness and palpitations. The common symptoms of acute mountain sickness (insomnia, headache, and nausea) frequently are associated with pregnancy, and it might be difficult to distinguish the cause of the symptoms. Most experts recommend a slower ascent with adequate time for acclimatization. No studies or case reports show harm to a fetus if the mother travels briefly to high elevations during pregnancy; recommend that pregnant people not sleep at elevations >12,000 ft (≈3,600 m) above sea level, if possible. Probably the greatest concern is that high-elevation destinations often are inaccessible and far from medical care (see Sec. 4, Ch. 5, High Elevation Travel & Altitude Illness).

TRANSPORTATION CONSIDERATIONS

Advise pregnant people to follow safety instructions for all forms of transport and to wear seat belts, when available, on all forms of transportation, including airplanes, buses, and cars (see Sec. 8, Ch. 5, Road & Traffic Safety). A diagonal shoulder strap with a lap belt provides the best protection. The shoulder belt should be worn between the breasts with the lap belt low across the upper thighs. When only a lap belt is available, pregnant people should wear it low, between the abdomen and across the upper thighs, not above or across the abdomen.

Air Travel

Most commercial airlines allow pregnant travelers to fly until 36 weeks' gestation. Some limit international travel earlier in pregnancy, and some require documentation of gestational age. Pregnant travelers should check with the airline for specific requirements or guidance, and should consider the gestational age of the fetus on the dates both of departure and of return.

Most commercial jetliner cabins are pressurized to an equivalent outside air pressure of 6,000–8,000 ft (≈1,800–2,500 m) above sea level; travelers might also experience air pressures in this range during travel by hot air balloon or on noncommercial aircraft. The lower oxygen tension under these conditions likely will not cause fetal problems in a normal pregnancy. People with pregnancies complicated by conditions exacerbated by hypoxia (e.g., preexisting cardiovascular problems, sickle cell disease, severe anemia [hemoglobin <8.0 g/dL], intrauterine fetal growth restriction) could, however, experience adverse effects associated with low arterial oxygen saturation.

7

Risks of air travel include potential exposure to communicable diseases, immobility, and the common discomforts of flying. Abdominal distention and pedal edema frequently occur. The pregnant traveler might benefit from an upgrade in airline seating and should seek convenient and practical accommodations (e.g., proximity to the lavatory). Pregnant travelers should select aisle seating when possible, and wear loose fitting clothing and comfortable shoes that enable them to move about more easily and frequently during flights.

Some experts report that the risk for deep vein thrombosis (DVT) is 5–10 times greater among pregnant than nonpregnant people, although the absolute risk is low. To help prevent DVT, pregnant travelers should stay hydrated, stretch frequently, walk and perform isometric leg exercises, and wear graduated compression stockings (see Sec. 8, Ch. 3, Deep Vein Thrombosis & Pulmonary Embolism).

Cosmic radiation during air travel poses little threat to the fetus but might be a consideration for pregnant travelers who fly frequently (see Sec. 9, Ch. 3, . . . *perspectives*: People Who Fly for a Living—Health Myths & Realities). Older airport security machines are magnetometers and are not harmful to the fetus. Newer security machines use backscatter x-ray scanners, which emit low levels of radiation. Most experts agree that the risk for complications from radiation exposure from these scanners is extremely low.

Cruise Ship Travel

Most cruise lines restrict travel beyond 24 weeks' gestation (see Sec. 8, Ch. 6, Cruise Ship Travel). Cruise lines might require pregnant travelers to carry a physician's note stating that they are fit to travel, including the estimated date of delivery. Pregnant people should check with the cruise line for specific requirements or guidance. For pregnant travelers planning a cruise, provide advice about gastrointestinal and respiratory infections, motion sickness (see Sec. 8, Ch. 7, Motion Sickness), and the risk for falls on a moving vessel, as well as the possibility of delayed care while at sea.

BIBLIOGRAPHY

Allotey J, Stallings E, Bonet M, Yap M, Chatterjee S, Kew T, et al.; PregCOV-19 Living Systematic Review Consortium. Clinical manifestations, risk factors, and maternal and perinatal outcomes of coronavirus disease 2019 in pregnancy: living systematic review and meta-analysis. BMJ. 2020;370:m3320.

Bisson DL, Newell SD, Laxton C; on behalf of the Royal College of Obstetricians and Gynaecologists. Antenatal and postnatal analgesia. BJOG. 2018;126(4):114–24.

Centers for Disease Control and Prevention. Guidelines for vaccinating pregnant women. Atlanta: The Centers; 2014. Available from: www.cdc.gov/vaccines/pregnancy/hcp-toolkit/guidelines.html.

Dotters-Katz S, Kuller J, Heine RP. Parasitic infections in pregnancy. Obstet Gynecol Surv. 2011;66(8):515–25.

Hezelgrave NL, Whitty CJ, Shennan AH, Chappell LC. Advising on travel during pregnancy. BMJ. 2011;342:d2506.

Irvine MH, Einarson A, Bozzo P. Prophylactic use of antimalarials during pregnancy. Can Fam Physician. 2011;57(11):1279–81.

Magann EF, Chauhan SP, Dahlke JD, McKelvey SS, Watson EM, Morrison JC. Air travel and pregnancy outcomes: a review of pregnancy regulations and outcomes for passengers, flight attendants, and aviators. Obstet Gynecol Surv. 2010;65(6):396–402.

Rasmussen SA, Jamieson DJ, Honein MA, Petersen LR. Zika virus and birth defects—reviewing the evidence for causality. N Engl J Med. 2016;374(20):1981–7.

Rasmussen SA, Watson AK, Kennedy ED, Broder KR, Jamieson DJ. Vaccines and pregnancy: past, present, and future. Semin Fetal Neonatal Med. 2014;19(3):161–9.

Roggelin L, Cramer JP. Malaria prevention in the pregnant traveller: a review. Travel Med Infect Dis. 2014;12(3):229–36.

TRAVEL & BREASTFEEDING

Erica Anstey, Katherine Shealy

The medical preparation of a traveler who is breastfeeding differs only slightly from that of other travelers and depends in part on whether the breastfeeding traveler and child will be separated or together during travel. Most travelers should be advised to continue breastfeeding their children throughout travel.

Before departure, travelers might benefit from compiling a list of local breastfeeding resources at their destination, to have on hand during travel. Clinicians and travelers can use the Find a Lactation Consultant Tool (www.FindALactationConsultant.com) to find contact information for experts at their destination. Clinicians and travelers can use La Leche League International's interactive map (www.llli.org/get-help) to find specific location and contact information for breastfeeding support group leaders and groups worldwide. Travelers who will need to store expressed milk while traveling can call ahead to their hotel or other place of lodging to request access to a refrigerator, if available.

TRAVEL WITH A BREASTFEEDING CHILD

Breastfeeding provides unique benefits to children while traveling. Explain clearly to breastfeeding travelers the value of continuing to breastfeed during travel. The American Academy of Pediatrics (AAP) recommends exclusive breastfeeding for the first 6 months of life. Exclusive breastfeeding means feeding only breast milk, no other food or drink, which potentially protects children from contaminants and pathogens in foods or liquids. Additionally, feeding only at the breast protects children from potential exposure to contaminants on bottles, containers, cups, and utensils.

During the first 6 months, breastfeeding children require no water supplementation, even in extreme heat environments. Breastfeeding protects children from eustachian tube collapse and pain during air travel, especially during ascent and descent, by allowing them to stabilize and gradually equalize internal and external air pressure.

Frequent, unrestricted breastfeeding opportunities ensure that the lactating traveler's milk supply remains sufficient, and that the child's nutrition and hydration are ideal. Travelers concerned about breastfeeding away from home might feel more comfortable breastfeeding the child in a fabric carrier or by using a nursing cover. In many countries, breastfeeding in public places is practiced more widely than in the United States. US federal legislation protects parents' and children's rights to breastfeed anywhere they are otherwise authorized to be while on federal property, including US Customs areas, embassies, and consulates overseas. The Consolidated Appropriations Act, 2021, SEC. 722 states, "Notwithstanding any other provision of law, a woman may breastfeed her child at any location in a Federal building or on Federal property, if the woman and her child are otherwise authorized to be present at the location" (see www.congress.gov/116/bills/hr133/BILLS-116hr133enr.pdf).

TRAVEL WITHOUT A BREASTFEEDING CHILD

Before departure, a breastfeeding person might decide to express and store a supply of milk to be fed to the child during the traveler's absence.

Building a supply takes time and patience, and is most successful when begun gradually, many weeks in advance of departure. Clinicians and others who provide lactation support should help travelers determine the best course for breastfeeding based on a variety of factors, including the amount of time available to prepare for the trip, the flexibility of time while traveling, options for expressing and storing milk while traveling, the duration of travel, and destination.

While away from the child, expressing milk can help the breastfeeding traveler maintain milk supply for when they return home. Expressing milk also can help avoid engorgement, which can increase the risk of developing a breast infection. Expressing milk by hand is a useful technique to learn prior to traveling because it does not require any equipment or a reliable power source, and detailed instructions are available at https://healthychildren.org/English/ages-stages/baby/breastfeeding/Pages/Hand-Expressing-Milk.aspx. Hand expressing can be helpful when travelers need to express milk while in transit (e.g., on a bus, car, plane, train). Travelers intending to use breast pumps should plan to pack multiple breast pump kits if they anticipate being unable to clean individual pump parts after each use (see the section on breast pump safety later in this chapter). A nursing cover can provide some privacy when expressing milk.

Travelers who return to a nursing child can continue breastfeeding and, if necessary, supplement with previously expressed milk or infant formula until milk supply returns to its prior level. Often, after returning from travel, several days of feeding at the breast will help bring milk supply back to its prior level. Prolonged separation from the nursing child might, however, increase the difficulty and time it takes to transition back to breastfeeding. A lactation consultant can help address breastfeeding challenges after a traveler reunites with their child.

MEDICATIONS, VACCINES & OTHER EXPOSURES

In almost all situations, clinicians can and should select medications and vaccines for the nursing traveler that are compatible with breastfeeding. In most circumstances, it is inappropriate to counsel travelers to wean to be vaccinated, or to withhold vaccination due to breastfeeding status.

Breastfeeding and lactation do not affect maternal or child dosage guidelines for any medication or vaccine; children always require their own medications and vaccines, regardless of maternal dose. In the absence of documented risk to the breastfeeding child associated with a particular maternal medication, the known risks of stopping breastfeeding generally outweigh a theoretical risk for exposure via breastfeeding.

Drugs & Chemicals

According to the AAP 2013 Clinical Report: The Transfer of Drugs and Therapeutics into Human Breast Milk, many parents are inappropriately advised to discontinue breastfeeding or to avoid taking essential medications because of fears of adverse effects on their breastfed infants. Only a few medications are contraindicated in people who are breastfeeding or are associated with adverse effects on their children.

The National Institutes for Health's Drugs and Lactation Database (LactMed; www.ncbi.nlm.nih.gov/books/NBK501922) is an online source for clinical information about drugs and chemicals to which breastfeeding travelers could be exposed. LactMed provides information about the levels of substances in breast milk and infant blood, potential effects on breastfeeding children and on lactation itself, and alternative drugs to consider.

Another resource, Hale's Medications and Mothers' Milk, is a regularly updated pharmaceutical reference guide that provides comprehensive, evidence-based information on the compatibility or effects of >1,300 drugs, diseases, vaccines, herbals, and syndromes on breastfeeding, and includes risk categories, pharmacologic properties, interactions with other drugs, and suitable alternatives. An online version is available by subscription and is printable.

MotherToBaby (https://mothertobaby.org) is a service of the nonprofit Organization of Teratology Information Specialists (OTIS) and provides evidence-based information on the safety of or risk from medications and other exposures during pregnancy and lactation. OTIS provides a free information and risk assessment service to mothers, health care providers, and the public via text, chat, phone, and email, in English and Spanish.

MALARIA CHEMOPROPHYLAXIS

Because chloroquine and mefloquine can be safely prescribed to infants, both are considered compatible with breastfeeding. Most experts consider short-term use of doxycycline compatible with breastfeeding. Primaquine can be used for breastfeeding people and for infants with normal glucose-6-phosphate dehydrogenase (G6PD) levels, but screen both for G6PD deficiency before prescribing this drug. Because data are not yet available on the safety of atovaquone-proguanil prophylaxis in infants weighing <11 lb (5 kg), the Centers for Disease Control and Prevention (CDC) does not recommend it to prevent malaria in people who are breastfeeding infants weighing <5 kg (see Sec. 5, Part 3, Ch. 16, Malaria, for more information).

The quantity of antimalarial drugs transferred to breast milk is not enough to provide protection against malaria for the infant. Breastfeeding infants need their own antimalarial drug. More information about malaria and breastfeeding is available at www.cdc.gov/breastfeeding/breastfeeding-special-circumstances/maternal-or-infant-illnesses/malaria.html.

TRAVELERS' DIARRHEA TREATMENT

Exclusive breastfeeding protects children against travelers' diarrhea (TD). Breastfeeding is ideal rehydration therapy. Children suspected of having TD should breastfeed more frequently and should not be offered other fluids or foods that replace breastfeeding. Breastfeeding travelers with TD should continue breastfeeding if possible, and increase their own fluid intake. The organisms that cause TD do not pass into breast milk.

Breastfeeding travelers should carefully check the labels of over-the-counter antidiarrheal medications to avoid using bismuth subsalicylate compounds, which can lead to the transfer of salicylate to the child via breast milk. Fluoroquinolones and macrolides, commonly used to treat travelers' diarrhea, are excreted in breast milk. Consult with the breastfed child's primary health care provider before deciding to prescribe antibiotics for breastfeeding travelers. Most experts consider the short-term use of azithromycin compatible with breastfeeding. Use of oral rehydration salts is fully compatible with breastfeeding.

Vaccinations

Vaccinate breastfeeding travelers and children according to routine, recommended vaccine schedules. Most live and inactivated vaccines do not affect breastfeeding, breast milk, or the process of lactation (see www.cdc.gov/breastfeeding/breastfeeding-special-circumstances/vaccinations-medications-drugs/vaccinations.html). Only 2 vaccines, smallpox (vaccinia) and yellow fever, require special consideration. Preexposure smallpox vaccine is contraindicated in breastfeeding people because of the risk for contact transmission to the breastfed child.

YELLOW FEVER VACCINE

Breastfeeding is a precaution against administering yellow fever vaccine. Three cases of yellow fever vaccine–associated neurologic disease (encephalitis) have been reported in infants exclusively breastfed by people who received yellow fever vaccine. All 3 infants were aged <1 month at the time of exposure.

Until specific research data are available, avoid vaccinating breastfeeding travelers against yellow fever. When a breastfeeding person must travel to a yellow fever endemic area, however, vaccination should be recommended. Although no data are available, some experts advise that breastfeeding travelers who receive yellow fever vaccine should temporarily suspend breastfeeding, and pump and discard milk for ≥2 weeks after vaccination before resuming breastfeeding (see Sec. 5, Part 2, Ch. 26, Yellow Fever, for more information). Refer the traveler to a lactation support provider for information on how to maintain milk production and how to best feed the child while not breastfeeding; options include using previously expressed milk, pasteurized donor human milk, infant formula, or a combination of these.

Zika Virus

CDC encourages people with Zika virus infection and those living in or traveling to areas with ongoing Zika virus transmission to breastfeed their children. Evidence suggests that the benefits of breastfeeding outweigh the risks of Zika virus transmission through breast milk. Current information is available at www.cdc.gov/pregnancy/zika/testing-follow-up/zika-in-infants-children.html.

AIR TRAVEL

Air travel should not be a barrier to breastfeeding or expressing breast milk. Being prepared and aware of available resources can help ease anxiety about traveling by air with breast milk, breast pump equipment, or a breastfeeding child.

Breast Pump Equipment & Breast Milk

Before departure, people who will be traveling by air and expect to have expressed milk with them during travel need to carefully plan how they will transport the expressed milk. Airport security regulations for passengers carrying expressed milk vary internationally and are subject to change.

In the United States, expressed milk and related infant and child feeding items are exempt from Transportation Security Administration (TSA) regulations limiting quantities of other liquids and gels (see www.tsa.gov/travel/special-procedures/traveling-children). Travelers can carry with them expressed milk, ice packs, gel packs (frozen or unfrozen), pumps and pump kits, and other accessories required to transport expressed milk through airport security checkpoints and onboard flights, regardless of whether the breastfeeding child is also traveling. At the beginning of the screening process, travelers should inform the TSA officer that they are carrying breastfeeding equipment, and separate the expressed milk and related accessories from the liquids, gels, and aerosols that are limited to 3.4 oz (100 mL) each, as subject to TSA's Liquids Rule, available at www.tsa.gov/travel/security-screening/liquids-rule.

Breast pumps are medical devices regulated by the US Food and Drug Administration (FDA), and most airlines allow passengers to carry breast pumps on board in addition to other permitted carry-on items. Travelers can check the airline's policies related to breastfeeding and breastfeeding equipment prior to travel.

X-rays used in airport screenings have no effect on breastfeeding, expressed milk, or the process of lactation. FDA states that no adverse effects are known from eating food, drinking beverages, or using medicine screened by x-ray. Travelers also should inform the TSA officer if they do not want expressed milk to be opened or irradiated in scanners. TSA officers might conduct additional screening procedures (e.g., pat down, and screening of other carry-on property). Travelers should plan for extra time at the airport to get through the airport security checkpoints when traveling with expressed milk and related supplies. Travelers might find that providing TSA officers with the related TSA regulations for expressed milk (available at www.tsa.gov/travel/special-procedures/traveling-children) can help facilitate the screening process.

Travelers carrying expressed milk in checked luggage should refer to cooler pack storage guidelines on the CDC website, Proper Storage and Preparation of Breast Milk (www.cdc.gov/breastfeeding/recommendations/handling_breastmilk.htm). Expressed milk is considered a food for individual use, and is not considered a biohazard. International Air Transport Authority regulations for shipping category B biological substances (UN 3373) do not apply to expressed milk.

Lactation Spaces

By 2023, all small, medium, and large hub airports in the United States are required by the Friendly Airports for Mothers Improvement Act (www.congress.gov/bill/116th-congress/senate-bill/2638) to provide a clean, private, non-bathroom lactation space in each terminal for breastfeeding or expressing milk. Travelers can check the airport's website to locate these spaces.

Packing & Shipping Breast Milk

Travelers shipping frozen milk should follow guidelines for shipping other frozen foods and liquids. Travelers planning to ship frozen milk might need to bring supplies (e.g., milk storage bags or resealable bags; paper lunch bags or newspaper for wrapping frozen milk; coolers; labels, packing tape, and shipping boxes; tongs or gloves for handling dry ice). Some shipping carriers provide temperature-controlled options that can be used for transporting expressed milk. Some employers will cover the cost of shipping expressed milk home for employees who are traveling for work. Travelers should make sure in advance that transporting expressed milk will meet customs regulations, because these can vary by country. Expressed milk does not need to be declared at US Customs upon return to the United States.

BREAST PUMP SAFETY

Travelers who plan to use an electric breast pump while traveling might need an electrical current adapter and converter, and should have a backup option available, including information on hand expression techniques or a manual pump. Travelers using a breast pump should be sure to follow proper breast pump cleaning guidance (see www.cdc.gov/healthywater/hygiene/healthychildcare/infantfeeding/breastpump.html) to minimize potential contamination. Related guidance for cleaning infant feeding items (e.g., bottles and the nipples, rings, and caps that go with them) is available at www.cdc.gov/healthywater/hygiene/healthychildcare/infantfeeding/cleansanitize.html.

Travelers should thoroughly wash hands with soap and water (see www.cdc.gov/handwashing/when-how-handwashing.html) prior to pumping and handling expressed milk; if safe water is not immediately available, travelers can use an alcohol-based hand sanitizer containing ≥60% alcohol (www.cdc.gov/handwashing/hand-sanitizer-use.html). If travelers are unable to clean pump parts between uses, they should bring extra sets of pump parts (e.g., connectors, flanges, membranes, valves) to use until they are able to thoroughly clean used parts. Travelers also could consider packing a cleaning kit for breast pump parts, including a cleaning brush, dish soap, and portable drying rack or mesh bag to hang items to air dry.

BIBLIOGRAPHY

Academy of Breastfeeding Medicine (ABM) Protocol Committee. ABM clinical protocol #8: human milk storage information for home use for full-term infants, revised 2017. Breastfeed Med. 2017;12(7):390–5.

Centers for Disease Control and Prevention. Travel recommendations for nursing families. Available from: www.cdc.gov/nutrition/infantandtoddlernutrition/breastfeeding/travel-recommendations.html.

Fleming-Dutra KE, Nelson JM, Fischer M, Staples JE, Karwowski MP, Mead P, et al. Update: interim guidelines for health care providers caring for infants and children with possible Zika virus infection—United States, February 2016. MMWR Morb Mortal Wkly Rep. 2016;65(7):182–7.

Hale TW, Rowe HE. Medications and mothers' milk, 17th edition. New York: Springer Publishing Company; 2017.

Kuhn S, Twele-Montecinos L, MacDonald J, Webster P, Law B. Case report: probable transmission of vaccine strain of yellow fever virus to an infant via breast milk. CMAJ. 2011;183(4):e243–5.

Sachdev HP, Krishna J, Puri RK, Satyanarayana L, Kumar S. Water supplementation in exclusively breastfed infants during summer in the tropics. Lancet. 1991;337(8747):929–33.

Sachs HC, AAP Committee on Drugs. The transfer of drugs and therapeutics into human breast milk: an update on selected topics. Pediatrics. 2013;132(3):e796–809.

Section on Breastfeeding. Breastfeeding and the use of human milk. Pediatrics. 2012;129(3):e827–41.

Staples JE, Gershman M, Fischer M. Yellow fever vaccine: recommendations of the Advisory Committee on Immunization Practices (ACIP). MMWR Recomm Rep. 2010;59(RR-7):1–27.

TRAVELING SAFELY WITH INFANTS & CHILDREN

Michelle Weinberg, Nicholas Weinberg, Susan Maloney

Children increasingly are traveling and living outside their home countries. Although data about the incidence of pediatric illnesses associated with international travel are limited, the risks that children face when traveling are likely similar to those faced by their adult travel companions.

Compared with adults, however, children are less likely to receive pretravel advice. In a review of children with posttravel illnesses seen at clinics in the GeoSentinel Global Surveillance Network, 51% of all children and 32% of children visiting friends and relatives (VFRs) had received pretravel medical advice, compared with 59% of adults. The most commonly reported health problems among child travelers are dermatologic conditions, including animal and arthropod bites, cutaneous larva migrans, and sunburn; diarrheal illnesses; respiratory disorders; and systemic febrile illnesses, especially malaria.

Motor vehicle and water-related injuries, including drowning, are other major health and safety concerns for child travelers. See Box 7-03 for recommendations on assessing and preparing children for planned international travel.

TRAVEL-ASSOCIATED INFECTIONS & DISEASES

Arboviral Infections

Pediatric VFR travelers with frequent or prolonged travel to areas where arboviruses (e.g., chikungunya, dengue, Japanese encephalitis, yellow fever, and Zika viruses) are endemic or epidemic could be at increased risk for infection. Children traveling to areas with arboviruses should use the same mosquito protection measures described elsewhere in this chapter (also see Sec. 4, Ch. 6, Mosquitoes, Ticks & Other Arthropods). Unlike

BOX 7-03 Assessing & preparing children for international travel: a checklist for health care providers

- ☐ Review travel-related and routine childhood vaccinations. The pretravel visit is an opportunity to ensure that children are up to date on their routine vaccinations.
- ☐ Assess all anticipated travel-related activities.
- ☐ Provide preventive counseling and interventions tailored to specific risks, including special travel preparations and any treatment required for infants and children with underlying health conditions, chronic diseases, or immunocompromising conditions.
- ☐ For children who require medications to manage chronic health conditions, caregivers should carry a supply sufficient for the trip duration.
- ☐ For adolescents traveling in a student group or program (see also Sec. 9, Ch. 8, Study Abroad & Other International Student Travel), consider providing counseling on the following:
    - Disease prevention
    - Drug and alcohol use
    - Empiric treatment and management of common travel-related illnesses
    - Risks of sexually transmitted infections and sexual assault
- ☐ Give special consideration to travelers visiting friends and relatives in low- and middle-income countries and assess risks for malaria, intestinal parasites, and tuberculosis.
- ☐ Consider advising adults traveling with children and older children to take a course in basic first aid before travel.
- ☐ For coronavirus disease 2019 (COVID-19) safety measures for children—including mask use, testing, and vaccination—see Sec. 5, Part 2, Ch. 3, COVID-19.

7

mosquitoes that transmit malaria, the *Aedes* mosquitoes that transmit chikungunya, dengue, yellow fever, and Zika are aggressive daytime biters; they also bite at night, especially in areas with artificial light. Consider dengue or other arboviral infections in children with fever if they recently returned from travel in endemic areas. Vaccination against dengue, tick-borne encephalitis, and yellow fever could be indicated for some children (see Sec. 7, Ch. 4, Vaccine Recommendations for Infants & Children, for details).

Diarrhea & Vomiting

Diarrhea and associated gastrointestinal illnesses are among the most common travel-related problems affecting children. Infants and children with diarrhea can become dehydrated more quickly than adults. The etiology of travelers' diarrhea (TD) in children is similar to that in adults (see Sec. 2, Ch. 6, Travelers' Diarrhea).

PREVENTION

Adults traveling with children should ensure the children follow safe food and water precautions and frequently wash their hands to prevent foodborne and waterborne illness. For infants, breastfeeding is the best way to reduce the risk for foodborne and waterborne illness (see Sec. 7, Ch. 2, Travel & Breastfeeding). Infant formulas available abroad might not have the same nutritional composition or be held to the same manufacturing safety standards as in the traveler's home country; parents feeding their child formula should consider whether they need to bring formula from home. If the infant is fed with formula, travelers should consider using liquid formula, which is sterile. Use of powdered infant formula has been associated with *Cronobacter* infection; infants <3 months old, infants born prematurely, and infants with weakened immune systems are at greatest risk. Parents should take extra precautions for preparing powdered infant formula (see www.cdc.gov/cronobacter/prevention.html).

Travelers should disinfect water served to young children, including water used to prepare infant formula (see Sec. 2, Ch. 8, Food & Water Precautions, and Sec. 2, Ch. 9, Water Disinfection, for details on safety practices). In some parts of the world, bottled water could be contaminated and should be disinfected to kill bacteria, viruses, and protozoa before consumption.

Similarly, travelers with children should diligently follow food precautions and ensure foods served to children are cooked thoroughly and eaten while still hot; caregivers should peel fruits typically eaten raw immediately before consumption. Additionally, adults should use caution with fresh dairy products, which might not be pasteurized or might be diluted with untreated water. For short trips, parents might want to bring a supply of safe snacks from home for times when children are hungry and available food might not be appealing or safe (see Sec. 2, Ch. 8, Food & Water Precautions, for more information).

Adult travelers with children should pay scrupulous attention that potable water is used for handwashing and cleaning bottles, pacifiers, teething rings, and toys that fall to the floor or are handled by others. After diaper changes, especially for infants with diarrhea, parents should be particularly careful to wash hands well to avoid spreading infection to themselves and other family members. When proper handwashing facilities are not available, hand sanitizer containing ≥60% alcohol can be used as a disinfecting agent. Because alcohol-based hand sanitizers are not effective against certain pathogens, however, adults and children should wash hands with soap and water as soon as possible. In addition, alcohol does not remove organic material, and people should wash visibly soiled hands with soap and water.

Chemoprophylaxis with antibiotics is not generally used in children; typhoid vaccine might be indicated, however (see Sec. 5, Part 1, Ch. 24, Typhoid & Paratyphoid Fever).

TREATMENT

ANTIBIOTICS

AZITHROMYCIN

Few data are available regarding empiric treatment of TD in children. Antimicrobial options for empiric treatment of TD in children are limited. In practice, when an antibiotic is indicated for moderate to severe diarrhea, some clinicians prescribe azithromycin as a single daily dose (10 mg/kg) for 3 days. Clinicians can prescribe unreconstituted azithromycin powder before travel, with instructions from the pharmacist for mixing it into an oral suspension prior to administration. Although resistance breakpoints have not yet been determined, elevated minimum inhibitory concentrations for azithromycin have been reported for some gastrointestinal pathogens. Therefore, counsel parents to seek medical attention for their children if they do not improve after empiric treatment. Before prescribing azithromycin for empiric TD treatment, review possible contraindications and the risks for adverse reactions (e.g., QT prolongation and cardiac arrhythmias).

FLUOROQUINOLONES

Although fluoroquinolones frequently are used for empiric TD treatment in adults, these medications are not approved by the US Food and Drug Administration (FDA) for this purpose in children aged <18 years because of cartilage damage seen in animal studies. The American Academy of Pediatrics (AAP) suggests that fluoroquinolones be considered for treatment of children with severe infections caused by multidrug-resistant strains of *Campylobacter jejuni*, *Salmonella* species, *Shigella* species, or *Vibrio cholerae*.

Fluoroquinolone resistance in gastrointestinal organisms has been reported from some countries, particularly in Asia. In addition, use of fluoroquinolones has been associated with tendinopathies, development of *Clostridioides difficile* infection, and central nervous system side effects including confusion and hallucinations. Routine use of fluoroquinolones for prophylaxis or empiric treatment for TD among children is not recommended.

RIFAXIMIN

Rifaximin is approved for use in children aged ≥12 years but has limited use for empiric treatment since it is only approved to treat noninvasive strains of *Escherichia coli*. Children with bloody diarrhea should receive medical attention, because antibiotic treatment of enterohemorrhagic *E. coli*, a cause of bloody diarrhea, has been associated with increased risk for hemolytic uremic syndrome (see Sec. 5, Part 1, Ch. 7, Diarrheagenic *Escherichia coli*).

ANTIEMETICS & ANTIMOTILITY DRUGS

Antiemetics generally are not recommended for self- or family-administered treatment of children with vomiting and TD. Because of the association between salicylates and Reye syndrome, bismuth subsalicylate (BSS), the active ingredient in both Pepto-Bismol and Kaopectate, is not generally recommended to treat diarrhea in children <12 years old. In certain circumstances, however, some clinicians use it off-label, with caution. Care should be taken if administering BSS to children with viral infections (e.g., influenza, varicella), because of the risk for Reye syndrome. BSS is not recommended for children aged <3 years.

Use of antiemetics for children with acute gastroenteritis is controversial; some clinical practice guidelines include the use of antiemetics, others do not. A Cochrane Collaboration Review of the use of antiemetics for reducing vomiting related to acute gastroenteritis in children and adolescents showed some benefits with dimenhydrinate, metoclopramide, or ondansetron. Guidelines from the Infectious Diseases Society of America suggest that an antinausea and antiemetic medication (e.g., ondansetron) can facilitate tolerance of oral rehydration in children >4 years of age, and in adolescents with acute gastroenteritis.

A recent systematic review and network meta-analysis comparing several antiemetics in acute gastroenteritis in children showed that ondansetron was the best intervention to reduce vomiting and prevent hospitalization and the need for intravenous rehydration. Routine use of these medications as part of self-treatment for emesis associated with TD in children has not yet been studied, however, and is not generally recommended.

Antimotility drugs (e.g., the opioid receptor agonists loperamide and diphenoxylate), generally should not be given to children <18 years of age with acute diarrhea. Loperamide is particularly contraindicated for children aged <2 years because of the risks for respiratory depression and serious cardiac events. Diphenoxylate and atropine combination tablets should not be used for children aged <2 years, and should be used judiciously in older children because of potential side effects (see Sec. 2, Ch. 6, Travelers' Diarrhea).

FLUID & NUTRITION MANAGEMENT

The biggest threat to an infant with diarrhea and vomiting is dehydration. Fever or increased ambient temperature increases fluid loss and accelerates dehydration. Advise adults traveling with children about the signs and symptoms of dehydration and the proper use of oral rehydration solution (ORS). Advise adults traveling with children to seek medical attention for an infant or young child with diarrhea who has signs of moderate to severe dehydration, bloody diarrhea, body temperature >101.3°F (38.5°C), or persistent vomiting (unable to maintain oral hydration). Adequate hydration is the mainstay of TD management.

ORAL REHYDRATION SOLUTION: USE & AVAILABILITY

Counsel parents that dehydration is best prevented and treated by ORS in addition to the infant's usual food. While seeking medical attention, caregivers should provide ORS to infants by bottle, cup, oral syringe (often available in pharmacies), or spoon. Low-osmolarity ORS is the most effective agent in preventing dehydration, although other formulations are available and can be used if they are more palatable to young children. Homemade sugar-salt solutions are not recommended.

Sports drinks are designed to replace water and electrolytes lost through sweat, and do not contain the same proportions of electrolytes as the solution recommended by the World Health Organization for rehydration during diarrheal illness. Drinks with a high sugar content (e.g., juice, soft drinks) can worsen diarrhea. If ORS is not readily available, however, offer children whatever safe liquid they will take until ORS is obtained. Breastfed infants should continue to breastfeed (for more details, see Sec. 7, Ch. 2, Travel & Breastfeeding).

ORS can be made from prepackaged glucose and electrolytes packets available at stores or pharmacies in almost all countries. Some pharmacies and stores that specialize in outdoor recreation and camping supplies also sell ORS packets.

ORS is prepared by adding 1 packet to boiled or treated water (see Sec. 2, Ch. 9, Water Disinfection). Advise travelers to check packet instructions carefully to ensure that the contents are added to the correct volume of water. Once prepared, ORS should be consumed or discarded within 12 hours if held at room temperature, or within 24 hours if kept refrigerated. A dehydrated child will usually drink ORS avidly and should continue to receive ORS if dehydration persists.

As dehydration lessens, the child might refuse the salty-tasting ORS, and adults can offer other safe liquids. An infant or child who has been vomiting will usually keep ORS down if it is offered by spoon or oral syringe in small sips; adults should offer these small sips frequently, however, so the child can receive an adequate volume of ORS. Older children will often drink well by sipping through a straw. Severely dehydrated children often will be unable to drink adequately. Severe dehydration is a medical emergency that usually requires administration of fluids by intravenous or intraosseous routes.

In general, children weighing <22 lb (10 kg) who have mild to moderate dehydration should be administered 2–4 oz (60–120 mL) of ORS for each diarrheal stool or vomiting episode. Children who weigh ≥22 lb (10 kg) should receive 4–8 oz (120–240 mL) of ORS for each diarrheal stool or vomiting episode. AAP provides detailed guidance on rehydration for vomiting and diarrhea at www.healthychildren.org/English/health-issues/conditions/abdominal/Pages/Treating-Dehydration-with-Electrolyte-Solution.aspx.

DIET MODIFICATION

Breastfed infants should continue nursing on demand. Formula-fed infants should continue their usual formula during rehydration and should receive a volume sufficient to satisfy energy and nutrient requirements. Lactose-free or lactose-reduced formulas usually are unnecessary. Diluting formula can slow resolution of diarrhea and is not recommended.

Older infants and children receiving semisolid or solid foods should continue to receive their usual diet during the illness. Recommended foods include cereals, fruits and vegetables, starches, and pasteurized yogurt. Travelers should avoid giving children food high in simple sugars (e.g., undiluted apple juice, presweetened cereals, gelatins, soft drinks) because these can exacerbate diarrhea by osmotic effects. In addition, foods high in fat tend to delay gastric emptying, and thus might not be well tolerated by ill children.

Travelers should not withhold food for ≥24 hours. Early feeding can decrease changes in intestinal permeability caused by infection, reduce illness duration, and improve nutritional outcome. Although highly specific diets (e.g., the BRAT [bananas, rice, applesauce, toast] diet) or juice-based and clear fluid diets commonly are recommended, such severely restrictive diets have no scientific basis and should be avoided.

Malaria

Malaria is among the most serious and life-threatening infections acquired by pediatric international travelers. Pediatric VFR travelers are at particularly high risk for malaria infection if they do not receive prophylaxis. Among people reported with malaria in the United States in 2017, 17% were children <18 years old; 89% had traveled to Africa. Seventy percent of the children who were US residents also were VFR travelers, and 61% did not take malaria chemoprophylaxis.

Children with malaria can rapidly develop high levels of parasitemia and are at increased risk for severe complications of malaria, including seizures, coma, and death. Initial symptoms can mimic many other common causes of pediatric febrile illness, which could delay diagnosis and treatment. Among 33 children with imported malaria diagnosed at 11 medical centers in New York City, 11 (32%) had severe malaria and 14 (43%) were initially misdiagnosed. Counsel adults traveling with children to malaria-endemic areas to use preventive measures, be aware of the signs and symptoms of malaria, and seek prompt medical attention if symptoms develop.

ANTIMALARIAL DRUGS

Pediatric doses for malaria prophylaxis are provided in Table 5-27. Calculate dosing based on body weight. Medications used for infants and young children are the same as those recommended for adults, except atovaquone-proguanil, which should not be used for prophylaxis in children weighing <5 kg because of lack of data on safety and efficacy. Doxycycline should not be recommended for malaria prophylaxis for children aged <8 years. Although doxycycline has not been associated with dental staining when given as a routine treatment for some infections, other tetracyclines might cause teeth staining.

Atovaquone-proguanil, chloroquine, and mefloquine have a bitter taste. Mixing pulverized tablets in a small amount of food or drink can facilitate the administration of antimalarial drugs to infants and children. Clinicians also can ask compounding pharmacists to pulverize tablets and prepare gelatin capsules with calculated pediatric doses. A compounding pharmacy can alter the flavoring of malaria medication tablets so that children are more willing to take them. The Find a Compounder section on the Alliance for Pharmacy Compounding website (http://a4pc.org/; 281-933-8400) can help with finding a compounding pharmacy. Because overdose of antimalarial drugs, particularly chloroquine, can be fatal, store medication in childproof containers and keep out of the reach of infants and children.

PERSONAL PROTECTIVE MEASURES & REPELLENT USE

Children should sleep in rooms with air conditioning or screened windows, or sleep under mosquito nets when air conditioning or screens are not available. Mosquito netting should be used over infant carriers. Children can reduce skin exposed to mosquitoes by wearing long pants and long sleeves while outdoors. Clothing and mosquito nets can be treated with an insect repellent/insecticide (e.g., permethrin) that repels and kills ticks, mosquitoes, and other arthropods. Permethrin remains effective through multiple washings. Clothing and mosquito nets should be retreated according to the product label. Permethrin should not be applied to the skin.

Although permethrin provides a longer duration of protection, recommended repellents that can be applied to skin also can be used on clothing and mosquito nets (see Sec. 4, Ch. 6, Mosquitoes, Ticks & Other Arthropods, for more details about these protective measures). The Centers for Disease Control and Prevention (CDC) recommends using US Environmental Protection Agency (EPA)–registered repellents (see www.epa.gov/insect-repellents/find-repellent-right-you) containing one of the following active ingredients: DEET (*N,N*-diethyl-*m*-toluamide); picaridin; oil of lemon eucalyptus (OLE); PMD (para-menthane-3,8-diol); IR3535; or 2-undecanone (methyl nonyl ketone). Repellent products must state any age restriction; if no age restriction is provided, EPA has not required a restriction on the use of the product. Most EPA-registered repellents can be used on children aged >2 months, except products containing OLE or PMD that specify they should not be used on children aged <3 years. Insect repellents containing DEET, picaridin, IR3535, or 2-undecanone can be used on children without age restriction.

Many repellents contain DEET as the active ingredient. DEET concentration varies considerably between products. The duration of protection varies with DEET concentration; higher concentrations protect longer; products with DEET concentration >50% do not, however, offer a marked increase in protection time.

The EPA has approved DEET for use on children without an age restriction. If used appropriately, DEET does not represent a health problem. The AAP states that the use of products with the lowest effective DEET concentrations (i.e., 20%–30%) seems most prudent for infants and young children, on whom it should be applied sparingly. For more tips on protecting babies and children from mosquito bites, see Box 7-04 and www.cdc.gov/mosquitoes/mosquito-bites/prevent-mosquito-bites.html.

Combination products containing repellents and sunscreen are generally not recommended because instructions for use are different, and sunscreen might need to be reapplied more often and in larger amounts than repellent. In general, apply sunscreen first, and then apply repellent. Mosquito coils should be used with caution in the presence of children to avoid burns and inadvertent ingestion. For detailed information about repellent use and other protective measures, see Sec. 4, Ch. 6, Mosquitoes, Ticks & Other Arthropods.

Rabies

Depending on travel destination and activities, animal exposures and bites might be a health risk for pediatric travelers. Worldwide, rabies is more common in children than adults. In addition to the potential for increased contact with animals, children also are more likely to be bitten on the head or neck, leading to more severe injuries. Counsel children and their families to avoid all stray or unfamiliar animals and to inform adults of any animal contact or bites. Bats throughout the world have the potential to transmit rabies virus.

Travelers should clean all bite and scratch wounds as soon as possible after the event occurs by using soap and water, or povidine iodine if available, for ≥20 minutes to prevent infections, (e.g., rabies). Wounds contaminated with necrotic tissue, dirt, or other foreign materials should be cleaned and debrided promptly by health care professionals, where possible. A course of antibiotics might be appropriate after animal bites or scratches, because these can lead to local or systemic infections. For mammal bites and scratches, children should be evaluated promptly to assess their need for rabies postexposure prophylaxis (see Sec. 4, Ch. 7, Zoonotic Exposures: Bites, Stings, Scratches & Other Hazards; and Sec. 5, Part 2, Ch. 18, Rabies).

7

BOX 7-04 Protecting infants & children from mosquito bites: recommendations for travelers

Dress children in clothing that covers arms and legs.
Cover strollers and baby carriers with mosquito netting.
Properly use insect repellent

- Always follow all label instructions.
- In general, do not use products containing oil of lemon eucalyptus (OLE) or para-menthane-diol (PMD) on children <3 years old.
- Do not apply insect repellent to a child's hands, eyes, mouth, cuts, or irritated skin.
- Adults should spray insect repellent onto their hands and then apply to a child's face.

Because rabies vaccine and rabies immune globulin might not be available in certain destinations, encourage families traveling to areas with high risk for rabies exposure to seriously consider preexposure rabies vaccination and to purchase medical evacuation insurance, depending on their destination and planned travel activities (see Sec. 7, Ch. 4, Vaccine Recommendations for Infants & Children, and Sec. 6, Ch. 1, Travel Insurance, Travel Health Insurance & Medical Evacuation Insurance).

Soil & Water Contact: Infections & Infestations

Children are more likely than adults to have contact with soil or sand, and therefore could be exposed to diseases caused by infectious stages of parasites in soil, including ascariasis, hookworm, cutaneous or visceral larva migrans, strongyloidiasis, and trichuriasis. Children and infants should wear protective footwear and play on a sheet or towel rather than directly on the ground. Clothing should not be dried on the ground. In countries with a tropical climate, clothing or diapers dried in the open air should be ironed before use to prevent infestation with fly larvae.

7

Schistosomiasis is a risk to children and adults in endemic areas. While in schistosomiasis-endemic areas (see Sec. 5, Part 3, Ch. 20, Schistosomiasis), children should not bathe, swim, or wade in fresh, unchlorinated water (e.g., lakes, ponds).

NONINFECTIOUS HAZARDS & RISKS

Air Travel

Although air travel is safe for most newborns, infants, and children, people traveling with children should consider a few issues before departure. Children with chronic heart or lung problems might be at risk for hypoxia during flight, and caregivers should consult a clinician before travel.

EAR PAIN

Ear pain can be troublesome for infants and children during descent. Pressure in the middle ear can be equalized by swallowing or chewing; thus, infants should nurse or suck on a bottle, and older children can try chewing gum. Antihistamines and decongestants have not been shown to be of benefit. No evidence suggests that air travel exacerbates the symptoms or complications associated with otitis media.

JET LAG

Travel to different time zones, jet lag, and schedule disruptions can disturb sleep patterns in infants and children, just as in adults (Sec. 8, Ch. 4, Jet Lag).

SAFETY RESTRAINTS

Travelers also should ensure that children can be restrained safely during a flight. Severe turbulence or a crash can create enough momentum that an adult cannot hold onto a child. The safest place for a child on an airplane is in a government-approved child safety restraint system (CRS) or device. The Federal Aviation Administration (FAA) strongly urges travelers to secure children in a CRS for the duration of the flight. Car seats cannot be used in all seats or on all planes, and some airlines might have limited safety equipment available. Travelers should check with the airline about specific restrictions and approved child restraint options. FAA provides additional information at www.faa.gov/travelers/fly_children.

Altitude Illness & Acute Mountain Sickness

Children are as susceptible to the deleterious effects of high elevation travel as adults (see Sec. 4, Ch. 5, High Elevation Travel & Altitude Illness). Slow ascent is the preferable approach for avoiding acute mountain sickness (AMS). Young children unable to talk can show nonspecific symptoms (e.g., loss of appetite or irritability, unexplained fussiness, changes in sleep and activity patterns). Older children might complain of headache or shortness of breath. If children demonstrate unexplained symptoms after an ascent, descent could be necessary.

Acetazolamide is not approved for pediatric use in children aged <12 years for altitude illness but is generally safe for use in children for other indications. Some providers prescribe acetazolamide to prevent AMS in pediatric travelers <12 years of age when a slow ascent is not feasible. The dose is 2.5 mg/kg every 12 hours, up to a maximum of 125 mg per dose, twice a day. No liquid formulation is available, but tablets can be crushed or packaged by a compounding pharmacy for a correct dose.

Drinking Water Contaminants

Drinking water disinfection does not remove environmental contaminants (e.g., lead or other metals). Travelers might want to carry specific filters designed to remove environmental contaminants, particularly for travel where the risk for exposure is greater due to larger amounts of water consumed (e.g., long-term travel or when living abroad). Filters should meet National Science Foundation (NSF) and American National Standards Institute (ANSI) standards 53 or 58 (see www.cdc.gov/nceh/lead/prevention/sources/water.htm).

Injuries

ACCOMMODATIONS: HOTELS & OTHER LODGINGS

Conditions at hotels and other lodgings abroad might not be as safe as those in the United States; adults traveling with children should carefully inspect accommodations for paint chips, pest poisons, inadequate balcony or stairway railings, or exposed wiring.

Adult caregivers should plan to provide a safe sleeping environment for infants during international travel. Caregivers should follow general recommendations from the AAP task force on preventing sudden infant death syndrome (SIDS) and other sleep-related causes of infant death (see https://services.aap.org/en/patient-care/safe-sleep). Cribs in some locations might not meet US safety standards. Additional information about crib safety is available from the US Consumer Product Safety Commission at www.cpsc.gov/SafeSleep.

MOTOR VEHICLES

Vehicle-related injuries are the leading cause of death in children who travel. Whenever traveling in an automobile or other vehicle, children should be properly restrained in a car seat, booster seat, or with a seat belt, as appropriate for their age, height, and weight. Information about child passenger safety is available at www.healthychildren.org/English/safety-prevention/on-the-go/Pages/Car-Safety-Seats-Information-for-Families.aspx. Car seats often must be brought from home because well-maintained and approved seats might not be available (or limited in availability) in other countries.

In general, children ≤12 years of age are safest when properly buckled in the rear seat of the car while traveling; no one should ever travel in the bed of a pickup truck. Advise families that cars might lack front or rear seatbelts in many low- and middle-income countries. Traveling families should attempt to arrange transportation or rent vehicles with seatbelts and other safety features.

All family members should wear helmets when riding bicycles, motorcycles, or scooters. Pedestrians should take caution when crossing streets, particularly in countries where cars drive on the left, because children might not be used to looking in that direction before crossing.

WATER-RELATED INJURIES & DROWNING

Drowning is the second leading cause of death in young travelers. Children might not be familiar with hazards in the ocean or in rivers. Swimming pools might not have protective fencing to keep toddlers and young children from accessing pool areas unattended. Adults should closely supervise children around water. An adult with swimming skills should be within an arm's length when infants and toddlers are in or around pools and other bodies of water; even for older children and better swimmers, the supervising adult should focus on the child and not be engaged with any distracting activities.

Water safety devices (e.g., personal flotation devices [lifejackets]) might not be available abroad, and families should consider bringing these from home. In addition, adults should ensure children wear protective footwear to avoid injury in many marine environments.

Sun Exposure

Sun exposure, and particularly sunburn before age 15 years, is strongly associated with melanoma and other forms of skin cancer (see Sec. 4, Ch. 1, Sun Exposure). Exposure to ultraviolet (UV) light is greatest near the equator, at high elevations, during midday (10 a.m.–4 p.m.), and where light is reflected off water or snow.

Physical, also known as inorganic, UV filters (sunscreens) generally are recommended for children aged >6 months. Less irritating to children's sensitive skin than chemical sunscreens, physical UV filters (e.g., titanium oxide, zinc oxide) should be applied as directed and reapplied as needed after sweating and water exposure. Babies aged <6 months require extra protection from the sun because of their thinner and more sensitive skin; severe sunburn in young infants is considered a medical emergency.

Advise parents that babies should be kept in the shade and dressed in clothing that covers the entire body. A minimal amount of sunscreen can be applied to small, exposed areas, including the infant's face and hands. For older children, sun-blocking shirts made for swimming preclude having to apply sunscreen over the entire trunk. Hats and sunglasses also reduce sun injury to skin and eyes.

If both sunscreen and a DEET-containing insect repellent are used, apply the sunscreen first and the insect repellent second (i.e., over the sunscreen). Because insect repellent can diminish the level of UV protection provided by the sunscreen by as much as one-third, children should also wear sun-protective clothing, reapply sunscreen, or decrease their time in the sun, accordingly.

7

OTHER CONSIDERATIONS

Identification

In case family members become separated, each infant or child should carry identifying information and contact numbers in their clothing or pockets. Because of concerns about illegal transport of children across international borders, parents traveling alone with children should carry relevant custody papers or a notarized permission letter from the other parent.

Insurance

As with adult travelers, verify insurance coverage for illnesses and injuries while abroad before departure. Travelers should consider purchasing special medical evacuation insurance for an airlift or air ambulance transport to facilities capable of providing adequate medical care (see Sec. 6, Ch. 1, Travel Insurance, Travel Health Insurance & Medical Evacuation Insurance).

Travel Stress

Changes in schedule, activities, and environment can be stressful for children. Travelers can help decrease these stresses by including children in planning for the trip and bringing along familiar toys or other objects. For children with chronic illnesses, make decisions regarding timing and itinerary in consultation with the child's health care providers.

BIBLIOGRAPHY

Ashkenazi S, Schwartz E. Traveler's diarrhea in children: new insights and existing gaps. Travel Med Infect Dis. 2020;34:101503.

Fedorowicz Z, Jagannath VA, Carter B. Antiemetics for reducing vomiting related to acute gastroenteritis in children and adolescents. Cochrane Database Syst Rev. 2011;2011(9):CD005506.

Goldman-Yassen AE, Mony VK, Arguin PM, Daily JP. Higher rates of misdiagnosis in pediatric patients versus adults hospitalized with imported malaria. Pediatr Emerg Care. 2016;32(4):227–31.

Hagmann S, LaRocque R, Rao S, Jentes E, Sotir M, Brunette G, et al.; Global TravEpiNet Consortium. Pre-travel health preparation of pediatric international travelers: analysis from the Global TravEpiNet Consortium. J Pediatric Infect Dis Soc. 2013;2(4):327–34.

Hagmann S, Neugebauer R, Schwartz E, Perret C, Castelli F, Barnett ED, et al. Illness in children after international travel: analysis from the GeoSentinel Surveillance Network. Pediatrics. 2010;125(5):e1072–80.

Han P, Yanni E, Jentes E, Hamer D, Chen L, Wilson M, et al. Health challenges of young travelers visiting friends and relatives compared with those traveling for other purposes. Pediatr Infect Dis J. 2012;31(9):915–9.

Herbinger KH, Drerup L, Alberer M, Nothdurft HD, Sonnenburg F, Loscher T. Spectrum of imported infectious diseases among children and adolescents returning from the tropics and subtropics. J Travel Med. 2012;19(3):150–7.

Hunziker T, Berger C, Staubli G, Tschopp A, Weber R, Nadal D, et al. Profile of travel-associated illness in children, Zurich, Switzerland. J Travel Med. 2012;19(3):158–62.

Mace K, Lucchi N, Tan K. Malaria surveillance—United States, 2017. MMWR Surveill Summ. 2021;70(2):1–40.

Niño-Serna LF, Acosta-Reyes J, Veroniki AA, Florez ID. Antiemetics in children with acute gastroenteritis: a meta-analysis. Pediatrics. 2020;145(4):e20183696.

VACCINE RECOMMENDATIONS FOR INFANTS & CHILDREN

Michelle Weinberg

Vaccinating children for travel requires careful evaluation. Whenever possible, children should complete routine childhood immunizations on a normal schedule. Travel at an earlier age, however, might require accelerated vaccine schedules. Not all travel-related vaccines are effective in infants, and some are specifically contraindicated.

Recommended childhood and adolescent immunization schedules are available at www.cdc.gov/vaccines/schedules/hcp/imz/child-adolescent.html. The Centers for Disease Control and Prevention (CDC) provides a catch-up schedule for children and adolescents who start a vaccination schedule late or who are >1 month behind (see www.cdc.gov/vaccines/schedules/hcp/imz/catchup.html). Tables also describe the recommended minimum intervals between doses for children who need to be vaccinated on an accelerated schedule, which could be necessary before international travel.

Country-specific vaccination recommendations and requirements for departure and entry vary over time. For example, proof of yellow fever vaccination is required for entry into certain countries. Meningococcal vaccination is required for travelers entering Saudi Arabia for Umrah or the annual Hajj pilgrimage. The World Health Organization (WHO) has issued temporary vaccination recommendations for residents of and long-term visitors to countries with active circulation of wild or vaccine-derived poliovirus. Some countries might require coronavirus disease 2019 (COVID-19) vaccine, testing, or both for entry. Check the CDC Travelers' Health website for current requirements and recommendations (https://wwwnc.cdc.gov/travel).

Additional information about diseases and routine vaccination is available in the disease-specific chapters in Section 5. Tools for determining routine and catch-up childhood vaccination are available at www.cdc.gov/vaccines/schedules/index.html.

MODIFYING IMMUNIZATION SCHEDULES FOR INFANTS & YOUNG CHILDREN BEFORE INTERNATIONAL TRAVEL

Several factors influence recommendations for the age at which a vaccine is administered, including age-specific risks for the disease and its complications, age-dependent ability to develop an adequate immune response to a vaccine, and potential interference with the immune response by passively transferred maternal antibodies.

Immunization schedules for infants and children in the United States do not provide guidance on modifications for people traveling internationally before the age when specific vaccines are routinely recommended. Age limits for vaccine administration are based on the risk for potential adverse events (e.g., yellow fever vaccine), lack of efficacy data or inadequate immune response (e.g., influenza vaccine, polysaccharide vaccines), maternal antibody interference and immaturity of the immune system (e.g., measles-mumps-rubella [MMR] vaccine), or lack of safety data.

To help parents decide when to travel with an infant or young child, advise them that the earliest opportunity to receive routinely recommended immunizations in the United States (except for doses of hepatitis B vaccine at birth and age 1 month) is when the baby is 6 weeks old. In general, live-virus vaccines (MMR, varicella, yellow fever) should be administered on the same day or spaced ≥28 days apart.

ROUTINE INFANT & CHILDHOOD VACCINES

Children should be vaccinated against diphtheria, *Haemophilus influenzae* type b (Hib), hepatitis A and hepatitis B virus, human papillomavirus, influenza, measles, mumps, *Neisseria meningitidis*, pertussis, polio, rotavirus, rubella, *Streptococcus pneumoniae*, tetanus, and varicella. To complete a vaccine series before travel, doses can be administered at the minimum ages and dose intervals. Inform parents that infants and children who have not received all recommended vaccine doses might not be fully protected. Rotavirus vaccine is unique among the routine vaccines given to infants in the United States because it has maximum ages for both the first and last doses; specifically consider the timing of travel so that the infant will be able to receive the complete vaccine series, if possible.

Coronavirus Disease 2019

The COVID-19 pandemic continues to evolve, and CDC's vaccination recommendations are updated regularly. For the most current recommendations for children and teens, see www.cdc.gov/coronavirus/2019-ncov/vaccines/stay-up-to-date.html. COVID-19 vaccines available for use in the United States can be administered simultaneously with all other vaccines.

7

Hepatitis A

Hepatitis A infection is usually mild or asymptomatic in infants and children <5 years old. Infected children can, however, transmit the infection to older children and adults, age groups at greater risk for severe disease. Ensure vaccination for all children traveling to areas with an intermediate or high risk for hepatitis A (see Sec. 5, Part 2, Ch. 7, Hepatitis A). Routine hepatitis A vaccination for children aged ≥12 months consists of 2 doses, separated by ≥6 months. Ideally, the first dose should be administered ≥2 weeks before travel. When protection against hepatitis A is recommended, infants aged 6–11 months should receive 1 dose of hepatitis A vaccine before travel outside the United States.

Hepatitis A vaccine is considered safe and immunogenic in infants; doses administered before 12 months of age, however, can result in a suboptimal immune response, particularly in infants with passively acquired maternal antibody. Therefore, doses administered to infants <12 months old are not considered to provide long-term protection; initiate the 2-dose hepatitis A vaccine series at age 12 months according to the routine immunization schedule.

HEPATITIS A IMMUNE GLOBULIN

When protection against hepatitis A is recommended, infants <6 months old should receive immune globulin (IG) before travel. One dose of 0.1 mL/kg intramuscularly provides protection for ≤1 month. Infants who do not receive vaccination who will be traveling for >1 month but ≤2 months should receive an IG dose of 0.2 mL/kg. If the traveler remains in a high-risk setting, IG (0.2 mL/kg) should be administered every 2 months until hepatitis A vaccine can be given at ≥6 months of age, if not contraindicated.

For optimal protection, children aged ≥1 year who are immunocompromised or who have chronic medical conditions, and who will be traveling to a high-risk area in <2 weeks, should receive the initial dose of hepatitis A vaccine and IG at separate anatomic injection sites.

RECOMMENDED DOSING INTERVALS FOR COADMINISTRATION OF LIVE-VIRUS VACCINES

Hepatitis A IG is an antibody-containing product that does not interfere with the immune response to yellow fever vaccine but can inhibit the response to other injected live-virus vaccines (e.g., MMR, varicella) for up to 6 months after administration (see Sec. 2, Ch. 3, Vaccination & Immunoprophylaxis—General Principles).

MMR vaccine is recommended for all infants aged 6–11 months traveling internationally. Because measles in infancy is a more severe disease than hepatitis A, administer hepatitis A vaccine and MMR vaccine simultaneously to infants aged 6–11 months to provide protection against hepatitis A and measles, but do not give hepatitis A IG.

If the interval between MMR or varicella vaccine administration and subsequent administration of an antibody-containing product is <14 days, repeat vaccination after the recommended interval unless serologic testing indicates a protective antibody response. For information about dosing intervals, see The Timing and Spacing of Immunobiologics, General Best Practice Guidelines for Immunization: Best Practices Guidance of the Advisory Committee on Immunization Practices, Table 3-4 (www.cdc.gov/vaccines/hcp/acip-recs/general-recs/timing.html#t-04) and Table 3-5 (www.cdc.gov/vaccines/hcp/acip-recs/general-recs/timing.html#t-05).

Hepatitis B

For certain age groups, hepatitis B vaccine can be administered with an accelerated schedule of 4 doses of vaccine given at 0, 1, 2, and 12 months; the last dose can be given after the child returns from travel (see Sec. 5, Part 2, Ch. 8, Hepatitis B, for details).

Influenza

Influenza viruses circulate predominantly in the winter months in temperate regions (typically November–April in the Northern Hemisphere and April–September in the Southern Hemisphere) but can occur year-round in tropical climates (see Sec. 5, Part 2, Ch. 12, Influenza). Because influenza viruses can circulate any time of the year, travelers aged ≥6 months who were not vaccinated during the influenza season in their country of residence should be vaccinated ≥2 weeks before departure if vaccine is available.

Children aged 6 months–8 years who have never received influenza vaccine, or who have not previously received a lifetime total of ≥2 doses, should receive 2 doses separated by ≥4 weeks. For annually updated recommendations about seasonal influenza vaccination, see www.cdc.gov/vaccines/hcp/acip-recs/vacc-specific/flu.html.

Measles-Mumps-Rubella or Measles-Mumps-Rubella-Varicella

Children traveling abroad need to be vaccinated against measles, mumps, and rubella at an age earlier than what is routinely recommended. Infants 6–11 months old should receive 1 MMR vaccine dose. Infants vaccinated before age 12 months must be revaccinated on or after their first birthday with 2 doses of MMR vaccine (separated by ≥28 days) or measles-mumps-rubella-varicella (MMRV) vaccine (separated ≥3 months). The minimum interval between any varicella-containing vaccine (MMRV or monovalent varicella) is 3 months.

MMRV vaccine is licensed for use in children aged 12 months–12 years and should not be given outside this age group. Recipients of a first dose of MMRV vaccine have a greater risk for febrile seizures compared with recipients of MMR and varicella vaccines administered concomitantly. Unless the caregiver expresses a preference for MMRV, CDC recommends administering separate MMR and varicella vaccine for the first dose of MMR and varicella vaccination for children 12–47 months.

Meningococcal

QUADRIVALENT CONJUGATE

Children aged 2 months–18 years who travel to or reside in areas of sub-Saharan Africa known as the meningitis belt during the dry season (December–June) should receive quadrivalent meningococcal conjugate (MenACWY) vaccine (see Sec. 5, Part 1, Ch. 13, Meningococcal Disease). In addition, travelers are required to have meningococcal vaccination to enter Saudi Arabia when traveling to Mecca for Umrah or the annual Hajj pilgrimage. The CDC Travelers' Health website (https://wwwnc.cdc.gov/travel) provides annual health requirements and recommendations for US travelers going to Mecca for Umrah or Hajj (also see Sec. 10, Part 1, Ch. 2, Saudi Arabia: Hajj & Umrah Pilgrimages).

The schedule for primary series meningococcal vaccine and booster doses varies depending on the vaccine administered (www.cdc.gov/vaccines/schedules/hcp/imz/child-adolescent.html#note-mening).

MENINGOCOCCAL B

Unless an outbreak of serogroup B disease has been reported, vaccination with a serogroup B meningococcal (MenB) vaccine is not routinely recommended for travel to the meningitis belt or other regions of the world. Although MenB vaccine is not licensed in the United States for children <10 years of age, some European countries recently introduced MenB vaccine as a routine immunization for infants. Some countries might have other meningococcal vaccines available. Consider meningococcal vaccination for infants residing in these countries according to the routine infant immunization recommendations of that country.

Polio

Polio vaccine is recommended for travelers going to countries with evidence of wild poliovirus (WPV) or vaccine-derived poliovirus circulating during the last 12 months, and for travelers with a high risk for exposure to someone with imported WPV infection when traveling to some countries that border areas with WPV circulation. Refer to the CDC Travelers' Health website destination pages for current polio vaccine recommendations (https://wwwnc.cdc.gov/travel/destinations/list).

Ensure that travelers complete the recommended age-appropriate polio vaccine series and receive a single lifetime booster dose, if necessary. Infants and children should receive an accelerated schedule to complete the routine series. See Sec. 5, Part 2, Ch. 17, Poliomyelitis, and CDC's Immunization Schedules website (www.cdc.gov/vaccines/schedules/hcp/imz/child-adolescent.html#note-polio) for information about accelerated schedules.

People ≥18 years of age traveling to areas where polio vaccine is recommended and who have received a routine series with either inactivated polio vaccine (IPV) or live oral polio vaccine in childhood should receive a single lifetime booster dose of IPV before departure. Available data do not indicate the need for more than a single lifetime booster dose with IPV. Requirements for long-term travelers might apply, however, when departing from certain countries.

7

LONG-TERM TRAVELERS TO COUNTRIES WITH POLIOVIRUS TRANSMISSION

In May 2014, the World Health Organization (WHO) declared the international spread of polio to be a Public Health Emergency of International Concern under the authority of the International Health Regulations (2005). To prevent further spread of disease, WHO issued temporary polio vaccine recommendations for long-term travelers (staying >4 weeks) and residents departing from countries with WPV transmission ("exporting WPV" or "infected with WPV") or with circulating vaccine-derived polioviruses types 1 or 3.

Long-term travelers and residents could be required to show proof of polio vaccination when departing from these countries for any destination. All polio vaccination administration should be documented on an International Certificate of Vaccination or Prophylaxis (ICVP). For ordering information and instructions on how to fill out the ICVP, see https://wwwnc.cdc.gov/travel/page/icvp. The polio vaccine must be received 4 weeks–12 months before the date of departure from the polio-infected country.

Country requirements can change, so clinicians should check for updates on the CDC Travelers' Health website (https://wwwnc.cdc.gov/travel/).

TRAVEL VACCINES FOR INFANTS & CHILDREN

Dengue

Dengue can cause mild to severe illness (see Sec. 5, Part 2, Ch. 4, Dengue). Although many people have asymptomatic infections, for some children dengue can be life-threatening. Travelers should adhere to mosquito protection measures during travel to dengue-endemic areas (see Sec. 4, Ch. 6, Mosquitoes, Ticks & Other Arthropods).

In June 2021, the Advisory Committee on Immunization Practices (ACIP) recommended the use of a live attenuated dengue virus vaccine, Dengvaxia (Sanofi Pasteur), to prevent disease in children aged 9–16 years. Children eligible to receive the vaccine include those with laboratory-confirmed previous dengue virus infection who live in areas of the United States, including the US territories of American Samoa, Puerto Rico, and the US Virgin Islands; and freely associated states, the Federated States of Micronesia, the Republic of Marshall Islands, and the Republic of Palau. Dengvaxia is not approved for use in US travelers who are visiting but who do not live in areas where dengue is endemic.

Only people who test positive for previous dengue infection or who have other laboratory-confirmed evidence of a previous dengue infection are eligible for vaccination with Dengvaxia (www.cdc.gov/dengue/vaccine/hcp/testing.html). In people without previous dengue infection, Dengvaxia can increase the risk for severe illness and hospitalization if the person gets infected after vaccination. Serodiagnostic tests recommended by health authorities with acceptable performance (≥75% sensitivity, ≥98% specificity) are available to test for evidence of previous dengue infection.

The vaccine is a series of 3 doses, administered 6 months apart at month 0, 6, and 12 months.

Japanese Encephalitis

Japanese encephalitis (JE) virus is transmitted by mosquitoes and is endemic throughout most of Asia and parts of the western Pacific. JE risk can be seasonal in temperate climates and year-round in more tropical climates. Risk to short-term travelers and those who confine their travel to urban centers is considered low. JE vaccine is recommended for travelers who plan to spend ≥1 month in endemic areas during JE virus transmission season. Consider JE vaccine for short-term (<1 month) travelers whose itinerary or activities could increase their risk for JE virus exposure. The decision to vaccinate a child should follow the more detailed recommendations found in Sec. 5, Part 2, Ch. 13, Japanese Encephalitis.

An inactivated Vero cell culture–derived JE vaccine (IXIARO) was licensed by the US Food and Drug Administration (FDA) in 2009 for use in the United States for travelers aged ≥17 years. In 2013, the recommendations were expanded, and the vaccine was licensed for use in children ≥2 months of age. For children aged 2 months–17 years, the primary series consists of 2 intramuscular doses administered 28 days apart. For travelers who received their primary JE vaccine series ≥1 year prior to potential JE virus exposure, ACIP recommends providing a booster dose before departure. Information on age-appropriate dosing is available at www.cdc.gov/japaneseencephalitis/vaccine/vaccineChildren.html.

Rabies

Rabies virus causes an acute viral encephalitis that is virtually 100% fatal. Traveling children can be at increased risk for rabies exposure, mainly from dogs that roam the streets in low- and middle-income countries. Bat bites carry a potential risk for rabies throughout the world. In addition to taking measures to avoid animal bites and scratches (see Sec. 4, Ch. 7, Zoonotic Exposures: Bites, Stings, Scratches & Other Hazards), preexposure and postexposure rabies prophylaxis is part of a broader approach to preventing this disease. Follow the recommendations in Sec. 5, Part 2, Ch. 18, Rabies, when making decisions about whether to provide rabies preexposure prophylaxis for children.

PREEXPOSURE PROPHYLAXIS

In June 2021, to align with the recently revised adult schedule, ACIP adjusted the number of recommended doses of rabies preexposure prophylaxis in children downward, from 3 to 2. For immunocompetent children <18 years old, administer the first dose of vaccine on day 0 and a second dose 7 days later (see Sec. 5, Part 2, Ch. 19, . . . *perspectives*: Rabies Immunization).

The advantages of the revised schedule are that it is both less expensive and easier to complete prior to travel. There are, however, no data on the duration of protection afforded by this 2-dose series. Because of this uncertainty, travelers with a sustained risk for rabies exposure should either have a titer drawn or receive a third dose of vaccine within 3 years of the initial series. Travelers unlikely to visit an at-risk destination after 3 years require no further titers or boosters unless they have a subsequent exposure.

POSTEXPOSURE PROPHYLAXIS

Children who have not received preexposure immunization and who might have been exposed to rabies require a weight-based dose of human rabies immune globulin (RIG) and a series of 4 rabies vaccine doses on days 0, 3, 7, and 14. Decisions about any changes in how to manage postexposure prophylaxis, schedule deviations for pre- or postexposure prophylaxis, and postexposure prophylaxis initiated abroad are expected from the ACIP.

Tick-Borne Encephalitis

Tick-borne encephalitis (TBE) is a viral disease transmitted by *Ixodes* ticks in parts of Asia and Europe. Rare in US travelers, TBE is usually asymptomatic but can appear as a biphasic illness with central nervous system involvement (see Sec. 5, Part 2, Ch. 23, Tick-Borne Encephalitis). Although TBE infection tends to be less severe in children, residual symptoms and neurologic deficits have been described.

Most infections result from the bite of infected tick, typically acquired when a person is bicycling, camping, hiking, or participating in other outdoor activities in brushy or forested areas. TBE also can be acquired by ingesting unpasteurized dairy products from infected animals, or, rarely, from direct person-to-person spread via blood transfusion, solid organ transplantation, or breastfeeding.

In August 2021, the FDA approved a TBE vaccine for people aged ≥1 year (www.fda.gov/vaccines-blood-biologics/ticovac); in February 2022, ACIP approved recommendations for vaccine use among people traveling or moving to a TBE-endemic area who will have extensive tick exposure based on planned outdoor activities and itinerary. Primary vaccination consists of 3 doses; the schedule varies by age. For children 1–15 years old, give the second dose 1–3 months after the first dose; for children aged ≥16 years, give the second dose 14 days–3 months after the first dose. All children should receive the third dose 5–12 months after receiving their second dose of the vaccine. A booster (fourth) dose can be given ≥3 years after completion of the primary immunization series if ongoing exposure or reexposure is expected.

Typhoid

Typhoid fever is caused by the bacterium *Salmonella enterica* serotype Typhi (see Sec. 5, Part 1, Ch. 24, Typhoid & Paratyphoid Fever). Travelers can avoid typhoid fever by following safe food and water precautions and frequently washing hands. Typhoid vaccine is recommended for travelers going to areas with a recognized risk for *Salmonella* Typhi exposure.

Two typhoid vaccines are licensed for use in the United States: Vi capsular polysaccharide vaccine (ViCPS) administered intramuscularly, and oral live attenuated vaccine (Ty21a). Both vaccines induce a protective response in 50%–80% of recipients. The ViCPS vaccine can be administered to children aged ≥2 years, who should receive a booster dose 2 years later if continued protection is needed. The Ty21a vaccine consists of a series of 4 capsules (1 taken orally every other day), which can be administered to children aged ≥6 years. Do not open capsules for administration; capsules must be swallowed whole. All 4 doses should be taken ≥1 week before potential exposure. A booster series for Ty21a should be taken every 5 years, if indicated.

Yellow Fever

Yellow fever, a disease transmitted by mosquitoes, is endemic to certain areas of Africa and South America (see Sec. 5, Part 2, Ch. 26, Yellow Fever). Proof of vaccination against yellow fever is required for entry into some countries (see Sec. 2, Ch. 5, Yellow Fever Vaccine & Malaria Prevention Information, by Country). Infants and children ≥9 months old and without contraindications should be vaccinated before traveling to countries where yellow fever is endemic.

Infants aged <9 months are at greater risk for developing encephalitis from yellow fever vaccine, which is a live-virus vaccine. Studies conducted during the early 1950s identified 4 cases of encephalitis out of 1,000 children aged <6 months who received yellow fever vaccine. An additional 10 cases of encephalitis associated with yellow fever vaccine administered to infants aged <4 months were reported worldwide during the 1950s.

Advise travelers with infants aged <9 months against traveling to areas where yellow fever is endemic. ACIP advises against administering yellow fever vaccine to infants aged <6 months. Infants aged 6–8 months should be vaccinated only if they must travel to areas of ongoing epidemic yellow fever, and if a high level of protection against mosquito bites is not possible. Clinicians considering vaccinating infants aged 6–8 months can consult their respective state health departments or CDC toll-free at 800-CDC-INFO (800-232-4636) or https://wwwn.cdc.gov/dcs/ContactUs/Form.

BIBLIOGRAPHY

Centers for Disease Control and Prevention. Japanese encephalitis vaccine: recommendations of the Advisory Committee on Immunization Practices. MMWR Recomm Rep. 2019;68(2):1–33.

Centers for Disease Control and Prevention. Meningococcal vaccination: recommendations of the Advisory Committee on Immunization Practices, 2020. MMWR Recomm Rep. 2020;69(9):1–41.

Centers for Disease Control and Prevention. Prevention of Hepatitis A virus infection in the United States: recommendations of the Advisory Committee on Immunization Practices. MMWR Recomm Rep. 2020;69(5):1–38.

Centers for Disease Control and Prevention. Use of a Modified Preexposure Prophylaxis Vaccination Schedule to Prevent Human Rabies: Recommendations of the Advisory Committee on Immunization Practices—United States, 2022. MMWR Morb Mortal Wkly Rep. 2022;71:619–27.

Centers for Disease Control and Prevention. Yellow fever vaccine: recommendations of the Advisory Committee on Immunization Practices (ACIP). MMWR Recomm Rep. 2015;64(23):647–50.

Global Polio Eradication Initiative. Public health emergency status: IHR public health emergency of international concern. Temporary recommendations to reduce international spread of poliovirus. Geneva: Global Polio Eradication Initiative; 2021. Available from: https://polioeradication.org/polio-today/polio-now/public-health-emergency-status.

Jackson BR, Iqbal S, Mahon B; Centers for Disease Control and Prevention (CDC). Updated recommendations for the use of typhoid vaccine—Advisory Committee on Immunization Practices, United States, 2015. MMWR Morb Mortal Wkly Rep. 2015;64(11):305–8.

Kimberlin DW, Barnett E, Lynfield R, Sawyer MH, editors. Red Book 2021–2024. Report of the Committee on Infectious Diseases, 32nd edition. Elk Grove Village (IL): American Academy of Pediatrics; 2021.

Paz-Bailey G, Adams L, Wong JM, Poehling KA, Chen WH, McNally V, et al. Dengue vaccine: recommendations of the Advisory Committee on Immunization Practices, United States, 2021. MMWR Recomm Rep. 2021;70(6);1–16.

INTERNATIONAL ADOPTION

Mary Allen Staat, Jennifer (Jenna) Beeler, Emily Jentes

Since 1999, >275,000 children have come to the United States to join families through international adoption. Children being adopted from other countries can have infectious (and environmental) diseases due to exposure to pathogens endemic to their birth country; they also might be underimmunized or unimmunized, have lacked access to clean water, lived in crowded or possibly unsanitary conditions, and be malnourished. Families traveling to unite with their adopted child, siblings who wait at home for the child's arrival, extended family members, and childcare providers are all at risk of acquiring infectious diseases secondary to travel or from contact with their new family member. Clinicians can play an important role in helping families prepare to travel and welcome adoptees safely.

PREPARING ADOPTIVE PARENTS & FAMILIES

Prospective adoptive parents should schedule a pretravel visit with a travel health clinic. To best prepare adoptive parents and families going to meet their new child, travel health providers should be aware of disease risks in the adopted child's country of origin, the medical and social history of the adoptee (if available), the medical and vaccination histories of family members traveling to meet the child, the season of travel, the length of stay in the country, and the itinerary. Provide prospective adoptive parents and any family members traveling with them with needed vaccinations, malaria prophylaxis, diarrhea prevention and treatment, advice on coronavirus disease 2019 (COVID-19) prevention measures and travel requirements, general advice on travel and food safety, and other travel-related health issues, as outlined elsewhere in the Centers for Disease Control and Prevention (CDC) Yellow Book.

Vaccinations

All family members should be up to date with all routine immunizations; this includes those who travel to meet the adopted child, those who remain at home, and all extended family members. Provided minimum age and dose intervals are followed, an accelerated dose schedule can be used to complete a vaccine series, if necessary.

Ensure all age-eligible people who will be in the household or in close contact with the adopted child (e.g., caregivers) are protected against diphtheria, hepatitis A virus (HAV), measles, pertussis, polio, tetanus, and varicella; include hepatitis B virus (HBV) vaccine if the adoptee has known infection or if the family is traveling to a country with high or intermediate levels of endemic HBV infection (see Sec. 5, Part 2, Ch. 8, Hepatitis B). Make sure all eligible family members are up to date with their COVID-19 vaccines (www.cdc.gov/coronavirus/2019-ncov/vaccines/stay-up-to-date.html).

HEPATITIS

Before the adopted child's arrival, immunize unprotected family members and close contacts against HAV. Because hepatitis B vaccine has only been routinely given since 1991, some adult family members and caretakers might need to be immunized if the adoptee has a known HBV infection.

MEASLES

Measles immunity or 2 doses of measles-mumps-rubella (MMR) vaccine separated by ≥28 days should be documented for all people born in or after 1957.

7

POLIO

If the adopted child is from a polio-endemic area (www.polioeradication.org, https://wwwnc.cdc.gov/travel/notices), ensure family members and caretakers have completed the recommended age-appropriate polio vaccine series. A one-time inactivated polio vaccine (IPV) booster for adults who completed the primary series in the past is recommended if they are traveling to polio-endemic areas; vaccination also can be considered for adults who remain at home but who will be in close contact caring for the child. Additional polio vaccine requirements for residents and long-term travelers (staying >4 weeks) departing from countries with polio transmission could affect outbound travel plans (see Sec. 5, Part 2, Ch. 17, Poliomyelitis).

TETANUS-DIPHTHERIA-PERTUSSIS

Adults who have not received the tetanus-diphtheria-acellular pertussis (Tdap) vaccine, including adults >65 years old, should receive a single dose to protect against diphtheria, pertussis, and tetanus.

VARICELLA

Administer varicella vaccine to people born in or after 1980 without a history of varicella disease, documented immunity (serology), or documentation of 2 doses of varicella vaccine.

OVERSEAS MEDICAL EXAMINATION

All immigrants, including children adopted internationally by US citizens, must undergo a medical examination in their country of origin, performed by a physician designated by the US Department of State. Additional information about the medical examination for internationally adopted children is available at https://travel.state.gov/content/travel/en/Intercountry-Adoption/Adoption-Process/how-to-adopt/medical-examination.html and https://eforms.state.gov/Forms/ds1981.pdf.

The explicit purpose of the overseas medical examination is to identify applicants with inadmissible health-related conditions. Prospective adoptive parents should not rely on this evaluation to detect all disabilities and illnesses a child might have. To understand more about possible health concerns for an individual child, prospective adoptive parents should consider a preadoption medical review with a pediatrician familiar with the health issues of internationally adopted children. That provider can review the available medical history and vaccination records for the child, thereby preparing parents for any potential health issues that might exist.

Prospective adoptive parents can then proactively schedule any recommended follow-up, including an initial medical examination that is recommended within 2 weeks of arrival to the United States (see www.cdc.gov/immigrantrefugeehealth/adoption/finding-doctor.html). Adoptive parents might receive a copy of the overseas examination, recorded on US Department of State medical forms, to give to clinicians at the initial follow-up medical examination.

FOLLOW-UP MEDICAL EXAMINATION

Providing health care to internationally adopted children can be challenging for several reasons (see Box 7-05). Adopted children should have a

BOX 7-05 Challenges to providing care to internationally adopted children

- Absence of a complete medical history
- Increased risk for developmental delays and psychological issues
- Lack of a biological family history
- Previously unidentified medical problems
- Questionable reliability of immunization records
- Variations in preadoption living standards
- Varying disease epidemiology in countries of origin

complete medical examination ≤2 weeks after their US arrival—earlier than that if they have anorexia, diarrhea, fever, vomiting, or other apparent health issues. In addition, a developmental screening examination conducted by an experienced clinician can help identify if immediate referrals should be made for a more detailed neurodevelopmental assessment and therapies. Clinicians might recommend further evaluation based on the age of the child, their country of origin, developmental status, nutritional status, previous living conditions, and the adoptive family's specific questions. Concerns raised during the preadoption medical review could dictate further investigation.

Infectious Diseases Screening

Screening recommendations for infectious diseases vary by organization. See Table 7-01 for the current panel of infectious disease screening tests recommended by the American Academy of Pediatrics (AAP) for internationally adopted children.

EOSINOPHILIA

All internationally adopted children should have a complete blood count with differential. An eosinophil count >450 cells/mL warrants further evaluation; intestinal parasite screening can identify some helminth infections. Investigation of eosinophilia also should include serologic evaluation for *Strongyloides stercoralis* and *Toxocara canis*; both are found worldwide. Perform serologic testing for filariasis and *Schistosoma* spp. in children arriving from endemic countries.

HEPATITIS A

Screening asymptomatic people for hepatitis A is generally not recommended; clinicians might, however, decide to test internationally adopted children for HAV IgG and IgM to identify those who are acutely infected and shedding virus. Vaccinate adopted children against HAV if they are not already immune.

In 2007 and early 2008, multiple cases of hepatitis A were reported in the United States secondary to exposure to newly arrived internationally adopted children. Some of these cases involved extended family members not living in the household. Identification of acutely infected toddlers new to the United States could prevent further transmission. If an acute infection is found in a child, close contacts can receive hepatitis A vaccine or immunoglobulin to prevent infection. In addition, serologic testing is a cost-effective way to identify children with past infection.

HEPATITIS B

With the widespread use of the hepatitis B vaccine, the prevalence of HBV infection has decreased overall, and lower rates of infection (1%–5%) have been reported in newly arrived international adoptees. In recent years, most children with HBV infection were known to be infected prior to adoption.

All internationally adopted children should be screened for HBV infection with serologic tests for hepatitis B surface antigen (HBsAg), hepatitis B surface antibody, and hepatitis B core antibody to determine past infection, current infection, or protection due to prior vaccination. For children positive for HBsAg, retest 6 months later to determine if they have chronic infection. Report results of a positive HBsAg test to the state health department.

HBV is highly transmissible within households; for this reason, all members of households adopting children with chronic HBV infection should be

Table 7-01 American Academy of Pediatrics (Red Book) recommended infectious disease screening for international adoptees[1,2]

INFECTIONS & DISEASES	RECOMMENDED TESTING	INDICATIONS
Filariasis, lymphatic	Serology	Eosinophilia; from endemic country
Hepatitis A	Serology	As appropriate (see text)
Hepatitis B	Serology	All children
Hepatitis C	Serology	As appropriate (see text)
HIV 1 & 2	Serology (antigen/antibody)	All children
Intestinal pathogens	Stool examination for O&P (1–3 specimens)	All children
	Cryptosporidium antigen testing (1 specimen)	All children
	Giardia duodenalis antigen testing (1 specimen)	All children
Schistosomiasis	Species serology	Eosinophilia or hematuria; from endemic country
Strongyloidiasis	Species serology	Eosinophilia
Syphilis	Serology (treponemal + nontreponemal testing)	All children
Toxocara canis	Serology	Eosinophilia
Trypanosoma cruzi	Serology	From endemic country
Tuberculosis[3]	TST	<2 years of age
	IGRA or TST	≥2 years of age
	IGRA	≥2 years of age previously vaccinated with BCG

Abbreviations: BCG, bacillus Calmette-Guérin; IGRA, interferon-γ release assay; O&P, ova and parasites; TST, tuberculin skin test

[1]Report all reportable diseases to the state or local health department.
[2]Collect a complete blood cell count with differential and red blood cell indices in addition to the disease-specific tests listed in the table.
[3]Repeat testing in 3–6 months if initial testing is negative.

immunized. Children with chronic HBV infection should receive additional tests for hepatitis e antigen (HBeAg), hepatitis B e antibody (anti-HBe), HBV viral load, hepatitis D virus antibody, and liver function, and should have a consultation with a pediatric gastroenterologist for long-term management.

Although not currently recommended by the CDC or the AAP, consider repeat screening 6 months after arrival for all children who initially test negative for hepatitis B surface antibody and surface antigen.

HEPATITIS C

The prevalence of hepatitis C in internationally adopted children is low. Most children with hepatitis C virus (HCV) infection are asymptomatic, and screening for risk factors (e.g., having an HCV-positive mother, surgery in the child's birth country, a history of transfusions, major dental work, intravenous drug use, tattoos, sexual activity or abuse, female genital cutting, traditional cutting) generally is not possible. But because effective treatments are available and infected patients need close follow-up to identify long-term complications, consider routine screening for HCV.

Use antibody testing (IgG ELISA) to screen children ≥18 months of age; use PCR testing for younger children. Refer children with HCV infection to a gastroenterologist for further evaluation, management, and treatment.

HIV

HIV screening is recommended for all internationally adopted children. HIV antibodies found in children aged <18 months could reflect maternal antibodies rather than infection of the infant. An HIV-1/HIV-2 antigen/antibody combination assay is used for standard screening, but some experts recommend PCR for any infant aged <6 months on arrival to the United States. A PCR assay for HIV DNA can confirm the diagnosis in an infant or child. If PCR testing is done, 2 negative results from assays administered 1 month apart, at least 1 of which is done after the age of 4 months, are necessary to exclude infection. Some experts recommend repeating screening for HIV antibodies 6 months after arrival if the initial test results are negative. Refer children with HIV infection to a specialist.

INTESTINAL PATHOGENS

Children treated for intestinal pathogens who have persistent growth delay, or who have ongoing or recurrent symptoms or unexplained anemia, merit a more extensive work-up. Notify public health authorities of reportable infections, and forward isolates for surveillance as appropriate.

PARASITIC

Gastrointestinal parasites commonly are seen in international adoptees, but prevalence varies by age and birth country. As children become older, the risk for parasitic infection and detection increases. The presence or absence of symptoms is not predictive of intestinal parasites; thus, screening is needed. In both past and more recent studies, the highest rates of parasite detection are reported among children adopted from Ukraine and from African, Latin American, and Asian countries, as compared to children coming from Russia and other countries in Eastern Europe. Unlike refugees, internationally adopted children are not treated for parasites before departure, and some clinicians opt to treat newly arrived adoptees with a single dose of albendazole.

Three stool samples collected in the early morning, 2–3 days apart, and placed in a container with preservative provides the highest yield for ova and parasite (O&P) detection. In addition, because routine O&P analysis is unlikely to include testing for either *Cryptosporidium* or *Giardia*, order the combined antigen test for these 2 parasites. *Giardia duodenalis* is the parasite most often identified.

BACTERIAL

Conduct additional stool testing for children with fever and diarrhea, especially acute-onset bloody diarrhea. Non-culture methods (e.g., gastrointestinal pathogen panels with PCR) commonly are used. If a bacterial pathogen is identified by a non-culture method, collect and culture samples to determine antimicrobial susceptibility and inform treatment decisions; bacterial pathogens can be resistant to antibiotics.

MALARIA

Routine malaria screening is not recommended for internationally adopted children. Instead, obtain thick and thin malaria smears immediately for any child coming from a malaria-endemic area who presents with fever or who has symptomatic splenomegaly (i.e., splenic enlargement plus fever or chills). Rapid diagnostic tests (RDTs) for malaria can help expedite the diagnosis, but microscopy is still required to confirm the results and to determine the degree of parasitemia (see Sec. 5, Part 3, Ch. 16, Malaria). PCR testing can confirm the species of parasite after the diagnosis has been established by either smear microscopy or RDT.

Further evaluation also is warranted in asymptomatic children with splenomegaly who come from areas endemic for malaria, as they could be exhibiting hyperreactive malaria splenomegaly.

This evaluation should include antibody titers for malaria, since asymptomatic children with splenomegaly caused by repeated malaria infections can have high titers but negative smears.

SEXUALLY TRANSMITTED INFECTIONS

CHLAMYDIA & GONORRHEA

Although screening for sexually transmitted infections other than HIV and syphilis is not routinely recommended, some experts will screen all children >5 years of age for chlamydia and gonorrhea. Regardless of age, if questions or concerns of sexual abuse are present, or if HIV or syphilis are diagnosed in the child, perform chlamydia and gonorrhea screening.

SYPHILIS

Screening for *Treponema pallidum* is recommended for all internationally adopted children. Initial screening is done with both nontreponemal and treponemal tests. Treponemal tests remain positive for life in most cases, even after successful treatment, and are specific for treponemal diseases, including syphilis and other diseases (e.g., bejel, pinta, yaws) found in some countries.

In children with a history of syphilis, documentation is rarely available for the initial evaluation (serology and lumbar puncture results with cell count, protein, VDRL), treatment (antibiotic used, dose, frequency, and duration), and follow-up serologic testing; therefore, conduct a full evaluation for disease, and provide treponemal treatment depending on the results.

TRYPANOSOMIASIS / CHAGAS DISEASE

Chagas disease is endemic to much of Mexico and throughout countries in Central and South America (see Sec. 5, Part 3, Ch. 25, American Trypanosomiasis / Chagas Disease). Infection risk varies by region within endemic countries. Although the risk for *Trypanosoma cruzi* infection is likely low in children adopted from endemic areas, consider screening.

Serologic testing when the child is aged 9–12 months will avoid possible false-positive results from maternal antibodies. PCR testing can be done for children <9 months of age. Refer children who test positive for Chagas disease to a specialist for further evaluation and management; treatment is effective.

TUBERCULOSIS

Internationally adopted children have 4–6 times the risk for tuberculosis (TB) compared to their US-born peers. TB screening is an integral part of the pretravel overseas medical examination; check with adoptive parents or with the local health department for screening results. If results are not immediately available, screen all internationally adopted children for TB after they arrive in the United States; report any positive cases to the state health department.

Screening for TB after US arrival is important because TB can be more severe in young children and can reactivate when the child gets older. To screen, AAP recommends a tuberculin skin test (TST) for children <2 years of age. For children ≥2 years of age, use either a TST or an interferon-γ release assay (IGRA). For children previously vaccinated with bacillus Calmette-Guérin (BCG), IGRAs appear to be more specific than the TST for *Mycobacterium tuberculosis* infection (see Sec. 5, Part 1, Ch. 23, . . . *perspectives*: Testing Travelers for *Mycobacterium tuberculosis* Infection). On arrival to the United States, some children might be anergic (i.e., have a false negative TB screen) due to malnutrition, stress, or untreated HIV infection, or they might have been infected just prior to travel. Thus, if the initial screen is negative, repeat testing 3–6 months after arrival.

If the TST or IGRA is positive, the child has TB infection, which requires additional evaluation to determine whether the child has TB disease. If a child has evidence of TB disease, consult with an infectious disease expert. Additional information is available at www.cdc.gov/tb/topic/treatment/ltbi.htm.

Vaccinations

The US Immigration and Nationality Act requires everyone seeking an immigrant visa for permanent residency to show proof of having received Advisory Committee on Immunization Practices (ACIP)-recommended vaccines before immigration (see www.cdc.gov/vaccines/schedules/hcp/imz/child-adolescent.html). This requirement extends to all immigrant infants and children entering the United States. Although internationally adopted children aged <10 years are exempt from the overseas immunization requirements, CDC encourages vaccination prior to travel to the United States. If an adopted child <10 years old is not vaccinated as part of their pretravel overseas medical examination, the adoptive parents must sign an affidavit indicating their intention to comply with the immunization requirements within 30 days of the child's arrival to the United States. The vaccination affidavit can be found at https://eforms.state.gov/Forms/ds1981.pdf.

VACCINATION RECORDS

Vaccination record reliability differs by, and even within, country of origin. Some children might have full documentation of vaccines received and dates given, while others have incomplete or no records. MMR is not given in most countries of origin because measles vaccine often is administered as a single antigen. In addition, some children might be immune to hepatitis A, measles, mumps, rubella, or varicella because of natural infection. A clinical diagnosis of any of these diseases, however, should not be accepted as evidence of immunity.

CATCH-UP VACCINATIONS

Most international adoptees arrive to the United States already having been vaccinated against diphtheria, hepatitis B, measles, pertussis, polio, tetanus, and tuberculosis (with BCG) in their country of birth. Because *Haemophilus influenzae* type b (Hib), hepatitis A, human papillomavirus, meningococcal, mumps, pneumococcal conjugate, rotavirus, rubella, and varicella vaccines are not given routinely in low- and middle-income countries, however, >90% of newly arrived internationally adopted children need catch-up vaccines to meet ACIP guidelines.

VACCINATION PLAN

Providers can choose 1 of 2 approaches for developing a vaccination plan for internationally adopted children. The first approach is to revaccinate regardless of the child's vaccination record from their birth country. The second approach, applicable to children ≥6 months of age, is to perform antibody testing and to revaccinate accordingly. One exception to this second approach is pertussis; *Bordetella pertussis* antibody titers do not correlate with immune status, although higher protective antibody levels for diphtheria and tetanus could be extrapolated to mean that a child has protection against pertussis, as well.

Hepatitis B is another exception. Anti-HBs as a correlate of vaccine-induced protection has only been determined for people who have completed an approved vaccination series. To be considered immune, ACIP recommends that children with positive hepatitis B surface antibody have documentation of 3 appropriately spaced doses of hepatitis B vaccine. For children with positive hepatitis B surface antibody and positive hepatitis B core antibody, vaccination is not required, as they are considered immune after natural infection.

For children ≥6 months of age, perform testing for diphtheria (IgG), hepatitis B (as outlined above), Hib, and tetanus (IgG). For children ≥12 months of age, also perform testing for hepatitis A, measles, mumps, rubella, and varicella. Since April 2016, many resource-poor countries have used bivalent oral polio vaccine; for children born on or after this date who do not have documentation of receiving IPV according to an approved (US or World Health Organization) schedule, administer the age-appropriate vaccine series. Revaccination with pneumococcal vaccine is recommended because the vaccine has 13 serotypes, and antibody testing would not be cost-effective.

Once the vaccination record has been assessed and antibody level results are available, give any indicated vaccines according to the current ACIP catch-up schedule. If an adopted child is <6 months old and uncertainty remains regarding their vaccination status or the validity of the vaccination record, administer vaccines according to the ACIP schedule.

Noninfectious Disease Screening

Several screening tests for noninfectious diseases should be performed in all or in select internationally adopted children. All children should have a complete blood count with a differential (as previously noted), hemoglobin electrophoresis, and glucose-6-phosphate-dehydrogenase

(G6PD) deficiency screening. Measure serum levels of thyroid-stimulating hormone, and obtain a blood lead level in all internationally adopted children. Consider testing for serum levels of iron, iron-binding capacity, transferrin, ferritin, and total vitamin D 25-hydroxy. Perform vision and hearing screening and a dental evaluation on all children. Consider neurologic and psychological testing if the child's clinical presentation raises concern.

BIBLIOGRAPHY

American Academy of Pediatrics. Immunizations received outside the United States or whose immunization status is unknown or uncertain. In: Kimberlin D, Barnett ED, Lynfield R, Sawyer MH, editors. Red Book 2021–2024: report of the Committee on Infectious Diseases, 32nd edition. Elk Grove Village (IL): American Academy of Pediatrics; 2021. pp. 96–8.

American Academy of Pediatrics. Medical evaluation for infectious diseases for internationally adopted, refugee, and immigrant children. In: Kimberlin D, Barnett ED, Lynfield R, Sawyer MH, editors. Red Book 2021–2024: report of the Committee on Infectious Diseases, 32nd edition. Elk Grove Village (IL): American Academy of Pediatrics; 2021. pp. 158–9.

American Academy of Pediatrics Committee on Infectious Diseases. Recommendations for administering hepatitis A vaccine to contacts of international adoptees. Pediatrics. 2011;128(4):803–4.

Centers for Disease Control and Prevention. CDC immigration requirements: technical instructions for tuberculosis screening and treatment: using cultures and directly observed therapy 2009. Available from: www.cdc.gov/immigrantrefugeehealth/exams/ti/panel/tuberculosis-panel-technical-instructions.html.

Mandalakas AM, Kirchner HL, Iverson S, Chesney M, Spencer MJ, Sidler A, et al. Predictors of *Mycobacterium tuberculosis* infection in international adoptees. Pediatrics. 2007;120(3):e610–6.

Marin M, Patel M, Oberste S, Pallansch MA. Guidance for assessment of poliovirus vaccination status and vaccination of children who have received poliovirus vaccine outside the United States. MMWR Morb Mortal Wkly Rep. 2017;66(1):23–5.

Staat MA, Rice M, Donauer S, Mukkada S, Holloway M, Cassedy A, et al. Intestinal parasite screening in internationally adopted children: importance of multiple stool specimens. Pediatrics. 2011;128(3):e613–22.

Staat MA, Stadler LP, Donauer S, Trehan I, Rice M, Salisbury S. Serologic testing to verify the immune status of internationally adopted children against vaccine preventable diseases. Vaccine. 2010;28(50):7947–55.

Wodi AP, Ault K, Hunter P, McNally V, Szilagyi PG, Bernstein H. Advisory Committee on Immunization Practices recommended immunization schedule for children and adolescents aged 18 years or younger—United States, 2021. MMWR Morb Mortal Wkly Rep. 2021;70(6):189–92.

7

TRAVELING WITH PETS & SERVICE ANIMALS

Emily Pieracci, Kendra Stauffer

International air and cruise travel with pets require advance planning. Travelers taking a companion or service animal to a foreign country must meet the entry requirements of that country and follow transportation guidelines of the airline or cruise company. Additionally, upon reentering the United States, pets that traveled abroad are subject to the same import requirements as animals that never lived in the United States (see Sec. 4, Ch. 9, Bringing Animals & Animal Products into the United States).

General information about traveling with a pet is available at www.cdc.gov/importation/traveling-with-pets.html. For destination country requirements, travelers should contact the country's embassy in Washington, DC, or the nearest consulate. The International Air Transportation Association also lists the requirements for pets to enter countries at www.iata.org/en/programs/cargo/live-animals/pets. Airline and cruise companies are another resource for travelers; most have webpages dedicated to traveling with pets.

TRAVELING WITH PETS OUTSIDE THE UNITED STATES

People planning to travel outside the United States with a pet should contact their local veterinarian well in advance of departure for assistance with completing all necessary paperwork and ensuring animal health and medical requirements are met. Depending on the destination country, pets might be required to have updated vaccinations and parasite treatments, International Standards Organization–compatible microchips implanted, and serologic tests prior to travel. Some countries require a coronavirus disease 2019 (COVID-19) test for pets prior to importation.

Completing the stringent testing and permit requirements for some countries (e.g., Australia) can take up to 6 months. People who plan to transport animals should consider the animals' species (e.g., cat, dog); mode of travel (e.g., airplane, cruise ship); season of travel (some carriers will not transport animals during the hottest or coldest parts of the year); and vaccination and testing requirements of the destination country and of transiting countries, if applicable. Transportation carriers might have additional requirements (e.g., breed restrictions for pets traveling in cargo, health certificates), so travelers intending to take pets outside the United States should contact air and cruise lines for information as soon as they are aware of their travel plans.

The US Department of Agriculture (USDA), Animal Plant and Health Inspection Service (APHIS) lists international export regulations for pets at www.aphis.usda.gov/aphis/pet-travel. Pet owners are responsible for making sure requirements of the destination country are met. USDA APHIS often is required to endorse a health certificate prior to an animal leaving the United States; certificates must be accurate, complete, and legible. Failure to meet destination country requirements can cause problems gaining certificate endorsement or difficulties upon arrival in the destination country (e.g., animal quarantine or retesting).

Travelers should be aware that long flights can be hard on pets, particularly older animals, animals with chronic health conditions, very young animals, and short-nosed breeds (e.g., Persian cats, English bulldogs) that can be predisposed to respiratory stress. The US Department of Transportation offers tips for traveling with animals by plane at www.transportation.gov/airconsumer/plane-talk-traveling-animals.

TRAVELING WITH SERVICE ANIMALS OUTSIDE THE UNITED STATES

The Department of Justice (DOJ) Americans with Disabilities Act (ADA) defines a service animal as any dog that is individually trained to do work or perform tasks for the benefit of a person with a disability, including an intellectual, mental, physical, psychiatric, or sensory disability. DOJ does not recognize emotional support animals as service animals, and airline carriers are not required to recognize emotional support animals as service animals.

Air Travel with Service Animals

The cabins of most commercial airplanes are highly confined spaces; passengers are seated in close quarters with limited opportunities to separate passengers from nearby disturbances. Animals on airplanes can pose a risk to the health, safety, and well-being of passengers and crew, and could disturb the safe and efficient operation of the aircraft. Accommodation of passengers traveling with service animals onboard a commercial airplane must be balanced against these concerns.

The Federal Aviation Administration (FAA) Reauthorization Act of 2018 developed minimum standards for service animals. Airline carriers can require passengers traveling with a service animal to document whether that animal has been individually trained to do work or perform tasks to assist the function of the passenger with a physical or mental disability; has been trained to behave in public; is in good health; and has the ability either not to relieve itself on a long (>8 hours) flight or to do so in a sanitary manner.

The US Department of Transportation (DOT) provides 2 forms to document a service animal's behavior, training, and health: Service Animal Air Transportation Form, available from www.transportation.gov/sites/dot.gov/files/2020-12/

Service%20Animal%20Health%20Behavior%20Training%20Form.pdf; and Service Animal Relief Attestation Form for Flight Segments Eight Hours or Longer, available from www.transportation.gov/sites/dot.gov/files/2020-12/Service%20Animal%20Relief%20Form.pdf.

In addition to the requirements already mentioned, airlines might require health certificates and vaccination records. Although airline carriers cannot restrict service dogs based solely on the breed or generalized type of dog, they might limit the number of service animals traveling with a single passenger with a disability, or require service animals be harnessed, leashed, or tethered unless the device interferes with the service animal's work or the passenger's disability prevents use of these devices; in which case, the carrier must permit the passenger to use signal, voice, or other effective means to maintain control of the service animal.

Cruise Ship Travel with Service Animals

7

Travelers should contact the cruise company they will be traveling with to learn more about each company's service animal policy. Some cruise lines are unable to accommodate animals onboard. Pets, service dogs in training, and emotional support dogs might not be allowed. People traveling aboard a ship with a service dog should consider rules or requirements at ports of call. For instance, many ports of call have strict entry requirements for animals. Travelers with service animals should visit the USDA's pet travel website (www.aphis.usda.gov/aphis/pet-travel) or their service animal's veterinarian to determine each destination country's policy regarding admission of service animals. Some locations do not recognize 3-year rabies vaccines, and annual vaccination might be required; consult with the service animal's veterinarian for more information.

Some locations require that service animals receive parasite treatment prior to arrival, and this information should be included in the service animal's health records. Some locations require that service animals travel with documentation (e.g., an import license), regardless of whether the service animal will disembark the ship. Check with the cruise company or country of destination for details.

Some locations have breed restrictions per the country's dog ordinances. Restricted-breed service animals might not be allowed to board the ship due to the destination country's laws. Travelers should check with the cruise line and country of destination for more information.

Travelers should hand-carry (i.e., not pack in baggage) all of their animals' required documents, including vaccination records. Service animals traveling without proper documentation might not be permitted to board the ship at embarkation.

REENTERING THE UNITED STATES WITH A PET OR SERVICE ANIMAL

Once a pet or service animal leaves the United States, it must meet all entry requirements to reenter, even if the animal has lived in the United States previously (see Sec. 4, Ch. 9, Bringing Animals & Animal Products into the United States).

BIBLIOGRAPHY

Centers for Disease Control and Prevention. Traveling with your pet. Available from: www.cdc.gov/importation/traveling-with-pets.html.

FAA reauthorization act of 2018; public law 115–254—Oct 5, 2018. Sec. 437: Harmonization of service animal standards. Available from: https://uscode.house.gov/statutes/pl/115/254.pdf.

Traveling by air with service animals. 85 FR 6448: 6448–76. Available from: www.federalregister.gov/documents/2020/02/05/2020-01546/traveling-by-air-with-service-animals.

US Department of Justice Civil Rights Division. Frequently asked questions about service animals and the ADA; July 20, 2015. Available from: www.ada.gov/regs2010/service_animal_qa.pdf.

Travel by Air, Land & Sea

AIR TRAVEL

Tai-Ho Chen, Araceli Rey, Clive Brown

In 2019, 4.5 billion passengers took nearly 47 million international flights. The following year, annual global passenger air travel volume decreased by nearly two-thirds (1.8 billion passengers took 22 million flights), a consequence of the coronavirus disease 2019 (COVID-19) pandemic. The pandemic reversed a trend of annually increasing air travel volume, attributable at least in part to the implementation of travel restrictions by many countries.

To promote safe travel during the pandemic, in July 2020 the US Department of Transportation and other government agencies, including the Centers for Disease Control and Prevention (CDC), collaborated to publish Runway to Recovery: The United States Framework for Airlines and Airports to Mitigate the Public Health Risks of Coronavirus. Runway to Recovery was based in part on the International Civil Aviation Organization (ICAO) report and guidance document, Take Off: Guidance for Air Travel through the COVID-19 Public Health Crisis, which includes a section on public health risk mitigation measures countries can use in the travel sector. These measures, among others, helped bolster passenger and aviation worker confidence that air travel could be conducted safely during the pandemic.

Travelers often have concerns about the health risks of flying on airplanes. Although illness might occur as a direct result of air travel, it is not commonly reported. Some main concerns include exacerbations of chronic medical conditions due to changes in air pressure and humidity; relative immobility during flights leading to thromboembolic disease; and risk for infection due to

CDC Yellow Book 2024. Jeffrey Nemhauser, Oxford University Press.
DOI: 10.1093/oso/9780197570944.003.0008

proximity to others on board who could have communicable diseases.

PREFLIGHT MEDICAL CONSIDERATIONS

The Aerospace Medical Association (www.asma.org) recommends evaluating chronic medical conditions and addressing instabilities prior to travel, particularly in people with underlying cardiovascular disease, diabetes, chronic lung disease, mental illness, seizures, stroke, recent surgery, or a history of deep vein thrombosis or pulmonary embolism. Travelers should be current on routine vaccinations and receive destination-specific vaccinations before travel.

Pregnant Travelers

For information on contraindications and precautions related to flying during pregnancy, see Sec. 7, Ch. 1, Pregnant Travelers.

Travelers with Disabilities

The US Transportation Security Administration (TSA) has information for travelers with disabilities and medical conditions that might affect their security screening (see www.tsa.gov/travel/special-procedures). Travelers with Disabilities (Sec. 3, Ch. 2) includes a table of useful online resources (see Table 3-05, Online resources for travelers with disabilities or chronic illnesses). For information on traveling with a service animal, see Sec. 7, Ch. 6, Traveling with Pets & Service Animals.

Travelers Who Require Supplemental Oxygen

Travelers who require supplemental in-flight oxygen should be aware that they must arrange for their own oxygen supplies while on the ground, at departure, during layovers, and upon arrival. Federal regulations prohibit passengers from bringing their own oxygen onboard flights; passengers should notify the airline ≥72 hours before departure if they require in-flight supplemental oxygen. In addition, airlines might not offer in-flight supplemental oxygen on all aircraft or flights, and some airlines permit only Federal Aviation Administration (FAA)–approved portable oxygen concentrators (for details, see www.faa.gov/about/initiatives/cabin_safety/portable_oxygen). Information about screening portable oxygen concentrators at US airports is available at www.tsa.gov/travel/security-screening/whatcanibring/items/portable-oxygen-concentrators.

CABIN AIR PRESSURE & CHRONIC DISEASE

During normal flight conditions, FAA requires that commercial aircraft maintain a cabin pressure equivalent to a maximum altitude of 8,000 ft (≈2,440 m) above sea level. Cabin pressures are typically maintained at an equivalent of 6,000–8,000 ft (≈1,830–2,440 m) above sea level, but newer aircraft can maintain cabin air pressures equivalent to lower altitudes. Most travelers without preexisting health conditions will not notice any effects from the decreased partial pressure of oxygen at these cabin pressures. By contrast, a traveler with anemia (including sickle cell disease), cardiopulmonary disease (especially people who normally require supplemental oxygen), or cerebrovascular disease can experience an exacerbation of their underlying medical condition. In addition, aircraft cabin air is typically dry, usually 10%–20% humidity, which can cause dryness of the mucous membranes of the upper airway and eyes.

Barotrauma

Barotrauma can occur when the pressure inside an air-filled, enclosed body space (e.g., abdomen, middle ear, sinuses) is not the same as the air pressure inside the aircraft cabin. Barotrauma most commonly occurs because of rapid changes in environmental pressure: during ascent, for example, when cabin pressure falls rapidly, and during descent, when cabin pressure quickly rises. Barotrauma most commonly affects the middle ear, and happens when the eustachian tube is blocked and a traveler is unable to equalize the air pressure in the middle ear with the outside cabin pressure.

Middle ear barotrauma is usually not severe or dangerous; rarely, though, it can cause complications (e.g., dizziness, hearing loss, a perforated tympanic membrane, permanent tinnitus). To help reduce the risks of barotrauma associated with cabin air pressure changes, travelers with ear, nose, and sinus infections or severe congestion might choose to postpone flying to prevent pain or injury, or use oral or nasal decongestants to help alleviate symptoms. Travelers with allergies should continue their regular allergy medications.

Travelers who have had recent surgery, particularly intra-abdominal, cardiothoracic, or intraocular procedures, should consult with their physician before flying. Travelers who participate in scuba diving should observe minimum recommended time intervals between diving and air travel to reduce the risk for altitude-induced decompression sickness (see Sec. 4, Ch. 4, Scuba Diving: Decompression Illness & Other Dive-Related Injuries, for details).

THROMBOEMBOLIC DISEASE

Decreased mobility during travel is associated with a small but measurable increased risk for venous thrombosis and pulmonary embolism, even in otherwise healthy travelers. The overall incidence of symptomatic venous thromboembolism in the month after travel is 1 in 4,600 flights of >4 hours in duration. Risk is increased by longer flight duration and is greater in people with known risk factors (e.g., clotting disorders, estrogen use, severe obesity, pregnancy, recent surgery or trauma, previous thrombosis). The American College of Chest Physicians recommends travelers on longer flights select aisle seats, walk frequently, and perform calf muscle exercises to reduce the risk for thrombosis. People with risk factors might benefit from wearing properly fitted graduated compression stockings (15–30 mmHg at the ankle) during flight. Aspirin has not been shown to decrease risk. See Sec. 8, Ch. 3, Deep Vein Thrombosis & Pulmonary Embolism, for more details).

IN-FLIGHT TRANSMISSION OF COMMUNICABLE DISEASES

Communicable diseases can be transmitted during air travel. People who are acutely ill or still within the infectious period for a specific disease should delay their travel until they are no longer contagious. For example, otherwise healthy adults can transmit influenza to others for 5–7 days, and transmission of respiratory viruses (e.g., measles) has been documented on commercial aircraft.

Travelers should wash their hands frequently and thoroughly or use an alcohol-based hand sanitizer containing ≥60% alcohol, especially after using the airplane lavatory and before eating meals. Some diseases spread by contact with infectious droplets (e.g., when an ill person sneezes or coughs and the secretions or droplets land on another person's face, mouth, nose, or eyes), or when an ill person touches communal surfaces (e.g., door handles, rest room faucets) with contaminated hands. Other people handling the contaminated surfaces can then be inoculated with the contaminant. Practicing good handwashing and respiratory hygiene (covering mouth with a tissue when coughing or sneezing) can help decrease the risk for infection by direct or indirect contact.

Cabin Ventilation & Air Filtration

Large commercial jet aircraft recirculate 35%–55% of the air in the cabin, mixed with outside air. The recirculated air passes through high-efficiency particulate air (HEPA) filters that capture 99.97% of particles (bacteria, larger viruses or virus clumps, fungi) ≥0.3 μm in diameter. Furthermore, laminar airflow generally circulates in defined areas within the aircraft, thus limiting the radius of distribution of pathogens spread by small-particle aerosols. As a result, the cabin air environment is less conducive to the spread of most infectious diseases than typical environmental systems in buildings.

Coronavirus Disease 2019 & Air Travel

COVID-19 transmission during air travel has been documented. In general, COVID-19 transmission risk on aircraft remains difficult to quantify and is likely to be affected by evolving administrative, engineering, and other controls being widely implemented in the commercial air travel sector. In 2020, as described in the introduction to this chapter, US government agencies and the ICAO each developed guidance for the airline industry to use in response to the pandemic. Recommendations included maximizing total cabin airflow on commercial aircraft during both ground and flight operations; implementing surface decontamination measures aimed at reducing risk for contact with infectious droplets; and modifying passenger movement patterns before, during, and after travel.

Travelers should familiarize themselves with the latest COVID-19–related requirements when planning air travel and, as their departure date approaches, follow the guidance of corresponding health authorities. People with confirmed or suspected COVID-19 should not travel until they are no longer thought to be contagious; similarly, those exposed might need to delay travel based on their history of infection or vaccination, according to current guidance.

IN-FLIGHT MEDICAL EMERGENCIES

Increasing numbers of travelers combined with an ever larger percentage of older passengers make the incidence of onboard medical emergencies likely to increase. Medical emergencies occur in ≈1 in 600 flights, or about 16 medical emergencies per 1 million passengers. The most common in-flight medical events are syncope or presyncope (37%); respiratory symptoms (12%); nausea or vomiting (10%); cardiac symptoms (8%); and seizures (6%).

Although in-flight medical emergencies occur, serious illness or death onboard a commercial aircraft is rare. Death was reported in ≈0.3% of medical emergencies, ≈2/3 were due to cardiac conditions. Most commercial airplanes that fly within the United States are required to carry ≥1 approved automated external defibrillator (AED) and an emergency medical kit.

Flight attendants are trained in basic first aid procedures (e.g., cardiopulmonary resuscitation [CPR], use of AEDs) but generally are not certified in emergency medical response. Many airlines use ground-based medical consultants to assist aircrew and volunteer passenger responders in managing medical cases. In nearly 50% of in-flight emergencies, physician volunteers have assisted (see the following chapter in this section, . . .*perspectives*: Responding to Medical Emergencies when Flying). The Aviation Medical Assistance Act, passed in 1998, provides some protection from liability to health care providers who respond to in-flight medical emergencies.

The goal of managing in-flight medical emergencies is to stabilize the passenger until the flight can safely reach ground-based medical care. When considering diversion to a closer airport, the captain must consider the needs of the ill passenger as well as other safety concerns (e.g., landing conditions, terrain, weather). Certain routes (e.g., transoceanic flights) and availability of definitive medical care might limit diversion options.

PREPARING AIRCREW

To better prepare aircrew for international travel, refer to Sec. 9, Ch. 2, Advice for Aircrew. The CDC Travelers' Health website (https://wwwnc.cdc.gov/travel) provides current information and travel health notices. Sec. 8, Ch. 8, Airplanes & Cruise Ships: Illness & Death Reporting & Public Health Interventions, provides advice for aircrew who might encounter passengers with potentially infectious diseases. The CDC Quarantine and Isolation webpage, Airline Guidance (www.cdc.gov/quarantine/air) provides requirements and tools for aircrew dealing with in-flight illness or death among passengers.

BIBLIOGRAPHY

Aerospace Medical Association. Medical considerations for airline travel. Available from: www.asma.org/publications/medical-publications-for-airline-travel/medical-considerations-for-airline-travel.

Bagshaw M, Illig P. The aircraft cabin environment. In: Keystone JS, Kozarsky PE, Connor BA, Northdurft HD, Mendelson M, Leder K, editors. Travel Medicine, 4th edition. Philadelphia: Elsevier; 2019. pp. 429–36.

Huizer YL, Swaanm CM, Leitmeyer KC, Timen A. Usefulness and applicability of infectious disease control measures in air travel: a review. Travel Med Infect Dis. 2015;13(1):19–30.

International Air Transport Association (IATA). Annual review 2021. Boston: The Association; 2021. Available from: www.iata.org/contentassets/c81222d96c9a4e0bb4ff6ced0126f0bb/iata-annual-review-2021.pdf.

International Civil Aviation Organization, Council on Aviation Recovery Taskforce. Aircraft module–air systems operations. Available from: www.icao.int/covid/cart/Pages/Aircraft-Module---Air-System-Operations.aspx.

International Civil Aviation Organization, Council on Aviation Recovery Taskforce. Guidance for air travel through the COVID-19 public health crisis. Available from: www.icao.int/covid/cart/Pages/CART-Take-off.aspx.

Nable JV, Tupe CL, Gehle BD, Brady WJ. In-flight medical emergencies during commercial travel. N Engl J Med. 2015;375(10):939–45.

Peterson DC, Martin-Gill C, Guyette FX, Tobias AZ, McCarthy CE, Harrington ST, et al. Outcomes of medical emergencies on commercial airline flights. N Engl J Med. 2013;368(22):2075–83.

Rosca EC, Heneghan C, Spencer EA, Brassy J, Plüddemann A, Onakpoya IJ, et al. Transmission of SARS-CoV-2 associated with aircraft travel: a systematic review. J Travel Med. 2021;28(7):taab133.

US Department of Transportation, US Department of Homeland Security, US Department of Health and Human Services. Runway to recovery: the United States framework for airlines and airports to mitigate the public health risks of coronavirus, version 1.1. Washington, DC: The Departments; 2020. Available from: www.transportation.gov/sites/dot.gov/files/2020-12/Runway_to_Recovery_1.1_DEC2020_Final.pdf.

8

RESPONDING TO MEDICAL EMERGENCIES WHEN FLYING

Kristina Angelo, Christopher Dalinkus

You find your seat, buckle up, and the plane takes off. An hour or so into the flight, you hear the flight attendant's request over the public address system, "If there are any medical personnel on the flight, please press your flight attendant call button." As a health care provider on the flight, you ask yourself, "Can I respond? Should I respond?"

Prior to the coronavirus disease 2019 (COVID-19) pandemic, the Federal Aviation Administration (FAA) reported that 2.7 million airline passengers traveled on >44,000 flights daily in the United States. In addition, >4 billion passengers traveled on commercial airlines globally each year, ≈10 million passengers per day. Medical emergencies occur on ≈1 of every 604 flights. The most common emergencies include syncope or presyncope, respiratory symptoms, or nausea and vomiting. For 90% of these emergencies, aircraft continue to their destination. For the remaining 10%, however, aircraft divert to an alternative landing site, most frequently for cardiac arrest, cardiac symptoms (e.g., chest pain), obstetric or gynecologic issues, or possible stroke. Despite the frequency of medical emergencies, the death rate is only ≈0.3%.

MEDICAL SUPPLIES ON AIRCRAFT

US Carriers

The FAA mandates which medical supplies US carrier aircraft flying domestically or internationally must have available onboard. Required medical supplies are listed in the Code of Federal Regulations (14 CFR, Part 121; subpart X, 121.803 and Appendix A). US carrier aircraft with ≥1 flight attendant are required to have a US Food and Drug Administration (FDA)–approved automated external defibrillator (AED), ≥1 first aid kit, and an emergency medical kit (EMK) in the passenger cabin. The number of first aid kits available on an aircraft corresponds to the number of seats: 1 kit for 0–50 seats; 2 for 51–150 seats; 3 for 151–250 seats; 4 for >250 seats.

A list of medications required in the EMK and equipment for administration (e.g., gloves, needles, syringes, adhesive tape, tourniquet) can be found in Box 8-01. A blood pressure cuff, stethoscope, cardiopulmonary resuscitation mask, oropharyngeal airways, and a manual resuscitation device are included for use in the event of a cardiac or pulmonary event.

BOX 8-01 Emergency medical kit (EMK) medication list

Antihistamine (25 mg tablets and 50 mg injectable)
Aspirin (325 mg)
Atropine
Bronchodilator, for inhalation
Dextrose (50%) and saline, for infusion
Epinephrine (1:1,000 and 1:10,000)
Lidocaine
Nitroglycerin tablets (0.4 mg)
Non-narcotic analgesic (325 mg)

International Carriers

EMK contents vary among international carriers, despite guidance from the International Civil Aviation Organization (ICAO). In a 2010 study of 12 European-based airlines, none complied with ICAO standards for EMKs.

LEGAL CONSIDERATIONS

US Domestic Flights

The 1998 Aviation Medical Assistance Act (AMAA) of the United States protects medical personnel from damages in federal or state court for providing good-faith medical care in the event of a medical emergency. The AMAA does not cover gross negligence or willful misconduct.

International Flights

Air carriers flagged in some countries (e.g., Canada, the United Kingdom, the United States) do not require clinicians to respond to in-flight medical emergencies. Other countries state that clinicians have an obligation to respond.

When responding to a medical emergency on an international flight, the AMAA might not apply. Furthermore, it is unclear what entity has jurisdiction over liability for care rendered; the country where the aircraft is registered might have jurisdiction, or jurisdiction could be based on the aircraft's geographic location at the time an incident occurs. In other cases, the medical responder's licensure country is the jurisdiction for liability. Jurisdiction might depend on whether the flight was in the air or on the ground when the incident occurred. Although most airlines and countries offer protection for Good Samaritans, a clinician responding to an emergency, even if an act of good will, might be at risk of litigation.

THINGS TO CONSIDER BEFORE RESPONDING

Have I consumed alcohol on the flight or before boarding? If you have, reconsider responding—you might be at risk for misconduct.

Am I familiar with how to work an AED?

What is my personal level of comfort and clinical competence to evaluate a person with a medical issue?

Am I flying on an international carrier whose flag is not the United States? The legal ramifications of delivering care to a fellow passenger are not always clear.

Box 8-02 provides a checklist for health care providers responding to in-flight medical emergencies.

8

BOX 8-02 Responding to in-flight medical emergencies: a checklist for health care providers

- ☐ Be calm and confident.
- ☐ Ask alert and oriented passengers for verbal consent to treat.
- ☐ Use flight attendants as assistants, as appropriate. Flight attendants are certified in cardiopulmonary resuscitation (CPR) and in the use of an automated external defibrillator (AED). Ask them for needed items from the first aid kit, EMK, and the AED.
- ☐ Obtain a medical history, check vital signs, and perform a physical examination appropriate to the problem.
- ☐ As necessary, ask for ground-based medical consultation for severely ill passengers; ask flight crew or other passengers to assist with translation; ask for medical equipment from other passengers (e.g., glucometer); and ask for other onboard clinician support (e.g., obstetrician if a pregnancy-related issue).
- ☐ Move patients to an area with more room (and privacy) if it can be done safely.
- ☐ Notify the crew immediately if the passenger is suspected to have a communicable disease or is severely ill.
- ☐ Document your clinical encounter on airline-specific forms.
- ☐ Communicate with the pilot via the cabin crew about the passenger's condition. The pilot has the responsibility to make the decision about diverting the flight.

(continued)

RESPONDING TO MEDICAL EMERGENCIES WHEN FLYING (CONTINUED)

ADDITIONAL CONSIDERATIONS

Deciding to Respond

For US-licensed health care providers, the decision to respond is a personal one, grounded in ethical obligation. Although the United States offers protections for medical personnel who aid ill passengers in good faith, the nature of the medical issue and the possibility that medications or equipment could be missing from the EMK could create a difficult situation. Always be honest with the flight attendants and the pilot regarding your assessment of the patient's condition and your degree of comfort with assisting; if needed supplies are not available aboard the aircraft, communicate this immediately. If traveling on an international carrier's flight, consider both ethics and the flight's legal jurisdiction.

Do Not Resuscitate

If a traveler has a "Do Not Resuscitate" order, you may choose to heed this. Be aware that individual airline policies might require flight attendants to attempt resuscitation despite this documentation.

BIBLIOGRAPHY

Aviation Medical Assistance Act of 1998, HR 2843, 105th Congress (1998). Available from: www.congress.gov/105/plaws/publ170/PLAW-105publ170.pdf.

Emergency medical equipment. 14 CFR §121.803 (2020). Available from: www.ecfr.gov/current/title-14/chapter-I/subchapter-G/part-121/subpart-X/section-121.803.

Federal Aviation Administration. Air traffic by the numbers. Available from: www.faa.gov/air_traffic/by_the_numbers.

Martin-Gill C, Doyle TJ, Yealy DM. In-flight medical emergencies, a review. JAMA. 2018;320(24):2580–90.

Nable JV, Tupe CL, Gehle BD, Brady WJ. In-flight medical emergencies during commercial travel. N Engl J Med. 2015;373(10):939–45.

Peterson DC, Martin-Gill C, Guyette FX, Tobias AZ, McCarthy CE, Harrington ST, et al. Outcomes of medical emergencies on commercial airline flights. N Engl J Med. 2013;368(22):2075–83.

Sand M, Gambichler T, Sand D, Thrandorf C, Altmeyer P, Bechara FG. Emergency medical kits on board commercial aircraft: a comparative study. Travel Med Infect Dis. 2010;8(6):388–94.

8

. . . *perspectives* chapters supplement the clinical guidance in this book with additional content, context, and expert opinion. The views expressed do not necessarily represent the official position of the Centers for Disease Control and Prevention (CDC).

DEEP VEIN THROMBOSIS & PULMONARY EMBOLISM

Nimia Reyes, Karon Abe

Deep vein thrombosis (DVT) is a condition in which a blood clot develops in the deep veins, usually in the lower extremities. A pulmonary embolism (PE) occurs when a part of the DVT clot breaks off and travels to the lungs, which can be life-threatening. Venous thromboembolism (VTE) refers to DVT, PE, or both. VTE is often recurrent and can lead to long-term complications (e.g., post-thrombotic syndrome after a DVT, chronic thromboembolic pulmonary hypertension after a PE).

Extended periods of limited mobility inherent to long-distance travel could increase a traveler's risk for VTE. An association between VTE and air travel was first reported in the early 1950s; since then, long-distance air travel has become more common, leading to increased concerns about travel-related VTE.

PATHOGENESIS

Virchow's classic triad for thrombus formation is venous stasis, vessel wall damage, and a hypercoagulable state. Prolonged, cramped sitting during long-distance travel interferes with venous flow in the legs, creating venous stasis. Seat-edge pressure to the popliteal area of the legs can aggravate venous stasis and contribute to vessel wall damage. Coagulation activation can result from an interaction between air cabin conditions (e.g., hypobaric hypoxia) and individual risk factors for VTE. Studies of the pathophysiologic mechanisms for the increased risk of VTE after long-distance travel have not produced consistent results, but venous stasis appears to play a major role. Other factors specific to air travel might increase coagulation activation, particularly in travelers with preexisting risk factors for VTE.

INCIDENCE

The annual incidence of VTE in the general population is estimated to be 0.1% but is greater in subpopulations with risk factors for VTE (Box 8-03). The actual incidence of travel-related VTE is difficult to determine because there is no national surveillance for VTE and no consensus on the definition of travel-related VTE, particularly regarding duration of travel and period of observation after travel.

AIR TRAVEL–RELATED VENOUS THROMBOEMBOLISM

Studies estimating the incidence of air travel–related VTE have used various criteria to determine risk factors and end points. For example, investigators have defined long-distance air travel as lasting anywhere from >3 hours to >10 hours. Although no standard definition exists, >4 hours is most often used. Post-flight observation period is similarly inconsistent and ranges from "hours after landing" to ≥8 weeks; 4 weeks, however, is most common. Finally, study outcomes range from asymptomatic DVT to symptomatic DVT/PE to severe or fatal PE. Asymptomatic DVT was estimated to be 5–20 times more common than symptomatic events, but asymptomatic DVT is of uncertain clinical significance and often resolves spontaneously.

In general, the incidence of air travel–related VTE appears to be low. For flights >4 hours, one study reported an absolute risk for VTE of 1 in 4,656 flights; another reported an absolute risk of 1 in 6,000 flights. People who travel on long-distance flights generally are healthier and therefore at a lower risk for VTE than the general population. Five prospective studies conducted to assess the incidence of DVT after travel >8 hours among travelers at low to intermediate risk for VTE yielded an overall VTE incidence of 0.5%; the incidence of symptomatic VTE was 0.3%.

Studies indicate that long-distance air travel might increase a person's overall risk for VTE by 2- to 4-fold. Some studies found that long-distance air travel increased the risk of VTE occurring, while others either found no definitive evidence of increased risk, or found that risk increased only if ≥1 additional VTE risk factors were present. Level of risk correlates with duration of travel and with

BOX 8-03 Venous thromboembolism (VTE) risk factors

- Cancer (active)
- Estrogen use (hormonal contraceptives or hormone replacement therapy)
- Hospitalization, surgery, or trauma (recent)
- Limited mobility (e.g., prolonged bed rest, paralysis, extended period of restricted movement [such as wearing a leg cast])
- Obesity (Body Mass Index [BMI] ≥30 kg/m^2)
- Older age (increasing risk after age 40)
- Pregnancy and the postpartum period
- Previous VTE
- Serious medical illness
- Thrombophilia (inherited or acquired) or a family history of VTE

preexisting risk factors for VTE. Risk decreases with time after air travel and returns to baseline by 8 weeks; most air travel–related VTE occurs within the first 1–2 weeks after the flight.

A similar increase in risk for VTE is noted with other modes of long-distance travel (bus, car, train), which implies that increased risk is due mainly to prolonged limited mobility rather than by the air cabin environment.

RISK FACTORS

Most travel-related VTE occurs in travelers with preexisting risk factors for VTE (Box 8-03). The combination of air travel with preexisting individual risk factors might synergistically increase risk. Some studies have shown that 75%–99.5% of people who developed travel-related VTE had ≥1 preexisting risk factor; one study showed that 20% had ≥5 risk factors. For travelers without preexisting risk factors, the risk of travel-related VTE is low.

For air travelers, height appears to be an additional risk factor; people <1.6 m (5 ft, 3 in) and those >1.9 m (6 ft, 3 in) tall were at increased risk. Because airline seats are higher than car seats and cannot be adjusted to a person's height, air travelers <1.6 m (5 ft, 3 in) tall might be more prone to seat-edge pressure to the popliteal area. Air travelers >1.9 m (6 ft, 3 in) tall are also at increased risk, possibly because taller travelers have less leg room.

CLINICAL PRESENTATION

Signs and symptoms of DVT/PE are nonspecific. Typical signs or symptoms of DVT in the extremities include pain or tenderness, swelling, warmth in the affected area, and redness or discoloration of the overlying skin. The most common signs or symptoms of acute PE include unexplained shortness of breath, pleuritic chest pain, cough or hemoptysis, and syncope.

DIAGNOSIS

Imaging studies are needed for diagnosis. Duplex ultrasonography is the standard imaging procedure for DVT diagnosis. Computed tomographic pulmonary angiography is the standard imaging procedure for diagnosis of PE. Ventilation-perfusion scan is the second-line imaging procedure.

TREATMENT

Anticoagulant medications commonly are used to treat DVT or PE; anticoagulants also are used for VTE prophylaxis. Bleeding can be a complication of anticoagulant therapy. The most frequently used injectable anticoagulants are unfractionated heparin, low molecular weight heparin (LMWH), and fondaparinux. Oral anticoagulants include apixaban, betrixaban, dabigatran, edoxaban, rivaroxaban, and warfarin.

PREVENTIVE MEASURES

The American College of Chest Physicians (ACCP) and the American Society of Hematology (ASH) each provide guidelines on the prevention of VTE in long-distance travelers.

American College of Chest Physicians Guidelines

ACCP 2012 guidelines (Grade 2C: weak recommendations, low- or very low-quality evidence): for long-distance travelers (>6 hours travel) at increased risk of VTE, the ACCP recommends frequent ambulation, calf muscle exercise, sitting in an aisle seat if feasible, and use of properly fitted below-the-knee graduated compression stockings (GCS) providing 15–30 mmHg of pressure at the ankle during travel. For long-distance travelers not at increased risk of VTE, use of GCS is not recommended. ACCP suggests against the use of aspirin or anticoagulants to prevent VTE in long-distance travelers.

American Society of Hematology Guidelines

ASH 2018 guidelines (conditional recommendations, very low certainty in the evidence of effects): for long-distance travelers (>4 hours travel) at substantially increased VTE risk (e.g., recent surgery, prior history of VTE, postpartum, active malignancy, or ≥2 risk factors, including combinations of the above with hormone replacement therapy, obesity, or pregnancy) the ASH guideline panel suggests GCS or prophylactic low molecular weight heparin (LMWH). If GCS or LMWH are not feasible, ASH suggests using aspirin rather than no VTE prophylaxis. For travelers without risk factors, ASH suggests not using GCS, LMWH, or aspirin for VTE prophylaxis.

Graduated Compression Stockings & Pharmacologic Prophylaxis

GCS appear to reduce asymptomatic DVT in travelers and are generally well tolerated. Decisions regarding use of pharmacologic prophylaxis for long-distance travelers at high risk should be made on an individual basis. When the potential benefits of pharmacologic prophylaxis outweigh the possible adverse effects, anticoagulants rather than antiplatelet drugs (e.g., aspirin) are recommended. People at increased risk should be evaluated with enough time before departure so that they understand how to take the medication; evaluate whether the traveler could have potential adverse effects from the combination of pharmacologic prophylaxis with any other medications they are taking.

Hydration

No evidence exists for an association between dehydration and travel-related VTE. Furthermore, no direct evidence exists to support the concept that drinking plenty of nonalcoholic beverages to ensure adequate hydration or avoiding alcoholic beverages has a protective effect. Therefore, maintaining hydration is reasonable and unlikely to cause harm, but it cannot be recommended specifically to prevent travel-related VTE.

In-Flight Mobility & Seat Assignment

Immobility while flying is a risk for VTE. Indirect evidence suggests that maintaining mobility could prevent VTE. In view of the role that venous stasis plays in the pathogenesis of travel-related VTE, recommending frequent ambulation and calf muscle exercises for long-distance travelers is reasonable.

An aisle seat also might be a protective factor to reduce the risk of developing VTE. In one study, travelers seated in window seats experienced a 2-fold increase in general risk for VTE compared with passengers in aisle seats; travelers with a body mass index ≥30 kg/m^2 who sat in window seats had a 6-fold increase in risk. Conversely, aisle seats are reported to have a protective effect compared with window or middle seats, probably because travelers are freer to move around.

RECOMMENDATIONS

General protective measures for long-distance travelers include calf muscle exercises, frequent ambulation, and aisle seating when possible. Additional protective measures for long-distance travelers at increased risk of VTE include properly fitted below-the-knee GCS and anticoagulant prophylaxis, but only in particularly high-risk cases where the potential benefits outweigh the risks.

8

BIBLIOGRAPHY

Aryal KR, Al-Khaffaf H. Venous thromboembolic complications following air travel: what's the quantitative risk? A literature review. Eur J Vasc Endovasc Surg. 2006;31(2):187–99.

Bartholomew JR, Schaffer JL, McCormick GF. Air travel and venous thromboembolism: minimizing the risk. Cleve Clin J Med. 2011;78(2):111–20.

Chandra D, Parisini E, Mozaffarian D. Meta-analysis: travel and risk for venous thromboembolism. Ann Intern Med. 2009;151(3):180–90.

Eklöf B, Maksimovic D, Caprini JA, Glase C. Air travel–related venous thromboembolism. Dis Mon. 2005;51(2–3):200–7.

Kahn SR, Lim W, Dunn AS, Cushman M, Dentali F, Akl EA, et al. Prevention of VTE in nonsurgical patients: antithrombotic therapy and prevention of thrombosis, 9th edition: American College of Chest Physicians evidence-based clinical practice guidelines. Chest. 2012;141(2 Suppl):e195S–226S.

Schobersberger W, Schobersberger B, Partsch H. Travel-related thromboembolism: mechanisms and avoidance. Expert Rev Cardiovasc Ther. 2009;7(12):1559–67.

Schreijer AJ, Cannegieter SC, Caramella M, Meijers JC, Krediet RT, Simons RM, et al. Fluid loss does not explain coagulation activation during air travel. Thromb Haemost. 2008;99(6):1053–9.

Schreijer AJ, Cannegieter SC, Doggen CJ, Rosendaal FR. The effect of flight-related behaviour on the risk of venous thrombosis after air travel. Br J Haematol. 2009;144(3):425–9.

Schünemann HJ, Cushman M, Burnett AE, Kahn SR, Beyer-Westendorf J, Spencer FA, et al. American Society of Hematology 2018 guidelines for management of venous thromboembolism: prophylaxis for hospitalized and nonhospitalized medical patients. Blood Adv. 2018;2(22):3198–225.

Watson HG, Baglin TP. Guidelines on travel-related venous thrombosis. Br J Haematol. 2011;152(1):31–4.

JET LAG

Greg Atkinson, Alan Batterham, Andrew Thompson

Jet lag results from a mismatch between a person's circadian (24-hour) rhythms and the time of day in the new time zone. When establishing risk of jet lag, first determine how many time zones a traveler will cross and what the discrepancy will be between time of day at home and at the destination at arrival. During the first few days after a flight to a new time zone, a person's circadian rhythms are still anchored to the time of day at their initial departure location. Rhythms then adjust gradually to the new time zone.

A useful web-based tool for world time zone travel information is available at www.timeanddate.com/worldclock/converter.html. For travelers crossing ≤3 time zones, especially if they are on a long-haul flight, symptoms (e.g., tiredness) are likely due to fatigue rather than jet lag, and symptoms should abate 1–3 days post-flight.

Many people flying >3 time zones for a vacation accept the risk for jet lag as a transient and mild inconvenience, but people traveling on business or to compete in athletic events might desire advice on prophylactic measures and treatments. If a traveler spends ≤2 days in the new time zone, they might prefer to anchor their sleep–wake schedule to the time of day at home as much as possible. Consider recommending short-acting hypnotics or alertness-enhancing drugs (e.g., caffeine) for such travelers to minimize total burden of jet lag during short round trips.

CLINICAL PRESENTATION

Jet lag symptoms can be difficult to define because of variation among people and because the same person can experience different symptoms after each flight. Jet-lagged travelers typically experience ≥1 of the following symptoms after flying across >3 time zones: gastrointestinal disturbances, decreased interest in food or enjoyment of meals; negative feelings (e.g., anxiety, depression, fatigue, headache, inability to concentrate, irritability); poor performance of physical and mental tasks during the new daytime; and classically, poor sleep, including (but not limited to) difficulty initiating sleep at the usual time of night (after eastward flights), early awakening (after westward flights), and fractionated sleep (after flights in either direction).

Symptoms are difficult to distinguish from the general fatigue resulting from international travel itself, as well as from other travel factors (e.g., hypoxia in the aircraft cabin). Validated multi-symptom measurement tools (e.g., Liverpool Jet Lag Index) can help distinguish between jet lag and fatigue. When travelers cross only 1–2 time zones, though, symptoms of and treatment for jet lag are not readily distinguishable from those for general travel fatigue.

In addition to jet lag symptoms, crossing multiple time zones can affect the timing of regular medication used for chronic conditions and illnesses. This can particularly affect patients taking medications with short half-lives that require >1 dose each day. Consider the destination and traveling time when evaluating travelers who take long-term medications, and recommend strategies to keep them on their dosing schedule.

PREVENTION & TREATMENT

Travelers use many approaches—before, during, and after flying—to reduce jet lag symptoms. In one survey, 460 long-haul travelers indicated that seat selection and booking a direct flight were primary strategies to reduce jet lag. Nearly all study participants used ≥1 behavioral strategy during their flight, including consuming or avoiding alcohol and caffeine (81%), altering food intake (68%), using light exposure (53%), periodic walking down the aisle of the plane (35%), and taking medication (15%), including melatonin (8%). Only 1 respondent used a jet lag application on a mobile device. Fewer people used all these strategies before takeoff and after arrival.

After arrival, light and social contacts influence the timing of internal circadian rhythms. A traveler staying in the time zone for >2 days should quickly try to adjust to the local sleep–wake schedule as much as possible.

Diet & Physical Activity

Most dietary interventions or functional foods have not been proven to reduce jet lag symptoms in randomized controlled trials and real flight conditions (see Sec. 2, Ch. 14, Complementary & Integrative Health Approaches to Travel Wellness). Most trials are in simulated flight conditions and have a high risk of bias, including studies looking at the effectiveness of *Centella asiatica*, elderberry, echinacea, pinokinase, and diets containing various levels of fiber, fluids, or macronutrients. In one study, long-haul flight crew who adopted more regular mealtimes showed a small improvement in their general subjective rating of jet lag, but not the separate symptoms of alertness or jet lag, on their days off work.

Because gastrointestinal disturbance is a common jet lag symptom, travelers might better tolerate smaller meals than larger ones before and during the flight; this strategy has not been investigated in a formal trial, however. Travelers might find caffeine and physical activity can help ameliorate daytime sleepiness at the destination, but little evidence exists to indicate that these interventions reduce overall feelings of jet lag. Any purported treatments based on use of acupressure, aromatherapy, or homeopathy have no scientific basis.

Hypnotic Medications

Prescription medications (e.g., temazepam, zolpidem, zopiclone) can reduce sleep loss during and after travel but do not necessarily help resynchronize circadian rhythms or improve overall jet lag symptoms. If indicated, prescribe the lowest effective dose of a short- to medium-acting compound for the initial few days of travel, bearing in mind these drugs do have adverse effects. In 2019, the US Food and Drug Administration (FDA) issued a warning about rare but serious adverse events (i.e., injuries caused by sleepwalking) occurring after patients took some sleep medications; adverse events were more commonly reported with eszopiclone, zaleplon, and zolpidem (see www.fda.gov/drugs/drug-safety-and-availability/fda-adds-boxed-warning-risk-serious-injuries-caused-sleepwalking-certain-prescription-insomnia).

Caution travelers about taking hypnotics during a flight because the resulting immobility could increase the risk for deep vein thrombosis. Travelers should not use alcohol as a sleep aid, because it disrupts sleep and can provoke obstructive sleep apnea.

Light

Exposure to bright light can advance or delay human circadian rhythms depending on when it is received in relation to a person's body clock time. Consequently, some researchers have proposed schedules for good and bad times for light exposure after arrival in a new time zone (www.caa.co.uk/Passengers/Before-you-fly/Am-I-fit-to-fly/Health-information-for-passengers/Jet-lag).

The best circadian time for light exposure might be at a time that is dark after crossing multiple time zones, raising the question of whether a light box is helpful. One small randomized controlled trial on supplementary bright light for reducing jet lag did not find clinically relevant effects of supplementary light on jet lag symptoms after a flight across 5 time zones going west.

Melatonin & Melatonin-Receptor Analogs

Probably the most well-known treatment for jet lag, melatonin, is secreted at night by the pineal gland. Melatonin delays circadian rhythms when taken during the rising phase of body temperature (usually the morning) and advances rhythms when ingested during the falling phase of body temperature (usually the evening). These effects are opposite to those of bright light.

The instructions on most products advise travelers to take melatonin before nocturnal sleep in the new time zone, irrespective of the number of time zones crossed or direction of travel. Studies published in the mid-1980s indicated a substantial benefit of taking melatonin just before sleep to reduce overall feelings of jet lag after flights. Subsequent larger studies did not replicate these earlier findings, however, and more research on melatonin's use in jet lag is needed.

Melatonin is a very popular sleep aid for jet lag in the United States, and no serious side effects have been linked to its use, although long-term studies have not been conducted. The American Academy of Sleep Medicine and the US National Center for Complementary and Integrative Health suggest that melatonin could be used to reduce symptoms of jet lag, although they caution that melatonin might not be safe when combined with some other medications. In addition, melatonin is considered a dietary supplement in the United States and is not regulated by the FDA. Therefore, the advertised concentration of melatonin has not been confirmed for most products on the market, and the presence of contaminants cannot be ruled out (see Sec. 2, Ch. 14, Complementary & Integrative Health Approaches to Travel Wellness).

A recent UK Drug and Therapeutics Bulletin stated that melatonin might increase the frequency of seizures in people with epilepsy. In addition, because it can potentially induce proinflammatory cytokine production, melatonin should not be taken by those with autoimmune diseases. Due to the potential for these problems, and the limited evidence from randomized controlled trials for any benefits, melatonin is not recommended in the United Kingdom.

8

Ramelteon, a melatonin-receptor agonist, is an FDA-approved treatment for insomnia. One milligram taken just before bedtime can decrease sleep onset latency after eastward travel across 5 time zones. Higher doses do not seem to lead to further improvements, and the effect of this medication on other symptoms of jet lag and the timing of circadian rhythms is unclear. In a well-designed multicenter trial involving simulated jet lag conditions, tasimelteon (a dual melatonin-receptor agonist) improved jet lag symptoms, including nighttime insomnia and daytime functioning; real-world evidence is needed to support or refute its use in the amelioration of jet lag.

Mobile Applications

Several mobile device applications (apps) can provide tailored advice to manage jet lag symptoms. Depending on how many time zones the traveler has passed through, Timeshifter (www.timeshifter.com) provides advice on when to use caffeine, light, melatonin, and sleep. Another app offering tailored advice was tested for use over several months of frequent flying. Participants reported reduced fatigue compared with the comparator group and improved aspects of health-related behavior (e.g., physical activity, snacking, and sleep quality) but not other measures of sleep (e.g., duration, latency, use of sleep-related medication). Although this and other apps are based on information from published laboratory-based experiments, they lack randomized controlled trials on their effectiveness for reducing jet lag symptoms after actual long-haul flights.

Combination Treatments

Multiple therapies to decrease jet lag symptoms can be combined into treatment packages. Marginal gains from multiple treatments could aggregate. In one small trial, a treatment package involving light exposure and sleep hygiene advice improved sleep quality and physical performance after an eastward flight across 8 time zones. The American Sleep Association offers general sleep hygiene advice at www.sleepassociation.org/about-sleep/sleep-hygiene-tips.

In general, no cure is available for jet lag. Instead, focus counseling on factors known from laboratory simulations to alter circadian timing. Until more randomized controlled trials of treatments prescribed before, during, or after transmeridian flights are published, focus on providing robust, evidence-based advice.

BIBLIOGRAPHY

Bin YS, Ledger S, Nour M, Postnova S, Stamatikis E, Cistulli PA, et al. How do travelers manage jetlag and travel fatigue? A survey of passengers on long-haul flights. Chronobiol Int. 2020;37(11):1621–8.

Herxheimer A. Jet lag. BMJ Clin Evid. 2014;2014:2303.

Janse van Rensburg DC, Fowler P, Racinais S. Practical tips to manage travel fatigue and jet lag in athletes. Br J Sports Med. 2021;55(15):821–2.

Ledger S, Bin YS, Nour M, Cistulli P, Bauman A, Allman-Farinelli M, et al. Internal consistency and convergent and divergent validity of the Liverpool jetlag questionnaire. Chronobiol Int. 2020;37(2):218–26.

Melatonin for jet lag. Drug Ther Bull. 2020;58(2):21–4.

Ruscitto C, Ogden J. The impact of an implementation intention to improve mealtimes and reduce jet lag in long-haul cabin crew. Psychol Health. 2016;32(1):61–77

Thompson A, Batterham AM, Jones H, Gregson W, Scott D, Atkinson G. The practicality and effectiveness of supplementary bright light for reducing jet-lag in elite female athletes. Int J Sports Med. 2013;34(7):582–9.

Van Drongelen A, Boot CR, Hlobil H, Twisk JW, Smid T, Van der Beek AJ. Evaluation of an mHealth intervention aiming to improve health-related behavior and sleep and reduce fatigue among airline pilots. Scand J Work Environ Health. 2014;40(6):557–68.

Waterhouse J, Reilly T, Atkinson G, Edwards B. Jet lag: trends and coping strategies. Lancet. 2007;369(9567):1117–29.

ROAD & TRAFFIC SAFETY

Erin Sauber-Schatz, Erin Parker, Michael Ballesteros

Around the world, thousands of people are killed every day in motor vehicle crashes involving bicycles, buses, cars, motorcycles, trucks, and pedestrians.

MOTOR VEHICLE CRASHES: BY THE NUMBERS

Annually, ≈1.35 million people are killed (≈3,740 people every day) and an additional 20–50 million are injured in motor vehicle crashes. Road traffic injuries have become the leading cause of death for children and young adults aged 5–29 years. Although only 60% of the world's vehicles are in low- and middle-income countries, 93% of the world's crash deaths occur in these countries. More than half of people who die on the world's roads each year are cyclists, motorcyclists, and pedestrians, also called vulnerable road users.

According to US Department of State data, motor vehicle crashes are the leading cause of nonnatural death among US citizens who die in a foreign country (see Sec. 4, Ch. 12, Injury & Trauma). In 2017 and 2018, 431 US citizens living or traveling internationally died following motor vehicle crashes; 62% of crash deaths occurred among drivers and passengers of passenger vehicles (cars, sport utility vehicles, trucks). Other traffic-related fatalities involved motorcycle drivers and passengers (21%) and pedestrians (8.8%).

Table 8-01 shows the top 30 countries visited by US citizens (2016–2017) based on the Survey of International Air Travelers from the US Department of Commerce. For each country, the table lists the estimated motor vehicle crash death rate per 100,000 population as an indicator for the risk of motor vehicle crash death and the number of US citizens who died in each country because of a crash death from 2017 through 2018.

MOTOR VEHICLE CRASHES: RISK FACTORS

Motor vehicle crashes are common among US citizens traveling abroad for many reasons. In many low- and middle-income countries, unsafe vehicles and an inadequate transportation environment contribute to the crash injury problem. According to the World Health Organization (WHO), vehicles sold in 80% of all countries worldwide fail to meet basic safety standards promoted by the United Nations World Forum for Harmonization of Vehicle Regulations. In addition, motor vehicles share the road with vulnerable road users, and the mix of traffic, including animals, buses, cars, rickshaws, taxis, and large trucks, increases the risk for crashes and injuries.

Speed is another risk factor for vehicular crashes, injuries, and deaths. According to the WHO, speed contributes to about a third of road fatalities in high-income countries and to nearly half in low- and middle-income countries, including fatalities among vulnerable road users (see www.who.int/publications/i/item/managing-speed). Other factors that contribute to the risk for motor vehicle crashes among travelers include

Table 8-01 Thirty most visited destinations for US citizens traveling abroad, 2016–2017 (US Department of Commerce), World Health Organization (WHO) estimated motor vehicle crash death rate (per 100,000 population) & number of US citizen crash deaths per country, 2017–2018[1]

COUNTRY	2016–2017 COUNTRY VISITATION RANK[2]	WHO ESTIMATED CRASH DEATH RATE (PER 100,000 POPULATION)[3]	NUMBER OF US CITIZEN CRASH DEATHS[4,5]
Mexico[6,7]	1	13.1	126
Canada[6]	2	5.8	8
United Kingdom[6]	3	3.1	NA
Dominican Republic	4	34.6	12
France	5	5.5	3
Italy[6]	6	5.6	5
Germany	7	4.1	8
Spain	8	4.1	NA
Jamaica	9	13.6	9
China[6]	10	18.2	6
Japan	11	4.1	3
Ireland	11	4.1	7
India	13	22.6	10
Netherlands[6]	13	3.8	NA
Costa Rica[6]	15	16.7	11
Bahamas	16	NA	1
Philippines[6]	17	12.3	14
Colombia	17	18.5	2
Aruba	19	NA	NA
Switzerland	20	2.7	NA
Israel	21	4.2	NA
Austria	22	5.2	NA

Table 8-01 **Thirty most visited destinations for US citizens traveling abroad, 2016–2017 (US Department of Commerce), World Health Organization (WHO) estimated motor vehicle crash death rate (per 100,000 population) & number of US citizen crash deaths per country, 2017–2018 (continued)**

COUNTRY	2016–2017 COUNTRY VISITATION RANK[2]	WHO ESTIMATED CRASH DEATH RATE (PER 100,000 POPULATION)[3]	NUMBER OF US CITIZEN CRASH DEATHS[4,5]
Peru	23	13.5	2
Hong Kong	23	NA	1
Thailand	23	32.7	29
Greece	26	9.2	5
Korea, South	26	9.8	3
Taiwan	26	NA	5
Australia	26	5.6	3
Iceland	30	6.6	NA

Abbreviation: NA, data not available.

[1]Most recent available complete data.
[2]US Department of Commerce, National Travel & Tourism Office. Top destinations of U.S. residents traveling abroad, 2016–2017. December 2018. Available from: https://travel.trade.gov/outreachpages/outbound.general_information.outbound_overview.asp
[3]World Health Organization. WHO global status report on road safety 2018. Geneva: World Health Organization; 2018.Available from: www.who.int/publications/i/item/9789241565684.
[4]US Department of State. Deaths of US citizens abroad by nonnatural causes, 2018. Available from: https://travel.state.gov/content/travel/en/international-travel/while-abroad/death-abroad1/death-statistics.html.
[5]A total of 158 crash deaths occurred in countries not included in the list of top-visited countries, including Vietnam (17 deaths) and Honduras (8 deaths). All other countries not listed reported ≤5 deaths in 2017–2018.
[6]2016 data not available for reported number of road travel deaths based on WHO global status report on road safety, 2018.
[7]Number of drivers and passengers combined for road user death percentage based on WHO global status report on road safety, 2018.

lack of familiarity with the roads, driving on the opposite side of the road, the influence of alcohol, poorly made or inadequately maintained vehicles, travel fatigue, poor road surfaces without shoulders, unprotected curves and cliffs, and absent lighting creating conditions of poor visibility.

Use of protective equipment significantly decreases the risk for injury and death during a vehicle crash. Seat belts, correctly installed children's booster and car seats, and helmets for bicycle and motorcycle riders reduce crash-related injury and death, but this equipment can be scarce in some countries. In addition, timely and effective emergency and hospital care might be unavailable in some locations. Trauma centers capable of providing optimal care for serious injuries are uncommon outside urban areas in many international destinations.

MOTOR VEHICLE CRASHES: RISK REDUCTION STRATEGIES

Strategies travelers can use to reduce the risks for motor vehicle crash injuries include remaining alert and avoiding distractions when cycling, driving, or walking; choosing transportation carefully (e.g., avoiding overcrowded buses); abstaining from alcohol before driving; and not accepting rides from an impaired driver (see Table 8-02 for more strategies). Travelers should always use seat belts and child safety seats and should rent vehicles with seat belts. Whenever possible, travelers

Table 8-02 Risk factors & recommended strategies to reduce risk for road traffic crashes and injuries while abroad

RISK FACTORS FOR CRASHES	RECOMMENDED RISK REDUCTION STRATEGIES
Alcohol-impaired driving	Alcohol increases the risk for all causes of injury. Do not drive after consuming alcohol or other drugs. Do not accept rides from drivers who have been drinking. Penalties for impaired driving (alcohol, drugs) can be severe overseas, and laws vary widely by country.
Bus travel	Avoid riding in overcrowded, overweight, or top-heavy buses or minivans, and avoid riding in mountainous terrain. Always avoid riding with an impaired (alcohol, drugs) or distracted driver.
Mobile telephones	Do not use a mobile or cellular telephone or text while driving. Distracted driving increases crash risk. Many countries have enacted laws banning cellular telephone use while driving and some countries have made using any kind of telephone, including hands-free, illegal while driving.
Country-specific driving hazards	Check the US Department of State Driving and Road Safety Abroad website (https://travel.state.gov/content/travel/en/international-travel/before-you-go/driving-and-road-safety.html) to learn more about driving in another country, and check the Association for Safe International Road Travel website (www.asirt.org) for driving hazards or risks by country.
General driving hazards	Avoid driving at night in low- and middle-income countries because adequate lighting is limited in many places. Always pay close attention to the correct side of the road when driving in countries that drive on the left. Speed is a major risk factor for crashes, injury, and death. Note speed limits and consider the driving conditions (road quality, infrastructure, weather).
Pedestrian hazards	Be alert when crossing streets, especially in countries where motorists drive on the left side of the road. Walk with a companion or someone from the host country. Use crosswalks and follow pedestrian signals when available. Pay full attention when crossing streets (i.e., don't walk distracted).
Taxis or hired drivers	Ride only in marked taxis, preferably those with working seat belts. If no seat belt is available or the vehicle is in disrepair, refuse the ride and wait for another taxi. Hire drivers familiar with the area and that have official status or credentials as taxis. Ask the US embassy or consulate for taxi company recommendations.

should only ride in taxis with seat belts, and opt for the rear seat. Travelers also should bring car seats or booster seats for their children from home, unless they can be assured of their availability and quality at the destination.

Discourage travelers from driving or riding on motorcycles or motorbikes, including motorcycle and motorbike taxis. For travelers who cannot be dissuaded, strongly recommend that they wear a helmet that meets US safety standards. A good-quality helmet can reduce the risk for death by 40% and for severe injury by 70%.

The Department of State has useful safety information for international travelers, including road safety and security alerts, international driving permits, and travel insurance (https://travel.state.gov/content/travel/en/international-travel/before-you-go/driving-and-road-safety.html), along with the Smart Traveler Enrollment Program (https://step.state.gov/step). In addition, the Association for International Road Travel (www.asirt.org) has useful safety information for international travelers, including road safety checklists and country-specific driving risks.

BIBLIOGRAPHY

Centers for Disease Control and Prevention. Motor vehicle safety. Available from: www.cdc.gov/motorvehiclesafety/index.html.

World Health Organization. 10 facts on global road safety. Available from: www.who.int/news-room/facts-in-pictures/detail/road-safety.

World Health Organization. Violence and injury prevention: developing global targets for road safety risk factors and service delivery mechanisms. Available from: www.who.int/activities/developing-global-targets-for-road-safety-risk-factors-and-service-delivery-mechanisms.

World Health Organization. Violence and injury prevention: road traffic injuries. Available from: www.who.int/news-room/fact-sheets/detail/road-traffic-injuries.

World Health Organization. WHO global status report on road safety 2015. Full report available from: www.afro.who.int/publications/global-status-report-road-safety-2015; summary report available from: www.who.int/violence_injury_prevention/road_safety_status/2015/GSRRS2015_Summary_EN_final2.pdf?ua=1.

World Health Organization. WHO global status report on road safety 2018. Geneva: World Health Organization; 2018. Available from: www.who.int/publications/i/item/9789241565684.

CRUISE SHIP TRAVEL

Kara Tardivel, Stefanie White, Aimee Treffiletti, Amy Freeland

Cruise ship travel presents a unique combination of health concerns. Travelers from diverse regions brought together in the often crowded, semi-enclosed shipboard environment can facilitate the spread of person-to-person, foodborne, and waterborne diseases. Outbreaks on ships can be sustained over multiple voyages by crewmembers who remain onboard, or by persistent environmental contamination. Port visits can expose travelers to local diseases and, conversely, be a conduit for disease introduction into shoreside communities.

Some people (e.g., those with chronic health conditions or who are immunocompromised, older people, pregnant people) merit additional considerations when preparing for a cruise. Because travelers at sea might need to rely on a ship's medical capabilities for an extended period, potential cruise passengers with preexisting medical needs should prepare accordingly by calling the cruise line's customer service center to learn what type and level of health care services are (and are not) available on specific ships.

CRUISE SHIP MEDICAL CAPABILITIES

Medical facilities on cruise ships can vary widely depending on ship size, itinerary, cruise duration, and passenger demographics. Generally, shipboard medical centers can provide medical care comparable to that of ambulatory care centers; some are capable of providing hospitalization services or renal dialysis. Although no agency officially regulates medical practice aboard cruise ships, the American College of Emergency Physicians (ACEP) published consensus-based guidelines for cruise ship medical facilities in 1995, and updated the guidelines in 2013. ACEP guidelines, which most major cruise lines follow, state that cruise ship medical facilities should be able to provide quality medical care for passengers and crew; initiate appropriate stabilization, diagnostic, and therapeutic maneuvers for critically ill or medically unstable patients; and assist in the medical evacuation of patients in a timely fashion, when appropriate (see www.acep.org/patient-care/policy-statements/health-care-guidelines-for-cruise-ship-medical-facilities).

ILLNESS & INJURY

Cruise ship medical centers deal with a wide variety of illnesses and injuries; ≈10% of conditions reported to cruise ship medical centers are an emergency or require urgent care. Approximately 95% of illnesses are treated or managed onboard, with the remainder requiring evacuation and shoreside consultation for dental, medical, or surgical issues. Roughly half of all passengers seeking medical care are >65 years old.

Medical center visits are primarily the result of acute illness or injury. The most frequently reported diagnoses include respiratory illnesses (30%–40%); injuries from slips, trips, or falls (12%–18%); seasickness (10%); and gastrointestinal (GI) illness (10%); 80% of onboard deaths are due to cardiovascular events.

Infectious Disease Outbreaks

The most frequently reported cruise ship outbreaks involve GI infections (e.g., norovirus), respiratory infections (e.g., coronavirus disease 2019 [COVID-19], influenza), and other vaccine-preventable diseases (VPDs), such as varicella. Although cruise ships do not have public health authority, to reduce the risk of introducing communicable diseases, some ships conduct medical screening during embarkation to identify ill passengers, prevent them from boarding, or require isolation if permission to board is given.

Before travel, to help limit the introduction and spread of communicable diseases on cruise ships, prospective cruise ship travelers and their clinicians should consult the Centers for Disease Control and Prevention (CDC) Travelers' Health website (https://wwwnc.cdc.gov/travel) for updates on outbreaks and destination-specific travel health notices. People who become ill with a communicable disease before a voyage should consult their health care provider and delay their travel until they are no longer contagious. When booking a cruise, travelers should check the trip cancellation policies and consider purchasing trip cancellation insurance (see Sec. 6, Ch. 1, Travel Insurance, Travel Health Insurance & Medical Evacuation Insurance).

Travelers who become ill during a voyage should seek care in the ship's medical center; the onboard staff will provide clinical management, facilitate infection-control measures, and take responsibility for reporting potential public health events. For information on how to report travelers who become ill with suspected communicable diseases after they return home from a cruise, see Sec. 8, Ch. 8, Airplanes & Cruise Ships: Illness & Death Reporting & Public Health Interventions.

8

INFECTIOUS DISEASE HEALTH RISKS

Gastrointestinal Illnesses

During 2006–2019, rates of GI illness among passengers on voyages lasting 3–21 days fell from 32.5 to 16.9 cases per 100,000 travel days. Despite the decrease, outbreaks continue to occur. CDC assists the cruise ship industry to prevent and control the introduction, transmission, and spread of GI illnesses on cruise ships. Information on cruise ship GI illnesses is available at www.cdc.gov/nceh/vsp; updates on GI illness outbreaks involving ships with US ports of call, specifically, are available from www.cdc.gov/nceh/vsp/surv/gilist.htm.

NOROVIRUS

On cruise ships, >90% of GI illness outbreaks with a confirmed cause are due to norovirus. Characteristics of norovirus that facilitate outbreaks include a low infective dose, easy person-to-person transmissibility, prolonged viral shedding, absence of long-term immunity, and the ability of the virus to survive routine cleaning procedures (see Sec. 5, Part 2, Ch. 16, Norovirus). For international cruise ships porting in the United States during 2006–2019, an average of 12 norovirus outbreaks occurred each year.

OTHER SOURCES OF GASTROINTESTINAL ILLNESS

GI outbreaks on cruise ships also have been caused by contaminated food or water; most outbreaks were associated with *Campylobacter*, *Clostridium perfringens*, or enterotoxigenic *Escherichia coli*.

PROTECTIVE MEASURES

Travelers can reduce the risk of acquiring a GI illness on cruise ships by frequently washing hands with soap and water, especially before eating and after using the restroom. Travelers should call the ship's medical center promptly, even for mild symptoms of a GI illness, and strictly follow cruise ship guidance regarding isolation and other infection-control measures.

Respiratory Illnesses

Respiratory illnesses are the most common medical complaint on cruise ships. During the pretravel visit, evaluate whether vaccines or boosters (e.g., COVID-19, influenza) are needed and emphasize the importance of practicing good respiratory hygiene and cough etiquette while onboard. As with GI illnesses, cruise ship passengers should report respiratory illness to the medical center promptly and follow isolation recommendations as instructed.

CORONAVIRUS DISEASE 2019

Severe acute respiratory syndrome coronavirus 2 (SARS-CoV-2), the virus that causes COVID-19, spreads more easily between people in close quarters, and multiple studies have concluded that transmission rates of SARS-CoV-2 among travelers on ships are much greater than in other settings. Cruise ship COVID-19 outbreaks can tax onboard medical and public health resources. Ship-to-shore medical evacuations to facilities capable of providing higher levels of medical care can present logistical challenges and pose additional risks to ill patients.

Cruise passengers and crewmembers who are not up to date with their COVID-19 vaccines are at increased risk for severe illness, hospitalization, medical evacuation, and death. Since cruising will always pose some risk of SARS-CoV-2 transmission, ensure that people planning cruise ship travel are up to date with their vaccinations, and assess their likelihood for developing severe COVID-19. For people at increased risk of severe COVID-19 regardless of their vaccination status (e.g., pregnant people, people who are immunocompromised), discuss the potential health hazards associated with cruise ship travel. CDC has developed recommendations and guidance designed to help cruise ship operators provide a safer and healthier environment for crewmembers, passengers, port personnel, and communities (www.cdc.gov/quarantine/cruise/covid-19-cruise-ship-guidance.html).

INFLUENZA

Historically, influenza has been among the most often reported VPDs occurring on cruise ships. Because passengers and crew originate from all regions of the globe, shipboard outbreaks of influenza A and B can occur year-round, with exposure to strains circulating in different parts of the world (see Sec. 5, Part 2, Ch. 12, Influenza). Thus, anyone planning a cruise should receive the current seasonal influenza vaccine ≥2 weeks before travel if vaccine is available and no contraindications exist. For people at high risk for influenza complications, health care providers should discuss chemoprophylaxis and how and when to initiate antiviral treatment.

Additional guidance on the prevention and control of influenza on cruise ships is available from www.cdc.gov/quarantine/cruise/management/guidance-cruise-ships-influenza-updated.html.

LEGIONNAIRES' DISEASE

Less common on cruise ships, Legionnaires' disease is nevertheless a treatable infection that can result in severe pneumonia leading to death (see Sec. 5, Part 1, Ch. 9, Legionnaires' Disease & Pontiac Fever). Approximately 10%–15% of all Legionnaires' disease cases reported to CDC occur in people who have traveled during the 10 days before symptom onset. Clusters of Legionnaires' disease associated with hotel or cruise ship travel can be difficult to detect, because travelers often disperse from the source of infection before symptoms begin. Data reported to CDC during 2014–2015 included 25 confirmed cases of Legionnaires' disease associated with cruise ship exposures.

In general, Legionnaires' disease is contracted by inhaling warm, aerosolized water containing the bacteria, *Legionella*. Transmission also can sometimes occur through aspiration of *Legionella*-containing water. Typically, people do not spread *Legionella* to others; a single episode of possible person-to-person transmission of Legionnaires' disease has been reported. Contaminated hot tubs are commonly implicated as a source of shipboard *Legionella* outbreaks, although potable water supply systems also have been culpable. Improvements in ship design and standardization of water disinfection have reduced the risk for *Legionella* growth and colonization.

DIAGNOSIS & REPORTING

People with suspected Legionnaires' disease require prompt antibiotic treatment. When evaluating cruise travelers for Legionnaires' disease, obtain a thorough travel history of all destinations during the 10 days before symptom onset to assist in identifying potential sources of exposure, and collect urine for *Legionella* antigen testing. Most cruise ships have the capacity to perform this test, which detects *L. pneumophila* serogroup 1, the most common serogroup.

Perform culture of lower respiratory secretions on selective media to detect non–*L. pneumophila* serogroup 1 species and serogroups. Culture also is used for comparing clinical isolates to environmental isolates during an outbreak investigation. Notify CDC of any travel-associated Legionnaires' disease cases by sending an email to travellegionella@cdc.gov. Quickly report all cases of Legionnaires' disease to public health officials, who can determine whether a case links to previously reported cases and work to stop potential clusters and new outbreaks.

Other Vaccine-Preventable Diseases

Although most cruise ship passengers come from countries with routine vaccination programs (e.g., Canada, the United States), many of the crew are from low- or middle-income countries where immunization rates can be low. Outbreaks of hepatitis A, measles, meningococcal disease, mumps, pertussis, rubella, and varicella have all been reported on cruise ships. The majority (82%) of these outbreaks occur among crewmembers; prior to the COVID-19 pandemic, varicella was the most frequently reported VPD. Other VPDs (e.g., pertussis) occur more often among passengers.

Each cruise line sets its own policies regarding vaccinations for its crew; some have limited or no requirements. Thus, all passengers should be up to date with routine vaccinations before travel, as well as any required or recommended vaccinations specific for their destinations. People of childbearing age should have documented immunity to measles, rubella, and varicella (either by vaccination or titer) before cruise ship travel.

Vectorborne Diseases

Some cruise ship ports of call include destinations where vectorborne diseases (e.g., dengue, Japanese encephalitis, malaria, yellow fever, Zika) are known to be endemic. In addition, new diseases can surface in unexpected locations; chikungunya was reported for the first time in the Caribbean in late 2013, with subsequent spread throughout the region and numerous other North, Central, and South American countries and territories. Zika was first reported in Brazil in 2015, and subsequently spread across the Caribbean and Latin America, sparking concern because of its association with microcephaly and other congenital abnormalities in the fetus. For disease-specific information, see the relevant chapters of Section 5.

For guidance on how to avoid bites from mosquitoes and other disease-transmitting arthropod vectors, both onboard and while on shore at ports of call, see Sec. 4, Ch. 6, Mosquitoes, Ticks & Other Arthropods. For specific details on yellow fever vaccination and malaria prevention, see Sec. 2, Ch. 5, Yellow Fever Vaccine & Malaria Prevention Information, by Country.

NONINFECTIOUS HEALTH RISKS

Stresses of cruise ship travel include varying weather and environmental conditions, and unaccustomed changes to diet and levels of physical activity. Despite modern stabilizer systems, seasickness is a common complaint, affecting up to 25% of travelers (see Sec. 8, Ch. 7, Motion Sickness). Note that travel is an independent risk factor for behaviors such as alcohol and illicit drug use and misuse (see Sec. 3, Ch. 5, Substance Use & Substance Use Disorders), and unsafe sex (see Sec. 9, Ch. 12, Sex & Travel).

TRAVEL PREPARATION

Cruise ship travelers have complex itineraries due to multiple short port visits. Although most port visits do not include overnight stays off ship, some trips offer travelers the opportunity to venture off the ship for ≥1 night. These excursions can complicate decisions about exposures and the need for specific antimicrobial prophylaxis, immunizations, and other prevention measures. Boxes 8-04 and 8-05 summarize recommended cruise travel preparations and healthy behaviors during travel for health care providers and cruise ship travelers.

Travelers with Additional Considerations

Travelers with chronic illnesses and travelers with disabilities who have additional needs

BOX 8-04 Healthy cruise travel preparation: a checklist for health care providers

RISK ASSESSMENT & RISK COMMUNICATION

- ☐ Discuss itinerary, including season, duration of travel, and activities at ports of call.
- ☐ Review the traveler's medical and immunization history, allergies, and any additional health needs.
- ☐ Discuss relevant travel-specific health hazards and risk reduction.
- ☐ Provide travelers with documentation of their medical history, immunizations, and medications.

VACCINATION & RISK MANAGEMENT

- ☐ Provide routinely recommended (age-specific), required (yellow fever), and recommended vaccines.
- ☐ Discuss safe food and water precautions.
- ☐ Discuss insect bite prevention.
- ☐ Provide older travelers with a baseline electrocardiogram, especially those with coronary artery disease.

MEDICATIONS BASED ON RISK & NEED

- ☐ Consider prescribing malaria chemoprophylaxis if itinerary includes stops in malaria-endemic areas.
- ☐ Consider prescribing motion sickness medications for self-treatment.

(e.g., dialysis, supplemental oxygen, wheelchairs) should inform their cruise line before traveling. Highly allergic travelers and travelers with underlying medical conditions should carry a file that contains essential, pertinent health information (e.g., allergies, blood type, chest radiograph [if abnormal], chronic conditions, electrocardiogram, medication list, primary and/or specialty care provider contact information). Travelers also should bring any medications recommended by their health care provider (e.g., an epinephrine auto-injector) to help facilitate care during a

BOX 8-05 Healthy cruise travel preparation: a checklist for travelers

PRETRAVEL

- ☐ Carry prescription drugs in original containers with a copy of the prescription and a physician's letter.
- ☐ Check the Centers for Disease Control and Prevention (CDC) Outbreak Updates for International Cruise Ships website (www.cdc.gov/nceh/vsp/surv/gilist.htm) for gastrointestinal outbreaks.
- ☐ Consider purchasing additional insurance coverage for overseas health care and medical evacuation.
- ☐ Consult medical and dental providers before cruise travel.
- ☐ Consult CDC Travelers' Health website (https://wwwnc.cdc.gov/travel/notices) for travel health notices.
- ☐ Defer travel while acutely ill.
- ☐ Evaluate the type and length of the planned cruise in the context of personal health requirements.
- ☐ Notify the cruise line of additional health needs (e.g., dialysis, supplemental oxygen, wheelchair).
- ☐ Pack Environmental Protection Agency (EPA)–registered insect repellent; consider treating clothes and gear with permethrin.
- ☐ Pack sunscreen.

DURING TRAVEL

- ☐ Avoid contact with people who are ill.
- ☐ Follow safe food and water precautions when eating off ship at ports of call.
- ☐ Maintain good fluid intake and avoid excessive alcohol consumption.
- ☐ Practice safe sex.
- ☐ Report all illnesses to ship's medical center and follow their recommendations.
- ☐ Use insect bite precautions during port visits, especially in vectorborne disease–endemic areas or areas experiencing outbreaks of vectorborne diseases (e.g., Zika, yellow fever)
- ☐ Use sun protection.
- ☐ Wash hands frequently with soap and water; if soap and water are not available, use ≥60% alcohol-based hand sanitizer.

POST TRAVEL

- ☐ See CDC's latest post-cruise health guidance regarding coronavirus disease 2019 at www.cdc.gov/coronavirus/2019-ncov/travelers/cruise-travel-during-covid19.html.

medical emergency. For detailed information on preparing travelers who have additional considerations for international travel, including severe allergies, chronic illness, disabilities, or immune compromise, see Section 3.

Pregnant Travelers

Most cruise lines have policies that do not permit people to board after their 24th week of pregnancy. Contact cruise lines directly for specific guidance before booking. For additional information on preparing pregnant people for international travel, see Sec. 7, Ch. 1, Pregnant Travelers.

Insurance Coverage

All prospective cruise travelers should verify coverage with their health insurance carriers and, if not included, consider purchasing additional insurance to cover medical evacuation and health services received onboard cruise ships and in foreign countries (see Sec. 6, Ch. 1, Travel Insurance, Travel Health Insurance & Medical Evacuation Insurance).

BIBLIOGRAPHY

Hill CD. Cruise ship travel. In: Keystone JS, Kozarsky PE, Connor BA, Nothdurft HD, Mendelson M, editors. Travel medicine, 4th edition. Philadelphia: Saunders Elsevier; 2019. pp. 377–82.

Jenkins KA, Vaughan GHJ, Rodriguez LO, Freeland AL. Acute gastroenteritis on cruise ships—United States, 2006–2019. MMWR Morb Mortal Wkly Rep. 2021;70(6):1–19.

Kordsmeyer A-C, Mojtahedzadeh N, Heidrich J, Militzer K, von Münster T, Belz L, et al. Systematic review on outbreaks of SARS-CoV-2 on cruise, navy and cargo ships. Int J Environ Res Public Health. 2021;18(10):5195.

Millman AJ, Kornylo Duong K, Lafond K, Green NM, Lippold SA, Jhung MA. Influenza outbreaks among passengers and crew on two cruise ships: a recent account of preparedness and response to an ever-present challenge. J Travel Med. 2015;22(5):306–11.

Mouchtouri VA, Lewis HC, Hadjichristodoulou C. A systematic review for vaccine-preventable diseases on ships: evidence for cross-border transmission and for pre-employment immunization need. Int J Environ Res Public Health. 2019;16(15):2713.

Payne DC, Smith-Jeffcoat SE, Nowak G, Chuwkwuma U, Geibe JR, Hawkins RJ, et al. SARS-CoV-2 infections and serologic responses from a Sample of U.S. Navy service members—USS Theodore Roosevelt, April 2020. MMWR Morb Mortal Wkly Rep 2020;69(23):714–21.

Peake DE, Gray CL, Ludwig MR, Hill CD. Descriptive epidemiology of injury and illness among cruise ship passengers. Ann Emerg Med. 1999;33(1):67–72.

Rice ME, Bannerman M, Marin M, Lopez AS, Lewis MM, Stamatakis CE, et al. Maritime varicella illness and death reporting, U.S., 2010–2015. Travel Med Infect Dis. 2018;23:27–33.

Rocklöv J, Sjödin H, Wilder-Smith A. COVID-19 outbreak on the Diamond Princess cruise ship: estimating the epidemic potential and effectiveness of public health countermeasures. J Travel Med. 2020;27(3):taaa030.

Stamatakis CE, Rice ME, Washburn FM, Krohn KJ, Bannerman M, et al. Maritime illness and death reporting and public health response, United States, 2010–2014. J Travel Med Inf Dis. 2017;19:16–21.

8

MOTION SICKNESS

Ashley Brown

Motion sickness describes the physiologic responses to travel by air, car, sea, train, and virtual reality immersion. Given sufficient stimulus, all people with functional vestibular systems can develop motion sickness. People vary in their susceptibility, however.

RISK FOR TRAVELERS

Risk factors for motion sickness include age, sex, preexisting medical conditions, and concurrent medications. Children aged 2–12 years are especially susceptible, but infants and toddlers are generally immune. Adults >50 years are less susceptible to motion sickness. Pregnancy, menstruation, and taking hormone replacement therapy or oral contraceptives have also been identified as potential risk factors. People with a history of migraines, vertigo, and vestibular disorders are more prone to motion sickness.

Some prescriptions can worsen motion sickness–associated nausea.

CLINICAL PRESENTATION

Motion sickness typically occurs after a triggering motion or event. People with motion sickness commonly experience dizziness; headache; nausea, vomiting, or retching; sweating. For a complete list of motion sickness–associated signs and symptoms, see Box 8-06.

NEUROPHYSIOLOGY

When sensory input does not align with expected patterns (neural mismatch), patients suffer dizziness and nausea. Sensory conflict theory (the most widely accepted explanation for motion sickness) proposes that the condition is caused by conflict between the visual, vestibular, and somatosensory systems, and involves complex neurophysiologic signaling between multiple nuclear regions, neurotransmitters, and receptors. Medications used to prevent and treat motion sickness are thought to work by suppressing the signals that contribute to neural mismatch.

NONPHARMACOLOGIC PREVENTION & INTERVENTIONS

Travelers can use nonpharmacologic interventions to prevent or treat motion sickness (see Box 8-07). Awareness and avoidance of situations that tend to trigger symptoms are the primary defenses against motion sickness.

TREATMENT

Medications used to treat motion sickness can vary in effectiveness and side effects; suggest travelers take a trial dose of medication at home before departure to find what works best for them. The most frequently used antihistamines to treat motion sickness include cyclizine, dimenhydrinate, meclizine, and promethazine (oral and suppository); nonsedating antihistamines appear to be less effective. Other commonly used motion sickness medications include anticholinergics (e.g., scopolamine [hyoscine, oral and transdermal]); benzodiazepines; dopamine receptor antagonists (e.g., metoclopramide, prochlorperazine); and sympathomimetics (often used in combination with antihistamines).

Complementary approaches with anecdotal evidence of effectiveness for preventing or treating motion sickness (e.g., acupressure and magnets, ginger, homeopathic remedies, pyridoxine [vitamin B6]) might be effective for individual travelers but cannot generally be recommended (see Sec. 2, Ch. 14, Complementary & Integrative Health Approaches to Travel Wellness). Clinical trials have shown that ondansetron, a commonly used antiemetic, is ineffective in preventing nausea associated with motion sickness.

Children & Motion Sickness

For children aged 2–12 years, dimenhydrinate (Dramamine), 1–1.5 mg/kg per dose, or diphenhydramine (Benadryl), 0.5–1 mg/kg per dose up to 25 mg, can be given 1 hour before travel and every 6 hours during the trip. Because some children have paradoxical agitation with these medications, encourage parents to try a test dose before departure. Oversedating young children with antihistamines can be life-threatening. Scopolamine can cause dangerous adverse effects in children and should not be used.

BOX 8-06 Motion sickness symptoms

Anorexia	Increased sensitivity to odors
Apathy	Loss of appetite
Cold sweats	Nausea
Drowsiness	Salivation, excessive
Generalized discomfort	Sweating
Headache	Vomiting or retching
Hyperventilation	Warm sensation

BOX 8-07 Non-pharmacologic prevention & interventions for motion sickness: a checklist for travelers

- ☐ Be aware. Try to avoid situations that tend to trigger your symptoms.
- ☐ Optimize your position to reduce motion or motion perception (e.g., drive a vehicle instead of riding in it; sit in the front seat of a car or bus; sit over the wing of an aircraft; hold your head firmly against the back of the seat; choose a window seat on flights and trains).
- ☐ Reduce sensory input. Lie face down, shut your eyes, try sleeping, look at the horizon.
- ☐ Maintain hydration by drinking water, eating small meals frequently, and limiting alcoholic and caffeinated beverages.
- ☐ Get plenty of sleep or rest. Being sleep-deprived can worsen motion sickness symptoms.
- ☐ Avoid smoking. Quitting (even short-term) reduces susceptibility to motion sickness.
- ☐ Try using distractions. Controlled breathing, listening to music, or using aromatherapy scents like mint, lavender, or ginger. Flavored lozenges also might help.
- ☐ Some people recommend using acupressure or magnets to prevent or treat nausea, although scientific data are lacking on how effective these interventions are for preventing motion sickness.
- ☐ Gradually expose yourself to continuous or repeated motion sickness triggers. Most people, in time, notice a reduction in motion sickness symptoms.

BIBLIOGRAPHY

Golding JF, Gresty MA. Pathophysiology and treatment of motion sickness. Curr Opin Neurol. 2015;28(1):83–8.

Leung AK, Hon KL. Motion sickness: an overview. Drugs Context. 2019;8:2019-9-4.

Priesol AJ. Motion sickness. Deschler DG, editor. Waltham (MA): UpToDate; 2021. Available from: www.uptodate.com/contents/motion-sickness.

Schmäl F. Neuronal mechanisms and the treatment of motion sickness. Pharmacology. 2013;91(3-4):229–41.

Zhang L, Wang J, Qi R, Pan L, Li M, Cai Y. Motion sickness: current knowledge and recent advance. CNS Neurosci Ther. 2016;22(1):15–24.

AIRPLANES & CRUISE SHIPS: ILLNESS & DEATH REPORTING & PUBLIC HEALTH INTERVENTIONS

Alida Gertz, Francisco Alvarado-Ramy

The Centers for Disease Control and Prevention (CDC) has a regulatory mission to protect the public health of the United States by preventing the introduction, transmission, and spread of communicable diseases from foreign countries into and within US states and territories. For diseases of concern that have received special designation by the President of the United States, CDC may issue federal public health orders for quarantine, isolation, and conditional release. Diseases falling under this specific federal public health authority (Table 8-03) include cholera, diphtheria, infectious tuberculosis, measles, plague, smallpox, yellow fever, viral hemorrhagic fevers, severe acute respiratory syndromes (e.g., Middle East respiratory syndrome [MERS], coronavirus disease 2019 [COVID-19]), and influenza due to novel or reemergent viruses that are causing (or have the potential to cause) a pandemic. The list of federally quarantinable diseases can be revised by executive order when a communicable disease becomes a significant public

Table 8-03 Executive Orders specifying diseases for which federal quarantine is authorized

EXECUTIVE ORDER	DATE	TITLE	REVISIONS, MODIFICATIONS, ADDITIONS	AVAILABLE FROM
13295	April 4, 2003	Revised List of Quarantinable Communicable Diseases	Specified the following diseases for the list of quarantinable communicable diseases: cholera; diphtheria; infectious tuberculosis; plague; smallpox; yellow fever; and viral hemorrhagic fevers (Lassa, Marburg, Ebola, Crimean-Congo, South American, and others not yet isolated or named); and severe acute respiratory syndrome (SARS)	www.federalregister.gov/d/03-8832
13375	April 1, 2005	Amendment to Executive Order 13295 Relating to Certain Influenza Viruses and Quarantinable Communicable Diseases	Added to the list, influenza caused by novel or reemergent influenza viruses that are causing, or have the potential to cause, a pandemic	www.federalregister.gov/d/05-6907
13674	July 31, 2014	Revised List of Quarantinable Communicable Diseases	Expanded the definition of severe acute respiratory syndromes	www.federalregister.gov/d/2014-18682
14047	September 17, 2021	Adding Measles to the List of Quarantinable Communicable Diseases	Added measles to the existing list, after infectious tuberculosis	www.federalregister.gov/documents/2021/09/22/2021-20629/adding-measles-to-the-list-of-quarantinable-communicable-diseases

health threat. For more information, see Specific Laws and Regulations Governing the Control of Communicable Diseases (www.cdc.gov/quarantine/specificlawsregulations.html).

PROTECTING THE PUBLIC'S HEALTH BEFORE, DURING & AFTER TRAVEL

In the United States, CDC conducts public health actions before, during, and after commercial flights and cruise travel to prevent or mitigate the introduction and spread of diseases of public health concern. Many of these actions are carried out by CDC quarantine station personnel working in collaboration with state, tribal, local, and territorial (STLT) public health officers. CDC quarantine stations are located at the 20 ports of entry, including land border crossings, where most travelers arrive to or transit through the United States. More information on CDC quarantine stations is available from www.cdc.gov/quarantine/quarantinestations.html.

Before Travel

In 2007, CDC and the US Department of Homeland Security (DHS) developed a public health Do Not Board (DNB) list to prevent people from boarding commercial aircraft if they are known to have, are suspected of having, or were exposed to a communicable disease of public health concern. A person placed on the DNB list will not be issued a boarding pass for any commercial airline flight originating from or arriving to a US airport.

STLT public health authorities notify CDC when people with communicable diseases of public health concern are at risk of traveling on a commercial flight; they also can recommend to CDC that people who meet certain criteria be added to the DNB list. For more information about the DNB list, see FAQs for Public Health Do Not Board and Lookout Lists (www.cdc.gov/quarantine/do-not-board-faq.html).

During Travel

Federal regulations mandate that before arrival, the person in charge of a conveyance destined for a US port of entry must report to the CDC quarantine station of jurisdiction (www.cdc.gov/quarantine/quarantine-stations-us.html) any death or "ill person" among passengers or crew. For the definition of an ill person, see CFR Title 42 §71.21: Report of death or illness (https://ecfr.io/Title-42/Section-71.21) and Box 8-08.

Airlines, DHS's US Customs and Border Protection, and emergency medical personnel at arriving airports can each provide CDC quarantine station staff with reports of illness and/or death that occurs during commercial air travel. Most reports of illness or death on commercial, seagoing vessels are received directly from the ship's medical staff or from a shipping agent. Airline and cruise ship illness and death reports also can originate from other federal partners or STLT health departments.

AIR TRAVEL RESPONSE

CDC's goals in responding to reports of illness during air travel are to determine whether the illness poses (or has the potential to pose) a public health threat and to take appropriate public health actions. When responding to reports of illness during air travel, public health officials can either allow ill air passengers to resume travel if their illness does not pose a meaningful public health risk; recommend ill air passengers

8

BOX 8-08 Regulatory definition of an "ill traveler" for the purposes of reporting illness on commercial airplanes and ships[1]

Fever,[2] plus ≥1 of the following
- Appears obviously unwell (applies to air travelers only)
- Breathing difficulty (or, for maritime travelers, suspected or confirmed pneumonia)
- Bruising or bleeding, new and unexplained, without a history of previous injury
- Consciousness decreased or confusion of recent onset
- Cough, persistent (or, for maritime travelers, cough with bloody sputum)
- Diarrhea, persistent (applies to air travelers only)
- Headache with stiff neck
- Vomiting, persistent (other than air or sea sickness)
- Rash

OR

Fever for >48 hours

OR

Acute gastroenteritis[3] (applies to maritime travelers only)

OR

Symptoms or other indications of a communicable disease, as the CDC may announce through posting of a notice in the Federal Register.

[1]Definition applies to all travelers, including passengers and crew, US citizens and non–US citizens.

[2]Measured temperature ≥100.4°F (≥38°C); feels warm to the touch; or provides a history of feeling feverish.

[3]Defined as diarrhea (≥3 episodes of loose stools in a 24-hour period or what is above normal for the person) OR vomiting accompanied by ≥1 of the following: ≥1 episode of loose stools in a 24-hour period, abdominal cramps, headache, muscle aches, or fever (temperature ≥100.4°F [≥38°C]).

with a suspected communicable disease seek medical care and delay further commercial travel until noninfectious; or require ill air passengers to be medically evaluated if they are suspected of having a quarantinable communicable disease.

Together with airport and public health response partners (e.g., emergency medical services, public health authorities), CDC staff board arriving airplanes to conduct public health assessments of ill travelers and to make recommendations regarding potentially exposed passengers. Potentially exposed travelers might be asked to provide their contact information before disembarking so that health authorities can follow up and provide additional health information if the ill traveler is diagnosed with a disease of public health concern.

CDC provides guidance to airlines on reporting and managing ill travelers on airplanes at Airline Guidance: Reporting Death/Illness (www.cdc.gov/quarantine/air/reporting-deaths-illness/index.html), and Airline Guidance: Managing Ill Passengers/Crew (www.cdc.gov/quarantine/air/managing-sick-travelers/index.html).

CRUISE SHIP RESPONSE

For public health responses to ill cruise ship passengers and crew, control measures typically are initiated while the ship is still at sea. CDC quarantine station personnel obtain clinical and epidemiologic information about the ill or deceased person(s), determine public health risk, and provide guidance to the ship's clinicians about case findings, infection control measures, and contact investigations.

CDC quarantine station personnel might respond by meeting a ship at the port of entry to further investigate or to assist the responding health department with surveillance and control measures. CDC personnel also might provide onsite response for outbreaks or clusters of disease, quarantinable communicable diseases, and some vaccine-preventable diseases (e.g., measles, rubella). CDC's Vessel Sanitation Program (www.cdc.gov/nceh/vsp/default.htm) is responsible for responding to reports of acute gastroenteritis on cruise ships.

CDC provides guidance to cruise lines on reporting and managing ill travelers at Cruise Ship Guidance: Reporting Death or Illness on Ships (www.cdc.gov/quarantine/cruise/reporting-deaths-illness/index.html), and Cruise Ship Guidance: Disease-specific Management of Ill Passengers/Crew (www.cdc.gov/quarantine/cruise/management/index.html).

After Travel

When a US or foreign public health authority notifies CDC of an illness of public health concern in airplane or cruise ship travelers who have reached their final destination, CDC conducts, or assists STLT health departments in conducting, a public health contact investigation. The primary purpose of the contact investigation is to identify and notify potentially exposed passengers and crew, so they can be offered clinical evaluation, postexposure prophylaxis (when necessary), and health education, including recommended quarantine periods.

REPORTING POSTTRAVEL ILLNESS

Travelers who become ill at their destination or after returning home should inform their health care providers of where, when, and on what type of conveyances they traveled. Report cases of communicable diseases of public health concern in returning travelers to appropriate public health authorities according to the state's specific reportable disease requirements.

When a risk for communicable disease transmission during travel is possible, health departments can notify CDC by contacting either the quarantine station with jurisdiction for their region (www.cdc.gov/quarantine/quarantinestations.html) or the CDC Emergency Operations Center (770-488-7100; eocreport@cdc.gov).

Report cases of travel-associated legionellosis to CDC to travellegionella@cdc.gov, and cases of acute gastroenteritis associated with cruise travel to vsp@cdc.gov.

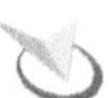

BIBLIOGRAPHY

Centers for Disease Control and Prevention. Vessel Sanitation Program operations manual, 2018. Available from: www.cdc.gov/nceh/vsp/pub/pub.htm.

Council of State and Territorial Epidemiologists. Cross cutting: border/international health. Available from: www.cste.org/members/group.aspx?code=BorderInternational.

Criteria for requesting federal travel restrictions for public health purposes, including for viral hemorrhagic fevers. Fed Regist. 2015;80(1640):16400–2. Available from: www.federalregister.gov/documents/2015/03/27/2015-07118/criteria-for-requesting-federal-travel-restrictions-for-public-health-purposes-including-for-viral.

Foreign quarantine. 42 CFR §71 (2000). Available from: www.ecfr.gov/current/title-42/chapter-I/subchapter-F/part-71.

Interstate quarantine. 42 CFR §70 (2000). Available from: www.ecfr.gov/current/title-42/chapter-I/subchapter-F/part-70.

Jungerman MR, Vonnahme LA, Washburn F, Alvarado-Ramy F. Federal travel restrictions to prevent disease transmission in the United States: An analysis of requested travel restrictions. Travel Med Infect Dis. 2017;18:30–5.

World Health Organization. Guide to hygiene and sanitation in aviation, 3rd edition. Geneva: The Organization; 2009. Available from: www.who.int/publications/i/item/9789241547772.

Travel for Work & Other Reasons

THE INTERNATIONAL BUSINESS TRAVELER

Davidson Hamer

In 2017, ≈4.8 million US residents traveled overseas for business. With an increasingly global economy, this number is expected to increase, although a major slowdown in business travel occurred due to the onset of the coronavirus disease 2019 (COVID-19) pandemic. Business travelers (also known as occupational travelers) include people traveling for conventions, research, work-related training, and volunteer work. Business travelers fall into several different categories according to duration and purpose of travel (see Table 9-01).

For international business travelers, the likelihood of an adverse health event increases with the number of trips made to at-risk areas and the length of time spent at the destination. Because most international business travelers take multiple trips each year, travel health providers should consider the cumulative risk to the traveler and not just the risks of the current trip.

HOW INTERNATIONAL BUSINESS TRAVELERS DIFFER FROM OTHER TRAVELERS

Unlike leisure travelers, international business travelers are usually employees, although some might be working as independent consultants. Business travelers' employers have a responsibility to protect their employees from health threats. Employers should cover the cost for all required and recommended vaccinations, prophylactic medications (e.g., antimalarials), and other health

CDC Yellow Book 2024. Jeffrey Nemhauser, Oxford University Press. © Oxford University Press 2023.
DOI: 10.1093/oso/9780197570944.003.0009

Table 9-01 **International business traveler categories**

CATEGORY	TRAVEL DURATION	TRAVEL DESCRIPTION	ADDITIONAL TRAVEL DETAILS	REPRESENTATIVE PROFESSIONS
Short-term traveler	≤2 weeks	Single destination for a specific meeting or event	Make presentations, attend conventions or association meetings	Academicians, business executives, health care professionals
Frequent traveler	2 weeks on average	Multiple trips per year to different locations	Most often over several years to same site but might repeat assignment	Auditors, business executives, engineers, managers (including financial managers), researchers, technical trainers, volunteer workers
Commuter or recurrent traveler	Varies	Regular international travel, multiple times per year	Special projects	Managers (e.g., financial, engineering), researchers
Assignee	3–12 months	Travels for specific, time-limited objectives	Does not relocate; might return home on a regular basis	Engineers, managers, specialists (e.g., legal, financial), volunteer workers
Expatriate	Long-term assignments (often 2–5 years or more)	Moves to host country	Usually relocates with family	Business executives, managers, researchers, technical experts

9

protection measures, either through in-house or contracted occupational health services or a sponsored health plan.

In the United States, employers are liable for tort suits for negligence and workers' compensation claims. Employers should have systems in place to evacuate employees traveling under their auspices; this typically requires a preexisting contractual relationship with an air medical evacuation provider or some form of comprehensive travel health insurance that includes medical evacuation coverage.

To better prepare their employees for healthy travel, businesses have developed international travel health programs (ITHPs). Primarily an innovation of larger corporations, ITHPs focus on disease prevention and health promotion activities before, during, and after international travel. Potential advantages of corporate travel health programs include fewer instances of urgent repatriations (including emergency medical evacuations) and hospital admissions for international business travelers; enhanced employee confidence; improved productivity overseas; and better public relations. Midsized and smaller businesses with large numbers of international business travelers might also benefit from the cost savings realized by an ITHP.

SPECIAL CONSIDERATIONS FOR INTERNATIONAL BUSINESS TRAVELERS

Risks for travel-related adverse health outcomes in international business travelers generally have been considered low. They have increased, however, as the number of people traveling for work (and the overall distance they travel) increases and as the time allotted for adjustment after arrival at destinations and after return home decreases. International business travelers are as likely as other travelers to develop some travel-related illnesses; a GeoSentinel analysis of 12,203 business travelers seen during 1997–2014 found that frequent diagnoses included malaria (9%), acute unspecified diarrhea (8%), viral syndrome (6%), and acute bacterial diarrhea (5%). Notably, only 45% of travelers in the analysis had had a pretravel encounter and, among the subset traveling to malaria-endemic regions for whom malaria prophylaxis data were available, 92% did not take prophylaxis or took an incomplete course of prescribed medication.

Extensive business travel also correlates with a higher body mass index and increased cholesterol, hypertension, and mental stress. A World Bank study showed overall health plan expenditures were 70% higher for international business travelers than for their nontraveling counterparts, and that the likelihood of developing a noncommunicable disease increased with travel frequency. The study also showed increased incidence for 20 noncommunicable disease categories among this employee group.

Although international business travelers should receive all indicated vaccines and prophylaxis prior to travel, gaps in care exist. For instance, not all practitioners adhere to the most current guidance, some clinicians provide insufficient pretravel counseling, and some travelers fail to follow recommendations when provided.

PRETRAVEL CONSIDERATIONS

Fitness for Travel

The pretravel consultation should determine and document fitness for travel. Fitness for travel, particularly the risk for adverse health events overseas, depends on several factors, including how well underlying medical conditions are controlled; how easily preexisting medical conditions can be managed during travel; duration of time spent away from home; destination-specific health risks; access to health care while away; and job tasks and activities. As much as possible, international business travelers, especially assignees, expatriates, and recurrent travelers—and their health care providers—should attempt to improve those factors within their control and to minimize the risks presented by factors outside their control.

Employers can authorize international travel for their employees after consideration of several factors including an assessment of health and safety risks. Although almost all medical risks can be managed, the health care provider must ascertain whether a health condition will, based on the medical resources expected to be available, prevent a traveler from performing their essential job functions. For example, diabetes monitoring and care could be challenging during international travel, particularly to more austere environments.

If a provider identifies underlying medical conditions during the pretravel consultation, it is their responsibility to have a full discussion with both the international business traveler and the employer regarding the added health risks imposed by international travel, and then carefully document these conversations. Disability laws apply to most employees. Tort suits and workers' compensation liability are considerations for situations in which a US standard of medical care is not readily available, or when an increased risk for accident, illness, or injury is expected.

Health Risks

Structure the pretravel consultation to identify and address risks to both physical and mental health. Administering vaccines, prescribing prophylactic medication, and educating travelers about how to mitigate health threats while traveling are key elements of the consultation. To best prepare an international business traveler for healthy travel, providers must have access to the traveler's full itinerary, including all work sites, stopovers, likely side trips, and potential itinerary changes. Do not assume that international business travelers will only visit major cities, stay in first-class hotels, and eat at 5-star restaurants.

Attempt to elicit information about conditions at worksites listed in the itinerary, going into as much detail as possible. International business travel can include visits to industrial sites where travelers can be exposed to chemical or physical hazards or poor air quality. Some work locations could pose slip, trip, and fall hazards or the possibility of other injuries. International business travelers visiting hospitals or medical environments might require protection from biological hazards. Providing requisite personal protective equipment (PPE) and education regarding its proper use is unique to the pretravel consultation for people preparing to work internationally.

Mental Health Assessment

A mental health assessment is another component of the pretravel consultation for international business travelers. Travel- and work-associated stressors can be additive and manifest as circadian rhythm disruption, sleep disorders, and increased alcohol or substance use. The ability to work effectively with people from other cultures is known as cultural adaptability; employers should consider providing cultural adaptability training for frequent travelers, particularly if the employee is being sent to work abroad for extended periods (assignees and expatriates). Predeployment testing can help measure whether an international business traveler has the requisite cultural adaptability skills, and a variety of assessment tools are available. Address mental health and adaptability issues before the international business traveler embarks on international travel or assignment.

Vaccines

Once mental health issues and risks associated with a particular travel itinerary have been identified and addressed, evaluate the traveler for needed vaccines. Update routine vaccines (e.g., influenza, measles, tetanus-diphtheria-pertussis), if indicated. Unlike the leisure traveler, the international business traveler typically needs to be fully productive when traveling overseas. The inability to perform one's job because of illness has serious implications for both employee and employer; recommend immunizations for international business travelers based on an individualized risk assessment of potential vaccine-preventable health risks.

Administer vaccinations with a view toward the international business traveler's total travel over the course of a year or next several years, not just a single trip. A single business trip of only 1 or 2 weeks' duration to a low-risk destination might not warrant immediate vaccination against a particular disease, but future work trips could present a risk for exposure. Consider offering a vaccine series even if the travel requiring it has not yet been planned. Because business travel often is scheduled last-minute, vaccinating the international business traveler for later trips when immunity against specific diseases is required is reasonable. This is true even if the traveler does not complete the full vaccine series in advance of the most current trip.

Malaria Chemoprophylaxis

Simply providing prescriptions for necessary prophylaxis against travel-related diseases, particularly malaria, is not sufficient. As a large GeoSentinel study recently noted, >90% of international business travelers who contracted malaria while traveling did not take their prescribed medication appropriately, or at all. Although international business travelers are aware of the need for prophylaxis, they demonstrate poor adherence that only worsens with the length of the trip. Reported reasons for nonadherence include the challenges posed by daily dosing, presumed immunity, busy schedules or forgetfulness, conflicting advice, and fear of side effects. The use of electronic reminders (e.g., software applications on handheld devices) can help.

Additional Considerations

CHANGES IN PLANS

Travel plans often change. Before departing, international business travelers should know where to access health and safety information for destinations not included on the original itinerary. Destination-specific health recommendations are available from the Centers for Disease Control and Prevention (CDC) Travelers' Health website (https://wwwnc.cdc.gov/travel/).

TRAVEL COMPANIONS

All family members accompanying the international business traveler also should visit a primary care provider for a pretravel physical and mental health screening; the inability of a child, companion, or spouse to adjust to an international environment is often a cause for early repatriation. Each family member should have their own consultation with a health care provider familiar with assessing the impact of travel on health and safety.

TRAVEL HEALTH ISSUES DURING TRAVEL & AT THE DESTINATION

Planning for and adhering to guidance provided by medical and human resources personnel can mitigate health and wellness risks posed by lengthy flights. These risks include deep vein thrombosis, dehydration, jet lag, and motion sickness (for more details on these conditions, see the relevant chapters in Section 8). Multiple-leg, complex itineraries can aggravate and increase the likelihood of these conditions occurring. To decrease a traveler's chances of experiencing adverse effects—which is particularly important when work duties are scheduled on or close to arrival—counsel travelers to limit or refrain from in-flight alcohol consumption, and caution against the use of hypnotic drugs to facilitate sleep while flying.

Coronavirus Disease 2019

Because of the COVID-19 pandemic, international travel guidance—ranging from alerts about the risk for COVID-19 in different countries to travel interdictions between certain countries—changes frequently. Countries might require proof of vaccination, quarantine on arrival, or documentation of negative test results before permitting entry. Quarantine can range from stays in a government-mandated facility, at one's home, or in a hotel; quarantine also could mean travelers need to be available by phone for a daily interview by government health authorities. Employers should check with their human resources office or publicly available references (e.g., CDC, US State Department, government websites in the destination country) for COVID-19 travel information, and work with their employees to help ensure they adhere to the latest requirements and recommendations.

Medication

Changing time zones can interfere with taking prescribed medicine on time, another potential threat to the health and wellness of international travelers. Adjusting the timing of regular medication during international travel might be a challenge for the international business traveler; help create schedules for travelers taking medication(s), both on the way overseas and when returning. Anticipating the possibility that checked luggage could be delayed, broken into, or lost during international travel, international business travelers should carry with them a travel health kit containing sufficient quantities of all necessary medications to last the duration of travel, and extra doses in case of delays.

Occupational & Environmental Hazards

On arrival, international business travelers should review with their hosts all safety, security, occupational, and environmental hazards specific to the destination. In low- and middle-income countries in particular, international business travelers could encounter occupational and environmental health risks much different from what they experience at home; chemicals used in some locations might no longer be used (or might never have been approved for use) in the United States because of their hazardous properties. Foreign governments might lack or not enforce exposure limits, requirements for PPE use, or worker safety laws.

Health Emergencies

Advise business travelers to use the Smart Traveler Enrollment Program (STEP), a free program offered through the US Department of State, in which international travelers and expatriates enroll their trip with the US embassy in the country of travel or residence. STEP benefits include receiving information alerts from the local embassy about health and safety issues, facilitating contact with the embassy if a problem arises, and helping family and friends reach international travelers through the embassy, in case of an emergency.

International business travelers should be well briefed on what to do in case of an overseas health emergency and which hospitals and health clinics in the vicinity provide the highest levels of medical care. This information might be available through the local US embassy and is another reason for travelers to consider enrolling in STEP. Details about how to access quality outpatient and inpatient care must be available to the international business traveler throughout the trip, and updated as needed.

POSTTRAVEL CARE

ITHPs provide international business travelers with both pretravel and posttravel care. Studies show that, upon returning home, 22%–64% of people traveling internationally for work will have an unresolved health issue meriting careful case management with referral to specialists. Because an international business traveler could be a sentinel for a health risk at an overseas facility or workplace, a correct diagnosis is important not only to the health and well-being of the traveler but also to that of the other workers at that jobsite.

Employers have a general duty to prevent occupational injuries. Returning workers can assist by notifying employers of any work-related incidents or on-the-job exposures. Such workplace hazards might require medical monitoring and referral to occupational health specialists for the person, and exposure mitigation by a hierarchy of controls at the location. International business travelers also should provide information about any changes in the quality of available medical care, accommodations, security, and any other medical or legal issues that could adversely affect the health of future travelers.

BIBLIOGRAPHY

Bunn WB. Assessing risk and improving travel vaccine programs for business travelers. J Occup Environ Med. 2014;56(11):1167–8.

Bunn W. Health and productivity in business/occupational travelers, assignees and expatriates. Int J Health Productivity. 2016;8(1):30–7.

Chen LH, Leder K, Barbre KA, Schlagenhauf P, Libman M, Keystone J, et al. Business travel-associated illness: a GeoSentinel analysis. J Travel Med. 2018;25(1):tax097.

Chen L, Leder K, Wilson M. Business travelers: vaccination considerations for this population. Expert Rev Vaccines. 2013;12(4):453–66.

Khan NM, Jentes ES, Brown C, Han P, Rao SR, Kozarsky P, et al. Pre-travel medical preparation of business and occupational travelers: an analysis of Global TravEpiNet Consortium, 2009 to 2012. J Occup Environ Med. 2016;58(1):76–82.

Richards C, Rundle A. Business travel and self-rated health, obesity, and cardiovascular disease risk factors. J Occup Environ Med. 2011;53(4):358–63.

Rogers B, Bunn W, Connor B. An update on travel vaccines and issues in travel and international medicine. Workplace Health Saf. 2016;64(7):462–8.

ADVICE FOR AIRCREW

Alan Kozarsky, Phyllis Kozarsky

As airlines expand their routes to include more destinations, particularly to low- and middle-income countries, aircrew (pilots and flight attendants) need to be prepared for travel-related exposures. Help aircrew protect themselves when traveling for their jobs and when off duty.

Aircrew are distinct from leisure travelers, and the nature of their work requires modifications to travel health recommendations. When consulting with aircrew, consider that they travel frequently; can have short layovers, often 24–48 hours; often travel to new destinations on short notice; might be more adventurous and exposed to more risks than typical tourists, despite short travel times; and that aircrew might perceive themselves to be low-risk since they mostly are healthy, and their in-country exposure time is short.

In general, air carriers that fly to low- and middle-income countries try to inform their crew about the health issues they face. Airlines do not necessarily employ occupational health providers or experts in travel medicine, however, and they can be unaware of special risks at the destinations they serve. Therefore, airlines should avail themselves of travel medicine professionals who can provide well-informed recommendations to their traveling employees.

GENERAL HEALTH MEASURES

When conducting a pretravel consultation for flight crew, ask each crewmember about their airline company's requirements. If in doubt regarding airline requirements, contact the medical director or occupational health department of the airline for guidance. For example, some airlines might require all aircrew without contraindications to be vaccinated against yellow fever, even those who fly primarily to regions without risk for the disease. Such a policy provides the employer with added flexibility to reassign employees to cover routes that include yellow fever–endemic regions and destinations. In addition, although pilots are required to have periodic medical examinations to ensure they are fit to fly, those visits do not typically address issues related to international travel, particularly to destinations in low-income countries.

Immunizations

ROUTINE VACCINES

Because of their travel frequency, aircrew could be exposed to various diseases that are uncommon in the United States. Measles can be life-threatening in adults and is more common in countries, including some in Europe, that lack mandatory childhood immunization requirements. Measles cases have increased in the United States, with exposures reported to have occurred in airports, and potentially on airplanes. The Centers for Disease Control and Prevention (CDC) has developed recommendations for airlines to help reduce the risk for measles transmission through air travel (see www.cdc.gov/quarantine/air/managing-sick-travelers/airline-recommendations.html).

Although US carriers generally do not require pilots and flight attendants to demonstrate adherence to the adult immunization schedule recommended by the Advisory Committee on Immunization Practices (www.cdc.gov/vaccines/schedules/hcp/imz/adult.html#vaccines-schedule), use the pretravel visit as an opportunity to ensure that aircrew are up to date with their vaccines. Check vaccination status for coronavirus disease 2019 (COVID-19), diphtheria-tetanus-pertussis, influenza, measles-mumps-rubella (MMR), polio, as well as age-appropriate vaccines (e.g., pneumococcal vaccine). International aircrew should use the pretravel health visit to ensure as complete protection as possible.

Aircrew also can be at risk for varicella infection. In tropical regions, chickenpox occurs in an older age group than in the United States. Contact with local populations in the tropics can increase the risk for varicella exposure among flight crew who do not have natural or vaccine-induced immunity.

TRAVEL VACCINES

No established guidelines are in effect for recommending travel vaccines to aircrew, but because of their frequent and at times unpredictable assignments to areas of risk, offering Japanese encephalitis, meningococcal, and typhoid vaccines is reasonable (see the relevant disease-specific chapters in Section 5 for details). In addition, consider yellow fever vaccine for aircrew whose unexpected reassignments might include countries that require proof of vaccination against yellow fever under the International Health Regulations (for details, see Sec. 2, Ch. 5, Yellow Fever Vaccine & Malaria Prevention Information, by Country, and Sec. 5, Part 2, Ch. 26, Yellow Fever). Ask about the possibility of itinerary changes so that vaccinations for upcoming trips can be given, or a series started early.

Hepatitis A vaccine is advisable for all travelers and should be stressed for aircrew, since most adults in the United States have not been immunized. Advise aircrew, particularly frequent travelers, to receive hepatitis B vaccine because of the unpredictability of exposure.

Aircrew are generally a group who travel frequently beyond work; during a consultation, always ask whether they are planning other travel, and address those risks at the same time. For example, some aircrew do relief work or fly to areas of natural disasters; consider vaccination against cholera.

Coronavirus Disease 2019

Many international carriers have offered their employees COVID-19 vaccination. The CDC, FAA, and US airlines strongly recommend vaccination against COVID-19 with a product approved or authorized by the US Food and Drug Administration. Pilots are prohibited from flying or serving as a required crewmember within 48 hours after immunization because of possible transient adverse effects (see FAA's FAQs on Use of COVID-19 Vaccines by Pilots and Air Traffic Controllers, at www.faa.gov/coronavirus/guidance_resources/vaccine_faq).

Advise aircrew not to report to work and to notify their airline's occupational health program if they are symptomatic or test positive for severe acute respiratory syndrome coronavirus 2 (SARS-CoV-2), the virus that causes COVID-19. Crewmembers should follow current guidance and company policies regarding testing, duration of isolation, mask wearing, and return to work. Aircrew also should contact their airline's occupational health program after exposure to a person with COVID-19; management guidance (e.g., testing, symptom monitoring, mask wearing, quarantine) should be based on their vaccination status and prior history of SARS-CoV-2 infection.

FAA's COVID-19 guidance and resources can be found at www.faa.gov/coronavirus/guidance_resources.

Malaria Prevention

Airlines typically inform crewmembers about which destinations report malaria transmission. Although malaria transmission might occur in some areas of destination countries, sometimes no transmission is reported in the capitals or the larger urban areas (e.g., Manila) where major American carriers fly. In sub-Saharan Africa, however, aircrew can have substantial exposure risk even during a short, 24-hour layover.

Unfortunately, aircrew awareness about malaria and prevention strategies might not be widespread; US and European aircrew traveling to malaria-endemic destinations continue to acquire malaria, including severe and complicated disease. Infections might result from lack of awareness of airline recommendations, failure to take precautions against mosquito bites, or lack of compliance with antimalarial prophylaxis. A small recent survey by Farag and colleagues from the Qatar Ministry of Health revealed that while most aircrew had heard of malaria, many were unaware of the route of transmission, and some were not even sure whether they had traveled to a destination where malaria risk was high.

Help aircrew learn as much as possible about malaria. Provide easy access to educational materials and chemoprophylaxis and, if desired, an individual risk assessment for preventive measures (see Sec. 5, Part 3, Ch. 16, Malaria). Aircrew should understand the importance of personal protective measures and how to use them properly (see Sec. 4, Ch. 6, Mosquitoes, Ticks & Other Arthropods). They should know how take chemoprophylaxis as prescribed; recognize that fever or chills after an exposure is a medical emergency; and know how to get medical assistance at their destinations or at home in the event of symptoms or signs of malaria.

At destinations where the prevalence of malaria is high, prescribe antimalarial medication for aircrew to take even during brief layovers. For some stops (e.g., in West Africa on the way to South Africa), aircrew are at some risk any time aircraft doors are open. Transmission can be focal and intermittent; prescribe chemoprophylaxis for every trip to regions highly endemic for malaria, and stress the importance of taking the full prescription as directed.

Several options are available for malaria prophylaxis depending on the destination, although duration of prophylaxis and adverse effect profiles of drugs make some options less optimal or prohibited for aircrew. Mefloquine, for example, is contraindicated for pilots due to its effects on the central nervous system. International airlines generally recommend that aircrew take the combination drug atovaquone-proguanil because of its minimal adverse effects and its dosing schedule. Country-specific recommendations for malaria chemoprophylaxis can be found in Sec. 2, Ch. 5, Yellow Fever Vaccine & Malaria Prevention Information, by Country, or on the CDC Travelers' Health website (https://wwwnc.cdc.gov/travel).

For destinations where crew are thought to be at low risk based on local intensity of transmission, accommodations, and personal behaviors, advise taking precautions to prevent mosquito bites without chemoprophylaxis. Few published data are available on the risk for malaria among aircrew with brief layovers, but some suggest that because of the typically shorter duration, risk for aircrew could be less than for tourists. Although risk for malaria transmission in hotels at a destination could be low, it might be greater at international airports due to layovers and unpredictable transit delays.

Other Vectorborne Diseases

During the past decade, several mosquito-borne viruses have emerged or reemerged, including chikungunya, dengue, and Zika (see the individual disease chapters in Section 5). Strict adherence to mosquito bite prevention in tropical and subtropical destinations is critical to preventing disease. Because Zika virus infection during pregnancy can cause severe birth defects, airlines should develop flight destination policies for pregnant aircrew based on CDC recommendations (https://wwwnc.cdc.gov/travel/page/zika-travel-information).

Food & Water Precautions: Travelers' Diarrhea

Aircrew should follow the same safe food and water precautions for prevention and management of travelers' diarrhea as other travelers (see Sec. 2, Ch. 8, Food & Water Precautions, and Sec. 2, Ch. 6, Travelers' Diarrhea). Aircrew should also be well versed in the recognition and self-treatment of moderate to severe travelers' diarrhea to shorten the duration of illness. Gastrointestinal illness can impair job performance and preclude safe operation of an airplane. In addition, pilots should be certain that any antidiarrheal medications they take are approved for use when flying. Loperamide, for example, is not permitted because it can cause drowsiness and dizziness.

Bloodborne & Sexually Transmitted Infections

Although bloodborne pathogen and sexually transmitted infection (STI) risks and preventions are addressed in more detail in other chapters of this book, note that frequent travelers have an increased likelihood of engaging in casual and unprotected sex, and that rates of HIV and other STIs are greater among travelers (see Sec. 9, Ch. 12, Sex & Travel). The risk of acquiring infections might be increased not only for STIs (e.g., chlamydia, gonorrhea), but also for viral illnesses (e.g., hepatitis B, hepatitis C). Because of the risk for bloodborne pathogen infections, discourage aircrew from having dental procedures or participating in activities during travel like acupuncture, piercing, or tattooing.

Tuberculosis Screening

Screen for tuberculosis (TB) exposure and symptoms and administer a periodic test for TB infection to aircrew who travel frequently to destinations where the prevalence of the disease is greater than in the United States, the incidence of drug resistance to usual TB treatment medication is high, or the crewmember will be in close contact with populations at risk for TB. For more details, see Sec. 5, Part 1, Ch. 23, . . . *perspectives*: Testing Travelers for *Mycobacterium tuberculosis* Infection.

Medications for Chronic Conditions

Instruct aircrew to carry extra quantities of all medications for chronic conditions; medications might not be available at some locations, and, even if available and less costly, might be counterfeit or of substandard quality. Counterfeit medications are readily available for purchase in many low- and middle-income countries, and travelers might not be able tell based on the packaging or pills whether drugs are genuine. Some counterfeit drugs contain little or no active ingredient, and others contain toxic contaminants (see Sec. 6, Ch. 3, . . . *perspectives*: Avoiding Poorly Regulated Medicines & Medical Products During Travel).

FITNESS TO FLY

Federal Aviation Administration (FAA)–certified aeromedical examiners (AMEs) examine pilots regularly and are responsible for certifying that they are fit to fly. Without prior clearance from the FAA, AMEs might not certify pilots taking prescription or over-the-counter medications known to cause drowsiness; the FAA provides a list at www.faa.gov/about/office_org/headquarters_offices/avs/offices/aam/ame/guide/pharm/dni_dnf. Sometimes medication approvals are made on a case-by-case basis. If questions arise, consult an AME (see www.faa.gov/pilots/amelocator to locate an AME).

Antihistamines

Do not prescribe medications for pilots that can affect their central nervous system while on duty. Pilots often are aware of some of the medications and classes of medications (e.g., antihistamines) that might interfere with their flight capacity.

Pilots who take sedating antihistamines, including chlorpheniramine and diphenhydramine, are not permitted to fly until >5 half-lives have elapsed after the last dose; this equates to a 9-day no-fly rule for chlorpheniramine and a 60-hour no-fly rule for diphenhydramine.

Pilots should not take new medications or drugs before or during travel, whether prescribed or over-the-counter, that have reported side effects known to interfere with judgment or the ability to safely operate a plane. Before providing pilots with nonsedating antihistamines (e.g., desloratadine, fexofenadine, loratadine), ensure the medications can be taken without adverse effect during a trial period.

Sleep Medication

The FAA prohibits the use of all prescription sleep medication other than zolpidem, which is permitted for use on an infrequent basis (only once or twice per month), and only to reset circadian rhythm. Taking zolpidem results in a 24 hour no-fly period and thus is more appropriate for use at the end of a trip than during a multiday international flight assignment.

Alcohol

Aircrew might have to follow individual airline requirements regarding the allowable time from most recent alcohol consumption to flight duty. The international regulatory expectation is zero alcohol level upon reporting for duty. Warn cabin crew that the alcohol content of beer and other alcohol-containing beverages could be considerably greater at international destinations than what they typically consume at home, which for pilot testing might result in a non–zero alcohol level after a layover overseas. US airline pilots are subject to random alcohol testing, and urine specimens could be collected before or after flights. Although cannabis and cannabinoids are legal in some US states for medical and recreational use, these are prohibited for pilots.

BIBLIOGRAPHY

Bagshaw M, Illig P. The aircraft cabin environment. In: Keystone JS, Kozarsky PE, Connor BA, Nothdurft HD, Mendelson M, Leder K, editors. Travel medicine, 4th edition. Philadelphia: Elsevier; 2019. pp. 429–36.

Byrne NJ, Behrens RH. Airline crews' risk for malaria on layovers in urban sub-Saharan Africa: risk assessment and appropriate prevention policy. J Travel Med. 2004;11(6):359–63.

Centers for Disease Control and Prevention. Notes from the field: malaria imported from West Africa by flight crews—Florida and Pennsylvania, 2010. MMWR Morb Mortal Wkly Rep. 2010;59(43):1412.

Schwartz MD, Macias-Moriarity LZ, Schelling J. Professional aircrews' attitudes toward infectious diseases and aviation medical issues. Aviat Space Environ Med. 2012;83(12):1167–70.

Selent M, de Rochars VMB, Stanek D, Bensyl D, Martin B, Cohen NJ, et al. Malaria prevention knowledge, attitudes, and practices (KAP) among international flying pilots and flight attendants of a US commercial airline. J Travel Med. 2012;19(6):366–72.

Soha A, Bansal D, Kokku SB, Al-Romaihi H, Khogali H, Farag E. Assessment of cabin crew awareness about malaria in a major airline. Mediterr J Hematol Infect Dis. 2019;11(1): e2019049.

Thole S, Kalhoefer D, an Der Heiden M, Nordmann D, Daniels-Haardt I, Jurke A. Contact tracing following measles exposure on three international flights, Germany, 2017. Euro Surveill. 2019;24(19):1800500.

US Department of Transportation, Federal Aviation Administration. Coronavirus guidance & resources from FAA. Available from: www.faa.gov/coronavirus/guidance_resources.

PEOPLE WHO FLY FOR A LIVING—HEALTH MYTHS & REALITIES

Raquel Velazquez-Kronen

Airline pilots and flight attendants might have concerns about long-term health risks related to their exposures in the workplace. Aircrew have the highest annual individual radiation dose of any occupation, work irregular hours, and can be at risk of exposure to infectious diseases when traveling. Here we answer some of the common health-related questions about people who fly for a living.

DO AIRCREW HAVE HIGHER RATES OF CANCER THAN THE GENERAL POPULATION?

Aircrew do not appear to be at higher risk for cancer than the general population. In the United States, 1 in 2 men and 1 in 3 women will develop some form of cancer in their lifetime. Many exposures can contribute to cancer risk, some of which could be related to a person's occupation. Airline pilots and flight attendants are exposed occupationally to certain known cancer risk factors (e.g., cosmic radiation, ultraviolet radiation, and circadian rhythm disruption).

Several studies of aircrew have shown that overall and cause-specific cancer mortality is low compared with the general population despite these additional occupational exposures. As compared to people who do not fly for a living, pilots and flight attendants might be more likely to develop skin and female breast cancers, but reasons for this are unclear. CDC provides more information on cancer in aircrew, including steps that might reduce skin and breast cancer risk, at www.cdc.gov/niosh/topics/aircrew/cancer.html.

ARE AIRCREW MORE LIKELY TO DEVELOP HEART DISEASE THAN THE GENERAL POPULATION?

Aircrew might be at greater risk for developing some forms of heart disease compared with the general population. Heart disease is the leading cause of death in the United States. Although occurrence is rare, aviation medical examiners need to consider the likelihood of an in-flight incapacitation event due to common medical conditions (e.g., some forms of heart disease). Among pilots, heart disease and related conditions are the leading cause of grounding due to medical disqualification.

The prevalence of peripheral artery disease also has been shown to increase with the number of years flight attendants have worked. Combined with lifestyle and genetic factors, numerous occupational exposures in aviation might contribute to heart disease risk (e.g., circadian rhythm disruption, fatigue, shift work, chronic stress). CDC has information on heart disease prevention at www.cdc.gov/heartdisease/prevention.htm.

ARE COMMERCIAL AIRCREW AT INCREASED RISK FOR CONTRACTING INFECTIOUS DISEASES?

Aircrew, especially flight attendants, interact with many people daily and can be exposed to infectious diseases when in contact with sick crewmembers, passengers, or their bodily fluids; by inhaling airborne pathogens; or by touching contaminated surfaces. Information on standard safety protections for aircrew, identifying potentially infectious travelers, and

(continued)

PEOPLE WHO FLY FOR A LIVING—HEALTH MYTHS & REALITIES (CONTINUED)

infection-control guidance are available at www.cdc.gov/niosh/topics/aircrew/communicablediseases.html and www.cdc.gov/quarantine/air/managing-sick-travelers/commercial-aircraft/infection-control-cabin-crew.html.

Aircrew can reduce their risk for becoming ill with infectious diseases by keeping up to date with routine vaccinations (e.g., diphtheria-tetanus-pertussis, influenza, measles-mumps-rubella) and by frequently washing hands with soap and water or using an alcohol-based hand sanitizer containing ≥60% alcohol when soap and water are not readily available. Aircrew should be trained to use appropriate personal protective equipment (e.g., disposable gloves, face masks) when assisting potentially infectious travelers (e.g., those with a fever or respiratory symptoms). For additional occupational health and safety information that might pertain to emerging infectious diseases or public health emergencies, aircrew also can review the Federal Aviation Administration (FAA)'s Safety Alerts for Operators (www.faa.gov/other_visit/aviation_industry/airline_operators/airline_safety/safo).

ARE WORKPLACE EXPOSURES LINKED TO REPRODUCTIVE HEALTH EFFECTS IN AIRCREW?

Some evidence suggests that cosmic radiation exposure, high physical job demands, and working during typical sleep hours might be associated with an increased risk for miscarriage among pregnant flight attendants. Flight attendants do not, however, appear to be at elevated risk for preterm birth, low infant birthweight, or female reproductive (e.g., ovarian, uterine) cancers. For breastfeeding aircrew members, exposure to external radiation while working will not expose a baby to radiation through the breastmilk.

The National Council on Radiation Protection and Measurements recommends a radiation dose limit of 0.5 mSv (millisievert) per month during pregnancy, and the National Oceanic and Atmospheric Administration (www.swpc.noaa.gov) provides information on current weather conditions and whether aircrew flying at higher altitudes could be exposed to higher radiation levels due to solar radiation activity.

Pregnant aircrew can take steps to reduce their exposure to other potential occupational hazards by limiting physically demanding job tasks (e.g., prolonged standing) and by following guidance on weight limits for lifting during pregnancy (see www.cdc.gov/niosh/topics/repro/images/Lifting_guidelines_during_pregnancy_-_NIOSH.jpg). More information on aircrew reproductive health issues is available at www.cdc.gov/niosh/topics/aircrew/reproductivehealth.html and www.cdc.gov/niosh/topics/repro/pregnancy.html.

WORK-RELATED FATIGUE OR SLEEP DISORDERS

As compared to the general population, aircrew report fatigue and sleep disorders more frequently, which could be due to high job stress, irregular sleep schedules, jet lag, and long work hours. Chronic fatigue and sleep disorders (e.g., insomnia) can have negative long-term effects on overall physical and mental health and represent a potential risk for workplace injury.

In addition to recommending regular sleep, FAA provides guidance for aircrew to help reduce fatigue and improve sleep. Because even short naps can help increase alertness and improve performance throughout the day, aircrew should consider taking a nap either before starting work or when an opportunity arises to take a break during work. Other strategies include engaging in a few minutes of light physical activity (e.g., stretching, walking) during work to break up continuous tasks, and minimizing exposure to sunlight (which can make it more difficult to get enough sleep) after working a night shift. The FAA has a free online fatigue prevention training available at www.faasafety.gov/gslac/ALC/CourseLanding.aspx?cID=174. CDC also offers a free fatigue prevention training for commercial pilots in Alaska at www.cdc.gov/niosh/docs/2016-162/default.html.

BIBLIOGRAPHY

Davenport ED, Gray G, Rienks R, Bron D, Syburra T, d'Arcy JL, et al. Management of established coronary artery disease in aircrew without myocardial infarction or revascularisation. Heart. 2019;105(Suppl 1):s25–s30.

Federal Aviation Administration. Basics of aviation fatigue. Available from: www.faa.gov/regulations_policies/advisory_circulars/index.cfm/go/document.information/documentID/244560.

Grajewski B, Whelan EA, Lawson CC, Hein MJ, Waters MA, Anderson JL, et al. Miscarriage among flight attendants. Epidemiology. 2015;26(2):192–203.

International Civil Aviation Organization. Part III medical assessment, chapter 1 cardiovascular system. In: Doc 8984 Manual of civil aviation medicine, 3rd edition. Montréal: The Organization; 2012. pp. III-1-1–82.

Jackson CA, Earl L. Prevalence of fatigue among commercial pilots. Occup Med (Lond). 2006;56(4):263–8.

Magann EF, Chauhan SP, Dahlke JD, McKelvey SS, Watson EM, Morrison JC. Air travel and pregnancy outcomes: a review of pregnancy regulations and outcomes for passengers, flight attendants, and aviators. Obstet Gynecol Surv. 2010;65(6):396–402.

McNeely E, Mordukhovich I, Tideman S, Gale S, Coull B. Estimating the health consequences of flight attendant work: comparing flight attendant health to the general population in a cross-sectional study. BMC Public Health. 2018;18(1):346.

Pinkerton LE, Hein MJ, Anderson JL, et al. Melanoma, thyroid cancer, and gynecologic cancers in a cohort of female flight attendants. Am J Ind Med. 2018;61(7):572–81.

. . . perspectives chapters supplement the clinical guidance in this book with additional content, context, and expert opinion. The views expressed do not necessarily represent the official position of the Centers for Disease Control and Prevention (CDC).

HEALTH CARE WORKERS, INCLUDING PUBLIC HEALTH RESEARCHERS & MEDICAL LABORATORIANS

Henry Wu, Eric Nilles

9

Health care workers practicing outside the United States face unique health hazards, including exposure to infectious diseases associated with patient contact or handling clinical specimens. Any type of health care worker (e.g., ancillary clinical staff, nurses, physicians, public health personnel, researchers, students and trainees on international rotations) working in clinical areas or handling specimens can be at risk (see Box 9-01).

Infectious agents can be spread through contact with blood, bodily fluids, respiratory secretions, or contaminated materials or surfaces. Health care workers might be exposed through dermal, ingestion, inhalation, or percutaneous routes of absorption. Risks vary depending on assigned duties, geographic location, and practice setting. Of note, health care workers working abroad can be at increased risk for exposure to patients with emerging, highly pathogenic, or uncommon, infectious diseases (e.g., Ebola virus disease, Middle East respiratory syndrome [MERS], or extensively drug-resistant tuberculosis [XDR-TB]).

PRETRAVEL VACCINATION & SCREENING

Before traveling or working abroad, all health care workers should be up to date with their routine age-appropriate vaccines, vaccines recommended for employment in health care settings (see Box 9-03), and coronavirus disease 2019 (COVID-19) vaccines (www.cdc.gov/coronavi

BOX 9-01 Risks for health care workers practicing outside the United States

Challenging practice conditions (e.g., extremely resource-limited settings, natural disasters, or conflict zones) can prevent health care providers from adhering to standard precautions.

Greater prevalence of transmissible infections (e.g., hepatitis B virus, hepatitis C virus, HIV, tuberculosis) with potentially increased transmission risk from untreated source patients.

Less stringent safety regulations or infection control standards.

Limited availability of personal protective equipment (PPE), safety-engineered devices, or postexposure management resources.

Unfamiliar practice conditions, equipment, or procedures.

rus/2019-ncov/vaccines/stay-up-to-date.html). In addition, ensure health care workers receive vaccinations specifically indicated for the country visited. Cholera vaccine, meningococcal vaccine, and inactivated polio vaccine (given as an adult booster dose) could be indicated for health care workers traveling to locations experiencing high incidence or outbreaks of these diseases.

Ebola Virus Disease

Consider vaccinating health care workers responding to Ebola virus outbreaks with the Ebola

BOX 9-02 Health care workers in extreme circumstances

Health care workers regularly provide care in a range of extreme circumstances, which can be characterized by limited or absent medical and public health infrastructure; lack of fundamental hygiene supplies (e.g., soap and water for handwashing); increased infectious disease transmission; extreme environmental conditions; and high levels of violence. In 2020, 484 attacks against aid workers were reported; 117 were killed.[1]

Because of the increased risks and consequences of severe disease or injury, adequate prevention and preparation are essential. Health problems for the health care worker can have serious implications, both for the person and for those who depend on the health care worker for provision of health care. Detailed instructions on how to prepare for travel or work in developing countries or humanitarian environments is covered in other sections, but additional key considerations for health care workers include the following:

RELIABLE COMMUNICATION EQUIPMENT, usually a satellite phone, ensuring service provider contract for duration of the mission. Consider portable solar recharging capabilities unless guaranteed a power supply, which is rare in most extreme circumstances.

EVACUATION INSURANCE AND A PLAN FOR ILL OR INJURED WORKERS. Not all deploying organizations provide evacuation insurance (see Sec. 6, Ch. 1, Travel Insurance, Travel Health Insurance & Medical Evacuation Insurance) or a detailed evacuation contingency plan. Both are critical, and the health care worker should be familiar with all details.

WORKERS' UNDERLYING HEALTH CONDITIONS. Monitor the provider's health closely, and initiate treatment early, if necessary. Any indication that a potentially serious condition is not responding to treatment should warrant rapid planning for potential medical evacuation.

WORKER PSYCHOLOGICAL STABILITY. Providers in conflict and disaster zones typically work long hours under dangerous conditions and are exposed to profound suffering. These experiences can be intensely stressful, leading to increased rates of depression, posttraumatic stress disorder, and anxiety (see Sec. 2, Ch. 12, Mental Health). Before deployment, providers should think about coping strategies and, as much as possible, stay in contact with a support network of family and friends.

CHEMICAL WARFARE AGENT ANTIDOTES. Although rare, health care workers could be exposed to chemical warfare agents while caring for patients. If exposure to these agents is a possibility, antidotes (e.g., atropine) should be immediately available.

[1]Source: Impunity must end: Attacks on health in 23 countries in conflict in 2016. Safeguarding Health in Conflict Coalition; 2017. Available from: www.safeguardinghealth.org/sites/shcc/files/SHCC2017final.pdf.

9

BOX 9-03 Recommended vaccinations or documented immunity for employment in health care settings abroad

Coronavirus disease 2019 (COVID-19)	Mumps
Diphtheria	Pertussis
Hepatitis B	Rubella
Influenza	Tetanus
Measles	Varicella

vaccine approved for use by the US Food and Drug Administration (FDA). For more details, see www.fda.gov/vaccines-blood-biologics/ervebo and www.cdc.gov/vhf/ebola/clinicians/vaccine.

Hepatitis B

Because hepatitis B immune globulin (HBIG) and urgent hepatitis B virus (HBV) infection testing might not be available in resource-poor or field practice settings, be certain traveling health care workers have documentation of post-vaccination antibodies to HBV. Health care workers without documented response to vaccination should receive ≥1 additional dose of hepatitis B vaccine and further serologic testing to assess response.

Hepatitis C & HIV

Pretravel baseline testing for hepatitis C virus (HCV) and HIV infection is not routinely recommended; consider performing baseline testing for people who will be working in areas with high incidence of disease where reliable testing will not be available locally in the event of an exposure.

Tuberculosis

The Centers for Disease Control and Prevention (CDC) recommends screening for latent tuberculosis infection (LTBI) with tuberculin skin test or interferon-γ release assay for US health care workers; baseline screening is particularly important for health care workers traveling to countries with greater TB transmission risk, or working in high-risk settings (e.g., health care facilities, prisons, refugee camps). For more details, see Sec. 5, Part 1, Ch. 22, Tuberculosis, and Sec. 5, Part 1, Ch. 23., . . . *perspectives*: Testing Travelers for *Mycobacterium tuberculosis* Infection.

For people without a documented history of LTBI, perform repeat testing 8–10 weeks after travel if they had known exposure to an infectious patient or worked for a prolonged period in an area with high incidence of disease or increased prevalence of multidrug resistant TB (MDR-TB). Routine vaccination of US health care workers with bacillus Calmette-Guérin (BCG) is not recommended; by contrast, some experts do advise vaccinating health care workers who will work in settings with high TB transmission risk and a high prevalence of isoniazid-resistant and rifampin-resistant strains. Currently, however, no FDA–approved BCG formulations are available in the United States.

PERSONAL PROTECTIVE EQUIPMENT

Health care workers should consistently follow standard precautions and apply other transmission-based precautions (e.g., airborne, contact, droplet) as needed; anyone untrained in infection-control practices should not participate in patient care or in activities with risk for exposure to infectious materials. For details, guidelines, and training materials on standard precautions and personal protective equipment (PPE), see www.cdc.gov/infection control/basics/index.html. PPE approved for single use only should not be reused. Health care workers should maintain strict safety standards, even if local practices are less stringent.

Aprons, gloves, gowns, surgical masks, protective eyewear, and air-purifying respirators (e.g., a National Institute for Occupational Safety and Health [NIOSH]–approved N95 filtering facepiece respirator fit-tested to the worker) might all be necessary to achieve an adequate level of personal protection. Specialized (enhanced) PPE and infection-control techniques might be indicated for infections (e.g., avian influenza, COVID-19, Ebola virus disease, MERS) that pose a high risk to health care workers. Current disease-specific epidemiology can be found on the CDC Travelers' Health website (https://wwwnc.cdc.gov/travel).

Because equipment and facilities for airborne isolation are limited or unavailable in many countries (whenever possible, local resources should be determined in advance), health care workers should consider bringing a personal supply of PPE. This includes NIOSH-approved respirators with a ≥N95 level of protection (e.g., a reusable elastomeric half-mask respirator, a supply of disposable filtering facepiece respirators). Considering the available equipment, health care workers should be properly trained for all anticipated procedures (e.g., PPE donning and doffing, respirator fit testing, reusable respirator decontamination).

Health care workers should anticipate environmental conditions (e.g., high heat, humidity) that can make PPE, particularly high-level PPE (e.g., gowns, respirators), challenging to wear and use for extended periods. In addition, identifying situations where enhanced PPE is needed can be difficult, especially when working in locations where TB is highly prevalent and patient isolation is suboptimal.

INFECTION TRANSMISSION ROUTES

Airborne & Respiratory Droplet–Transmitted Infections

Although some airborne or respiratory droplet–transmitted infections (e.g., COVID-19, seasonal influenza, measles, varicella) are vaccine-preventable, others (e.g., MERS, pneumonic plague, TB) do not have routine or even available vaccines. TB infection is a particular concern for health care workers going to areas with high incidence of disease or an increased prevalence of MDR-TB (see Sec. 5, Part 1, Ch. 22, Tuberculosis).

Infections Transmitted by Blood & Body Fluids

Health care workers are at risk for infections transmitted through blood or body fluids via mucous membrane, percutaneous, or nonintact skin exposures. Bloodborne pathogens (e.g., HBV, HCV, HIV) can be transmitted through these routes. Other bodily fluid sources of infection for hepatitis viruses and HIV include amniotic fluid, cerebrospinal fluid, pericardial fluid, peritoneal fluid, pleural fluid, semen, synovial fluid, and vaginal secretions.

Other pathogens transmitted to health care workers via blood or bodily fluids include several not endemic to the United States (e.g., *Brucella* species, the bacteria that cause brucellosis; viruses like dengue and Ebola; and parasitic infections, such as malaria).

PERCUTANEOUS & DERMAL EXPOSURE

Typically, exposure to bloodborne pathogens occurs as a result of percutaneous exposure to contaminated sharps, including lancets, needles, scalpels, and broken glass from capillary or test tubes. Infection risk is increased after percutaneous exposures to larger blood volumes (e.g., deeper injuries, hollow-bore needles, procedures involving direct cannulation of an artery or vein, or visible blood on the injuring device).

Needlestick injuries are a common mode of percutaneous exposure to bloodborne pathogens; health care workers should avoid practices known to increase risk for needlestick injuries (e.g., recapping or using needles to transfer a bodily fluid between containers). Health care workers should be aware that safety-engineered medical devices and biosafety equipment (e.g., sharps containers) might not be available.

Skin exposures to potentially infectious bodily fluids are only considered a risk for bloodborne pathogen infection if skin integrity is compromised (e.g., through dermatitis, abrasion, open wounds). Higher circulating viral load in the source patient is also thought to increase transmission risk, which can be of particular concern in resource-poor settings where treatments for viral hepatitis and HIV are limited.

INFECTION RISK

Health care workers who have received hepatitis B vaccine and have developed immunity to the virus are at virtually no risk for infection. Reported risk for HCV transmission after a percutaneous exposure to HCV-infected blood or body fluid varies; recent studies report rates around 0.2%. The risk for HIV transmission is ≈0.3% after a percutaneous exposure to HIV-infected blood, and ≈0.09% after a mucous membrane exposure. Unless visibly bloody, feces, nasal secretions, saliva, sputum, sweat, tears, urine, and vomitus, are not considered infectious for HCV or HIV.

POSTEXPOSURE INTERVENTION

IMMEDIATE ACTIONS

Health care workers with occupational exposures to blood or body fluids should thoroughly wash the exposed area with soap and water. If mucous membrane exposure has occurred, the area should be flushed with copious amounts of water or saline.

If possible, assess both HCV and HIV infection status of the source patient; rapid HIV testing of the source patient is preferred. Exposures originating from source patients who test HIV negative are considered not to pose HIV transmission risk unless they have clinical evidence of primary HIV infection or HIV-related disease (see Sec. 5, Part 2, Ch. 11, Human Immunodeficiency Virus / HIV). HBV testing of the source patient might be indicated if the health care worker is not a documented responder to hepatitis B vaccination.

Perform baseline testing of the exposed health care worker for HCV and HIV infection immediately after exposure. In addition, if the exposed health care worker has no documented serologic response to hepatitis B vaccination, perform baseline testing for HBV infection. Seek qualified medical evaluation as soon as possible to guide decisions for postexposure prophylaxis (PEP).

POSTEXPOSURE PROPHYLAXIS

A decision to initiate PEP is based on the timing, nature, and source of the exposure. Regimen choice is affected by available drugs, the exposed person's medical history and pregnancy status, potential drug interactions, and the possibility of exposure to a drug-resistant strain. Expert consultation is important when considering PEP. When expert advice is not immediately available, contact the National Clinician Consultation Center (888-448-4911; http://nccc.ucsf.edu/clinician-consultation/pep-post-exposure-prophylaxis) for assistance in managing occupational exposures to HBV, HCV, and HIV.

HEPATITIS B

If the source patient is not confirmed to be HBV surface antigen (HBsAg) negative, begin PEP with hepatitis B immune globulin and vaccination for health care workers who do not have documented serologic response to hepatitis B vaccination or who are incompletely vaccinated against hepatitis B.

HIV

To reduce the chance of HIV transmission after percutaneous or mucous membrane exposures to potentially infectious bodily fluids from patients with known or potential HIV infection, PEP is recommended. A number of medication combinations are available for PEP (see HIV and Occupational Exposure at www.cdc.gov/hiv/workplace/healthcareworkers.html). Before travel, employers and health care workers should determine whether HIV PEP regimens are available at their practice locations; if not, they should consider bringing their own reliable supply for emergency use.

HIV PEP should be initiated as soon as possible after exposure. PEP efficacy is thought to decrease with increasing time after exposure, particularly if initiated >72 hours after exposure, and PEP can be stopped if new information changes the decision to treat. Counsel PEP recipients about drug interactions, drug toxicities, and the importance of adherence.

TESTING & COUNSELING

Postexposure testing and counseling are important follow-up measures for exposed health care workers, whether hepatitis B immune globulin or HIV PEP have been administered or not (see Box 9-04 for details).

BOX 9-04 Postexposure testing & counseling

POSTEXPOSURE TESTING

Hepatitis B virus (HBV): If the health care worker is not a documented serologic responder to hepatitis B vaccination or is incompletely vaccinated, conduct baseline and follow-up testing for HBV infection for those with known or potential HBV exposure.

- Perform a baseline test for total antibodies to HBV core antigen (HBcAg) as soon as possible after exposure.
- Perform follow-up testing for HBV surface antigen (HBsAg) and HBcAg at 6 months after exposure.

Hepatitis C virus (HCV): Conduct baseline and follow-up testing for HCV infection for those with known or potential exposure to HCV.

- Perform a baseline test for HCV antibody; if the baseline test is positive, perform an HCV RNA test.
- Perform follow-up testing for HCV RNA at 3–6 weeks after exposure.
- Test for HCV antibody at 4–6 months after exposure; if positive, perform a confirmatory RNA test.

HIV: Conduct baseline and follow-up testing for HIV infection for those with known or potential HIV exposure.

- Follow-up testing at 6 weeks, 3 months, and 6 months.
- Follow-up testing at 6 weeks and 4 months is acceptable if a 4th-generation, combination HIV p24 antigen-HIV antibody test is used.
- Extended HIV follow-up testing for ≤12 months, for people infected with HCV (after exposure to a co-infected source).

POSTEXPOSURE COUNSELING

Advise exposed health care workers to take precautions to avoid secondary transmission (e.g., abstain from sexual contact, use condoms or other barrier methods to prevent sexual transmission, avoid blood or tissue donations, and refrain from breastfeeding, if possible) especially during the first 12 weeks after exposure

Psychological counseling is essential because the emotional impact of occupational exposures can be substantial and can be exacerbated by stressors inherent to the overseas work environment.

BIBLIOGRAPHY

Centers for Disease Control and Prevention. Infection control basics. Available from: www.cdc.gov/infectioncontrol/basics/index.html.

Choi MJ, Cossaboom CM, Whitesell AN, Dyal JW, Joyce A, Morgan RL, et al. Use of Ebola vaccine: recommendations of the Advisory Committee on Immunization Practices, United States, 2020. MMWR Recomm Rep. 2021;70(1):1–12.

Humanitarian Outcomes. Aid Worker Security Database (AWSD): figures at a glance 2021. Available from: www.humanitarianoutcomes.org/sites/default/files/publications/figures_at_glance_2021.pdf.

Kuhar DT, Henderson DK, Struble KA, Heneine W, Thomas V, Cheever LW, et al. Updated US Public Health Service guidelines for the management of occupational exposures to human immunodeficiency virus and recommendations for postexposure prophylaxis. Infect Control Hosp Epidemiol. 2013;34(9):875–92.

Lyon RM, Wiggins CM. Expedition medicine—the risk of illness and injury. Wilderness Environ Med. 2010;21(4):318–24.

Moorman AC, de Perio MA, Goldschmidt R, Chu C, Kuhar D, Henderson DK, et al. Testing and clinical management of health care personnel potentially exposed to hepatitis C virus—CDC guidance, United States, 2020. MMWR Recomm Rep. 2020;69(6):1–8.

National Clinicians Consultation Center. Post-exposure prophylaxis (PEP): timely answers for urgent exposure management. Available from: http://nccc.ucsf.edu/clinician-consultation/pep-post-exposure-prophylaxis.

Safeguarding Health in Conflict Coalition. Impunity must end: Attacks on health in 23 countries in conflict in 2016. 2017. Available from: www.safeguardinghealth.org/sites/shcc/files/SHCC2017final.pdf.

Schillie S, Vellozzi C, Reingold A, Harris A, Haber P, Ward JW, et al. Prevention of hepatitis B virus infection in the United States: recommendations of the Advisory Committee on Immunization Practices. MMWR Recomm Rep. 2018;67(RR-1):1–31.

Sosa LE, Njie GJ, Lobato MN, Bamrah Morris S, Buchta W, Casey ML, et al. Tuberculosis screening, testing, and treatment of U.S. health care personnel: recommendations from the National Tuberculosis Controllers Association and CDC, 2019. MMWR Morb Mortal Wkly Rep. 2019;68(19):439–43.

HUMANITARIAN AID WORKERS

Sean Kivlehan, Stephanie Kayden

Humanitarian aid workers assist people forced from their homes because of conflict or natural disasters. Assistance begins within hours after a disaster and often continues for years. Humanitarian relief deployments can last for weeks to years; the work can be rewarding and adventurous but requires preparation. During deployments, humanitarian aid workers must plan to be self-sufficient and to face unique challenges, including insecure environments and emotional stress.

Each year hundreds of thousands of professional aid workers are deployed worldwide to support people affected by disaster and conflict. Many of these efforts are coordinated by the United Nations Office for the Coordination of Humanitarian Affairs, whose appeals in 2021 identified 235 million people in 34 countries or regions in need, a number that continues to grow (Figure 9-01).

Professional aid workers often deploy with large specialist organizations (e.g., Doctors Without Borders) that have infrastructure and resources to properly support their personnel. Many more people (e.g., doctors, civic and religious groups) participate as amateur responders to international disasters. In contrast with professional aid workers, amateur responders might deploy with smaller, less prepared groups and little experience in providing humanitarian aid (Box 9-05).

UNIQUE CHALLENGES

Aid workers experience situations and specific risks (e.g., safety, security, mental health) related to providing humanitarian relief. Safety and security challenges include exposure to the conflict or disaster environment that precipitated or sustained the crisis; damaged or absent infrastructure (e.g., living accommodations, sanitation facilities); and high levels of insecurity. Mental health risks

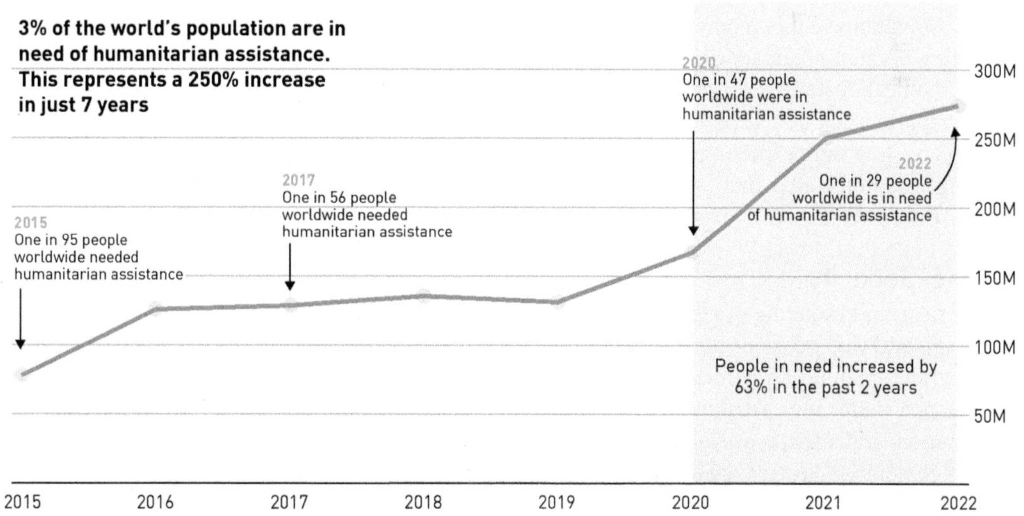

3% of the world's population are in need of humanitarian assistance. This represents a 250% increase in just 7 years
2015
One in 95 people worldwide needed humanitarian assistance
2017
One in 56 people worldwide needed humanitarian assistance
2020
One in 47 people worldwide were in humanitarian assistance
2022
One in 29 people worldwide is in need of humanitarian assistance
People in need increased by 63% in the past 2 years
300M
250M
200M
150M
100M
50M
2015
2016
2017
2018
2019
2020
2021
2022

FIGURE 9-01 **Trends in the global number of people in need of humanitarian assistance (2015–2022)**

Source: Global Humanitarian Overview 2022. United Nations Office for the Coordination of Humanitarian Affairs. Inter-Agency Coordinated Appeals: Overview for 2022. Available from: https://gho.unocha.org/appeals/inter-agency-coordinated-appeals-overview-2022.

BOX 9-05 Voluntourism

Volunteer tourism (also called "voluntourism") describes tourists volunteering for a charity or development organization, usually for short periods, in low- and middle-income countries. Although largely well intentioned, the impact of short-term visits—often by volunteers lacking specific understanding of the local context and lacking requisite training or skills—is variable and might be harmful in certain settings.

Voluntourism in humanitarian emergencies can be particularly problematic given dynamic and often dangerous humanitarian environments that require professional knowledge, organizational infrastructure, and understanding of the humanitarian response coordination system. Without the necessary individual competencies and organizational support, voluntourists in these settings expose themselves to unnecessary personal risks and can create a burden on the broader humanitarian response operations.

include living in stressful environments; working long hours under adverse or extreme conditions; and challenges to reentering home life and post-deployment activities.

Humanitarian service can have an adverse effect on personal health. Studies of long-term humanitarian aid workers indicate that >35% report a deterioration in their personal health during the mission. Injuries from accidents and violence are risks for humanitarian aid workers and cause more deaths than disease or natural causes. Recent estimates place the risk for medical evacuations, hospitalizations, and violence-related deaths at ≈6 per 10,000 person-years among aid workers. Conditions and outcomes vary by location, nature of the humanitarian event, and time spent in the field. A study of American Red Cross workers reported that 10% experienced accident or injury and 16% were exposed to violence. The same study demonstrated that >40% found the experience more stressful than expected.

9

Safety & Security

Security risks and targeting of aid workers with kidnapping and violence continues to be a concern for the humanitarian community. Risks to staff are not uniformly distributed across the humanitarian landscape, however. Ongoing surveillance of violence directed against humanitarian aid and disaster relief workers continues to demonstrate that most of these events occur in a few insecure locations, including Afghanistan, Cameroon, Central African Republic, Democratic Republic of the Congo, Ethiopia, Mali, Nigeria, Somalia, South Sudan, and Syria.

Injuries and motor vehicle accidents are common risks for travelers, including humanitarian aid workers, throughout the world. Aid workers should be sensitive to their surroundings and carefully select the type of transportation and hour of travel, if possible (see Sec. 8, Ch. 5, Road & Traffic Safety).

In disaster and emergency situations, aid workers should be aware of physical hazards (e.g., debris, downed power lines, unstable structures, and other environmental hazards). Workers in certain conflict and post-conflict settings should be educated on improvised explosive devices, landmines, and other unexploded ordnance. Although less common, some environments might involve unusual exposures, such as radiation (e.g., after the 2011 earthquake and tsunami in Japan) or chemical agents (e.g., mustard gas and sarin used on civilians in the Syrian conflict). Humanitarian aid and disaster relief workers who will be deployed to insecure areas, including active conflict zones, should undergo specialized security briefings by the deploying agency or private sources. Reputable and free resources exist for basic security training (e.g., the United Nations BSAFE course [https://training.dss.un.org/thematicarea/category?id=6]).

In situations associated with damage or destruction to local services and facilities, humanitarian aid workers should anticipate and plan for limited accommodations and logistical and personal support. Humanitarian aid and disaster relief workers destined for low-resource areas or situations can benefit from pretravel training and counseling regarding the moral complexities of providing service in these environments.

Encourage humanitarian aid workers from the United States to enroll in the Department of State's Smart Traveler Enrollment Program (STEP, https://step.state.gov/step) to register with the US embassy in their destination country. Enrollment before departure will ensure that the local consulate is aware of their presence and can provide them with notifications, account for them, and include them in evacuation plans.

Travelers providing humanitarian assistance should review and understand medical, evacuation, and life insurance provided by their employing agency. They also should consider supplemental travel, travel health, and medical evacuation insurance to cover medical care and evacuation should they become ill or injured (see Sec. 6, Ch. 1, Travel Insurance, Travel Health Insurance & Medical Evacuation Insurance). Travelers should carefully review evacuation policies for any exclusions, such as from higher risk countries or potential exposure to certain infectious diseases (e.g., Ebola, coronavirus disease 2019 [COVID-19]).

Mental Health

Studies suggest that aid workers returning from humanitarian missions, particularly missions characterized by high or chronic stress, have increased symptoms of anxiety, depression, and posttraumatic stress disorder. People with preexisting mental health issues, including anxiety and depression, could be predisposed to worse outcomes.

Generally, humanitarian aid and disaster relief workers demonstrate considerable resilience and adapt to the stressful environments, but elevated and chronic stress can lead to deterioration in mental health and decompensation in some people. Predeployment briefings can increase an aid worker's ability to cope with highly stressful environments; data are lacking, however, on the effectiveness of postdeployment debriefings to decrease adverse mental health impacts of deployment.

A detailed evaluation of risk factors (e.g., preexisting mental illness, family history of mental illness, history of alcohol or substance use disorder) might identify previously unrecognized chronic mental health conditions. Identifying alcohol or substance dependence or underlying mental health issues (e.g., depression) is particularly important because stressful humanitarian environments frequently exacerbate these conditions, which are often the reason for emergency repatriation (see Sec. 2, Ch. 12, Mental Health, and Sec 3, Ch. 5, Substance Use & Substance Use Disorders).

PREPARATION

Careful attention to pretravel evaluation, both physical and mental health, can reduce the likelihood of illness and the need for emergency repatriation of humanitarian aid workers. Comprehensive medical and—for those planning long-term assignments—dental evaluations can prepare aid workers by identifying previously unrecognized conditions, enabling treatment before travel. Medical illness or injury among deployed staff, particularly serious conditions that require repatriation, are not only burdensome and potentially dangerous for the affected staff member, but these events redirect limited organizational resources from the intended beneficiaries.

Most of the core elements of the pretravel evaluation and counseling are discussed in detail in Sec. 2, Ch. 1, The Pretravel Consultation, and in Sec. 9, Ch. 4, Health Care Workers, Including Public Health Researchers & Medical Laboratorians. Administer routine vaccinations and prescribe malaria prophylaxis or medications to prevent altitude sickness, as appropriate. COVID-19 risk and related guidance can vary based on the individual and the destination, but the Centers for Disease Control and Prevention recommends vaccination for all travelers. Additional COVID-19 guidance is discussed in Sec. 5, Part 2, Ch. 3, COVID-19. Give guidance on food and water precautions; self-treatment for travelers' diarrhea; protection from insect bites; environmental protection from the elements including sun exposure; behavioral risk avoidance; and injury prevention. Several of these topics listed here are covered in detail in Section 2 and Section 4.

For health care workers providing medical care as part of their humanitarian activities, evaluate occupational risk and the need for preventive preexposure or postexposure interventions. Medical humanitarian aid workers responding to outbreaks of communicable diseases are often at increased risk for exposure and infection by specific infectious pathogens, which requires meticulous attention to infection control and personal protective measure protocols. Medical workers (see Sec. 9, Ch. 4, Health Care Workers, Including Public Health Researchers & Medical Laboratorians) should ensure their organization provides adequate safety protocols and personal protective equipment (e.g., gloves, gowns, masks, eye protection).

In humanitarian emergencies, direct infrastructure damage; lack of equipment, supplies, and human resources; or a surge in medical need can all contribute to a medical facility becoming compromised or overwhelmed. Counsel volunteers with significant underlying medical conditions, who are likely to require care themselves, against travel; encourage them to support the response in other ways. Similarly, a person who is pregnant should discuss their plans with their obstetrician and should typically be advised to defer deployment.

For travelers planning to participate in animal rescue activities, share information available in Sec. 4, Ch. 9, Bringing Animals & Animal Products into the United States, and discuss rabies preexposure prophylaxis (see Sec. 5, Part 2, Ch. 18, Rabies).

Travel Health Kits

In general, because aid workers will need a more comprehensive travel health kit than the typical traveler (Sec. 2, Ch. 10, Travel Health Kits), they should consult with their deploying organization to determine how extensively to tailor their packed supplies. For example, health care workers deployed by a medical organization will usually be able to access basic pharmacologic and other medical supplies for acute care treatment from the organization and should be familiar with basic first aid to self-treat any injury until they can obtain medical attention.

Conversely, people with chronic medical conditions requiring treatment should ensure they travel with prescriptions and medications sufficient for the duration of their service. They also should consider bringing along treatment for exacerbations of diseases or conditions they might not usually experience (e.g., asthma, back pain). Because not all pharmaceuticals are globally available, travelers on extended deployments should review safe alternatives to their regular medication (see Sec. 6, Ch. 3, . . . *perspectives*: Avoiding Poorly Regulated Medicines & Medical Products During Travel). Aid workers should store medications in 2 separate allotments in case of loss or theft. Sec. 2, Ch. 10, Travel Health Kits, provides additional information on preparing, storing, and traveling with medications.

People with dental crowns or bridgework should consider taking temporary dental adhesive for short-term management of a dislodged dental appliance. In addition to a basic travel health kit, humanitarian aid workers should consider bringing the items listed in Box 9-06.

BOX 9-06 International humanitarian aid travel health kit checklist: additional items

- ☐ Cash (new or crisp bills can often be exchanged at better rates)
- ☐ Contact lenses, prescription glasses (extra pairs, if applicable)
- ☐ Gloves (leather gloves if physical labor will be performed)
- ☐ Headlamp and spare batteries
- ☐ Insect repellent
- ☐ Insecticide-impregnated mosquito net (if traveling to areas endemic for insect-borne diseases)
- ☐ Long pants, shirts that cover the shoulders
- ☐ Menstrual supplies
- ☐ Mobile telephone, equipped to work internationally (or preferably unlocked)
- ☐ Money belt
- ☐ Safety goggles
- ☐ Sewing kit
- ☐ Sturdy work boots (particularly in disaster or rudimentary settings)
- ☐ Sunglasses
- ☐ Sunscreen

Personal Items

Loss of life, serious injuries, missing and separated families, and destruction of communities are often associated with humanitarian emergencies; aid workers should recognize they are likely to encounter stressful situations as part of their work. Keeping a personal item nearby (e.g., a family photo, favorite music, religious or spiritual material) can offer comfort. Communicating with family members and close friends from time to time can be an important means of support.

Access to mobile phones and internet services are frequent challenges in humanitarian emergencies. Global mobile coverage continues to improve, however, and free applications (e.g., WhatsApp) have expanded accessibility. For more remote regions, satellite telephones are an option, although some government authorities might prohibit or limit their importation and use, particularly in conflict zones. Before travel, aid workers should clarify any restrictions to telephone, internet, or satellite technology in the destination country.

Documents

Aid workers should carry extra passport-style photos, which might be required for certain types of security passes, visas, and work permits. Travelers should bring photocopies of documents (e.g., credit cards, passports) and copies of their medical, nursing, or other professional licenses, if applicable.

Aid workers also should have medical information (e.g., blood type, immunization records), available. Travelers should carry physical copies of all these documents, leave copies with their main contact at home, scan and email copies to their smartphones (if appropriate), and ensure the documents are securely stored and available in a cloud storage service. In addition, aid workers should carry information for their emergency contacts written on paper, and not rely exclusively on an electronic device.

POSTTRAVEL

Returning humanitarian aid and disaster relief workers should seek medical care if they sustained injuries during their travel or become ill after returning home. To ensure a thorough assessment, returning aid workers should advise their providers of the nature and location of their recent travel. Depending on the duration and nature of the deployment, including if they were providing direct medical care, returning aid workers might benefit from a comprehensive medical review. Educate workers involved in responding to infectious disease outbreaks on posttravel illness monitoring recommendations or requirements, if applicable.

Homecoming can be psychologically challenging, and aid workers should seek treatment or counseling if they have concerns about transitioning to postdeployment life. Consider referring workers who witnessed or were involved in mass casualties, deaths, or serious injuries or who have been victims of violence (e.g., assault, kidnapping, serious road traffic crash) for critical incident counseling. Educate returning aid workers that the onset of adverse psychological effects after exposure to traumatic experiences can be delayed, sometimes by several months or longer.

9

BIBLIOGRAPHY

Brooks SK, Dunn R, Sage CA, Amlot R, Greenberg N, Rubin GJ. Risk and resilience factors affecting the psychological wellbeing of individuals deployed in humanitarian relief roles after a disaster. J Ment Health. 2015;24(6):385–413.

Costa M, Oberholzer-Riss M, Hatz C, Steffen R, Puhan M, Schlagenhauf P. Pre-travel health advice guidelines for humanitarian workers: a systematic review. Travel Med Infect Dis. 2015;13(6):449–65.

Humanitarian Outcomes. Aid Worker Security Database (AWSD): figures at a glance 2021. Available from: www.humanitarianoutcomes.org/sites/default/files/publications/figures_at_glance_2021.pdf.

Macpherson RIS, Burkle FM. Humanitarian aid workers: the forgotten first responders. Prehosp Disaster Med. 2021;36(1):111–4.

United Nations Office for the Coordination of Humanitarian Affairs (OCHA). Global humanitarian overview 2021. Geneva: OCHA; 2020. Available from: https://reliefweb.int/sites/reliefweb.int/files/resources/GHO2021_EN.pdf.

Young T, Pakenham KI. The mental health of aid workers: risk and protective factors in relation to job context, working conditions, and demographics. Disasters. 2021;45(3):501–26.

UNITED STATES MILITARY DEPLOYMENTS

Sherry Gracey, Alexander Keller, Gary Montgomery, Gregory Raczniak, Bryan Schumacher, Nicholas Studer

In 2021, ≈1.4 million Americans served on active duty in the military, and approximately 800,000 were in the reserve forces. The United States Armed Forces follow most of the recommendations in the Centers for Disease Control and Prevention (CDC) Yellow Book as a matter of policy. Certain situations apply only to military personnel, however, and some policies or recommendations differ from what is recommended for civilian travel in this text.

Military physicians generally manage military-unique aspects of medical care for service members, but civilian physicians might interact with people on reserve status, on leave from duty, recently discharged from active duty, or veterans. Less commonly, active-duty service members not stationed near military hospitals or clinics must use civilian physicians for their care. Deployments can vary depending on the service branch, so understanding the type of deployment or work travel the service member participated in is essential because not all deployments or work travel are alike.

FORCE HEALTH PROTECTION

Force health protection (FHP) is an important concept in military medicine. FHP is defined as all measures taken by commanders, supervisors, individual service members, and the Military Health System to conserve, improve, promote, protect, and restore the mental and physical well-being of service members across the range of military activities and operations. Delivery of vaccines, use of malaria chemoprophylaxis agents, and mental health screening are examples of the many measures employed under the umbrella of FHP and are likely the most common scenarios that civilian providers will encounter. Medical and mental health screenings, both pre- and postdeployment, also support FHP to identify, track, and treat concerns.

Medical interventions for FHP are the responsibility of the unit commander, with advice from the unit medical officer. When predeployment vaccines or malaria chemoprophylaxis are indicated, the commander includes such requirements in the mission plan. Service members are then required to receive these interventions under proper medical supervision. If a particular vaccine or drug is medically contraindicated, alternative agents might be used if available. The unit medical officer documents which military personnel have not received standard preventive measures so these people can receive additional monitoring or treatment if they become ill.

FHP policy positions in the Department of Defense (DoD) are issued as directives and instructions. All directives and instructions can be found online at www.esd.whs.mil/dd. The Policy and Program for the Department of Defense Immunization Program is found in directive 6205.02 (July 23, 2019) at www.esd.whs.mil/Portals/54/Documents/DD/issuances/dodi/620502p.pdf?ver=2019-07-23-085404-617.

Although policy is made at higher levels in Washington, DC, the final decision to use vaccines or malaria chemoprophylaxis under FHP is made by commanders in the field, guided by their medical staff. In certain circumstances, individual service members might be exempt from vaccination. The 2 types of exemptions from immunization are administrative and medical. Granting administrative exemptions is a nonmedical function, usually controlled by the unit commander with input from other sources (e.g., religious counsel). Granting medical exemptions is a medical function that can be validated only by a health care professional.

IMMUNIZATIONS

DoD policy states that the recommendations for immunization from CDC and the Advisory Committee on Immunization Practices generally shall be followed, consistent with requirements and guidance developed by the US Food and Drug Administration (FDA) and with consideration for the unique needs of military settings and exposure risks. Specific assignment-dependent vaccines given prior to deployment are summarized at the Military Health System website (https://health.mil/Military-Health-Topics/Health-Readiness/Immunization-Healthcare/Vaccine-Recommendations/Vaccine-Recommendations-by-AOR).

The Defense Health Agency (DHA) Immunization Healthcare Branch (IHB) enhances military medical readiness by coordinating DoD vaccination programs worldwide. A valuable source of service-specific information on immunizations for all branches of the United States Armed Forces is available on the DHA IHB website (www.health.mil/vaccines).

MALARIA PROPHYLAXIS

Preventing malaria in military units deployed to endemic areas is essential. Medical commanders must designate trained staff to provide comprehensive malaria prevention counseling to military and civilian personnel considered at risk of contracting malaria.

Several features of malaria prophylaxis are specific to the US military because of the unique activities and stressors of military deployments. When antimalarial drugs are used, the military can only use FDA-approved agents in accordance with the specific FDA-approved indications for population-based approaches. If off-label use is felt to be in the best interest of the person or unit, trained and knowledgeable clinicians must provide one-on-one medical evaluations, document in the medical record the rationale for such use, and provide a prescription for the drug or vaccine to each service member.

Primary Prophylaxis

Atovaquone-proguanil (Malarone) is the recommended malaria prophylaxis option for all personnel for both short- and long-term deployments in high-transmission areas of Africa. For practical purposes, this includes most of sub-Saharan Africa. For people unable to receive atovaquone-proguanil because of intolerance or contraindication, doxycycline is the preferred second-line therapy.

Use of mefloquine prophylaxis is a third-line recommendation for those unable to receive either atovaquone-proguanil or doxycycline. Before prescribing mefloquine for prophylaxis, consider the absolute and relative contraindications as described in the approved product label.

Atovaquone-proguanil and doxycycline are both first-line choices in areas other than sub-Saharan Africa. Reserve the use of mefloquine for people with intolerance or contraindications to first-line medications.

Although primaquine is included as an acceptable alternative by CDC for primary prophylaxis in some countries where the risk for malaria is exclusively or mostly due to *Plasmodium vivax*, primaquine is not FDA-approved for primary prophylaxis. Because use of primaquine for primary prophylaxis constitutes off-label use, it cannot be prescribed for a deploying group. It can, however, be prescribed by a licensed medical provider on an individual basis as part of medical practice.

Terminal Prophylaxis (Presumptive Antirelapse Therapy)

PRIMAQUINE

To prevent the late relapse of *P. vivax* or *P. ovale* malaria in returning military populations, the United States Armed Forces routinely use primaquine for terminal prophylaxis (also referred to as presumptive antirelapse therapy [PART]). As a matter of policy, primaquine is given to otherwise healthy people on their departure from an endemic area. Primaquine is used for this indication much more frequently in the military than in most civilian travelers. For more information on terminal prophylaxis, see Sec. 5, Part 3, Ch. 16, Malaria.

DOSING

The FDA-approved regimen for terminal prophylaxis is 15 mg (base) given daily for 14 days. In 2003, CDC recommended 30 mg (base) of primaquine daily for 14 days for terminal prophylaxis based on available evidence, but the FDA-approved regimen remains the lower dose. Adherence to the daily 14-day regimen is poor unless primaquine is given under

9

directly observed therapy, which is rarely done. As a result of noncompliance and subtherapeutic dosing with the 15-mg/day regimen, periodic outbreaks of relapsed *P. vivax* malaria continue to occur in returning military personnel. Use of the higher-dose primaquine regimen for terminal prophylaxis is now recommended for military personnel.

TIMING

A recurrent issue for military medicine is the correct timing of primaquine when given as terminal prophylaxis in conjunction with the standard prescribed primary prophylaxis. Primaquine can be given at any time after personnel leave an endemic area. For convenience and for enhancing adherence to the 14-day regimen, it is often best for military units to prescribe primaquine in the immediate 2 weeks after return. During this time, units are often still at their home base completing in-processing before "block leave." Once personnel depart on leave, adherence and monitoring for side effects becomes more challenging, and civilian physicians might encounter service members who were prescribed terminal prophylaxis.

HEMOLYTIC ANEMIA

The most crucial risk of primaquine use is the potential for hemolytic anemia in people who are glucose-6-phosphate-dehydrogenase (G6PD)–deficient. Current policy is for all US military personnel to be screened for G6PD deficiency on entry into military service. Some (e.g., reservists) might have deployed without testing, however, or clinicians might not be able to confirm results for all people in a unit requiring terminal prophylaxis. Hemolytic reactions to primaquine can occur in people with an unrecognized G6PD deficiency.

9

TAFENOQUINE

In 2018, the FDA approved tafenoquine for malaria prophylaxis and treatment, including terminal prophylaxis for *P. vivax* and *P. ovale* malaria. As with primaquine, the most important risk of tafenoquine is hemolytic anemia in people who are G6PD-deficient. As of 2019, tafenoquine is considered a second-line drug for both chemoprophylaxis of chloroquine-resistant malaria and terminal prophylaxis in military populations. This guidance for tafenoquine use in members of the US military differs from recommendations for use in civilian populations; see Sec. 5, Part 3, Ch. 16, Malaria, for CDC guidance regarding civilian use of tafenoquine.

UNIQUE MILITARY NEEDS

US military personnel can encounter threats (e.g., biological warfare agents) that are not usually considered for civilian travelers. Drug prophylaxis, drug treatment, immunoglobulins, and vaccines can be given only in accordance with FDA-licensed products and regimens and for FDA-approved indications. Products not approved by the FDA are given to service members only with voluntary informed consent under an institutional review board–approved protocol and in accordance with a current and FDA-approved investigational new drug application.

Only under exceptional circumstances would products not approved by the FDA be given to military personnel without their informed consent. The FDA Commissioner can authorize the use of an unapproved medical product or an unapproved use of an approved medical product during a declared emergency involving a heightened risk of attack on the public or US military forces or when national security could be affected.

RETURNING SERVICE MEMBERS WITH HEALTH CONCERNS

Although symptoms and health concerns after a deployment can be similar to health issues reported from nonmilitary returning travelers, deployments present a different set of circumstances for service members than does civilian travel. These circumstances include differential vaccination recommendations, physical and psychological impact from deployment experiences, environmental exposures, and infections that create distinct health concerns. Civilian providers can help members of the United States Armed Forces access medical services, but providers should reference service-specific standards to help ensure that the treatments and medications they offer are appropriate.

The authors of this chapter are all uniformed service members of the United States Government (USG). The views expressed in this section are those of the authors and do not necessarily reflect the official policy or position of any USG Department.

BIBLIOGRAPHY

Food and Drug Administration. Emergency use authorization of medical products and related authorities, January 2017. Available from: www.fda.gov/regulatory-information/search-fda-guidance-documents/emergency-use-authorization-medical-products-and-related-authorities.

Office of the Assistant Secretary of Defense (Health Affairs). HA-Policy 13-002. Guidance on medications for prophylaxis of malaria, 2013. Available from: https://health.mil/Reference-Center/Policies/2013/04/15/Guidance-on-Medications-for-Prophylaxis-of-Malaria.

US Department of Defense. Department of Defense directive: Force Health Protection (FHP), no. 6200.04. Washington, DC: Department of Defense; 2004. Available from: www.esd.whs.mil/Portals/54/Documents/DD/issuances/dodd/620004p.pdf.

US Department of Defense. Department of Defense instruction: application of Food and Drug Administration (FDA) rules to Department of Defense Force Health Protection programs, no 6200.02. Washington, DC: US Department of Defense; 2008. Available from: www.esd.whs.mil/Portals/54/Documents/DD/issuances/dodi/620002p.pdf.

LONG-TERM TRAVELERS & EXPATRIATES

Lin Hwei Chen, Davidson Hamer

The risk for illness or injury increases with duration of travel, so travelers planning long-term (commonly considered ≥6 months) visits to low- or middle-income countries require special consideration regardless of whether they are expatriates with definite plans or adventurers with open itineraries. Points to discuss in the pretravel consultation include accessing routine and emergency care at the destination, vaccines, infectious diseases not prevented by vaccines, injury prevention, and cultural and mental health issues that long-term travelers might encounter.

ACCESSING CARE ABROAD

Before departure, all long-term travelers should undergo complete medical and dental examinations. For expatriates, a mental health evaluation prior to travel could identify and help address underlying issues that often cause early repatriation. Travelers should anticipate that they will need care at some point during their stay and plan where they will obtain it and how they will pay for it.

People traveling for work or with an organization (e.g., a nongovernmental organization, Peace Corps, a university) might have a predetermined source for care; some might access advice from the international expatriate community. By contrast, other travelers should identify a health care source in advance (see Sec. 6, Ch. 2, Obtaining Health Care Abroad). Long-term travelers also should determine whether they will need supplemental travel health insurance and evacuation insurance (see Sec. 6, Ch. 1, Travel Insurance, Travel Health Insurance & Medical Evacuation Insurance).

In some countries, travelers are likely to encounter medications of poor quality that are substandard, falsified, counterfeit, or expired. Because the pills and packaging could be nearly indistinguishable from their legitimate counterparts, travelers should bring a sufficient supply of their routine medications (e.g., antihypertensive or antihyperlipidemic drugs) from the United States (see Sec. 6, Ch. 3, . . . *perspectives*: Avoiding Poorly Regulated Medicines & Medical Products During Travel).

Controlled substances and certain over-the-counter and commonly prescribed medications are illegal to bring into some countries. The International Society of Travel Medicine Pharmacist Professional Group offers the Database on International Regulations on Importation of Medicines for Personal Use (Table 9-02). The International Narcotic Control Board website includes guidelines provided by

Table 9-02 Importing medications for personal use

INFORMATION SOURCE	RESOURCE	AVAILABLE FROM
International Society of Travel Medicine (ISTM) Pharmacist Professional Group	ISTM Pharmacist Professional Group Database on International Regulations on Importation of Medicines for Personal Use	www.istm.org/pharmacistgroup
International Narcotics Control Board (INCB)	Country Regulations for Travelers Carrying Medicines Containing Controlled Substances	www.incb.org/incb/en/travellers/country-regulations.html
	General Information for Travelers Carrying Medicines Containing Controlled Substances	www.incb.org/incb/en/travellers/general-information.html
	Travelling Internationally with Medicines Containing Controlled Substances	www.incb.org/incb/en/travellers/index.html

each country and is a good reference for travelers looking for information about whether they can legally import their medications to their destinations (Table 9-02).

Options for obtaining sufficient medications include requesting an override from the insurance company to dispense the entire quantity of medication; paying out-of-pocket for the full amount of medication needed and then submitting to the insurance company for reimbursement; refilling prescriptions during trips home; or relying on visiting friends or family members to bring refilled medication supplies.

VACCINES

Long-term travelers should be aware of any vaccine requirements for entry, employment, or schooling at their destination. Update routine vaccines, including influenza vaccine, before travelers depart, and consider disease risk in surrounding areas because long-term travelers are likely to travel locally. A short-term traveler to Seoul, for example, would not be considered at risk for Japanese encephalitis (JE), but expatriates living in Seoul might have opportunities to visit the Korean countryside or other areas in Asia where they could be exposed to the JE virus. Similarly, consider yellow fever vaccination even if the posting location is not in an endemic area, because the traveler might journey to endemic areas while living abroad.

Hepatitis A & Typhoid Fever

Given the cumulative risk for hepatitis A and typhoid fever infection among long-term travelers, vaccination against these two diseases is appropriate (see Sec. 5, Part 2, Ch. 7, Hepatitis A, and Sec. 5, Part 1, Ch. 24, Typhoid & Paratyphoid Fever). Neither of the US Food and Drug Administration (FDA)–approved typhoid vaccines, however, effectively prevents infection in all recipients; the injectable (ViCPS) and the oral (Ty21a) vaccine are each estimated to protect ≈50%–80% of recipients from infection. Thus, travelers who receive these vaccines should still adhere to safe food and water precautions (see Sec. 2, Ch. 8, Food & Water Precautions). Moreover, duration of protection afforded by each vaccine is limited; a repeat dose of ViCPS is recommended every 2 years for travelers at continued risk of infection. For Ty21a recipients, a booster is recommended every 5 years.

Hepatitis B

Travel-associated hepatitis B infections are rare, but the risk for travelers might be greater than for nontravelers, especially for long-term travelers and expatriates, so consider hepatitis B vaccine for this population (see Sec. 5, Part 2, Ch. 8, Hepatitis B).

Japanese Encephalitis

Infection with JE virus is associated with longer stays in endemic areas. JE vaccine is recommended for travelers who plan longer stays or residence in endemic areas, travelers anticipating outdoor activities in endemic areas after dusk, and travelers who are uncertain of specific destinations or activities (see Sec. 5, Part 2, Ch. 13, Japanese Encephalitis).

Meningococcal

Meningococcal disease is more likely in travelers with prolonged exposure to local populations in endemic or epidemic areas; consider quadrivalent conjugate vaccine for at-risk travelers (see Sec. 5, Part 1, Ch. 13, Meningococcal Disease)

Rabies

Rabies preexposure prophylaxis is an important consideration for people spending prolonged time in endemic countries, especially in places where rabies immune globulin is not available, which is true of many low- and middle-income countries (see www.cdc.gov/rabies/resources/countries-risk.html). Prioritize vaccination for children who will be living in high-risk areas (see Sec. 5, Part 2, Ch. 18, Rabies, and Sec. 5, Part 2, Ch. 19, . . . *perspectives*: Rabies Immunization).

Yellow Fever

Yellow fever vaccination might be required by some countries or recommended for endemic areas (see Sec. 2, Ch. 5, Yellow Fever Vaccine & Malaria Prevention Information, by Country, and Sec. 5, Part 2, Ch. 26, Yellow Fever). For instance, numerous unvaccinated Chinese expatriates became ill with yellow fever while working in Angola during the outbreak there in 2016, illustrating the importance of yellow fever vaccination for people who will be living or working in endemic areas.

INFECTIOUS DISEASES NOT PREVENTED BY VACCINES

Dengue & Other Arboviral Diseases

Dengue seroconversion among long-term travelers from the Netherlands with median travel duration of 20 weeks found an attack rate of 6.5% or incidence rate of 13.9 per 1,000 person-months travel in endemic areas. Other mosquito-borne viral illnesses (e.g., chikungunya, Zika), also pose potential risk. Advise long-term travelers and expatriates to protect themselves from mosquito vectors (see Sec. 4, Ch. 6, Mosquitoes, Ticks & Other Arthropods); most travelers are not candidates to receive dengue vaccine (for details, see Sec. 5, Part 2, Ch. 4, Dengue). Section 5 also provides disease-specific information on chikungunya and Zika virus infections.

Hepatitis C & Hepatitis E

Transfusion is a potential source of hepatitis C virus infection in expatriates. Hepatitis E virus is spread by the fecal–oral route; the risk for infection is greatest in Asia, although it has been transmitted in many different tropical locations. Pregnant people are at greatest risk for fulminant disease from hepatitis E. For more information on these infections, see the relevant chapters in Section 5.

HIV & Sexually Transmitted Infections

Travelers and expatriates are at increased risk for HIV and sexually transmitted infections (STIs), and the consistency of condom use among expatriates is low (see Sec. 9, Ch. 12, Sex & Travel). Educate long-term travelers about the risk for HIV and STIs at their destination, as well as preventive measures. Consider the potential for occupational exposure to HIV among health care workers, and during the pretravel consultation include discussions of postexposure prophylaxis with antiretroviral therapy and risk avoidance (see Sec. 5, Part 2, Ch. 11, Human Immunodeficiency Virus / HIV, and Sec. 9, Ch. 4, Health Care Workers, Including Public Health Researchers & Medical Laboratorians).

Malaria

For long-term travelers, emphasize the importance of adjuncts to prophylaxis (see Sec. 4, Ch. 6, Mosquitoes, Ticks & Other Arthropods). Even when urged to adhere to personal protective measures and reassured that long-term prophylaxis is safe and effective, traveler adherence likely will decline over time. Consequently, the pretravel consultation for a long-term traveler to malaria-endemic areas should stress the severity of the disease, its signs and symptoms, and the need to seek care immediately if signs and symptoms develop. Travelers also can consider bringing a reliable supply of drugs to treat malaria (atovaquone-proguanil or artemether lumefantrine) if they are diagnosed with the disease (see Sec. 2, Ch. 5, Yellow Fever Vaccine & Malaria Prevention Information, by Country, and Sec. 5, Part 3, Ch. 16, Malaria).

RISK FACTORS CONTRIBUTING TO INFECTION

Data suggest that malaria incidence increases, and use of preventive measures decreases, with increasing length of stay abroad. Among expatriate corporate employees in Ghana, adherence to malaria prophylaxis deteriorated with increasing duration of stay, and all employees who had been on the site for >1 year had abandoned prophylaxis. About half of the cohort only intermittently used insect repellent, and more than one-third never used repellent.

Even though most British expatriates from the UK Foreign and Commonwealth Office had good knowledge about malaria and its prevention strategies, they adhered to malaria prophylaxis <25% of the time; only 25% reported rigorous compliance, and 13% reported having contracted malaria. A recent GeoSentinel Global Surveillance Network analysis found that *Plasmodium falciparum* malaria was the most frequent diagnosis among ill returned expatriate workers, occurring in 6%, and was acquired most commonly in sub-Saharan Africa. Given the high risk for malaria among travelers in Africa, these data on long-term travelers and expatriates highlight worrisome risks and practices.

French service members deployed to the Central African Republic for 4 months in 2013 experienced malaria at a rate of 150 cases per 1,000 person-years. A survey found that prophylaxis compliance correlated positively with use of other prophylactic measures against malaria (e.g., insecticide-treated clothing, mosquito net use, taking prophylaxis at the same time every day), correct perception of malaria risk, favorable perception of prophylaxis effectiveness, and peer-to-peer reinforcement.

CHEMOPROPHYLAXIS

A traveler residing in an area of continuous malaria transmission should continue to use malaria prophylaxis for the entire stay. Doxycycline has been well tolerated for long-term malaria prophylaxis in the military, and the Centers for Disease Control and Prevention (CDC) has no recommended limits on its duration of use for malaria prophylaxis. Peace Corps volunteers frequently use mefloquine during prolonged stays and have a discontinuation rate of 0.9%. Mefloquine might be appropriate for long-term prophylaxis in chloroquine-resistant areas because of its convenient weekly dosing, but concern has increased regarding its neuropsychiatric side-effect profile, especially because the FDA label indicates that neurologic side effects could persist.

Atovaquone-proguanil has shown good long-term tolerability in post-marketing surveillance, with a discontinuation rate of only 1% because of diarrhea; for long-term use, however, atovaquone-proguanil can be a more expensive option than other antimalarial drugs. Peace Corps volunteers prescribed atovaquone-proguanil adhered to prophylaxis better than did people given doxycycline and mefloquine. If extended (>5 years) use of chloroquine is planned, a baseline ophthalmic examination with biannual follow-up is recommended to screen for potential retinal toxicity.

Because of its convenient weekly dosing, the antimalarial drug tafenoquine appears to be a promising choice for long-term travelers; an association with vortex keratopathy might limit its use. Moreover, tafenoquine use should be avoided in people with documented glucose-6-phosphate-dehydrogenase (G6PD) deficiency, as well as in those who have not been tested for G6PD deficiency. It is also not recommended for use in people with a history of psychotic disorder. Pregnancy is a contraindication to tafenoquine use.

PREGNANCY

The possibility of pregnancy requires careful consideration for travelers to areas where malaria is endemic (see Sec. 5, Part 3, Ch. 16, Malaria, and Sec. 7, Ch. 1, Pregnant Travelers). Malaria infection during pregnancy can result in severe complications to both mother and fetus. When pregnancy is anticipated, prophylaxis options might need to be adjusted; explore the possibility of pregnancy with all long-term travelers of childbearing age before departure.

For a person who is pregnant or who plans to become pregnant during long-term travel, mefloquine is considered safe in all trimesters. Data from published studies in pregnant people have shown no increase in the risk for teratogenic effects or adverse pregnancy outcomes after mefloquine prophylaxis during pregnancy. Chloroquine also has been used long-term without ill effects on pregnancy. If a person traveling long-term is taking atovaquone-proguanil, doxycycline, or primaquine, they should discontinue their medication and begin weekly mefloquine (or chloroquine in those areas where it remains efficacious) for at least 3–4 weeks to build up a therapeutic blood level of mefloquine before attempting to conceive.

During the pretravel consultation, advise people of the potential risks associated with becoming pregnant while taking antimalarial drugs. Doxycycline, for example, is associated with fetal toxicity in animal studies, and its use is contraindicated during pregnancy. Primaquine and tafenoquine can harm a G6PD-deficient fetus, so should not be used. The effect of atovaquone-proguanil on the fetus is unknown.

Other Parasitic Infections

Parasitic infections vary with location and include amebiasis, filariasis, giardiasis, cutaneous leishmaniasis, schistosomiasis, and strongyloidiasis; vectorborne infections (e.g., filariasis, cutaneous leishmaniasis) can be prevented by using insect bite precautions and protective clothing, and by avoiding locations where the vectors are prevalent (see Sec. 5, Part 3, Ch. 9, Lymphatic Filariasis, and Sec. 5, Part 3, Ch. 14, Cutaneous Leishmaniasis). For travelers with appropriate (or potential) geographic exposure risks, consider the possibility of filariasis and cutaneous leishmaniasis.

Travelers can avoid schistosomiasis by not bathing, swimming, or wading in fresh water, guidance that can be difficult to communicate to long-term travelers who, for example, might be living in sub-Saharan Africa and looking forward to river rafting or vacationing at a lake. Travelers can prevent *Strongyloides stercoralis* and hookworm infections by not walking barefoot through soil or on sandy beaches. The risks for schistosomiasis and strongyloidiasis can increase with long-term travel; consider screening travelers on their return, and suggest that people with access to health care also seek screening during long-term expatriate assignments (for details, see Sec. 11, Ch. 3, . . . *perspectives*: Screening Asymptomatic Returned Travelers). Although seropositivity appears to be generally low for many parasitic infections, seroconversion for *Schistosoma* spp. occurred in 6% of Dutch long-term travelers to endemic areas.

Avoiding unwashed or uncooked foods, including greens and vegetables, can help reduce a travelers' chances of ingesting foodborne parasites (e.g., *Ascaris*).

Travelers' Diarrhea

Because diarrhea and gastrointestinal diseases occur commonly, educate long-term travelers about ways to manage gastrointestinal illnesses (see Sec. 2, Ch. 6, Travelers' Diarrhea), including rehydration, use of antimotility agents, empiric antimicrobial therapy, and knowing when to seek care.

Compared with short-term travelers, long-term travelers experience more chronic diarrhea and postinfectious irritable bowel syndrome, possibly because some become less adherent to food and water precautions over time. Advise travelers of the need to continue food and water precautions to reduce the risk for these conditions (see Sec. 2, Ch. 8, Food & Water Precautions).

Tuberculosis

In destinations where the burden of tuberculosis (TB) is high, the risk of infection in travelers can rise to that of the local population, depending on their length of stay and closeness of contact with the local population. For long-term travelers, consider a baseline interferon-γ release assay or a tuberculin skin test before travel, and repeat the same test after travel. TB screening is particularly important for health care workers or people working in hospitals, prisons, or refugee camps (see Sec. 5, Part 1, Ch. 23, . . . *perspectives*: Testing Travelers for *Mycobacterium tuberculosis* Infection).

INJURY

Because injuries are the leading cause of preventable death in travelers, educate long-term travelers about safety. Stress the importance of road and vehicle safety, and emphasize that travelers should choose the safest vehicle options available (see Sec. 8, Ch. 5, Road & Traffic Safety). Roads are often poorly constructed and maintained, traffic laws might not be enforced, vehicles might not have seatbelts or be kept in good condition, and local drivers might be reckless and minimally trained. See Sec. 4, Ch. 12, Injury & Trauma, for strategies to reduce the risk of traffic and other injuries.

MENTAL HEALTH

Culture shock and the stress of long-term travel can trigger or exacerbate mental illness. Assess long-term travelers for a preexisting diagnosis of mental illness, depressed mood, recent major life stressors, and use of medications that can adversely affect mental health. Any of these conditions suggest a need for further screening.

Warn all long-term travelers against illicit drug use, and urge them to take care of their physical and mental health by exercising regularly and eating healthfully. Travelers should be able to recognize signs of anxiety and depression and have a plan for coping. Having photographs or other mementos of friends and family at hand, and staying in close contact with loved ones at home, can alleviate the stress of long-term travel (see Sec. 2, Ch. 12, Mental Health).

LONG-TERM TRAVELERS WITH OPEN ITINERARIES

Offering pretravel care to long-term travelers, especially travelers with no itinerary or who have only vague travel plans, presents unique challenges. These travelers benefit from broad immunization coverage for all potential exposures to vaccine-preventable diseases.

Because their plans are unclear, these travelers must understand that they might need to diagnose and treat themselves for common ailments, including musculoskeletal problems, upper respiratory tract infections, skin disorders, travelers' diarrhea, urinary tract infections, and vaginitis. For travelers (e.g., backpackers) who might go in and out of malaria-endemic areas, a sensible approach is to provide a supply of atovaquone-proguanil with instructions on how to take it when they visit risk areas.

In addition to strategies to prevent health problems and injuries during their long sojourns, traveler education is imperative regarding health resources, signs and symptoms that require urgent medical evaluation, and medical evacuation.

SCREENING LONG-TERM TRAVELERS & EXPATRIATES AFTER RETURN

After returning to their country of origin, long-term travelers (e.g., highly adventurous travelers, expatriate workers, Peace Corps volunteers) ideally should have a thorough medical interview to assess potential infectious exposures. A careful itinerary-specific history with detailed questioning about potential high-risk exposures including animal, food and water, and human contacts is the foundation of the posttravel evaluation.

Conduct a physical examination focused on specific signs and symptoms, and a selected array of tests. These tests include a complete blood count with differential, hepatic transaminases, stool ova and parasite examination, and serologic markers depending on types of exposure, but most importantly for schistosomiasis and strongyloidiasis. Serologic testing can detect subclinical infections and help identify instances where treatment would be advised (see Sec. 11, Ch. 3, . . . *perspectives*: Screening Asymptomatic Returned Travelers). The posttravel evaluation also provides an opportunity for preventive counseling for potential future travel.

BIBLIOGRAPHY

Chen LH, Leder K, Barbre KA, Schlagenhauf P, Libman M, Keystone J, et al. Business travel–associated illness: a GeoSentinel analysis. J Travel Med. 2018;25(1):tax097.

Créach M-A, Velut G, de Laval F, Briolant S, Aigle L, Marimoutou C, et al. Factors associated with malaria chemoprophylaxis compliance among French service members deployed in Central African Republic. Malaria J. 2016;15:174.

Cunningham J, Horsley J, Patel D, Tunbridge A, Lalloo DG. Compliance with long-term malaria prophylaxis in British expatriates. Travel Med Infect Dis. 2014;12(4):341–8.

Hamer DH, Ruffing R, Callahan MV, Lyons SH, Abdullah AS. Knowledge and use of measures to reduce health risks by corporate expatriate employees in western Ghana. J Travel Med. 2008;15(4):237–42.

Landman KZ, Tan KR, Arguin PM; Centers for Disease Control and Prevention (CDC). Knowledge, attitudes, and practices regarding antimalarial chemoprophylaxis in U.S. Peace Corps Volunteers—Africa, 2013. MMWR Morb Mortal Wkly Rep. 2014;63(23):516–7.

Lim PL, Han P, Chen LH, MacDonald S, Pandey P, Hale D, et al. Expatriates ill after travel: results from the Geosentinel Surveillance Network. BMC Infect Dis. 2012;12:386.

National Academies of Sciences, Engineering, and Medicine; Health and Medicine Division; Committee to Review Long-Term Health Effects of Antimalarial Drugs; Board on Population Health and Public Health Practice. Assessment of long-term health effects of antimalarial drugs when used for prophylaxis. Styka AN, Savitz DA, editors. Washington (DC): National Academies Press; 2020.

Overbosch FW, Schinkel J, Stolte IG, Prins M, Sonder GJB. Dengue virus infection among long-term travelers from the Netherlands: A prospective study, 2008–2011. PLoS One. 2018;13(2):e0192193.

Pierre CM, Lim PL, Hamer DH. Expatriates: special considerations in pretravel preparation. Curr Infect Dis Rep. 2013;15(4):299–306.

Soonawala D, van Lieshout L, den Boer MA, Claas EC, Verweij JJ, Godkewitsch A, Ratering M, et al. Post-travel screening of asymptomatic long-term travelers to the tropics for intestinal parasites using molecular diagnostics. Am J Trop Med Hyg. 2014;90(5):835–9.

Whelan J, Belderok S, van den Hoek A, Sonder G. Unprotected casual sex equally common with local and Western partners among long-term Dutch travelers to (sub)tropical countries. Sex Transm Dis. 2013;40(10):797–800.

STUDY ABROAD & OTHER INTERNATIONAL STUDENT TRAVEL

Kristina Angelo, Sarah Kohl

Students travel internationally for many reasons, including studying abroad, leisure travel during a gap year, providing health care, or participating in humanitarian activities. During the 2018–2019 academic year, nearly 350,000 US students studied abroad, an increase of 1.6% from the previous year. Study abroad notably declined by 53.1% the following academic year (2019–2020) because of the coronavirus disease 2019 (COVID-19) pandemic. The most common destination for US students to study abroad is Europe, but they also study in low- or middle-income countries, placing them at risk for acquiring infectious diseases that are not endemic at home.

Gap year travel, or travel during a year off from academic studies, is increasingly popular and can also be associated with travel-related health risks. Medical, nursing, or veterinary students studying abroad can be at increased risk for acquiring bloodborne pathogens or zoonotic infections, and students participating in humanitarian activities could experience stress-related problems and environmental hazards. The purpose of travel and the student's planned activities should be captured at the pretravel consultation as part of the risk assessment.

Resources for students preparing to travel abroad include their institution's study abroad program administrators, health care providers at a pretravel consultation, and other students who have returned from a similar trip (see Table 9-03 for additional, online study abroad resources). Appropriate preparation can help students stay healthy during travel and reduce the chances they will become ill or engage in behaviors abroad that can place their health at risk.

Table 9-03 **Online health & safety information for students, health care providers & study abroad program professionals**

ORGANIZATION/SOURCE	RESOURCES PROVIDED	AVAILABLE FROM
Centers for Disease Control and Prevention	Country-specific health information	https://wwwnc.cdc.gov/travel
	Before, during, and after travel tips for students	https://wwwnc.cdc.gov/travel/page/studying-abroad
The Center for Global Education, SAFETI (Study Abroad First-Educational Travel Information)	Videos on health issues (alcohol awareness) A–Z index on health and safety issues Course and workshops	http://globaled.us/SAFETI
NAFSA: Association of International Educators	Study abroad program guidance	www.nafsa.org
Pathways to Safety International	Interpersonal and gender-based violence assistance	https://pathwaystosafety.org
US Department of State Bureau of Consular Affairs	Country-specific safety guidance Travel advisories with safety and security information	https://travel.state.gov
	Special considerations for US students abroad	https://travel.state.gov/content/travel/en/international-travel/before-you-go/travelers-with-special-considerations/students.html
US Department of State Overseas Security Advisory Council	Crime and safety reports Travel guidance Traveler toolkit	www.osac.gov

9

PREDEPARTURE PREPARATION

Health Care Providers: Roles & Responsibilities

When conducting pretravel consultations with student travelers, cover the core topics of risk assessment, risk mitigation, and preparation to respond effectively to health and safety problems while abroad (see Sec. 2, Ch. 1, The Pretravel Consultation). Make recommendations about vaccines, prophylaxis and self-treatment medications, provide information on country-specific health risks, and give guidance on how to obtain medical and dental care while abroad. Remind students who will be traveling abroad for >90 days to fill any prescriptions for the duration of their trip before they leave the United States and to pack a travel health kit (see Sec. 2, Ch. 10, Travel Health Kits).

Other relevant topics to discuss include alcohol and illicit drug use and dependency; bloodborne pathogen precautions (e.g., avoiding acupuncture, blood products, needles, piercings and tattoos, surgeries) while traveling; gender and sex-related health issues, including information for lesbian, gay, bisexual, transgender, queer (LGBTQ+) students; managing stress and other mental health issues associated with international travel (e.g., culture shock, altered sleep patterns, jet lag); and practicing safe sex, including what to do in the event of pregnancy. Share information on how to prevent unintentional injuries (see Sec. 4, Ch. 12, Injury & Trauma). Provide additional recommendations for students with disabilities or special needs (see Sec. 3, Ch. 2, Travelers with Disabilities), students with preexisting health conditions (see Sec. 3, Ch. 3, Travelers with Chronic Illnesses), and students participating in humanitarian activities (see Sec. 9, Ch. 5, Humanitarian Aid Workers).

Students should purchase travel insurance that covers major medical, evacuation, and repatriation (see Sec. 6, Ch. 1, Travel Insurance, Travel Health Insurance & Medical Evacuation Insurance); "study abroad" insurance plans might be available through the school or parent institution and could provide a reasonable, cost-effective option. Encourage student travelers planning adventure activities (e.g., kayaking, skydiving) to include extreme sports coverage on their health insurance policy (see Sec. 9, Ch. 11, Adventure Travel). All students should register with the Department of State's Smart Traveler Enrollment Program (STEP, https://step.state.gov/step) and check the Centers for Disease Control and Prevention Travelers' Health website destination pages (https://wwwnc.cdc.gov/travel/destinations/list) for destination-specific advice (e.g., best practices for disease prevention, outbreak information) before departure.

Study Abroad Programs: Roles & Responsibilities

Study-abroad professionals should share instructions with students about whom to contact in the study abroad program in the event of emergency and nonemergency situations. If telehealth services are planned, the program should address internet connectivity and concerns about legal health jurisdiction prior to departure (see Sec. 2, Ch. 16, Telemedicine). The program might need contingency plans in the event of a disease outbreak or civil unrest. Study-abroad staff also should encourage students to familiarize themselves with codes of conduct for their home and host institutions, as well as local health and safety issues, cultural norms, laws, and political climate. Additionally, program staff should inform students and families about the responsibilities and qualifications of chaperones accompanying a study abroad program.

SPECIFIC ISSUES

Alcohol & Illicit Drugs

A lower minimum drinking age and cultural acceptability of alcohol consumption in the host country, combined with stress or mental health issues, can lead to increased alcohol consumption among students when abroad. Use and abuse of alcohol and illicit drugs pose serious health consequences, can increase the risk for accidents and injuries, and make students potential targets for crime and incarceration (see Sec. 3, Ch. 5, Substance Use & Substance Use Disorders). Moreover, availability or use of recreational drugs (e.g., cannabis) by citizens of host countries might not necessarily mean their use is legal for international travelers.

Although cannabis is legal under certain US state laws, its use continues to be illegal under US federal law. US airports and airlines operate under federal jurisdiction and, as such, do not recognize the medical marijuana laws or cards of any state. In countries outside the United States where cannabis is illegal, students found in possession of the drug—even those with a valid US prescription—can be arrested; if found guilty, they could be deported, fined, or imprisoned. The International Narcotics Control Board (www.incb.org/incb/en/travellers/index.html) has country-specific information for students with prescription medications containing controlled substances.

Both health care providers and study abroad program personnel should counsel students about the consequences of alcohol and illicit drug use. Study abroad programs should strongly discourage all illicit drug use. Advise students to drink alcohol responsibly and in moderation, and to seek medical attention if they feel ill after drinking.

Bloodborne Pathogens

Students planning to provide medical, nursing, or veterinary care overseas should receive hepatitis B vaccination or have evidence of immunity. Inform these travelers about what to do in the event of a needlestick injury. At the pretravel consultation, consider providing postexposure HIV prophylaxis for students to take with them in the event of a bloodborne exposure if they will be providing care in a country with high HIV prevalence (see Sec. 9, Ch. 4, Health Care Workers, Including Public Health Researchers & Medical Laboratorians). Psychological counseling is essential after an occupational bloodborne exposure. Provide information on blood safety in the event the traveler has an emergency or needs a blood transfusion (see Sec. 6, Ch. 2, Obtaining Health Care Abroad). Warn students of the risks associated with getting acupuncture, piercings, or tattoos while abroad; sterility of needles or ink cannot be guaranteed.

Emergency Contact Information Card

Students should always carry their personal information and important telephone numbers as hard copies and electronically in their mobile devices. The Center for Global Education offers a printable sample emergency contact card at http://studentsabroad.com/handbook/emergency-card.php?country=General. For students with additional mental health or physical needs, provide written documentation of all health issues, prescribed medications, and recommended care plans; students should ensure that this letter gets translated accurately into the local language(s). Students should leave photocopies of all travel documents at home with their emergency contacts and the study abroad program office.

9

Gender-Related Issues

Students, including those who self-identify as LGBTQ+, should familiarize themselves with cultural attitudes, local laws, and tolerance of gender identification and sexuality in their host country (see Sec. 2, Ch. 13, LGBTQ+ Travelers). Check the US Department of State website (http://travel.state.gov) and specific US embassy or consulate websites in countries and cities around the world (www.usembassy.gov) to obtain information on host country laws.

The International Lesbian, Gay, Bisexual, Trans, and Intersex Association (ILGA World) publishes a map of sexual orientation laws by country, including protection against discrimination and criminalization of same-sex sexual acts (https://ilga.org/maps-sexual-orientation-laws). Additional research and planning might be needed to identify health care providers in the host country with experience working with LGBTQ+ people, if needed.

Mental Health

International travel can be stressful for students who might be inexperienced travelers, reliant on their home support systems, or traveling for longer periods of time. Culture shock, fear, insecurity, isolation, and loneliness can exacerbate existing mental health issues or unveil new ones (see Sec. 2, Ch. 12, Mental Health). When deciding on a destination for study, students should consider their preexisting level of mental (and physical) well-being and the availability of local resources. Encourage students to take an active role in planning for care abroad by disclosing all chronic mental health conditions and support needs during the pretravel consultation, and to the study abroad program office before departure.

Advise students to continue their routine medications while abroad; assist with developing a plan to manage a flare of symptoms while traveling (e.g., seeking local care, consulting with current providers, repatriation in the event of severe mental health issues). Students should confirm that mental health services are covered by their travel health insurance. Recommend that students engage in self-care abroad by getting regular exercise, establishing good sleep patterns, joining interest groups, and maintaining contact with family and friends at home.

Safer Sex

Discuss safer sex practices (e.g., birth control, condom use, emergency contraception, HIV preexposure prophylaxis [PrEP]) with international student travelers and provide information about the prevalence of sexually transmitted infections (STIs) at their destination. Students should follow local social norms about public displays of affection and dating to avoid possible adverse consequences; they also should be empowered to report any episode of sexual harassment or assault to local authorities, emergency contacts, and the study abroad program.

DURING & AFTER TRAVEL CONSIDERATIONS

During their time abroad, students should seek health care immediately if they become ill, injured, or have a bloodborne pathogen exposure. Students should adhere to food and water precautions (see Sec. 2, Ch. 8, Food & Water Precautions), and use insect repellent (see Sec. 4, Ch. 6, Mosquitoes, Ticks & Other Arthropods) to prevent vectorborne diseases.

Students who become ill after returning home should alert health care providers about their international travel. Students with fever ≤1 year after returning from study or travel in malaria-endemic areas (see Sec. 2, Ch. 5, Yellow Fever Vaccine & Malaria Prevention Information, by Country, and Sec. 5, Part 3, Ch. 16, Malaria) merit testing for malaria. Students with new sexual partners while abroad should be tested for STIs, including chlamydia, gonorrhea, HIV, and syphilis if they develop symptoms while abroad; they also should be screened for STIs when they return home.

After returning home, students will undergo a period of readjustment. All students should have access to mental health services after return to help cope with events that occurred overseas and to assist with reverse culture shock.

BIBLIOGRAPHY

Angelin M, Evengård B, Palmgren H. Illness and risk behavior in health care students studying abroad. Med Educ. 2015;49(7):684–91.

Aresi G, Moore S, Berridge DM, Marta E. A longitudinal study of European students' alcohol use and related behaviors as they travel abroad to study. Subst Use Misuse. 2019;54(7):1167–77.

Furuya-Kanamori L, Mills D, Sheridan S, Lau C. Medical and psychological problems faced by young Australian gap year travelers. J Travel Med. 2017;24(5):tax052.

Open Doors. U.S. students study abroad data; 2022. Available from: https://opendoorsdata.org/

VISITING FRIENDS & RELATIVES: VFR TRAVEL

Danushka Wanduragala, Christina Coyle, Kristina Angelo, William Stauffer

In this book, a "visiting friends and relatives (VFR) traveler" is defined as a person who currently resides in a higher-income country who returns to their former home (in a lower-income country) for the purpose of visiting friends and/or relatives. More broadly, family members (e.g., children, partners) born in the VFR traveler's higher-income country of residence are also included in this traveler category.

Migration patterns to the United States over the past 30 years have resulted in increasing numbers of immigrants arriving from Africa, Latin America, and Asia. Approximately 14% of US residents (≈45 million people) are foreign born, and ≈45% of all overseas international travelers coming from the United States list VFR as their reason for travel.

DISPROPORTIONATE INFECTIOUS DISEASE RISKS

Compared to other groups of international travelers, VFR travelers experience a greater incidence of travel-associated infectious diseases (e.g., hepatitis A, malaria, sexually transmitted infections, tuberculosis, typhoid fever). Several underlying reasons for this observation have been identified (see Box 9-07). VFR travelers are a heterogeneous and complex group, however, and assumptions based on population generalizations are not appropriate.

BOX 9-07 Reported reasons travelers visiting friends and relatives (VFR) are at increased risk for travel-associated infections & diseases

CULTURAL & SOCIETAL BARRIERS

Cultural and language discordance between local travel health care providers and members of the VFR community.
Immigration status concerns among members of the VFR community.
Lack of awareness of travel medicine among members of the VFR community.
Mistrust of the local medical system among members of the VFR community.

HEALTH CARE PROVIDER-DEPENDENT BARRIERS

Lack of knowledge of malaria prevention, identification, and treatment.
Underlying unconscious bias and racism (negative social-political determinants of health).

LOGISTICAL BARRIERS

Financial barriers, including lack of insurance coverage.
Lack of access (travel health clinics not located in areas where VFR travelers live; less marketing and outreach to VFR communities).

UNIQUE ELEMENTS OF VFR TRAVEL

Duration: VFR travelers might stay at their destination longer than tourists or other travelers going to the same area.
Infectious diseases: VFR travelers might travel more frequently to destinations with high disease endemicity and increased exposure risk.
Last-minute and emergency travel: VFR travelers might need to make sudden travel plans to visit ill family members or attend funerals.
Other features that place VFR travelers at increased risk for travel-associated illness:

- Less likely to use insect bite precautions (e.g., insect repellent, mosquito nets, protective clothing).
- More likely to stay in the community and at homes of friends and relatives.
- Participation in daily family and community activities (e.g., drinking tap or untreated water, sharing locally prepared foods).

As with any other international traveler, conduct individualized counseling and recommendations after thoroughly discussing and evaluating the VFR traveler's existing knowledge and beliefs about travel health, in combination with their specific travel characteristics and plans. Exploring the nuanced cultural considerations of the individual traveler is instrumental to providing more effective travel recommendations.

Malaria

As noted, several travel-associated infectious diseases occur at disproportionately high rates in VFR travelers. Box 9-07 highlights multiple reasons for this (e.g., barriers to receiving appropriate pretravel care, unique features of VFR travel), reasons that have been best studied for malaria. Although the global burden of malaria has been decreasing, malaria importation into the United States has been increasing in recent years; 2,161 confirmed imported cases were reported in 2017, the highest number in 45 years. Of these cases, 73% occurred among VFR travelers; 86% were imported from Africa, and 67% of African cases originated in West Africa. These figures are supported by data collected from the GeoSentinel global surveillance network clinics during 2003–2016, which showed that 53% of returned travelers diagnosed with malaria were VFR travelers, 83% of whom acquired their disease in sub-Saharan Africa.

Although VFR travelers who were born abroad experience a greater incidence of malaria infection than other international travelers, severe disease and death from malaria among this population has historically been lower than in tourists and business travelers, possibly because of preexisting immunity. VFR travelers are, however, still vulnerable to severe malaria; 55% of malaria hospitalizations in 2017 occurred in this population, and deaths also are reported. For instance, VFR travelers accounted for 5/5 reported malaria deaths in 2014 and 5/11 deaths in 2015.

Timely recognition and prompt delivery of appropriate treatment are critical to improving outcomes in malaria patients. Misdiagnoses by health care providers from nonendemic regions who lack familiarity with the disease have been reported, leading to delays in therapy. Potential misdiagnosis underscores the need for VFR travelers to carefully adhere to chemoprophylaxis and other malaria prevention strategies.

The same factors that lead to a greater incidence of travel-associated infectious diseases among VFR travelers generally, also contribute to an increased risk for malaria in VFR travelers going to Africa. Although VFR travelers' knowledge, attitudes, and practices (KAPs) have been widely reported in the literature, little systematic or rigorous data are published that provide evidence that KAPs differ substantially between VFR and other traveler groups. More recent studies contradict the traditional narrative that VFR travelers are less concerned than other travelers about the possibility of malaria infection. In fact, VFR travelers have equal or more concern about malaria, but existing barriers mean they are less able to act on those concerns.

Other Infections & Conditions

During 2012–2016, about half of all typhoid and paratyphoid A cases in the United States occurred in VFR travelers, mostly those returning from southern Asia. Most isolates were resistant or showed decreased susceptibility to antimicrobial agents like fluoroquinolones.

VFR travelers aged <15 years are at greatest risk for hepatitis A; children and adolescents often have asymptomatic infections. A Canadian study found that 65% of hepatitis A cases occurred in VFR travelers aged <20 years; and in a Swedish study of 636 cases of imported infection, 52% were in VFR travelers, of whom 90% were <14 years old. Other travel-associated infections (e.g., hepatitis B, measles) also occur more commonly in young VFR travelers.

As a group, VFR travelers may be more likely than others to travel internationally while pregnant or at extremes of age, risk factors that can predispose to more severe outcomes from certain infections. For example, malaria during pregnancy is associated with higher morbidity and mortality, and exposure to Zika virus during pregnancy can result in serious fetal and infant complications. The very young and the elderly can have unusual clinical presentations of infections and worse outcomes. For instance, infants develop tuberculosis meningitis more commonly than people in other age groups, and older age is associated with more severe coronavirus disease 2019 (COVID-19) outcomes.

PRETRAVEL HEALTH COUNSELING

VFR travelers are more likely to seek travel health advice from a primary care clinic than from a travel medicine specialty clinic. Primary care clinics should ensure clinical staff are able to provide basic travel health information and services, and should create systems and working relationships with travel health experts for consultation and referral when appropriate. Primary care and travel clinics can employ various strategies to reach and better serve VFR populations (Box 9-08).

In addition, certain health risks and prevention recommendations might vary or deserve special attention for VFR travelers. Increase awareness among VFR travelers regarding their unique risks for travel-associated infections, and develop strategies to help overcome the barriers they face in accessing and acquiring travel health services. One possible approach is to provide VFR travelers with a comparison of the effect and cost of contracting certain diseases versus the cost of taking preventive measures.

Malaria Prevention

Encourage VFR travelers going to malaria-endemic areas to take prophylactic medications, but also remind them of the benefits of barrier methods of prevention (e.g., insect repellents, mosquito nets, protective clothing), particularly for children (see Sec. 4, Ch. 6, Mosquitoes, Ticks & Other Arthropods). Social pressures from host families can dissuade VFR travelers from implementing effective prevention techniques (e.g., using insect repellents and mosquito nets, staying indoors during periods of peak mosquito feeding). Discuss any potential concerns, and provide viable alternative options (e.g., clothing pre-treated

BOX 9-08 Improving outreach & service to VFR travelers: recommendations for clinics

PRIMARY CARE CLINICS (VFR travelers disproportionately seek care at primary care clinics vs. travel medicine clinics)

Ensure clinicians receive continuing education in travel health and travel medicine.

Provide clinicians access to essential travel medicine information (e.g., CDC Yellow Book, Heading Home Healthy, UpToDate).[1]

Establish systems and relationships with travel medicine experts and infectious diseases specialists for consultation and referral.

TRAVEL MEDICINE SPECIALTY CLINICS

Conduct outreach to local communities:

- Give talks to community or faith groups on travel medicine with Q&A sessions.
- Meet with VFR community leaders.
- Use various forms of media for outreach (e.g., volunteer for community radio call-in programs to discuss travel health).

Consider adding evening and weekend appointments to the clinic schedule; reserve time slots for last-minute, emergency travel, and returned travelers who are ill.

Create a welcoming clinic environment:

- Decorate with artwork and provide reading materials from countries and cultures of the VFR communities being served.
- Provide an area for prayers.
- Provide language-accessible educational materials.

Encourage patients to "shop around" for the lowest price medications and to purchase in the United States before departing.

Encourage local pharmacies and health systems in areas with greater need to stock appropriate chemoprophylaxis agents.

Ensure VFR travelers have adequate supplies of travel medicines (e.g., malaria chemoprophylaxis):

- Direct pharmacists to call if the VFR traveler is not filling the entire prescription.
- Include travel duration on all travel medicine prescriptions.
- Provide cards to help patients advocate for themselves at pharmacies.[2]

BOTH PRIMARY CARE & TRAVEL MEDICINE CLINICS

Help patients navigate the healthcare system (e.g., assist in making appointments at appropriate clinics, help arrange transportation).

Increase access to professional medical interpreters; train staff how to use interpreters.

Provide culturally and linguistically appropriate educational materials in audio, video, and written formats.

Train clinical staff and health care providers about conscious and unconscious bias, health equity, and to practice cultural humility.

[1]Centers for Disease Control and Prevention Yellow Book (https://wwwnc.cdc.gov/travel/page/yellowbook-home); Heading Home Healthy (www.HeadingHomeHealthy.org); UpToDate (www.uptodate.com).

[2]See the self-advocacy information card developed by the Minnesota Department of Health in collaboration with a West Africa Community Advisory Board to help VFR travelers obtain affordable antimalarial drugs. Available from: www.health.state.mn.us/diseases/travel/medcost.pdf.

9

with insect repellents, odorless repellents, freestanding mosquito nets).

MALARIA CHEMOPROPHYLAXIS

Due to cost and other disincentives to purchasing malaria chemoprophylaxis in the United States, VFR travelers frequently report they plan to buy these drugs overseas. Substandard malaria chemoprophylaxis drugs are common, however, in certain low- and middle-income countries; in addition, these drugs are a frequent target for drug counterfeiting (see Sec. 6, Ch. 3, . . . *perspectives*: Avoiding Poorly Regulated Medicines & Medical Products During Travel). Moreover, because of greater familiarity with products available for purchase at their destination, VFR travelers might favor or endorse a drug that is either inappropriate or contraindicated for use. Counsel against using drugs for which there is documented resistance (e.g., chloroquine, proguanil monotherapy) or that are used for malaria treatment (e.g., artesunate, quinine-based drugs) and not prophylaxis.

For all the above reasons, educate travelers about the risks associated with taking medicines acquired abroad, and advise them to obtain their medications in the United States prior to travel. Recent research has shown the price for the exact same prescription of most common antimalarial drugs can vary greatly among different pharmacies in the same area. Encourage VFR travelers to comparison shop and assist them in finding the best drug price. The Minnesota Department of Health has developed a self-advocacy information card (see www.health.state.mn.us/diseases/travel/medcost.pdf) with a West Africa Community Advisory Board to help VFR travelers obtain affordable antimalarial drugs.

Patients also can contact their health insurance provider to learn whether prescription coverage can be extended due to a longer trip. Clinicians can include a note to "notify the prescriber if entire prescription is not filled," and assist the pharmacy and patient to resolve any issues.

Vaccinations

Travel vaccine recommendations and requirements for VFR travelers are the same as those for other travelers. In addition, establish whether VFR travelers, particularly those born outside the United States, have had routine childhood immunizations (e.g., diphtheria-tetanus-pertussis; measles-mumps-rubella) or a clinical history of vaccine-preventable diseases (e.g., varicella).

In the absence of documentation of immunizations, consider adult travelers susceptible and offer age-appropriate vaccinations. Alternatively, perform serologic studies to demonstrate proof of immunity when documentation is lacking (but suspicion of a completed vaccination series is high), or when clinical or epidemiological evidence to suspect prior infection is present.

Although vaccine recommendations for VFR travelers do not differ substantially from those

BOX 9-09 Vaccinating VFR travelers: caveats & recommendations

HEPATITIS A

Hepatitis A infection is common in childhood in low- and middle-income countries (see Sec. 5, Part 2, Ch. 7, Hepatitis A). After infection, natural immunity is life-long. Due to changing epidemiology, however, do not assume immunity to hepatitis A; many young adults and adolescents from low- and middle-income countries are susceptible and should be vaccinated.

HEPATITIS B

Hepatitis B infection is common in most immigrant groups. Because of routine immunization recommendations in the United States, at-risk immigrants might have a record of receiving hepatitis B vaccination but might not have been screened for chronic infection prior to vaccination. If a patient is at risk for hepatitis B (born or resided in a country with ≥2% prevalence), and no record of a negative test for hepatitis B chronic infection is available, screen for chronic infection (hepatitis B antigen testing) regardless of vaccine status (see Sec. 5, Part 2, Ch. 8, Hepatitis B).

VARICELLA

Varicella infection occurs later in life in the tropics, and rates of death and complications from varicella disease are higher in adults than in children. Do not assume immunity; perform immunization or antibody testing if no clear clinical history of infection is apparent.

OFF-LABEL VACCINE USE

Experienced providers familiar with the literature may consider off-label use of vaccines for high-risk pediatric VFR travelers when the benefit is felt to outweigh the risk (e.g., measles-mumps-rubella in children <12 months old, typhoid in children <2 years old). See Sec. 7, Ch. 3, Traveling Safely with Infants & Children, and Sec. 7, Ch. 4, Vaccine Recommendations for Infants & Children.

PRETRAVEL SCREENING FOR CHRONIC INFECTIONS

Use pretravel VFR consultations as an opportunity to screen for common chronic infections (e.g., hepatitis B, hepatitis C, HIV, schistosomiasis, strongyloidiasis, latent tuberculosis). For more information, see Guidance for the US Domestic Medical Examination for Newly Arriving Refugees (www.cdc.gov/immigrantrefugeehealth/guidelines/domestic-guidelines.html) and Sec. 11, Ch. 11, Newly Arrived Immigrants, Refugees & Other Migrants.

ROUTINE HEALTH CARE VISITS: PLANNING AHEAD

Use routine health care visits for children and adults as an opportunity to ask about future travel plans. Offer travel vaccines, advice, and recommendations.

of other travelers, important specific caveats are listed in Box 9-09.

RESOURCES FOR HEALTH CARE PROVIDERS

Heading Home Healthy

The Heading Home Healthy program (www.HeadingHomeHealthy.org), supported by the Centers for Disease Control and Prevention, focuses on reducing travel-related illnesses in VFR travelers. The program was developed to provide VFR travelers with resources for safe travel and includes videos, informational resources, and health tools in multiple languages. Heading Home Healthy also offers a clinical support tool for primary care health providers who are preparing their patients to travel home safely.

BIBLIOGRAPHY

Angelo KM, Libman M, Caumes E, Hamer DH, Kain KC, Leder K, et al. Malaria after international travel: a GeoSentinel analysis, 2003–2016. Malar J. 2017;16(1):293.

Bruneel F, Tubach F, Corne P, Megarbane B, Mira JP, Peytel E, et al.; Severe Imported Malaria in Adults (SIMA) Study Group. Severe imported falciparum malaria: a cohort study in 400 critically ill adults. PLoS One. 2010;5(10):e13236.

Centers for Disease Control and Prevention. National typhoid and paratyphoid fever Surveillance annual summary, 2015. Available from: www.cdc.gov/typhoid-fever/reports/annual-report-2015.html.

Goldman-Yassen AE, Mony VK, Arguin PM, Daily JP. Higher rates of misdiagnosis in pediatric patients versus adults hospitalized with imported malaria. Pediatr Emerg Care. 2016;32(4):227–31.

Hendel-Paterson B, Swanson SJ. Pediatric travelers visiting friends and relatives (VFR) abroad: illnesses, barriers and pre-travel recommendations. Travel Med Infect Dis. 2011;9(4):192–203.

Volkman HR, Walz EJ, Wanduragala D, Schiffman E, Frosch A, Alpern JD, et al. Barriers to malaria prevention among immigrant travelers in the United States who visit friends and relatives in sub-Saharan Africa: a cross-sectional, multi-setting survey of knowledge, attitudes, and practices. PLoS ONE 2020;15(3):e0229565.

Walz EJ, Volkman HR, Adedimeji AA, Abella J, Scott LA, Angelo KM, et al. Barriers to malaria prevention in US-based travellers visiting friends and relatives abroad: a qualitative study of West African immigrant travellers. J Travel Med. 2019:1;26(2):tay163.

9

MASS GATHERINGS

Joanna Gaines, Kristina Angelo

Mass gatherings are typically defined as large numbers of people (>1,000) at a specific location, for a specific purpose. Practically speaking, a mass gathering can be any assembly of people large enough to strain local resources. Travelers to mass gatherings face unique risks because these events are associated with environmental hazards, challenging security situations, and increased opportunity for infectious disease transmission due to the influx of attendees, crowding, and poor hygiene from temporary food and sanitation facilities. Although the coronavirus disease 2019 (COVID-19) pandemic caused the cancellation or postponement of numerous mass gatherings, a growing number are being held, with mixed public health consequences.

MASS GATHERING CHARACTERISTICS

International travelers and their medical providers should understand the characteristics of mass gatherings. Some can be spontaneous (e.g., political protests); others are planned events. Some mass gatherings regularly occur at different locations (e.g., the Olympic Games, the Fédération Internationale de Football Association [FIFA] World Cup); other gatherings recur in the same location (e.g., Hajj, the annual Islamic pilgrimage to Mecca [see Sec. 10, Part 1, Ch. 2, Saudi Arabia:

Table 9-04 Examples of international mass gathering events

EVENT TYPE	EVENT NAME	HOST COUNTRY	TYPICAL ATTENDANCE
Religious	Hajj	Saudi Arabia	2.5 million
Sporting	FIFA World Cup 2022	Qatar	3 million
Cultural (arts/music)	Carnival	Brazil (also worldwide)	7 million
Business	EXPO 2023	Argentina	>5 million

Hajj & Umrah Pilgrimages]). Table 9-04 provides a brief representative list of mass gatherings, including type (religious observance, sporting event, or art and music festival), location, and typical attendance numbers. Most mass gatherings can be described effectively in terms of their activities, capacity, duration, location, participants, purpose, size, timing, and venue (see Table 9-05).

MASS GATHERING–ASSOCIATED HEALTH CONCERNS

Attendance at a mass gathering can exacerbate a traveler's existing medical conditions. Emergency medical services often are involved in preparations for gatherings, and are usually equipped to address acute medical conditions (e.g., asthma, gastrointestinal issues, injuries, myocardial infarction). Onsite healthcare providers are usually capable of handling gathering-associated conditions (e.g., dehydration, heat exhaustion, hypothermia, sunburn).

Catastrophic Incidents

Catastrophic incidents are of particular concern during mass gatherings, especially with extremely dense crowds. Numerous casualties have occurred at mass gatherings due to poor crowd management, structural collapses, fires, and violence. Crush injuries and death can result from crowding and stampedes. At the 2015 Hajj pilgrimage in Saudi Arabia, for example, thousands of pilgrims died in a stampede; in 2021, dozens of pilgrims, including children, were killed during a stampede at an annual Lag BaOmer festival in Israel.

Ensuring personal safety during mass gatherings is necessary. Travelers should remain aware of their surroundings. Although the risk for large-scale incidents (e.g., terror attacks) are low, they are impossible to predict or eliminate (see Sec. 4, Ch. 11, Safety & Security Overseas).

Infectious Diseases

Mass gathering attendees are at risk for infections, including vaccine-preventable illnesses (e.g., COVID-19, influenza, pneumococcus). Past mass gatherings have been associated with outbreaks of influenza, meningococcal disease, and norovirus. Mass gatherings also have implications for global health security.

Travelers who import infectious diseases to mass gathering host sites can infect both their fellow attendees and local organizers who, in turn, can become sources of infection to others. In this way (and depending on routes of transmission, incubation periods, and other disease-specific factors) concentrations of people attending mass gatherings facilitate the amplification of a disease. Participants can then export the illness internationally to destinations other than the host location. For emerging diseases, little might be known at first about all the various routes of transmission or consequences of infection. When Zika initially emerged in 2015 in Brazil, for example, shortly before the country hosted the Olympic and Paralympic Games, the potential for sexual and vertical transmission of the virus was unknown.

CORONAVIRUS DISEASE 2019

COVID-19 poses a unique risk for both travelers to mass gatherings and for the countries hosting mass gathering events, due to the influx of international attendees, varied country-specific immunization practices and vaccine access, and difficulty enforcing mask use or physical

Table 9-05 Mass gatherings: characteristic features & potential risks

FEATURE	POTENTIAL RISK CONSIDERATIONS
ACTIVITIES	Some activities can be risky or strenuous (e.g., walking long distances in extreme temperatures) or could involve alcohol or drug use.
CAPACITY	Hosts differ in their ability to detect, respond to, and prevent public health emergencies. Understanding health outcomes previously associated with a recurring mass gathering can help travelers prepare for future events. Security arrangements vary.
DURATION	The longer an event lasts, the more likely local resources will be depleted and become strained.
LOCATION	Environment and infrastructure affect health and safety of events; some host countries and cities have better natural or engineered resources to handle large numbers of people than others.
PARTICIPANTS	Attendees can represent a unique demographic (e.g., religious, political groups), or vary by gender or age (e.g., older adults attempting to complete a religious pilgrimage toward the end of their life).
PURPOSE	Mass gatherings can be political, religious, social, or athletic events. The purpose of an event can determine the activities and affect the mood of participants.
SIZE	The density of crowds, not just the number of attendees, contribute to health and safety risks. More densely packed crowds can facilitate disease spread or induce riots or crowd crush disasters.
TIMING	Mass gatherings and local capacity are affected by the timing of an event. Season / weather can influence the number in attendance which affects the host's ability to organize a safe mass gathering.
VENUE	Indoor versus outdoor events create different sets of challenges for mass gathering organizers. Food, water, housing, and sanitation, can be of varying quality.

distancing. Logistics related to staff safety, visitor safety, site circulation (e.g., queuing), event location (e.g., indoor vs. outdoor), commerce (e.g., food and beverage venues), and sanitation (e.g., availability, location, and number handwashing stations) are among the issues to be considered when planning or visiting an event during the pandemic.

COVID-19 has impacted recommendations and requirements for all international travelers, including mass gathering attendees. Some countries require travelers to demonstrate proof of vaccination (including ≥1 booster dose) against COVID-19, prior to entry. Others may require mandatory quarantine periods for those not vaccinated. Travelers should check with local health authorities at their intended destination to ensure they are aware of the most current requirements.

CLINICIAN GUIDANCE

Risk Assessment

ACTIVITIES & ITINERARIES

Ask travelers about their activities and itineraries. Verify a traveler's itinerary to identify risks at the destination, in addition to those associated with the event itself. Travelers might add side trips or extend travel beyond the mass gathering.

PATIENT CHARACTERISTICS

Consider the patient's unique characteristics. Chronic health conditions can be exacerbated while participating in a mass gathering. Counsel patients on the importance of having adequate supplies of medication for the duration of their trip, and documentation for any prescriptions.

Risk Mitigation

VACCINES

Encourage vaccination. Ensure that travelers have all appropriate pretravel vaccinations, including routine and required vaccines, and are up to date with their vaccinations against COVID-19 (www.cdc.gov/coronavirus/2019-ncov/vaccines/stay-up-to-date.html).

REQUIREMENTS

Identify requirements for mass gathering attendees beyond those required for entry to a country. For example, whereas Saudi Arabia mandates that all participants in the Hajj be vaccinated against meningococcal disease, this requirement does not apply to other travelers visiting the country.

RECOMMENDATIONS

In addition to any host-country requirements, some destinations and venues can have additional recommendations for mass gathering attendees based on public health concerns (e.g., demonstrating proof of COVID-19 vaccination). Be prepared to identify and provide needed pretravel health services based on host-site recommendations.

PROVIDE EDUCATION & GUIDANCE TO TRAVELERS

Educate travelers on preventive measures, including regular application of sunscreen and insect repellent or advice on how to choose safe food and water from vendors. Emphasize the importance of regular handwashing with soap and water and the use of hand sanitizer with ≥60% alcohol content when sanitation facilities are not available. Box 9-10 is a checklist for travelers to use as they plan to attend a mass gathering.

BOX 9-10 Mass gathering events: a planning checklist for travelers

☐ CHECK HOST NATION REQUIREMENTS

In addition to the entry requirements of the host nation, become informed about all requirements for participating in the mass gathering (e.g., medical tests, proof of vaccination, use of smartphone applications).

☐ SEE A TRAVEL MEDICINE PROVIDER

Make an appointment to see a travel medicine specialist at least 4–6 weeks before travel—this should allow enough time for you to receive most of your necessary vaccinations.

Discuss your itinerary and any planned activities with the provider—this will allow your provider to make more accurate recommendations to ensure your health and safety.

Discuss your medical history with the travel medicine specialist—some travel medicines might not be safe to take with medicines you take regularly.

If a travel medicine provider is not locally available, a primary care provider should be able to ensure you have adequate vaccinations and the health information necessary.

☐ SEE YOUR REGULAR HEALTH CARE PROVIDER

Work with your regular health care provider to make sure existing medical conditions are well controlled before you leave.

Ensure you have an adequate supply of all your regular prescription medicines prior to departure.

☐ REGISTER WITH THE US DEPARTMENT OF STATE'S SMART TRAVELER ENROLLMENT PROGRAM (STEP, https://step.state.gov/step)

STEP provides travelers with notifications (e.g., travel warnings, travel alerts, other destination-specific information).

STEP also makes sure that the State Department can find you if you experience serious legal, medical, or financial difficulties overseas.

In case of emergency at home, STEP can help friends and family contact you.

☐ VISIT THE CENTERS FOR DISEASE CONTROL AND PREVENTION (CDC) TRAVELERS' HEALTH WEBSITE (https://wwwnc.cdc.gov/travel)

Learn more about health and safety issues at specific destinations.

Find out if CDC has posted any Travel Health Notices for your destination or mass gathering event.

STAY CURRENT

The Centers for Disease Control and Prevention regularly updates its Travelers' Health website (https://wwwnc.cdc.gov/travel) with Travel Health Notices (notifications of disease outbreaks in countries around the world) and information on select mass gatherings (e.g., Hajj, the Olympic Games).

BIBLIOGRAPHY

Abubakar I, Gautret P, Brunette GW, Blumberg L, Johnson D, Poumerol G, et al. Global perspectives for prevention of infectious diseases associated with mass gatherings. Lancet Infect Dis. 2012;12(1):66–74.

Gautret P, Angelo KM, Asgeirsson H, Duvignaud A, van Genderen PJJ, Bottieau E, et al. International mass gatherings and travel-associated illness: a GeoSentinel cross-sectional, observational study. Travel Med Infect Dis. 2019;32:101504.

Lombardo JS, Sniegoski CA, Loschen WA, Westercamp M, Wade M, Dearth S, et al. Public health surveillance for mass gatherings. Johns Hopkins APL Tech Dig. 2008;27(4):1–9.

McCloskey B, Endericks T. Learning from London 2012: a practical guide to public health and mass gatherings. London: Public Health England; 2013. Available from: www.ifv.nl/kennisplein/Documents/2013-Health-Protection-Agency-Learning-from-london-2012.pdf.

Ranse J, Beckwith D, Khan A, Yexli S, Hertenlendy AJ, Hutton A, et al. Novel respiratory viruses in the context of mass-gathering events: a systematic review to inform event planning from a health perspective. Prehosp Dis Med. 2021; 36(5):599–604.

Steffen R, Bouchama A, Johansson A, Dvorak J, Isla N, Smallwood C, et al. Non-communicable health risks during mass gatherings. Lancet Infect Dis. 2012;12(2):142–9.

World Health Organization. Public Health for Mass Gatherings. Geneva: The Organization; 2015. Available from: www.who.int/publications/i/item/public-health-for-mass-gatherings-key-considerations.

ADVENTURE TRAVEL

Christopher Van Tilburg

9

Adventure travel is unique because of challenging terrain, extreme weather, remote locales, and longer durations. Popular adventure travel destinations include trekking to Everest Base Camp, climbing Mount Kilimanjaro, hiking the Inca Trail, sailing the South Pacific, touring the Galápagos, and exploring the North and South Poles. Adventure travel can include activities like backpacking, cycling, diving, mountaineering, river rafting, skiing, and surfing. Adventure travelers could be conducting scientific research, providing humanitarian relief, or climbing mountains or driving overland as part of an expedition.

As compared to other types of travel, risk for illness and injury with adventure travel is much greater for several reasons (see Box 9-11). Risk for

BOX 9-11 Adventure travel–associated risk factors for illness & injury

Climate, terrain, and weather can be extreme.

Communication often is limited, even with modern technology.

Destinations can be remote and lack access to care.

Travelers exert themselves physically, increasing caloric, fluid, and sleep requirements.

Trips are often long, spanning several weeks, months, or years.

Trips are often goal oriented, which can cause travelers to exceed safety limits and take increased risks.

Unexpected complications can occur with flight schedules, vehicle breakdowns, weather delays, and other factors.

travel-associated illness and injury is a function of 2 variables: probability and consequence. The probability of a mishap occurring is based on the frequency ("how often"), duration ("how long"), and severity ("how bad") of the hazards encountered; during adventure travel, each is increased. Objective hazards include difficult environmental conditions (e.g., terrain, weather). Dehydration, poor nutrition, and insufficient sleep are examples of subjective or human-controlled hazards.

Consequence, the second variable, is a measure of the outcome or result of an illness or injury. In adventure travel, where conditions are often austere and access to definitive care is remote, even if the probability of a mishap occurring is low, the consequences are nearly always magnified. Minor injuries or illnesses happening in the wrong setting can be disastrous.

Major accidents are rarely due to a single event. Multiple events usually occur in sequence preceding an accident. Travelers should be vigilant about the probability and consequence of risk, and try to make good decisions before they get into trouble.

PRETRAVEL CONSIDERATIONS

During the pretravel consultation, in addition to providing routine travel medicine advice, gather extra information and discuss precautions for wilderness and expedition travel. Several excellent wilderness medicine resources exist, including conferences, journals and textbooks, and professional societies (e.g., the Wilderness Medical Society; www.wms.org).

Trip Type

When talking with adventure travelers, obtain details about the type, length, and remoteness of the trip. Guided trips could eliminate some of the need for complex logistics planning on the part of the traveler. Even with guided trips, though, participants should still ask trip organizers about guide experience and medical training; types of medical kits and safety equipment carried by guides; contingency plans for emergencies; recommendations for medications and medical supplies to be carried by participants; and types of recommended insurance.

In a few cases (e.g., Mount Everest expeditions, polar cruises), a formal medical officer with a comprehensive medical kit might accompany the participants. By contrast, for self-planned trips, travel health providers might need to offer more support with logistics, insurance, evacuation planning, and to augment a comprehensive medical kit with prescription medications.

Confirm that the experience, fitness, and skill level of the participant matches the trip type. Novices at diving, mountaineering, sailing, or skiing should participate in instructional trips. Encourage people with less experience or who are visiting a location for the first time to go on a guided trip. Because many people will consult a travel medicine professional only after they have selected and paid for their adventure, some might need a medical waiver or letter to change the trip to be more in line with their skill, experience, and fitness.

Personal Health Requirements

Travelers might need medical clearance to participate in a guided trip. For travelers with chronic diseases, the primary care provider (PCP) should complete the medical clearance and provide prescriptions for regular medications, if possible (see Sec. 3, Ch. 3, Travelers with Chronic Illnesses). Travel health practitioners can complete pretravel medical clearance if it is a usual function of their practice, and the patient has no underlying chronic diseases or medications; even so, consider consulting with the traveler's PCP to help determine medical clearance.

Screen travelers for conditions that can be exacerbated by exertion or environmental hazards (e.g., high elevation, temperature extremes). Ask travelers whether they have a history of anaphylaxis-level allergies, asthma, cardiac disease, cerebrovascular disease (e.g., stroke, transient ischemic attack), chronic pain treated with opiates, deep vein thrombosis, diabetes, oxygen-dependent emphysema, joint replacement, pulmonary embolism, recent surgery, or sleep apnea. Any of these conditions could indicate a traveler is at risk for adverse outcomes under physiological stressful conditions. Travelers with a previous history of environmental illness (e.g., altitude illness, anaphylaxis, frostbite, heat exhaustion, hypothermia) could be at risk for recurrence.

Travelers with chronic or major medical issues should carry a medication list, printed copies of their most recent electrocardiogram, chest x-ray, and their medical history; or download electronic copies to their phone in PDF or JPG format. Caution travelers who rely on battery-operated devices (e.g., continuous positive airway pressure [CPAP] machine, insulin pump) about the possibility of device failure, and discuss the need for a backup plan or the possibility that they should avoid adventure travel altogether. Some people with chronic illness, especially those who are medically dependent on electronic devices, who have difficulty ambulating, and who are medically frail, likely are not good candidates for adventure travel.

Adequate hydration, nutrition, and sleep could be in short supply, especially with increased demands due to exertion, weather, and terrain. During the planning stages, travelers should pay attention to how they will obtain water, food, and rest on their journey.

Travel Insurance

Insurance is widely variable and comes in many forms, and having insurance does not guarantee rescue (see Sec. 6, Ch. 1, Travel Insurance, Travel Health Insurance & Medical Evacuation Insurance). Travelers might need to pay in advance for rescue, evacuation, and repatriation, which can be expensive, especially for aeromedical transport from remote locations. Travelers should bring sufficient emergency cash and a credit card with high credit and cash advance limits.

Coverage can be contingent on preexisting conditions, deductibles, maximum expenditures, and medical control approval. Insurers also might not authorize aeromedical transport. Insurance companies might deny claims involving alcohol or drugs, chronic illness, mental health, pregnancy, and acts of war or civil unrest. Travelers should read policies carefully before purchasing and departing on their trip.

DOMESTIC HEALTH INSURANCE

Domestic health insurance might or might not be effective outside a home country. Often, travelers need to pay up front for medical care and get reimbursed from health insurance providers once they return home.

TRAVEL INSURANCE

Travel insurance, which often includes medical, trip cancellation, evacuation, and repatriation benefits, might exclude coverage for wilderness rescue and adventure sports like diving, mountaineering, and skiing. An adventure sports rider is available with some travel insurance policies.

WILDERNESS RESCUE INSURANCE

Usually purchased separately from travel insurance, wilderness rescue insurance policies are available through specialty clubs, outdoor and professional associations, and organizations (e.g., the American Alpine Club [https://americanalpineclub.org], Divers Alert Network [https://dan.org]).

SHORT-TERM RESCUE INSURANCE

Short-term rescue insurance is available in some destination countries through local helicopter rescue companies, mountaineering clubs, and ski resorts. In Switzerland, for example, travelers can become a member of Rega (www.rega.ch/en/), the aeromedical rescue service.

COMPREHENSIVE EXPEDITION POLICIES

Comprehensive expedition policies can include travel, medical, rescue, repatriation, and security services.

First Aid & Safety Training

If travelers have time, they should consider completing basic life support and first aid courses before departure. These can be particularly helpful for regular adventure travelers. Such courses can be found through local community colleges and fire departments, the American Heart Association (https://cpr.heart.org/en), and the American Red Cross (www.redcross.org/take-a-class/cpr/cpr-training/cpr-classes).

Emergency Resources

Travelers should always keep their credit cards, money, passport, and other documents on their person because they might need to seek medical care or evacuate urgently without their luggage.

BOX 9-12 Adventure travel health & safety tips

ALLERGIES & ANAPHYLAXIS

Bites, stings, food, and other allergens can cause anaphylaxis. Epinephrine and corticosteroids can be lifesaving if administered immediately. See Sec. 3, Ch. 4, Highly Allergic Travelers.

ALTITUDE ILLNESS

Travelers to high elevations might require acetazolamide, dexamethasone, or other medications to prevent or treat altitude illness. Mental status changes and ataxia are warning signs for high-altitude cerebral edema. Breathlessness at rest is the sign of life-threatening high-altitude pulmonary edema. See Sec. 4, Ch. 5, High Elevation Travel & Altitude Illness.

BASIC WOUND CARE

Travelers should be aware of basic wound care and self-treatment with antibiotics. Redness, swelling, pus, and warmth are signs of infection that might require medical attention.

FROSTBITE

Frostbite is treated with rapid rewarming with non-scalding warm water. Warn travelers not to allow a thawed extremity to refreeze (see Sec. 4, Ch. 2, Extremes of Temperature).

HEAT STROKE

Heat stroke marked by a temperature of 40°C and mental status changes is a medical emergency (see Sec. 4, Ch. 2, Extremes of Temperature).

HYPOTHERMIA

For hypothermia, cessation of shivering and mental status changes are dangerous signs (see Sec. 4, Ch. 2, Extremes of Temperature).

RABIES

Rabies is prevalent around the world, and preexposure (pretravel) vaccination should be considered because rabies immune globulin and vaccine might be difficult to find in certain countries (see Sec. 5, Part 2, Ch. 18, Rabies).

VENOMOUS CREATURES

Jellyfish, scorpions, snakes, spiders, and ticks can deliver toxic venom, inoculate microbes, and cause anaphylaxis. Region-specific antivenoms can be found for certain venomous species around the world (see Sec. 4, Ch. 7, Zoonotic Exposures: Bites, Stings, Scratches & Other Hazards).

Travelers also can store backup copies as a PDF or JPG on a mobile phone.

Before leaving on their adventure, travelers should know embassy contacts, emergency escape routes, local medical facilities, and local rescue resources. Travel medicine practitioners willing to accept emails, phone calls, and text messages from travelers abroad should make sure that travelers understand this is not a substitute for local emergency care (see Sec. 2, Ch. 16, Telemedicine). In a pretravel medicine encounter, physicians might have only a few minutes to educate travelers. Depending on the type, duration, and location of trip, a few key adventure travel health and safety tips (see Box 9-12) might be worth discussing.

WILDERNESS SUPPLIES

Adventure travelers should pack and carry the following clothing, supplies, and gear.

Clothing

Remind travelers that clothing helps prevent heat and cold illness as well as bites and stings from insects and other arthropods. Cold weather clothing should be made of polyester, nylon, Merino wool, or, in some circumstances, down. Layering typically consists of a base layer, insulating layers of heavy-pile polyester or nylon-encased polyester (down suffices if traveling to a location that is dry and cold, but does not function well when it gets wet), and a windproof, waterproof outer layer of tightly woven nylon with a durable water-repellent coating. Gloves, hat, neck warmer, warm socks, and goggles are vital to cover all exposed skin.

For hot weather, sun- and insect-protective clothing is important, including loose-fitting, lightweight clothing made from nylon, polyester, or a cotton blend. Long-sleeve shirts and long pants offer the most protection. A wide-brim sun hat, a sun shirt with a hood, and a bandana or buff protect the head and neck; sunglasses protect eyes. For more details on protection from sun exposure and extreme temperatures during travel, see the respective chapters in Section 4. Clothing should be sprayed with permethrin to ward off insects and arthropods (see Sec. 4, Ch. 6, Mosquitoes, Ticks & Other Arthropods).

Footwear should be activity-specific boots or shoes, equally important in a marine or mountain environment. Because even a minor foot injury can be debilitating, advise travelers to never go without footwear.

Communication & Route-Finding Equipment

Travelers should carry a mobile phone enabled with a global positioning system (GPS). Phones can be used to store electronic versions of documents (e.g., embassy and hospital contact information, insurance policies, medical data, passport copies, plane tickets) in email, JPG, or PDF format. Because not all North American mobile phones and service plans are compatible with international networks, travelers should check with their local (i.e., domestic) carrier before departing.

Alternatively, an unlocked (not restricted to any carrier) global-compatible mobile phone can be used with a local SIM card in the country of travel. Inexpensive phones and SIM cards are usually available at stores in airports and major cities. In some countries, registration to obtain a local SIM card requires fingerprinting and a passport.

An emergency satellite communication device is an excellent tool to carry. This device can synch with a mobile phone to send routine and emergency messages, usually via text. Where cellular phone service is not available, travelers might consider an unlocked (no frequency restrictions) VHF/UHF radio or a satellite phone. Several countries worldwide require users of handheld radios and satellite phones to have permits, however; advise travelers that restrictions might exist at their destination, and to learn what they are before departing.

Remind travelers that electronics are not foolproof; often they are limited by battery power, deep canyons, dense cloud cover, government restrictions, and physical damage caused by extreme temperatures, impact, or water exposure. A backup external battery and external power source (e.g., a solar or dynamo charger) are useful.

For extreme terrain and remote locations, adventurers should carry a GPS app installed on their mobile phone. Alternatively, they can carry a separate GPS device. Suggest that travelers upload maps to their phones or GPS devices prior to departure. They also might choose to learn how to use and to bring an altimeter, compass, and local topographic map (the latter might need to be acquired in-country).

Emergency Kits

Adventure travelers often require a comprehensive, yet compact, personal emergency kit for medical care and survival and equipment repair. Beyond a basic travel health kit (see Sec. 2, Ch. 10, Travel Health Kits), adventure travelers should consider packing additional items due to the remote nature of their travel. Standard kits might need to be augmented for specific types of travel (e.g., high elevation, jungle, open ocean, polar, undersea).

If travelers are on guided trips, they might only need a small personal medical kit. Before they depart, travelers should determine whether guides provide group emergency equipment (e.g., comprehensive medical kit, automatic external defibrillator, portable hyperbaric chamber and oxygen, portable stretcher). Be cautious if asked to prescribe medications for guides to stock in the expedition medical kit intended for clients. Third-party use of prescription medication is unlawful in most jurisdictions and best left for the guide company medical director. If prescribing to a guide as a patient, clarify that the medication is for the guide's personal use.

MEDICATIONS

Provide prescriptions and guidance for self-treatment for febrile illness, gastroenteritis (travelers' diarrhea), respiratory illness, and wound infections. In addition to routine travel medications (e.g., analgesics, antiemetics, motion sickness medication), consider prescribing ophthalmologic antibiotics and anesthetic, nonsedating antihistamines, and altitude illness medicines. Instruct travelers on self-treatment of anaphylaxis, because this can be lifesaving; epinephrine auto injectors are common, but a less-expensive alternative is a vial of epinephrine and a syringe. Diabetics should carry glucagon and glucose gel for hypoglycemia.

BOX 9-13 Additional safety equipment: a checklist for adventure travelers

- ☐ Antibacterial wipes
- ☐ Chemical heat packs
- ☐ Duct tape
- ☐ Earplugs and eyeshade
- ☐ Emergency sleeping sack or tarp
- ☐ Eyeglasses (spare pair)
- ☐ Hand sanitizer
- ☐ Headlight with extra batteries
- ☐ Insect repellent
- ☐ Laundry detergent
- ☐ Mobile phone with global positioning system (GPS) app
- ☐ Multi-tool
- ☐ Oral rehydration salts
- ☐ Perlon cord
- ☐ Polyurethane straps and plastic cable ties
- ☐ Rain poncho and umbrella
- ☐ Safety pins
- ☐ Satellite communication device
- ☐ Spare phone power pack or solar/dynamo charger
- ☐ Sun hat, bandana, and sunglasses
- ☐ Sunscreen and lip balm
- ☐ Water purification tablets
- ☐ Whistle
- ☐ Toilet paper

Consider opioid and prescription nonsteroidal anti-inflammatory pain medication, bearing in mind that in some countries, travelers might be restricted from bringing in opioid drugs, even for their own use. A patient on chronic opioids might consider bringing naloxone for emergency reversal of opioid overdose.

SAFETY SUPPLIES

In addition to items typically included in a general travel health kit, adventure travelers should consider packing safety equipment that can help in an emergency (see Box 9-13).

BIBLIOGRAPHY

Iserson KV. Medical planning for extended remote expeditions. Wilderness Environ Med. 2013;24(4):366–77.

Lipnick MS, Lewin M. Wilderness preparation, equipment, and medical supplies. In: Auerbach PS, editor. Auerbach's wilderness medicine, 7th edition. Philadelphia: Elsevier; 2017. pp. 2272–305.

Mellor A, Dodds N, Joshi R, Hall J, Dhillon S, Hollis S, et al. Faculty of Prehospital Care, Royal College of Surgeons Edinburgh guidance for medical provision for wilderness medicine. Extrem Physiol Med. 2015;4:22.

9

SEX & TRAVEL

Melanie Taylor, Ina Park

A natural human desire for novel experiences, coupled with the often-experienced loss of inhibition associated with being away from home, can lead some travelers to take greater than usual sexual behavioral risks (e.g., engaging in sex with new, unknown partners; having sex with multiple partners; connecting with sex networks) while abroad. Any of these behaviors can increase the traveler's risk for exposure to sexually transmitted infections (STIs), including HIV. Use of alcohol or drugs (which further decrease inhibition), or geosocial networking applications ("apps" which increase the efficiency of meeting sexual partners while abroad) can amplify a traveler's chances of having an at-risk exposure, in some cases substantially.

Clinicians have an opportunity to help patients reduce their risk of exposure to STIs through pretravel behavioral-prevention and risk-reduction counseling and medical care. Elements of the pretravel preparation include STI prevention guidance (e.g., advocating for the use of condoms or other barrier methods); STI screening, treatment, and vaccines; and a discussion about HIV pre- and postexposure prophylaxis. Consider providing preexposure prophylaxis (PrEP) to prevent HIV infection in travelers planning to have condomless sex. The pretravel consultation also gives clinicians a chance to review safety recommendations to prevent sexual assault during travel.

SEX WHILE TRAVELING

Sex while traveling encompasses the categories of casual consensual sex, sex tourism, sexual violence or assault, connection to sex trafficking, and sexual exploitation of children.

Casual Consensual Sex

Casual consensual sex during travel describes informal, non-transactional sexual encounters with other travelers or locals. Longer duration of travel, traveling alone or with friends, alcohol or drug use, younger age, and being single are factors associated with engaging in casual sex while traveling internationally. Other associations with casual sex are listed in Box 9-14. Two meta-analyses estimated that 20%–34% of male international travelers engage in casual sex abroad, and that 43%–49% of all travelers participating in casual sex abroad have condomless sex.

MEN WHO HAVE SEX WITH MEN

For men who have sex with men (MSM), conclusions from the literature regarding their sexual behavior when traveling are conflicting. Some studies examining MSM sexual behavior when traveling have concluded that this population is more likely to engage in condomless anal intercourse with partners of unknown HIV status; to have concurrent or multiple sex partners; or to have sex in conjunction with substance use while traveling. These can be particularly true if the reason for travel is to attend group sex events or gatherings (e.g., cruises, circuit parties). Other reports, however, indicate that MSM might adapt their behaviors when traveling to destinations perceived to have a higher risk for HIV. One study found that MSM who travel internationally were less likely to have condomless anal intercourse with partners abroad compared to partners encountered at home or during domestic travel.

Sex Tourism

Travel for the specific purpose of procuring sex is considered "sex tourism," and sex tourism destinations frequently are countries where commercial sex is legal. In some countries, sex tourism supports sex trafficking, among the largest and most lucrative criminal industries in the world. Sex tourists have traditionally been men from high-income countries who travel to low- and middle-income countries to pay for sex with local women, including commercial sex workers. Sex tourism among American and European women also has been described, particularly to the Caribbean.

Having condomless sex with commercial sex workers is associated with an increased risk for

BOX 9-14 Factors associated with higher frequency of casual or unprotected sex abroad

- Casual sex at home and during a previous travel experience
- Expectation of casual sex while abroad
- History of previous sexually transmitted infection
- Illicit drug use, alcohol abuse, tobacco use
- Long-term travel (expatriates, military, Peace Corps volunteers)
- Male
- Single
- Traveling without a partner (either alone or with friends)
- Younger age
- ≥2 sex partners in the last 2 years

9

STIs. Multidrug-resistant gonorrhea infections have been linked to encounters with sex workers. High rates of HIV are also frequently found among sex workers, with a systematic review describing a global prevalence of 11.8%. Among sex workers in Thailand, however, HIV rates of up to 44% have been described; in Kenya, the rate among sex workers has been reported to be even higher (up to 88%).

Sexual Violence & Assault

People of any age, gender, or sexual orientation can be victims of sexual violence during travel and should be aware of this risk. The risk for sexual assault is greater among young women traveling alone and in regions of high sexual violence prevalence (e.g., central and southern sub-Saharan Africa, Andean Latin America, Australasia). In addition, some studies have identified that young gay and bisexual males (MSM) traveling internationally might be victims of sexual violence more frequently than females or heterosexual males. Sexual violence can occur more often in association with international recreational travel, but it is also reported in travelers participating in humanitarian aid work. Alcohol and drug use have been shown to increase vulnerability for sexual assault. Unfamiliar cultural norms, environments, language barriers, and safety concerns might also increase the risk.

POST-SEXUAL ASSAULT MEDICAL CARE

Victims of sexual violence (particularly rape) should seek immediate medical attention. Health care sought after 72 hours could negate the benefits of postexposure prophylaxis for HIV and STIs, lower the effectiveness of emergency contraception, and reduce the value of any collected forensic evidence. Seeking medical care following a sexual assault can, however, be difficult in places where safety is a concern, where health care is not easily accessed, and where language and other barriers might not facilitate appropriate evaluation.

In addition to HIV and other STI postexposure prophylaxis, emergency contraception, and the forensic examination, medical attention after sexual assault should include treatment of injuries and provision of mental health and other supportive care. Adolescent-adapted services should be available and sought to address the related but different needs of youth who have been victims of sexual violence.

Sex Trafficking & Sexual Exploitation of Children

Although commercial sex work is legal in some parts of the world, sex trafficking, sex with a minor, and child pornography are always criminal activities according to US law, and travelers can be prosecuted in the United States even if they participated in such activities abroad. The Trafficking Victims Protection Act (www.state.gov/international-and-domestic-law) makes it illegal to recruit, entice, or obtain a person of any age to engage in commercial sex acts or to benefit from such activities.

SEX WITH MINORS

Federal law bars US residents traveling abroad from having sex with minors; this applies to all travelers, both adult and youth. Travel health providers should inform student travelers and other young people going abroad that according to US law, it is illegal for a US resident to have sex with a minor in another country. The legal age of consent varies around the world, from 11–21 years old. Some countries have no legal age of consent, with local laws forbidding all sexual relations outside of marriage.

CHILD PORNOGRAPHY

Regardless of the local age of consent, participation in child pornography anywhere in the world is illegal in the United States. US Code Title 18, Chapter 110, (www.law.cornell.edu/uscode/text/18/part-I/chapter-110) prohibits sex with minors, as well as the purchase, procurement, holding, or storage of material depicting such acts. These crimes are subject to prosecution with penalties of up to 30 years in prison. Victims of child pornography suffer multiple forms of abuse (emotional, physical, psychological, as well as sexual), poverty and homelessness, and health problems, including physical injury, STIs, other infections and illnesses, drug and alcohol addiction, and malnourishment.

SEXUAL EXPLOITATION OF CHILDREN

Sexual exploitation of children in travel and tourism affects all countries of the world regardless of income level. Offenders can include expatriates, humanitarian aid workers, international business travelers, military personnel, people attending large-scale sporting and cultural events, teachers, travelers and tourists, and volunteers. Financial vulnerabilities of families and communities resulting from the millions of travel and tourism jobs lost due to the coronavirus disease 2019 pandemic, the availability of cheap and accessible travel, and expanding access to information and communication technologies are expected to increase opportunities for child sexual exploitation.

COMBATTING SEXUAL EXPLOITATION OF CHILDREN

To combat sexual exploitation of children, some international hotels and other tourism services have voluntarily adopted a code of conduct that includes training their employees to recognize and report suspicious activities. Tourist establishments supporting this initiative to protect children from sex tourism are listed online (www.thecode.org). Providers and travelers who suspect child sexual exploitation occurring abroad can report tips anonymously by calling the Homeland Security Investigations Tip Line (toll-free at 866-347-2423), or by submitting information online to US Immigration and Customs Enforcement (www.ice.gov/tips) or the International Centre for Missing & Exploited Children (www.icmec.org).

In the United States, the National Center for Missing & Exploited Children's Cyber Tipline collects reports of child prostitution and other crimes against children (toll-free at 800-843-5678, https://report.cybertip.org).

PROTECT ACT

Since 2003, when Congress passed the federal PROTECT Act, US Immigrations and Customs Enforcement has arrested >11,000 offenders for child sex tourism and exploitation, including 1,100 outside of the United States. The PROTECT Act strengthens the US government's ability to prosecute and punish crimes related to sex tourism, including incarceration of ≤30 years for acts committed at home or abroad.

Cooperation of the host country is required to open an investigation of criminal activity, resulting in a much lower than hoped for conviction rate. In some places, the judicial system might be prone to bribery and corruption, or the government is otherwise willing to expand tourism and the money it brings at the expense of children being trafficked for sex. The US Department of State has published a list of 20 ways to fight human trafficking, including recommendations for youth and their parents, attorneys, health care providers, journalists, and other stakeholders (www.state.gov/j/tip/id/help).

SEXUALLY TRANSMITTED INFECTIONS

See Sec. 11, Ch. 10, Sexually Transmitted Infections, for details regarding the management of STIs in returned travelers.

Epidemiology

In 2019, the World Health Organization estimated that 376 million new infections with curable sexually transmitted pathogens (chlamydia, gonorrhea, trichomoniasis, and syphilis) occur annually. Globally, >500 million adults are estimated to be infected with a genital herpes virus; ≈40 million people are infected with HIV; and >300 million with human papillomavirus infections, the cause of cervical cancer. Over 30 infections are sexually transmitted, several of which are neither curable nor vaccine preventable.

The distribution of STI prevalence and STI resistance to available treatment varies, and some countries and regions have very high rates of STIs. International travelers having sex with new partners while abroad are exposed to different "sexual networks" than at home and can serve as a conduit for importing novel or antimicrobial-resistant STIs into parts of the world where they are unknown or rare. For example, gonorrhea (among the more common STIs globally with ≈78 million new cases in 2016) has become extensively drug resistant in some parts of the world. Multidrug-resistant gonorrhea infections have been associated with unprotected sex and commercial sex during travel. Patients presenting with antimicrobial-resistant gonococcal infections should prompt providers to inquire about their travel history and the travel history of their sex partners.

Prevention

STI incidence is increased ≤3-fold in people who experience casual sex while traveling internationally, a consequence of new sexual partnerships and unprotected intercourse. Condoms prevent both STIs and unwanted pregnancy. Preventive vaccines (which can be considered as part of pretravel care) are available for some infections transmitted through intercourse (e.g., hepatitis A, hepatitis B, human papillomavirus). HIV PrEP might be appropriate for travelers planning to engage in condomless sex during travel. Travelers should consider packing condoms from their home country to avoid the need to search for them in the countries visited during travel. Women carrying condoms in luggage might need to conceal these to avoid questions related to sexual activity or assumed behaviors.

MONKEYPOX

In May 2022, a multinational outbreak of monkeypox began; 3 months later (by the end of August) it involved people from >90 countries (www.cdc.gov/poxvirus/monkeypox/response/2022/world-map.html). During the outbreak, the causative agent, monkeypox virus (see Sec. 5, Part 2, Ch. 22, Smallpox & Other Orthopoxvirus-Associated Infections), spread person-to-person primarily through close (both sexual and non-sexual) skin-to-skin contact. Most cases occurred among gay, bisexual, and other men who have sex with men; international travel played a role in introducing the virus to new countries. Remind all travelers that sex with new partners can increase their risk of contracting infections, including monkeypox.

BIBLIOGRAPHY

End Child Prostitution and Trafficking (ECPAT). Summary paper on sexual exploitation of children in travel and tourism. Bangkok: ECPAT; 2020. Available from: www.ecpat.org/wp-content/uploads/2020/12/ECPAT-Summary-paper-on-Sexual-Exploitation-of-Children-in-Travel-and-Tourism-2020.pdf.

Kennedy KM, Flaherty GT. The risk of sexual assault and rape during international travel: implications for the practice of travel medicine. J Travel Med. 2015;22(4):282–4.

Lee VC, Sullivan PS, Baral SD. Global travel and HIV/STI epidemics among MSM: what does the future hold? Sex Health. 2017;14(1):51–8.

Lu TS, Holmes A, Noone C, Flaherty GT. Sun, sea and sex: a review of the sex tourism literature. Trop Dis Travel Med Vaccines. 2020;6(1):24.

Minhaj FS, Ogale YP, Whitehill F, Schultz J, Foote M, Davidson W, et al. Monkeypox Outbreak—Nine States, May 2022. MMWR Morb Mortal Wkly Rep. 2022;71(23):764–9.

Newman WJ, Holt BW, Rabun JS, Phillips G, Scott CL. Child sex tourism: extending the borders of sexual offender legislation. Int J Law Psychiatry. 2011;34(2):116–21.

Svensson P, Sundbeck M, Persson KI, Stafstrom M, Östergren P-O, Mannheimer L, et al. A meta-analysis and systematic literature review of factors associated with sexual risk-taking during international travel. Travel Med Infect Dis. 2018;24:65–88.

Truong HM, Fatch R, Grasso M, Robertson T, Tao L, Chen YH, et al. Gay and bisexual men engage in fewer risky sexual behaviors while traveling internationally: a cross sectional study in San Francisco. Sex Transm Infect. 2015;91(3):220–5.

US Department of Justice. Extraterritorial sexual exploitation of children. Available from: www.justice.gov/criminal-ceos/extraterritorial-sexual-exploitation-children.

Vivancos R, Abubakar I, Hunter PR. Foreign travel, casual sex, and sexually transmitted infections: systematic review and meta-analysis. Int J Infect Dis. 2010;14(10):e842–51.

World Health Organization. Health care for women subjected to intimate partner violence or sexual violence. Available from: www.who.int/reproductivehealth/publications/violence/vaw-clinical-handbook/en.

10 Popular Itineraries

THE RATIONALE FOR POPULAR ITINERARIES

In this section of the CDC Yellow Book, experts who have lived in or frequently visited destinations share their insider's knowledge of those places. Each chapter is intended to help travel health providers feel more comfortable giving advice about destinations they might never have visited. Editorial decisions about which popular itineraries to include are guided by a variety of factors, including volume of US travel and uniqueness of health risks.

CDC Yellow Book 2024. Jeffrey Nemhauser, Oxford University Press. © Oxford University Press 2023.
DOI: 10.1093/oso/9780197570944.003.0010

PART 1: AFRICA & THE MIDDLE EAST

AFRICAN SAFARIS

Kate Varela, Juliet Kasule, Joseph Ojwang, Aimee Geissler, Karl Neumann

DESTINATION OVERVIEW

Arguably the ultimate in adventure travel, an African safari is the experience of a lifetime. Safari-goers have options to view wildlife from different vantages: on land (traditional savannah guided car safaris, open trucks, air-conditioned vans, personal vehicles), on the water (in a dugout canoe), or from the air (private aircraft, hot air balloon). Hiking with trained, licensed guides in well-scouted settings offers another opportunity to see wildlife up close; treks to view chimpanzees or gorillas, for example, are highly popular.

With >150 game parks and reserves across the continent, individual travelers, families, backpackers, and people with similar interests (e.g., serious photographers) have a range of choices and budget options. Some parks are remote and rustic, with long drives to see the animals but with fewer tourists. Other parks are easily accessible with self-drive options. Many safaris accept young children and adolescent participants; gorilla trekking and other more strenuous activities require participants to be ≥15 years of age.

Map 10-01 and Map 10-02 show several major African game parks. In East Africa, the Maasai Mara National Reserve in Kenya is the northern extension of Tanzania's Serengeti National Park game reserve. Together these 2 parks are home to the complete collection of the so-called big 5—Cape buffalo, elephants, leopards, lions, and rhinoceros—the large wild animals for which Africa is most famous. Other East African game parks that offer exceptional wildlife viewing include Tsavo National Park (Kenya); Akagera National Park (Rwanda); Ngorongoro Crater (Tanzania); and Ngamba Island Chimpanzee Sanctuary, Murchison Falls National Park, Queen Elizabeth National Park, and Ziwa Rhino Sanctuary (Uganda). Travelers can trek to see gorillas at the Virunga National Park (Democratic Republic of the Congo), Volcanoes National Park (Rwanda), and Bwindi Impenetrable National Park (Uganda); "impenetrable" refers to the challenging hiking required in this park.

Game park destinations in Southern Africa include Moremi Game Reserve, Chobe National Park, and Kalahari Desert (Botswana); Etosha National Park (Namibia); Kruger National Park (South Africa); Lower Zambezi National Park and South Luangwa National Park (Zambia); and the Hwange National Park (Zimbabwe). Pendjari National Park in Benin, home to West African lions and elephants, is a major part of the largest intact ecosystem in West Africa, the transnational W-Arly-Pendjari (WAP) complex, which spans Benin, Burkina Faso, and Niger. Mole National Park (Ghana) boasts >93 mammal species, including elephants and hippos.

Although the centerpiece of safari-going remains viewing majestic animals in their natural habitat, many tour operators now also offer programs on local culture and history, ecosystems, and geology. Conservation-based tours promoting responsible tourism give travelers an

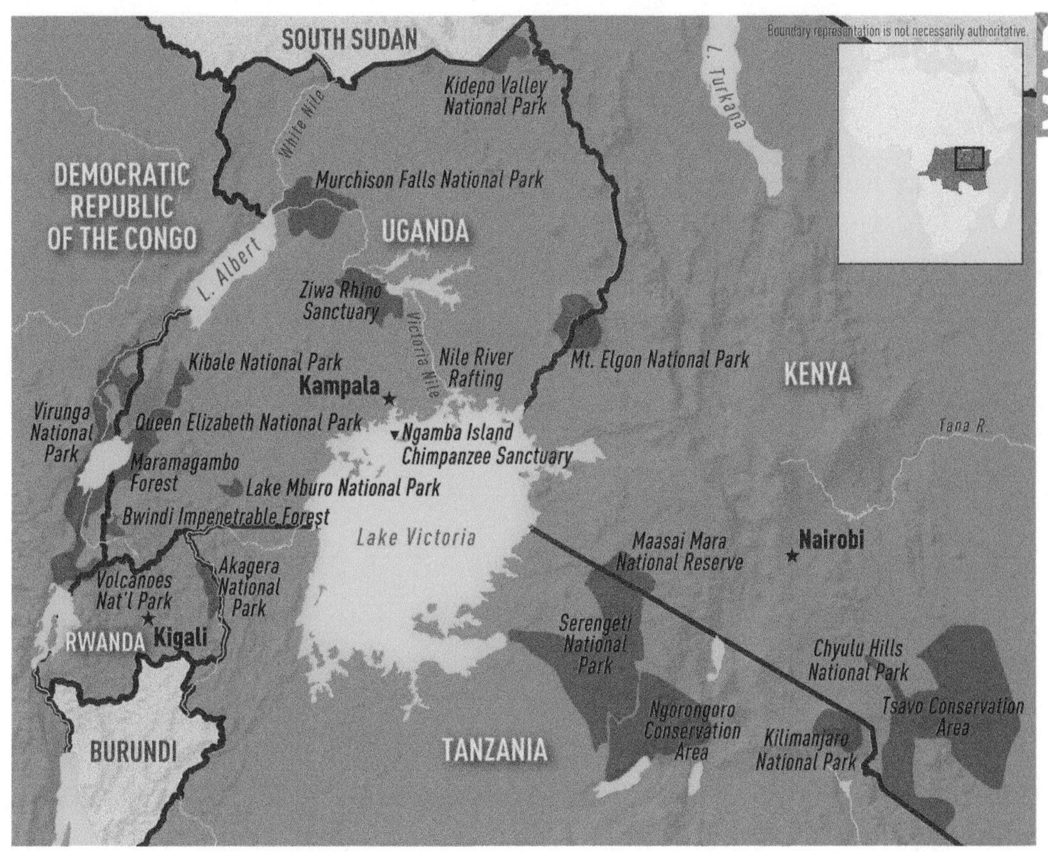

MAP 10-01 African game parks & reserves (North)

opportunity to help safeguard wildlife, protect vital habitat, and benefit local people.

INFECTIOUS DISEASE RISKS

Health, safety, and comfort issues that safari-goers are likely to encounter are mostly predictable and largely avoidable. A pretravel consultation with a travel health care provider is essential. Multiple vaccinations might be required for healthy safari travel. Provide advice specific to each traveler's itinerary, country, and game park. Because vaccines take time to become effective, advise travelers to seek vaccination as early as possible prior to planned departure. For people trekking to see gorillas, certain vaccines are recommended to protect both travelers and animals, including coronavirus disease 2019 (COVID-19), diphtheria-tetanus-pertussis, hepatitis A and hepatitis B, influenza, measles-mumps-rubella, polio, and yellow fever.

Enteric Infections & Diseases

HEPATITIS A

Hepatitis A virus is transmitted through ingestion of contaminated food or water or through direct contact with an infectious person. Hepatitis A is among the most common vaccine-preventable infections acquired during travel. Risk is greatest for people who live or visit rural areas, trek in backcountry areas, or frequently eat or drink in settings of poor sanitation. Vaccination is recommended for travelers to sub-Saharan Africa, including safari-goers (see Sec. 5, Part 2, Ch. 7, Hepatitis A).

TRAVELERS' DIARRHEA

Travelers' diarrhea (TD) is the most predictable travel-related illness and is common on safaris. Prepare travelers by explaining the risks for TD and how best to prevent it through appropriate hand hygiene and careful selection of

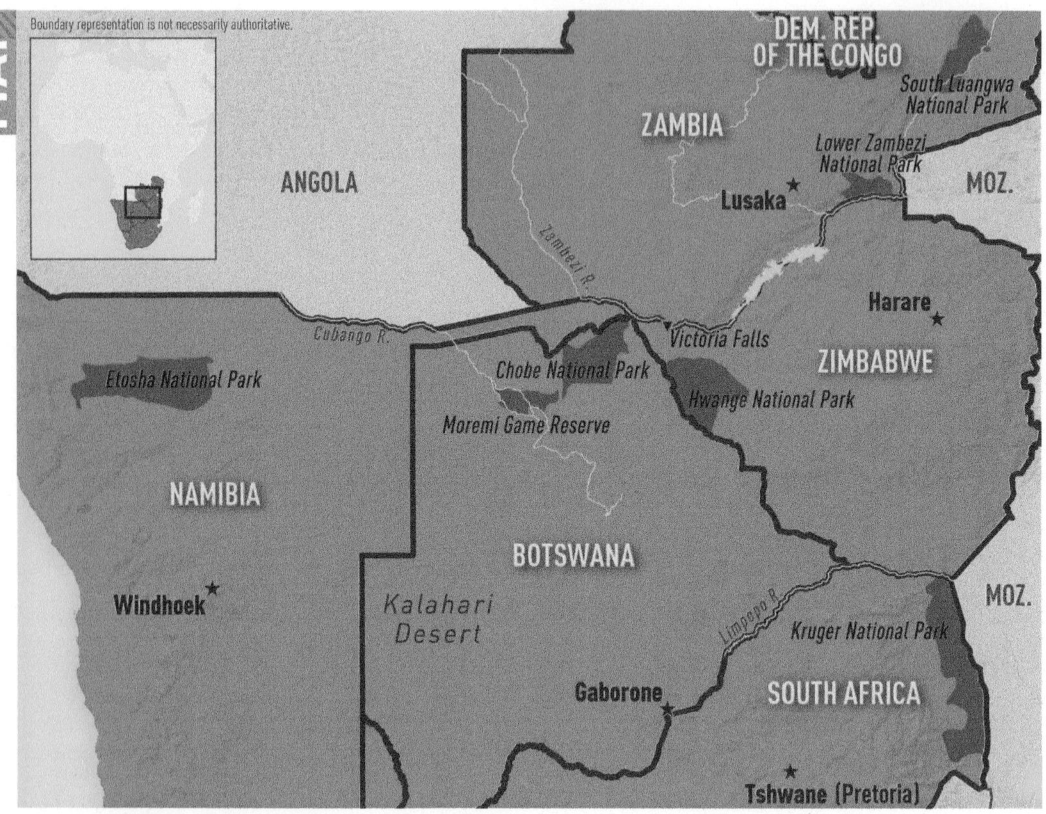

MAP 10-02 African game parks & reserves (South)

foods and beverages (see Sec. 2, Ch. 6, Travelers' Diarrhea). Infectious causes of TD include bacteria (e.g., *Campylobacter jejuni*, *Escherichia coli*, *Salmonella* spp., *Shigella* spp.), viruses (e.g., norovirus, rotavirus), and protozoa (e.g., *Cryptosporidium*, *Giardia*).

Most TD cases are mild and self-limiting. Advise travelers to carry antimotility medicine for symptomatic relief of mild TD. Consider prescribing antibiotic therapy to treat moderate to severe TD and providing travelers with clear written guidance about TD prevention and step-by-step instructions about how and when to use medications. Travelers should carry any medications with them on safari, because access to authentic drugs is not guaranteed in remote locations (see Sec. 6, Ch. 3, . . . *perspectives*: Avoiding Poorly Regulated Medicines & Medical Products During Travel). Travelers should consult a physician for moderate, severe, or persistent TD.

No vaccines are available for most pathogens that cause TD. Cholera vaccine is not needed for safari-goers unless they are planning a side trip to work in a refugee camp or do humanitarian aid work in an affected country. Advise travelers to carry alcohol-based hand sanitizer with ≥60% alcohol for use when water and soap are scarce or unsafe, or conditions are generally unhygienic. Travelers should avoid drinking tap water while on safari and only consume adequately disinfected (e.g., commercially bottled) water from an unopened, factory-sealed container (see Sec. 2, Ch. 8, Food & Water Precautions).

TYPHOID FEVER

Typhoid fever is a bacterial disease caused by *Salmonella typhi* (see Sec. 5, Part 1, Ch. 24, Typhoid & Paratyphoid Fever). Typhoid fever vaccine generally is recommended for safari-goers. Because vaccination does not confer 100% protection, however, even vaccinated travelers should avoid consumption of potentially contaminated food and water.

Respiratory Infections & Diseases

Respiratory illnesses (e.g., COVID-19, influenza, tuberculosis [TB]) can spread between people and from people to the wildlife they encounter.

CORONAVIRUS DISEASE 2019

In zoos and animal sanctuaries, big cats (cougars, lions, pumas, tigers, snow leopards) and mountain gorillas have tested positive for severe acute respiratory syndrome coronavirus 2 (SARS-CoV-2), the virus that causes COVID-19. Special operating procedures are in now place to protect wildlife and travelers; these include mandatory COVID-19 testing, limited group capacity, and required mask use to enter Volcanoes National Park and other gorilla parks; several game parks, including Kruger National Park in South Africa, also require entrants to provide a negative COVID-19 test result before permitting entry. Travelers should check with tour operators and park websites ahead of travel for up-to-date requirements, and follow park requirements to help keep both wildlife and people safe and healthy.

Advise travelers to closely adhere to all international travel guidance for COVID-19 testing, vaccination, and quarantine, including countries transited through and upon return to the United States (www.cdc.gov/coronavirus/2019-ncov/travelers/international-travel/index.html). For current information on COVID-19 at their destination(s), travelers to Africa should consult the US Embassy website (https://travel.state.gov/content/travel/en/traveladvisories/COVID-19-Country-Specific-Information.html). For the US government's COVID-19 international travel requirements and recommendations, see www.cdc.gov/coronavirus/2019-ncov/travelers/international-travel/index.html. All travelers going to Africa should be up to date with their COVID-19 vaccines (www.cdc.gov/coronavirus/2019-ncov/vaccines/stay-up-to-date.html).

INFLUENZA & TUBERCULOSIS

While on safari, when trekking, or when visiting local communities, travelers can potentially encounter livestock species susceptible to influenza (e.g., chickens, pigs, waterfowl) and TB (e.g., cows).

Chimpanzees, gorillas, and other wildlife also are susceptible to influenza virus and *Mycobacterium tuberculosis* infection. Responsible tourism requires ill people to refrain from wildlife trekking or other activities that involve close contact with wildlife.

Soil- & Waterborne Infections

SCHISTOSOMIASIS

Freshwater lakes, ponds, and rivers all pose a risk for exposure to *Schistosoma* species, a parasite found in freshwater snails (see Sec. 5, Part 3, Ch. 20, Schistosomiasis). Travelers should consider all freshwater sources to be contaminated and avoid bathing, swimming, wading, or other freshwater contact in disease-endemic countries. River trips (e.g., Nile River white-water rafting) present a risk for schistosomiasis (bilharzia). Swimming in the ocean or well-chlorinated pools is not a risk for schistosomiasis.

Vectorborne Diseases

Travelers should take steps to avoid arthropod bites to reduce their risk for vectorborne infections (for detailed recommendations, see Sec. 4, Ch. 6, Mosquitoes, Ticks & Other Arthropods).

CHIKUNGUNYA, DENGUE, ZIKA

Chikungunya, dengue, and Zika are arboviruses transmitted by *Aedes* species mosquitoes in game parks throughout Africa (for details on each of these diseases, see the relevant chapters in Section 5). *Aedes* mosquitoes are aggressive daytime biters, but also bite at night.

MALARIA

Malaria is endemic in sub-Saharan Africa, and transmission occurs in most game parks. Most infections are caused by *Plasmodium falciparum.* All *P. falciparum* in sub-Saharan Africa is considered chloroquine-resistant. Safari activities often include sleeping in tents and observing animals at dusk or after dark, sometimes near water holes, all of which increase the risk for exposure to malaria-carrying *Anopheles* mosquitoes. Appropriate malaria chemoprophylaxis and personal protection—wearing long-sleeved shirts and pants, using insect repellents, and sleeping under permethrin-impregnated mosquito netting—are essential (see Sec. 2, Ch. 5, Yellow Fever Vaccine & Malaria Prevention Information, by Country, and Sec. 5, Part 3, Ch. 16, Malaria).

RICKETTSIAL DISEASES

African tick-bite fever (ATBF) is endemic to much of sub-Saharan Africa; among returning travelers, it is the most commonly diagnosed rickettsial disease (see Sec. 5, Part 1, Ch. 18, Rickettsial Diseases). Travel-associated cases of ATBF often occur in clusters of people exposed while participating in common activities (e.g., bush hiking, game hunting, safari tours). Travelers can protect themselves from infection by taking precautions to prevent tick bites.

TRYPANOSOMIASIS

Day-biting tsetse flies (*Glossina* species) transmit African trypanosomiasis (sleeping sickness), a disease only rarely seen in travelers (see Sec. 5, Part 3, Ch. 24, African Trypanosomiasis). Several reports document trypanosomiasis in travelers returning from visits to national parks or game reserves, including Kenya's Maasai Mara National Reserve. Advise travelers that neutral-colored clothing seems to deter the flies, and that permethrin-impregnated clothing and insect repellant can reduce fly bites.

WEST NILE

West Nile virus is an arbovirus transmitted by *Culex* species mosquitoes that are typically more active at dusk and dawn.

10

YELLOW FEVER

Travelers going on an African safari should consult a travel medicine professional for the very latest information regarding yellow fever at their destination. Currently, the World Health Organization and the Centers for Disease Control and Prevention recommend yellow fever vaccination for much of sub-Saharan Africa (see Sec. 2, Ch. 5, Yellow Fever Vaccine & Malaria Prevention Information, by Country, and Sec. 5, Part 2, Ch. 26, Yellow Fever).

Some countries require proof of yellow fever vaccination in the form of a valid International Certificate of Vaccination or Prophylaxis (ICVP), also known as the yellow card, as a condition of entry. Moreover, some safaris cross international borders to include ≥1 country. Assist travelers by checking the requirements for each country on their itinerary, including countries they only transit through on the way to their destination.

Viral Hemorrhagic Fevers

Crimean-Congo hemorrhagic fever (CCHF), Ebola virus disease (EVD), Lassa fever, Marburg virus disease (MVD), and Rift Valley fever (RVF) are viral hemorrhagic fevers (VHFs) found in and around some game parks in sub-Saharan Africa. Although travelers are rarely affected, zoonotic exposure to VHFs can occur through direct contact with wildlife (e.g., bats, nonhuman primates, rodents), insect (e.g., mosquito) or tick bites, and contact with blood or body fluid of livestock (see Sec. 5, Part 2, Ch. 25, Viral Hemorrhagic Fevers).

Travelers who touch or come into proximity of bats (e.g., spelunking, visiting bat caves) are at greatest risk for Ebola virus or Marburg virus exposure. Four confirmed cases of MVD occurred in travelers visiting Kitum Cave in Kenya and Python Cave in Maramagambo Forest, Uganda. Caution travelers against visiting locations where VHF outbreaks are occurring, to avoid contact with bats and rodents, and to avoid blood or body fluids of livestock or animal carcasses.

ENVIRONMENTAL HAZARDS & RISKS

Animal Bites & Wildlife-Related Injuries

Wild animals are unpredictable. Travelers should follow verbal and written instructions provided by safari operators and guides and should take extra precautions if camping or traveling without a guide in a national park. Wildlife-related injuries usually occur when travelers disregard rules (e.g., when they approach animals too closely to feed or photograph them). People should never try to feed, handle, or pet unfamiliar animals, whether domestic or wild. If bitten or scratched by a monkey, travelers should be evaluated for B virus postexposure prophylaxis (see Sec. 5, Part 2, Ch. 1, B Virus).

Rabies exists throughout Africa; dogs and bats are the primary animal reservoirs (see Sec. 5, Part 2, Ch. 18, Rabies). The estimated rate of rabies exposures in travelers ranges from 16–200 per 100,000 travelers globally. Warn travelers not to enter caves where bats roost and shelter. Advise travelers to consult a physician for rabies post-exposure prophylaxis in case of animal bites or scratches or suspected bat exposures (e.g., sleeping in a cabin or tent where bats are found).

Consider preexposure prophylaxis for people whose planned activities will increase their chances of direct animal encounters (e.g., adventure travelers, animal sanctuary visitors, campers, cave explorers [spelunkers], participants in veterinary care or wildlife management programs). Additional considerations for preexposure prophylaxis might include whether rabies immunoglobulin (RIG) and rabies vaccination are available in the visited country in case of exposure (see www.cdc.gov/rabies/resources/countries-risk.html).

Climate & Sun Exposure

Some parks are located at higher elevations and closer to the equator, making proper sun precautions imperative for avoiding sunburn, heat exhaustion, heat stroke, and dehydration. Advise travelers to seek shade, when possible, to avoid the sun during midday hours, and to carry water. In addition, advise travelers to wear sunglasses, protective clothing, and hats, and to use a broad-spectrum (protects against both ultraviolet A and ultraviolet B) sunscreen, SPF ≥15. Recommend travelers bring sunscreen and sunburn remedies with them, because selection can be limited and expensive once in country (see Sec. 4, Ch. 1, Sun Exposure).

Natural Disasters

Natural disasters (e.g., earthquakes, flooding, landslides, volcanic eruptions) have all occurred and affected international travelers in recent years. During the rainy season, floods and landslides can be more common. Safari-goers should expect sudden road closures, plan alternative routes, and take precautions during storms. Dust storms might occur during the dry season. Poor air quality can exacerbate asthma or other lung diseases. Encourage all travelers to enroll in the US Department of State's Smart Traveler Enrollment Program (https://step.state.gov/step) to receive up-to-date information in the event of a disaster.

SAFETY & SECURITY

Crime

Within the game parks, crime is unusual; robberies and car-jackings are more common in urban areas (see Sec. 4, Ch. 11, Safety & Security Overseas). Travelers should check with the US Department of State's Bureau of Consular Affairs (http://travel.state.gov/travelsafely) ahead of travel to learn more about safety and security risks before traveling.

Traffic-Related Injuries

In sub-Saharan African countries, the rates of fatal motor vehicle crashes are among the highest in the world. Travelers should fasten seat belts when riding in motor vehicles, and wear a helmet when riding bicycles or motorbikes (see Sec. 8, Ch. 5, Road & Traffic Safety). Within game parks, serious motor vehicle crashes are rare because poor road conditions generally discourage speeding. Travel in rural areas between parks is high risk, however, especially after dark. If possible, travelers should avoid nighttime driving in sub-Saharan Africa, and pedestrians should take extra care to watch for speeding vehicles. Travelers should avoid boarding overcrowded buses, and avoid driving or riding on motorcycles and motorbikes.

AVAILABILITY & QUALITY OF MEDICAL CARE

Travelers should work with their primary care provider to ensure any underlying illnesses are managed before travel. Before leaving the United States, each traveler also should be certain they have international health insurance coverage; and because surgical support or other advanced health care might not be available in the destination country, encourage travelers to purchase an additional medical evacuation insurance policy (see Sec. 6, Ch. 1, Travel Insurance, Travel Health Insurance & Medical Evacuation Insurance, and Sec. 6, Ch. 2, Obtaining Health Care Abroad).

Recommend travelers carry a personal medical kit with sufficient medication to treat allergies, chronic conditions, routine health needs, and emergencies (see Sec. 2, Ch. 10, Travel Health Kits). Warn travelers with food allergies that food labels might not reliably indicate potential allergens, and that lack of emergency services and language barriers can compound the risk for any severe allergic reaction that requires emergency medical care (see Sec. 3, Ch. 4, Highly Allergic Travelers). Prescribe an epinephrine autoinjector for highly allergic travelers. Options for feminine hygiene products can be limited on safari—advise travelers to pack an adequate supply.

Symptoms of many diseases acquired in Africa can surface weeks and occasionally months after exposure, sometimes long after the traveler has returned home. Obtain a travel history from all patients presenting for care.

BIBLIOGRAPHY

Angelo KM, Libman M, Caumes E, Hamer DH, Kain KC, Leder K, et al. Malaria after international travel: a GeoSentinel analysis, 2003–2016. Malar J. 2017;16(1):293.

Clerinx J, Van Gompel A. Schistosomiasis in travellers and migrants. Travel Med Infect Dis. 2011;9(1):6–24.

Cornel AJ, Lee Y, Almeida A, Johnson T, Mouatcho J, Ventner M, et al. Mosquito community composition in South Africa and some neighboring countries. Parasit Vectors. 2018;11(1):331.

Jensenius M, Fournier P, Kelly P, Myrvang B, Racoult D. African tick bite fever. Lancet Infect Dis. 2003;3(9):557–64.

Kading RC, Borland EM, Cranfield M, Powers AM. Prevalence of antibodies to alphaviruses and flaviviruses in free-ranging game animals and nonhuman primates in the greater Congo Basin. J Wildl Dis. 2013;49(3):587–99.

Lankau EW, Montgomery JM, Tack DM, Obonyo M, Kadivane S, Blanton JD, et al. Exposure of US travelers to rabid zebra, Kenya, 2011. Emerg Infect Dis. 2012;18(7):1202–4.

Macfie EJ, Williamson EA. Best practice guidelines for great ape tourism. Gland, Switzerland: International Union for Conservation of Nature and Natural Resources, Species Survival Commissioner Primate Specialist Group (PSG); 2010. Available from: https://portals.iucn.org/library/sites/library/files/documents/ssc-op-038.pdf.

Makhulu EE, Villinger J, Adunga VO, Jeneby MM, Kimathi EM, Mararo E, et al. Tsetse blood-meal sources, endosymbionts and trypanosome-associations in the Maasai Mara National Reserve, a wildlife-human-livestock interface. PLoS Negl Trop Dis. 2021;15(1):e0008267.

Morgan OW, Brunette G, Kapella BK, McAuliffe I, Katongole-Mbidde E, Li W, et al. Schistosomiasis among recreational users of upper Nile River, Uganda, 2007. Emerg Infect Dis. 2010;(16)5:866–8.

World Health Organization. Vaccines and vaccination against yellow fever. WHO position paper—June 2013. Wkly Epidemiol Rec. 2013;88(27):269–83.

SAUDI ARABIA: HAJJ & UMRAH PILGRIMAGES

Salim Parker, Joanna Gaines

DESTINATION OVERVIEW

Hajj and Umrah are religious pilgrimages to Mecca, Saudi Arabia. Islamic religious doctrine dictates that every able-bodied adult Muslim who can afford to do so is obligated to make Hajj at least once in their lifetime. Hajj takes place from the 8th through the 12th day of the last month of the Islamic year (Dhul Hijjah). The timing of Hajj is based on the Islamic lunar calendar; its dates shift relative to the Gregorian calendar, occurring ≈11 days earlier each successive year. In 2021, for example, Hajj took place from July 17–22, but in 2022, Hajj occurred from July 7–12. Muslims can perform Umrah, the "minor pilgrimage," any time of the year; unlike Hajj, Umrah is not compulsory.

Normally, ≈2–3 million Muslims from >183 countries perform Hajj each year, and the Kingdom of Saudi Arabia (KSA) continues its efforts to allow an even greater number of pilgrims (hajjis) attend. In a typical year, >11,000 pilgrims travel from the United States. Due to the coronavirus disease 2019 (COVID-19) pandemic, however, only 1,000 pilgrims received permission to perform Hajj in 2020. In 2021, 60,000 were allowed, and in 2022, 1 million pilgrims made the pilgrimage. In both 2020 and 2021, because no cross-border entry into the country was permitted, KSA limited Hajj pilgrims to residents of Saudi Arabia.

PERFORMING THE PILGRIMAGE

Most international pilgrims fly into Jeddah or Medina and take a bus to Mecca. Although the actual pilgrimage lasts only 5 days, most foreign pilgrims visit Saudi Arabia for 2–7 weeks.

Day 1

On the first day of Hajj (8th day of Dhul Hijjah), hajjis travel by foot or by bus ≈5.5 miles (9 km) to Mina, the largest temporary city in the world, where most stay in air-conditioned tents.

Day 2

At dawn on the 9th day of Dhul Hijjah, hajjis begin an ≈7.75-mile (12.5-km) trip by foot, shuttle bus, or train to the Plain of Arafat (Map 10-03 [all distances shown are approximate]). During the summer months, daytime temperatures can reach 122°F (50°C). The walking route features mist sprinklers, but the risk for heat-related illnesses is high, and ambulances and medical stations are positioned along the way to provide medical assistance.

Hajj climaxes on the Plain of Arafat, a few miles east of Mecca. Pilgrims spend the day in supplication, praying and reading the Quran. Being on Arafat on the 9th of Dhul Hijjah, even for only a few moments, is an absolute rite of Hajj. Any hajji who fails to reach the Plain of Arafat on that day must repeat their pilgrimage. After sunset, pilgrims begin the ≈6.5-mile (10.5-km) journey to Muzdalifah, where most sleep in the open air. Potential health threats in Muzdalifah include breathing the thick dust and inadequate or overcrowded washing and sanitation facilities.

Day 3

At sunrise on the 10th day of Dhul Hijjah, pilgrims collect small pebbles to carry to Jamaraat, the site of multiple deadly crowd crush disasters. At Jamaraat, hajjis throw 7 tiny pebbles at the largest of 3 white pillars—the stoning of the effigy of the Devil. Afterwards, pilgrims traditionally sacrifice an animal. Some purchase vouchers to have licensed abattoirs perform this ritual on their behalf, thereby limiting potential exposure to zoonotic diseases. Other pilgrims visit farms where they sacrifice an animal themselves or have it done by an appointed representative.

Day 4

The next morning, on the 11th day of Dhul Hijjah, hajjis go to the Grand Mosque, which houses the Ka'aba ("The Cube"), and which Muslims consider the house of God. Pilgrims perform *tawaf*, 7 complete counterclockwise circuits around the Ka'aba. Because each floor of the 3-level mosque can hold 750,000 people, performing *tawaf* can take hours. In addition to *tawaf*, pilgrims have the option of performing *sa'i*, walking (sometimes running) 7 times between the hills of Safa and Marwah, then drinking water from the Well of Zamzam. Hajjis can travel between Safa and Marwah via air-conditioned tunnels, which have separate sections for walkers and disabled pilgrims. At the end of the day, pilgrims return to Mina (via Jamaraat) pelting all 3 pillars with pebbles.

Day 5

The next day, the 12th day of Dhul Hijjah, pilgrims pelt all 3 pillars in Mina with pebbles again and then, after performing a final *tawaf*, some leave Mecca, ending their Hajj. Other pilgrims stay an additional night, pelt the 3 pillars with pebbles once more the next day, perform their final *tawaf*, and end the pilgrimage. Although not required, some hajjis include a trip to Medina, where they visit the Mosque of the Prophet, home to the tomb of Mohammed.

INFECTIOUS DISEASE RISKS

KSA can elect to restrict the entry of travelers coming from countries experiencing infectious disease outbreaks. In 2012, for example, KSA did not permit anyone from Uganda to attend Hajj

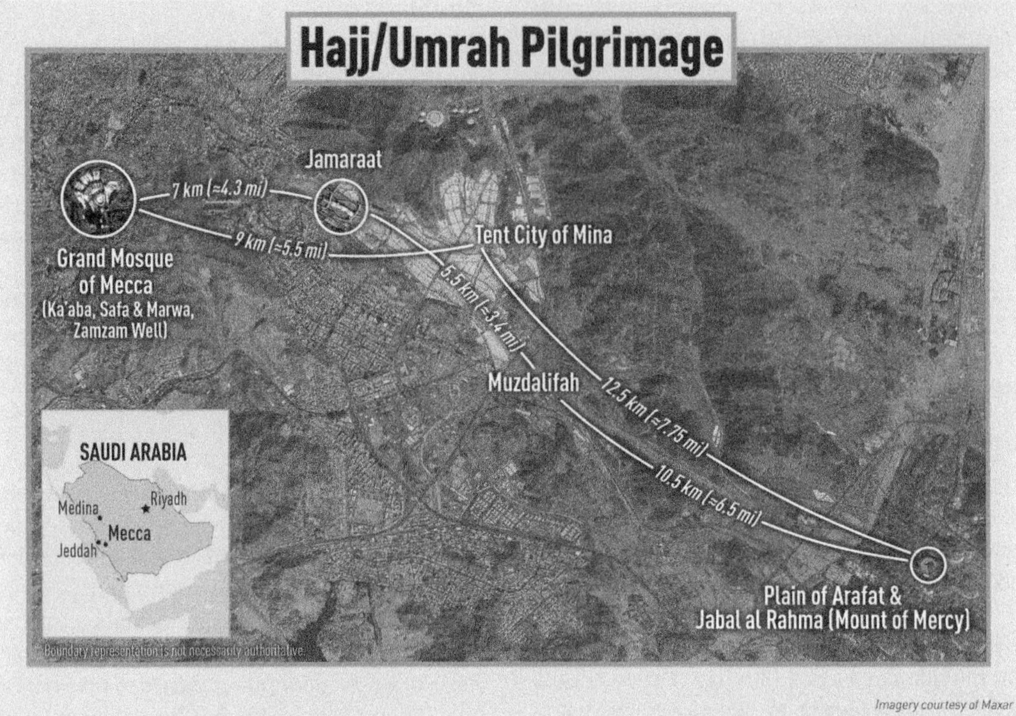

MAP 10-03 Hajj / Umrah pilgrimage

due to an Ebola outbreak in that country; the same restriction applied to Guinea, Liberia, and Sierra Leone in 2014 and 2015.

Required Vaccines

Current Hajj vaccination requirements are available from the Embassy of the Kingdom of Saudi Arabia in the United States (www.saudiembassy.net/hajj-and-umrah-health-requirements). As part of the Hajj and Umrah visa application process, KSA requires proof of vaccination against COVID-19 and meningococcal disease (for all pilgrims), polio (for pilgrims coming from countries where the disease is reported), and yellow fever (for all pilgrims arriving from yellow fever–endemic countries).

CORONAVIRUS DISEASE 2019

In 2020 and 2021, KSA only permitted Saudi residents <65 years old to apply for pilgrimage permits. In 2022, the Saudi government reopened Hajj to pilgrims (<65 years old) from countries outside KSA. Priority was granted to those who had not previously performed the pilgrimage. For the 2020 Hajj, because COVID-19 vaccines were not yet available, KSA required Hajj pilgrims to have a negative PCR test. In 2021 and 2022, hajjis also had to provide proof of immunization with an approved COVID-19 vaccine. The Kingdom recognizes vaccines produced by Johnson & Johnson, Moderna, Oxford/Astra Zeneca, and Pfizer/BioNTech.

For current information on COVID-19 in Saudi Arabia, consult the US Embassy & Consulates in Saudi Arabia website (https://sa.usembassy.gov/). For the US government's COVID-19 international travel requirements and recommendations, see www.cdc.gov/coronavirus/2019-ncov/travelers/international-travel/index.html. All travelers going to Saudi Arabia should be up to date with their COVID-19 vaccines (www.cdc.gov/coronavirus/2019-ncov/vaccines/stay-up-to-date.html).

MENINGOCOCCAL

The Hajj has been associated with meningococcal outbreaks. In 1987, serogroup A was responsible for an outbreak and carriage by returning pilgrims to certain countries that resulted in disease among local contacts. Serogroup W was responsible for similar occurrences in 2000 and 2001.

KSA requires all pilgrims to submit a certificate of vaccination with the quadrivalent (ACYW135) vaccine against meningitis, issued no more than 3 years and no less than 10 days before arrival in Saudi Arabia. The conjugate vaccine is preferred because it is associated with reduced carriage, unlike the polysaccharide vaccine.

The KSA Ministry of Health currently advises people who are pregnant and children not to travel to the Hajj; if these groups choose to travel, however, they should receive meningococcal vaccination according to licensed indications for their age. For more details on meningococcal disease and its prevention, see Sec. 5, Part 1, Ch. 13, Meningococcal Disease.

POLIO

Although KSA's requirement for polio vaccine does not apply to adult pilgrims from the United States, ensuring full vaccination before travel is best. All pilgrims traveling from countries where polio is reported are required to show proof of vaccination ≤6 weeks prior to departure. KSA also administers a single dose of the oral polio vaccine to pilgrims coming from countries where polio has been reported, this in addition to any polio vaccine the hajji might have received in their country of origin. About 500,000 doses of polio vaccine are given at ports of entry, representing >90% of eligible pilgrims.

Bloodborne Pathogens

After completing Hajj, men shave their heads. KSA limits barber licenses and requires barbers to use only disposable, single-use blades, to limit transmission of bloodborne pathogens between customers. Remind male travelers to patronize only officially licensed barbers whose establishments are clearly marked. The Centers for Disease Control and Prevention (CDC) recommends all travelers to KSA, particularly health care workers or other caretakers participating in Hajj, be up to date with routine immunizations, including hepatitis B vaccine.

Enteric Infections & Diseases

Diarrheal disease is common during Hajj. During the pretravel consultation, inform travelers about prevention, oral rehydration strategies, proper use of antimotility agents, and self-treatment of travelers' diarrhea (TD) with antibiotics. Most TD in hajjis is bacterial (≤83%), with smaller proportions caused by viruses and parasites. More information on TD can be found in Sec. 2, Ch. 6, Travelers' Diarrhea.

The World Health Organization recommends that travelers visiting farms, or other areas where animals are present, practice general hygiene measures, including avoiding contact with sick animals and regular handwashing before and after touching animals. Travelers should avoid consuming raw or undercooked animal products, including milk and meat.

Respiratory Infections & Diseases

Respiratory tract infections are common during Hajj, and pneumonia is among the most common causes of hospital admission. The risk for respiratory infections underscores the need to follow recommendations from the Advisory Committee on Immunization Practices for pneumococcal conjugate and polysaccharide vaccines for pilgrims aged ≥65 years and for younger travelers with comorbidities.

Although not a requirement, the CDC strongly recommends that hajjis be fully vaccinated against seasonal influenza. Behavioral interventions, including regular handwashing with soap and water, properly wearing a facemask, cough etiquette, and, if possible, physical distancing and contact avoidance, can help mitigate the risk for respiratory illnesses among pilgrims. Assess travelers for respiratory fitness, administer necessary vaccines, and prescribe adequate supplies of portable respiratory medications (inhalers are easier to transport than nebulizers) as needed.

Crowded conditions, even outdoors (densities can reach 9 pilgrims per square meter), can increase the probability of respiratory disease transmission during Hajj, including COVID-19 and Middle East respiratory syndrome (MERS). At the time of writing, no Hajj-associated cases of COVID-19 or MERS have been reported. Many pilgrims come from areas highly endemic for tuberculosis (TB); some arrive for Hajj with active pulmonary disease. Educate pilgrims about the risk for TB, and instruct them to follow up with their doctor if they develop symptoms of active TB.

MIDDLE EAST RESPIRATORY SYNDROME

MERS, caused by the Middle East respiratory syndrome coronavirus (MERS-CoV), was identified in Saudi Arabia in 2012 (see Sec. 5, Part 2, Ch. 14, Middle East Respiratory Syndrome / MERS). Domestic cases in and around the Arabian Peninsula and exported cases, including in the United States, have ranged from mild to severe; ≈35% of reported cases have been fatal. Close contact with someone who has confirmed MERS-CoV infection, exposure to camels, and consuming raw or undercooked camel products (e.g., milk, urine, meat) are all considered risk factors for human infection with MERS-CoV.

Skin Infections

Chafing caused by long periods of standing and walking in the heat can lead to bacterial or fungal skin infections. Advise travelers to keep their skin dry, use talcum powder, and to be aware of any pain or irritation caused by garments. Travelers should disinfect open sores and blisters and keep them covered. As a sign of respect, pilgrims enter the Grand Mosque with the tops of their feet uncovered; while most hajjis perform *tawaf* in their bare feet, encourage travelers with diabetes to wear appropriate, protective footwear.

10

Vectorborne Diseases

Aedes mosquitoes, vectors for dengue, and *Anopheles* mosquitoes, vectors for malaria, are present in Saudi Arabia. Travelers should follow mosquito bite prevention measures outlined in Sec. 4, Ch. 6, Mosquitoes, Ticks & Other Arthropods. Dengue has been documented in Mecca and Jeddah, but not in association with Hajj. KSA conducts extensive spraying campaigns before Hajj, and especially targets the housing units of pilgrims from malaria- and dengue-endemic areas. The cities of Jeddah, Mecca, Medina, Riyadh (the capital of KSA), and Ta'if have no malaria transmission, and prophylaxis against malaria is neither recommended nor required for pilgrims.

ENVIRONMENTAL HAZARDS & RISKS

Animal Bites

Pilgrims bitten by animals should seek immediate medical attention to address any potential rabies exposure (see Sec. 4, Ch. 7, Zoonotic Exposures: Bites, Stings, Scratches & Other Hazards, and Sec. 5, Part 2, Ch. 18, Rabies).

Climate & Sun Exposure

Heat is a threat to the health and well-being of all travelers; both heat exhaustion and heatstroke can cause incapacitation and death among pilgrims (see Sec. 4. Ch. 2, Extremes of Temperature). Travelers are particularly at risk when Hajj occurs during summer months; the average high temperatures during June–September are ≥110°F. High temperatures combined with high humidity can lead to a heat index indicative of an extreme heat warning. High heat alone can exacerbate chronic conditions.

Depending on the exact location of their lodgings within Mina and whether they use trains or shuttle buses to get from one location to another, hajjis might walk up to ≈35–40 miles (≈55–65 km) over the 5 days; about 45% of pilgrims walk during the Hajj rituals. Counsel pilgrims to stay well hydrated, wear sunscreen, and seek shade or use umbrellas when possible. Religious leaders have ruled that it is permissible for hajjis to perform some rituals after dark. In addition, except for a pilgrim's required presence on Arafat on the 9th day of Dhul Hijjah, most other compulsory rituals can be postponed, done by proxy, or redeemed by paying a penalty.

OTHER HEALTH CONSIDERATIONS

Chronic Health Conditions

Hajj is arduous, even for young, healthy pilgrims. Because many Muslims wait until they are older before performing Hajj, they are more likely to have chronic health conditions. Travelers caught up in the experience of Hajj or Umrah might forget to take their usual medications. People with chronic medical conditions should have a health assessment before traveling to Hajj. Tailor a plan for each traveler's unique risks, including adjusting the usual medical regimen if necessary, ensuring an adequate supply of medications, and providing education about symptoms that indicate a condition requiring urgent attention.

Pilgrims with diabetes should have a customized management plan that enables them to meet the arduous physical challenges of the Hajj. They should bring adequate amounts of all medications, plus syringes and needles if they are insulin dependent. They also should carry an emergency kit with them on their pilgrimage; the kit should include easily accessible carbohydrate sources, glucagon, a glucometer and test strips, urine ketone sticks to evaluate for ketoacidosis, and a list of medications and care plans. Emphasize the importance of wearing durable and protective footwear to reduce the incidence of minor foot trauma, which can lead to infections.

Menstruation

Muslim law prohibits a person who is menstruating from performing *tawaf*. All other rituals are independent of menses. Because pilgrims generally know well in advance that they will be making a pilgrimage, those who intend to manipulate their menstrual cycle should consult with a physician 2–3 months before the journey.

SAFETY & SECURITY

Fire

Fire is a potential risk during Hajj. In 1997, open stoves set tents on fire, and the resulting blaze killed 343 pilgrims and injured >1,500. In 2015, a hotel caught fire and >1,000 pilgrims were evacuated. KSA no longer allows pilgrims to erect their own lodgings or prepare their own food; permanent fiberglass structures have replaced formerly makeshift accommodations.

Traffic-Related Injuries

As in other countries, motor vehicle crashes are the primary safety risk for US travelers to KSA. Remind Hajj pilgrims of the importance of seatbelt use in any vehicle, including buses (see Sec. 8, Ch. 5, Road & Traffic Safety). Encourage pilgrims to be mindful of their own safety when they walk long distances through or near dense traffic.

Trauma

Trauma is a major cause of injury and death during Hajj. Hajj is associated with dense crowding, leading to crush disasters or stampedes. Thousands of pilgrims were killed during a crush at Mina in 2015, making it the deadliest Hajj disaster on record. Death usually results from asphyxiation or head trauma, and large crowds limit the movement of emergency medical services, making prompt rescue and treatment difficult.

AVAILABILITY & QUALITY OF MEDICAL CARE

Travelers who become ill during Hajj have access to medical facilities located in and around the holy sites. An estimated 25,000 health care workers are typically in attendance, and medical services are offered free of charge to all pilgrims. For safety reasons, KSA advises that children, the frail elderly, seriously ill, and pregnant people postpone Hajj and Umrah.

10

BIBLIOGRAPHY

Aldossari M, Aljoudi A, Celentano D. Health issues in the Hajj pilgrimage: a literature review. East Mediterr Health J. 2019;25(10):744–9.

Alsafadi H, Goodwin W, Syed A. Diabetes care during Hajj. Clin Med. 2011;11(3):218–21.

Alzahrani AG, Choudhry AJ, Al Mazroa MA, Turkistani AH, Nouman GS, Memish ZA. Pattern of diseases among visitors to Mina health centers during the Hajj season, 1429 H (2008 G). J Infect Public Health. 2012;5(1):22–34.

Assiri A, Al-Tawfiq JA, Al-Rabeeah AA, Al-Rabiah FA, Al-Hajjar S, Al-Barrak A, et al. Epidemiological, demographic, and clinical characteristics of 47 cases of Middle East respiratory syndrome coronavirus disease from Saudi Arabia: a descriptive study. Lancet Infect Dis. 2013;13(9):752–61.

Benkouiten S, Al-Tawfiq JA, Memish ZA, Albarrak A, Gautret P. Clinical respiratory infections and pneumonia during the Hajj pilgrimage: a systematic review. Travel Med Infect Dis. 2019;28:15–26.

Memish ZA. Saudi Arabia has several strategies to care for pilgrims on the Hajj. BMJ. 2011;343:d7731.

Memish ZA. The Hajj: communicable and noncommunicable health hazards and current guidance for pilgrims. Euro Surveill. 2010;15(39):19671.

Memish ZA, Al-Rabeeah AA. Health conditions of travellers to Saudi Arabia for the pilgrimage to Mecca (Hajj and Umra) for 1434 (2013). J Epidemiol Glob Health. 2013;3(2):59–61.

Memish Z, Zumla A, Alhakeem R, Assiri A, Turkestani A, Al Harby KD, et al. Hajj: infectious disease surveillance and control. Lancet. 2014;383(9934):2073–82.

Yezli S. The threat of meningococcal disease during the Hajj and Umrah mass gatherings: a comprehensive review. Travel Med Infect Dis. 2018;24:51–8.

SOUTH AFRICA

Lucille Blumberg, Amy Herman-Roloff

DESTINATION OVERVIEW

South Africa is "a world in one country." Diverse geography that ranges from lush subtropical regions, old hardwood forests, and sweeping Highveld vistas to the deep desert of the Kalahari, along with expansive game reserves, are one part of this world. The people who live in South Africa, whose origins are in Africa, Europe, India, and Southeast Asia, make up another; they bring a vibrant, artistic, and culinary global culture to the country. All these, combined with access to the modern conveniences of a developed infrastructure, make the country truly unique.

South Africa is the only country in the world with 3 capital cities. Cape Town, the seat of Parliament, is the legislative capital. The president and cabinet and most foreign embassies have their offices in the administrative capital, Tshwane (Pretoria). South Africa's Supreme Court of Appeal is in Bloemfontein, the judicial capital. And although not considered a capital, Johannesburg, the most populous city in the country, is the seat of the Constitutional Court of South Africa.

South Africa has experienced a surge in both business and pleasure travel in the past 2 decades; visitors arrive from within the African continent as well as from North America and Europe. Business travelers typically head to the commercial centers of Cape Town, Durban, and Johannesburg. Tourist itineraries are as diverse as the country itself. From Cape Town, for example, visitors can follow the wine route of the Western Cape, exploring the many vineyards along the way, or they can drive along the spectacular coast. Going east from Cape Town, travelers can visit the southernmost point of Africa at Cape Agulhas—where the Indian and Atlantic Oceans meet in a roar of foam—and continue on to the small scenic towns of Knysna and Plettenberg Bay. South Africa is also a common destination for humanitarian aid workers, missionaries, and students. A sizable number of South Africans live outside the country; those returning home for a visit are considered VFR travelers (see Sec. 9, Ch. 9, Visiting Friends & Relatives: VFR Travel).

Game reserves located throughout the country attract many tourists (see Map 10-04). The largest, the Kruger National Park, is a world famous, highly accessible game reserve in the far northeast of the country along the border with Mozambique. KwaZulu-Natal has a fair number of game parks, including Hluhluwe Imfolozi Park and Saint Lucia, set inland from Durban; and the Eastern Cape has several parks, including Addo Elephant Park and Shamwari Private Game Reserve, easily accessed from Gqeberha (Port Elizabeth) on the southern coast. Many small, luxury game reserves have emerged to cater to high-end travelers.

INFECTIOUS DISEASE RISKS

All travelers to South Africa should be up to date on routine vaccinations, including diphtheria-tetanus-pertussis and measles-mumps-rubella.

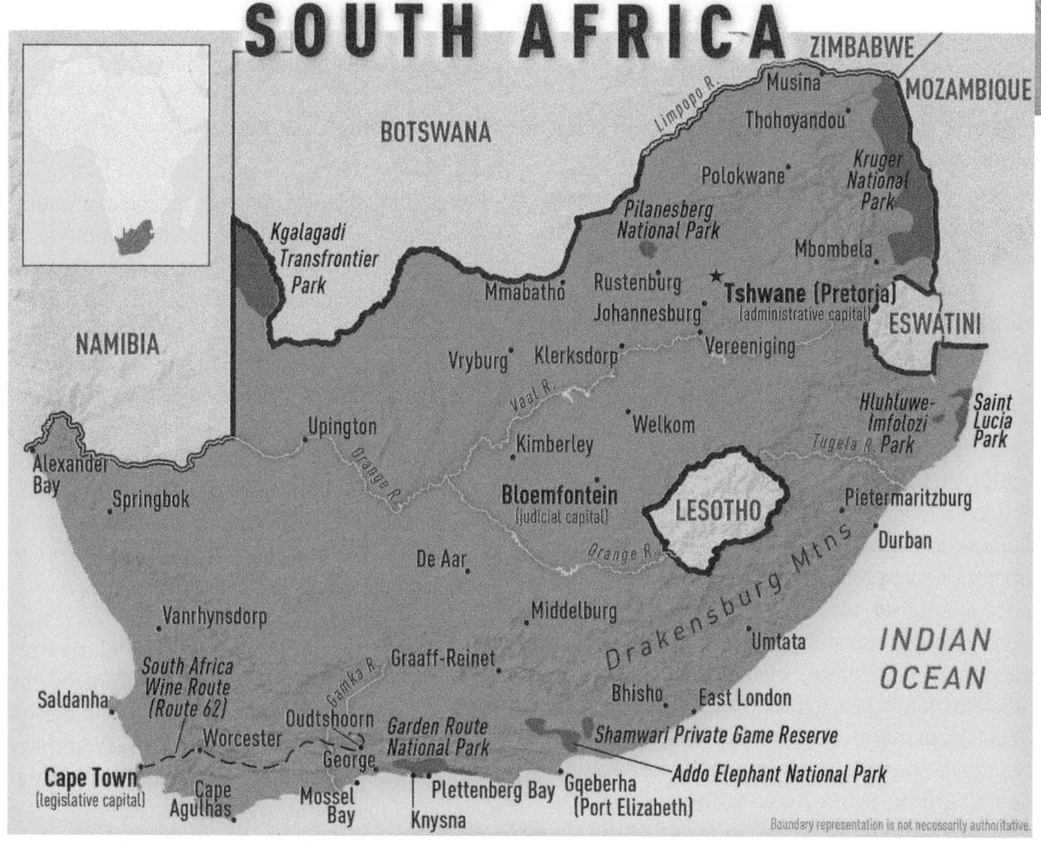

MAP 10-04 South Africa

Enteric Infections & Diseases

LISTERIOSIS

During 2017–2018 a very large outbreak of listeriosis was linked to a contaminated processed meat product from a single producer. The outbreak ended after the plant was closed, decontaminated, and refurbished.

TRAVELERS' DIARRHEA

As with most destinations, the risk for travelers' diarrhea in South Africa depends on style of travel and travelers' food choices (see Sec. 2, Ch. 6, Travelers' Diarrhea, and Sec. 2, Ch. 8, Food & Water Precautions). In most major cities, tap water is safe to drink, but in more rural areas, travelers should consume only bottled water. The usual spectrum of bacterial, viral, and parasitic infections exists in South Africa. Educate travelers about the prevention and self-treatment of travelers' diarrhea.

TYPHOID FEVER

Sporadic cases of typhoid are reported in South Africa, but overall, the risk for this disease to travelers is low.

Respiratory Infections & Diseases

CORONAVIRUS DISEASE 2019

People planning travel to South Africa can review the most current coronavirus disease 2019 (COVID-19) situation information and guidance from the National Institute for Communicable Diseases (www.nicd.ac.za). They also should consult the US Embassy & Consulates in South Africa website (https://za.usembassy.gov/). For the US government's COVID-19 international travel requirements and recommendations, see www.cdc.gov/coronavirus/2019-ncov/travelers/international-travel/index.html. All travelers going to South Africa should be up to date with their

COVID-19 vaccines (www.cdc.gov/coronavirus/2019-ncov/vaccines/stay-up-to-date.html).

INFLUENZA

Influenza viruses typically circulate during the winter months in South Africa, with peak transmission occurring during June–August. The burden of influenza in South Africa is significant, with ≈40,000 hospitalizations and ≈12,000 deaths each year. Travelers should have an influenza vaccination with the recommended Southern Hemisphere formulation, if available.

Sexually Transmitted Infections & HIV

South Africa has the largest estimated number of people living with HIV of any country in the world. The prevalence of HIV infection is ≈19% among people aged 15–49 years, and the prevalence among sex workers is considerably higher. Other sexually transmitted infections (STIs) also are present at high rates, including antimicrobial-resistant gonorrhea (ciprofloxacin resistance in 70%–80% of cases). Dual therapy with azithromycin and ceftriaxone is recommended for travelers returning from South Africa who are diagnosed with gonorrhea. Make travelers aware of the significant HIV and STI risks in South Africa and the importance of using condoms when having sex with someone whose HIV or STI status is unknown. Additionally, counsel travelers planning to engage in high-risk sexual encounters while in South Africa about preexposure prophylaxis (PrEP). For more information see Sec. 5, Part 2, Ch. 11, Human Immunodeficiency Virus / HIV; Sec. 9, Ch. 12, Sex & Travel; and Sec. 11, Ch. 10, Sexually Transmitted Infections.

Soil- & Waterborne Infections

SCHISTOSOMIASIS

Schistosoma spp. parasites, found throughout Africa, can be present in any body of unchlorinated, fresh water (see Sec. 5, Part 3, Ch. 20, Schistosomiasis). *Schistosoma haematobium* is the dominant species in South Africa, but *S. mansoni* occasionally has been detected. Advise travelers to avoid swimming in lakes, streams, and along dams in Limpopo, Mpumalanga, North West, KwaZulu-Natal, the Eastern Cape, and Gauteng provinces. By contrast, the provinces of Western Cape, Northern Cape, and most of Free State are considered schistosomiasis-free.

Vectorborne Diseases

MALARIA

Plasmodium falciparum malaria occurs along the border with Zimbabwe and Mozambique in the Mopani and Vhembe Districts of Limpopo Province; in the Ehlanzeni District of Mpumalanga Province; and in the uMkhanyakude District of KwaZulu-Natal Province. Kruger National Park spans 2 provinces, Mpumalanga and Limpopo, and is considered endemic for malaria with seasonal transmission. Visitors to these areas should take malaria chemoprophylaxis and use mosquito bite precautions; preventing mosquito bites is the first line of defense against malaria (see Sec. 4, Ch. 6, Mosquitoes, Ticks & Other Arthropods; Sec. 5, Part 3, Ch. 16, Malaria).

In March 2017, after a seasonal malaria outbreak in Limpopo Province, the Centers for Disease Control and Prevention (CDC) received reports of malaria in the western Waterberg District, an area with historic malaria transmission. Subsequent sporadic cases have been reported there (see Sec. 2, Ch. 5, Yellow Fever Vaccine & Malaria Prevention Information, by Country).

The South African National Department of Health recommends that travelers practice mosquito avoidance year-round in malaria risk areas and take malaria chemoprophylaxis during September–May. CDC, however, recommends chemoprophylaxis at all times of the year. Artemisinin combination therapy remains effective for treatment; artemether lumefantrine is the first-line therapy for uncomplicated infection, and artesunate is widely available for severe malaria treatment. Rare cases of so-called Odyssean, "taxi," or "suitcase" malaria have been reported in Gauteng province, likely related to relocation of infected mosquitoes from endemic areas.

RICKETTSIAL DISEASES

African tick-bite fever is common in South Africa (see Sec. 5, Part 1, Ch. 18, Rickettsial Diseases). The disease is characterized by an acute febrile illness, eschar at the bite site, regional adenopathy, and in some cases a maculopapular or petechial rash. The spectrum of illness varies from mild to, rarely, more severe disease resulting in hemorrhage and multisystem pathology. Campers and hikers in rural areas are especially at risk and should take measures to prevent tick bites (see Sec. 4, Ch. 6, Mosquitoes, Ticks & Other Arthropods). Travelers taking doxycycline for malaria chemoprophylaxis might have some protection against tick-bite fever, but no studies exist to support or refute this viewpoint. Taking doxycycline solely as prophylaxis for tick-bite fever (as opposed to taking it for malaria chemoprophylaxis) is not recommended.

YELLOW FEVER

There is no risk for yellow fever in South Africa.

YELLOW FEVER VACCINE REQUIREMENTS

South Africa requires a valid International Certificate of Vaccination or Prophylaxis (ICVP; https://wwwnc.cdc.gov/travel/page/icvp) documenting yellow fever vaccination ≥10 days before arrival in South Africa for all travelers aged ≥1 year, traveling from or transiting for >12 hours through the airport of a country with risk for yellow fever virus transmission. South Africa considers a one-time dose of yellow fever vaccine (properly documented with an ICVP) to be valid for the life of the traveler. Any traveler not meeting this requirement can be refused entry to South Africa or quarantined for ≤6 days. Unvaccinated travelers presenting a medical waiver signed by a licensed health care provider are generally allowed entry.

Travelers going to, or transiting through, South Africa are advised to seek the most current information by consulting the CDC Travelers' Health website (https://wwwnc.cdc.gov/travel/), the websites of the US embassy and consulates in South Africa (https://za.usembassy.gov), and the embassy of South Africa in Washington, DC (www.saembassy.org).

Viral Hemorrhagic Fevers

Rare cases of Crimean-Congo hemorrhagic fever have been reported in travelers visiting farms and rural areas of South Africa. It remains an occupational disease in animal health workers, farmers, and hunters.

ENVIRONMENTAL HAZARDS & RISKS

Animal Bites & Rabies

Rabies is endemic to South Africa and dogs are the major source for human rabies cases. The KwaZulu-Natal and Eastern Cape provinces have the highest incidence of rabies. Travelers have no way of telling whether an animal is rabid and should avoid all contact with animals. Instruct travelers to wash any bite or scratch from an animal with soap and water immediately and to see a clinician as soon as possible.

Rabies vaccine and rabies immunoglobulin are available for postexposure prophylaxis in the main centers, but access and availability will vary, and these treatments will likely be less available in rural areas. Consider preexposure rabies prophylaxis for travelers spending time in rural areas (see Sec. 4, Ch. 7, Zoonotic Exposures: Bites, Stings, Scratches & Other Hazards, and Sec. 5, Part 2, Ch. 18, Rabies). Most of the new formulations of equine rabies immune globulin (RIG) used in the South African public health system are potent, highly purified, and safe. Some private medical centers stock human RIG.

Climate & Sun Exposure

Latitude and elevation are major factors in the amount of solar ultraviolet radiation (UVR) that reaches the Earth's surface. South Africa's latitude spans 22°S to 34°S, and its elevation ranges from sea level to 3,482 m (≈11,500 ft), although the average height of Highveld plateau in the interior of the country is around 1,200 m (≈4000 ft). In some areas of South Africa (e.g., Durban, Pretoria), the UV index exceeds 11 in the summer months, which is considered very high. Given the frequent cloud-free skies, travelers should wear a broad-brimmed hat, sunglasses, a broad-spectrum sunscreen of ≥30 SPF on exposed skin, and sun-protective clothing to lessen the likelihood of sun damage and sun burn (see Sec. 4, Ch. 1, Sun Exposure, for more guidance).

SAFETY & SECURITY

Crime

Over the past several years, South Africa has experienced a rise in violent crime, including armed robberies, car jackings, home invasions, and rape (see Sec. 4, Ch. 11, Safety & Security Overseas). Stress awareness for personal safety and security with all travelers. Travelers should also seek local guidance on appropriate security precautions to take in specific areas.

Political Unrest

In mid-2021, in the context of a struggling economy, made worse by the COVID-19 pandemic and the arrest of former President Jacob Zuma, South Africa experienced major political unrest. Violent clashes between protesters and police, along with looting, occurred primarily in metropolitan areas, especially Durban and Johannesburg.

With a significant unemployment rate, especially among youth, unrest is a perpetual threat. To stay informed and avoid being accidently caught in areas of potential unrest, travelers should enroll in the US Department of State's Smart Traveler Enrollment Program (https://step.state.gov/step) before traveling, and follow the local news while in South Africa.

Traffic-Related Injuries

South Africa has a modern road system, which frequently leads to travel at high speeds. Drivers should be alert for dangerous driving practices, stray animals, and poor-quality roads in remote rural areas (see Sec. 8, Ch. 5, Road & Traffic Safety).

AVAILABILITY & QUALITY OF MEDICAL CARE

Although South Africa has a wide range of living standards, most visitors experience standards comparable to those in high-income countries. Fewer visitors go to rural areas or to the lower-income townships found outside most towns and cities. Adventure-seekers, hikers, and missionaries will experience a wider range of living standards. Similarly, the availability and quality of health care is variable. Middle- and upper-income South Africans have a standard of health comparable to that of North Americans, with access to private sector, world-class medical facilities, many of which also cater to an increasing number of visitors coming to South Africa for medical tourism. By contrast, many South Africans live in areas with limited amenities, experience significant disease transmission, and rely on frequently under-resourced public sector facilities for treatment.

Medical Tourism

Because of the affordable and high-quality private health sector in South Africa, medical tourism is steadily on the rise. Travelers to South Africa for medical tourism frequently access cancer treatment, cosmetic surgery, dental, fertility, or transplant services (see Sec. 6, Ch. 4, Medical Tourism).

BIBLIOGRAPHY

De Boni L, Msimang V, De Voux A, Frean J. Trends in the prevalence of microscopically-confirmed schistosomiasis in the South African public health sector, 2011–2018. PLoS Negl Trop Dis. 2021;15(9):e0009669.

Frean J, Grayson W. South African tick bite fever: an overview. Dermatopathology (Basel). 2019;6(2):70–6.

Kularatne R, Maseko V, Gumede L, Kufa T. Trends in *Neisseria gonorrhoeae* antimicrobial resistance over a ten-year surveillance period, Johannesburg, South Africa, 2008–2017. Antibiotics (Basel). 2018 Jul 12;7(3):58.

Moodley I, Kleinschmidt I, Sharp B, Craig M, Appleton C. Temperature-suitability maps for schistosomiasis in South Africa. Ann Trop Med Parasitol. 2003;97(6):617–27.

National Department of Health. Addendum to the South African guidelines for the prevention and treatment of malaria updated 2018. Pretoria: The Department; 2019. Available from: www.nicd.ac.za/wp-content/uploads/2019/03/National-Guidelines-for-prevention-of-Malaria_updated-08012019-1.pdf.

National Department of Health. National guidelines for the prevention of malaria, South Africa 2018. Pretoria: The Department; 2018. Available from: www.mic.uct.ac.za/sites/default/files/image_tool/images/51/2018_NDOH_Malaria%20Prophylaxis_0.pdf.

National Department of Health. National guidelines for the treatment of malaria, South Africa 2019. Pretoria: The Department; 2020. Available from: https://health.gov.za/wp-content/uploads/2020/11/national-guidelines-for-the-treatment-of-malaria-south-africa-2019.pdf.

The South African National Travel Health Network. SaNTHNet. Available from: www.santhnet.co.za.

Thomas J, Govender N, McCarthy KM, Erasmus LK, Doyle TJ, Allam M, et al. Outbreak of listeriosis in South Africa associated with processed meat. N Engl J Med. 2020;382(7):632–43.

Weyer J, Dermaux-Msimang V, Grobbelaar A, Le Roux C, Moolla N, Paweska J, et al. Epidemiology of human rabies in South Africa, 2008–2018. S Afr Med J. 2020;110(9):877–81.

TANZANIA & ZANZIBAR

Rachel Eidex, Peter Mmbuji

DESTINATION OVERVIEW

Tanzania, land of the Serengeti and Zanzibar, can offer in a single destination what cannot be found anywhere in the world, either through tailored packages or independent visits. Boasting >32 national parks and reserves, each region of Tanzania offers a unique experience; the country is a top destination for travelers interested in aquatic recreation, mountaineering, or seeing wildlife.

In 2008, the *New York Times* named the snow and ice–capped Mount Kilimanjaro as a world "Place to Go" and a must-see destination. Climbing the tallest free-standing mountain in the world is like a virtual climatic world tour, hiking from the tropics through to the arctic. In addition to Mount Kilimanjaro, travelers can visit Serengeti National Park, one of the Seven Natural Wonders of Africa; Ngorongoro Conservation Area, a World Heritage Site; Mahale and Gombe National Parks on the shores of Lake Tanganyika, famous for their chimpanzees; and swim with the whale sharks in the Indian Ocean off Mafia Island (see Map 10-05).

Dar es Salaam is Tanzania's most populous city and its former capital; it is also the country's commercial center and home to its largest international airport. To get from Dar es Salaam (located on the Indian Ocean coast) to the islands of Zanzibar, one can take a 2-hour ferry ride or a 25-minute flight. Dodoma, designated Tanzania's national capital in 1996, is ≈450 km (280 mi) inland, west of Dar es Salaam.

Travelers can visit Tanzania throughout the year. April is often the wettest month, and many popular resorts, guest houses, and tented camps close during this time. Tanzania can be safe and easy to navigate, but all travelers should plan in advance. Unprepared travelers can struggle with travelers' diarrhea, vectorborne diseases, or altitude illness when attempting to summit Tanzania's beautiful peaks. People traveling anywhere in Tanzania should be advised about the risk for vaccine-preventable diseases, foodborne and waterborne illnesses, malaria and other vectorborne diseases, and traffic injuries. With appropriate preparation, however, Tanzania is a rewarding and unforgettable destination.

INFECTIOUS DISEASE RISKS

Travelers to Tanzania should be up to date on essential immunizations and carefully advised on recommendations for travel vaccines, including coronavirus disease 2019 (COVID-19), hepatitis A, polio, and tetanus. Proof of vaccination against yellow fever is required for travelers entering from yellow fever–endemic countries; carefully review each traveler's full travel itinerary to determine whether they will need yellow fever vaccine.

Enteric Infections & Diseases

CHOLERA

Caused by the bacterium *Vibrio cholerae*, cholera is characterized by abdominal cramps, profuse watery diarrhea, and vomiting (see Sec. 5, Part 1, Ch. 5, Cholera). In Tanzania, cholera outbreaks occur mostly during the rainy season and are due to poor sanitation and an inadequate supply of clean and safe drinking water. The last outbreak (2015–2019), totaling 33,702 cases and 556 deaths, affected all regions of the country.

Cholera can cause severe dehydration within a few hours; travelers should practice safe food and water precautions (see Sec. 2, Ch. 8, Food & Water Precautions) and careful hand hygiene. Travelers also should know the location of the nearest facility to seek medical care (see the US embassy in Tanzania website, https://tz.usembassy.gov/). The Advisory Committee on Immunization Practices recommends that adults traveling to areas with active cholera transmission be vaccinated with cholera vaccine. Because most travelers from the United States do not visit areas with active cholera transmission, they can avoid infection by adhering carefully to preventive measures (food and water precautions, scrupulous hand hygiene) without vaccination.

MAP

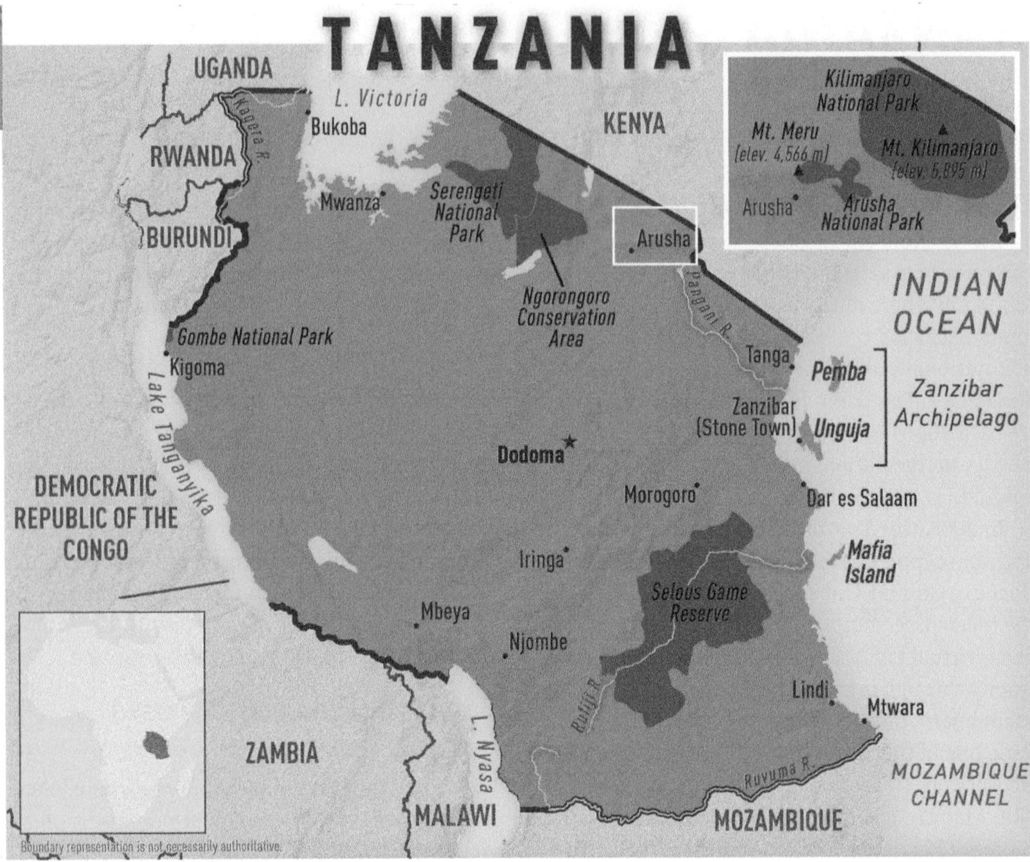

MAP 10-05 Tanzania & Zanzibar

10

GIARDIASIS

Giardiasis is endemic to Tanzania with high infection rates among young children. *Giardia* infection is acquired primarily by swallowing contaminated water, particularly untreated water from lakes, streams, and swimming pools; people also can get infected from eating contaminated food (see Sec. 5, Part 3, Ch. 12, Giardiasis). As with cholera, the best way to prevent giardiasis is to consume only safe food and water, and to practice good hygiene, including frequent handwashing.

TRAVELERS' DIARRHEA

Travelers' diarrhea (TD) is the most common health complaint among travelers to Tanzania. Because TD commonly is due to consuming contaminated food or water, educate travelers on prevention measures and personal hygiene. Travelers should avoid consuming tap water in Tanzania. Travelers affected by TD should hydrate to replace lost body fluids and minerals. Most TD cases are mild and self-limiting, but travelers should still carry with them antimotility medications (e.g., Imodium or loperamide) to provide relief. Travelers also can carry antimicrobial drugs to treat moderate to severe TD (see Sec. 2, Ch. 6, Travelers' Diarrhea, and Sec. 2, Ch. 8, Food & Water Precautions).

TYPHOID FEVER

Typhoid fever (see Sec. 5, Part 1, Ch. 24, Typhoid & Paratyphoid Fever) is prevalent in Tanzania; the annual incidence rate between 2003 and 2007 was 580–1,400 cases/100,000 persons. Infected people can show symptoms 1–3 weeks after exposure. Travelers, especially long-term travelers, should get vaccinated; because the vaccine is not 100% effective, however, and because vaccine-induced immunity can be overwhelmed by a large bacterial inoculum, travelers should ensure they practice safe food precautions (e.g., eating foods that are well cooked and served hot, making sure fruits and vegetables are washed with clean water and cooked or peeled before consuming). Advise travelers to observe personal hygiene with regular and thorough handwashing or use of hand sanitizer with ≥60% alcohol when soap and safe water are unavailable.

Respiratory Infections & Diseases

Respiratory illnesses account for a high proportion of morbidity and mortality in Tanzania; >75% of hospital deaths are due to pneumonia and tuberculosis. Encourage travelers to Tanzania to take preventive measures against respiratory infections, including being vaccinated against COVID-19 and influenza, washing hands, avoiding sick people, and practicing respiratory etiquette.

CORONAVIRUS DISEASE 2019

For current information on COVID-19 in Tanzania, consult the US Embassy in Tanzania website (https://tz.usembassy.gov/). For the US government's COVID-19 international travel requirements and recommendations, see www.cdc.gov/coronavirus/2019-ncov/travelers/international-travel/index.html. All travelers going to Tanzania should be up to date with their COVID-19 vaccines (www.cdc.gov/coronavirus/2019-ncov/vaccines/stay-up-to-date.html).

Sexually Transmitted Infections & HIV

Over the past 10 years, Tanzania has implemented many measures to control its HIV epidemic. As of 2018, ≈1.6 million people were still living with HIV across Tanzania. In addition to HIV, prevalence of sexually transmitted infections is common, including chlamydia, gonorrhea, syphilis, and trichomoniasis. Educate travelers on the necessary precautions to prevent STIs, including HIV (see Sec. 5, Part 2, Ch. 11, Human Immunodeficiency Virus / HIV, and Sec. 9, Ch. 12, Sex & Travel).

Soil- & Waterborne Infections

SCHISTOSOMIASIS

Travelers who bathe, swim, or wade in unchlorinated freshwater sources in Tanzania, including Lake Tanganyika and Lake Victoria, are at risk for schistosomiasis (bilharzia).

Vectorborne Diseases

DENGUE

In recent years, the incidence of dengue in Tanzania has increased, particularly along the coastal regions, including in Dar es Salaam and the islands of Zanzibar. As with other mosquito-borne diseases, travelers taking steps to prevent bites (including proper use of mosquito nets and insect repellent) is key to preventing infections (see Sec. 4, Ch. 6, Mosquitoes, Ticks & Other Arthropods).

MALARIA

Chloroquine-resistant *Plasmodium falciparum* is endemic throughout Tanzania (see Sec. 2, Ch. 5, Yellow Fever Vaccine and Malaria Prevention Information, by Country). The islands of Zanzibar have been targeted for malaria elimination; although authorities have met with some success, malaria transmission still occurs on islands throughout the archipelago. In addition, climate change has expanded the range of suitable habitats for *Anopheles* spp. mosquitoes; thus, consider malaria prophylaxis for all travelers going to Tanzania, and educate all travelers, regardless of their itinerary, on mosquito avoidance techniques.

The tropical malaria-endemic location of Mount Kilimanjaro means that many trekkers will be taking malaria prophylaxis during their climb and will likely need to continue taking malaria prophylaxis after descent, particularly if they are visiting game parks or staying overnight at elevations below 1,800 m (≈5,900 ft).

TRYPANOSOMIASIS

Although cases of African trypanosomiasis are rare, they have been reported among travelers to Tanzanian national parks. Educate travelers on ways to reduce tsetse fly exposure (see Sec. 5, Part 3, Ch. 24, African Trypanosomiasis).

YELLOW FEVER

Yellow fever has never been reported from Tanzania. Due to the presence of the mosquito vector and the risk in neighboring countries, however, Tanzania has been designated low risk for yellow fever by the World Health Organization. Travelers ≥1 year of age arriving from a country with risk of yellow fever virus transmission, including transit >12 hours in an airport located in a country with risk of yellow fever virus transmission, are required to show proof of vaccination on an International Certificate of Vaccination or Prophylaxis (https://wwwnc.cdc.gov/travel/page/icvp) to enter the country (see Sec. 2, Ch. 5, Yellow Fever Vaccine and Malaria Prevention Information, by Country).

ENVIRONMENTAL HAZARDS & RISKS

Altitude Illness & Acute Mountain Sickness

Many travelers visit Tanzania for the opportunity to summit Mount Meru (4,566 m; 14,980 ft) or Mount Kilimanjaro (5,895 m; 19,340 ft), both located in northern Tanzania. Mountain climbing is physically demanding, requiring a good fitness level and preparation for the elements. Weather in these locations is characterized by extremes; travelers should be prepared for tropical heat, heavy rains, and bitter cold, and they should store gear in waterproof bags.

Altitude illness is a major reason why only about half of those who attempt to summit Kilimanjaro reach the crater rim, Gilman's Point at 5,685 m (18,651 ft), and ≤10% reach the top, Uhuru (Freedom) Peak at 5,895 m (19,340 ft). Travelers with signs and symptoms of altitude illness must stop their ascent. If symptoms worsen, descent is mandatory. Climbers should have a flexible itinerary and consider employing an extra guide who can accompany any members of the group down the mountain if they become ill.

Prevalence rates of acute mountain sickness (AMS) were 75%–77% in recent studies of 4- and 5-day ascents of Kilimanjaro. People using the carbonic anhydrase inhibitor acetazolamide were much less likely to develop AMS on 5-day ascents, but ≥40% of people taking this medication still reported AMS symptoms. For any traveler planning to ascend to elevations >8,000 ft, be sure to discuss the signs and symptoms of altitude illness and provide guidance on its prevention and treatment (for details, see Sec. 4, Ch. 5, High Elevation Travel & Altitude Illness). Climbers can prevent altitude illness and enhance their enjoyment of the experience by allowing more time to acclimatize (see Box 10-01).

MEDICAL MANAGEMENT

People with some preexisting health conditions can be more susceptible to problems associated with travel to high elevations, or their medications can interact with those taken to prevent AMS. For travelers in higher risk categories, a pretravel consultation with a travel health provider who has specialized knowledge of altitude illness is critical.

Anyone with a history of AMS susceptibility, and for those in whom adequate acclimatization is not possible, use of medications to prevent altitude illness (e.g., acetazolamide) is recommended. Acetazolamide accelerates acclimatization and is effective in preventing AMS when started the day before ascent, and can also be used in treating

BOX 10-01 Acclimatization tips for high elevation hiking in Tanzania

Before attempting to climb Mt. Kilimanjaro (5,895 m, ≈19,340 ft), travelers can acclimatize by first hiking ≥1 of the following

- Ngorongoro crater (2,286 m; 7,500 ft); try to spend the last few nights here prior to climbing Mt. Kilimanjaro
- Mt. Meru (4,566 m; 14,980 ft); 70 km (≈43 miles) away from Mt. Kilimanjaro, Mt. Meru is considered a good "warm up" hike
- Point Lenana (4,895 m; 16,059 ft) on Mt. Kenya; combined Mt. Kenya and Mt. Kilimanjaro climbing trips are available

Add ≥1–2 days to the planned ascent of Mt. Kilimanjaro

- Taking additional time facilitates acclimatization, regardless of the route taken to the top
- Extra time for acclimatization is beneficial for travelers taking routes normally promoted as 4- to 6-day trips

AMS. Children can take it safely. Dexamethasone is an alternative for AMS prevention in people intolerant of or allergic to acetazolamide. Climbers also can use dexamethasone to prevent high-altitude pulmonary edema (HAPE) and to prevent and treat high-altitude cerebral edema (HACE).

TRAVEL HEALTH KITS & TRAVEL HEALTH INSURANCE

Advise travelers planning to climb the mountains in Tanzania to carry a personal first aid kit that includes, among other necessary items, altitude illness medication, analgesics, antibacterial and antifungal cream, antibiotics for travelers' diarrhea, antiemetics, antihistamines, antimalarials, bandages and tape, a blister kit, oral rehydration salts, and throat lozenges (see Sec. 2, Ch. 10, Travel Health Kits). Include information on potential drug–drug interactions between medications used for altitude illness and routine or travel-related medications. In addition, discuss the need for adequate health insurance, including medical evacuation insurance, with travelers planning climbs (see Sec. 6, Ch. 1, Travel Insurance, Travel Health Insurance & Medical Evacuation Insurance). Encourage travelers to confirm that their purchased policies cover the cost of evacuation or rescue from the top of a mountain and any associated care.

Animal Bites & Rabies

Canine rabies is prevalent throughout Tanzania, and travelers should avoid animal bites (see Sec. 5, Part 2, Ch. 18, Rabies). Advise travelers to avoid petting or handling wild animals and unfamiliar dogs, including puppies. Instruct travelers to seek care if bitten or scratched. Because both rabies vaccine and rabies immunoglobulin can be difficult to access, opportunities for postexposure prophylaxis might be limited. Depending on the itinerary and planned activities, discuss with travelers the merits of preexposure vaccination and purchasing medical evacuation insurance coverage (see Sec. 6, Ch. 1, Travel Insurance, Travel Health Insurance & Medical Evacuation Insurance).

Sun Exposure & Ocean Sports

Snorkeling, scuba diving, and other ocean sports are popular among travelers to Tanzania. Include information on sun exposure (see Sec. 4, Ch. 1, Sun Exposure) and water safety (see Sec. 4, Ch. 4, Scuba Diving: Decompression Illness & Other Dive-Related Injuries) as part of the pretravel consultation. For less experienced scuba divers, be certain to discuss the risks of barotrauma and decompression illness. Inform travelers that broad-spectrum sunscreen (protects against both ultraviolet A and ultraviolet B) might not be readily available in country; advise that they carry an adequate supply from home.

SAFETY & SECURITY

Crime

Crime in Tanzania is more common in urban settings, and tourists often can be targets for petty theft and scams. Common sense can prevent most crimes, but travelers should check with the US Department of State Bureau of Consular Affairs (http://travel.state.gov/travelsafely) and Overseas Security Advisory Council (www.osac.gov) ahead of time to learn more about safety and security risks at their destination.

Traffic-Related Injuries

Road traffic accidents occur often in Tanzania. Major contributors to risk include poor road quality, improperly maintained vehicles, and reckless driving habits. Counsel travelers to wear seat belts, use reputable transportation operators, and to avoid traveling at night. Pedestrians should have heightened awareness when crossing streets; traffic laws might be different from expected or disregarded by drivers.

AVAILABILITY & QUALITY OF MEDICAL CARE

Although health care can be accessed throughout the country, clinics and hospitals similar to those in high-income countries are found primarily in larger cities, and specialized care is limited (see Sec. 6, Ch. 2, Obtaining Health Care Abroad). Many medications are available over the counter, but quality might be unreliable (see Sec. 6, Ch. 3, . . . *perspectives*: Avoiding Poorly Regulated Medicines & Medical Products During Travel). Encourage travelers to carry with them any medications they anticipate needing, including malaria prophylaxis and prescription medications.

BIBLIOGRAPHY

Ahmed S, Reithinger R, Kaptoge SK, Ngondi JM. Travel is a key risk factor for malaria transmission in pre-elimination settings in sub-Saharan Africa: a review of the literature and meta-analysis. Am J Trop Med Hyg. 2020;103(4):1380–7.

Boniface R, Museru L, Kiloloma O, Munthali V. Factors associated with road traffic injuries in Tanzania. Pan Afr Med J. 2016;23:46.

Jackson SJ, Varley J, Sellers C, Josephs K, Codrington L, Duke G, et al. Incidence and predictors of acute mountain sickness among trekkers on Mount Kilimanjaro. High Alt Med Biol. 2010;11(3):217–22.

Jelinek T, Bisoffi Z, Bonazzi L, van Thiel P, Bronner U, de Frey A, et al. Cluster of African trypanosomiasis in travelers to Tanzanian national parks. Emerg Infect Dis. 2002; 8(6):634–5.

Kulkarni MA, Desrochers RE, Kajeguka DC, Kaaya RD, Tomayer A, Kweka EJ, et al. 10 years of environmental change on the slopes of Mount Kilimanjaro and its associated shift in malaria vector distributions. Front Public Health. 2016;4:281.

Luks AM, Swenson ER, Bartsch P. Acute high-altitude sickness. Eur Respir Rev. 2017;26(143):160096.

Morgan AP, Brazeau NF, Ngasala B, Mhamilawa LE, Denton M, Msellem M, et al. Falciparum malaria from coastal Tanzania and Zanzibar remains highly connected despite effective control efforts on the archipelago. Malar J. 2020;19(1):47.

Rack J, Wichmann O, Kamara B, Günther M, Cramer J, Schönfeld C, et al. Risk and spectrum of diseases in travelers to popular tourist destinations. J Travel Med. 2005;12(5):248–53.

Schönenberger S, Hatz C, Bühler S. Unpredictable checks of yellow fever vaccination certificates upon arrival in Tanzania. J Travel Med. 2016;23(5):taw035.

Vilkman K, Pakkanen SH, Lääveri T, Siikamäki H, Kantele A. Travelers' health problems and behavior: prospective study with post-travel follow-up. BMC Infect Dis. 2016;16:328.

PART 2: THE AMERICAS & THE CARIBBEAN

BRAZIL

Alexandre Macedo de Oliveira

DESTINATION OVERVIEW

At nearly 3.3 million square miles in size, Brazil is the fifth largest country in the world and the largest country in South America, occupying nearly half the land area of the continent. With >210 million people, Brazil is home to the world's largest Portuguese-speaking population. The world's eighth largest economy, Brazil is classified as an upper-middle-income country. Nearly 85% of Brazilians live in urban areas.

Brazil is the most popular tourist destination in South America, and the second most popular in all Latin America. In 2018, >6 million international visitors traveled to Brazil; the country hosted the Fédération Internationale de Football Association (FIFA) World Cup in 2014 and the Summer Olympic and Paralympic Games in 2016. Rio de Janeiro, Brazil's second-largest city (population >7 million) and most frequently visited tourist destination, is famous for its beaches, landmarks, and annual Carnival festivities. São Paulo, one of the world's largest cities with >21 million people in the greater metropolitan area, is the economic center of Brazil and the most visited destination for business travel. Brazilian people prize many of their major cities, including Florianópolis, Fortaleza, Manaus, Recife, and Salvador, for their coastlines and regional culture.

The country also boasts multiple UNESCO World Heritage sites, including Iguaçu National Park in Paraná, home to the largest waterfalls in the Americas; the historic towns of Olinda (Pernambuco), Ouro Preto (Minas Gerais), Salvador (Bahia), and São Luis (Maranhão); the modern capital of Brasília; and natural areas of the Amazon Forest and the Pantanal Conservation Area, which extends from one state (Mato Grosso do Sul) into another (Mato Grosso) and into portions of two countries (Bolivia and Paraguay). The Atlantic forests and the archipelago of Fernando de Noronha in the Atlantic Ocean are World Heritage sites (see Map 10-06).

The Amazon Forest, large portions of which extend into the countries that neighbor Brazil, attracts travelers in search of exotic adventures. The region presents unique risks, and careful planning and attention to travelers' health needs before, during, and after the trip is critical. Because mosquito-borne diseases (chikungunya, dengue, malaria, yellow fever, and Zika) are endemic throughout the Amazon, advise travelers to complete all relevant vaccinations and provide them with detailed instruction on the proper use of chemoprophylaxis and mosquito avoidance. The hot and humid climate throughout the forest increases the risks for dehydration and heat stroke; travelers should practice extreme caution and, whenever possible, resist the temptation to consume potentially unsafe food and beverages.

INFECTIOUS DISEASE RISKS

Travelers to Brazil should be up to date on routine vaccines, including coronavirus disease 2019 (COVID-19), influenza, measles-mumps-rubella (MMR), and diphtheria-tetanus-pertussis.

BRAZIL

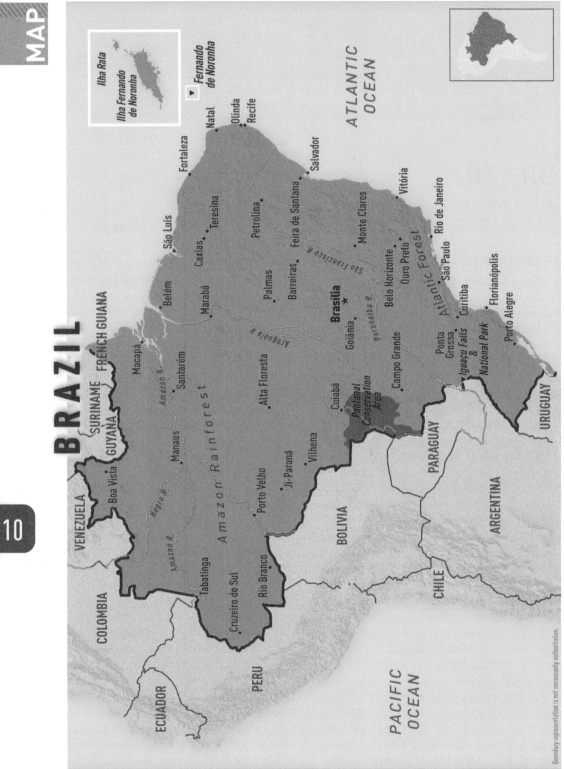

MAP 10-06 Brazil

Hepatitis A vaccination also is recommended. Consider hepatitis B vaccination for most travelers, but especially for anyone who could be exposed to blood or other body fluids (e.g., through medical services, sexual contact, tattooing).

Enteric Infections & Diseases

TRAVELERS' DIARRHEA

Travelers should take food and water precautions throughout Brazil, including in the big cities (see Sec. 2, Ch. 8, Food & Water Precautions). Travelers' diarrhea (TD) is the most common travel-related ailment, and visitors consuming raw fruits and vegetables, unpasteurized dairy products, and food from street vendors increase their risk for foodborne infections. Oral rehydration salts are available from public health clinics and in almost all pharmacies in Brazil. For further information about travelers' diarrhea, see Sec. 2, Ch. 6, Travelers' Diarrhea.

TYPHOID FEVER

Consider vaccinating "adventurous eaters" against typhoid, along with travelers who stay with friends or relatives or who visit smaller cities, villages, or rural areas (see Sec. 5, Part 1, Ch. 24, Typhoid & Paratyphoid Fever).

Respiratory Infections & Diseases

CORONAVIRUS DISEASE 2019

For current information on COVID-19 in Brazil, consult the US Embassy & Consulates in Brazil website (https://br.usembassy.gov). For the US government's COVID-19 international travel requirements and recommendations, see www.cdc.gov/coronavirus/2019-ncov/travelers/international-travel/index.html. All travelers going to Brazil should be up to date with their COVID-19 vaccines (www.cdc.gov/coronavirus/2019-ncov/vaccines/stay-up-to-date.html).

ENDEMIC FUNGI

A variety of fungi (e.g., *Paracoccidioides* in the south and southeast) are endemic to Brazil. Inhaling the spores of fungi typically present in the soil (e.g., *Coccidioides*, *Cryptococcus neoformans*, *Histoplasma*, *Paracoccidioides*) can cause respiratory illness and occasionally more severe disease (e.g., meningitis, bone infections). For more details, see Sec. 5, Part 4, Ch. 1, Coccidioidomycosis / Valley Fever, and Sec. 5, Part 4, Ch. 2, Histoplasmosis. Travelers should beware of bat guano in caves and use caution before disturbing soil, particularly if contaminated by bat or bird feces.

INFLUENZA

Peak influenza circulation occurs during April–September in most of Brazil but can occur throughout the year in tropical areas. The influenza vaccine recommended for use in the Northern Hemisphere each year confers protection against the virus strains circulating in the Southern Hemisphere that same year. The Centers for Disease Control and Prevention (CDC) recommends seasonal influenza vaccination ≥2 weeks before travel, and pneumococcal vaccination for people ≥65 years of age, and for younger adults and children with chronic medical conditions.

TUBERCULOSIS

Tuberculosis (TB) is prevalent in Brazil, but short-term travelers are not considered to be at high risk for infection unless visiting specific crowded environments. Before they leave the United States, consider TB testing for travelers who anticipate prolonged exposure to people known to have, or at high risk for having, TB (e.g., people in clinics, hospitals, prisons, homeless shelters). For more detailed information, see Sec. 5, Part 1, Ch. 22, Tuberculosis, and Sec. 5, Part 1, Ch. 23, . . . *perspectives*: Testing Travelers for *Mycobacterium tuberculosis* Infection.

10

Sexually Transmitted Infections & HIV

The HIV infection rate in Brazil is 0.5% among adults aged 15–49 years, comparable to other countries in South America. Discuss options for preexposure prophylaxis with travelers at greater risk for acquiring HIV infection (see www.cdc.gov/hiv/prep, and Sec. 5, Part 2, Ch. 11, Human Immunodeficiency Virus / HIV). In Brazil, people who use drugs, men who have sex with men, and female sex workers are more likely than the general population to be infected with HIV.

In Brazil, condoms are available free of charge in public health clinics, tourist service centers, and other distribution points in many cities. Male condoms are also available throughout Brazil in pharmacies, convenience stores, and supermarkets; female condoms are available in some locations.

Soil- & Waterborne Infections

LEPTOSPIROSIS

In urban areas of Brazil, outbreaks of leptospirosis have occurred after heavy flooding (see Sec. 5, Part 1, Ch. 10, Leptospirosis). Travelers who have contact with standing water or mud after heavy rainfall are at increased risk. Advise travelers to avoid entering bodies of freshwater potentially contaminated with animals' body fluids.

SCHISTOSOMIASIS

Schistosoma spp. are parasites found in freshwater lakes and rivers in many states of Brazil, especially in the northeast. Advise travelers to avoid bathing, swimming, or wading in fresh, unchlorinated water, where they could contract schistosomiasis (see Sec. 5, Part 3, Ch. 20, Schistosomiasis). Bathing or swimming in saltwater is not a source of infection.

Vectorborne Diseases

Vectorborne diseases (bacterial, viral, parasitic) are present in many areas of Brazil; these infections are among the leading causes of febrile illness in travelers returning from South America.

CHIKUNGUNYA & DENGUE

Risk for chikungunya and dengue infection is increased in many large Brazilian cities due to large populations of *Aedes* mosquitoes, which transmit these viruses (see Sec. 5, Part 2, Ch. 2, Chikungunya, and Sec. 5, Part 2, Ch. 4, Dengue). During 2000–2015, cases of dengue surged throughout Brazil, with epidemics reported in large cities, including Rio de Janeiro and Salvador. Preliminary data show that in 2019, Brazil recorded ≈132,000 cases of chikungunya and ≈1.5 million probable cases of dengue. Travelers to Brazil should take measures to protect themselves from mosquito bites (see Sec. 4, Ch. 6, Mosquitoes, Ticks & Other Arthropods).

LEISHMANIASIS

Cutaneous and visceral leishmaniasis occur in Brazil and are most common in the Amazon and northeast regions (see Sec. 5, Part 3, Ch. 14, Cutaneous Leishmaniasis, and Sec. 5, Part 3, Ch. 15, Visceral Leishmaniasis). The risk for transmission is greatest from dusk to dawn because the sand fly vector typically feeds (bites) at night and during twilight hours. Ecotourists and adventure travelers might be at increased risk, but even short-term travelers in endemic areas have developed leishmaniasis. Travelers should take measures to avoid insect bites (see Sec. 4, Ch. 6, Mosquitoes, Ticks & Other Arthropods).

LYMPHATIC FILARIASIS

Brazil is actively participating in the global program to eliminate lymphatic filariasis (LF); LF is considered endemic to only 4 cities in Brazil, all located in the Recife Metropolitan Region (northeastern coast) of the country. As of 2020, all regions had achieved the targets set by the World Health Organization (WHO) to stop annual treatment, suggesting low likelihood of ongoing disease transmission and minimal risk to travelers. Brazil is still working to achieve all targets demonstrating elimination of LF as a public health problem (see Sec. 5, Part 3, Ch. 9, Lymphatic Filariasis, and the WHO website, www.who.int/en/news-room/fact-sheets/detail/lymphatic-filariasis#).

MALARIA

Almost all malaria in Brazil occurs in the Amazon Basin, although less competent malaria vector species are present in other parts of the country. *Plasmodium vivax* is the main malaria species; only ≈10%–20% of malaria cases are caused by *P. falciparum*. CDC recommends chemoprophylaxis for travelers going to malaria-endemic areas of Brazil (see Sec. 2, Ch. 5, Yellow Fever Vaccine & Malaria Prevention Information, by Country; Map 2-04; and the CDC Malaria webpage, www.cdc.gov/parasites/malaria/index.html). No malaria transmission occurs in the cities of Brasília (the capital), Rio de Janeiro, or São Paolo, or at Iguaçu Falls.

RICKETTSIAL DISEASES

Tickborne rickettsial diseases in Brazil include *febre maculosa* and Brazilian spotted fever, which are caused by etiologic agents from the same genus (*Rickettsia*) that causes Rocky Mountain spotted fever in the United States (see Sec. 5, Part 1, Ch. 18, Rickettsial Diseases). Travelers should take precautions (e.g., wearing appropriate clothing, applying insect repellants on clothes and skin) to avoid tick bites both indoors and outdoors (see Sec. 4, Ch. 6, Mosquitoes, Ticks & Other Arthropods).

TRYPANOSOMIASIS

Except in the north of the country where cases continue to rise, most states in Brazil have eliminated Chagas disease (American trypanosomiasis) through improved housing conditions and insecticide spraying for the vector. Although the risk is extremely low, travelers and ecotourists staying in poor-quality housing, especially in the Amazon region, might be at greater risk for this disease.

Outbreaks have been associated with consuming food or beverages containing açaí, an Amazonian fruit eaten throughout Brazil, and sugar cane juice (*caldo de cana*). Oral transmission occurs when people consume food or beverages contaminated with triatomines—the bloodsucking insects that transmit the etiologic agent of Chagas disease (*Trypanosoma cruzi*)—or their feces (see Sec. 5, Part 3, Ch. 25, American Trypanosomiasis / Chagas Disease).

YELLOW FEVER

Mosquitoes that transmit yellow fever virus can be found throughout the Amazon Basin and in forested regions along all major river basins in Brazil, including Iguaçu Falls and as far south as Rio Grande do Sul. During 2016–2017, outbreaks of sylvatic yellow fever extended to the southeastern coast of Brazil, including the cities of Rio de Janeiro and São Paulo, areas with historically low risk for transmission. Several unvaccinated travelers visiting these areas became ill with the disease, and some died.

Evidence of an expanded range of yellow fever transmission in Brazil led WHO and CDC to broaden their vaccination coverage recommendations for the country in 2017. Although Brazil does not require proof of vaccination against yellow fever for entry into the country, CDC recommends yellow fever vaccination for all travelers aged ≥9 months going to areas with risk for transmission. Updated information on areas of risk can be found on the CDC Travelers' Health website (https://wwwnc.cdc.gov/travel/destinations/traveler/none/brazil); see Sec. 2, Ch. 5, Yellow Fever Vaccine & Malaria Prevention Information, by Country.

People planning travel to other countries in South America (e.g., Colombia) could be required to show proof of yellow fever vaccination at airline counters before exiting Brazil.

ZIKA

Zika virus is an arbovirus (genus *Flavivirus*) transmitted mainly by mosquitoes, typically, although not exclusively, *Aedes aegypti*. Zika virus also can be sexually transmitted and transmitted during pregnancy to a fetus. First reported in Brazil in 2015, Zika was likely introduced to the country 2 years prior. A large Zika outbreak occurred in 2016, and >215,000 probable cases were reported. By 2019, the number of cases had dropped to 10,000.

Most Zika infections are asymptomatic and, when present, symptoms are mild. Commonly reported signs and symptoms include arthralgia, conjunctivitis, fever, and maculopapular rash; Guillain-Barré syndrome and encephalopathy have also been reported (see Sec. 5, Part 2, Ch. 27, Zika).

Vertical transmission leads to congenital Zika virus infection; sequelae can include microcephaly with central nervous system anomalies, other serious neurologic consequences, and fetal loss. Because of the risk for birth defects in infants born to people infected with Zika during pregnancy, CDC encourages a pretravel discussion of risks with anyone who is pregnant or trying to become pregnant. Zika travel information is available at the CDC Travelers' Health website (https://wwwnc.cdc.gov/travel/page/zika-information).

ENVIRONMENTAL HAZARDS & RISKS

Animal Bites

RABIES

Overall, the risk for rabies infection in Brazil is very low. Preexposure rabies vaccination is recommended for travelers with extended itineraries, particularly children, and people planning trips to rural areas (see Sec. 5, Part 2, Ch. 18, Rabies). For shorter stays, preexposure rabies vaccination is recommended for adventure travelers, those who might be occupationally exposed to animals, and people staying in locations >24 hours away from access to rabies immune globulin (e.g., the Amazon Forest).

SNAKES

Poisonous snakes are a hazard in many places in Brazil, although deaths from snake bites are rare (see Sec. 4, Ch. 7, Zoonotic Exposures: Bites, Stings, Scratches & Other Hazards). Counsel travelers to seek immediate medical attention any time a bite wound breaks the skin, or if a snake sprays venom into their eyes. In some areas of the country, specific antivenoms are available, and being able to identify the snake species (or taking a picture) might prove critical to delivery of optimal medical care. The national toll-free number for intoxication and poisoning assistance is 0800-722-6001 (in Portuguese only).

Climate & Sun Exposure

Ensure travelers to Brazil are familiar with climatic conditions at their destinations before they go. Except in the south, where temperatures peak at 85°F (30°C), temperatures >104°F (40°C) are common in cities along the coast and in the Amazon region during October–March (see Sec. 4, Ch. 2, Extremes of Temperature).

SAFETY & SECURITY

Crime

Travel in Brazil is generally safe, although crime remains a problem in urban areas and has spread to rural areas. The incidence of crime against tourists is greater in areas surrounding beaches, hotels, nightclubs, and other tourist destinations (see Sec. 4, Ch. 11, Safety & Security Overseas). Drug-related violence has resulted in clashes with police in tourist areas. Several Brazilian cities have established specialized police units that patrol areas frequented by tourists and provide assistance to crime victims.

Political Unrest

Political demonstrations might disrupt public and private transportation. Encourage travelers to register with the US Department of State's Smart Traveler Enrollment Program (STEP; https://step.state.gov/step) to receive advisories and alerts for areas they plan to visit.

Prostitution

Although commercial sex work is legal in Brazil, operating a brothel and financial exploitation of sex workers are both against the law.

Traffic-Related Injuries

As in many foreign countries, motor vehicle accidents in Brazil are a leading cause of injury and death among US travelers (see Sec. 8, Ch. 5, Road & Traffic Safety). Road conditions in Brazil differ significantly from those in the United States, and driving at night can be dangerous. The national toll-free number for emergency roadside assistance (193) is in Portuguese only. Driving after drinking alcohol, even small quantities, is illegal, and travelers can expect police checkpoints during evenings and nights in many urban areas. Seatbelt use is mandatory, and motorcyclists are required by law to wear helmets.

Children aged ≤10 years must be seated in the back seat. Brazilian federal law requires infants ≤1 year of age to use rear-facing car seats, children 1–4 years of age to use forward-facing car seats, and children 4–7.5 years of age to use booster seats. Anyone traveling with small children should bring their own car or booster seats, in the event these are limited or unavailable.

AVAILABILITY & QUALITY OF MEDICAL CARE

Quality health care is available in most sizable Brazilian cities. Brazilian public health services are free, even for visitors. Foreign visitors can seek treatment in the emergency care network of Brazil's public health system, known as the Unified Health System, or by its Portuguese acronym, SUS, or through private facilities. A non-comprehensive list of private medical services can be found on the US Embassy in Brazil website (https://br.usembassy.gov). The toll-free emergency number for ambulance services throughout Brazil is 192. The Brazilian Ministry of Health provides information in Portuguese for international visitors (see www.gov.br/anvisa/pt-br/assuntos/paf/saude-do-viajante), including a list of reference hospitals for mass gathering events in Brazil.

Medical Tourism

Brazil has a growing number of private clinics that cater to international clientele and offer medical procedures using advanced technologies. Travel to Brazil for cosmetic surgery, assisted reproductive technology, or other elective medical procedures has increased in recent years, becoming a major part of the medical industry. Although the quality of care overall can vary widely, Brazil has many cosmetic surgery facilities on par with those found in the United States. Travelers seeking cosmetic surgery or other elective procedures should do their research and make sure that emergency medical services are available at their clinic of choice (see Sec. 6, Ch. 4, Medical Tourism).

BIBLIOGRAPHY

Hamer DH, Angelo K, Caumes E, van Genderen PJJ, Florescu SA, Popescu CP, et al. Fatal yellow fever in travelers to Brazil, 2018. MMWR Morb Mortal Wkly Rep. 2018;67(11):340–1.

Malaria Atlas Project. Country profile: Brazil. Available from: https://malariaatlas.org/trends/country/BRA.

Melo CFCAE, Vasconcelos PFDC, Alcantara LCJ, Araujo WN. The obscurance of the greatest sylvatic yellow fever epidemic and the cooperation of the Pan American Health Organization during the COVID-19 pandemic. Rev Soc Bras Med Trop. 2020;53:e20200787.

Ministry of Health. Epidemiological bulletin: special issue. Chagas disease World Day, 14 April; year 2 [in Portuguese]. Brasilia: The Ministry; 2021. Available from: www.gov.br/saude/pt-br/centrais-de-conteudo/publicacoes/boletins/boletins-epidemiologicos/especiais/2021/boletim_especial_chagas_14abr21_b.pdf.

Ministry of Health. Ministry of Health. Epidemiological bulletin 41. Monitoring of cases of urban arboviruses transmitted by *Aedes aegypti* (dengue, chikungunya and Zika), epidemiological weeks 01 to 52 [in Portuguese]. Brasilia: The Ministry; 2020. Available from: www.gov.br/saude/pt-br/centrais-de-conteudo/publicacoes/boletins/boletins-epidemiologicos/edicoes/2020/boletim_epidemiologico_svs_41.pdf.

Nobrega AA, Garcia MH, Tatto E, Obara MT, Costa E, Sobel J, et al. Oral transmission of Chagas disease by consumption of acai palm fruit, Brazil. Emerg Infect Dis. 2009;15(4):653–5.

Petersen E, Wilson ME, Touch S, McCloskey B, Mwaba P, Bates M, et al. Rapid spread of Zika virus in the Americas—implications for public health preparedness for mass gatherings at the 2016 Brazil Olympic Games. Int J Infect Dis. 2016;44:11–5.

Possas C, Lourenço-de-Oliveira R, Tauil PL, Pinheiro FP, Pissinatti A, Cunha RVD, et al. Yellow fever outbreak in Brazil: the puzzle of rapid viral spread and challenges for immunisation. Mem Inst Oswaldo Cruz. 2018;113(10):e180278.

Sabino EC, Buss LF, Carvalho MPS, Prete CA Jr, Crispim MAE, Fraiji NA, et al. Resurgence of COVID-19 in Manaus, Brazil, despite high seroprevalence. Lancet. 2021;397(10273):452–5.

Silva MMO, Tauro LB, Kikuti M, Anjos RO, Santos VC, Gonçalves TSF, et al. Concomitant transmission of dengue, chikungunya, and Zika viruses in Brazil: clinical and epidemiological findings from surveillance for acute febrile illness. Clin Infect Dis. 2019;69(8):1353–9.

DOMINICAN REPUBLIC

Macarena García, Luis Bonilla, Bianca Alvarez

DESTINATION OVERVIEW

The Dominican Republic—the second-largest Caribbean nation, both by area and by population—covers the eastern two-thirds of the Caribbean Island of Hispaniola; Haiti comprises the western third. The capital city, Santo Domingo, is located on the southern coast of the island (see Map 10-07). Although English is spoken in most tourist areas, Spanish is the official language. Approximately 250,000 US citizens call the Dominican Republic home. Average temperatures range from 73.5°F (23°C) in January to 80°F (26.5°C) in August. The island receives more rain during May–November, and tropical storms or hurricanes are possible.

DOMINICAN REPUBLIC

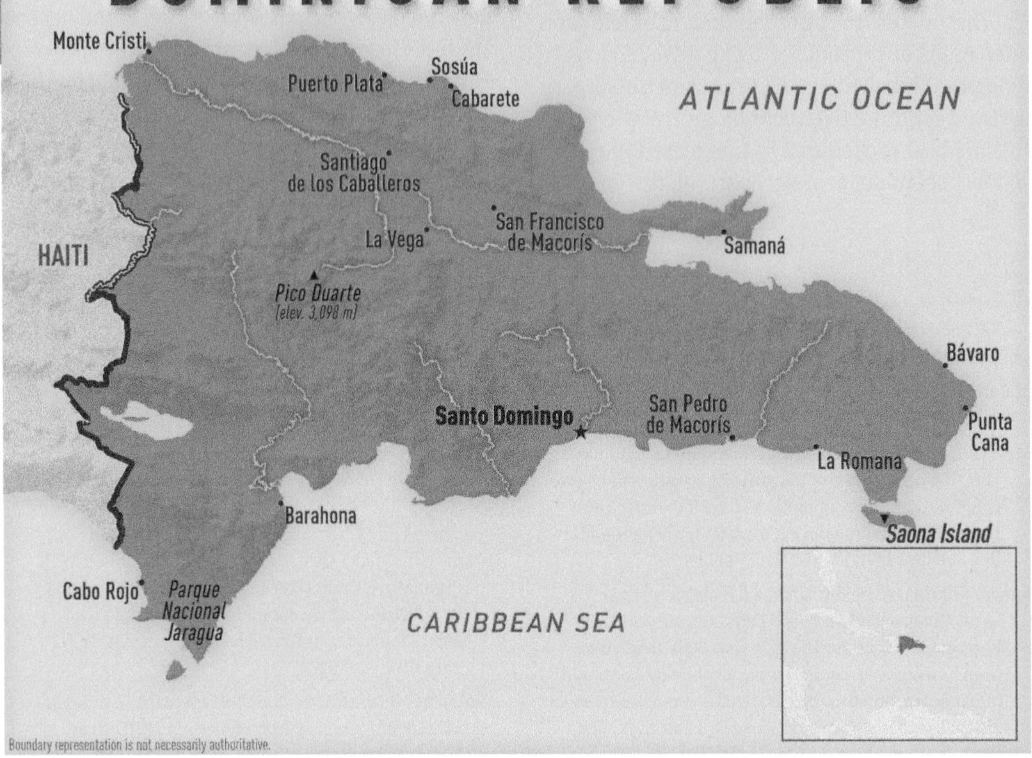

Boundary representation is not necessarily authoritative.

MAP 10-07 Dominican Republic

In 2018, >6.5 million foreign tourists, including ≈3 million from Canada and the United States, visited the Dominican Republic, making it the most visited destination in the Caribbean. The Dominican Republic offers a diverse geography of beaches, mountain ranges (including the highest point in the Caribbean, Pico Duarte [3,098 m; 10,164 ft]), sugar cane and tobacco plantations, and farmland. Most tourism is concentrated in the east of the country around Bávaro and Punta Cana, which offer all-inclusive beach resorts.

Whale watching is popular seasonally near the northeastern area, Samaná, and kitesurfing and windsurfing attract visitors to the northern areas of Puerto Plata, Sosúa, and Cabarete. Santo Domingo has an attractive colonial district that contains many historical sites dating back to Christopher Columbus's arrival in the New World. Few travelers visit other parts of the country, where tourist infrastructure is limited or nonexistent.

INFECTIOUS DISEASE RISKS

All travelers should be up to date on routine vaccinations, including coronavirus disease 2019 (COVID-19) and seasonal influenza. Cases of vaccine-preventable diseases have been reported among the local population and unvaccinated tourists from Europe and other parts of the world. Travelers also should be vaccinated against hepatitis A.

Enteric Infections & Diseases

CHOLERA

The most recent cholera outbreak in the Dominican Republic occurred in 2018 in Independencia Province and was readily contained. Since then, no cholera cases have been reported. For current recommendations for travelers to the Dominican Republic, visit the Centers for Disease Control and Prevention Travelers' Health website, https://wwwnc.cdc.gov/travel/destinations/traveler/none/dominican-republic.

TRAVELERS' DIARRHEA

Although food hygiene at large, all-inclusive resorts and popular tourist locations has improved in the past few years, travelers' diarrhea (TD) continues to be the most common health problem for visitors to the Dominican Republic (see Sec. 2, Ch. 6, Travelers' Diarrhea). Food purchased on the street or sold on beaches by informal sellers presents a greater risk for illness (see Sec. 2, Ch. 8, Food & Water Precautions). Advise travelers not to eat raw or undercooked seafood, and remind them to drink only purified, bottled water. Ice served in well-established tourist locations is usually made from purified water and safe to consume. Ice might not be safe in remote or non-tourist areas, however.

TYPHOID FEVER

Travelers should be vaccinated against typhoid fever, especially anyone visiting friends or relatives (see Sec. 5, Part 1, Ch. 24, Typhoid & Paratyphoid Fever).

Respiratory Infections & Diseases

CORONAVIRUS DISEASE 2019

For current information on COVID-19 in the Dominican Republic, consult the US Embassy in the Dominican Republic website (https://do.usembassy.gov/). For the US government's COVID-19 international travel requirements and recommendations, see www.cdc.gov/coronavirus/2019-ncov/travelers/international-travel/index.html. All travelers going to the Dominican Republic should be up to date with their COVID-19 vaccines (www.cdc.gov/coronavirus/2019-ncov/vaccines/stay-up-to-date.html).

TUBERCULOSIS

In 2019, the National Tuberculosis (TB) Control Program reported an incidence of 30.4 TB cases per 100,000 inhabitants. Although there is community spread of TB, no reports exist of travelers or tourists becoming infected with TB while visiting the Dominican Republic.

Sexually Transmitted Infections & HIV

Although illegal, commercial sex workers (CSW) are found throughout the Dominican Republic; Samaná, Sosúa, and Puerto Plata are known sex tourism destinations. HIV prevalence among female CSW is ≈3%, and up to 6% in some areas; syphilis (12%), hepatitis B virus (2.4%), and hepatitis C virus (0.9%) are also concerns. Among men who have sex with men, HIV prevalence is ≤4.5% and active syphilis ≤13.9%. Travelers should avoid sexual intercourse with CSW and always use condoms with any partner whose HIV or sexually transmitted infection status is unknown (see Sec. 9, Ch. 12, Sex & Travel). Hepatitis B vaccine is recommended for people who could be exposed to blood through needles or medical procedures, or body fluids during sexual intercourse with a new partner.

Soil- & Waterborne Infections

LEPTOSPIROSIS

Leptospirosis is prevalent on the island; in 2020, 210 leptospirosis cases and 38 deaths were reported. *Leptospira* contamination can be attributed to climatic conditions (e.g., heavy rainfall, flooding) and to environmental factors, including agricultural practices, animal husbandry, inadequate disposal of waste, and poor sanitation. Travelers should avoid recreational activities in lakes and rivers, and other unprotected exposures to fresh water potentially contaminated with animal urine (see Sec. 5, Part 1, Ch. 10, Leptospirosis).

SCHISTOSOMIASIS

Based on the results of a 2013 serological survey conducted in provinces with a history of schistosomiasis transmission, the Dominican Republic has likely eliminated schistosomiasis transmission. This status has not yet been verified according to World Health Organization (WHO) criteria.

Vectorborne Diseases

Vectorborne viral diseases (e.g., dengue), as well as parasitic diseases (e.g., malaria) are potential concerns for travelers to the Dominican Republic. All travelers should take precautions to prevent mosquito bites by wearing long-sleeved shirts and long pants and by using insect repellent (see Sec. 4, Ch. 6, Mosquitoes, Ticks & Other Arthropods).

ARBOVIRUSES: CHIKUNGUNYA, DENGUE & ZIKA

Dengue is widespread in the Dominican Republic; 3,964 cases and 38 deaths were reported in 2020. Although cases of dengue are reported year-round, transmission frequently increases during the rainy season, May–November. The principal mosquito vector of the dengue virus, *Aedes aegypti*, is found in both rural and urban areas in the Dominican Republic (see Sec. 5, Part 2, Ch. 4, Dengue). Neither chikungunya nor Zika have been detected in the Dominican Republic for several years.

LYMPHATIC FILARIASIS

The Dominican Republic is actively participating in the global program to eliminate lymphatic filariasis (LF). LF is considered endemic to some smaller foci in the east and southwest regions of the country. As of 2020, the country had achieved targets set by the WHO to stop annual treatment, suggesting low likelihood of ongoing disease transmission and minimal risk to travelers. The Dominican Republic is still working to achieve all targets demonstrating elimination of LF as a public health problem (see Sec. 5, Part 3, Ch. 9, Lymphatic Filariasis, and the WHO website, www.who.int/en/news-room/fact-sheets/detail/lymphatic-filariasis#).

MALARIA

10

Malaria is endemic to the Dominican Republic (see Sec. 2, Ch. 5, Yellow Fever Vaccine & Malaria Prevention Information, by Country, and Sec. 5, Part 3, Ch. 16, Malaria). During 2020, a total of 822 cases of malaria were reported; 2 were fatal.

Malaria transmission occurs primarily in the provinces near the border with Haiti, and the provinces of La Altagracia (including the resort areas of Bávaro and Punta Cana), San Cristóbal, San Juan, and Santo Domingo. In the Distrito Nacional, city of Santo Domingo (the capital), transmission has been reported in the Los Tres Brazos and La Ciénaga areas. Transmission is rare in other places. The malaria species found in the Dominican Republic, *Plasmodium falciparum*, remains sensitive to all known antimalarial drugs, including chloroquine. Malaria chemoprophylaxis is recommended for travelers to provinces of the Dominican Republic with documented transmission.

ENVIRONMENTAL HAZARDS & RISKS

Animal Bites & Rabies

Reports of animal rabies in the Dominican Republic are not uncommon, and the last reported case of human rabies was in 2019. In 2020, no cases of animal rabies or human rabies were reported. Postexposure rabies prophylaxis is available in specialized and regional hospitals. Consider preexposure vaccination for travelers potentially at risk for animal bites (e.g., people spending extended time outdoors, anyone handling animals). Advise travelers to avoid petting or playing with animals.

Climate & Sun Exposure

Visitors to the Dominican Republic often underestimate the strength of the sun and the dehydrating effect of the humid environment. Encourage travelers to take precautions to avoid sunburn by wearing hats and suitable clothing, along with proper application of a broad-spectrum sunscreen with a sun protection factor (SPF) ≥15 that protects against both ultraviolet A and B (see Sec. 4, Ch. 1, Sun Exposure). Travelers should drink plenty of hydrating fluids throughout the day.

Toxic Exposures

METHANOL

Poisonings from consuming methanol-contaminated ethanol in fermented beverages occur in both resort areas and in the community in the Dominican Republic. In December 2017, an outbreak involved 41 vacationers in the resort areas of Punta Cana. In December 2019, 4 people became sick and 2 died from methanol poisoning. In a community outbreak in November 2020, 9 men in the Santo Domingo Este municipality suffered methanol poisoning after consuming a contaminated drink. During January–April 2021, an outbreak involving >300 people, predominantly in the northern and northeastern regions of the country, was traced to drinking adulterated ethanol; >100 died. The majority of cases occurred the week after the long Easter weekend.

SAFETY & SECURITY

Crime

The risk for crime in the Dominican Republic is like that of major cities in the United States. Although most crime affecting tourists involves robbery or pickpocketing, more serious assaults occasionally occur, and perpetrators might react violently if resisted (see Sec. 4, Ch. 11, Safety & Security Overseas). Visitors to the Dominican Republic should follow normal safety precautions (e.g., going out in groups, especially at night; using only licensed taxi drivers; drinking alcohol in moderation; and being cautious of strangers). Criminal activity often is higher during the Christmas and New Year season, and additional caution during that time is warranted.

Traffic-Related Injuries

Driving in the Dominican Republic is hazardous (see Sec. 8, Ch. 5, Road & Traffic Safety). Traffic laws are rarely enforced, and drivers commonly drive while intoxicated, text while driving, exceed speed limits, do not respect red lights or stop signs, and drive without seatbelts or helmets. According to WHO statistics, the Dominican Republic has the highest number of traffic deaths per capita in the world (110 per 100,000 population in 2019).

Many fatal or serious traffic crashes involve motorcycles and pedestrians. Motorcycle taxis, used throughout the country, including in tourist areas, frequently carry ≥2 passengers riding without helmets. Remind visitors to avoid motorcycle taxis, to use only licensed taxis, and to always wear a seatbelt.

AVAILABILITY & QUALITY OF MEDICAL CARE

In the Dominican Republic, public medical clinics lack basic resources and supplies, and few or no English-speaking staff are available. In addition, only minimal staff are available overnight in non-emergency wards; if hospitalized, travelers should consider hiring a private nurse to spend the night.

Private hospitals and doctors might offer a more comprehensive range of services but typically require advance payment or proof of adequate insurance before providing medical services or admitting a patient. Some hotels and resorts have preestablished, exclusive arrangements with select medical providers; these can have additional, associated costs, and might also limit choices for emergency medical care.

Psychological and psychiatric services are limited, even in the larger cities, with hospital-based care available only through government institutions.

Medical Tourism

The market for medical tourism, including plastic surgery and dental care, is growing in the Dominican Republic. Thousands of patients travel to the country each year to access medical services that cost a fraction of what they do in the United States. Several companies and clinics offer package deals that include postsurgical recovery at local tourist resorts. Most health care facilities catering to medical tourists have not, however, met the standards required by international accrediting bodies.

Some medical tourists to the Dominican Republic have experienced a substandard quality of care, health care–associated infections, and even death. Anyone considering the Dominican Republic as a destination for medical procedures should consult with a US health care provider before travel, and research whether the health care providers and facilities in the Dominican Republic meet accepted standards of care (see Sec. 6, Ch. 4, Medical Tourism). Legal options in case of malpractice are very limited in the Dominican Republic.

10

BIBLIOGRAPHY

Dominican Republic Ministry of Public Health. Annual national TB bulletin 2019 [in Spanish]. Santo Domingo (DR): The Ministry; 2019. Available from: https://repositorio.sns.gob.do/download/17/boletines-tuberculosis/786/boletin-tuberculosis-2019.pdf.

Dominican Republic Ministry of Public Health. Weekly epidemiological bulletin #16-2021 [in Spanish]. Santo Domingo (DR): The Ministry; 2021. Available from: www.digepisalud.gob.do/docs/Boletines%20epidemiologicos/Boleti

nes%20semanales/2021/Boletin%20Semanal%20 16-2021.pdf.

Dominican Republic Ministry of Public Health. Weekly epidemiological bulletin #19-2021 [in Spanish]. Santo Domingo (DR): The Ministry; 2021. Available from: www.digepisalud.gob.do/docs/Boletines%20epidemio logicos/Boletines%20semanales/2021/Boletin%20Sema nal%2019-2021.pdf.

Dominican Republic Ministry of Public Health. Weekly epidemiological bulletin #42-2021 [in Spanish]. Santo Domingo (DR): The Ministry; 2021. Available from: www.digepisalud.gob.do/docs/Boletines%20epidemio logicos/Boletines%20semanales/2021/Boletin%20Sema nal%2042-2021.pdf.

Ekdahl K, de Jong B, Andersson Y. Risk of travel-associated typhoid and paratyphoid fevers in various regions. J Travel Med. 2005;12(4):197–204.

Hewitt R, Willingham AL. Status of schistosomiasis elimination in the Caribbean region. Trop Med Infect Dis. 2019;4(1):24.

International Federation of Red Cross and Red Crescent Societies. Disaster Response Emergency Fund (DREF) Emergency Plan of Action (EPoA), Dominican Republic: cholera outbreak. DREF no. MDRDO011, 2018. Available from: https://reliefweb.int/sites/reliefweb.int/files/resources/MDRDO011do.pdf.

National Council for HIV AIDS. Third survey of behavioral surveillance with serological linkage in key populations [in Spanish]. Santo Domingo (DR): CONIVISIDA; 2018. Available from: www.conavihsida.gob.do/images/phocadownload/MYE/Encuestas_comportamiento_vin culacion_serologica/Tercera_Encuesta_Vigilancia%20 3EVCVS_2018.pdf.

Presidency of the Dominican Republic. Under the slogan "For zero cases of human rabies in the Dominican Republic," government begins National Day of Vaccination against rabies; Oct 29, 2021 [in Spanish]. Available from: https://presidencia.gob.do/noticias/bajo-el-lema-por-cero-casos-de-rabia-humana-en-republica-dominicana-gobierno-inicia.

HAITI

Stanley Juin, Macarthur Charles, Timbila Koama, Chung (Ken) Chen

10

DESTINATION OVERVIEW

The Republic of Haiti is a country located on the island of Hispaniola in the Greater Antilles archipelago of the Caribbean Sea (see Map 10-08). The shared border between Haiti and the Dominican Republic is porous; migrant workers move readily between the 2 countries, and cultural influences are shared. North America and France have large Haitian diaspora communities. Travelers visiting friends and relatives (VFR) make up a large proportion of visitors to Haiti each year. Other reasons people come to Haiti include foreign diplomacy, international business, missionary and humanitarian aid work, and tourism.

Port-au-Prince, Haiti's capital, is often the main entry point for international arrivals. Haiti has many tourist destinations, including a popular cruise ship destination in Labadie (Port Labadee), which has white sand beaches and scenery that attract visitors year-round. Historical architecture sites (e.g., Cathédrale Notre-Dame in the city of Cap-Haïtien; Citadelle Laferrière, reputedly the largest fortress in the Americas and a UNESCO World Heritage Site, located on top of mountain Bonnet à l'Evèque) are popular tourist destinations. The annual Haitian Carnival, which takes place in February or March, draws crowds from around the world. Haiti has strong economic and social ties with international organizations; as such, business travelers, foreign diplomats, humanitarian aid workers, and missionaries often visit Haiti.

Travelers can find various types of accommodations in Haiti, ranging from dormitory-style to bed-and-breakfast inns to house rentals and upscale hotels in major cities. Most accommodations include internet, but signal and reliability are often poor due to interruptions of services within the country.

INFECTIOUS DISEASE RISKS

Environmental degradation has contributed to Haiti's poor sanitation and water quality. As a result,

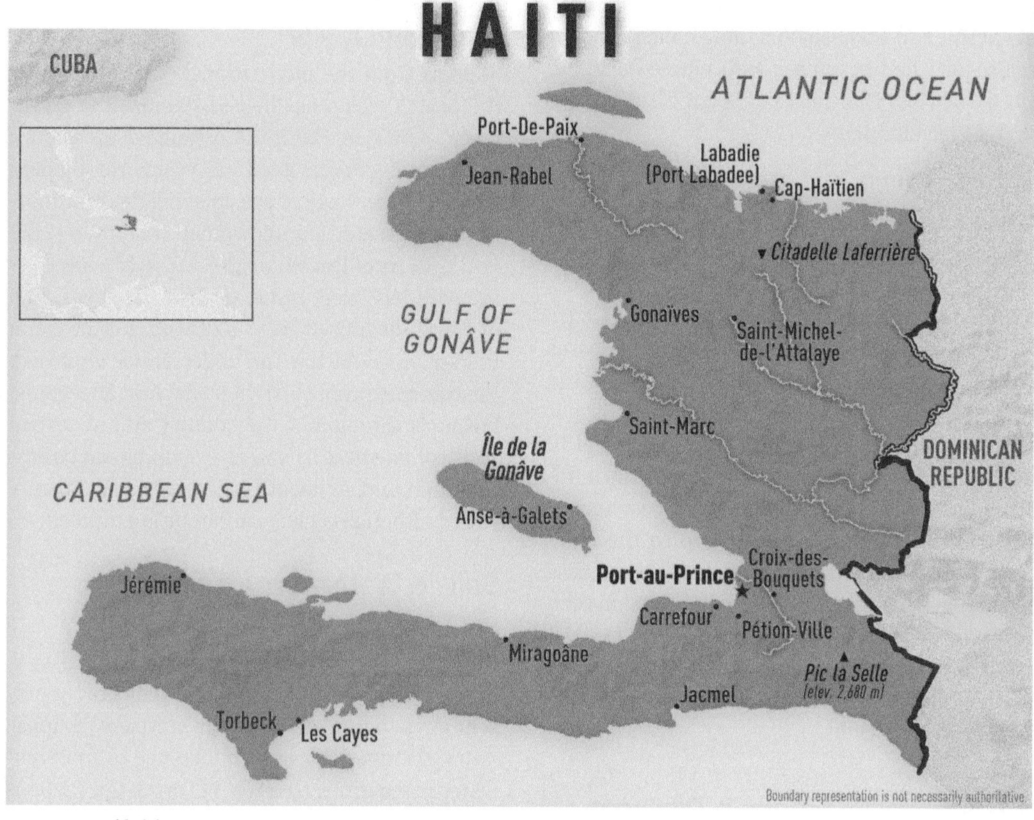

MAP 10-08 Haiti

multiple public health risks exist for Haitians and for travelers to Haiti. Anyone traveling to Haiti should be up to date on routine vaccinations, including diphtheria (cases have increased in recent years) and tetanus boosters, seasonal influenza, and measles. Although measles has been eliminated in Haiti, the risk for reintroduction is ever-present.

Enteric Infections & Diseases

CHOLERA

As of February 2021, the cholera outbreak that started after the 2010 earthquake had caused 820,555 suspected cases of illness and 9,792 deaths. The epidemic curve peaked in 2011, with declining incidence and mortality rates annually due to improved access to clean water and sanitation and the efforts of cholera treatment centers. In 2019, 9 years after the outbreak started, Haiti reported 720 suspected cholera cases and only 3 deaths. In October 2022, after 3 years of no reports of culture-confirmed cholera, Haiti's National Public Health Laboratory identified new cases of culture-confirmed disease and was investigating additional suspect cases.

Despite declining cases, cholera remains a persistent public health threat in Haiti. Oral cholera vaccine has been implemented as part of a complementary set of ongoing control measures that include improved diarrheal disease surveillance and enhanced laboratory capacity. Travelers should adhere to food and water precautions, and—depending on their planned itinerary—consider cholera vaccine (see Sec. 5, Part 1, Ch. 5, Cholera). For current recommendations, see the Centers for Disease Control and Prevention (CDC) Travelers' Health destination page for Haiti (https://wwwnc.cdc.gov/travel/destinations/traveler/none/haiti).

TRAVELERS' DIARRHEA

Visitors to Haiti are at high risk for travelers' diarrhea (TD). Travelers who want to experience the local flavorful cuisine (e.g., *griot* [seasoned fried pork], plantains, rice with red beans, and a variety of fish and shellfish, including conch), should select food and beverages with care (see Sec. 2, Ch. 6, Travelers' Diarrhea, and Sec. 2, Ch. 8, Food & Water Precautions).

TYPHOID FEVER

Without prompt treatment, *Salmonella enterica* serotype Typhi infection can cause serious morbidity and mortality (Sec. 5, Part 1, Ch. 24, Typhoid & Paratyphoid Fever). On average, Haiti's Ministry of Health reports 1,200 suspected cases weekly throughout the country. Although the true extent of typhoid infection in Haiti is not fully known, cases are reported regularly in all 10 departments. Due to major public health infrastructure investments (sanitation, access to safe drinking water) made in response to the cholera outbreak, the number of typhoid fever cases has been decreasing, but disease transmission remains active. Urge all travelers to adhere to strict food and water precautions, and—depending on their planned itinerary—to consider receiving typhoid fever vaccine.

Respiratory Infections & Diseases

CORONAVIRUS DISEASE 2019

For current information on coronavirus disease 2019 (COVID-19) in Haiti, consult the US Embassy in Haiti website (https://ht.usembassy.gov). For the US government's COVID-19 international travel requirements and recommendations, see www.cdc.gov/coronavirus/2019-ncov/travelers/international-travel/index.html. All travelers going to Haiti should be up to date with their COVID-19 vaccines (www.cdc.gov/coronavirus/2019-ncov/vaccines/stay-up-to-date.html).

TUBERCULOSIS

Tuberculosis (TB) is more prevalent in Haiti than in neighboring countries. Using appropriate and effective strategies, the Programme National de Lutte contre la Tuberculose (PNLT) has been able to improve case detection and treatment throughout the country. Short-term travelers are not at high risk of tuberculosis unless they are residing or spending extended time in specific crowded environments (e.g., shared room hostels, prisons).

Sexually Transmitted Infections & HIV

Support from the international community over the past 20 years has helped stabilize the prevalence of HIV in Haiti; the estimated prevalence is 2% among adults aged >15 years. Among people 15–24 years age of age, infection is disproportionately greater among women than men (2.3% vs. 1.6%). As of December 2020, 85% of people living with HIV were aware of their diagnosis, 83% of those diagnosed were receiving antiretroviral therapy, and 72% have an undetectable viral load. Preexposure prophylaxis is available at all regional hospitals throughout the country and at several high-volume health centers. Condoms can be easily purchased at local pharmacies and grocery stores, although quality cannot be guaranteed.

Soil- & Waterborne Infections

HELMINTHS

Although the prevalence of helminthiasis is diminishing in Haiti, intestinal parasites represent a potential concern for travelers, emphasizing the need for strict adherence to food and water precautions (see Sec. 5, Part 3, Ch. 13, Soil-Transmitted Helminths).

Vectorborne Diseases

Vectorborne diseases, both viral and parasitic, are common in Haiti and include dengue and *Plasmodium falciparum* malaria. Travelers to Haiti should take measures to protect themselves from mosquito bites (see Sec. 4, Ch. 6, Mosquitoes, Ticks & Other Arthropods).

ARBOVIRUSES: CHIKUNGUNYA, DENGUE & ZIKA

In 2021, ongoing dengue surveillance in Haiti confirmed 18 cases out of >5,000 specimens tested through October of that year. Seroprevalence studies conducted in 2017 found ≈72% of Haitians had been exposed to dengue, confirming the results of a previous study conducted in 2012. Advise longer-term travelers to Haiti to select accommodations with air conditioning or well-screened windows and doors; to wear clothes that cover the arms and legs; and to use insect repellent. No confirmed cases of chikungunya or Zika have been documented in Haiti since June 2014.

LYMPHATIC FILARIASIS

Haiti actively participates in the global program to eliminate lymphatic filariasis (LF). LF is considered endemic to Hispaniola, including many parts of Haiti. As of 2020, several areas of the country, including Port-au-Prince, still require annual mass treatment campaigns aimed at reducing parasite transmission (see www.who.int/en/news-room/fact-sheets/detail/lymphatic-filariasis#). Prevention involves adherence to insect bite precautions (see Sec. 5, Part 3, Ch. 9, Lymphatic Filariasis).

MALARIA

Chloroquine-sensitive *P. falciparum* malaria is endemic to Haiti (see Sec. 2, Ch. 5, Yellow Fever Vaccine and Malaria Prevention Information, by Country). The incidence of malaria has been decreasing since 2016; current incidence is ≈70 cases per 100,000 people, annually. The highest transmission rates are reported to occur after the rainy seasons, March–May and October–November. Malaria is a localized infection in Haiti and is reported primarily from the Southern region. Nevertheless, CDC recommends that all travelers to Haiti, regardless of itinerary, take malaria chemoprophylaxis (see Sec. 5, Part 3, Ch. 16, Malaria).

ENVIRONMENTAL HAZARDS & RISKS

Animal Bites & Rabies

Haiti is more affected by rabies than any other nation in the Americas. Prevention efforts in the country have increased, but with a high number of stray dogs, the number of cases of human rabies is not yet clearly defined. Preexposure rabies vaccination is recommended for travelers anticipating contact with animals. Travelers with high-risk exposures for rabies generally require medical evacuation to the United States to receive definitive care and management, including appropriate postexposure prophylaxis (see Sec 5, Part 2, Ch. 18, Rabies).

Ciguatera Fish Poisoning

Ciguatera fish poisoning commonly occurs in Haiti. Outbreaks can happen seasonally or sporadically, particularly after storms. Not all fish of a given species or from a given area will necessarily be toxic. Travelers to Haiti should avoid eating reef fish weighing >2.7 kg (6 lbs) or the filets of large fish (see Sec. 4, Ch. 10, Food Poisoning from Marine Toxins).

Climate & Sun Exposure

With some variation depending on elevation, the climate in Haiti is tropical and hot, and remains so throughout the year. Haiti has an average monthly temperature range of 77°F–84°F. Humidity is often high, and microclimates exist depending on the geographic location. Travelers should minimize sun exposure and use a broad-spectrum sunscreen (see Sec. 4, Ch. 1, Sun Exposure). Sunscreen products are not always available in local markets, however, and travelers should pack enough to last them for the duration of their travel.

Natural Disasters

Natural disasters are common in Haiti, including earthquakes, floods, hurricanes, and tropical storms. Hurricane season lasts from June–November. In 2008, Haiti experienced a series of 4 hurricanes and tropical storms within 2 months. Hurricane Matthew, the first Category 4 hurricane to hit the island since 1964, struck Haiti in October 2016; 546 people died and >120,000 were displaced. Strong winds and heavy rain caused flash floods, mudslides, river floods, crop and vegetation loss, and destruction of homes and businesses. One year later, rain and flooding from Hurricane Irma compounded the losses to Haiti's agricultural sector. These combined disasters further weakened an already fragile infrastructure.

In January 2010, Haiti experienced a 7.0 magnitude earthquake that killed >220,000 people and displaced 1.5 million people from their homes. More recently, on August 14, 2021, a magnitude 7.2 earthquake struck southwest Haiti, about 70 miles west of the capital of Port-au-Prince, killing ≈2,200 people and injuring >12,000. In addition, 28 of the 66 health facilities in the region were severely damaged or destroyed. Two days later, tropical storm Grace made landfall causing flooding and complicating relief efforts. Together, these emergencies have strained Haiti's health care system immensely.

SAFETY & SECURITY

Crime

The crime rate in Haiti is high, particularly in Port-au-Prince, presenting persistent safety concerns for travelers. Although much of the violent crime is perpetrated by Haitians against Haitians, American citizens also have been victims (see Sec. 4, Ch. 11, Safety & Security Overseas). Travelers arriving on flights from the United States have been targeted for robbery and attack.

During Carnival, crime, disorderly conduct, and general congestion increase. Advise travelers to maintain awareness of their surroundings, avoid nighttime travel, keep valuables well hidden (not left in parked vehicles), and to lock all doors and windows.

Political Unrest

Political and civil unrest represents a safety concern for visitors to Haiti. Frequent and sometimes spontaneous protests occur in Port-au-Prince. Demonstrations—which travelers should avoid, when possible—can turn violent. The US Department of State's Smart Traveler Enrollment Program (STEP; https://step.state.gov/step) electronically pushes information to travelers about safety conditions at their destination and provides direct embassy contact in case of man-made emergencies (political unrest and demonstrations, rioting, terrorist activity) or natural disasters.

10

Traffic-Related Injuries

Motor vehicle injuries are the most common cause of death for healthy US residents traveling abroad (see Sec. 8, Ch. 5, Road & Traffic Safety). The risk for death from road injuries in Haiti is high; the 2019 average rate was 18.77 per 100,000 population, compared with an average rate of 15.33 for the Americas region. Road conditions in Haiti differ greatly from those in the United States; roads and lanes are generally unmarked, speed limits are seldom posted or adhered to, rights of way are not observed, and animals, carts, and vendors all share the roads with motor vehicles. Some roads are unpaved or have large potholes. Lack of streetlights significantly compounds the risk of being on roads at night.

Traffic is usually chaotic and congested in urban areas. Vibrantly painted *tap taps* are open-air vehicles (buses or pick-up trucks), mechanically unsound, and often overloaded with passengers. Although *tap taps* are a common form of public transportation for Haitians, advise travelers to avoid using them because of safety concerns (crashes, kidnappings, robberies). Remind travelers to remain alert when walking, to choose safe vehicles, and to observe safety practices when operating vehicles. Travelers should fasten seat belts when riding in cars, and wear a helmet when riding bicycles or motorbikes.

AVAILABILITY & QUALITY OF MEDICAL CARE

According to the World Health Organization, delivery of primary health care services was already challenged in Haiti before the 2021 earthquake. Since then, the health care situation has become even more complicated; many facilities, primarily in the south, are unable to function because of physical damage, and medical facilities can close without notice due to social unrest.

The Haitian health care system faces multiples shortages (e.g., limited availability of essential medicines and supplies, lack of trained health professionals) and is costly. Over 40% of the population report not having used the public health care system, even in cases of serious injury or illness, principally due to the cost. Thus, access to health care, especially for medical emergencies remains a challenge in Haiti, and medical evacuation often is necessary for patients who require immediate attention. Consequently, people planning travel to Haiti should purchase travel health insurance and medical evacuation insurance (see Sec. 6, Ch. 1, Travel Insurance, Travel Health Insurance & Medical Evacuation Insurance) and bring a travel first aid kit (see Sec. 2, Ch. 10, Travel Health Kits).

BIBLIOGRAPHY

Institute for Health Metrics and Evaluation. Haiti. Available from: www.healthdata.org/haiti.

Institut Haïtien de l'Enfance (IHE) and ICF. Haiti mortality, morbidity and service utilization survey (EMMUS-VI) 2016–2017 [in French]. Pétion-Ville, (Haiti) and Rockville (MD): Institut Haïtien de l'Enfance and ICF; 2018. Available from: www.dhsprogram.com/pubs/pdf/FR326/FR326.pdf.

International Association for Medical Assistance to Travellers. Ciguatera fish poisoning. Available from: www.iamat.org/risks/ciguatera-fish-poisoning.

Ministère de la Santé Publique et de la Population (MSPP). Sitrep COVID-19 08-07-21 [in French]. Available from: www.mspp.gouv.ht/page-covid-19.

National Oceanic and Atmospheric Administration. National Hurricane Center tropical cyclone report: Hurricane Matthew (AL142016). Miami: The Center; 2017. Available from: www.nhc.noaa.gov/data/tcr/AL142016_Matthew.pdf.

United Nations Development Programme (UNDP) Human Development Report Office. Human development report 2013. The rise of the South: human progress in a diverse world. New York: The Programme; 2013. Available from: http://hdr.undp.org/sites/default/files/reports/14/hdr2013_en_complete.pdf.

US Department of State. Haiti 2017 crime and safety report. Washington, DC: Bureau of Diplomatic Security, Overseas Security Advisory Council; 2017. Available from: www.osac.gov/Content/Report/fcbed0b9-1eda-45a8-b6f4-15f4ae15ebaa.

Weppelmann TA, Burne A, von Fricken ME, Elbadry MA, Beau De Rochars M, Boncy J, et al. A tale of two flaviviruses: a seroepidemiological study of dengue virus and West Nile virus transmission in the Ouest and Sud-Est Departments of Haiti. Am J Trop Med Hyg. 2017;96(1):135–40.

World Food Programme. Haiti. Available from: www.wfp.org/countries/haiti.

World Health Organization. Haiti. Available from: www.who.int/countries/hti/en.

MEXICO

Sonia Montiel, Alba Phippard, Kathleen Moser

DESTINATION OVERVIEW

Mexico, the second most populous country in Latin America (population >120 million), is the country most often visited by US tourists. Many US residents, particularly in the border region, frequent Mexico to visit friends and relatives, contributing to the nearly 200 million US–Mexico land border crossings annually. The capital, Mexico City, is one of the world's largest cities (population >20 million) and is a popular destination for business and mass gathering events.

Mexico's diverse geography throughout its 32 states attracts travelers for nature, recreation, and sport (Map 10-09). The country's rich history, diverse cuisine, and proud culture reflects its pre-Columbian and Hispanic past. In the past decade, travelers to Mexico have increasingly sought health and wellness services throughout the country.

INFECTIOUS DISEASE RISKS

All travelers should be up to date on their routine immunizations. Varicella is endemic to Mexico, and measles and mumps outbreaks in Mexico have coincided with worldwide and regional outbreaks. Hepatitis A is also endemic to Mexico; visitors should receive ≥1 dose of the hepatitis A vaccine series before travel.

Enteric Infections & Diseases

CHOLERA

Isolated cases and outbreaks of *Vibrio cholera* occur occasionally in Mexico. Risk for infection is low, however, and cholera vaccination is not recommended for travelers to Mexico.

GIARDIASIS

Giardia is endemic throughout the world. In addition to drinking water precautions, remind travelers to avoid swallowing water when

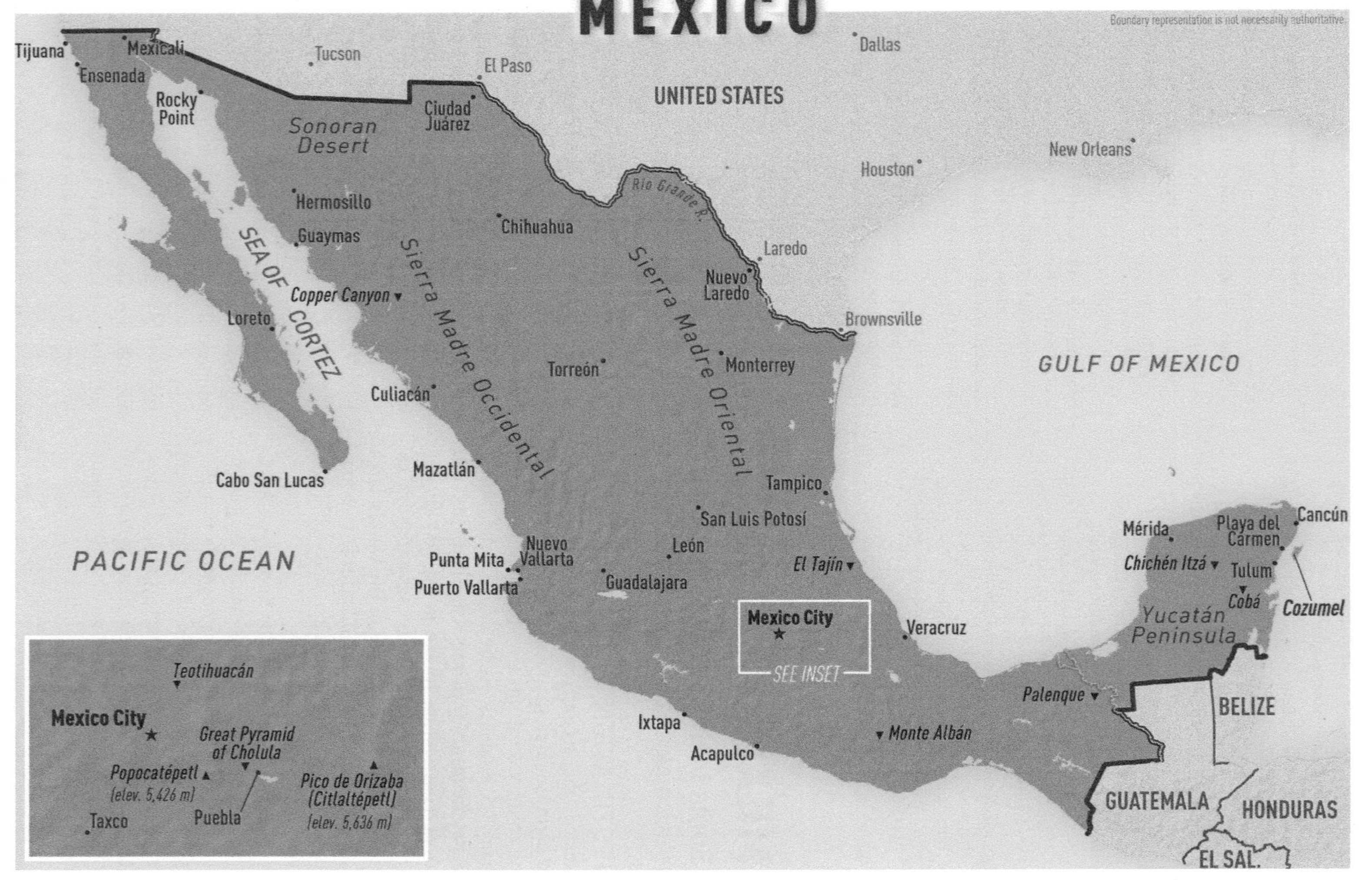
MEXICO
Boundary representation is not necessarily authoritative.
UNITED STATES
Tijuana
Ensenada
Mexicali
Rocky Point
Tucson
Sonoran Desert
Hermosillo
Guaymas
SEA OF CORTEZ
Loreto
Copper Canyon
Cabo San Lucas
Culiacán
Mazatlán
Sierra Madre Occidental
Ciudad Juárez
El Paso
Chihuahua
Torreón
Río Grande R.
Sierra Madre Oriental
Nuevo Laredo
Laredo
Monterrey
Brownsville
Dallas
Houston
New Orleans
GULF OF MEXICO
Tampico
San Luis Potosí
León
Guadalajara
Nuevo Vallarta
Punta Mita
Puerto Vallarta
PACIFIC OCEAN
El Tajín
Mexico City
SEE INSET
Ixtapa
Acapulco
Veracruz
Monte Albán
Palenque
Mérida
Chichén Itzá
Yucatán Peninsula
Playa del Carmen
Cancún
Tulum
Cobá
Cozumel
BELIZE
GUATEMALA
HONDURAS
EL SAL.
Mexico City
Teotihuacán
Great Pyramid of Cholula
Popocatépetl (elev. 5,426 m)
Pico de Orizaba (Citlaltépetl) (elev. 5,636 m)
Puebla
Taxco

MAP 10-09 Mexico

swimming or wading in recreational waters, including pools and lakes (see Sec. 5, Part 3, Ch. 12, Giardiasis).

TAENIASIS & CYSTICERCOSIS

Taeniasis in humans, a tapeworm infection, is caused by ingestion of the eggs of 3 *Taenia* parasite species in raw or undercooked beef or pork (see Sec. 5, Part 3, Ch. 22, Taeniasis). Taeniasis can present as a mild or asymptomatic intestinal infection. Cysticercosis, a more serious infection of muscle, brain, or other tissues, is caused by ingestion of the larval cysts of *Taenia solium* excreted by human carriers (see Sec. 5, Part 3, Ch. 6, Cysticercosis). Over months to decades, the infection can progress to neurocysticercosis, a rare but potentially disabling or fatal infection. *T. solium* is endemic to Mexico. Undercooked vegetables contaminated with *T. solium* larvae could be the major source of cysticercosis infection.

TRAVELERS' DIARRHEA

Travelers' diarrhea commonly affects visitors to Mexico. Education is key to prevention; provide travelers with instructions on safe food and water precautions (see Sec. 2, Ch. 8, Food & Water Precautions). Remind travelers that tap water in Mexico is not potable; that they should avoid consuming unpasteurized, often artisanal, dairy products, particularly soft or fresh cheeses; and that they should avoid eating raw or undercooked meat or fish, leafy greens, or raw vegetables. For further information about travelers' diarrhea, see Sec. 2, Ch. 6, Travelers' Diarrhea.

TYPHOID FEVER

Typhoid fever is endemic to Mexico and can be life-threatening (see Sec. 5, Part 1, Ch. 24, Typhoid & Paratyphoid Fever). The Centers for Disease Control and Prevention (CDC) recommends that most travelers to Mexico get the typhoid vaccine, especially people planning to stay with friends or relatives, and those visiting smaller cities or rural areas. Vaccinated travelers also should follow food and water precautions to prevent typhoid fever and other enteric infections.

Respiratory Infections & Diseases

CORONAVIRUS DISEASE 2019

For current information on coronavirus disease 2019 (COVID-19) in Mexico, consult the US Embassy & Consulates in Mexico website (https://mx.usembassy.gov/). For the US government's COVID-19 international travel requirements and recommendations, see www.cdc.gov/coronavirus/2019-ncov/travelers/international-travel/index.html. All travelers going to Mexico should be up to date with their COVID-19 vaccines (www.cdc.gov/coronavirus/2019-ncov/vaccines/stay-up-to-date.html).

ENDEMIC FUNGI

Coccidioides is endemic to the soil of northwestern Mexico and *Histoplasma* is found mainly in Mexico's central and southeast regions (see Sec. 5, Part 4, Ch. 1, Coccidioidomycosis / Valley Fever, and Sec. 5, Part 4, Ch. 2, Histoplasmosis). Anyone planning to participate in soil disrupting activities (e.g., construction or farming) should be aware of the risks for and symptoms of fungal lung infection, and practice mitigation techniques. For prevention measures, see www.cdc.gov/niosh/topics/valleyfever/default.html and www.cdc.gov/niosh/topics/histoplasmosis/default.html.

INFLUENZA

Influenza strains circulate in Mexico, just as they do in the United States. Pretravel influenza vaccination ≥2 weeks before departure is a prudent health protection measure.

LEGIONNAIRES' DISEASE

Consider legionellosis in the differential diagnosis of travelers who develop pneumonia within 14 days of travel, especially older and immunocompromised people (see Sec. 5, Part 1, Ch. 9, Legionnaires' Disease & Pontiac Fever). Travel histories for people returning from Mexico who were diagnosed with Legionnaires' disease periodically identify associations between the disease and stays at specific hotels and resorts in Mexico.

TUBERCULOSIS

Mexico is considered a moderate-incidence country for tuberculosis (TB). TB incidence in Mexico is lower than in Africa, Asia, and Eastern Europe, but incidence is several-fold greater than in the United States. Help travelers determine their potential for exposure to *Mycobacterium tuberculosis.* Risk for infection is greatest among people intending to remain in Mexico ≥6 months; anyone planning to work in places where they could be exposed to patients with untreated TB (e.g., drug rehabilitation centers, health care settings, prisons, shelters); people planning extended or frequent visits home to spend time with friends and relatives; or people eating unpasteurized dairy products (see Sec. 5, Part 1, Ch. 22, Tuberculosis).

Sexually Transmitted Infections & HIV

HIV prevalence in Mexico is low, except among high-risk populations (e.g., sex workers, injection drug users, men who have sex with men). Other sexually transmitted infections, including chlamydia, gonorrhea, and syphilis, also are more prevalent in these populations. Travelers should avoid condomless sex with unknown or unfamiliar partners (condoms are easily available for purchase in Mexico) and injection drug use.

For people expecting to stay in Mexico ≥6 months, medical tourists, or anyone who might be exposed to blood or other body fluids, including through sexual contact, hepatitis B vaccine is recommended.

Soil- & Waterborne Infections

CUTANEOUS LARVA MIGRANS

More remote (i.e., less visited) beaches pose a risk for cutaneous larva migrans (CLM), a creeping skin eruption commonly associated with dog hookworm infection (see Sec. 5, Part 3, Ch. 4, Cutaneous Larva Migrans, and Sec. 11, Ch. 8, Dermatologic Conditions). Resort areas implementing stray cat and dog removal programs have reduced the chances of infection on their beaches. CLM is preventable by wearing shoes and avoiding direct skin contact with soil and sand.

Vectorborne Diseases

ARBOVIRUSES: CHIKUNGUNYA, DENGUE & ZIKA

Counsel all travelers to Mexico, including those visiting friends or relatives frequently or for extended periods, to take steps to prevent mosquito bites by using insect repellent, wearing long-sleeved shirts and long pants, and staying in accommodations with air conditioning or screens (see Sec. 4, Ch. 6, Mosquitoes, Ticks & Other Arthropods).

Chikungunya has been reported in Mexico since 2014 (see Sec. 5, Part 2, Ch. 2, Chikungunya). Dengue is endemic throughout Mexico; virus transmission is a risk year-round, and large outbreaks occur periodically (see Sec. 5, Part 2, Ch. 4, Dengue). Zika also is a risk in Mexico (see Sec. 5, Part 2, Ch. 27, Zika). Because of the risk for birth defects in infants born to mothers infected with Zika during pregnancy, people who are pregnant or trying to become pregnant, and their sex partners, should be aware of the most recent CDC recommendations at https://wwwnc.cdc.gov/travel/page/zika-information.

LEISHMANIASIS

Sand flies that transmit cutaneous leishmaniasis are found in southern Mexico and along parts of both the Pacific and Gulf coasts (see Sec. 5, Part 3, Ch. 14, Cutaneous Leishmaniasis). Risk for infection is greatest for ecotourists, field biologists, and long-term travelers. Travelers can reduce their risk for sand fly bites by avoiding outdoor activities at night, wearing protective clothing and applying insect repellent to exposed skin and under the edges of clothing; and sleeping in air-conditioned or well-screened areas.

MALARIA

Dramatic decreases in malaria incidence in recent decades mean risk for infection among travelers to Mexico is low. Major resorts are free of the disease, as is the US–Mexico border region. *Plasmodium vivax* malaria prophylaxis is currently recommended only for travelers going to Chiapas and the southern part of Chihuahua (see Sec. 2, Ch. 5, Yellow Fever Vaccine and Malaria Prevention Information, by Country). Mosquito avoidance (but not chemoprophylaxis) is recommended for travelers visiting Campeche, Durango, Nayarit, Quintana Roo, Sinaloa, Sonora, and Tabasco.

RICKETTSIAL DISEASE

In Mexico, rickettsial diseases include tickborne Rocky Mountain spotted fever (RMSF), which potentially is fatal unless treated promptly with a tetracycline; and fleaborne typhus, a disease with dengue-like symptoms (see Sec. 5, Part 1, Ch. 18, Rickettsial Diseases). Mexico's large urban and rural stray dog population is a reservoir for the RMSF vector, *Rhipicephalus sanguineus*, the brown dog tick. Risk for infection is greatest among people who have contact with dogs, and visitors to grassy, brushy, or wooded areas, particularly in states along the US–Mexico border, including Baja California, Sonora, Chihuahua, and Coahuila. Provide travelers with information about how to avoid flea and tick bites, both indoors and outside (Sec. 4, Ch. 6, Mosquitoes, Ticks & Other Arthropods).

TRYPANOSOMIASIS

Chagas disease, transmitted by triatomine insects infected with *Trypanosoma cruzi*, is endemic throughout Mexico (see Sec. 5, Part 3, Ch. 25, American Trypanosomiasis / Chagas Disease). In 2017, the national incidence was reported to be 0.70 cases (<1 case) per 100,000 population, varying by year and state. Most cases occur along the Pacific Coast and the Gulf of Mexico, and in central and southern Mexico. The risk for travelers is believed to be extremely low; risk might be heightened for travelers staying in poor-quality housing in endemic regions.

ENVIRONMENTAL HAZARDS & RISKS

Air Pollution

Air pollution in Mexico City has decreased in recent years. It can still be particularly severe during the dry winter months, however, exacerbating asthma and aggravating chronic lung and heart conditions (see Sec. 4, Ch. 3, Air Quality & Ionizing Radiation).

Altitude Illness

Mexico City is over a mile high (2,250 m; 7,382 ft). Healthy travelers coming from lower elevations and people with heart and lung conditions might require an acclimatization period (see Sec. 4, Ch. 5, High Elevation Travel & Altitude Illness).

Animal Bites

RABIES

In late 2019, the World Health Organization declared Mexico free from human rabies transmitted by dogs. Other animals, including bats, coatis (also known as coatimundi, cholugo, moncún, or tejón), coyotes, foxes, and skunks, are reported carriers of rabies virus. Preexposure rabies prophylaxis is recommended for adventure travelers, ecotourists, field biologists, and others participating in activities where they are at increased risk for wildlife exposure, and also for those visiting less developed, remote areas of the country where access to medical care is limited. Rabies immune globulin for postexposure prophylaxis is available in Mexico (see Sec. 5, Part 2, Ch. 18, Rabies).

SCORPIONS, SNAKES & OTHER VENOMOUS WILDLIFE

When visiting rural areas or participating in outdoor activities, especially during spring and summer, travelers should be aware of Mexico's diverse venomous creatures. Injuries and deaths caused by *Centruroides* genus (bark) scorpions have been reported from states along the Pacific Coast and in the central states of Durango, Guanajuato, State of Mexico, and Morelos. Other potential exposures include bites from pit vipers (*Agkistrodon*, *Bothrops*, and *Crotalus* spp.), coral snakes (*Micruroides* spp.), and spiders (*Latrodectus* and *Loxosceles* spp.), and stings from fire ants, bees, and wasps (see Sec. 4, Ch. 7, Zoonotic Exposures: Bites, Stings, Scratches & Other Hazards). Antidotes and antivenoms are available at some locations in Mexico.

Beach & Ocean Exposures

SARGASSUM SEAWEED

Sargassum (brown seaweed) season occurs during the warmer months, typically April–August along Mexico's Caribbean coastline. Exposure to decomposing seaweed can result in difficulty breathing, headaches, nausea, and skin eruptions called "swimmers' dermatitis." Advise travelers to avoid direct skin exposure to Sargassum seaweed and, if exposed, to rinse themselves with copious amounts of fresh water and to seek medical attention if they experience respiratory trouble.

Climate & Sun Exposure

Mexico's climate varies by region, season, and elevation. Longer wavelength ultraviolet (UV) A and shorter wavelength UVB rays intensify at southern latitudes. Travelers engaging in outdoor activities should use broad-spectrum sunscreen (readily available for purchase in Mexico) and use caution with prolonged or repetitive sun exposure to avoid sunburn (see Sec. 4, Ch. 1, Sun Exposure).

Natural Disasters

EARTHQUAKES

Sitting atop 3 large tectonic plates, Mexico is one of the most seismically active countries in the world; 80% of earthquakes are registered in the southeastern region. Travelers should follow the audible earthquake early warning system and evacuation instructions, typically posted in large buildings.

HURRICANES

Hurricane season extends from mid-May–November. Travelers, especially to coastal regions, should be alert to weather reports. After tropical storms or hurricanes, travelers should be mindful of the potential increased incidence of diarrheal illnesses and mosquito-borne diseases.

Toxic Exposures

LEAD

Lead can be present in traditional Mexican pottery. Although many traditional potters have switched to lead-free glazes, their kilns might remain contaminated from past use. Lead can leach into food and into beverages prepared, stored, and served in these dishes. The effects of lead poisoning depend on the amount and duration of exposure, and the age of the person intoxicated. The US Food and Drug Administration (FDA) strongly advises against using pottery with leachable lead for cooking, serving, or storing food and drink (www.fda.gov/food/metals-and-your-food/questions-and-answers-lead-glazed-traditional-pottery). Lead-testing kits can help assess safety.

MERCURY

Occasional reports of severe mercury poisoning associated with use of Mexican skin-lightening creams should serve as a warning against the purchase of any cosmetics that claim to treat acne, lighten the skin, or fade freckles or age spots.

SAFETY & SECURITY

Crime

Although travel to Mexico is generally considered safe, thefts and robberies do occur, and drug-related violence exists (see Sec. 4, Ch. 11, Safety & Security Overseas). Travelers should consult the US Department of State website (https://travel.state.gov/content/travel/en/international-travel/International-Travel-Country-Information-Pages/Mexico.html) for relevant safety and security alerts pertaining to their intended destinations within Mexico.

Political Unrest

Frequent protests occur in the big cities. Demonstrations are usually peaceful but can be large and worsen already congested traffic. When possible, travelers should avoid protests and the surrounding areas.

Traffic-Related Injuries

Injuries, not infectious diseases, pose the greatest life threat to healthy travelers in Mexico. In one review, about half (51%) of all US traveler deaths in Mexico were injury-related, with 18% due to motor vehicle crashes (see Sec. 8, Ch. 5, Road & Traffic Safety). Mexico's highway system and roads are mostly modern, well-maintained, and safe. Toll highways are often of higher quality. Nevertheless, driving in city traffic and at night through the countryside can be dangerous. Remind travelers to use seat belts when riding in cars. Helmet use when riding a bicycle or motorbike is highly recommended, although not strictly enforced.

AVAILABILITY & QUALITY OF MEDICAL CARE

Good health care is available in most cities in Mexico, and tourist hotels and resorts usually have physicians available. Payment (cash or credit card) might be required before any care is given. Most providers do not accept US health insurance or Medicare/Medicaid plans.

Medical Tourism

Many US residents visit Mexico to receive health services. Medical tourists going to Mexico primarily seek cosmetic surgery, dental, and eye care services from providers in northern border cities. Increasingly, a complete range of services and specialized procedures for medical tourists are being made available in Cancún, Guadalajara, Mérida, Mexico City, Monterrey, and Tijuana, cities that feature a more robust infrastructure.

Some people who travel to Mexico for medical care have become infected with antimicrobial-resistant strains of bacteria not commonly found in the United States (see Sec. 11, Ch. 5, Antimicrobial Resistance). In 2019, for example, CDC warned medical tourists against having invasive medical procedures performed in specific hospitals and cities due to risk for infection with carbapenem-resistant *Pseudomonas aeruginosa*. People considering travel to Mexico for medical procedures are advised to consult with a US health professional ≥1 month before departure and to verify provider qualifications and facility credentials in Mexico. Local standards for facility accreditation and provider certification differ from those in the United States. Make potential medical tourists aware of the additional inherent risks associated with surgery, medical procedures, and traveling while being treated for a medical condition or during recovery (see Sec. 6, Ch. 4, Medical Tourism).

Many people also travel to Mexico to purchase more affordable prescription drugs. The FDA recommends only purchasing medications from legal sources in the United States because the safety and effectiveness of drugs purchased in other countries cannot be assured (see Sec. 6, Ch. 3, . . . *perspectives*: Avoiding Poorly Regulated Medicines & Medical Products During Travel). The agency has posted guidance regarding the importation of drug or device products into the United States from other countries at www.fda.gov/industry/import-basics/personal-importation#whatis.

BIBLIOGRAPHY

Hotez PJ, Bottazzi ME, Dumonteil E, Buekens P. The Gulf of Mexico: a "hot zone" for neglected tropical diseases? PLoS Negl Trop Dis. 2015;9(2):e0003481.

Ibáñez-Cervantes G, León-García G, Castro-Escarpulli G, Mancilla-Ramírez J, Victoria-Acosta G, Cureño-Díaz M, et al. Evolution of incidence and geographical distribution of Chagas disease in Mexico during a decade (2007–2016). Epidemiol Infect. 2018;147:e41.

Kracalik I, Ham C, Smith AR, Vowles M, Kauber K, Zambrano M, et al. Notes from the field: Verona integron-encoded metallo-β-lactamase–producing carbapenem-resistant *Pseudomonas aeruginosa* infections in U.S. residents associated with invasive medical procedures in Mexico, 2015–2018. MMWR Morb Mortal Wkly Rep. 2019;68(20):463–4.

Nunez EO, Arias RMB, Martinez MEA, Larios JAR, Crooks VA, Labonté R, et al. An overview of Mexico's medical tourism industry: the cases of Mexico City and Monterrey. Vancouver: SFU Medical Tourism Research Group, Simon Fraser University; 2014.

Pan American Health Organization AHO. Mexico is free from human rabies transmitted by dogs. Available from: www.paho.org/hq/index.php?option=com_content&view=article&id=15585:mexico-is-free-from-human-rabies-transmitted-by-dogs&Itemid=1926&lang=en.

Rodriguez-Morales AJ, Villamil-Gómez WE, Franco-Paredes C. The arboviral burden of disease caused by co-circulation and co-infection of dengue, chikungunya and Zika in the Americas. Travel Med Infect Dis. 2016;14(3):177–9.

Sosa-Gutierrez CG, Vargas-Sandoval M, Torres J, Gordillo-Pérez G. Tick-borne rickettsial pathogens in questing ticks, removed from humans and animals in Mexico. J Vet Sci. 2016;17(3):353–60.

Toda M, Gonzalez FJ, Fonseca-Ford M, Franklin P, Huntington-Frazier M, Gutelius B, et al. Notes from the field: multistate coccidioidomycosis outbreak in U.S. residents returning from community service trips to Baja California, Mexico—July–August 2018. MMWR Morb Mortal Wkly Rep. 2019;68(14):332–333.

World Health Organization. Mercury in cosmetics and skin lightening products. 2019. Available from: www.who.int/publications-detail/mercury-in-cosmetics-and-skin-lightening-products.

PERU

Rodolfo Bégué, Miguel Cabada

DESTINATION OVERVIEW

Peru (Map 10-10) is the third largest country in South America. Peru's varied microclimates and ecologic diversity, which ranges from coastal beaches to Amazon rainforest to the snow-capped peaks of the Andes Mountains, made the land hospitable to pre-Inca and Inca peoples. Today, Peru is an attractive destination for tourists interested in history, recreation, and adventure. Many Peruvians who work in the tourist industry have a reasonable understanding of English.

Peru lies almost entirely between 70° and 80° longitude (as do the mid-Atlantic and New England states in the United States). Peru has a single time zone and does not change its clocks during the year. Jetlag is not normally a problem for US travelers to Peru, regardless of season.

US citizens visiting Peru do not need a visa. Most tourists fly into the capital, Lima, a mega-metropolis with nearly 10 million people and multiple neighborhoods (districts). Most visitors to Lima stay in Miraflores, Barranco, or occasionally, downtown (el Centro). The US Embassy office is in Surco; contact information is available on their website (https://pe.usembassy.gov). Popular activities in Lima include historic city tours, night life, and sampling the many local cuisines.

10

About 90 minutes away by plane is the former capital of the Inca empire, Cusco. A cosmopolitan city with a population of ≈400,000, Cusco is at a much higher elevation (3,339 m; ≈11,000 ft) than Lima (154 m; ≈500 ft) and is surrounded by many archeological sites, each a short bus ride away, including Sacsayhuamán, Q'enco, Písac, Ollantaytambo, Puka Pukara, Tambomachay, and others. The city itself has multiple cultural attractions that travelers can visit on foot (e.g., the Inca Museum, the Qorikancha Temple, the Barrio de los Artesanos in the San Blas neighborhood, and numerous churches). The 4-hour train trip to the ancient city of Machu Picchu (2,430 m; ≈8,000 ft) is extremely popular. South of Cusco is the highest navigable lake in the world, Lake Titicaca (3,812 m; ≈12,500 ft). Shared by Peru with neighboring Bolivia, Lake Titicaca is home of the Uru people and the man-made floating islands on which they live.

Along its long Pacific Ocean coast, Peru has amazing beaches from north (Catacaos, Piura) to south (Ica). Other cities near the coast include Trujillo, Nazca with its mysterious pre-Inca lines etched into desert sands, and Arequipa, a starting point for travelers wishing to explore the world's second deepest canyon, Valle de Colca.

In the Andes, high-elevation destinations include Cajamarca, Huaraz (with the Cordillera Blanca Mountain range and Huascarán National Park both nearby), Huancayo, and Ayacucho. East of the Andes is the Amazon rainforest; Iquitos, bathed by the Amazon River and reachable only by plane or boat, is the largest and best-known city in the region; other cities include Pucallpa and Puerto Maldonado. Adventure and nature tourists often visit Manú National Park in Madre de Dios.

INFECTIOUS DISEASE RISKS

Peru follows the World Health Organization's Expanded Program on Immunization, which includes many (but not all) vaccines used in the United States. Although vaccination rates in Peru are relatively high, recent outbreaks of vaccine-preventable diseases have occurred, including diphtheria (2020), measles (2018–2019), and varicella (endemic). Thus, travelers should be up to date with all routine vaccines. For adults, additional booster doses might be indicated; for young children, an accelerated schedule could be indicated to assure protection (see www.cdc.gov/vaccines/schedules). Hepatitis A and hepatitis B are hyperendemic in provinces throughout the country, and travelers should be appropriately vaccinated.

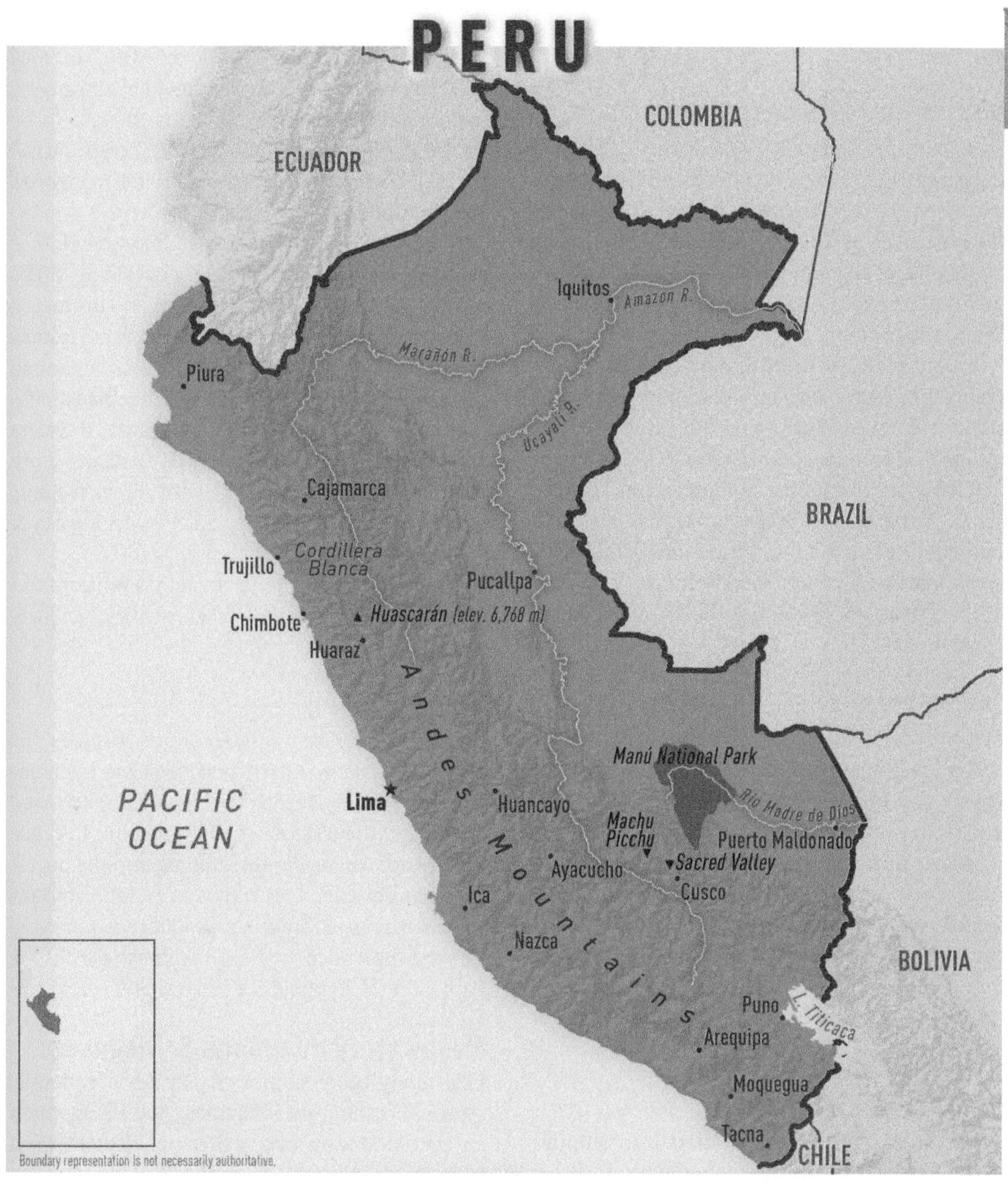

MAP 10-10 Peru

Enteric Infections & Diseases

Peru has one of the richest and most exotic cuisines in the world, suitable for all palates. Cooked, hot dishes mostly are safe from foodborne pathogens, but fresh produce, fruits, and vegetables can be easy vehicles for infection. Although not the bulk of Peruvian cuisine, raw or partially cooked fish or meat (e.g., ceviche, tiradito, carpaccio), are popular in Peru and pose a risk for foodborne illness. Sauces added to some dishes might carry infectious pathogens.

CHOLERA

In the early 1990s, after a century of absence, *Vibrio cholerae* O1 was reintroduced into the Americas via Peru. Since then, cholera has all but disappeared from the Americas. Some endemic strains are occasionally detected, but epidemic cholera is not a risk, and cholera vaccine is not indicated for travel to Peru.

CYCLOSPORIASIS & CRYPTOSPORIDIOSIS

Cyclospora cayetanensis, named after the local Universidad Peruana Cayetano Heredia, is endemic to Peru. *C. cayetanensis* infection shares many features with giardiasis (described next), but treatment is different, requiring trimethoprim-sulfamethoxazole (see Sec. 5, Part 3, Ch. 5, Cyclosporiasis).

Cryptosporidium parvum and *C. hominis* follow a similar epidemiology; treatment is typically not attempted unless symptoms are protracted, or the host is immunocompromised. Oral rehydration is the most effective supportive therapy (see Sec. 5, Part 3, Ch. 3, Cryptosporidiosis). Travelers can reduce their risk for cyclosporiasis and cryptosporidiosis by carefully adhering to food and water precautions (see Sec. 2, Ch. 8, Food & Water Precautions).

GIARDIASIS

Transmitted by ingestion of contaminated water and sometimes vegetables, *Giardia duodenalis* infection presents with abdominal pain, bloating, "sulfur" belching, and vomiting. Giardiasis is more frequent among hikers, travelers to rural areas, or people who consume fresh juices. Travelers should avoid potential sources of infection, including drinking and recreational water that could be contaminated. No vaccine against giardiasis is available. For further information, see Sec. 5, Part 3, Ch. 12, Giardiasis.

10

HEPATITIS A

Hepatitis A virus is transmitted by contaminated food and water and is endemic to Peru; vaccination is highly effective and strongly recommended for all unvaccinated travelers. Whereas hepatitis A vaccine is routinely given to US children, most adults have not received the vaccine. Immune globulin is an alternative for people in whom the vaccine is contraindicated, including infants <6 months of age and anyone allergic to the vaccine or vaccine components (for prescribing details, including precautions and contraindications, see Sec. 5, Part 2, Ch. 7, Hepatitis A).

TRAVELERS' DIARRHEA

Anecdotal information suggests travelers' diarrhea (TD) among tourists to Peru is frequent and grossly underreported. The main cause is thought to be bacterial (primarily enterotoxigenic *Escherichia coli* strains). Less frequent causes are viral (norovirus, rotavirus) and parasitic (giardiasis).

Travelers should practice frequent hand-cleaning with hand sanitizer containing ≥60% alcohol, and avoid uncooked foods and untreated water, including tap water at hotels and restaurants. Bottled water is usually safe, as is canned soda, but ice is not safe. For infants, breastfeeding is safest; if feeding infant formula, travelers should use bottled or boiled water to reconstitute formula (see Sec. 7, Ch. 2, Travel & Breastfeeding, and Sec. 7, Ch. 3, Traveling Safely with Infants & Children).

For more information about prevention and treatment of travelers' diarrhea, see Sec. 2, Ch. 6, Travelers' Diarrhea.

TYPHOID FEVER

Before the 1990s, typhoid fever (caused by *Salmonella enterica* serotype Typhi) was hyperendemic to Peru. Since then, incidence has decreased greatly, but the disease remains endemic. Because the disease can be life-threatening and the bacterium has developed resistance to multiple antimicrobial agents, all travelers should receive one of the recommended typhoid vaccines (see Sec. 5, Part 1, Ch. 24, Typhoid & Paratyphoid Fever).

Respiratory Infections & Diseases

Like many other countries, Peru has endemic, seasonal respiratory infections, not all of which are preventable by routine vaccines. Because Peru is in the Southern Hemisphere, the seasons are opposite to seasons in the United States, which is relevant to the epidemiology of influenza. The influenza vaccine recommended for use in the Northern Hemisphere each year confers protection against the virus strains circulating in the Southern Hemisphere that same year.

CORONAVIRUS DISEASE 2019

For current information on coronavirus disease 2019 (COVID-19) in Peru, consult the US Embassy in Peru website (https://pe.usembassy.

gov). For the US government's COVID-19 international travel requirements and recommendations, see www.cdc.gov/coronavirus/2019-ncov/travelers/international-travel/index.html. All travelers going to Peru should be up to date with their COVID-19 vaccines (www.cdc.gov/coronavirus/2019-ncov/vaccines/stay-up-to-date.html).

TUBERCULOSIS

Tuberculosis (TB) is endemic to Peru. Multidrug-resistant and extensively drug-resistant TB strains frequently are detected, making treatment difficult and avoidance and prevention crucial. Infection risk is greatest among long-term travelers, especially people who visit friends and family, expatriates, missionaries, voluntourists (for a definition, see Sec. 9, Ch. 5, Humanitarian Aid Workers, Box 9-05), and health care workers. For management recommendations, see Sec. 5, Part 1, Ch. 22, Tuberculosis, and Sec. 5, Part 1, Ch. 23, . . . *perspectives*: Testing Travelers for *Mycobacterium tuberculosis* Infection.

Sexually Transmitted Infections & HIV

Although all sectors of the population are affected, HIV is more prevalent among commercial sex workers (prostitution is legal in Peru) and men who have sex with men, particularly in major cities (e.g., Iquitos, Lima). Some strains of HIV circulating in Peru are resistant to antiretroviral therapy, but probably not more than what is seen in other parts of the world (see Sec. 5, Part 2, Ch. 11, Human Immunodeficiency Virus / HIV). Antimicrobial-resistant strains of *Chlamydia trachomatis* and *Neisseria gonorrhoeae* are well described in Peru. Advise travelers to practice safe sex and to use barrier protection (e.g., condoms), especially with partners whose HIV or sexually transmitted infection status is unknown. Condoms are available for purchase in Peru.

Vectorborne Diseases

Mosquitoes and other biting insects are part of the experience in Peru, mainly in rural areas and the Amazon. Exposure depends largely on where a traveler is going, for how long, and their accommodations. Prevention is the best policy. Advise travelers to avoid areas at high risk for insect bites, to minimize exposed skin, and to use insect repellents properly (see Sec. 4, Ch. 6, Mosquitoes, Ticks & Other Arthropods). For travelers going to malaria- or yellow fever–endemic areas of Peru, chemoprophylaxis or vaccination might be indicated (see the following sections for details).

ARBOVIRUSES: CHIKUNGUNYA, DENGUE & ZIKA

Three important vectorborne illnesses in Peru, chikungunya, dengue, and Zika, can range in severity from mild to severe. The epidemiology of each is cyclical and only partly understood, but outbreaks occur frequently. The viruses that cause these diseases are transmitted by "day-biting" *Aedes* mosquito species, whose habitats are <2,300 m (≈7,500 ft) elevation. Vertical Zika virus infection from a pregnant person to a developing fetus can be especially devastating (see virus-specific chapters in Section 5, and on the Centers for Disease Control and Prevention (CDC) Travelers' Health website, https://wwwnc.cdc.gov/travel/page/zika-information).

CARRIÓN DISEASE

Bartonella bacilliformis, the cause of Oroya Fever and verruga peruana (together known as Carrión disease), is a bacterium transmitted by *Lutzomyia* sandflies (see Sec. 5, Part 1, Ch. 2, Bartonella Infections). Endemic to some areas in Ancash (Caraz), Cajamarca, and Cusco (Urubamba), *Bartonella* infection is a low risk for most tourists. Nevertheless, travelers to the listed areas should practice insect bite precautions.

LEISHMANIASIS

Cutaneous leishmaniasis, which manifests as chronic ulcers, is a parasitic infection transmitted by the bite of certain sandflies endemic to many valleys in the Andes and tropical Amazon rainforest. Travelers visiting the Manú National Park in Madre de Dios are at greatest risk. No vaccine or chemoprophylaxis is available. Advise travelers to carefully adhere to insect bite precautions (see Sec. 4, Ch. 6, Mosquitoes, Ticks & Other Arthropods; and Sec. 5, Part 3, Ch. 14, Cutaneous Leishmaniasis).

MALARIA

Malaria is a risk on the eastern side of the Andes in areas <2,500 m (≈8,200 ft) elevation, including all of the Amazon rainforest and a few isolated areas on the northern Pacific Coast. Malaria is not a risk along most of the Pacific Coast, Lima Province, or the high Andes, including Cusco, Machu Picchu, and Lake Titicaca. The most common malaria species in Peru are *Plasmodium vivax* (80%) and *P. falciparum* (20%). Prepare travelers planning to enter endemic areas to take malaria chemoprophylaxis (i.e., atovaquone-proguanil, doxycycline, mefloquine, or tafenoquine) that protects against chloroquine-resistant malaria. For prescribing details, see Sec. 2, Ch. 5, Yellow Fever Vaccine & Malaria Prevention Information, by Country; Sec. 5, Part 3, Ch. 16, Malaria; and the CDC Malaria webpages (www.cdc.gov/parasites/malaria/index.html).

YELLOW FEVER

In Peru, areas of yellow fever endemicity overlap areas of malaria endemicity. CDC recommends vaccination for all travelers aged ≥9 months going to areas with a risk for yellow fever transmission (see Sec. 2, Ch. 5, Yellow Fever Vaccine & Malaria Prevention Information, by Country). Peru does not require proof of yellow fever vaccination for entry.

ENVIRONMENTAL HAZARDS & RISKS

10

Altitude Illness & Acute Mountain Sickness

Travelers who visit Cusco (3,339 m; ≈11,000 ft), Machu Picchu (2,430 m; ≈8,000 ft), Lake Titicaca (3,812 m; ≈12,500 ft), or who go hiking or climbing in the Andes Mountains (e.g., Huascarán [6,768 m; ≈22,200 ft] in the Cordillera Blanca range) are at risk for altitude illness and acute mountain sickness. See Sec. 4, Ch. 5, High Elevation Travel & Altitude Illness, for details regarding altitude illness and its medical management.

Animal Bites & Rabies

Although rabies is endemic among dogs and wild animals (bats and others) in Peru, preexposure prophylaxis is generally not recommended except for adventure travelers, veterinarians working in-country, or people planning on spending time in the open wilderness. Travelers should not approach or pet unknown animals. Although rabies vaccine is widely available in Peru, rabies immune globulin is not; thus, CDC recommends emergency return home or evacuation to the nearest destination that can deliver appropriate postexposure prophylaxis for anyone bitten or scratched by a potentially rabid animal (see Sec. 5, Part 2, Ch. 18, Rabies). Medical evacuation insurance can cover the cost of emergency travel (see Sec. 6, Ch. 1, Travel Insurance, Travel Health Insurance & Medical Evacuation Insurance).

Climate & Sun Exposure

Beach time in Peru brings the risk for sun exposure. Sun exposure is also a risk during visits to high mountain peaks and the Amazon rainforest. Travelers should bring and use sunscreen, but sunscreen is available for purchase in Peru. Travelers to areas where sunscreen and insect repellent are both needed should apply sunscreen first, then repellent, and avoid combination products because these are not as effective (see Sec. 4, Ch. 1, Sun Exposure).

SAFETY & SECURITY

As a norm, Peruvians are friendly and try their best to accommodate newcomers. That said, tourists are easy prey for petty criminals. Travelers should always go out with a group or tour guide. In addition, travelers should avoid carrying large sums of money, keep their money in a secure pocket (not a purse), and show only small amounts of cash at a time. Most restaurants and major venues accept major credit cards. Whenever possible, travelers should make advance arrangements and payments.

Travelers also should make certain they are in safe company when drinking Pisco Sour (20%–30% alcohol content), the traditional drink of Peru.

Crime

Major crime is common in Peru but is a domestic problem; tourists are not normally implicated. Urge travelers to stay with a group or chaperone. Drug trafficking or consumption is illegal. Marijuana, in small amounts and with a prescription (which must be locally obtained or validated) is allowed for medicinal purposes. Ayahuasca, a hallucinogenic preparation, is commonly offered to tourists in Peru. The ayahuasca rituals are not illegal, but the safety and regulations for recreational use have not been established. Travelers taking psychoactive medications (e.g., antidepressants) who try ayahuasca could be at increased risk for adverse outcomes; consultation with a physician knowledgeable about potential drug interactions is advised.

Political Unrest

Peru is a Republic with a democratic government. The political situation is very fragile, however, and can change at any moment. Travelers should avoid getting involved in activism or political discussions (see Sec. 4, Ch. 11, Safety & Security Overseas).

Terrorism

Peru experienced a long period of terrorism during the 1980s and 1990s. The groups involved have been mostly defeated or have retreated to small cells in isolated areas of the country not normally visited by travelers.

Traffic-Related Injuries

Travelers should not drive in Peru. Roads are treacherous and traffic rules loosely followed. Travelers should avoid hailing informal taxicabs and instead opt to make a reservation through the hotel or tour guide. Tipping cab drivers is not customary and will identify travelers as tourists. Advise travelers to always wear a seat belt in vehicles. When on foot, travelers should pause to make certain traffic has stopped completely before stepping into the street.

AVAILABILITY & QUALITY OF MEDICAL CARE

Peru has a mixed public and private health care system. Travelers who need health care should access the private system of clinics (*clínicas privadas*) located throughout Lima and the major cities; lists of these clinics are available from hotels that cater to tourists or the US Embassy in Peru (https://pe.usembassy.gov). Private clinic personnel usually understand English well, and many of their doctors have received part of their training in the United States. Treatment is relatively inexpensive, and most credit cards are accepted. Purchasing medication in Peru can be challenging; counterfeit medication is sold, and some medicines might not be available or could have different or unrecognizable names (see Sec. 6, Ch. 3, *perspectives*: Avoiding Poorly Regulated Medicines & Medical Products During Travel).

Travelers visiting friends or relatives should identify health care sources through their local acquaintances.

Medical Tourism

Peru is not a common destination for medical tourism. Medical tourism is not recognized or regulated by the local medical college, which makes it both dangerous and illegal.

10

BIBLIOGRAPHY

Cabezas C, Trujillo O, Gonzales-Vivanco A, Benites Villafane CM, Balbuena J, Borda-Olivas AO, et al. Seroepidemiology of hepatitis A, B, C, D and E virus infections in the general population of Peru: a cross sectional study. PLoS One. 2020;15(6): e0234273

Garcia PJ, Cárcamo CP, Chiappe M, Holmes KK. Sexually transmitted and reproductive tract infections in symptomatic clients of pharmacies of Lima, Peru. Sex Transm Infect. 2007;83(2):142–6.

Munayco C, Chowell G, Tariq A, Undurraga EA, Mizumoto J. Risk of death by age and gender from COVID-19 in Peru, March–May, 2020. Aging (Albany NY). 2020;12(14):13869–81.

Solano-Villarreal E, Valdivia W, Pearcy M, Linard C, Pasapera-Gonzales J, Moreno-Gutierrez D, et al. Malaria risk assessment and mapping using satellite imagery and boosted regression trees in the Peruvian Amazon. Sci Rep. 2019;9(1):15173.

Soria J. Mugruza R, Levine M, León SR, Arévalo J, Ticona E, Beck IA, Frenkel LM. Pretreatment HIV drug resistance and virologic outcomes to first-line antiretroviral therapy in Peru. AIDS Res Hum Retroviruses. 2019;35(2):150–4.

Villegas L, Otero L, Sterling TR, Huaman MA, Van der Stuyft P, Gottuzzo E, et al. Prevalence, risk factors and treatment outcomes of isoniazid- and rifampicin-mono-resistant pulmonary tuberculosis in Lima, Peru. PLoS One. 2016;11(4):e0152933.

Winnicka L, Abdullah A, Yang T, Norville K, Irizarry-Acosta M. Yellow fever in an unvaccinated traveler to Peru. Open Forum Infect Dis. 2017;4(4):ofx205.

PART 3: ASIA

BURMA (MYANMAR)

Wai Yan Aung

DESTINATION OVERVIEW

Burma (also called Myanmar) offers travelers a mix of traditional and modern culture. Nearly all visitors to this country come to see the classic golden temples of Rangoon (Yangon), Burma's former capital and its largest city. Visitors also enjoy strolling colonial-era parks and shopping at Bogyoke Aung San Market. The city includes British, Chinese, and Indian influences. Travelers wanting a glimpse of rural life can do so with a short ferry ride across the Yangon River to Dala, or by riding the circle train that makes a loop just north of the city.

Many travelers take advantage of the improving domestic air and bus service to explore other parts of the country. International flights to Mandalay are available from neighboring China, Singapore, and Thailand. Burma's varied geography includes highlands, plains, beaches, and >800 islands. Several climate zones are found along its river basins and mountain ranges.

10

The people of Burma are diverse—the country has 135 officially recognized ethnic groups speaking >100 different languages. Of the country's >56 million people, about two-thirds can speak or understand Burmese. English is widely spoken in popular visitor destinations, where travelers often remark on the hospitality and generosity of their hosts.

Religious sites and ancient cities, with their temples and festivals, attract many visitors to Burma. Unique architecture and heritage combine at places like Bagan, Bago, Kyaiktiyo Pagoda, and Mrauk U. Travelers can easily arrange outdoor activities (e.g., boating, cycling, trekking) around Inle Lake, Hsipaw, or Kalaw in hilly Shan State, home to a thrilling train ride across the Goteik viaduct. River cruises along the Ayeyarwady begin or end in Mandalay (Map 10-11). Meditation retreats are also widely available.

INFECTIOUS DISEASE RISKS

Travelers to Burma should be up to date on routine vaccines, including diphtheria-tetanus-pertussis, hepatitis A, measles-mumps-rubella (MMR), polio, and varicella (chickenpox). Influenza exhibits a seasonal pattern that peaks during June–September, overlapping with the typical rainy season; influenza vaccine is recommended for travelers.

Bloodborne Pathogens

The prevalence of hepatitis B infection in Burma has been estimated as low to intermediate. Hepatitis B vaccination is especially crucial for anyone engaging in activities that increase their chances of exposure to blood or body fluids (e.g., people who might use injection drugs, those traveling to provide or receive medical care, and people who plan to get a tattoo or engage in condomless sexual contact). For more details, see Sec. 5, Part 2, Ch. 8, Hepatitis B.

Enteric Infections & Diseases

Local dishes such as *mohinga* (rice noodles in fish soup), curries, and salads appeal to many visitors. Travelers should observe safe food and water precautions, however, especially in secondary towns and in rural areas, where cleanliness during food preparation, utensil washing, and safe waste disposal might be lacking or not practiced. See Sec. 2,

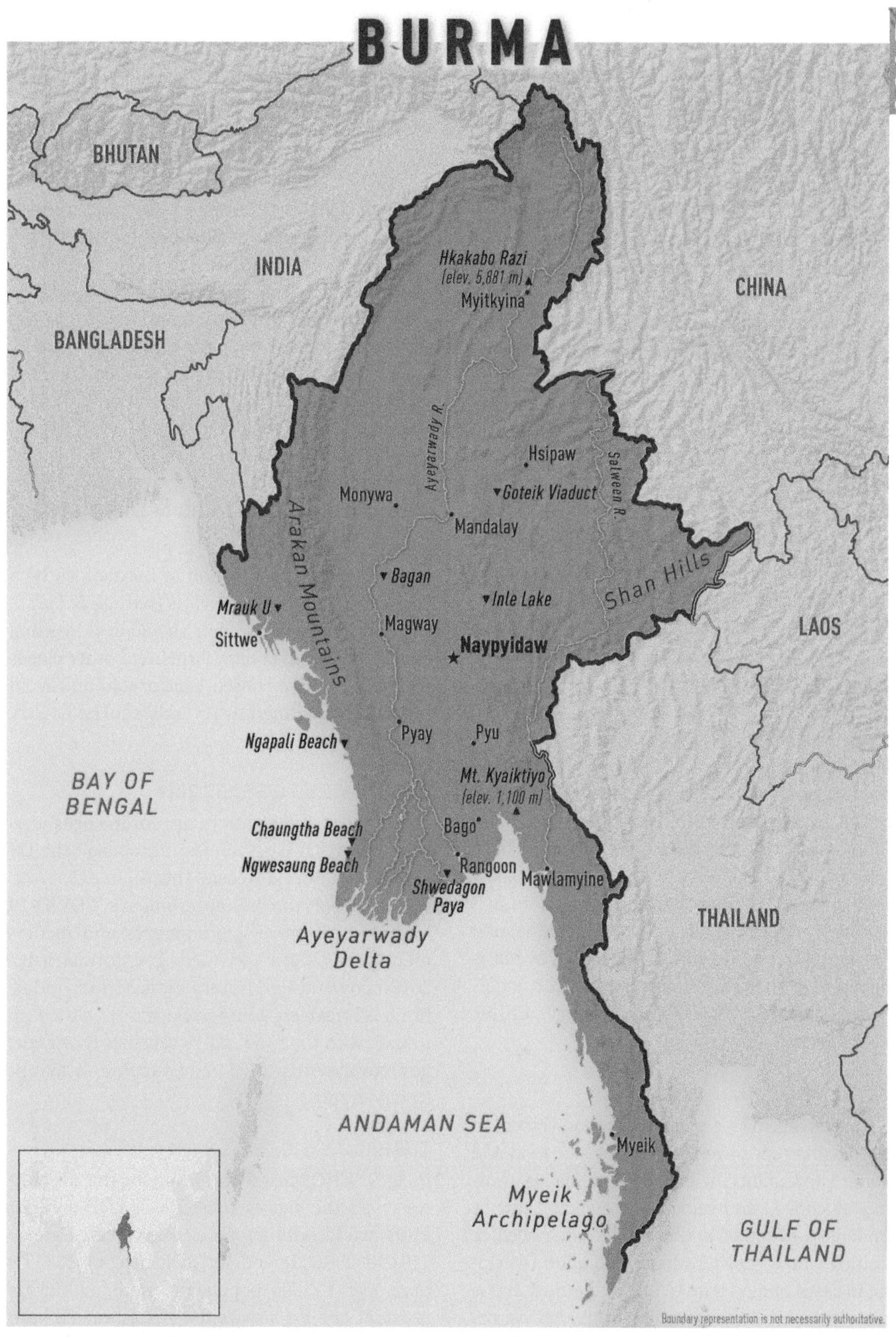
BURMA
BHUTAN
INDIA
CHINA
BANGLADESH
Hkakabo Razi
(elev. 5,881 m)
Myitkyina
Ayeyarwady R.
Hsipaw
Salween R.
Monywa
Goteik Viaduct
Mandalay
Arakan Mountains
Bagan
Inle Lake
Shan Hills
Mrauk U
Magway
LAOS
Sittwe
Naypyidaw
Ngapali Beach
Pyay
Pyu
BAY OF BENGAL
Mt. Kyaiktiyo
(elev. 1,100 m)
Chaungtha Beach
Bago
Ngwesaung Beach
Rangoon
Mawlamyine
Shwedagon Paya
THAILAND
Ayeyarwady Delta
ANDAMAN SEA
Myeik
Myeik Archipelago
GULF OF THAILAND
Boundary representation is not necessarily authoritative.

MAP 10-11 Burma (Myanmar)

Ch. 6, Travelers' Diarrhea, and Sec. 2, Ch. 8, Food & Water Precautions, for additional recommendations. Tap water in Burma is considered not safe for drinking.

CHOLERA

Burma last reported cholera data to the World Health Organization (WHO) for 2016. Nonetheless, WHO believes Burma to be a country that remains at risk for the disease. For a list of countries reporting active cholera transmission, see the Centers for Disease Control and Prevention (CDC) Travelers' Health website (https://wwwnc.cdc.gov/travel/diseases/cholera#areas). For recommendations regarding use of cholera vaccine in international travelers, see Sec. 5, Part 1, Ch. 5, Cholera.

HEPATITIS A

As in much of Asia, hepatitis A virus is endemic to Burma (Sec. 5, Part 2, Ch. 7, Hepatitis A). Travelers can reduce their risk for hepatitis A infection by following safe food and water precautions (see Sec. 2, Ch. 8, Food & Water Precautions) and by getting vaccinated before travel.

OPISTHORCHIASIS

Opisthorchiasis—caused by *Opisthorchis viverrini*—has long been endemic in the Greater Mekong subregion in Southeast Asia. Although information on human liver fluke infection in Burma has not been published until very recently, data now show that *O. viverrini* human infection is prevalent in 3 southern regions of the country, Bago, Mon, and Yangon. Risk to most travelers is likely low but is increased among people who eat raw or undercooked freshwater fish (see Sec. 5, Part 3, Ch. 10, Liver Flukes).

TRAVELERS' DIARRHEA

Travelers' diarrhea is common among visitors to Burma. Instruct travelers to follow safe food and water precautions by eating food that is thoroughly cooked and served hot, avoiding raw or undercooked foods, and drinking only boiled or bottled water. Oral rehydration solution is helpful in cases of moderate to severe diarrhea and is usually available in pharmacies. Although visitors can receive treatment from clinics or hospitals in major cities, consider prescribing antibiotics for travelers to carry for self-treatment of moderate to severe diarrhea (see Sec. 2, Ch. 6, Travelers' Diarrhea).

TYPHOID FEVER

Typhoid fever is common in Burma. Although only limited data are available on the prevalence of drug-resistant typhoid infections in Burma, studies conducted in Rangoon demonstrate a high prevalence of first-line antimicrobial drug resistance in other bacterial infections, suggesting the same could be true for typhoid. Typhoid vaccine is recommended for travel to Burma (see Sec. 5, Part 1, Ch. 24, Typhoid & Paratyphoid Fever).

Respiratory Infections & Diseases

AVIAN INFLUENZA

Live bird markets, common in Burma, can be a source of avian influenza virus (see Sec. 5, Part 2, Ch. 12, Influenza). Travelers should avoid visiting bird markets and poultry farms, and other places where live birds are raised, kept, or sold, and avoid preparing or eating raw or undercooked poultry products.

CORONAVIRUS DISEASE 2019

For current information on coronavirus disease 2019 (COVID-19) in Burma, consult the US Embassy in Burma website (https://mm.usembassy.gov/). For the US government's COVID-19 international travel requirements and recommendations, see www.cdc.gov/coronavirus/2019-ncov/travelers/international-travel/index.html. All travelers going to Burma should be up to date with their COVID-19 vaccines (www.cdc.gov/coronavirus/2019-ncov/vaccines/stay-up-to-date.html).

TUBERCULOSIS

In 2019, WHO ranked Burma among the 20 countries with the highest tuberculosis (TB) burdens in the world, with a total of 181,000 cases (range 119,000–256,000) and an incidence of 338 TB cases per 100,000 population. Both multidrug-resistant and extensively drug-resistant TB have been reported in Burma. Overall, however, risk to travelers is low.

Sexually Transmitted Infections & HIV

The prevalence of HIV among people ≥15 years old living in Burma is 0.6%. According to the most recent official estimates (www.who.int/docs/default-source/searo/myanmar/hiv-aids-(english).pdf), ≈220,000 people in Burma were living with HIV in 2017; ≈66% were receiving antiretroviral therapy (ART). More recent (unpublished) estimates are that as of late 2020, ≈240,000 people were living with HIV, almost 83% of whom were receiving ART. Advise travelers on correct and consistent use of external or internal latex condoms to reduce the risk for HIV infection and other sexually transmitted infections with any new sex partners (see Sec. 9, Ch. 12, Sex & Travel, and Sec. 11, Ch. 10, Sexually Transmitted Infections). Good quality condoms are widely available for purchase in Burma, both at local pharmacies and at grocery stores.

Soil- & Waterborne Infections

LEPTOSPIROSIS

Leptospirosis (see Sec. 5, Part 1, Ch. 10, Leptospirosis) is common in Burma and most often occurs during the rainy season. Risk for contracting leptospirosis is associated with participating in outdoor activities (e.g., kayaking, rafting, swimming, wading) that bring people in contact with contaminated freshwater sources.

SCHISTOSOMIASIS

A low risk for schistosomiasis exists in Bago Region, and in Rakhine and Shan states (including Inle Lake). Widespread distribution is presumed in the Ayeyarwady Delta, and travelers should avoid bathing, swimming, wading, or other contact with freshwater in this region (see Sec. 5, Part 3, Ch. 20, Schistosomiasis).

Vectorborne Diseases

CHIKUNGUNYA, DENGUE & ZIKA

Vectorborne diseases endemic to Burma include chikungunya, dengue, and Zika (see the respective disease chapters in Section 5). Risk for chikungunya and dengue exists throughout Burma; peak transmission occurs during the rainy season, May/June–October. Because of the risk for birth defects in infants born to people infected with Zika during pregnancy, people who are pregnant or trying to become pregnant should review the most recent recommendations available on the CDC Travelers' Health website (https://wwwnc.cdc.gov/travel/page/zika-information).

JAPANESE ENCEPHALITIS

Japanese encephalitis (JE) is presumed to be endemic throughout Burma, and travelers should take precautions to avoid mosquito bites (see Sec. 4, Ch. 6, Mosquitoes, Ticks & Other Arthropods). Consider recommending JE vaccine for travelers who will be in country for >1 month or whose itineraries include higher-risk activities (e.g., spending substantial time in rural areas; participating in outdoor activities like camping, farming, or hiking; staying in accommodations without air conditioning, window or door screens, or mosquito nets). See Sec. 5, Part 2, Ch. 13, Japanese Encephalitis, for more details.

MALARIA

Malaria is endemic in all areas of Burma below 1,000 m (≈3,300 ft) elevation, including the ancient capital city of Bagan. Malaria incidence in Burma exceeds that of neighboring countries in the Greater Mekong subregion and is concentrated in and around forested areas. Chloroquine- and mefloquine-resistant malaria has been and continues to be a concern, and chemoprophylaxis recommendations vary accordingly. For malaria prevention recommendations, see Sec. 2, Ch. 5, Yellow Fever Vaccine & Malaria Prevention Information, by Country, and Sec. 5, Part 3, Ch. 16, Malaria.

ENVIRONMENTAL HAZARDS & RISKS

Animal Bites

RABIES

Among the >150 countries reporting cases of rabies, Burma has an increasing number of dog bites and one of the highest rates of disease. Rabies vaccination is recommended for travelers participating in outdoor activities (e.g., camping, caving) that could increase their risk of animal bites. Vaccination is also recommended for travelers working with animals (e.g., veterinarians), people taking long trips or moving to Burma, and young children, for whom it can be difficult to prevent interaction with dogs or other animals (see Sec. 5, Part 2, Ch. 18, Rabies). Rabies immune globulin is available at tertiary and international hospitals in Burma for postexposure prophylaxis.

SNAKES

Snake species in Burma vary by location. Many snakes are non-venomous; others are only mildly venomous and not particularly dangerous to humans. A few snakes are highly venomous, however, and their bites are potentially lethal. Estimates of >10,000 snakebites and >1,000 snakebite deaths are reported each year in Burma, which has one of the highest rates of venomous snakebites in the world.

Burma produces antivenom specific for Russell's viper (*Daboia russelii*) and cobra venom. These locally produced products are more effective than imported products not specific for Burma's indigenous snake species. Most local hospitals in Burma are stocked with antivenoms. Advise travelers to seek medical attention immediately if bitten.

In addition, educate travelers that snakebites are preventable and avoiding snakes is key. Travelers should not aggravate or provoke snakes. When walking through brushy areas or undergrowth, travelers should wear tall boots to protect their legs; using a flashlight at night also can be helpful. Travelers should avoid sleeping on the ground; advise those who do to use a well-tucked-in mosquito net.

10

Climate & Sun Exposure

Climate in Burma varies depending on season and elevation. During the dry months, November–February, Rangoon and southern Burma average 80°F (27°C) during the day, but farther north, nighttime temperatures can drop to 45°F–50°F (8°C–10°C).

Hot season, March–May, and rainy season, May/June–October, are appropriately named. Average high temperatures during the hot season can exceed 95°F (35°C) in many parts of the country, including popular tourist destinations like Rangoon and central Burma (Bagan and Mandalay). Prolonged heat exposure poses a risk for various forms of heat-related illness, especially for travelers in poor physical condition, very old or very young travelers, people participating in strenuous activities, and those unaccustomed to heat (see Sec. 4, Ch. 2, Extremes of Temperature). During periods of high heat, travelers should seek shade, drink ample water, and wear lightweight, loose-fitting, light-colored clothing. Sunscreen products are widely available for purchase (see Sec. 4, Ch. 1, Sun Exposure).

Natural Disasters

Flooding is always a possibility during the rainy season in Burma, and various regions are prone to flash floods.

SAFETY & SECURITY

Political Unrest

Since February 2021, after a military coup in Burma, political unrest and anti-coup protests have occurred throughout the country. Travelers to Burma should register with the Department of State's Smart Traveler Enrollment Program (STEP; https://step.state.gov/step).

Traffic-Related Injuries

Vehicular crashes are a leading cause of injury and death among travelers (see Sec. 8, Ch. 5, Road & Traffic Safety). Remind people visiting Burma to use only reputable taxi or public transportation companies and to always wear seat belts. Motorcycles account for a high percentage of road traffic deaths and should be avoided. Pedestrians and bicyclists are also common victims of road traffic deaths and should exercise caution; right-of-way rules and infrastructure improvements (e.g., bike lanes, crosswalks) to protect these groups are often not in place or not followed. When sidewalks are not available, travelers should walk on the side of the road facing oncoming traffic. Advise anyone who plans to ride a bicycle in Burma to bring and wear a helmet.

AVAILABILITY & QUALITY OF MEDICAL CARE

Travelers with chronic medical conditions should not rely on being able to purchase or refill medications in Burma; counterfeit and substandard medications are common (see Sec. 6, Ch. 3, . . . *perspectives*: Avoiding Poorly Regulated Medicines & Medical Products During Travel).

Hospitals providing an international standard level of care are located only in major cities like Mandalay and Rangoon; local treatment for acute severe injuries or chronic disease exacerbations can be suboptimal. Encourage travelers going to Burma to strongly consider purchasing medical evacuation insurance coverage (see Sec. 6, Ch. 1, Travel Insurance, Travel Health Insurance & Medical Evacuation Insurance).

BIBLIOGRAPHY

Cui L, Yan G, Sattabongkot J, Cao Y, Chen B, Chen X, et al. Malaria in the Greater Mekong subregion: heterogeneity and complexity. Acta Trop. 2012;121(3):227–39.

Dapat C, Saito R, Kyaw Y, Naito M, Hasegawa G, Suzuki Y, et al. Epidemiology of human influenza A and B viruses in Myanmar from 2005 to 2007. Intervirology. 2009;52(6):310–20.

Hotez PJ, Bottazzi ME, Strych U, Chang LY, Lim YA, Goodenow MM, et al. Neglected tropical diseases among the Association of Southeast Asian Nations (ASEAN): overview and update. PLoS Negl Trop Dis. 2015;9(4):e0003575.

Lo E, Nguyen J, Oo W, Hemming-Schroeder E, Zhou G, Yang Z, et al. Examining *Plasmodium falciparum* and *P. vivax* clearance subsequent to antimalarial drug treatment in the Myanmar–China border area based on quantitative real-time polymerase chain reaction. BMC Infect Dis. 2016;16(1):154.

Myanmar Information Management Unit: MIMU. The 2014 Myanmar population and housing census. Available from: http://themimu.info/census-data.

Ngwe Tun MM, Kyaw AK, Hmone SW, Inoue S, Buerano CC, Soe AM, et al. Detection of Zika virus infection in Myanmar. Am J Trop Med Hyg. 2018;98(3):868–71.

Schweitzer A, Horn J, Mikolajczyk RT, Krause G, Ott JJ. Estimations of worldwide prevalence of chronic hepatitis B virus infection: a systematic review of data published between 1965 and 2013. Lancet. 2015;386(10003):1546–55.

Tun Win Y, Gardner E, Hadrill D, Su Mon CC, Kyin MM, Maw MT, et al. Emerging zoonotic influenza A virus detection in Myanmar: surveillance practices and findings. Health Secur. 2017;15(5):483–93.

World Health Organization. Global status report on road safety 2018. Geneva: The Organization; 2018. Available from: www.who.int/publications/i/item/9789241565684.

CHINA

Sarah Borwein, Kate Gaynor

DESTINATION OVERVIEW

China, the world's most populous country (>1.4 billion people), is the fourth largest geographically, behind Russia, Canada, and the United States. Divided into 23 provinces, 5 autonomous regions, 4 municipalities, and 2 Special Administrative Regions (Map 10-12), China is home to diverse customs, languages, and topographies. The climate varies from tropical in the south to subarctic in the north, with wide variations between regions and seasons.

The long history and varied natural beauty of China can be traced through its 56 UNESCO World Heritage sites, including the Forbidden City and Temple of Heaven, the Great Wall, the terracotta warriors of Xi'an, and the spectacular mountainous sanctuaries of the west. Recent additions include Quanzhou; Emporium of the World in Song-Yuan; Mount Fanjing in southwest China; the archeological ruins of Liangzhu City in the Yangtze River Delta; the migratory bird sanctuaries along the coast of the Bohai Gulf; the Tusi tribal domains in

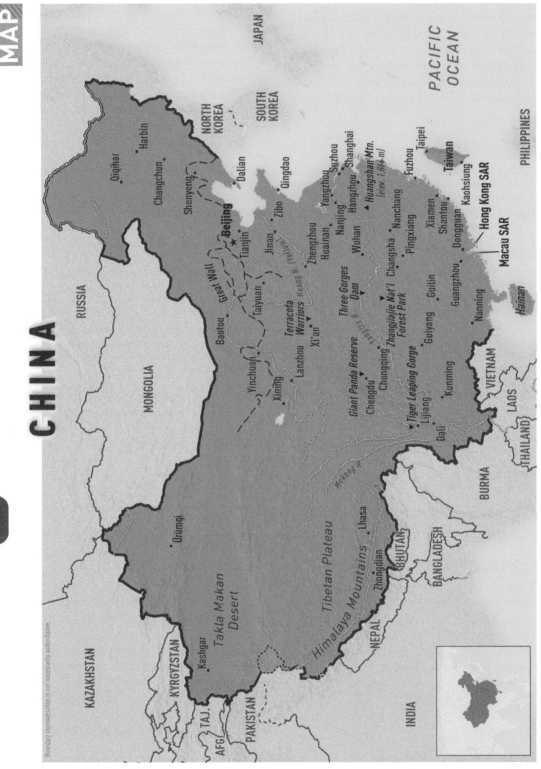

MAP 10-12 China

western China; and the Grand Canal, the oldest (dating back to 468 BCE) and longest (1,115 miles; 1,794 km) man-made canal in the world.

In 2019, >145 million people visited China, and the number of outbound travelers reached nearly 155 million, 3 times more than in 2010. Tourism in China has grown at an extraordinary pace over the past decade, although the coronavirus disease 2019 (COVID-19) pandemic that began in 2020 has, as everywhere, drastically reduced both inbound and outbound travel. By early 2022, China's borders remained effectively closed to international tourism; domestic travel, however, had rebounded sharply, reaching (or even exceeding) 2019 levels. Domestic travelers have been flocking to the usual tourist destinations, including sightseeing in Beijing and the Great Wall, touring Shanghai, cruising the Yangtze River, and visiting the Huangshan (Yellow Mountain) site in Anhui Province (see Box 10-02 for a list of other popular tourist destinations).

Aside from tourism, increasing numbers of people travel to China to visit friends and relatives, to study, to adopt children, or to do humanitarian aid work. These non-tourist travelers might be at greater risk of becoming ill because they underestimate health hazards, are less likely to seek pretravel advice, and are more likely to stay in local or rural accommodations. People traveling to China to adopt often worry about the health of the child (see Sec. 7, Ch. 5, International Adoption), sometimes neglecting their own health.

China has the world's second largest economy and more billionaires (658) than any other country in the world. At the same time, per capita income is still below the world average, with wide disparity in wealth and development between the more urban east and the rural west. Health risks vary accordingly.

INFECTIOUS DISEASE RISKS

Travelers should be up to date on routine vaccinations, including seasonal influenza vaccine. Travelers also should be current on vaccines against diphtheria-tetanus-pertussis, measles-mumps-rubella, and varicella. China began a massive measles vaccination campaign in September 2010 that has decreased the number of reported measles cases; a brief resurgence occurred during 2013–2015, but high measles vaccination coverage has resulted in historically low numbers of measles cases since 2017. Nonetheless, a few travelers made news headlines by triggering outbreaks in their home countries after returning from China. The reported incidence of rubella has fallen, but availability of data is patchy. Cases of pertussis and varicella occur regularly.

Vaccine Quality & Availability in China

China is making considerable advances in vaccine production, working with established pharmaceutical companies in a joint venture approach or by developing and manufacturing vaccines locally. One example is the recent introduction of the Sinovac-CoronaVac COVID-19 vaccine produced by Sinovac Biotech Ltd., a Chinese biopharmaceutical company based in Beijing.

BOX 10-02 Popular tourist destinations in China

GUILIN: uniquely shaped limestone karst mountains, featured in paintings
HAINAN ISLAND: tropical beaches, luxury resorts
HARBIN: spectacular annual winter ice festival
HONG KONG: futuristic architecture, East-meets-West mystique
MACAU: giant modern casinos contrast with a fascinating Portuguese heritage
SICHUAN PROVINCE: home to China's iconic symbol, the giant panda (for more details, see Box 10-03)
TIBET: accessible by the world's highest railroad (maximum elevation 5,072 m; ≈16,600 ft)
YUNNAN PROVINCE: attractions include the Stone Forest outside Kunming, the historic cobblestone city of Lijiang, the Shangri-La valley, and the Tiger Leaping Gorge
ZHANGJIAJIE NATIONAL FOREST PARK (HUNAN PROVINCE): dizzying glass-bottomed canyon bridge, the tallest and longest glass bridge in the world; mountains inspired the setting for the movie *Avatar*

In the past, counterfeit and improperly stored vaccines were a major issue, but China has waged a robust response to recent vaccine scandals and these issues are now rare, at least in major urban areas. Vaccine shortages are, however, frequent. For example, meningococcal vaccines were in short supply in parts of China during 2017–2018, and as of late 2021, tetanus-diphtheria-pertussis (Tdap) vaccine for adults was not available anywhere on the mainland. Travelers should not assume they can complete an unfinished vaccination series once in China; thus, ensure that all travelers going to China are up to date with routine vaccination series before travel. By contrast, circumstances in Hong Kong are different; international vaccines are in use there and are generally available.

Bloodborne Pathogens

HEPATITIS B

Hepatitis B infection is endemic to China (see Sec. 5, Part 2, Ch. 8, Hepatitis B). Nearly one-third of the 350 million people worldwide infected with the hepatitis B virus reside in China. The Advisory Committee on Immunization Practices recommends hepatitis B vaccine for all US adults aged 19–59 years; hepatitis B vaccine should be considered for nonimmune travelers to China.

Enteric Infections & Diseases

BRUCELLOSIS

Brucellosis occurs in pastoral areas of China, particularly the northwest. Travelers should strictly avoid raw or unpasteurized milk products and undercooked meat products (see Sec. 5, Part 1, Ch. 3, Brucellosis).

HEPATITIS E

Hepatitis E is highly endemic in China and can be acquired by drinking untreated water, eating undercooked meats, or staying in areas with poor sanitation (see Sec. 5, Part 2, Ch. 10, Hepatitis E). Pregnant people in their third trimester are at particular risk for severe disease. Because no routine vaccine is available, advise travelers to practice good hand hygiene and to adhere to safe food and water precautions (see Sec. 2, Ch. 8, Food & Water Precautions).

POLIO

The Xinjiang Uygur Autonomous Region borders Pakistan, a polio-endemic country. Adults traveling to this region who will be working in health care facilities, humanitarian aid settings, or refugee camps should be vaccinated against polio, including a single lifetime booster dose of polio vaccine as an adult (see Sec. 5, Part 2, Ch. 17, Poliomyelitis).

TRAVELERS' DIARRHEA

The risk for travelers' diarrhea (see Sec. 2, Ch. 6, Travelers' Diarrhea) appears to be low in so-called "luxury" accommodations in China but moderate elsewhere. Travelers should adhere to safe food and water precautions, and strictly avoid undercooked fish and shellfish and (as noted previously) unpasteurized milk (see Sec. 2, Ch. 8, Food & Water Precautions).

Other than in Hong Kong, tap water is not safe to drink, even in major cities. Most hotels provide boiled or bottled water, and bottled water is readily available.

TYPHOID FEVER

Typhoid fever is not a significant risk in China's major urban areas. Consider vaccinating travelers planning visits to rural areas, adventure travelers, and travelers visiting friends and relatives. Advise them to adhere to safe food and water precautions.

Respiratory Infections & Diseases

CORONAVIRUS DISEASE 2019

Located in central China at the confluence of the Han and Yangtze rivers, Wuhan is a city of 11 million people and a major travel hub accessible by air, land, and water. On December 31, 2019, Chinese officials reported to the World Health Organization (WHO) an outbreak of unusual pneumonia cases linked to a seafood market there. The outbreak spread globally, and on March 11, 2020, WHO officially declared COVID-19 a pandemic.

In response to the outbreak, officials in China combined a swift and stringent lockdown of Wuhan and Hubei Province, with public health messaging, widespread testing, contact tracing, and isolation of all cases and quarantine of contacts. They also built several brand new, full-service COVID-19 hospitals within a matter of days, and established a network of *fangcang* (makeshift) hospitals in public venues (e.g., convention centers, sports stadiums).

Patients with mild illness were isolated in these newly established facilities, thereby reducing the risk of infecting household members. Confirmed or suspected cases were required to be seen at a small number of government-designated fever clinics. Indoor mask-wearing was strictly enforced. Tracking mobile phone applications assigned users a color-coded QR code based on their risk for infection. A green QR code became mandatory for entry into many facilities including stores, restaurants, and public transportation.

As of early 2022, China had partially vaccinated >1 billion of its people using 1 of 6 locally produced vaccines. For current information on COVID-19 in China, consult the US Embassy & Consulates in China website (https://china.usembassy-china.org.cn/). For the US government's COVID-19 international travel requirements and recommendations, see www.cdc.gov/coronavirus/2019-ncov/travelers/international-travel/index.html. All travelers going to China should be up to date with their COVID-19 vaccines (www.cdc.gov/coronavirus/2019-ncov/vaccines/stay-up-to-date.html).

TUBERCULOSIS

China remains moderately endemic for tuberculosis (TB). Travelers can become infected through exposure to a person with active *Mycobacterium tuberculosis* infection. Consuming unpasteurized milk products poses a risk for infection with *Mycobacterium bovis*, another mycobacterium that can cause TB disease in people. For long-term travelers or travelers whose itineraries place them at increased risk for exposure, consider predeparture TB testing with retesting upon their return home. For more details, see Sec. 5, Part 1, Ch. 22, Tuberculosis, and Sec. 5, Part 1, Ch. 23, . . . *perspectives*: Testing Travelers for *Mycobacterium tuberculosis* Infection.

Sexually Transmitted Infections & HIV

Sexually transmitted infections (STIs), including chlamydia, gonorrhea, HIV, and syphilis, are a growing problem in China, particularly along the booming eastern seaboard. Drug-resistant gonorrhea is increasingly prevalent. Make travelers aware of STI risks and the importance of using condoms when having sex with anyone whose HIV or STI status is unknown. As previously noted, travelers also should receive hepatitis B vaccination before travel.

Soil- & Waterborne Infections

SCHISTOSOMIAS & LEPTOSPIROSIS

Although eradication programs have been quite successful, schistosomiasis (see Sec. 5, Part 3, Ch. 20, Schistosomiasis), primarily due to *Schistosoma japonicum*, continues to be reported in various areas, including the Yangtze and Mekong River basins. Advise travelers to avoid freshwater swimming, which also decreases their risk of contracting the bacterial illness, leptospirosis (Sec. 5, Part 1, Ch. 10).

Vectorborne Diseases

CHIKUNGUNYA & DENGUE

Chikungunya has been reported in China, but the level of risk is not well quantified. Dengue, however, is known to be a more significant health risk (see Sec. 5, Part 2, Ch. 4, Dengue). In 2014, China experienced its worst dengue outbreak in decades; Guangdong province reported >40,000 cases in just 2 months. Dengue epidemics occur in China every 4–6 years, mostly in the southern provinces. Travelers should practice insect bite precautions during the summer months (see Sec. 4, Ch. 6, Mosquitoes, Ticks & Other Arthropods).

JAPANESE ENCEPHALITIS

Japanese encephalitis (JE) occurs in all regions of China except Qinghai, Xinjiang, and Xizang (Tibet) (see Table 5-13). China has successfully reduced the incidence of JE through vaccination and, as of 2008, included JE in its expanded national immunization program; JE remains a potential threat to unvaccinated travelers, however.

Although JE season varies by region, most cases occur in local residents during June–October. In addition to season of travel, the risk to travelers depends on their activities, destination, and duration of stay. JE vaccine is recommended for travelers planning to spend ≥1 month in endemic (mainly rural) areas during June–October, when risk for transmission is greatest.

Consider vaccinating shorter-term travelers (<1 month) who plan to visit rural areas, and travelers at increased risk for JE virus exposure based on anticipated activities or itineraries (e.g., those spending substantial time outdoors or staying in accommodations without air conditioning, mosquito nets, or window screens). Sporadic JE cases have occurred on an unpredictable basis in short-term travelers, including in peri-urban Beijing and Shanghai. See Sec. 5, Part 2, Ch. 13, Japanese Encephalitis, for more detailed information.

MALARIA

In the 1940s, China reported >30 million cases of malaria per year. A 70-year eradication campaign progressively reduced numbers, and in 2021, WHO declared China malaria-free. Travelers should still follow insect bite precautions, however, because of the risk for infection with other vectorborne diseases (see Sec. 4, Ch. 6, Mosquitoes, Ticks & Other Arthropods).

PLAGUE

Plague outbreaks occur sporadically in the northern and southwestern areas of the country (see Sec. 5, Part 1, Ch. 15, Plague). Plague is rarely seen

BOX 10-03 Visiting a giant panda reserve in Sichuan Province: health considerations for travelers

The giant panda (*Ailuropoda melanoleuca*) is China's national emblem and one of its most iconic images. Native to south central China, the giant panda's natural habitat has been greatly encroached upon and only a small number of these animals now exist in the wild, in remote areas where seeing them is almost impossible. In response, the Chinese government established over 60 giant panda reserves across southwestern China. Travel to Sichuan province to visit one or more of these habitats and to see the stunning scenery has become increasingly popular. In some locations, especially during the hot summer months, giant pandas spend much time inside, viewable only through glass. The Sichuan giant panda reserves were designated a UNESCO World Heritage Site in 2006.

CHENGDU RESEARCH BASE OF GIANT PANDA BREEDING

Located just 10 km (≈6 mi) north of the city of Chengdu, the Chengdu Research Base of Giant Panda Breeding is a well-developed park.

In some reserves (including the Chengdu Research Base), visitors can get closer to the animals by joining a Panda Volunteer program. Participation in these programs is generally available only to adults and must be arranged and paid for in advance. Programs can vary from one day to one month in length and some might require participants to provide certification of good health. Opportunities to photograph the wildlife can be limited.

ANIMAL BITES

Sichuan Province has a large population of free-roaming dogs. Consider any dog bite a rabies risk. Because of the distance from definitive medical care, including postexposure prophylaxis, encourage travelers planning to visit Sichuan to consider rabies preexposure prophylaxis.

Despite their cute and cuddly appearance, giant pandas are wild animals with a very powerful bite. They can also be infected with rabies. Travelers should avoid any temptation to get close to giant pandas for a "selfie" or a hug.

ELEVATION & TERRAIN OF GIANT PANDA RESERVES

The terrain harboring the giant panda reserves is often rugged and at elevations ranging from 1,100 m (≈3,600 ft) to 4,400 m (≈14,400 ft). Advise tourists visiting reserves at high elevation to acclimatize slowly, and to consider carrying acetazolamide.

The region has many smaller reserves, some of which are peri-urban, others of which can be quite remote and require considerable travel or trekking, making them inaccessible to physically challenged or less physically fit travelers.

ROAD TRAVEL RISKS APPLY TO THESE MORE REMOTE RESERVES.

Travelers to less urban reserves should be prepared for remoteness and travel with a well-stocked travel health kit.

FOOD & WATER PRECAUTIONS AND SANITATION

Travelers to Sichuan Province should follow safe food and water precautions.

Flush toilets are unlikely to be available.

in tourists but is a risk to campers, hikers, hunters, spelunkers, and others exposed to wild rodents or flea-infested cats and dogs.

TICK-BORNE ENCEPHALITIS

Tick-borne encephalitis (TBE) is present in northeastern parts of China and is a risk during March–November. Consider recommending TBE vaccination for travelers engaging in outdoor activities (e.g., camping, hiking) in endemic areas (see Sec. 5, Part 2, Ch. 23, Tick-Borne Encephalitis). Even among vaccinated travelers, reinforce the importance of taking preventive measures (e.g., wearing long pants tucked into socks, using insect repellent, regularly checking for ticks).

ENVIRONMENTAL HAZARDS & RISKS

Air Pollution

Rapid economic expansion and industrialization since 1978 has resulted in serious air pollution issues, along with water and soil contamination, that peaked in 2013. Regional haze triggered public anxiety and official concern, leading to the Air Pollution and Control Plan, which was implemented in 2013; subsequently a series of other initiatives to control soil, water, and plastic waste pollution began.

To tackle air pollution, China introduced several policies and measures targeted at reducing emissions and promoting alternative energy production. Increased use of natural gas and restrictions against burning coal are key to these plans. Other measures included closing highly polluting factories, moving factories farther away from population centers, afforestation projects (planting trees in areas where there had been no trees before), and promoting the use of electric vehicles. These measures have resulted in a dramatic reduction in air pollution, particularly in fine particulate matter ($PM_{2.5}$).

Once renowned for its toxic haze, Beijing is no longer among the 10 most polluted cities in the world. Nonetheless, pollution remains a problem in many parts of the country; and China still accounts for over half of the world's 200 most polluted cities. In the spring of 2021, several large sandstorms originating in southern Mongolia blanketed eastern China in hazardous dust. These sandstorms are unpredictable and are likely to continue. Travelers can check 5-day air quality forecasts at https://aqicn.org/map/china.

Short-term exposure to the levels of air pollution in China's megacities can irritate the eyes and throat. Travelers with underlying cardiorespiratory diseases, including asthma, chronic obstructive pulmonary disease, or congestive heart failure, might find their condition exacerbated. In addition, exposure to high levels of air pollution significantly increases the risk for upper and lower respiratory tract infections, including otitis, sinusitis, bronchitis, and pneumonia. Children and older people are most vulnerable.

Even before the COVID-19 pandemic, surgical-style facemasks were fashionable in China's large cities, especially Beijing, Hong Kong, and Shanghai; facemasks provide wearers no protection from air pollution, however. Properly fitted N95 masks can filter out particulates and might be advisable for people determined to engage in outdoor exercise at times when air quality is very poor (see Sec. 4, Ch. 3, Air Quality & Ionizing Radiation). Many facilities, particularly schools, have installed sophisticated central air-filtering devices and constructed enclosed sports venues.

Altitude Illness

Western China is home to some of the tallest mountains in the world. Some popular destinations are Xining (2,295 m; ≈7,500 ft), Lijiang (2,418 m; ≈7,900 ft), Shangri-La (3,280 m; ≈11,000 ft), and Lhasa (3,658 m; ≈12,000 ft). Preparation and gradual ascent to acclimatize are the mainstays travelers should follow to prevent the onset of altitude illness (see Sec. 4, Ch. 5, High Elevation Travel & Altitude Illness).

Visitors planning high elevation travel whose itineraries do not permit gradual acclimatization—or people otherwise known to be at risk for developing acute mountain sickness (AMS)—should carry their own supply of acetazolamide, because it is not reliably available in China. Dexamethasone, used to both prevent and treat AMS and high-altitude cerebral edema, and to potentially prevent high-altitude pulmonary edema (HAPE), reportedly is available in China. Similarly, nifedipine (as a prevention and treatment for HAPE) reportedly is available. The quality and ready availability of either of these drugs is unknown; thus, as with acetazolamide, travelers should carry a personal supply in a travel health kit.

Animal Bites & Rabies

An analysis of data collected by the GeoSentinel Surveillance Network showed that dog bites are surprisingly common among tourists to China. In addition, in China (as in much of Asia) rabies remains a serious problem. Animal rabies is endemic in China and might even be increasing, especially in the dog population. Thus, travelers should consider any dog or other mammal bite received anywhere in China, including urban areas, a high risk for rabies infection (see Sec. 5, Part 2, Ch. 18, Rabies).

Because international-standard rabies immune globulin is often unavailable, animal bites can be trip-enders, requiring evacuation to Bangkok, Hong Kong, or home, to receive appropriate post-exposure prophylaxis (PEP). Rabies is a particular risk for younger children, who are more likely to approach animals and less likely to report bites or scratches. Incorporate a discussion of rabies risk and prevention during pretravel consultations, and develop a strategy with travelers for dealing with possible exposures, including purchasing medical evacuation insurance coverage (see Sec. 6, Ch. 1, Travel Insurance, Travel Health Insurance & Medical Evacuation Insurance). Consider providing long-term travelers and expatriates going to live in China with the rabies preexposure vaccination series.

Human rabies deaths in China peaked at 3,300 cases in 2007 and decreased to 290 cases in 2019; the decline in human rabies deaths is mainly attributable to widespread use of PEP and public PEP awareness.

Natural Disasters

Five of the 10 deadliest natural disasters in history have occurred in China. In the last few decades, almost every type of major hazard except volcanic eruption has hit China, including cold waves, droughts, earthquakes, forest and grassland fires, hailstorms, heat waves, red tides, sandstorms, and torrential rains resulting in debris flows and landslides. Typhoons and storm surges occur regularly along the southern and eastern seaboards.

Earthquakes cause significant death and destruction. For instance, devastating earthquakes struck the western provinces of Qinghai in 2010 and Sichuan in 2019. Advise US citizen travelers to enroll with the Department of State's Smart Traveler Enrollment Program (STEP; https://step.state.gov/step); STEP will provide travelers with information and alerts from local US embassies or consulates about disasters, safety, and security issues at their destination.

Vitamin D Deficiency

Vitamin D deficiency is a major issue in the northern provinces of China, where (despite the progress in reducing air pollution noted previously) smog blocks out sunlight, leading to inadequate vitamin D absorption even during the summer months. To decrease the risk of osteomalacia and osteoporosis in travelers spending >6 months in China, prescribe vitamin D supplementation.

Wet Markets

So-called "wet markets" are common throughout China, south Asia, and southeast Asia. The term wet market is a generic one, encompassing many types of marketplaces selling perishable goods; some sell only fruit and vegetables, but others sell live animals that are slaughtered on-site after purchase. Most do not sell wild or exotic animals, and the tendency to lump all wet markets together has fueled Sinophobia related to the origins of the COVID-19 pandemic.

The exotic animal trade has been banned in China, but smuggling of animals (e.g., pangolins) is highly profitable and difficult to control. A coordinated international response will be required to curb the exotic animal trade. Travelers should avoid visiting markets selling live animals because these have been linked with many zoonotic outbreaks, including monkeypox and severe acute respiratory syndrome (SARS). Avian influenza transmission is another reason for travelers to avoid live animal markets.

SAFETY & SECURITY

Crime

Rates of violent crime are low in China, but minor theft, pickpocketing, and various forms of scams and fraud do occur, especially in densely populated and more heavily touristed areas. Scams targeting foreign businesses also have been reported. Travelers should remain vigilant about their personal belongings, and avoid responding to emails from, or giving out sensitive information to, unknown sources.

Political Unrest

Travelers should be aware of and avoid involvement in protests and flare-ups of unrest in places as diverse as Hong Kong, Tibet, and Xinjiang Province. Travelers also should avoid public criticism of the Communist Party or the government. The internet is censored, and many widely used social media sites might be unavailable.

Traffic-Related Injuries

Traffic in China is often chaotic. The rate of traffic crashes, including fatal ones, is among the highest in the world (see Sec. 8, Ch. 5, Road & Traffic Safety). Traffic crashes, even minor ones, can create major traffic jams and sometimes turn into violent altercations, particularly when foreign travelers are involved (see Sec. 4, Ch. 11, Safety & Security Overseas).

China has not signed the convention that created the International Driving Permit and requires travelers to have a Chinese license to drive. Recent regulations have allowed foreign travelers to obtain a temporary (≤3 months) driver's license, if they have a valid overseas driver's license *and* a notarized copy translated into Chinese; in addition, travelers are required to attend lessons on Chinese road safety regulations.

Driving is on the right side of the road in mainland China and Taiwan, but on the left in Hong Kong and Macau. If travelers choose to drive, advise them to avoid driving at night or when weather conditions are bad, and to not assume that traffic rules or rights-of-way will be respected. Despite national seatbelt legislation being in effect since 2004, seatbelt use is inconsistent, and rear seatbelts often are unavailable. Use of child safety seats recently become mandatory. For all these reasons, travelers likely will find it safer and simpler to hire a local driver or to use public transportation than to drive themselves. Travelers should take care when opening the door of a taxi or private vehicle, to avoid hitting cyclists or pedestrians.

ELECTRONIC BICYCLES

Electronic bicycles (E-bikes) are popular in China and do not have to be registered. E-bike riders often travel in pedestrian and bicycle lanes as well as with traffic. Because E-bikes have no engine noise, pedestrians might not readily identify an oncoming E-bike. Motor vehicles and E-bikes often drive without lights, making night travel dangerous. Bicycle helmets are rarely worn in China; a new 2020 law requiring helmet use for riders of motorcycles and E-bikes has resulted in a shortage of available helmets.

AVAILABILITY & QUALITY OF MEDICAL CARE

Strongly encourage travelers to invest in travel health insurance, including medical evacuation insurance coverage (see Sec. 6, Ch. 1, Travel Insurance, Travel Health Insurance & Medical Evacuation Insurance). Many hospitals do not accept foreign medical insurance, and patients are expected to pay a deposit to cover the anticipated cost of treatment before care is delivered. Many major cities, including Beijing, Guangzhou, Hong Kong, Shanghai, and Shenzhen have medical facilities that meet international standards. Hospitals in other cities might have "VIP wards" (*gaogan bingfang*) with English-speaking staff. The standard of care in such facilities is somewhat unpredictable, however, and cultural and regulatory differences can cause difficulties for travelers. In rural areas, rudimentary medical care might be all that is available.

Blood & Blood Product Safety

Hepatitis B and hepatitis C virus transmission from poorly sterilized medical equipment remains a risk in remote areas. The blood supply is heavily regulated and generally deemed safe, but is very limited, especially for rare types, including Rhesus negative blood; hospitals usually have only a few units of blood on hand. Rhogam legally is available only in Hong Kong, and recently in Shenzhen, under a new program permitting drugs and medical equipment already marketed in Hong Kong to be used in the Guangdong–Hong Kong–Macau "Greater Bay Area" after approval.

Emergency Medical Services

Emergency medical services are scarce in many parts of China, most acutely in rural areas. In major cities, 2 types of ambulance are available: general ambulances and ambulances that carry more advanced medical equipment. No recognized paramedic profession exists in China, and ambulances might be staffed instead with doctors or nurses with variable levels of training. In many rural areas, rather than waiting for an ambulance to arrive, injured travelers might be better off taking a taxi or other immediately available vehicle to the nearest major hospital.

Medical Tourism

Most people who choose to try traditional Chinese remedies do so uneventfully, albeit not without accepting some risk. Remind travelers that acupuncture needles can be a source of bloodborne and skin infections; acupressure might be preferable. Herbal medicine products can be contaminated with heavy metals or pharmaceutical agents.

China is currently witnessing an influx of patients coming from Africa seeking treatment not available in their home countries. Medical tourists from high-income countries looking for as-yet unapproved experimental treatments are also a growing market (see Sec. 6, Ch. 4, Medical Tourism).

Pharmacies

Pharmacies often sell prescription medications over the counter, but these can be counterfeit, substandard, or contaminated (see Sec. 6, Ch. 3, . . . *perspectives*: Avoiding Poorly Regulated Medicines & Medical Products During Travel). Advise travelers to bring all their regular medications in sufficient quantity. If travelers need more or other medications, recommend that they visit a reputable clinic or hospital. China allows travelers to bring controlled medications into the country in quantities "reasonable for personal use." Especially for controlled medications, travelers are expected to carry a copy of the written prescription with them and, whenever possible, a signed note from the prescribing physician written on letterhead stationery.

BIBLIOGRAPHY

Amicizia D, Zangrillo F, Lai PL, Iovine M, Panatto D. Overview of Japanese encephalitis disease and its prevention. Focus on IC51 vaccine (IXIARO®). J Prev Med Hyg. 2018;59(1):E99–107.

Burki T. China's successful control of COVID-19. Lancet Infect Dis. 2020;20(11):1240–1.

Davis XM, MacDonald S, Borwein S, Freedman DO, Kozarsky PE, von Sonnenburg F, et al. Health risks in travelers to China: the GeoSentinel experience and implications for the 2008 Beijing Olympics. Am J Trop Med Hyg. 2008;79(1):4–8.

Li Z, Xu Jindong, Xu J, Tan H, Zhang C. Current situation, causes, and countermeasures to NIP vaccine shortages in Guangzhou, China. Hum Vaccin Immunother. 2020;16(1):76–9.

Lu X, Zhang S, Xing J, Wang Y, Chen W, Ding D, et al. Progress of air pollution control in China and its challenges and opportunities in the ecological civilization era. Engineering. 2020;6(12):1423–31.

Miao F, Li N, Yang J, Chen T, Liu Y, Zhang S, et al. Neglected challenges in the control of animal rabies in China. One Health. 2021;12:100212.

Shaw MT, Leggat PA, Borwein S. Travelling to China for the Beijing 2008 Olympic and Paralympic games. Travel Med Infect Dis. 2007;5(6):365–73.

United Nations World Tourism Organization. UNWTO tourism highlights: 2018 Edition. Madrid: The Organization; 2018. Available from: www.e-unwto.org/doi/book/10.18111/9789284419876.

World Health Organization. Global hepatitis report 2017. Geneva: The Organization; 2017. Available from: www.who.int/publications/i/item/global-hepatitis-report-2017.

Xia J, Min L, Shu J. Dengue fever in China: an emerging problem demands attention. Emerg Microbes Infect. 2015;4(1):e3.

Yu X, Li N. Understanding the beginning of a pandemic: China's response to the emergence of COVID-19. J Infect Public Health. 2021;14(3):347–52.

INDIA

Kristin VanderEnde, Meghna Desai

DESTINATION OVERVIEW

India is approximately one-third the size of the United States but has 4 times the population—almost 1.4 billion people—making it the second most populous country in the world, behind China. Rich in history, culture, and diversity, India is the birthplace of 4 of the world's religions: Buddhism, Hinduism, Jainism, and Sikhism. India is experiencing rapid urbanization, as noted in the growth of megacities (e.g., Delhi, Mumbai). India's topography is varied, ranging from tropical beaches to deserts, foothills, and the Himalaya Mountains. Northern India has a more temperate climate; the south is more tropical year-round. Many travelers prefer India during the winter (November–March), when temperatures are more agreeable.

Because of India's size, short-term travelers usually select a region of the country to visit for any given trip. A typical itinerary to the north includes the cities of Agra, Delhi, Varanasi, and cities in Rajasthan State (e.g., Jaipur [the Pink City] and Udaipur). More southern routes might swing through the beaches of Goa and the cities of Bengaluru (Bangalore) and Mumbai. In the east, Kolkata (Calcutta) is considered the cultural capital of the country.

Despite the many and varied itineraries, most health recommendations for travelers to India are similar. The incidence of some illnesses (e.g., those transmitted by mosquitoes) is greater during the monsoon season (June–September), which has high temperatures, heavy rains, and the risk of flooding. Travelers visiting friends and relatives (VFRs) require extra consideration. Because they might stay in rural areas not often visited by tourists or businesspeople, live in homes, and eat and drink with their families, VFR travelers are at greater risk for many travel-related illnesses (see Sec. 9, Ch. 9, Visiting Friends & Relatives: VFR Travel). Some VFR travelers might not seek pre-travel health advice since they are returning to their land of origin.

INFECTIOUS DISEASE RISKS

All travelers to India should be up to date with routine immunizations (see www.cdc.gov/vaccines/schedules). Infants 6–11 months old should get 1 dose of measles-mumps-rubella (MMR) vaccine before travel to India; this dose does not count as part of the routine childhood vaccination series. Vaccination against hepatitis A, hepatitis B, and coronavirus disease 2019 (COVID-19) is recommended for travelers to India; specific guidance varies by age of the traveler (see the disease-specific chapters in Section 5). Additionally, India requires travelers coming from countries reporting cases of polio to show proof of oral polio vaccination; travelers should check with the Ministry of Health to learn if there is a requirement for a dose of polio vaccine prior to entry into India.

Enteric Infections & Diseases

CHOLERA

Active cholera transmission has been reported from India in recent years and might be underreported. For current cholera vaccine recommendations for travel to India, refer to the destination page on the Centers for Disease Control and Prevention (CDC) Travelers' Health website (https://wwwnc.cdc.gov/travel/destinations/traveler/none/india). For more information on cholera, see Sec. 5, Part 1, Ch. 5, Cholera.

10

GIARDIASIS

Giardiasis (see Sec. 5, Part 3, Ch. 12, Giardiasis) is a major cause of diarrheal disease and is associated with morbidity in both children and adults in India. Travelers should maintain good hand hygiene, avoid drinking tap water, and should exclusively consume boiled, bottled, or filtered water (see Sec. 2, Ch. 9, Water Disinfection).

HEPATITIS E

Hepatitis E virus is transmitted through fecally contaminated water and person-to-person through the fecal–oral route (see Sec. 5, Part 2, Ch. 10, Hepatitis E). Highly endemic to India, hepatitis E is a major cause of acute viral hepatitis and acute liver failure. Infection during pregnancy puts people at greater risk for severe disease as well as adverse pregnancy outcomes (e.g., miscarriage, neonatal demise).

Travelers drinking untreated water or going to areas with poor sanitation are at risk for infection. Travelers should maintain good hand hygiene; avoid tap water; drink only boiled, bottled, or filtered water; and eat thoroughly cooked meats (see Sec. 2, Ch. 8, Food & Water Precautions). Travelers immunized against hepatitis A who develop symptomatic hepatitis likely have hepatitis E.

TRAVELERS' DIARRHEA

Travelers' diarrhea (TD) is acquired through ingestion of contaminated food, water, or beverages, particularly in places where basic hygiene and sanitation infrastructure is poor. Both cooked and uncooked foods are potential vehicles for infection if handled improperly. The risk for TD is high in India; travelers have >60% likelihood of developing TD during a 2-week journey. Discuss self-treatment for diarrheal illness with travelers (see Sec. 2, Ch. 6, Travelers' Diarrhea, and Sec. 2, Ch. 8, Food & Water Precautions).

TYPHOID & PARATYPHOID FEVER

In the United States, ≈85% of cases of typhoid fever are in people who traveled to India or other countries in South Asia (see Sec. 5, Part 1, Ch. 24, Typhoid & Paratyphoid Fever). Thus, even for short-term travel, typhoid vaccine is recommended. Patients hesitant to be vaccinated might be persuaded by learning that typhoid fever acquired in South Asia is typically multidrug-resistant, and in a growing number of instances extensively drug-resistant. Remind all travelers to India to also practice good hand hygiene and follow safe food and water precautions.

Paratyphoid fever, a clinically similar disease caused by *Salmonella enterica* serotypes Paratyphi A, B, and C, has become increasingly prevalent in South Asia, but typhoid vaccines are not protective against this infection.

Respiratory Infections & Diseases

CORONAVIRUS DISEASE 2019

Nationwide, COVID-19 vaccine coverage in India is low. For current information on COVID-19 in India, consult the US Embassy & Consulates in India website (https://in.usembassy.gov/). For the US government's COVID-19 international travel requirements and recommendations, see www.cdc.gov/coronavirus/2019-ncov/travelers/international-travel/index.html. All travelers going to India should be up to date with their COVID-19 vaccines (www.cdc.gov/coronavirus/2019-ncov/vaccines/stay-up-to-date.html).

ENDEMIC FUNGI

Four environmentally transmitted fungal pathogens are predominant to India; risk to travelers varies by activity and underlying health conditions.

ASPERGILLOSIS

Aspergillus spp. are airborne fungi that cause a broad array of illnesses ranging from mild to severe. Azole resistance and unavailability of amphotericin B complicate treatment. Most severe aspergillosis illness occurs in patients who are severely immunocompromised or critically ill.

CRYPTOCOCCOSIS

Cryptococcus neoformans exists in the environment worldwide. The fungus is typically found in soil, on decaying wood, in tree hollows, or in bird droppings (see www.cdc.gov/fungal/diseases/cryptococcosis-neoformans/causes.html). When inhaled, *C. neoformans* can cause a pneumonia-like illness. *C. neoformans* also is known to cause meningitis, especially in people who are immunocompromised or living with HIV. Diagnostic testing is limited in India.

HISTOPLASMOSIS

In areas where *Histoplasma* spp. are endemic, occupational and recreational (e.g., bat or bird-watching, cave exploration) activities that disrupt the soil surface can release infectious mold spores into the air. If inhaled, these spores can cause acute pulmonary disease and, more rarely, focal or disseminated extrapulmonary infection (see Sec. 5, Part 4, Ch. 2, Histoplasmosis).

MUCORMYCOSIS

Various modes of transmission (inhalation being most common) for *Mucorales* spp. have been described. Underlying diabetes mellitus and glucocorticoid steroid use are among the major risk factors for mucormycosis in India. Mucormycosis has become a risk among patients recovering from COVID-19 and is associated with poor outcomes in these patients.

INFLUENZA

Influenza virus circulation in India usually peaks during the monsoon season (June–September) with secondary peaks during winter (November–February). Furthermore, the actual timing of the influenza season varies across the country due to differences in regional climates. Influenza vaccine coverage in India is assumed to be very low (no official data are available). Travelers who receive the Northern Hemisphere influenza vaccine might not be fully protected from the viral strain circulating in India and should observe all necessary behavioral precautions to protect themselves from influenza, including frequent handwashing and respiratory etiquette. Travelers to India are strongly encouraged to receive an influenza vaccine directed against the Southern Hemisphere influenza strains from their health care providers, either in the United States (if available) or in India.

TUBERCULOSIS

Approximately 25% of all tuberculosis (TB) cases worldwide are reported from India. Travelers planning to work in high-risk settings or in crowded institutions (e.g., homeless shelters, hospitals, medical clinics, prisons) are at risk for exposure. Travelers visiting ill friends or relatives or engaging in congregate activities (e.g., religious gatherings) also can face TB exposure risk.

Discuss the importance of testing before and after travel, and measures travelers can take to prevent disease. Travelers with anticipated exposure risks should undergo tuberculin skin testing have an interferon-γ release assay (IGRA) before leaving the United States (see Sec. 5, Part 1, Ch. 23, . . . *perspectives*: Testing Travelers for *Mycobacterium tuberculosis* Infection). If a tuberculin skin test is used, CDC recommends the 2-step method for establishing a baseline. If the predeparture test results are negative, repeat the same type of test 8–10 weeks after the traveler returns from India.

Use of bacillus Calmette-Guérin (BCG) vaccine in health care workers who will have increased risk of exposure during travel has been proposed, although this recommendation remains controversial (see Sec. 5, Part 1, Ch. 22, Tuberculosis). US Food and Drug Administration–approved BCG formulations are no longer available in the United States.

Sexually Transmitted Infections & HIV

As of 2019, an estimated 2.3 million people in India were living with HIV infection. Although the reported adult HIV prevalence in India is low, prevalence is much greater in specific locations (e.g., in the states of Manipur, Mizoram, Nagaland) and among high-risk populations (e.g., people who inject drugs, transgender people, men who have sex with men, and female sex workers). Condomless sex increases a traveler's risk for HIV and other sexually transmitted infections, including chlamydia, gonorrhea, and syphilis.

Indian law penalizes acts related to prostitution, including running a brothel, soliciting, and trafficking. High-quality condoms and other barrier methods are available for sale in drugstores in India. Homosexuality is not illegal in India.

Skin Infections

SUPERFICIAL DERMATOPHYTOSIS

In addition to emerging viral and multidrug-resistant bacterial pathogens, superficial dermatophytosis has become a significant problem for travelers to India, largely due to the presence of a widespread fungal strain that is highly resistant to treatment. Indiscriminate use of topical antifungal + highly potent steroid combination preparations is believed to have contributed to the rise of the fungal strain (see www.cdc.gov/fungal/diseases/ringworm/steroids.html). Travelers who develop a rash they think is ringworm should be aware that creams sold widely in drugstores in India can worsen the infection and cause other health problems. Consider prescribing a product that travelers can take in their travel health kit. For severe or recurrent infections, consider posttravel molecular testing for species identification (see Sec. 11, Ch. 8, Dermatologic Conditions).

Soil- & Waterborne Infections

HELMINTHS

India accounts for 65% of soil-transmitted helminth infections in Southeast Asia, and 27% of all cases globally. Pathogens are found in both urban and rural areas, and include roundworm (*Ascaris lumbricoides*), hookworm (*Ancylostoma duodenale* and *Necatur americanus*), and whipworm (*Trichuris trichiura*). Symptoms might be nonspecific and include abdominal pain, diarrhea (with blood or mucous), fatigue, nausea, vomiting, and weight loss. To reduce the risk for infection, travelers should pay attention to hand hygiene, safe food and water precautions, and always wear shoes (see Sec. 5, Part 3, Ch. 13, Soil-Transmitted Helminths).

Vectorborne Diseases

CHIKUNGUNYA, DENGUE & ZIKA

During the last several years, India has experienced outbreaks of chikungunya, transmitted by infected *Aedes* species (*Ae. aegypti* or *Ae. albopictus*) mosquitoes. Chikungunya symptoms are similar to those of dengue and malaria, but often with severe and persistent arthralgia (see Sec. 5, Part 2, Ch. 2, Chikungunya).

Dengue is transmitted by infected *Aedes* species (*Ae. aegypti* or *Ae. albopictus*) mosquitoes and is endemic to all of India except at high elevation in mountainous regions (see Sec. 5, Part 2, Ch. 4, Dengue). Large outbreaks can occur, including in many urban areas. Incidence is greatest during the wet summer season, which includes the monsoon season (June–September). *Aedes* mosquitoes bite both indoors and outdoors. Travelers to India should take measures to protect themselves from mosquito bites (see Sec. 4, Ch. 6, Mosquitoes, Ticks & Other Arthropods).

Zika is a risk in India. Because of the possibility for birth defects in infants born to mothers infected with Zika during pregnancy, people who are pregnant or trying to become pregnant should review the most recent recommendations at https://wwwnc.cdc.gov/travel/page/zika-information.

JAPANESE ENCEPHALITIS

Japanese encephalitis (JE) virus is present throughout the country. Transmission occurs mostly from May–October in northern states and year-round in southern states. The JE virus is transmitted to humans who live and work in rural areas (typically around rice paddies and irrigation systems), primarily by *Culex* mosquitoes that feed on infected birds, pigs, and other mammals. Symptoms include diarrhea, fever, severe headache, vomiting, general weakness, and neurological symptoms. Vaccination is recommended for people traveling extensively in rural areas, long-term travelers, and people assigned to work in endemic areas (see Sec. 5, Part 2, Ch. 13, Japanese Encephalitis).

LEISHMANIASIS (KALA AZAR)

Visceral leishmaniasis (VL), transmitted by sandflies (*Phlebotomus argentipes*), presents with acute fever and splenomegaly (see Sec. 5, Part 3, Ch. 15, Visceral Leishmaniasis). Travelers to India should take measures to protect themselves from both day- and night-biting sandflies (see Sec. 4, Ch. 6, Mosquitoes, Ticks & Other Arthropods).

LYMPHATIC FILARIASIS

Lymphatic filariasis (LF) is transmitted by several mosquito vectors that bite during day, evening, and night, including *Aedes*, *Anopheles*, and *Culex* mosquito spp. (see Sec. 5, Part 3, Ch .9, Lymphatic Filariasis). LF presents with lymphedema and elephantiasis many years after the infection; in men, LF can present with hydrocele (swelling of the scrotum). In most instances, short-term travelers are at low risk because multiple bites over time are necessary for infection. Long-term travelers and expatriates are at greater risk.

MALARIA

Malaria remains a public health problem in India. Both *Plasmodium vivax* and chloroquine-resistant *P. falciparum* are found throughout India, including the cities of Mumbai and New Delhi; most cases occur in 7 states: Chhattisgarh, Gujarat, Jharkhand, Madhya Pradesh, Odisha, Uttar Pradesh, and West Bengal. Malaria-transmitting mosquitoes bite primarily between dusk and dawn. For recommended prophylaxis and mosquito bite precautions, see Sec. 2, Ch. 5, Yellow Fever Vaccine & Malaria Prevention Information, by Country; Sec. 4, Ch. 6, Mosquitoes, Ticks & Other Arthropods; and Sec. 5, Part 3, Ch. 16, Malaria.

RICKETTSIAL DISEASES

Rickettsial infections, including outbreaks, are present across India; scrub typhus is the most common (see Sec. 5, Part 1, Ch. 18, Rickettsial Diseases). Infection is seasonal (after the rainy season), more prevalent in rural areas, and often presents with nonspecific signs and symptoms. Travelers should wear long sleeves and pants and protect exposed skin with insect repellents when visiting potential vector-infested areas, especially areas with forest and vegetation (see Sec. 4, Ch. 6, Mosquitoes, Ticks & Other Arthropods). Counsel travelers to seek prompt medical care for acute fever onset, rash, or eschar (tan, brown, or black tissue) around an insect bite.

YELLOW FEVER

India has no risk for yellow fever (YF), and CDC has no recommendations for travelers to receive YF vaccine before going to India. The Government of India, however, has strict and carefully defined country entry requirements for proof of vaccination against yellow fever from travelers ≥9 months old (infants <9 months old exempted) arriving from areas with risk of yellow fever virus transmission (for details, see Sec. 2, Ch. 5, Yellow Fever Vaccine and Malaria Prevention Information, by Country).

ENVIRONMENTAL HAZARDS & RISKS

Air Quality

Air pollution is a major public health problem across India, and travelers might encounter high-level exposures to various pollutants in urban, peri-urban, and rural settings. All travelers to India should be aware of local air pollution concerns and any advisories in effect on a day-to-day basis (see Sec. 4, Ch. 3, Air Quality & Ionizing Radiation). Vulnerable groups (e.g., children, older people) and people with preexisting health conditions (e.g., asthma, chronic lung disease, coronary artery disease) are particularly at risk for adverse outcomes. When air quality is poor or expected to deteriorate, travelers should avoid outdoor activities and follow local health guidance from the Government of India, Ministry of Environment and Forests (MOEF), Central Pollution Control Board (www.moef.gov.in), and the US Embassy and US Consulates in India (https://in.usembassy.gov/).

Altitude Illness & Acute Mountain Sickness

Popular tourist destinations in India include the high-elevation Himalayas. Inform travelers visiting these areas about the early symptoms of altitude illness and acute mountain sickness, to not ascend to higher elevations when experiencing symptoms, and to descend if symptoms become worse while resting at the same elevation (see Sec. 4, Ch. 5, High Elevation Travel & Altitude Illness). Travelers with certain underlying medical problems can be at increased risk for adverse events associated with travel to high elevations and should consult a physician familiar with this topic prior to departure.

Animal Bites & Rabies

India has the highest burden of rabies in the world; rabid dogs are common (see Sec. 5, Part 2, Ch. 18, Rabies). Travelers bitten or scratched by a dog or other mammal in India might have limited or no access to postexposure rabies treatment; rabies immune globulin is generally not available in India. Encourage travelers to consider purchasing a medical evacuation insurance policy that will cover travel to receive recommended rabies postexposure prophylaxis. Discuss preexposure rabies vaccination with travelers who have high exposure risk, including adventure travelers, campers, cave explorers, children, people for whom there is an occupational exposure risk (e.g., veterinarians, wildlife biologists), and people visiting rural areas.

Animal bites and wounds can transmit diseases other than rabies. Cellulitis, fasciitis, and wound infections can result from the scratch or bite of any animal. Potentially fatal to humans, B virus is carried by macaques (see Sec. 5, Part 2, Ch. 1, B Virus). These Old World monkeys inhabit many of the temples in India, scatter themselves in many tourist gathering places, and are kept as pets. Macaques can be aggressive and often seek food from people. When visiting temples, travelers should not carry any food in their bags, hands, or pockets. Stress to travelers that they should not approach or attempt to handle monkeys or other animals. If bitten, travelers should seek immediate medical care.

Travelers, particularly those going to rural areas, should be aware of the risk for snake bites, and should take precautions to wear solid shoes or boots and use a flashlight when walking outside at night.

Climate & Sun Exposure

Sun exposure and heat-related illnesses are concerns for travelers in India, particularly during summer months and at high elevations (see Sec. 4, Ch. 1, Sun Exposure, and Sec. 4, Ch. 2, Extremes of Temperature). Travelers should eat and drink regularly, wear loose and lightweight clothing, and limit physical activity at times when temperatures are high.

Natural Disasters

Natural disasters, including cyclones, droughts, earthquakes, floods, and landslides, are not uncommon in India. Travelers should become aware of the natural disaster risks at their destination. Encourage US citizens and nationals traveling and living in India to enroll in the US Department of State's Smart Traveler Enrollment Program (https://step.state.gov/step) to receive information from the US embassy on safety conditions, and to help the US embassy in India contact them in an emergency, including during natural disasters.

SAFETY & SECURITY

Crime

Crime does occur in India, but rarely is it directed toward foreign travelers; verbal and sometimes physical harassment of female foreign travelers is a concerning exception. Although most victims of harassment are locals, attacks in tourist areas highlight the fact that visitors to India are also at risk and should exercise vigilance and situational awareness. Petty crimes (e.g., pickpocketing, purse snatching) are very common when using public transportation, while out walking, and in heavily populated tourist areas.

Mass Gatherings

Drawing tens of millions of people, Kumbh Mela is the largest mass gathering event / religious pilgrimage in the world. Celebrated according to the Hindu calendar, Kumbh Mela occurs 4 times over an approximately 12-year cycle. During each observance of this normally 4-month long festival, pilgrims ritually bathe in one of 4 sacred rivers in India; in 2021, Kumbh Mela was limited to 30 days due to the COVID-19 pandemic. Mass casualty trauma (e.g., crush injuries, stampedes) and transmission of antimicrobial-resistant organisms and enteric and respiratory pathogens are among the more serious risks to health and safety associated with attendance (see Sec. 9, Ch. 10, Mass Gatherings).

Political & Religious Unrest

Demonstrations and general strikes (*bandh*) often cause inconvenience. Religious violence occurs occasionally. Travelers should obey curfews and travel restrictions, and avoid demonstrations and rallies because of the potential for violence.

Terrorism

India continues to experience terrorist and insurgent activities that can affect US citizens directly or indirectly. Terror attacks have targeted public places (e.g., cinemas, hotels, markets, mosques, restaurants in large urban areas, trains and train stations), including some places frequented by tourists. Although an attack can occur at any time, they generally take place during the busy evening hours in markets and other crowded places. Travelers should pay attention to US Department of State advisories regarding issues that arise at some borders, religious tensions, or terrorist activities. In times of instability, travelers should seek guidance from the US Embassy or Consulates in India website (https://in.usembassy.gov/) for appropriate action (see Sec. 4, Ch. 11, Safety & Security Overseas).

Traffic-Related Injuries

India's roadways are some of the most hazardous in the world, and have large numbers of traffic-related deaths, including among pedestrians (see Sec. 8, Ch. 5, Road & Traffic Safety). Animals, bicycles, overcrowded buses, motor scooters, people, rickshaws, and trucks all compete for space on streets and roads, increasing the risk for crashes. Travelers should fasten seat belts when riding in cars, and wear a helmet when riding bicycles or motorbikes. Advise travelers to avoid boarding overcrowded buses and not to travel by bus into the interior of the country or on curving, mountainous roads. Discourage nighttime driving (long-distance travel in particular), even with a hired, paid driver.

AVAILABILITY & QUALITY OF MEDICAL CARE

While India ranks highly in the international quality standards maintained at its major private hospitals that employ the bulk of the country's doctors, it lags in postoperative care (e.g., environment, hygiene, infection control) and regulations (e.g., facilitators, hospitals, insurance, medicolegal issues) as compared to regional competitors.

Travelers needing medical care while traveling can contact the US embassy in India (https://in.usembassy.gov/) for referrals, speak to a hotel concierge, or check www.indiahealthcare.org, which includes links to find medical treatment by category, and a list of hospitals accredited by the National Accreditation Board for Hospitals & Healthcare Providers (Constituent Board of the Quality Council of India). Most major hospitals in big cities accept payment by major credit cards; hospitals and doctors in smaller cities might only accept cash.

Medical Tourism

Well-trained English-speaking health care practitioners and low cost for high-quality treatment make India a health care destination for a mix of alternative (ayurveda, homeopathy, yoga), curative (cosmetic, surgical), and wellness medicine.

ACKNOWLEDGMENTS

The authors would like to acknowledge substantial contributions to the sections on vectorborne, foodborne, and waterborne diseases from Dr. Kayla Laserson, Bill & Melinda Gates Foundation, India. We thank the following people for their expert review and contributions across various sections of the chapter: Dr. Syed Asrafuzzaman, Department of Health and Human Services (Availability & Quality of Medical Care); Mr. Yvon Guillaume, US Department of State (Safety & Security); Dr. John Jereb, CDC (Tuberculosis); Dr. Deepika Joshi and Dr. Melissa Nyendak, CDC India (HIV & Sexually Transmitted Infections); Dr. Vikas Kapil, CDC (Air Quality); Dr. Siddhartha Saha, CDC India (Influenza); and Dr. Anoop Velayudhan, Indian Council of Medical Research (Fungal Infections and Superficial Dermatophytosis).

BIBLIOGRAPHY

Banerjee S, Denning DW, Chakrabarti A. One Health aspects & priority roadmap for fungal diseases: a mini-review. Indian J Med Res. 2021;153(3):311–9.

Children's Investment Fund Foundation. Worms in India: the scale up and success of a world-leading deworming program. 2019. Available from: https://ciff.org/news/worms-india-scale-and-success-world-leading-deworming-programme.

Date KA, Newton AE, Medalla F, Blackstock A, Richardson L, McCollough A, et al. Changing patterns in enteric fever incidence and increasing antibiotic resistance of enteric fever isolates in the United States, 2008–2012. Clin Infect Dis. 2016;63(3):322–9.

de Saussure PPH. Management of the returning traveler with diarrhea. Ther Adv Gastroenterol. 2009;2(6):367–75.

Federation of Indian Chambers of Commerce and Industry. FICCI knowledge paper: building best practices in healthcare services globally. New Delhi: The Federation; 2019.

National AIDS Control Organization. Sankalak: status of national AIDS response, second edition. New Delhi: NACO, Ministry of Health and Family Welfare, Government of India; 2020. Available from: http://naco.gov.in/sites/default/files/Sankalak%20Status%20of%20National%20AIDS%20Response,%20Second%20Edition%20(2020).pdf.

Sharma A, Mishra B. Rickettsial disease existence in India: resurgence in outbreaks with the advent of 20th Century. Indian J Health Sci Biomed Res. 2020;13:5–10.

Sudarshan M, Narayana DA. Providing evidence for effective prevention and control of rabies in India. Indian J Public Health. 2019 Sep;63(Suppl 1):S1.

Verma R, Khanna P, Chawla S. Recommended vaccines for international travelers to India. Hum Vaccin Immunother. 2015;11(10):2455–7.

World Health Organization. World malaria report 2019. Geneva: The Organization; 2019. Available from: www.who.int/publications/i/item/9789241565721.

NEPAL

David Shlim

DESTINATION OVERVIEW

Home to >29 million people, Nepal stretches for 805 km (500 mi) along the Himalayan mountains that form its natural border with China (see Map 10-13). The topography rises from low plains at 70 m (≈230 ft) elevation to the highest point in the world at 8,848 m (≈29,029 ft), the summit of Mount Everest. Kathmandu, the capital city with a population of >2 million people, sits in a lush valley at 1,324 m (≈4,344 ft) elevation.

Nepal's latitude of 28°N (the same as Florida) means that its non-mountainous areas are temperate year-round. Most annual rainfall comes during the monsoon season (June–September). The main tourist seasons are the spring (March–May) and fall (October–November). The winter months, December–February, are pleasant in the lowlands but can be too cold to make trekking enjoyable in the high mountains.

Approximately 30% of travelers to Nepal go to trek into the mountains; others go to experience the country's culture and stunning natural beauty. Lumbini, in the Terai region, is the birthplace of the Buddha and has become an increasingly popular and beautifully developed pilgrimage destination for Buddhists from around the world. In recent years, trekkers have begun traveling to the Manaslu area, which offers a hiking experience featuring less-developed lodges and extended time away from roads. Notable in this area is the Nubri Valley, which also has many sacred Buddhist sites.

10

In addition to trekking, Nepal has some of the best rafting and kayaking rivers in the world. Jungle lodges in Chitwan National Park allow visitors to see a wide range of wildlife, including crocodiles, rhinoceros, tigers, and a huge variety of exotic birds. Less adventurous travelers can drive to comfortable hotels offering commanding views of the Himalayas, both near Kathmandu and near Pokhara. The airport near Lumbini is being upgraded to an international airport. Pokhara airport also is scheduled to become an international airport in the future, giving visitors more options for traveling in and out of Nepal.

INFECTIOUS DISEASE RISKS

Enteric Infections & Diseases

Travelers to Nepal are at high risk for enteric diseases. Hepatitis A vaccine and typhoid vaccine are the 2 most important pretravel immunizations. The risk for typhoid fever and paratyphoid fever among visitors to Nepal is among the highest in the world, and the prevalence of fluoroquinolone resistance also is high (see Sec. 5, Part 1, Ch. 24, Typhoid & Paratyphoid Fever). Tap water in Nepal is not considered safe for drinking, and travelers should only drink boiled or bottled water (see Sec. 2, Ch. 8, Food & Water Precautions, and Sec. 2, Ch. 9, Water Disinfection).

CYCLOSPORIASIS

Cyclospora cayetanensis, an intestinal protozoal pathogen, is highly endemic to Nepal (see Sec. 5, Part 3, Ch. 5, Cyclosporiasis). Risk for infection is distinctly seasonal; transmission occurs almost exclusively during May–October, with a peak in June and July. Because transmission occurs outside the main tourist seasons, cyclosporiasis primarily effects expatriates who stay through the monsoon. In addition to watery diarrhea, profound anorexia and fatigue are the hallmark symptoms of *Cyclospora* infection. The treatment of choice is trimethoprim-sulfamethoxazole; no highly effective alternatives have been identified.

HEPATITIS E

Hepatitis E virus is endemic in Nepal, and several cases each year are diagnosed in visitors or expatriates. No vaccine against hepatitis E is commercially available; travelers should follow safe food and water precautions (see Sec. 5, Part 2, Ch. 10, Hepatitis E).

TRAVELERS' DIARRHEA

Travelers' diarrhea is a risk, and the risk during the spring trekking season (March–May) is double that of the fall trekking season (October–November). Because many visitors head to remote areas that do not have available medical care, provide

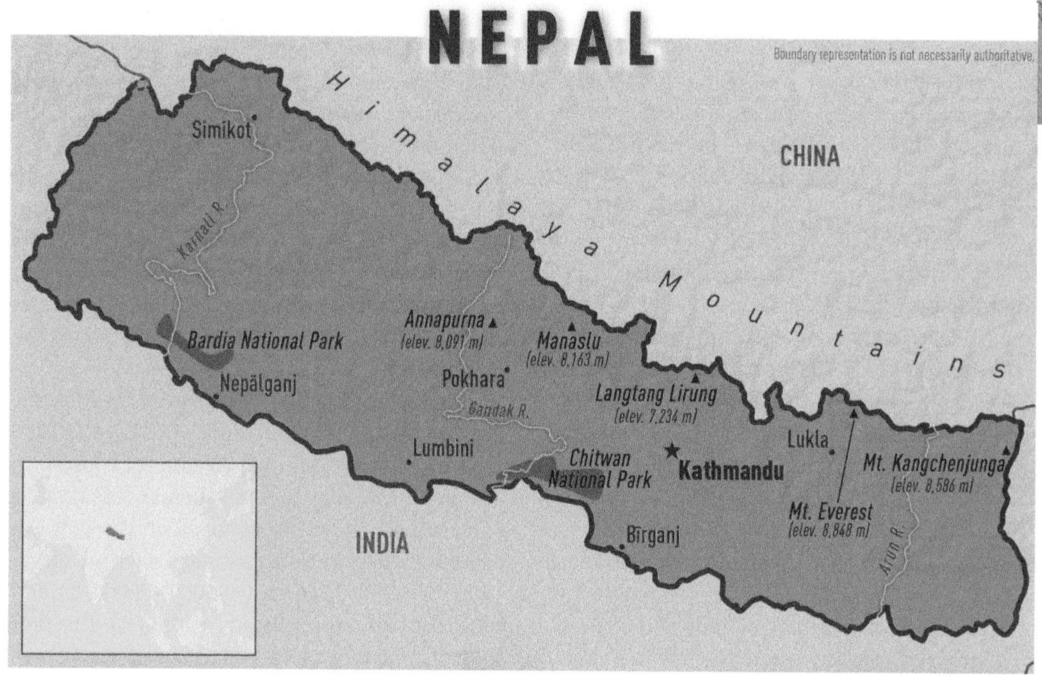

MAP 10-13 Nepal

travelers with medications for self-treatment (see Sec. 2, Ch. 6, Travelers' Diarrhea). Extensive resistance to fluoroquinolones has been documented among bacterial diarrheal pathogens in Nepal.

Respiratory Infections & Diseases

Respiratory illnesses among travelers are common, both in Kathmandu and on trekking routes. The advent of coronavirus disease 2019 (COVID-19) makes it more difficult to assume the etiology of a respiratory infection. Prolonged symptoms beyond 7–10 days often requires a medical assessment.

CORONAVIRUS DISEASE 2019

For current information on COVID-19 in Nepal, consult the US Embassy in Nepal website (https://np.usembassy.gov/). For the US government's COVID-19 international travel requirements and recommendations, see www.cdc.gov/coronavirus/2019-ncov/travelers/international-travel/index.html. All travelers going to Nepal should be up to date with their COVID-19 vaccines (www.cdc.gov/coronavirus/2019-ncov/vaccines/stay-up-to-date.html).

INFLUENZA

Influenza is a risk in Nepal, particularly in crowded teahouses at higher elevations. Trekkers should receive a current influenza immunization before travel.

TUBERCULOSIS

Tuberculosis (TB) disease that exists among local people can be due to drug-resistant strains of *Mycobacterium tuberculosis*. Both multidrug-resistant and extensively–drug resistant TB have been reported in Nepal. Overall, however, risk to travelers is low.

Vectorborne Diseases

DENGUE

In 2019, the Ministry of Health in Nepal reported ≈18,000 cases of dengue, and in 2022, >46,000 cases. Counsel all travelers going to Nepal during the warmer, wetter months to pack an Environmental Protection Agency–registered insect repellent in their travel health kit and to practice insect bite precautions (see Sec. 4, Ch. 6, Mosquitoes, Ticks & Other Arthropods).

JAPANESE ENCEPHALITIS

Japanese encephalitis (JE) is endemic to Nepal; the greatest disease risk is in the Terai region during and immediately after monsoon season (June–October). JE has been identified in local residents of the Kathmandu Valley, but only 1 case of JE acquired in Nepal has been reported in a foreign traveler, a tourist who spent time in the Terai region in August. JE vaccine is not routinely recommended for people trekking to higher elevation areas or spending short periods in Kathmandu or Pokhara en route to such treks. JE vaccine is recommended for expatriates living in Nepal (see Sec. 5, Part 2, Ch. 13, Japanese Encephalitis).

MALARIA

Although targeted for complete elimination of malaria by 2020, Nepal continues to report low (and decreasing) numbers of indigenous cases, primarily *Plasmodium vivax*. No malaria transmission occurs in Kathmandu or Pokhara, and all the main Himalayan trekking routes are free of malaria, but documented transmission persists in some areas of the country. For this reason (and until malaria is eliminated from Nepal), the Centers for Disease Control and Prevention continues to recommend chemoprophylaxis for travelers visiting destinations below 2,000 m (≈6,500 ft) elevation.

ENVIRONMENTAL HAZARDS & RISKS

10

Air Quality

Air pollution problems in the Kathmandu valley are frequent. People with underlying cardiorespiratory illness, including asthma, chronic obstructive pulmonary disease, or congestive heart failure can suffer exacerbations in Kathmandu, particularly after a viral upper respiratory infection. Short-term exposure to these levels of air pollution can irritate the eyes and throat. In addition, exposure to high levels of air pollution greatly increases the risk for both upper and lower respiratory tract infections, including otitis, sinusitis, bronchitis, and pneumonia (see Sec. 4, Ch. 3, Air Quality & Ionizing Radiation). Children and older people are the most vulnerable.

Altitude Illness & Acute Mountain Sickness

The destinations for most trekkers are the Annapurna region west of Kathmandu, the Langtang trekking area north of Kathmandu, and the Mount Everest region east of Kathmandu. In the Annapurna region, short-term trekkers can choose to hike to viewpoints in the foothills without reaching any high elevations. Others can undertake a longer trek around the Annapurna massif, going over a 5,416 m (≈17,769 ft) pass, the Thorung La.

The highest point in the Langtang region (the summit of Langtang Lirung) is 7,245 m (23,770 ft); overall, however, high-elevation exposure in Langtang National Park is generally less than in the Everest region. By contrast, trekkers in the Mount Everest region routinely sleep at elevations of 4,267–4,876 m (≈14,000–16,000 ft) and hike to elevations >5,486 m (≈18,000 ft). This prolonged exposure to very high elevations means that travelers must be knowledgeable about the risk for altitude illness and might need to carry specific medications to prevent and treat the problem (see Sec. 4, Ch. 5, High Elevation Travel & Altitude Illness).

Most trekkers in the Mount Everest region arrive by flying to a tiny airstrip at Lukla at 2,860 m (≈9,383 ft) elevation; they then reach Namche Bazaar at 3,440 m (≈11,286 ft) elevation the next day. Acetazolamide prophylaxis can substantially decrease the chances of developing acute mountain sickness in Namche.

Animal Bites & Rabies

Rabies is highly endemic among the dogs in Nepal, but in recent years Kathmandu has had fewer stray dogs. Half of all traveler exposures to a possibly rabid animal occur near Swayambunath, a beautiful hilltop shrine also known as the monkey temple. Advise travelers to be extra cautious with dogs and monkeys in this area. Monkeys can be aggressive if approached, and will jump on a person's back if they smell food in a backpack. Clinics in Kathmandu that specialize in the care of foreign travelers almost always have complete postexposure rabies prophylaxis, including human rabies immune globulin. Private helicopter companies in Nepal provide rescue; thus, most people can return to Kathmandu from a trek within 1–2 days. Even in the absence of helicopter rescue, trekkers bitten in the mountains have been able to return to Kathmandu in an average of 5 days.

Natural Disasters

In April 2015, a major earthquake in Nepal caused extensive damage and killed >9,000 people. Most of the damage occurred in non-tourist areas and the infrastructure for tourism has largely been repaired. The Langtang trekking area, north of Kathmandu, was virtually destroyed by a landslide triggered by the earthquake; since then, many services have been rebuilt, and tourism is returning to the area.

Large glacial lakes formed by melting glaciers can fail massively and cause intense downstream destructive flooding. Sudden snowstorms have occasionally occurred during trekking seasons, resulting in some deaths and numerous stranded trekkers. Ordinarily, though, the weather during the trekking seasons is mild.

SAFETY & SECURITY

Road Construction Issues

In recent years, Nepal has seen a frenzy of motorable road construction. Once the most roadless country in the world, much of Nepal is now connected by roads that vary in quality from well-constructed and maintained to terrifying. Hasty planning and construction have resulted in many road washouts and landslides, especially during the heavy rains of the monsoon, and road travel in general is an uncomfortable experience.

Motor roads have been constructed up the 2 major valleys of the Around-Annapurna Trek, shortening the trip from 21 to 5 days for people traveling by vehicle. In many cases, traditional trekking trails are no longer being maintained or have been subsumed by the road, substantially changing the nature of the experience and leading trekkers to seek out the few remaining roadless areas for a more traditional hiking experience. Encourage trekkers to inquire about road construction in areas where they intend to hike, because many have found that hiking on dusty or muddy roads, alongside buses, jeeps, and motorcycles, is not the experience they were anticipating.

AVAILABILITY & QUALITY OF MEDICAL CARE

Contact information for 2 clinics in Kathmandu specializing in the care of foreign travelers in Nepal is available on the International Society of Travel Medicine website (www.istm.org). Hospital facilities have improved steadily over the years, and general and orthopedic emergency surgery are available and reliable in Kathmandu. Acute cardiac care also is available, including the placement of coronary artery stents. Modern hospitals tend to compete for foreign patients, and travelers should carry the names of reliable clinics and hospitals so they can request the hospital of their choice. Occasionally, patients are taken to an alternative hospital without their consent; when reaching a hospital, patients or their companions should ascertain whether they are indeed in the hospital they requested. Medical evacuation points providing definitive care outside of Nepal include locations in India and in Thailand.

Medical Evacuation

Helicopter evacuation from most areas is readily available. Communication has improved from remote areas because of satellite and cellular telephones, and private helicopter companies accept credit cards and are eager to perform evacuations for profit. Evacuation can often take place on the same day as the request, weather permitting. Helicopter rescue is usually limited to morning hours because of afternoon winds in the mountains. Helicopter rescue is billed at ≈$4,000 per hour, with an average total cost of $8,000–$10,000 US. Evacuation insurance policies generally require that rescues be arranged through the insurance provider; if not, the cost of the rescue will be borne by the traveler. Because of ready access to helicopter evacuation, trekkers have sometimes requested rescues for trivial conditions. Due to the potential for abuse of unnecessary helicopter rescue, some international evacuation insurance companies no longer provide coverage for Nepal or impose an additional surcharge for coverage there.

BIBLIOGRAPHY

Cave W, Pandey P, Osrin D, Shlim DR. Chemoprophylaxis use and the risk of malaria in travelers to Nepal. J Travel Med. 2003;10(2):100–5.

Government of Nepal, Ministry of Health and Population, Department of Health Services, Epidemiology and Disease Control Division. Situation update of dengue 2022. Available from: http://edcd.gov.np/news/download/situation-update-of-dengue-2022.

Hoge CW, Shlim DR, Echeverria P, Rajah R, Herrmann JE, Cross JH. Epidemiology of diarrhea among expatriate residents living in a highly endemic environment. JAMA. 1996;275(7):533–8.

Murphy H, Bodhidatta L, Sornsakrin S, Khadka B, Pokhrel A, Shakya S, et al. Traveler's diarrhea in Nepal—changes in etiology and antimicrobial resistance. J Travel Med. 2019;26(8):taz054.

Pandey P, Lee K, Amatya B, Angelo KM, Shlim DR, Murphy H. Health problems in travellers to Nepal visiting CIWEC clinic in Kathmandu—a GeoSentinel analysis. Travel Med Infect Dis. 2021;40:101999.

Schwartz E, Shlim DR, Eaton M, Jenks N, Houston R. The effect of oral and parenteral typhoid vaccination on the rate of infection with *Salmonella typhi* and *Salmonella paratyphi* A among foreigners in Nepal. Arch Intern Med. 1990;150(2):349–51.

THAILAND

James Heffelfinger, Joshua Mott, Sopon Iamsirithaworn

10

DESTINATION OVERVIEW

Thailand, a geographically diverse country a little smaller than the state of Texas (see Map 10-14), is a popular destination for tourists, offering beaches, a wide range of cultures and cuisine, eco-adventure opportunities, nightlife, and shopping. Thailand is also a regional business hub. In 2019, ≈40 million visitors spent >1 night in Thailand—the number of visitors to Thailand increased annually during each of the 5 years before the onset of the coronavirus disease 2019 (COVID-19) pandemic. During 2020, Thailand had <7 million visitors, an 80% reduction compared with 2019, mainly due to COVID-19 travel restrictions.

Of a total population of 70 million people, >10 million live in the capital city of Bangkok, a major commercial center. Tourists to Bangkok visit historic and cultural sites including Buddhist temples, the Grand Palace, and the Emerald Buddha. The main arteries of Bangkok are the Chao Phraya River and its canals, which provide access to tourist sites, the floating market, and restaurants. Bangkok includes many culinary options, from sidewalk noodle stands to 4- and 5-star restaurants representing a variety of global cuisines. Although Thai is a tonal language that can be difficult for Americans to learn, English is commonly spoken at most popular destinations. Maps, road signs, and tourist guides frequently provide information in both English and Thai.

Many visitors to Thailand also visit Chiang Mai in the north. The old city is surrounded by a moat and defensive wall; beyond the wall are >300 temples, a popular night bazaar for shopping, and easy access to handicraft villages, elephant nature parks, and other popular outdoor adventures.

Thailand's central location and major international airport in Bangkok make it an easy access point for other destinations in Asia. In addition, the country has become a popular retirement destination for people from around the world, including many US citizens. The warm climate and low cost of living make Thailand an attractive place to live.

INFECTIOUS DISEASE RISKS

All travelers should be up to date on their routine vaccinations, including seasonal influenza. In addition, vaccination against hepatitis A and hepatitis B is strongly recommended. Consider Japanese encephalitis (JE) and typhoid fever vaccines based on the traveler's potential risk during a visit to, or residence in, Thailand.

Enteric Infections & Diseases

CHOLERA

Active cholera transmission has been infrequently reported from Thailand in recent years.

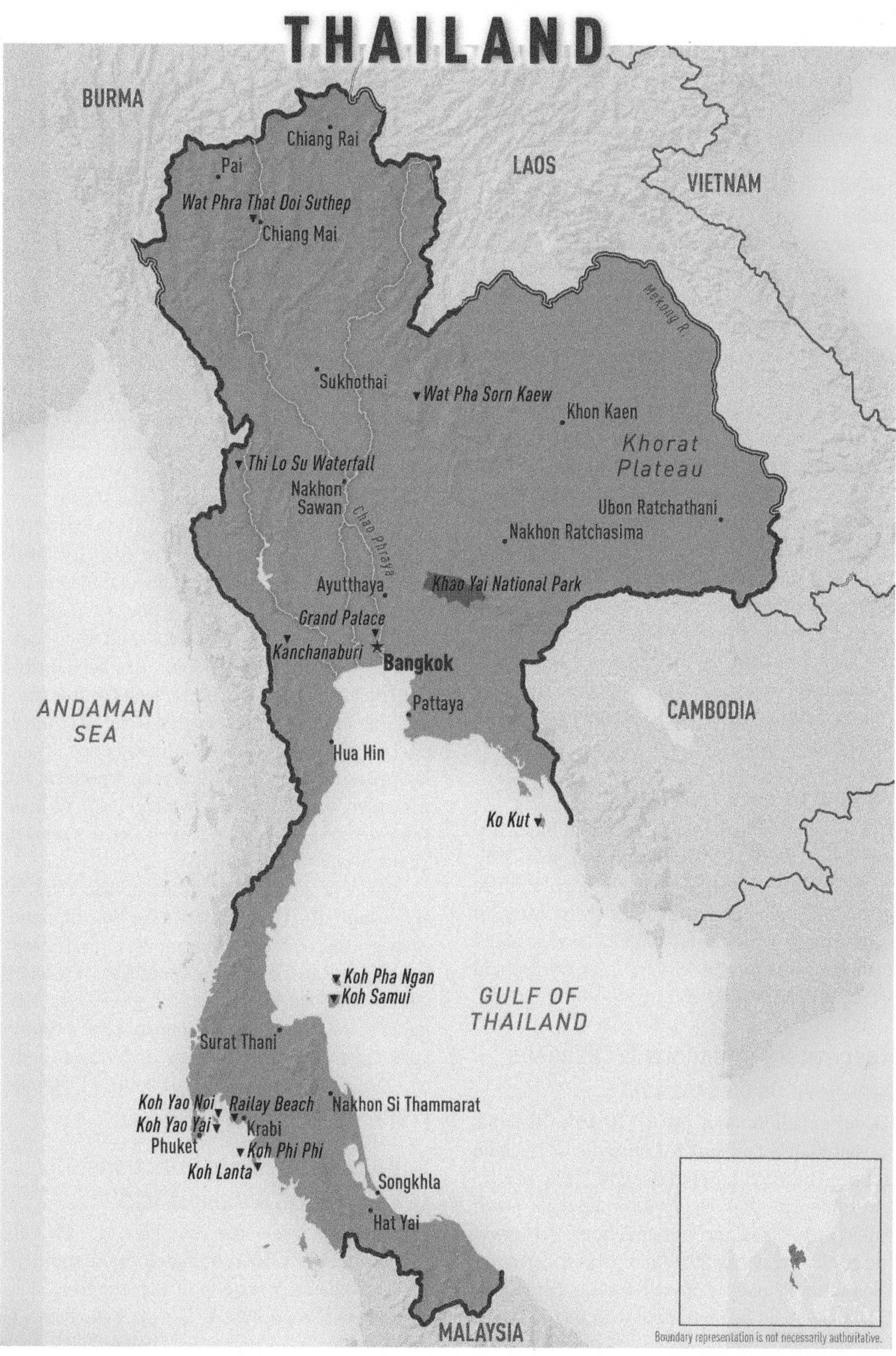
THAILAND
BURMA
LAOS
VIETNAM
CAMBODIA
MALAYSIA
ANDAMAN SEA
GULF OF THAILAND
Chiang Rai
Pai
Wat Phra That Doi Suthep
Chiang Mai
Mekong R.
Sukhothai
Wat Pha Sorn Kaew
Khon Kaen
Khorat Plateau
Thi Lo Su Waterfall
Nakhon Sawan
Chao Phraya
Ubon Ratchathani
Nakhon Ratchasima
Ayutthaya
Khao Yai National Park
Grand Palace
Kanchanaburi
Bangkok
Pattaya
Hua Hin
Ko Kut
Koh Pha Ngan
Koh Samui
Surat Thani
Koh Yao Noi
Railay Beach
Nakhon Si Thammarat
Koh Yao Yai
Krabi
Phuket
Koh Phi Phi
Koh Lanta
Songkhla
Hat Yai
Boundary representation is not necessarily authoritative.

MAP 10-14 Thailand

For current recommendations for travelers to Thailand, see the Centers for Disease Control and Prevention (CDC) Travelers' Health website (https://wwwnc.cdc.gov/travel/destinations/traveler/none/thailand).

TRAVELERS' DIARRHEA

Thailand's street food is convenient, delicious, and inexpensive. Unfortunately, it also can be a source of travelers' diarrhea (TD) because lack of clean running water in outdoor eateries precludes good hand and food preparation hygiene. For travelers determined to experience Thai street food, the risk for foodborne illness might be mitigated to some degree by following some basic food and water safety precautions. For instance, visit only restaurants or food stalls that cook food to order, avoid raw or undercooked food, eat only steaming hot food served on new disposable dishes, avoid raw garnishes, eat fruit that you peel yourself, and only drink beverages from sealed containers (see Sec. 2, Ch. 8, Food & Water Precautions). For further information about travelers' diarrhea, see Sec. 2, Ch. 6, Travelers' Diarrhea. Fluoroquinolone-resistant enteric pathogens are widespread in Thailand and other areas of Southeast Asia.

TYPHOID FEVER

Typhoid fever is endemic to Thailand. Incidence has been declining, however, and was estimated to be 3 cases per 100,000 population in 2014. People planning extended stays or travel to remote parts of the country should be vaccinated against typhoid (see Sec. 5, Part 1, Ch. 24, Typhoid & Paratyphoid Fever).

Respiratory Infections & Diseases

CORONAVIRUS DISEASE 2019

For current information on COVID-19 in Thailand, consult the US Embassy & Consulate in Thailand website (https://th.usembassy.gov/). For the US government's COVID-19 international travel requirements and recommendations, see www.cdc.gov/coronavirus/2019-ncov/travelers/international-travel/index.html. All travelers going to Thailand should be up to date with their COVID-19 vaccines (www.cdc.gov/coronavirus/2019-ncov/vaccines/stay-up-to-date.html).

TUBERCULOSIS

Thailand has a high burden of tuberculosis (TB). Immunocompromised travelers who visit Thailand for extended visits could be at increased risk for TB. Travelers should avoid people known to have active TB, and refrain from consuming unpasteurized dairy products (see Sec. 5, Part 1, Ch. 22, Tuberculosis).

Sexually Transmitted Infections & HIV

Thailand is a destination for tourists seeking sex (see Sec. 9, Ch. 12, Sex & Travel). Although commercial sex work is illegal, it is practiced in many places in Thailand. Visitors to Thailand's red-light districts should be aware that these areas have been associated with human trafficking.

In 2019, ≈470,000 people were living with HIV/AIDS in Thailand. The number of new HIV infections reported nationwide each year decreased during 2010–2019. A 100% condom program, which encourages sex workers and their customers to always use condoms, has helped slow the spread of HIV and other sexually transmitted infections (STIs). Nonetheless, HIV infection remains concentrated in many populations. In 2020, an estimated 12% of men who have sex with men, and 3% of sex workers (≈4% of male sex workers and 1.7% of female sex workers) in Thailand were living with HIV.

Travelers should be aware of the risks of acquiring HIV and other STIs in Thailand, always use condoms during sex, and avoid injecting drugs or sharing needles. Travelers whose practices put them at high risk for HIV infection should discuss preexposure prophylaxis with their primary care and travel medicine providers (see Sec. 5, Part 2, Ch. 11, Human Immunodeficiency Virus / HIV).

Soil- & Waterborne Infections

LEPTOSPIROSIS & MELIOIDOSIS

Leptospirosis (see Sec. 5, Part 1, Ch. 10, Leptospirosis) cases occur mainly in the southern and northeastern regions of the country; melioidosis (see Sec. 5, Part 1, Ch. 12, Melioidosis) is highly endemic to northeast Thailand. For both diseases, most cases occur during the rainy season, July–October. Adventure travelers can be at increased risk for these diseases because their activities expose them to soil and surface water. Advise travelers visiting endemic areas to avoid contact with soil and water and to ensure that any open wounds are covered to prevent exposure. When contact cannot be avoided, travelers should wear protective clothing and footwear to reduce their exposure risk. Counsel travelers to immediately and thoroughly clean abrasions, burns, or lacerations contaminated with soil or surface water.

Vectorborne Diseases

DENGUE & ZIKA

Dengue (see Sec. 5, Part 2, Ch. 4, Dengue) is endemic throughout Thailand. Large epidemics occur every several years. Peak transmission is during the rainy season, although cases are reported year-round even in non-epidemic years. Travelers to Thailand should take measures to protect themselves from mosquito bites to prevent dengue (see Sec. 4, Ch. 6, Mosquitoes, Ticks & Other Arthropods).

Transmission of Zika virus (see Sec. 5, Part 2, Ch. 27, Zika) has occurred in Thailand, but no evidence suggests recent outbreaks. Because of the risk for birth defects in infants born to people infected with Zika during pregnancy, however, travelers who are pregnant or trying to become pregnant should review the most recent CDC recommendations at https://wwwnc.cdc.gov/travel/page/zika-information.

JAPANESE ENCEPHALITIS

JE is endemic to many parts of Thailand outside the capital. Transmission occurs year-round, with seasonal epidemics occurring in the northern provinces during May–October. Although most outbreaks occur in the Chiang Mai valley, cases have occurred in travelers who visited resorts or coastal areas in southern Thailand. JE vaccine is recommended for travelers who plan to visit Thailand for ≥1 month and should be considered for people visiting for a shorter period who have an increased risk for JE virus exposure due to their itineraries or activities (see Sec. 5, Part 2, Ch. 13, Japanese Encephalitis).

MALARIA

Malaria is endemic to specific areas in Thailand, particularly the rural, forested areas bordering Burma (Myanmar), Cambodia, and Laos, and the provinces of the far south along the border with Malaysia. Transmission is year-round, peaking during the rainy season, with a second, smaller peak in December. Approximately 80% of cases are due to *Plasmodium vivax*; <20% are due to *P. falciparum*. CDC recommends protection against mosquito bites and antimalarial prophylaxis for travelers visiting any of the endemic areas (see Sec. 2, Ch. 5, Yellow Fever Vaccine and Malaria Prevention Information, by Country; Sec. 4, Ch. 6, Mosquitoes, Ticks & Other Arthropods; and Sec. 5, Part 3, Ch. 16, Malaria). Atovaquone-proguanil, doxycycline, or tafenoquine are the recommended prophylactic antimalarial drugs for travelers going to malaria-endemic areas in Thailand; mosquito avoidance only (no chemoprophylaxis) is recommended for people traveling to areas where cases of malaria transmission are rare to few (e.g., Bangkok, Chiang Mai, Phuket).

ENVIRONMENTAL HAZARDS & RISKS

Air Quality

Air quality in Thailand varies by province and fluctuates throughout the year, with seasonal smog becoming an increasing health concern in some areas of the country (see Sec. 4, Ch. 3, Air Quality & Ionizing Radiation). The air quality in several provinces (Bangkok, Chiang Mai, Chiang Rai, Khon Kaen, Lampang, Lamphun, Mae Hong Son, Nan, and Samut Sakhon) has exceeded Thai and US government daily standards for fine particulate matter ($PM_{2.5}$) during parts of the year. In Chiang Mai and other northern provinces, air quality is frequently poor during February–April because of agricultural burning and forest fires.

Animal Bites & Rabies

Government-sponsored mass vaccination campaigns for cats and dogs have reduced the prevalence of rabies in Thailand, but a small risk persists. Preexposure vaccination is recommended only for travelers whose occupation puts them at risk for exposure (e.g., veterinarians) or people who will be traveling to areas where immediate access to care and rabies biologics will be difficult (see Sec. 5, Part 2, Ch. 18, Rabies). Rabies vaccine for preexposure and postexposure prophylaxis and human rabies immune globulin are readily available in all provincial and most district hospitals throughout Thailand.

Climate & Sun Exposure

Because Thailand is close to the equator, the climate is often hot and humid (see Sec. 4, Ch. 1, Sun Exposure, and Sec. 4, Ch. 2, Extremes of Temperature). Flooding is always a possibility, and various regions are prone to flash floods. Monsoon rains typically fall during July–October and can last until relatively cooler, drier weather begins in November, making November–February a popular time of year to visit.

Natural Disasters

Tsunamis are a risk in Thailand; the 2004 tsunami was the deadliest on record. Two other tsunamis have hit Thailand since 2004, resulting in ≈8,000 deaths.

SAFETY & SECURITY

Crime

The crime rate in Thailand exceeds that of some other countries in Asia. Although most crime involves petty theft, crime related to drug use and the illegal drug trade, gambling, and human trafficking and prostitution also occur. And while more violent crime (e.g., homicide, rape) involving visitors is uncommon in Thailand, it has happened.

Political Unrest

Thailand has experienced political unrest throughout the country and ethnonationalist violence in the southern provinces. In 2014, a caretaker military government was established to maintain peace, develop a constitution, and facilitate democratic elections. The country remains politically divided, however, and demonstrations and government protests continue. Prudent travelers should avoid these gatherings because no one can predict whether they will stay peaceful or turn violent (see Sec. 4, Ch. 11, Safety & Security Overseas).

To find out if, when, and where political protests might occur, travelers should monitor the local news, social media outlets, and the US Embassy & Consulate in Thailand website (https://th.usembassy.gov/). In addition, by enrolling with the US Department of State's Smart Traveler Enrollment Program (https://step.state.gov/step), US citizens and nationals traveling and living in Thailand receive safety alerts from the US embassy; it also enables the US embassy to contact them in the event of an emergency.

Terrorism

Recent terrorism-related incidents in Thailand have been related to the South Thailand insurgency, a separatist group with roots in ethnic and religious tensions. The insurgency has been ongoing for several decades and is concentrated in 4 provinces (Narathiwat, Pattani, Songkhla, Yala) in the far south of the country, near the Malaysian border. Martial law is enforced in these provinces. Due to safety concerns, US government employees need official authorization to travel to these areas, and the US embassy in Thailand strongly discourages all other Americans from going. The Royal Thai Government has taken active measures to counter terrorism through legislation, capacity-building, and communication and collaboration with other countries in the region.

Traffic-Related Injuries

Traffic accidents are common in Thailand. According to the World Health Organization, in 2018, Thailand had one of the world's highest traffic-related fatality rates, due in large part to reckless driving (see https://travel.state.gov/content/travel/en/international-travel/International-Travel-Country-Information-Pages/Thailand.html#ExternalPopup). Approximately 20,000 motor vehicle deaths occur in Thailand each year. Motorcycles, a cheap and popular mode of travel, are among the most vulnerable vehicles on the road. During 2019–2021, 85% of road accidents involved motorcycles or scooters, and a substantial proportion (73% in 2012) of motor vehicle deaths are due to motorcycle and scooter crashes. Travelers should avoid riding motorbikes, including motorbike taxis, but if they must ride, they should wear a helmet. Travelers also should fasten seat belts when riding in cars (see Sec. 8, Ch. 5, Road & Traffic Safety).

AVAILABILITY & QUALITY OF MEDICAL CARE

Health care in Thailand is generally considered to be of good quality and less costly than in many high-income countries. Approximately 20% of hospitals are private, and many accept online registration and have English-speaking staff. Most major medical centers are in larger metropolitan areas. In rural areas, availability and quality of medical care is more limited.

Medical Tourism

Medical tourism to Thailand increased during 2010–2019. The cost of medical or surgical treatment is lower, and the level of care is considered comparable to that of many places in the United States. Thailand is among the top medical tourism destinations worldwide. Travelers intending to obtain medical care abroad should research the facilities at their destination; learn about health insurance coverage, travel regulations, and requirements for visitors seeking medical care in Thailand; and consult with their primary care physician and a travel medicine specialist in advance of their trip (see Sec. 6, Ch. 4, Medical Tourism).

BIBLIOGRAPHY

AIDSinfo. Global dataset on HIV epidemiology and response. Available from: https://aidsinfo.unaids.org.

Hinjoy S, Hantrakun V, Kongyu S, Kaewrakmuk J, Wangrangsimakul T, Jitsuronk S, et al. Melioidosis in Thailand: present and future. Trop Med Infect Dis. 2018;32(2):38.

US Central Intelligence Agency. The world fact book 2021; East and Southeast Asia: Thailand. Washington, DC: The Agency; 2021. Available from: www.cia.gov/the-world-factbook/countries/thailand.

US Department of State, Bureau of Consular Affairs. Travel and transportation: Thailand. Available from: https://travel.state.gov/content/travel/en/international-travel/International-Travel-Country-Information-Pages/Thailand.html.

World Health Organization. Global status report on road safety 2018. Geneva: The Organization; 2018. Available from: www.who.int/publications/i/item/9789241565684.

World Health Organization. Towards a rabies-free Thailand by 2020. Available from: www.who.int/news-room/feature-stories/detail/towards-a-rabies-free-thailand-by-2020.

10

11 Posttravel Evaluation

GENERAL APPROACH TO THE RETURNED TRAVELER

Jessica Fairley

As many as 43%–79% of travelers to low- and middle-income countries become ill with a travel-associated health problem. Although most of these illnesses are mild, some travelers become sick enough to seek care from a health care provider. Most posttravel infections become apparent soon after returning from abroad, but incubation periods vary, and some syndromes can present months to years after initial infection or after travel.

When evaluating a patient with a probable travel-associated illness, approach the differential diagnosis by incorporating both the patient presentation and risk factors related to travel (e.g., destination, duration of travel, and exposures; see Table 11-01). Salient points of the history of present illness and the travel and medical history, descriptions of common nonfebrile syndromes, and initial management steps are outlined below. The differential diagnosis and management for a traveler with fever (or febrile syndrome) is discussed in detail in Sec. 11, Ch. 4, Fever in the Returned Traveler.

THE POSTTRAVEL EVALUATION

History of the Present Illness

As with any medical evaluation, the history of the present illness and associated clinical factors are the first considerations when approaching an ill returned traveler. Information about the timing of illness, immunization and prophylaxis history, itinerary, exposures, and comorbidities can help refine the diagnosis.

TIMING OF ILLNESS IN RELATION TO TRAVEL

Because most common travel-associated infections have short incubation periods, most ill travelers will seek medical attention ≤1 month

CDC Yellow Book 2024. Jeffrey Nemhauser, Oxford University Press. © Oxford University Press 2023.
DOI: 10.1093/oso/9780197570944.003.0011

Table 11-01 Elements of a complete travel history in an ill returned traveler

ELEMENT	DETAILS
HISTORY OF THE PRESENT ILLNESS	Symptoms: primary & associated Date of symptom or illness onset Geographic location at time of symptom onset (e.g., while away, in transit, after return) Healthcare received while abroad and after return (e.g., medications, hospitalizations)
TRAVEL DETAILS	Destinations visited and itineraries Duration of travel (date of departure and date of return) Reason for travel • Business (include details about possible exposures and type of work done) • Immigration • Leisure • Missionary, volunteer, humanitarian aid work • Providing or receiving medical care • Research or education • Visiting friends & relatives Accommodations and sleeping arrangements • Camping • Hostel • Hotel with or without air conditioning, window screens, or mosquito nets • Safari, including camping outdoors, in a lodge, in a luxury tent • Someone's home Transportation used
RECREATIONAL ACTIVITIES	Camping and hiking Safari Sightseeing Water exposures • Boating or rafting • Fresh water (lake, river, stream) bathing, boating, swimming, wading • Hot springs • Hot tubs, swimming pools • Ocean (diving, snorkeling, surfing; consider marine life exposure) Other activities
EXPOSURES	Animal or arthropod bites, stings, scratches Drinking water (bottled, purified, tap, use of ice) Foods • Raw fruits, vegetables • Undercooked meat • Unpasteurized dairy products • Seafood Insect bites (mosquito, tick, sand fly, tsetse fly) Medical or dental care (planned or unplanned) Disease outbreaks in visited destinations Sexual activity during travel (document condom use, new partner[s]) Tattoos or piercings while traveling
VECTORBORNE DISEASE PRECAUTIONS	Adherence to malaria prophylaxis Insect repellent use (25%–40% DEET or other Environmental Protection Agency–registered product) Mosquito nets

Table 11-01 Elements of a complete travel history in an ill returned traveler (continued)

ELEMENT	DETAILS
VACCINES RECEIVED	Coronavirus disease 2019 (COVID-19) Hepatitis A Hepatitis B Influenza Japanese encephalitis Measles-mumps-rubella (MMR) Meningococcal disease Polio Rabies Tetanus-diphtheria-acellular pertussis (Tdap) Typhoid Varicella Yellow fever
MEDICATIONS TAKEN	Malaria prophylaxis All medicines taken (whether routinely or for symptomatic treatment), including antibiotics • Herbal, complementary, alternative • Over the counter • Prescription
PAST MEDICAL HISTORY	Chronic medical conditions • Autoimmune disease • Cancer • Diabetes • Heart disease • Immunosuppressive conditions Recent illnesses or surgeries
ADDITIONAL INFORMATION	Alcohol, tobacco, illicit drug use Family history Recent travel, domestic or international, especially ≤6 months

of returning from their destinations. Dengue and other arboviral infections, influenza, and travelers' diarrhea are examples of infections with shorter incubation periods (<2 weeks). Diseases with slightly longer incubation periods, ≤4–6 weeks, include viral hepatitis, acute HIV, leishmaniasis, malaria, and typhoid fever, among others. Occasionally, some infections (e.g., leishmaniasis, malaria, schistosomiasis, tuberculosis) might become manifest months or even years after a traveler returns. Consider malaria in the differential diagnosis of any traveler who traveled to a malaria-endemic area ≤1 year of presentation. A detailed travel history that extends beyond a few months before presentation is important. The most common travel-associated infections by incubation period are listed in Table 11-02, Table 11-03, and Table 11-04.

IMMUNIZATION & PROPHYLAXIS HISTORY

When evaluating an ill returned traveler, review the traveler's vaccination history and malaria prophylaxis used. Fewer than half of US travelers who visit low- and middle-income countries seek pretravel medical advice, increasing the likelihood that they did not receive pretravel vaccines and did not receive or take antimalarial drugs. Although adherence to malaria prophylaxis does not rule out the possibility of malaria,

Table 11-02 **Common travel-associated infections by incubation period: <14 days**

DISEASE	USUAL INCUBATION PERIOD	INCUBATION PERIOD (RANGE)	DISTRIBUTION
Chikungunya	2–4 days	1–14 days	Tropics, subtropics
Coronavirus disease 2019 (COVID-19)	3–7 days, or less, depending on the predominate, circulating variant		Worldwide
Dengue	4–8 days	3–14 days	Tropics, subtropics
Encephalitis, arboviral (e.g., Japanese encephalitis, tick-borne encephalitis, West Nile)	3–14 days	1–20 days	Agents vary by region
Enteric (typhoid or paratyphoid) fever	7–18 days	3–60 days	Especially in South Asia
HIV infection, acute	10–28 days	10 days–6 weeks	Worldwide
Influenza	1–3 days		Worldwide, can be acquired during travel
Legionellosis	5–6 days	2–10 days	Worldwide
Leptospirosis	7–12 days	2–26 days	Worldwide, most common in tropical areas
Malaria, *Plasmodium falciparum*	6–30 days	98% have onset within 3 months of travel	Tropics, subtropics
Malaria, *Plasmodium vivax*	8 days–12 months	≈50% have onset >30 days after completion of travel	Widespread in tropics and subtropics
Spotted fever rickettsiosis	Few days to 2–3 weeks		Causative species vary by region
Zika	3–14 days		Widespread in Latin America; endemic through much of Africa, Southeast Asia, and Pacific Islands

it substantially reduces the risk and increases the possibility of an alternative diagnosis.

Likewise, history of vaccination against hepatitis A and yellow fever would make these diseases unlikely causes of hepatitis or jaundice in a returning traveler. Remember to ask about routine vaccinations like measles-mumps-rubella (MMR) and tetanus-diphtheria-pertussis (Tdap). The most common vaccine-preventable diseases among returned travelers seeking care at GeoSentinel clinics during 1997–2010 included hepatitis A, hepatitis B, influenza, and typhoid

Table 11-03 Common travel-associated infections by incubation period: 14 days–6 weeks

DISEASE	USUAL INCUBATION PERIOD	INCUBATION PERIOD (RANGE)	DISTRIBUTION
Encephalitis, arboviral Enteric (typhoid or paratyphoid) fever HIV infection, acute Leptospirosis Malaria	See Table 11-02 for usual incubation periods		See Table 11-02 for global distribution
Amebic liver abscess	Weeks–months		Most common in low- and middle-income countries
Hepatitis A	28–30 days	15–50 days	Most common in low- and middle-income countries
Hepatitis E	26–42 days	2–9 weeks	Worldwide
Schistosomiasis, acute (Katayama syndrome)	4–8 weeks		Most common in sub-Saharan Africa

fever. More than half of these patients with vaccine-preventable diseases were hospitalized.

ITINERARY & TRAVEL DURATION

A traveler's itinerary is crucial to formulating a differential diagnosis because exposures differ depending on the region of travel and the specific areas (e.g., rural vs. urban). A febrile illness with nonspecific symptoms could be dengue, malaria, rickettsial disease, or typhoid fever, among others, depending on the itinerary and endemicity of these infections. Being able to exclude certain infections based on the travel itinerary can help avoid unnecessary testing.

A 2013 study from the GeoSentinel Surveillance Network found that the frequency of certain

Table 11-04 Common travel-associated infections by incubation period: >6 weeks

DISEASE	USUAL INCUBATION PERIOD	INCUBATION PERIOD (RANGE)	DISTRIBUTION
Amebic liver abscess Hepatitis E Malaria Schistosomiasis, acute	See Table 11-03 for usual incubation periods		See Table 11-03 for global distribution
Hepatitis B	90 days	60–150 days	Worldwide
Leishmaniasis, visceral	2–10 months	10 days–years	Africa, Latin America, Asia, southern Europe, and the Middle East
Tuberculosis	Primary, weeks Reactivation, years		Worldwide, rates and resistance levels vary widely

diseases varied depending on the region of the world visited; among travelers with fevers, for example, dengue was diagnosed most frequently among travelers coming from Asia, while malaria was diagnosed most frequently among travelers returning from Africa.

Travel duration is also a factor because the risk for a travel-associated illness increases with the length of the trip. A tropical medicine specialist can assist with the differential diagnosis and might be aware of outbreaks or the current prevalence of an infectious disease in an area. The 2014–2015 Ebola virus epidemic in West Africa highlighted the importance of epidemiologic factors and travel itineraries in managing patients and protecting staff and the community.

EXPOSURES

Knowing a patient's exposures during travel (e.g., consumption of contaminated food or water, insect bites, freshwater swimming) also can assist with the differential diagnosis. In addition to malarial parasites, mosquitoes transmit viruses (e.g., chikungunya, dengue, yellow fever, Zika) and filarial parasites (e.g., *Wuchereria bancrofti*). Depending on the clinical syndrome, a history of a tick bite could suggest a diagnosis of tick-borne encephalitis, African tick-bite fever, or other rickettsial infections. Tsetse flies are the vector for transmission of *Trypanosoma brucei*, a protozoan that causes African sleeping sickness. Tsetse flies are large, and their bites are painful; patients often recall being bitten. Freshwater bathing, swimming, wading, or other contact can put travelers at risk for leptospirosis, schistosomiasis, and other diseases.

11

Accommodations and activities also can influence the risk of acquiring certain diseases while abroad. Travelers who visit friends and relatives are at greater risk for malaria, typhoid fever, and other diseases, often because they stay longer, travel to more remote destinations, have more contact with local water sources, and typically do not seek pretravel advice (see Sec. 9, Ch. 9, Visiting Friends & Relatives: VFR Travel). Travelers backpacking and camping in rural areas have a greater risk for certain diseases than those staying in luxury, air-conditioned hotels.

COMORBIDITIES

Underlying illnesses can affect a traveler's susceptibility to infection as well as the clinical manifestations and severity of disease. An increasing number of international travelers are immunosuppressed, whether due to HIV infection, treatment with immune-modulating medications, being an organ transplant recipient, or other primary or acquired immunodeficiencies (see Sec. 3, Ch. 1, Immunocompromised Travelers). In addition, several factors associated with travel can exacerbate underlying conditions (e.g., chronic lung disease, inflammatory bowel disease, ischemic heart disease).

Symptoms & Illness Severity

Although the symptoms of many infectious and travel-associated syndromes overlap, the initial symptoms and presentation should ultimately guide the differential diagnosis: gastrointestinal symptoms and febrile illnesses are the most common syndromes in returning travelers. Remember that conditions such as appendicitis, urinary tract infections, and domestically acquired viral infections also can present in returning travelers.

Severity of illness is not only important for patient triage but also can help clinicians distinguish certain infections. Is the traveler hemodynamically stable? Is the infection potentially life-threatening (e.g., malaria)? Does the traveler have a severe respiratory syndrome or signs of hemorrhagic fever? Some suspected illnesses might necessitate prompt involvement of public health authorities. For more details, see General Management, later in this chapter.

COMMON SYNDROMES

The 3 most common clinical syndromes after travel to low- and middle-income countries are dermatologic conditions, diarrheal diseases, and systemic febrile illnesses, each of which is described in more detail elsewhere in this section (see Dermatologic Conditions, Persistent Diarrhea in Returned Travelers, and Fever in the Returned Traveler). Evaluate febrile travelers returning from malaria-endemic destinations immediately. Other common clinical presentations and findings include animal bites and scratches, asymptomatic eosinophilia, and respiratory illnesses.

Animal Bites & Scratches

Promptly evaluate any traveler who reports animal exposures during travel (see Sec. 4, Ch. 7, Zoonotic Exposures: Bites, Stings, Scratches & Other Hazards). Consider travelers with animal bites and scratches as high-risk for rabies exposure, and provide rabies postexposure prophylaxis, as indicated (see Sec. 5, Part 2, Ch. 18, Rabies). If the traveler was exposed to a macaque, herpes B postexposure prophylaxis might be indicated (see Sec. 5, Part 2, Ch. 1, B Virus).

Asymptomatic Eosinophilia

Eosinophilia in a returning traveler suggests possible helminth infection. Allergic diseases, hematologic disorders, and a few other viral, fungal, and protozoan infections also can cause eosinophilia. Eosinophilia can be present during pulmonary migration of parasites (e.g., *Ascaris*, hookworm, schistosomiasis, *Strongyloides*).

Other parasitic infections associated with eosinophilia include lymphatic filariasis, chronic strongyloidiasis, acute trichinellosis, and visceral larva migrans. These infections might be asymptomatic, but also could have associated symptoms (e.g., rash, swelling). In an outbreak of sarcocystosis among travelers returning from Tioman Island, Malaysia, those affected presented with eosinophilia and myalgias and had eosinophilic myositis on muscle biopsy (see Sec. 5, Part 3, Ch. 18, Sarcocystosis).

Parasitic infections are rare in most travelers, so consider other etiologies for eosinophilia; for instance, eosinophilia can be a sign of a hematologic malignancy. See Section 5 for more information on specific diseases.

Respiratory Illnesses

Respiratory illnesses are frequent among returned travelers and are typically associated with common respiratory viruses, including influenza and now, severe acute respiratory syndrome coronavirus 2, the cause of coronavirus disease 2019 (COVID-19). Since the pandemic began in early 2020, coronavirus disease (COVID-19) has overtaken influenza in overall global incidence. And although historically influenza has been the most common vaccine-preventable disease associated with international travel, COVID-19 could surpass it in that regard. To make that determination, however, a better understanding of the epidemiology of travel-associated COVID-19 transmission is needed (see Sec. 5, Part 2, Ch. 3, COVID-19).

If the travel history is appropriate and respiratory symptoms do not have a clear alternative diagnosis, include other emerging respiratory infections (e.g., avian influenza, Middle East respiratory syndrome [MERS]) in the differential diagnosis. In suspected cases of an emerging respiratory infection, alert local public health authorities and the Centers for Disease Control and Prevention (CDC) immediately. See relevant chapters in Section 5 for more information on these emerging infections; for a list of febrile respiratory illnesses that can occur after exposures in tropical destinations, see Table 11-10 in the chapter, Fever in the Returned Traveler.

Delayed illness onset and chronic cough after travel could be tuberculosis, especially in a long-term traveler or health care worker. Helminths and helminth infections associated with pulmonary symptoms include *Ascaris*, hookworms (*Ancylostoma* or *Necator*), paragonimiasis, schistosomiasis, and strongyloidiasis.

GENERAL MANAGEMENT

Triage

Most posttravel illnesses can be managed on an outpatient basis, but some patients, especially those with systemic febrile illnesses, might need to be hospitalized. Furthermore, potentially severe, transmissible infections (e.g., COVID-19, Ebola, MERS) require enhanced infection control measures and often, higher levels of care. Severe clinical presentations (e.g., acute respiratory distress, hemodynamic instability, mental status changes) require inpatient care. Have a low threshold for admitting a febrile patient if malaria is suspected; complications can occur rapidly. Management in an inpatient setting is especially vital for patients unlikely to follow up reliably or who have no one at home to assist if symptoms quickly worsen.

Initial Evaluation

After conducting a thorough physical exam, paying particular attention to skin manifestations or evidence of prior insect bites, order tests based on chief complaint and exposure history. Frequently useful tests include complete blood count with differential (to look for anemia, eosinophilia, leukocytosis, leukopenia, thrombocytopenia); blood cultures and malaria rapid diagnostic tests (depending on the presence of fever and travel itinerary); a complete metabolic profile (to identify electrolyte, renal, or liver dysfunction); serologic or PCR tests for arboviral infections (as needed); and stool cultures and ova and parasite exams. These tests often can help narrow the differential diagnosis and determine disease severity.

Antimicrobial Resistance

Be aware of the risk to international travelers for acquiring antimicrobial resistant organisms. Carefully consider travel history when caring for patients, both to identify effective treatments for infections and to ensure infection control interventions are in place to prevent spread of antimicrobial resistance (see Sec. 11, Ch. 5, Antimicrobial Resistance).

Consultation

Consult an infectious disease specialist when managing complicated or severe travel-associated infections, or when the diagnosis remains unclear. A tropical medicine or infectious disease specialist should be involved in cases that require specialized treatment (e.g., leishmaniasis, severe malaria, and neurocysticercosis).

Involve local, state, and federal public health authorities whenever managing transmissible, high-consequence infections. CDC provides on-call assistance with the diagnosis and management of parasitic infections at 404-718-4745 (for parasitic infections other than malaria) or 770-488-7788 (toll-free at 855-856-4713) for malaria, during business hours. After business hours or for other conditions, call the CDC Emergency Operations Center at 770-488-7100.

BIBLIOGRAPHY

Angelo KM, Kozarsky PE, Ryan ET, Chen LH, Sotir MJ. What proportion of international travellers acquire a travel-related illness? A review of the literature. J Travel Med. 2017;24(5):tax046.

Boggild AK, Castelli F, Gautret P, Torresi J, von Sonnenburg F, Barnett ED, et al. Vaccine preventable diseases in returned international travelers: results from the GeoSentinel Surveillance Network. Vaccine. 2010;28(46):7389–95.

Centers for Disease Control and Prevention. Notes from the field: acute muscular sarcocystosis among returning travelers—Tioman Island, Malaysia, 2011. MMWR Morb Mortal Wkly Rep. 2012;61(2):37–8.

Chen LH, Wilson ME, Davis X, Loutan L, Schwartz E, Keystone J, et al. Illness in long-term travelers visiting GeoSentinel clinics. Emerg Infect Dis. 2009;15(11):1773–82.

Fairley JK, Kozarsky PE, Kraft CS, Guarner J, Steinberg JP, Anderson E, et al. Ebola or not? Evaluating the ill traveler from Ebola-affected countries in West Africa. Open Forum Infect Dis. 2016;3(1):ofw005.

Hamer DH, Connor BA. Travel health knowledge, attitudes and practices among United States travelers. J Travel Med. 2004;11(1):23–6.

Hendel-Paterson B, Swanson SJ. Pediatric travelers visiting friends and relatives (VFR) abroad: illnesses, barriers and pre-travel recommendations. Travel Med Infect Dis. 2011;9(4):192–203.

Leder K, Torresi J, Libman MD, Cramer JP, Castelli F, Schlagenhauf P, et al. GeoSentinel surveillance of illness in returned travelers, 2007–2011. Ann Intern Med. 2013;158(6):456–68.

Ryan ET, Wilson ME, Kain KC. Illness after international travel. N Engl J Med. 2002;347(7):505–16.

Schulte C, Krebs B, Jelinek T, Nothdurft HD, von Sonnenburg F, Loscher T. Diagnostic significance of blood eosinophilia in returning travelers. Clin Infect Dis. 2002;34(3):407–11.

RAPID DIAGNOSTIC TESTS FOR INFECTIOUS DISEASES

Elizabeth Rabold, Jesse Waggoner

Rapid diagnostic tests (RDTs) refer to a group of diagnostics categorized by performance characteristics rather than the specific analyte or test platform. Such assays have relatively short performance times, provide results to inform clinical decision making, and enable management at the point-of-care (POC). RDTs are available in a variety of test formats and platforms and for various detection targets. RDTs are designed for detecting pathogen-specific antigens or nucleic acid sequences, as well as host antibody responses against certain pathogens (Table 11-05).

To select an appropriate RDT, factor in the pros and cons of the different analytes, timing of patient presentation, and specifics of the disease or syndrome under investigation (e.g., acute versus chronic infection). RDTs described here include any pathogen-specific or syndrome-based test that can be incorporated into a POC testing protocol for a given infection or clinical syndrome.

Tests that meet the definition of an RDT may be performed under a certificate of waiver (so-called "waived" tests) indicating they are simple to perform with a low risk for yielding an incorrect result. The certificate of waiver is specific to the United States. Nevertheless, some of its requirements are useful when considering using RDTs in international settings. For example, although

Table 11-05 Common rapid diagnostic test analytes & testing formats: advantages & disadvantages

RDT ANALYTE	ADVANTAGES	DISADVANTAGES	FORMAT	EXAMPLES
Antibody	IgM+ in late-acute/early convalescent phase IgG+ in chronic infections or after previous exposure Rapid and inexpensive	Antibodies from prior exposure and cross-reactivity limit specificity Insensitive in acute disease	Lateral flow Latex agglutination	Dengue Hepatitis B Hepatitis C HIV Syphilis
Antigen	Direct detection of pathogen antigens Detected in acute/active infection Rapid and inexpensive	Less sensitive than nucleic acid testing Does not provide type/strain information	Lateral flow Latex agglutination Solid phase "dipstick"	Dengue Ebola HIV Influenza Malaria SARS-CoV-2
Nucleic acid (RNA or DNA)	Sensitive and specific in acute phase Can provide quantitative information	Expensive Requires specific instrumentation Longer performance time	PCR/RT-PCR LAMP/RT-LAMP RPA/RT-RPA	Chlamydia Multiplex respiratory and gastrointestinal panels *Neisseria* SARS-CoV-2

Abbreviations: LAMP, loop-mediated amplification; PCR, polymerase chain reaction; RPA, recombinase polymerase amplification; RT, reverse transcription; SARS-CoV-2, severe acute respiratory syndrome coronavirus 2 mandated personnel requirements for such tests are minimal, testers must be trained and document proficiency on use of the assay. Waived tests can only be performed on unmodified specimens (whole blood, saliva, urine) according to the most recent manufacturer recommendations. Deviations from the specimen type or manufacturer protocol make the test high-complexity and require that it be performed in a dedicated laboratory setting. Finally, RDT reagents might have specific storage requirements and a limited shelf life. These factors impact accuracy of the test and necessitate oversight and quality assessments to ensure proper performance.

Some tests with performance characteristics of an RDT might not be readily compatible with POC testing. For instance, an increasing number of waived, sample-to-answer molecular diagnostics (nucleic acid amplification tests) are becoming available. At a given institution, these assays might only be performed in a central laboratory at specific times, thereby limiting their applicability at the POC. These assays typically must be performed with dedicated bench-top equipment; adding this capacity at clinical sites, therefore, might not be feasible.

RAPID DIAGNOSTIC TESTS FOR CLINICAL SYNDROMES

RDTs, including multiplex molecular panels (Table 11-06 and Table 11-07), are available for many common clinical syndromes among travelers, the etiologies of which can overlap substantially with those of non-travel–associated syndromes. Thus, clinics might augment RDT diagnosis of common pathogens with specialized or follow-up testing for rare pathogens or positive results.

In general, RDTs for antigen and antibody detection are less sensitive than standard laboratory assays. Rapid HIV tests that use blood and cheek swab samples are widely available and perform well in identifying individuals with chronic infections. Even later-generation antigen/antibody tests remain less sensitive than molecular testing for acute HIV infection, however, and in high-risk patients, molecular testing or repeat testing is warranted. The sensitivity of rapid antigen tests for influenza and certain gastrointestinal pathogens (e.g., norovirus, rotavirus) are notably poor. Negative results should not dictate therapy decisions, and positive results should be confirmed with molecular testing.

Multiplex molecular panels are becoming more common for central nervous system (CNS), gastrointestinal, and respiratory infections, and new panels are under evaluation for febrile returning travelers. These panels often are very sensitive and can test for many pathogens in a single sample. These tests are expensive, however, and results must be interpreted in the clinical context; certain pathogens might require additional testing when there is high clinical suspicion. Notably, available multiplex assays do not test for common bacterial causes of pneumonia. Also, detection of emerging or novel pathogens is not feasible with large, preconstructed testing panels. When interpreting results provided by multiplex molecular panels, consider the prolonged shedding periods of certain pathogens, the possibility of multiple positive results or co-infections, the detection of asymptomatic carriage, and the variable accuracy for different agents on the panel (e.g., cryptococcus in CNS panels, adenovirus in respiratory panels).

Undifferentiated acute febrile illness is a common and potentially life-threating clinical presentation among returning travelers that poses a diagnostic challenge and requires prompt evaluation, diagnosis, and management. RDTs might be unavailable or insufficient to diagnose the many possible causes of febrile illness. For example, a commercial RDT for malaria has been cleared for use in hospitals and laboratories but not for individual clinics; microscopy is still the diagnostic tool of choice in malaria cases to identify the species and calculate the level of parasitemia (see Sec. 5, Part 3, Ch. 16, Malaria). Furthermore, patients with malaria can be co-infected with other pathogens that can contribute to and complicate diagnosis and management. RDTs are not available in the United States for other common causes of undifferentiated acute febrile illness in travelers (e.g., dengue, leptospirosis).

Coronavirus Disease 2019

High demand for diagnostics for severe acute respiratory syndrome coronavirus 2 (SARS-CoV-2), the virus that causes coronavirus disease

Table 11-06 Lateral-flow immunochromatographic tests & small panels for pathogens in returning international travelers: selected features

SYNDROME	PATHOGENS	SPECIMEN TYPES	ADDITIONAL INFORMATION
SYSTEMIC FEBRILE ILLNESS	Dengue virus	Serum	Not FDA-cleared; highly variable performance; antibodies may cross-react between flaviviruses
	Ebola virus	Whole blood	Received Emergency Use Authorization from FDA and Emergency Use Listing from WHO
	Plasmodium spp.	Whole blood	Best performance characteristics for *Plasmodium falciparum* infections
GASTROINTESTINAL INFECTIONS	*Vibrio cholerae*	Stool sample	Not FDA-cleared; may be accurate for 01- and/or 0139-positive strains
	Norovirus, rotavirus	Stool sample	Available in the United States separately or in combination
RESPIRATORY INFECTIONS	Influenza virus	Nasopharyngeal or throat swab	Rapid test sensitivity 50%–70%; negative testing should not direct treatment
	SARS-CoV-2	Nasal or nasopharyngeal swabs	RDT and "at home" test availability increasing; performance with variants under investigation
SEXUALLY TRANSMITTED INFECTIONS	*Chlamydia trachomatis* and *Neisseria gonorrhea*	Urine, vaginal swab	Molecular tests remain gold standard; a sample-to-answer molecular assay is available
	HIV	Whole blood, oral fluids	Antibody and antibody/antigen kits available; molecular testing preferred for acute infection
	Treponema pallidum	Whole blood	Antibody detection; may not be appropriate for acute infection

Abbreviations: FDA, US Food and Drug Administration; IDSA, Infectious Disease Society of America; RDT, rapid diagnostic test; SARS-CoV-2, severe acute respiratory syndrome coronavirus 2; WHO, World Health Organization

2019 (COVID-19), combined with an emphasis on decreasing exposures to people infected with the virus, led the US Food and Drug Administration (FDA) to issue an Emergency Use Authorization for several RDTs and multiplex panels that include SARS-CoV-2. RDTs include rapid antigen diagnostics and the first molecular diagnostic for home use. These can be performed with self- or caregiver-collected samples. Some home test kits require that users download a smartphone application that provides test interpretation for the user and reports de-identified data for public health surveillance. These diagnostic kits perform best in symptomatic people; results in asymptomatic people should be interpreted with caution.

Table 11-07 Multiplex molecular panels for pathogens in returning international travelers: selected features

SYNDROME	PATHOGENS	SPECIMEN TYPES	ADDITIONAL INFORMATION
ACUTE FEBRILE ILLNESS	Bacteria, viruses, and parasites from different regions	Whole blood	Research use only; clinical performance for many targets has not been determined.
GASTROINTESTINAL PATHOGENS	Includes common bacteria, viruses, and parasites	Stool sample	Sensitive; certain positive results might be unrelated to active infection.
MENINGITIS & ENCEPHALITIS	Includes common bacteria, viruses, and fungi	CSF	Not a replacement for CSF bacterial culture; negative results do not exclude an infectious etiology of meningitis or encephalitis.
RESPIRATORY PATHOGENS	Includes atypical bacteria, common viruses, and SARS-CoV-2	Nasopharyngeal swab	Pathogens can have prolonged shedding time; positive results might not rule out infection from other pathogens.

Abbreviations: CSF, cerebrospinal fluid; SARS-CoV-2, severe acute respiratory syndrome coronavirus 2

DIAGNOSTIC TESTING PERFORMED DURING TRAVEL

People who become ill while traveling might seek medical care abroad; development and availability of RDTs for diagnosis of tropical infectious diseases has expanded greatly in recent years, and travelers might return home having been diagnosed based on results from these tests. RDTs for tropical infections typically are lateral-flow immunochromatographic tests that detect antigens from or antibodies to certain pathogens. Because only 1 such test (for malaria) is cleared for use in the United States, the diagnostic characteristics of RDTs used overseas are unfamiliar to most providers. Additionally, a variety of RDTs might be available for certain pathogens (e.g., dengue) in other countries, with widely varying or poorly studied performance characteristics. Institutions that do not have continuous access to a single brand of test further complicates interpretation of results provided by the laboratory.

The following is an illustrative, though by no means exhaustive, list of several common infections for which RDTs are available.

Dengue. Rapid, lateral-flow assays are available to detect the dengue nonstructural protein 1 (NS1) antigen, and IgM and IgG. Dengue tests have widely variable performance characteristics depending on the manufacturer, circulating dengue types, a patient's past medical history, and symptom duration.

Emerging Infections. Emerging pathogens represent a diagnostic challenge. Rapid assays became available after outbreaks of chikungunya, Ebola, and Zika. Such assays might not be available or well-studied at the peak of an outbreak, however.

Leishmaniasis. Assays to detect antibodies against the rK39 antigen (visceral leishmaniasis) have demonstrated good specificity in endemic regions, and highest sensitivity for detecting disease in South Asia.

Leptospirosis. Because of the many pathogenic and intermediate *Leptospira* serotypes that result in human disease worldwide, the usefulness of serologic assays for diagnosing leptospirosis is limited.

Malaria. An FDA-cleared RDT for malaria is available, and malaria RDTs are widely used throughout the world. In general, these tests perform best for *Plasmodium falciparum*, with variable or poor performance for other *Plasmodium* species.

Typhoid. Rapid serologic tests have demonstrated only moderate accuracy to diagnose typhoid. Additionally, these tests are designed to detect *Salmonella enterica* serotype Typhi only.

FUTURE DIRECTIONS

The number of assays compatible with POC testing will undoubtedly continue to increase. Building upon testing milestones achieved during the COVID-19 pandemic, "at home" testing, including molecular testing, is expected to increase in the coming years for both respiratory viruses and other pathogens. Because of the wide breadth and diversity of infecting pathogens in returned travelers, use of POC testing for nondomestic infectious diseases might not be practical for most centers once test volume, personnel training, and cost are taken into consideration. POC testing for common syndromes that affect travelers and nontravelers alike (e.g., respiratory tract and gastrointestinal infections) could provide rapid diagnosis, inform triage decisions, and limit unnecessary laboratory testing.

BIBLIOGRAPHY

Babady NE. The FilmArray respiratory panel: an automated, broadly multiplexed molecular test for the rapid and accurate detection of respiratory pathogens. Expert Rev Mol Diagn. 2013;13(8):779–88.

Centers for Disease Control and Prevention. Ready? Set? Test! Patient testing is important. Get the results right. Atlanta: The Centers; 2019. Available from: www.cdc.gov/labquality/images/waived-tests/RST-Booklet_Dec-2019.pdf.

Gonzalez MD, McElvania E. New developments in rapid diagnostic testing for children. Infect Dis Clin North Am. 2018;32(1):19–34.

Hunsperger EA, Yoksan S, Buchy P, Nguyen VC, Sekaran SD, Enria DA, et al. Evaluation of commercially available diagnostic tests for the detection of dengue virus NS1 antigen and anti-dengue virus IgM antibody. PLoS Negl Trop Dis. 2014;8(10):e3171.

Infectious Disease Society of America. IDSA practice guidelines. Available from: www.idsociety.org/practice-guideline/practice-guidelines.

Pai NP, Vadnais C, Denkinger C, Engel N, Pai M. Point-of-care testing for infectious diseases: diversity, complexity, and barriers in low- and middle-income countries. PLoS Med. 2012;9(9):e1001306.

US Food and Drug Administration. CLIA—Clinical Laboratory Improvement Amendments—currently waived analytes. Available from: www.accessdata.fda.gov/scripts/cdrh/cfdocs/cfClia/analyteswaived.cfm.

US Food and Drug Administration. In vitro diagnostics EUAs. Available from: www.fda.gov/medical-devices/coronavirus-disease-2019-covid-19-emergency-use-authorizations-medical-devices/in-vitro-diagnostics-euas.

SCREENING ASYMPTOMATIC RETURNED TRAVELERS

Michael Libman, Sapha Barkati

Except for coronavirus disease 2019 (COVID-19), CDC has no official guidance or recommendations for screening asymptomatic international travelers in the absence of specific risk factors for infectious diseases. Nevertheless, screening travelers returning from developing countries represents a substantial portion of the activity of many travel health and tropical medicine clinics.

The scientific literature on the clinical utility and cost effectiveness of screening asymptomatic travelers is sparse. Asymptomatic travelers can harbor many infections acquired during travel, some of which have the potential to cause serious sequelae or have public health implications. In some cases, these will include pathogens rarely found in the traveler's country of origin. US medical practitioners might have little familiarity with these travel-associated diseases, and specific diagnostic tests might not be readily available or will require expertise in their proper interpretation.

DECIDING TO SCREEN

The decision to screen an asymptomatic person for travel-acquired pathogens depends on their exposure history, itinerary, type of travel, and the public health implications of identifying infection. Screening healthy short-term travelers for infectious diseases other than COVID-19, especially people who do not report a particular exposure, is usually not necessary. On the other hand, consider obtaining specific tests for long-term travelers (e.g., adventure travelers, expatriates, humanitarian aid workers, missionaries, travelers visiting friends and relatives) who might have prolonged or heavy exposure to epidemiologically relevant pathogens with potential for long-term consequences. A traveler's exposure history might be unreliable or not predictive of infection, however, and the value of a detailed itinerary can be limited by incomplete information. Finally, the type of travel might not provide a practical assessment of risk.

For the long-term traveler on hiatus from a continuing assignment abroad, the periodic travel health consultation offers the clinician a chance to screen for infectious diseases, conduct a general health evaluation, and to review health behaviors, malaria prophylaxis, and vaccination status. Promote and reinforce primary prevention by discussing behavioral or other risk factors that could predispose the traveler to ill health (e.g., exposures to contaminated food and drink, arthropods, and freshwater sources; drug use; high-risk sex). The usual recommendations for a periodic health exam, which might include screening for cardiovascular disorders, diabetes, hypertension, and malignancy, also apply.

Benefit & Risk of Screening Asymptomatic Travelers

Before scheduling screening tests for asymptomatic returned travelers, evaluate the sensitivity and specificity of the test, and the risk and cost to the patient. The low prevalence of tropical infections in asymptomatic travelers will heavily influence the positive predictive value of the screening tests, leading to an increased likelihood of false-positive results. As a result, the asymptomatic traveler could be subjected to further investigations, generating greater costs, anxiety, and other possible harms related to diagnostic follow-up, creating complex considerations of benefit versus risk.

Screening traditionally has been viewed as a secondary prevention intervention, that is, an attempt to identify occult illnesses or health risks. Cost effectiveness of screening depends on the disease of interest, potential outcomes associated with the disease both for the individual traveler and the public's health, and whether an early intervention could reduce morbidity or mortality. One exception regarding asymptomatic screening is newly arrived immigrants and refugees; for recommendations regarding these individuals see Sec. 11, Ch. 11, Newly Arrived Immigrants, Refugees & Other Migrants.

SCREENING FOR NONPARASITIC INFECTIONS

Arboviruses

CHIKUNGUNYA & DENGUE

Screening for chikungunya and dengue in asymptomatic travelers typically is not recommended because there are no specific treatments for infection once identified. Travelers concerned about the risk for complications after a secondary dengue infection sometimes request screening. The absolute risk elevation is minimal, however, and generally there is no specific intervention. The exception are children 9–16 years old living in dengue-endemic areas; Dengvaxia vaccine is a prevention option for those presenting with laboratory-confirmed previous dengue infection (see Sec. 5, Part 2, Ch. 4, Dengue).

ZIKA

The prevalence of Zika virus infection in many countries has decreased dramatically since 2017; as a result, the likelihood of a false-positive test result has increased. Moreover, Zika virus IgM antibody persists months after infection, making it difficult to determine the date of infection, which is crucial information for judging the risk in a pregnant person. Nonetheless, remain vigilant for the potential reemergence of Zika, and review screening guidelines for travelers, including pregnant people and their partners (see Sec. 5, Part 2, Ch. 27, Zika, and www.cdc.gov/zika/hc-providers/index.html).

Coronavirus Disease 2019

The COVID-19 pandemic, caused by the severe acute respiratory syndrome coronavirus 2 (SARS-CoV-2) virus, has had vast health, social, and economic effects. The emergence of variants makes the evolution of this pandemic unpredictable. As the pandemic progresses, guidance for populations and travelers evolve, as do requirements and recommendations for crossing international borders (see www.cdc.gov/coronavirus/2019-ncov/travelers/international-travel/index.html). For patients who test positive for SARS-CoV-2 after international travel, consider prioritizing specimens for whole genome sequencing, as applicable.

Sexually Transmitted Infections & Bloodborne Pathogens

High rates of sexual activity with new partners, including sex workers, have been documented in overseas backpackers, military personnel, expatriate workers, and people doing volunteer work. Of concern are the low rates of reported condom use. Moreover, travelers might engage in other high-risk activities (e.g., getting a tattoo or piercing, using injection or intranasal drugs, receiving medical or dental care). Returning travelers with acute hepatitis B, hepatitis C, HIV, monkeypox, or syphilis infection pose public health risks and might be hesitant to volunteer a relevant exposure history.

A detailed questionnaire on risk factors for sexually transmitted infections and bloodborne pathogens is recommended for all travelers; always consider screening according to published guidelines. Screening people with relevant exposures should include HIV and syphilis serologic tests, and nucleic acid amplification testing for chlamydia and gonorrhea in urine and at sites of contact (e.g., pharynx, rectum). For travelers with an identified specific risk factor (e.g., blood exposure, condomless sex) who have not been previously vaccinated against

(continued)

SCREENING ASYMPTOMATIC RETURNED TRAVELERS (CONTINUED)

hepatitis B virus (HBV), perform HBV testing; hepatitis C virus (HCV) testing also is indicated. Test all travelers born between 1945 and 1965 for HCV if not previously tested.

Tuberculosis

The incidence of tuberculosis (TB) infection related to travel is difficult to estimate. Those with a history of work in high-prevalence settings (e.g., health care institutions, refugee camps) merit screening. Pretravel and posttravel tuberculin skin testing (TST) can require as many as 4 visits to a health care provider—2 pretravel visits for a 2-step test, and 2 posttravel visits after potential exposure. The TB screening process can be simplified by using the interferon-γ release assay (IGRA), which is more expensive but less likely to yield false-positive results in people who received a previous bacillus Calmette-Guérin (BCG) vaccination.

Studies assessing IGRA use for serial testing demonstrated large variations in the rate of conversion and reversion. Fully investigate any positive TST or IGRA result, assess symptoms suggestive of active TB disease, and obtain a chest x-ray. For more information, see Sec. 5, Part 1, Ch. 23, . . . *perspectives*: Testing Travelers for *Mycobacterium tuberculosis* Infection.

SCREENING FOR PARASITIC INFECTIONS

Travelers often are most concerned about the possibility of an occult parasitic infection (see also Sec. 11, Ch. 9,. . . *perspectives*: Delusional Parasitosis). Unfortunately, the literature shows that patient questionnaires and common laboratory testing used to screen for parasitic diseases have poor sensitivity and specificity. Studies have shown that even an exhaustive risk-factor history in asymptomatic patients is unable to reliably detect those who would or would not have evidence of parasitic infection. Physical examination is equally unrevealing.

Most commonly, a stool examination is performed, typically microscopy. Several molecular assays are commercially available to detect a panel of bacterial, viral, and parasitic pathogens. In some cases, these panels are more sensitive than traditional testing methods, and even asymptomatic people often are found to harbor pathogens. The clinical implications of asymptomatic carriage, sometimes at a low level, are unknown for most of these agents, and the risks and benefits of treatment are not well studied. Serologic tests typically are more sensitive for parasitic infections; some have performance limitations related to specificity, but are often preferred for screening asymptomatic travelers.

For questions about parasites and screening for parasitic infections, see www.cdc.gov/parasites/, or contact the CDC at www.cdc.gov/parasites/contact.html.

Helminths

Travelers often are concerned about "worms," by which they usually mean intestinal helminths (see Sec. 5, Part 3, Ch. 13, Soil-Transmitted Helminths). Infections of travelers with large burdens of the common nematodes (e.g., *Ascaris*, hookworm, *Trichuris*) are rare, however. Questioning returning expatriates infected with intestinal helminths has disclosed no attributable symptoms compared with uninfected controls. The life cycles of almost all helminths preclude any real risk of ongoing person-to-person transmission from asymptomatic hosts in high-income countries; helminths generally have a natural lifespan of months to a few years, which ensures eventual spontaneous clearance. In addition, low-intensity infections are of limited clinical importance, though in rare cases aberrant migration of *Ascaris* spp. can result in clinical disease. The exception to this is *Strongyloides stercoralis*.

STRONGYLOIDIASIS

For *Strongyloides* infections, serious complications are well known, nonspecific symptoms can easily be overlooked, duration of carriage after infection is unlimited due to its autoinfection cycle, and the original burden of infection is irrelevant (see Sec. 5, Part 3, Ch. 21, Strongyloidiasis). Specific types of immune suppression (e.g., corticosteroid therapy, hematologic malignancy, hematopoietic stem cell transplant, human T-lymphotropic virus type 1 [HTLV-1] infection, solid organ transplant) are risk factors for developing a potentially lethal hyperinfection syndrome or disseminated strongyloidiasis. The COVID-19 pandemic has prompted widespread, urgent dexamethasone use, which could lead to an increased risk for severe strongyloidiasis in exposed travelers and migrants.

Consider screening for strongyloidiasis in select high-risk travelers with potential skin exposure to human feces, usually a result of walking barefoot in areas without proper sanitation facilities. Unfortunately, the sensitivity of stool-based biomolecular and parasitological methods is low. Molecular detection of helminths is more sensitive and specific compared to microscopy, but sensitivity is still insufficient for screening purposes. Moreover, molecular techniques are not widely available outside the reference laboratory and research setting. Serologic methods are often required, as discussed elsewhere in this chapter.

SCHISTOSOMIASIS

There is no evidence to demonstrate that the low-burden *Schistosoma* infections typically found in travelers lead to the types of complications found in endemic areas (e.g., liver fibrosis, malignancy). Nevertheless, the possibility of complications cannot be entirely ruled out, particularly in people who have more intense exposures (see Sec. 5, Part 3, Ch. 20, Schistosomiasis). Even brief exposures to freshwater lakes and rivers in known endemic areas in Africa are associated with substantial seroconversion rates. In addition, complications due to ectopic egg migration occasionally can occur in light infections and without warning.

Consider serologic screening in asymptomatic travelers who bathed or swam in freshwater canals, lakes, or rivers in areas endemic for schistosomiasis. Other types of fresh water (e.g., adequately chlorinated swimming pools) carry minimal exposure risk because they do not support the larval parasitic forms. Screening becomes most sensitive only 8–10 weeks after potential exposure and is useful only in those who have not been infected with a schistosome previously. *Schistosoma* antigens (e.g., circulating anodic antigen [CAA]) can be detected in blood and urine in active infection and can be used to monitor cure after treatment, but sensitivity in asymptomatic travelers is not well studied, and these tests are not widely available.

Interpreting traditional tests for the parasites that cause schistosomiasis and strongyloidiasis can be challenging. Urine and stool examination for *Schistosoma* spp. and stool examination for *Strongyloides* lack sensitivity, particularly in low-burden infection; thus, serologic testing has been advocated as the best screening tool. Problems inherent to serologic screening include expense, lack of easy availability, and lack of standardization. Serologic tests often are designed to maximize sensitivity, typically at the expense of specificity. Unfortunately, specificity is almost impossible to define. Seropositivity in the absence of direct pathogen detection is common, and its clinical significance can be difficult to determine.

Fortunately for patients with schistosomiasis (or strongyloidiasis), treatment is easy and effective; for people deemed at risk of strongyloidiasis who require immediate immunosuppression, consider empiric treatment. The common antihelminthic agents used for short-course therapy (e.g., albendazole, ivermectin, praziquantel) have excellent safety profiles. Be aware, however, that rare but severe adverse events can occur when using certain antihelminthics in patients who have occult, unsuspected co-infection with other parasites. Of note, albendazole can cause increased intracranial pressure with focal signs, seizures, and retinal damage in people infected with *Taenia solium*; diethylcarbamazine can provoke ocular damage in people infected with *Onchocerca*; and

(continued)

11

SCREENING ASYMPTOMATIC RETURNED TRAVELERS (CONTINUED)

ivermectin can cause encephalopathy in people infected with *Loa loa*.

FILARIASIS

Reports of travelers with late complications from asymptomatic filarial infections are virtually nonexistent, and filarial screening (blood or skin snips for microfilaria) is generally not recommended for asymptomatic travelers.

OTHER HELMINTHIC INFECTIONS

Helminth parasitic infections rarely seen in returning travelers include fascioliasis, neurocysticercosis, and paragonimiasis, among others. Screening asymptomatic travelers for these infections is generally not appropriate. Primary care providers should refer patients to an infectious disease specialist when biological, clinical, or radiologic abnormalities increase suspicion for these infections. Intestinal helminths (e.g., *Ascaris*, *Enterobius*, hookworms, *Strongyloides*, *Trichuris*) rarely cause severe illness in travelers. Other than for *Strongyloides* in select high-risk travelers, screening is not recommended for intestinal helminth infections.

Protozoa

BLOOD- & TISSUE-DWELLING

MALARIA

No justification can be made for screening most asymptomatic travelers for malaria, whether by blood film, molecular methods, or serologic tests. No available tests can detect the latent hepatic forms (hypnozoites) of *Plasmodium vivax* or *P. ovale*. Remind travelers to seek evaluation for unexplained fever and to notify practitioners of international travel within the past 12 months.

Immigrants with frequent and regular exposure to malaria might gradually develop partial immunity, which can result in low-level parasitemia with minimal symptoms. Immigrants from malaria-endemic areas might later recrudesce with more severe illness, but this phenomenon is rare in non-immigrant travelers. Of note, in rare cases, travelers compliant with prophylaxis might still acquire malaria; often they will present with low parasitemia infections, and their symptoms can manifest after ending prophylaxis. In these cases, testing asymptomatic travelers is generally inadequately sensitive and not recommended. Rather, advise travelers to remain vigilant for symptoms, particularly unexplained fever.

TRYPANOSOMIASIS

Occult trypanosomiasis in asymptomatic travelers (as opposed to immigrants) appears to be extremely rare. Screening tests (e.g., molecular diagnostics, serology) are of unknown value. Consider *Trypanosoma cruzi* testing for travelers who lived for >6 months in rustic housing (e.g., shelters with mud walls and thatched roofs) in endemic areas of Latin America, especially if they report having seen triatomine bugs inside their dwelling. Also consider testing in people who received blood products in an endemic area, or in travelers with clinical manifestations compatible with acute Chagas disease (see Sec. 5, Part 3, Ch. 25, American Trypanosomiasis / Chagas Disease).

East African trypanosomiasis has affected travelers but typically causes acute symptoms. West African trypanosomiasis generally is not reported in travelers. Refer patients to an infectious disease specialist when these infections are suspected based on biological, clinical, or radiologic abnormalities.

INTESTINAL

Treat symptomatic intestinal protozoa infections, particularly *Entamoeba histolytica* which can cause severe disease and ectopic infections (e.g., liver abscess). Except for *E. histolytica* infection (which is only rarely asymptomatic), the finding of pathogenic protozoa in asymptomatic patients is of questionable significance.

The most common protozoa found in asymptomatic travelers are *Blastocystis* and *Giardia* species. History of exposure to contaminated food or water has poor predictive value. No evidence suggests that asymptomatic carriers are likely to develop symptoms later, and the medications used to treat these protozoa can have adverse effects. In theory, asymptomatic carriers pose a public health risk, but transmission by asymptomatic travelers appears to be rare. In addition, stool microscopy for protozoa is expensive, not very sensitive, not highly reproducible, and many laboratories have limited expertise; thus, screening is not recommended unless evidence of onward transmission is present.

Microscopy cannot distinguish *Entamoeba histolytica* from *E. dispar*. Differentiation requires further specimen collection and testing. Studies reveal that most travelers with *Entamoeba* on microscopy are carrying *E. dispar*. Antigen testing for *E. histolytica* and *Giardia* (among others) is fairly reliable but lacks the potential to screen for all intestinal parasites with a single test, and only some antigen tests are able to differentiate *E. histolytica* from *E. dispar*.

Commercial molecular methods to screen stool specimens for multiple pathogens simultaneously typically include several protozoa, generally with better sensitivity than microscopy. These assays also can specifically distinguish potentially pathogenic *E. histolytica* from nonpathogenic amoebae. They offer rapid turnaround times and, although costs remain high, these assays are increasingly being used in returned travelers with suspected protozoal infections. Some of these panels detect organisms for which pathogenicity remains controversial, (e.g., *Blastocystis* and *Dientamoeba*). Identifying these pathogens can lead to patient anxiety and unnecessary treatment; thus, screening asymptomatic travelers for intestinal protozoa is not routinely recommended.

GENERAL GUIDELINES

Eosinophilia

Screening for eosinophilia is a common test because it is quick, universally available, and theoretically of value in detecting invasive helminths, if not protozoa. Multiple studies have shown, however, that testing for eosinophilia has poor sensitivity for identifying parasitic infections; the low prevalence of infection in asymptomatic travelers means that the positive predictive value is poor, and the finding of eosinophilia can lead to an extensive and often fruitless search for a cause, generating patient anxiety and high costs. Many cases of eosinophilia resolve spontaneously, possibly because of infection with nonpathogenic organisms or a noninfectious cause (e.g., allergy, drug reaction). Repeat eosinophil counts after several weeks or months before embarking on an extensive investigation.

A recent study in travelers and migrants showed that those with helminthic infection (as compared to other diagnoses) had much higher eosinophil counts. Counts can be highly variable, though, even within a single day, and are suppressed by endogenous or exogenous steroids. Using absolute eosinophil counts, rather than eosinophils as a percentage of leukocytes, is more reproducible and predictive.

Duration of Travel & Other Risk Factors

Table 11-08 and the following traveler classification scheme provide general guidelines for screening asymptomatic returned travelers for imported infections.

ALL TRAVELERS

For guidance regarding international travel and posttravel COVID-19 testing, refer to www.cdc.gov/coronavirus/2019-ncov/travelers/international-travel/index.html.

SHORT-TERM TRAVELERS

Screening asymptomatic short-term (<3–6 months) travelers is usually low-yield and should be directed by specific risk factors revealed in the history. A history of prolonged (>2 weeks) digestive symptoms during travel can suggest protozoal infection. Consider serologic testing of travelers who bathed or swam in unchlorinated freshwater sources in regions

(continued)

11

SCREENING ASYMPTOMATIC RETURNED TRAVELERS (CONTINUED)

Table 11-08 Considerations for screening asymptomatic travelers

RISK FACTOR OR EXPOSURE	SUGGESTED SCREENING TESTS
All travelers Short stay (<3–6 months) No identified risk factor/exposure	COVID-19[1] No additional screening
Long-stay (>3–6 months) Poor sanitation or hygiene	CBC with eosinophil count Creatinine CRP Liver transaminases Consider stool ova and parasites
Sexual contact	Chlamydia Gonorrhea HBV, if not previously vaccinated (for men who have sex with men, people who have sex with unknown partners) HCV (if risk factors present or if born between 1945–1965) HIV Syphilis
Injection or intranasal drug use Medical or dental care Piercing Tattoo	HBV, if not previously vaccinated (for injection drug use) HCV (for injection or intranasal drug use, unregulated tattoos) HIV
Pregnant people who traveled in known current Zika virus–endemic or epidemic area or sexual contact with a partner who traveled in these areas	Screening asymptomatic pregnant travelers who have potential exposure (but without ongoing risk) is not routinely recommended outside an outbreak situation NAAT ≤12 weeks after potential exposure in endemic or epidemic regions can be considered in pregnant people
Health care worker	TB screening (TST or IGRA)
Prolonged residence (>6 months) with population in a highly TB-endemic area	TB screening (TST or IGRA)
Walking barefoot on soil potentially contaminated with human feces or sewage	*Strongyloides* serology
Exposure to freshwater rivers, lakes, or irrigation canals	*Schistosoma* serology

Abbreviations: CBC, complete blood count; COVID-19, coronavirus disease 2019; CRP, C-reactive protein; HBV, hepatitis B virus; HCV, hepatitis C virus; NAAT, nucleic acid amplification test; TB, tuberculosis; TST, tuberculin skin test; IGRA, interferon-γ release assay

[1]Recommendation might change with the evolution of the pandemic. Refer to the updated recommendations available from: www.cdc.gov/coronavirus/2019-ncov/travelers/international-travel/index.html.

with known schistosomiasis risk, especially sub-Saharan Africa.

In addition, consider serology testing for *Strongyloides* in select high-risk travelers who have skin exposure to soil likely to be contaminated with human feces, usually individuals with a history of frequently walking barefoot outdoors. Obtain a sexual history; screen for

11

sexually transmitted and bloodborne infections, if warranted. Zika virus testing for asymptomatic travelers (including pregnant people) with potential exposure is generally not recommended (see Sec. 5, Part 2, Ch 27, Zika). Consider TB screening for those returning from work in health care or other high-risk settings.

LONG-TERM TRAVELERS & EXPATRIATES

The overall yield of screening increases for longer-stay (>3–6 months) travelers. The emphasis should be on those with the longest stays and the most problematic sanitary conditions or other exposures. In some cases, employers require certain tests, partly for liability reasons. Performing stool examinations mostly provides psychological reassurance. Consider obtaining serologic testing for schistosomiasis and strongyloidiasis in people with recent or remote travel histories to endemic areas and who report some level of risk.

A complete blood count with white blood cell differential and eosinophil counts, liver transaminases, creatinine, and C-reactive protein are usually the basic set of tests performed. Interpret results cautiously; abnormalities might trigger further testing. Zika virus testing for asymptomatic travelers with potential exposure, including pregnant people, is generally not recommended outside of a recognized outbreak. Limit TST or IGRA testing to travelers who worked in a health care or similar setting or who had intimate and prolonged contact with residents of a highly TB-endemic area for ≥6 months. Only perform other screening based on exceptional exposures or knowledge about local outbreaks.

BIBLIOGRAPHY

Baaten GG, Sonder GJ, van Gool T, Kint JA, van den Hoek A. Travel-related schistosomiasis, strongyloidiasis, filariasis, and toxocariasis: the risk of infection and the diagnostic relevance of blood eosinophilia. BMC Infect Dis. 2011;11:84.

Casacuberta-Partal M, Janse JJ, van Schuijlenburg R, de Vries JJC, Erkens MAA, Suijk K, et al. Antigen-based diagnosis of *Schistosoma* infection in travellers: a prospective study. J Travel Med. 2020;27(4):1–9.

Centers for Disease Control and Prevention. International travel during COVID-19; 2020. Available from: www.cdc.gov/coronavirus/2019-ncov/travelers/international-travel-during-covid19.html.

Centers for Disease Control and Prevention. Zika virus for health care providers; 2022. Available from: www.cdc.gov/zika/hc-providers.

MacLean JD, Libman M. Screening returning travelers. Infect Dis Clin North Am. 1998;12(2):431–43.

Overbosch FW, van Gool T, Matser A, Sonder GJB. Low incidence of helminth infections (schistosomiasis, strongyloidiasis, filariasis, toxocariasis) among Dutch long-term travelers: A prospective study, 2008–2011. PLoS ONE. 2018;13(5):e0197770.

Salzer HJF, Rolling T, Vinnemeir CD, Tannich E, Schmiedel S, Addo MM, et al. Helminthic infections in returning travelers and migrants with eosinophilia: diagnostic value of medical history, eosinophil count and IgE. Travel Med Infect Dis. 2017;20:49–55.

Smith BD, Morgan RL, Beckett GA, Falck-Ytter Y, Holtzman D, Teo CG, et al. Recommendations for the identification of chronic hepatitis C virus infection among persons born during 1945–1965. MMWR Recomm Rep. 2012;61(RR-4):1–18.

Soonawala D, van Lieshout L, den Boer MA, Claas EC, Verweij JJ, Godkewitsch A, et al. Post-travel screening of asymptomatic long-term travelers to the tropics for intestinal parasites using molecular diagnostics. Am J Trop Med Hyg. 2014;90(5):835–9.

US Preventive Services Task Force. Final recommendation statement. Hepatitis C: screening; 2022. Available from: www.uspreventiveservicestaskforce.org/Page/Document/RecommendationStatementFinal/hepatitis-c-screening.

Weinbaum CM, Williams I, Mast EE, Wang SA, Finelli L, Wasley A, et al. Recommendations for identification and public health management of persons with chronic hepatitis B virus infection. MMWR Recomm Rep. 2008;57(RR-8):1–20.

Yansouni CP, Merckx J, Libman MD, Ndao M. Recent advances in clinical parasitology diagnostics. Curr Infect Dis Rep. 2014;16(11):434.

. . . *perspectives* chapters supplement the clinical guidance in this book with additional content, context, and expert opinion. The views expressed do not necessarily represent the official position of the Centers for Disease Control and Prevention (CDC).

FEVER IN THE RETURNED TRAVELER

Mary Elizabeth Wilson

Fever often accompanies serious illness in returned travelers. The most common life-threatening tropical disease associated with fever in returned travelers is malaria. Because an increased temperature can signal a rapidly progressive infection, initiate early evaluation, especially in people who have visited areas with malaria in recent months (see Sec. 5, Part 3, Ch. 16, Malaria).

The initial focus in evaluating a febrile returned traveler should be on identifying infections that are potentially life-threatening, treatable, or transmissible. In some instances, public health officials must be alerted if the traveler was possibly contagious while traveling or infected with a pathogen of public health concern (e.g., Ebola virus, yellow fever virus) at the origin or destination. During an outbreak (e.g., the Ebola epidemic in West Africa), special screening protocols could be needed. A specific cause for fever might not be identified in ≥25% of returned travelers.

NARROWING THE DIFFERENTIAL DIAGNOSIS

Most illnesses in returned travelers (e.g., diarrhea, pneumonia, or pyelonephritis) are caused by common and cosmopolitan infections that must be considered along with the more unusual ones. Because the geographic area of travel determines the relative likelihood of major causes of fever, identifying where the febrile patient traveled and/or lived is essential (see Table 11-09). Ask about travel-related activities (e.g., cave exploration, dental or medical care, sexual activity, newly acquired tattoos); exposures (e.g., animal bites, freshwater exposure in schistosomiasis-endemic areas); and living arrangements (e.g., dwelling type, use of mosquito nets, air conditioning, window screens), any of which might elicit useful clues. Pretravel preparation (e.g., vaccinations, malaria prophylaxis) will markedly reduce (although not eliminate) the likelihood of some infections, so this is also a relevant part of the history.

Because each infection has a characteristic incubation period (the range is extremely wide for some), define timing of exposure for different geographic areas; this can help exclude some infections from the differential diagnosis. Most serious febrile infections manifest within the first month after return from tropical travel, yet infections related to travel exposures occasionally occur months or even >1 year after return. In the United States, >90% of reported cases of *Plasmodium falciparum* malaria manifest ≤30 days of return, but almost half of cases of *P. vivax* malaria manifest >30 days after return.

FINDINGS REQUIRING URGENT ATTENTION

Presence of fever plus certain associated signs, symptoms, or laboratory findings can suggest specific infections (see Table 11-10). Findings that should prompt urgent attention include hemorrhage, low blood pressure, altered consciousness, and high respiratory rate. Even if an initial physical examination is unremarkable, repeat the exam if the diagnosis is not clear, because new findings might appear that will help in the diagnostic process (e.g., skin lesions, a tender liver). Although most febrile illnesses in returned travelers are related to infections, bear in mind that other conditions, including pulmonary emboli and drug hypersensitivity reactions, also can be associated with fever.

Fever accompanied by a syndrome (see Table 11-11) deserves further scrutiny, because it could indicate a disease of public health concern, for which immediate infection containment and control measures are indicated.

Travelers visiting friends and relatives (VFR) often do not seek pretravel medical advice and are at greater risk for some diseases than other

Table 11-09 Common causes of fever in the tropics by geographic area

GEOGRAPHIC AREA	COMMON FEVER-CAUSING TROPICAL DISEASES	OTHER INFECTIONS CAUSING OUTBREAKS OR CLUSTERS OF DISEASE AMONG TRAVELERS
CARIBBEAN	Chikungunya Dengue Malaria (on the island of Hispaniola) Zika	Histoplasmosis, acute Leptospirosis
CENTRAL AMERICA	Chikungunya Dengue Malaria (primarily *Plasmodium vivax*) Typhoid or paratyphoid fever Zika	Coccidioidomycosis Histoplasmosis Leishmaniasis Leptospirosis
SOUTH AMERICA	Chikungunya Dengue Malaria (primarily *P. vivax*) Zika	Bartonellosis Histoplasmosis Leptospirosis Yellow fever
SOUTH-CENTRAL ASIA	Dengue Malaria (primarily non-*P. falciparum*) Typhoid or paratyphoid fever	Chikungunya Scrub typhus
SOUTHEAST ASIA	Dengue Malaria (primarily non-*P. falciparum*)	Chikungunya Leptospirosis
SUB-SAHARAN AFRICA	Dengue Malaria (primarily *P. falciparum*) Tickborne rickettsia (main cause of fever in southern Africa) Schistosomiasis, acute (Katayama fever)	Chikungunya Meningococcal meningitis Trypanosomiasis, African Typhoid or paratyphoid fever

travelers. GeoSentinel Surveillance Network data showed that a larger proportion of VFR travelers than tourist travelers presented with serious (requiring hospitalization), potentially preventable travel-related illnesses (see Sec. 9, Ch. 9, Visiting Friends & Relatives: VFR Travel).

CHANGES OVER TIME

Clinicians have access to online resources that provide information about geographic-specific risks, disease activity, and other useful information (e.g., drug-susceptibility patterns for pathogens). Infectious disease outbreaks are dynamic, as demonstrated by the Ebola epidemics in West Africa, spread of chikungunya virus in the Americas beginning in late 2013, nosocomial spread of travel-associated Middle East respiratory syndrome in Korea in 2015, the rapid spread of Zika virus in the Americas in 2015 and 2016, and the global spread of coronavirus disease 2019 (COVID-19). In contrast, because of the wide use of vaccine, hepatitis A infection is now infrequently seen in US travelers.

Infections with typical seasonal transmission in the United States might occur at different times of the year, or throughout the year in the tropics and subtropics. For example, influenza transmission can occur throughout the year in tropical areas, and the peak season in the Southern Hemisphere is late spring/early summer into the fall; clinicians in the Northern Hemisphere should be alert to the possibility of influenza outside the usual wintertime influenza season.

Table 11-10 Clinical findings & fever-associated infectious diseases after tropical travel

CLINICAL FINDING & FEVER	INFECTIOUS DISEASES TO CONSIDER			
	BACTERIAL	VIRAL	PARASITIC	FUNGAL OR OTHER
ABDOMINAL PAIN	Typhoid or paratyphoid fever	None	Liver abscess (amebic or pyogenic)	None
ALTERED MENTAL STATUS OR CENTRAL NERVOUS SYSTEM INVOLVEMENT	Meningococcal meningitis Scrub typhus	Arboviral encephalitides (e.g., JE, WNV) Rabies Tick-borne encephalitis	Angiostrongyliasis Malaria, cerebral Trypanosomiasis, African	None
ARTHRALGIA OR MYALGIA (SOMETIMES PERSISTENT)	None	Chikungunya Dengue Ross River virus Zika	Sarcocystosis, muscular Trichinellosis	None
EOSINOPHILIA	None	None	Angiostrongyliasis Fascioliasis Sarcocystosis Schistosomiasis, acute Trichinellosis Other parasites (rare)	Drug hypersensitivity reaction
FEVER ONSET >6 WEEKS AFTER TRAVEL	Melioidosis Tuberculosis	Acute hepatitis B, hepatitis C, hepatitis E	Liver abscess, amebic Malaria (*Plasmodium ovale*, *P. vivax*) Trypanosomiasis, African	None
FEVER >2 WEEKS (PERSISTENT)	Brucellosis Q fever Tuberculosis Typho id or paratyphoid fever	Cytomegalovirus Epstein-Barr virus HIV, acute	Leishmaniasis, visceral (rare) Malaria Schistosomiasis, acute Toxoplasmosis	None
HEMORRHAGE	Leptospirosis Meningococcemia Rickettsial infections (Spotted fever group)	Viral hemorrhagic fevers (e.g., dengue, Ebola, Lassa, yellow fever)	None	None

JAUNDICE	Leptospirosis	Acute hepatitis A, hepatitis B, hepatitis C, hepatitis E Viral hemorrhagic fevers (including yellow fever)	Malaria, severe	None
MONONUCLEOSIS SYNDROME	None	Cytomegalovirus Epstein-Barr virus HIV, acute	Toxoplasmosis	None
NORMAL OR LOW WHITE BLOOD CELL COUNT	Rickettsial infections Typhoid or paratyphoid fever	Chikungunya Dengue HIV, acute Zika	Malaria	None
RASH	Meningococcemia Rickettsial infections (Spotted fever or Typhus group) Typhoid or paratyphoid fever (rash may be sparse–absent)	Chikungunya Dengue HIV, acute Measles Varicella Zika	None	None
RESPIRATORY SYMPTOMS & PULMONARY INFILTRATES	Legionellosis Leptospirosis Melioidosis Plague, pneumonic Pneumococcus and other common bacterial respiratory pathogens Psittacosis Q fever Tuberculosis	Coronavirus infections (including COVID-19, MERS) Influenza and other common viral respiratory pathogens	Schistosomiasis, acute	Coccidioidomycosis, acute Histoplasmosis, acute

Abbreviations: COVID-19, coronavirus disease 2019; JE, Japanese encephalitis; MERS, Middle East respiratory syndrome; WNV, West Nile virus.

Table 11-11 Febrile syndromes in travelers: potential diseases of public health concern requiring immediate infection containment & control

FEBRILE SYNDROMES (i.e., SYMPTOMS & FEVER)	POTENTIAL DISEASES OF PUBLIC HEALTH SIGNIFICANCE
BRUISING OR UNUSUAL BLEEDING (EASILY, WITHOUT PREVIOUS INJURY)	Viral hemorrhagic fever
COUGH (PERSISTENT)	Pertussis
DECREASED CONSCIOUSNESS	Meningococcal meningitis
DIARRHEA (PERSISTENT, VOLUMINOUS)	Cholera
FLACCID PARALYSIS (RECENT ONSET)	Polio Other enteroviruses
JAUNDICE	Hepatitis A
RAPID RESPIRATORY RATE	Coronavirus disease 2019 (COVID-19) Influenza Middle East respiratory syndrome (MERS) Pneumonic plague
RASH (WITH OR WITHOUT CONJUNCTIVITIS)	Measles Meningococcemia Viral hemorrhagic fevers
VOMITING (PERSISTENT, OTHER THAN AIR OR MOTION SICKNESS)	Norovirus

Travelers can become colonized or infected by bacteria resistant to commonly used antibiotics (see Sec. 11, Ch. 5, Antimicrobial Resistance). Bacteria that produce extended-spectrum β-lactamases and carbapenem-resistant Enterobacterales, including bacteria expressing the metalloprotease NDM-1, have been found in infections acquired during travel, sometimes related to elective or emergency medical care. Travelers to South and Southeast Asia are at high risk of acquiring multidrug-resistant Enterobacterales. Enteric fever (typhoid or paratyphoid fever) has become increasingly resistant to fluoroquinolones, third-generation cephalosporins, and azithromycin, especially in Asia (see Sec. 5, Part 1, Ch. 24, Typhoid & Paratyphoid Fever).

CLINICAL TIPS

For more clinical tips about fever in returning travelers, see Box 11-01.

BOX 11-01 Fever in returning travelers: clinical tips

ANTIMICROBIAL RESISTANT ORGANISMS (see Sec. 11, Ch. 5, Antimicrobial Resistance)

Travelers could be infected or colonized with drug-resistant pathogens, especially travelers who were hospitalized abroad or who took antimicrobial agents to treat travelers' diarrhea.

ARBOVIRAL INFECTIONS (see the chapters in Section 5: Chikungunya, Dengue, Zika)

Dengue is the most common cause of febrile illness among people who seek medical care after travel to Latin America or Asia.

Other arboviral infections are emerging as causes of fever in travelers, including chikungunya and Zika viruses.

COMMON INFECTIONS

Do not overlook common infections (e.g., diarrhea, pneumonia, pyelonephritis) in the search for exotic diagnoses.

FEVER & BLEEDING (see Sec. 5, Part 1, Ch. 10, Leptospirosis; Sec. 5, Part 1, Ch. 13, Meningococcal Disease; Sec. 5, Part 1, Ch. 18, Rickettsial Diseases; and Sec. 5, Part 2, Ch. 25, Viral Hemorrhagic Fevers)

Viral hemorrhagic fevers other than dengue (e.g., Ebola, Lassa fever, Marburg hemorrhagic fever) are important to identify but rare in travelers.

Because of the need to institute prompt, specific treatment, always consider the possibility of bacterial infections (e.g., leptospirosis, meningococcemia, rickettsial infections) that can also cause fever and hemorrhage.

INFECTION CONTROL & PUBLIC HEALTH

Keep in mind infection control, public health implications, and requirements for reportable diseases.

MALARIA (see Sec. 5, Part 3, Ch.16, Malaria)

Malaria is the most common cause of acute undifferentiated fever after travel to sub-Saharan Africa and some other tropical areas.

Malaria can progress rapidly (especially *Plasmodium falciparum*); evaluate promptly and initiate treatment immediately, if diagnosed.

A history of taking malaria chemoprophylaxis does not exclude the possibility of malaria.

Patients with malaria can be afebrile at the time of evaluation, but typically give a history of fever or chills; have prominent respiratory (including acute respiratory distress syndrome), gastrointestinal, or central nervous system findings.

SEXUALLY TRANSMITTED INFECTIONS (see Sec. 11, Ch. 10, Sexually Transmitted Infections)

Sexually transmitted infections, including acute HIV, can cause acute febrile infections.

BIBLIOGRAPHY

Bottieau E, Clerinx J, Schrooten W, Van den Enden E, Wouters R, Van Esbroeck M, et al. Etiology and outcome of fever after a stay in the tropics. Arch Intern Med. 2006;166(15):1642–8.

Jensenius M, Han PV, Schlagenhauf P, Schwartz E, Parola P, Castelli F, et al. Acute and potentially life-threatening tropical diseases in western travelers—a GeoSentinel multicenter study, 1996–2011. Am J Trop Med Hyg. 2013;88(2):397–404.

Leder K, Torresi J, Libman MD, Cramer JP, Castelli F, Schlagenhauf P, et al. GeoSentinel surveillance of illness in returned travelers, 2007–2011. Ann Intern Med. 2013;158(6):456–68.

Ryan ET, Wilson ME, Kain KC. Illness after international travel. N Engl J Med. 2002;347(7):505–16.

Thwaites GE, Day PJ. Approach to fever in the returning traveler. N Engl J Med. 2017;376(6):548–60.

Wilson ME, Weld LH, Boggild A, Keystone JS, Kain KC, von Sonnenburg F, et al. Fever in returned travelers: results from the GeoSentinel Surveillance Network. Clin Infect Dis. 2007;44(12):1560–8.

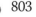

ANTIMICROBIAL RESISTANCE

D. Cal Ham, Joseph Lutgring, Diya Surie, Louise Francois Watkins, Cindy Friedman

Antimicrobial resistance enables microbes to avoid or diminish the effects of antimicrobial agents and is acquired through either genetic mutation or the acquisition of resistance genes. Antimicrobial-resistant organisms can cause infections that are difficult to treat, often requiring the use of agents that are more expensive, less effective, or more toxic (see www.cdc.gov/drugresistance/about.html).

Resistance can occur in bacterial, viral, parasitic, and fungal pathogens. The epidemiology of resistant organisms can vary from country to country (and region to region) and might differ from that seen in the United States. International travelers should be aware of their risk of acquiring resistant organisms when abroad, and medical professionals should consider travel history when caring for patients, both to identify effective treatments for infections and to ensure infection-control interventions are in place to prevent the spread of antimicrobial resistance.

This chapter discusses resistant bacteria and an emerging fungal pathogen; these microbes can be acquired from community and health care exposures during international travel and can cause illness or asymptomatic colonization. Additional information about organism-specific resistance is available in the disease-specific chapters of Section 5, Travel-Associated Infections & Diseases. The topic of antimicrobial resistance is also addressed in Sec. 6, Ch. 4, Medical Tourism.

INFECTIOUS AGENTS & EPIDEMIOLOGY

Antimicrobial-Resistant Organisms in the Community

Globally, the emergence and spread of resistance have been linked to widespread use of antimicrobials in agriculture and in animal (veterinary) and human health care. Inadequate sanitation and water purification infrastructure also plays a role. At the community level, antimicrobial resistance can take many forms; two of relevance to travelers are diarrhea-causing bacteria, and bacteria that result in long-term intestinal colonization and (sometimes) extraintestinal infections.

DIARRHEA-CAUSING BACTERIA

Bacteria that cause diarrhea include a variety of enteric pathogens (e.g., *Campylobacter jejuni*, enterotoxigenic *Escherichia coli*, *E. coli* O157, *Salmonella* spp., *Shigella* spp.). Among these enteric pathogens, resistance to recommended treatment agents has risen worldwide in recent years, posing challenges for medical management. Refer to Section 5 for details of antimicrobial resistance in specific bacterial species.

INTESTINAL COLONIZATION & EXTRAINTESTINAL INFECTIONS

Bacterial colonization of the intestine is influenced and facilitated by a person's diet; their use of agents that disrupt normal microbial flora (e.g., antacids, antibiotics); and their interactions with animals, other humans, and the environment. Enteric bacteria that commonly inhabit the human intestine (e.g., *E. coli*, *Klebsiella pneumoniae*) can be transmitted between close contacts (e.g., household members). Similarly, people who become colonized with antimicrobial-resistant bacteria during international travel can pass these to others. If present, intestinal colonization with antibiotic-resistant bacteria can last from a few weeks to >1 year post-travel; rates of colonization typically decline after 2–3 months, however.

Intestinal colonization with bacteria resistant to carbapenems, extended-spectrum cephalosporins, or colistin can also result in a range of difficult-to-treat extraintestinal infections.

SOURCES OF INFECTION

Bacteria resistant to critically important antibiotics (e.g., carbapenems, extended-spectrum cephalosporins, colistin, macrolides, quinolones) have been isolated from a wide range of community sources, including animals and people, drinking water, meat, and produce. Consuming foods prepared by street vendors, taking antibiotics during travel, and having travelers' diarrhea have all been associated with intestinal colonization with antibiotic-resistant bacteria. People with comorbidities (e.g., chronic bowel disease) also are more likely to become colonized with resistant bacteria during travel.

RISK TO TRAVELERS

The risk for intestinal colonization with antimicrobial-resistant enteric bacteria during travel is related to the prevalence of resistant organisms in the countries visited. Studies have identified that travelers returning from countries in East Africa, northern Africa, South America, South Asia, Southeast Asia, and the Middle East are at risk for colonization with bacteria resistant to extended-spectrum cephalosporins; risk for acquisition was greatest, however, after travel to India, Peru, and Vietnam. Acquisition of carbapenem-resistant Enterobacterales (CRE) has been reported in travelers returning from South Asia and Southeast Asia.

Colonization with *E. coli* carrying a novel gene that confers colistin resistance has been reported in travelers returning from countries in northwest Africa, South America and the Caribbean, East and Southeast Asia, Europe, and the Middle East. Although not used routinely to treat gram-negative infections in the United States, colistin is one of few remaining therapeutic options for extensively resistant infections. Emergence of colistin resistance, then, is of public health concern. In a study of 412 US international travelers, the rate of acquisition of bacteria with the mobile colistin resistance (*mcr*) gene was ≈5%. Bacteria harboring an *mcr* gene (e.g., *mcr*-1) appear to be primarily community-associated; *mcr* genes are often found in extended-spectrum β-lactamase (ESBL)–producing Enterobacterales.

Antimicrobial-Resistant Organisms in Health Care Settings

This section describes organisms of concern associated with overseas health care exposures (e.g., hospitalization, surgery). Recent hospitalization in another country can put travelers and medical tourists at risk for colonization or infection with organisms (bacteria, fungi) that possess antimicrobial resistance mechanisms that are rare in the United States. Resistance reports for specific organisms by country are available at https://resistancemap.cddep.org/AntibioticResistance.php.

Gram-negative bacteria resistant to broad-spectrum antibiotics can cause difficult-to-treat infections. Some of the more concerning genetically mediated mechanisms of antibiotic resistance (mechanisms that can confer resistance to carbapenems, extended-spectrum cephalosporins, or colistin) have the potential for rapid spread to other bacteria. ESBL-producing gram-negative bacteria, for example, originally described in health care settings, are now present outside of health care globally, including in the United States.

CARBAPENEMASE-PRODUCING BACTERIA

Carbapenemase-producing bacteria inactivate all or nearly all β-lactam antibiotics and are often highly antibiotic-resistant, making them difficult to treat. In some countries, as compared to the United States, carbapenemase production is the more frequent mechanism of carbapenem resistance, especially for *Pseudomonas aeruginosa*. Around the world, New Delhi Metallo-β-lactamase (NDM) is the most common carbapenemase; in the United States, however, where *K. pneumoniae* carbapenemase (KPC) predominates, NDM is still relatively uncommon.

In the United States, infections with carbapenemase-producing bacteria occur almost exclusively in people who were recently hospitalized or who had other health care exposures, and in residents of long-term care facilities. Among international travelers, infection with carbapenemase-producing bacteria similarly has been linked to hospitalizations and to medical tourism. In 2018, for example, a large outbreak of carbapenem-resistant *P. aeruginosa* occurred among medical tourists from several countries, including the United States, who traveled to Tijuana, Mexico, for elective bariatric surgery. The mechanism of antibiotic resistance was identified as Verona Integron-encoded Metallo-β-lactamase (VIM) carbapenemase. Also in 2018, the European Centre for Disease Prevention and Control reported an outbreak of carbapenem-resistant *K. pneumoniae* among travelers from 3 countries hospitalized in Gran Canaria, Spain; in this instance, resistance was due to bacterial production of the oxacillinase-48-like (OXA-48-like) carbapenemase.

In some countries, carbapenemase-producing bacteria cause both health care–associated and community-associated infections. In the aforementioned study of 412 US international travelers, the authors identified a low rate (<1%) of carbapenemase-producing CRE acquisition among travelers to South and Southeast Asia who did not have health care exposure.

MOBILE COLISTIN RESISTANCE

While bacteria harboring the *mcr* gene appear to be primarily community-associated, 2 hospital-based outbreaks of *K. pneumoniae* with *mcr* have been reported (one in China, the other in Portugal); the strain in the Portugal outbreak also produced a carbapenemase. Cases of colistin-resistant, carbapenemase-producing Enterobacterales have been associated with health care in other countries as well. Emergence of *mcr* in carbapenemase-producing CRE might result in the rapid spread of strains with extremely limited treatment options in health care settings.

ANTIMICROBIAL-RESISTANT GRAM-POSITIVE BACTERIA

Antimicrobial-resistant gram-positive bacteria are a major cause of health care–associated infections. Methicillin-resistant *Staphylococcus aureus* and vancomycin-resistant enterococci (VRE) are endemic to the United States, and travelers hospitalized outside the United States also can become colonized or infected by these organisms. Transmissible linezolid resistance has been identified in gram-positive bacilli, including *S. aureus*, coagulase-negative *Staphylococcus*, and *Enterococcus* spp. from several countries worldwide, particularly in South America. This resistance is of particular concern in VRE, for which treatment options are already limited.

CANDIDA AURIS

The fungal pathogen *Candida auris* has rapidly emerged worldwide; >40 countries have reported cases, but broader spread is suspected. *C. auris* is distinct from other *Candida* species because it tends to cause outbreaks in health care facilities, can result in long-term asymptomatic skin colonization, persists in health care environments, and has high levels of resistance to multiple classes of antifungal agents. Strains of *C. auris* resistant to the 3 main classes of antifungal medications have been identified in several countries, including the United States.

Since *C. auris* was first reported in 2016, the number of cases in the United States has increased greatly. Many of the initial cases reported in the United States occurred in patients who had received health care previously in countries with documented *C. auris* transmission. Currently, however, most cases are the result of local spread in US health care settings, particularly long-term care facilities for high-acuity patients.

C. auris can be misidentified by some laboratory diagnostics, which might contribute to under-detection of cases, both domestically and outside the United States. Improved laboratory detection and targeted colonization screening, especially among health care contacts of known cases, can facilitate earlier identification of *C. auris* and its spread. Notify public health agencies and implement infection-control measures if *C. auris* is identified or suspected.

PREVENTION

In the Community

Contaminated food is the most common source of enteric pathogen exposures among travelers. Foods grown or prepared under unhygienic conditions can be a source of enteric bacteria. Bacteria harboring *mcr* genes have been identified in foods and food animals (e.g., camels, cattle, pigs, poultry) in multiple countries. Contaminated water is another potential source of antibiotic-resistant enteric bacteria (e.g., *Campylobacter* spp., *E. coli*, *Salmonella* spp., *Shigella* spp.). See Sec. 2, Ch. 9, Water Disinfection, for recommendations regarding water treatment. Insects (e.g., flies) also can serve as vectors in the spread of resistant bacteria.

Safe food choices and careful attention to good hand hygiene can reduce the risk for exposure to pathogens, including those that harbor antimicrobial resistance genes. See Sec. 2, Ch. 8, Food & Water Precautions, for recommendations regarding food consumption and guidance on hand hygiene. In addition, discourage travelers from purchasing or obtaining antibiotics for self-treatment in countries where drugs are available without prescription. Not only can these medications be ineffective for treating the traveler's condition, but their use carries additional risks of unforeseen and untoward side effects. Antibiotics can disrupt the traveler's healthy microbiota and promote acquisition of resistant organisms that can be carried in the traveler's gastrointestinal tract for many months and transfer resistance to other organisms.

Management of mild cough, stomach upset, mild diarrhea, and other minor ailments usually does not require antibiotics. International travelers should include over-the-counter medications in their travel health kit (see Sec. 2, Ch. 10, Travel Health Kits), and clinicians can prescribe antibiotics during a pretravel clinic visit and instruct travelers on self-treatment of moderate diarrheal illness. Educate travelers about health issue warning signs that should prompt them to seek care. More information on management of travelers' diarrhea during travel is available in Sec. 2, Ch. 6, Travelers' Diarrhea.

Travelers and their treating clinicians should be aware that common bacterial infections in destination countries might be resistant to first-line antimicrobial drugs typically used in the United States. For example, fluoroquinolone-resistant enteric pathogens are now found globally. Therefore, if travelers need antibiotics to treat moderate to severe diarrhea, an alternative antibiotic (e.g., azithromycin) might be required. Evidence regarding effective therapies to prevent colonization or infection with resistant enteric organisms in travelers is lacking; investigations into the utility of probiotics and bismuth-containing compounds are under way.

In Health Care Settings

Patients admitted to health care facilities outside the United States, especially in low- and middle-income countries, might be at a greater risk for acquiring antimicrobial-resistant organisms due to a higher prevalence of these organisms and differences in infection-control standards and practices. Exposures can be facilitated by inadequate hand hygiene among staff and personnel, insufficient environmental cleaning, and irregular supply or use of personal protective equipment by health care workers. These gaps are more common in low-resource settings. In addition, access to newer combination therapies (e.g., ceftazidime-avibactam, imipenem-cilastatin-relebactam, meropenem-vaborbactam) used to treat infections caused by highly resistant carbapenemase-producing bacteria can be limited in some low- and middle-income countries.

Information about infection prevention and control services in international health care settings often is limited. When possible (e.g., for non-emergency procedures), people traveling overseas, particularly to low- and middle-income countries, can reduce their risk for health care–associated exposures by choosing facilities with active infection-prevention and control programs (see Sec. 6, Ch. 2, Obtaining Health Care Abroad, and Sec. 6, Ch. 4, Medical Tourism for more details and recommendations). Travelers should opt to receive health care at facilities that have been accredited for their infection-prevention and control programs by national and international authorities. Joint Commission International, an accreditation body used by US facilities, maintains a website of accredited hospitals globally (www.worldhospitalsearch.org/hospital-search). Although accredited health care facilities might have better infection-control practices than non-accredited facilities, accreditation does not necessarily guarantee absence of risk for pathogen transmission.

POSTTRAVEL CONSIDERATIONS

Depending on their travel destination, some patients might be at greater risk for colonization and infection with resistant organisms. Strive to obtain an international travel history going back ≥12 months from patients presenting for care. Travel-related information can play an important role in the clinical care provided and infection control practices employed during clinical encounters.

Health Care Provider Guidance for Returning Travelers

For patients who recently stayed overnight in a health care facility outside the United States, the Centers for Disease Control and Prevention (CDC) has pathogen-specific guidance for CRE and *C. auris.*

CARBAPENEM-RESISTANT ENTEROBACTERALES

When CRE is identified in a patient with a history of an overnight stay in a health care facility outside the United States in the past 6 months, send the CRE isolate for confirmatory susceptibility testing and to determine the carbapenem-resistance mechanism. For patients admitted to health care facilities in the United States after hospitalization in facilities outside the United States within the past 6 months, consider rectal screening to detect CRE colonization; place patients in contact precautions while awaiting the screening cultures. Additional recommendations for patients infected or colonized with CRE can be found in the CRE Toolkit (www.cdc.gov/hai/pdfs/cre/CRE-guidance-508.pdf) and https://stacks.cdc.gov/view/cdc/25250/cdc_25250_DS1.pdf.

CANDIDA AURIS

Consider screening for *C. auris* colonization in patients who have had an overnight stay in a health care facility outside the United States in the previous 12 months, especially if the stay occurred in a country with documented *C. auris* cases (see www.cdc.gov/fungal/candida-auris/tracking-c-auris.html#world). CDC recommendations on how to screen are available from www.cdc.gov/fungal/candida-auris/c-auris-screening.html. All isolates of *Candida* collected from the bloodstream or other normally sterile sites should be identified to the species level. Also consider species identification for *Candida* isolates from nonsterile sites when the patient had an overnight stay in a health care facility outside the United States in the previous 12 months in a country with documented *C. auris* transmission.

Closely monitor patients being treated for *C. auris* for treatment failure. Susceptibility testing can help guide treatment selection. Additional recommendations for providers caring for patients infected or colonized with *C. auris* is available at www.cdc.gov/fungal/candida-auris/health-professionals.html.

BIBLIOGRAPHY

Arcilla MS, van Hattem JM, Haverkate MR, Bootsma MCJ, van Genderen PJJ, Goorhuis A, et al. Import and spread of extended-spectrum β-lactamase-producing *Enterobacteriaceae* by international travellers (COMBAT study): a prospective, multicentre cohort study. Lancet Infect Dis. 2017;17(1):78–85.

Centers for Disease Control and Prevention. Antibiotic resistance threats in the United States, 2019. Atlanta: The Centers; 2019. Available from: www.cdc.gov/drugresistance/pdf/threats-report/2019-ar-threats-report-508.pdf.

Chen L, Todd R, Kiehlbauch J, Walters M, Kallen A. Notes from the field: pan-resistant New Delhi Metallo-beta-lactamase-producing *Klebsiella pneumoniae*—Washoe County, Nevada, 2016. MMWR Morb Mortal Wkly Rep. 2017;66(1):33.

Friedman DN, Carmeli Y, Walton AL, Schwaber MJ. Carbapenem-resistant *Enterobacteriaceae*: a strategic roadmap for infection control. Infect Control Hosp Epidemiol. 2017;38(5):580–94.

Liu YY, Wang Y, Walsh TR, Yi LX, Zhang R, Spencer J, et al. Emergence of plasmid-mediated colistin resistance mechanism MCR-1 in animals and human beings in China: a microbiological and molecular biological study. Lancet Infect Dis. 2016;16(2):161–8.

Mellon G, Turbett SE, Worby C, Oliver E, Walker AT, Walters M, et al. Acquisition of antibiotic-resistant bacteria by U.S. international travelers. N Engl J Med. 2020;382(14):1372–4.

Peirano G, Bradford PA, Kazmierczak KM, Badal RE, Hackel M, Hoban DJ, et al. Global incidence of carbapenemase-producing *Escherichia coli* ST131. Emerg Infect Dis. 2014;20(11):1928–31.

Weersma RK, Zhernakova A, Fu Jingyuan. Interaction between drugs and the gut microbiome. Gut. 2020;6(8):1510–9.

Woerther PL, Andremont A, Kantele A. Travel-acquired ESBL-producing *Enterobacteriaceae:* impact of colonization at individual and community level. J Travel Med. 2017;24(Suppl 1):S29–34.

World Health Organization. Global Antimicrobial Resistance and Use Surveillance System (GLASS) report 2021. Geneva: The Organization; 2021. Available from: www.who.int/publications/i/item/9789240027336.

11

RESPIRATORY INFECTIONS

Regina LaRocque, Edward Ryan

Respiratory infections are a major reason for returning travelers seeking medical care. Upper respiratory infection is more common than lower respiratory infection. In general, the respiratory infections that affect travelers are like those in non-travelers, and exotic causes are rare. When evaluating a returning traveler with a respiratory infection, inquire about the details of travel, including type of travel and travel destinations.

INFECTIOUS AGENTS

Bacteria

Bacterial causes of respiratory illnesses include *Bordetella pertussis, Burkholderia pseudomallei, Chlamydophila pneumoniae, Corynebacterium diphtheriae, Haemophilus influenzae, Mycoplasma pneumoniae*, and *Streptococcus pneumoniae. Coxiella burnetii* and *Legionella pneumophila* can cause outbreaks and sporadic cases of respiratory illness.

Viruses

Viral pathogens are the most common cause of respiratory infection in travelers. Causative agents include adenoviruses, coronaviruses (e.g., severe acute respiratory syndrome coronavirus 2 [SARS-CoV-2], the cause of coronavirus disease 2019 [COVID-19], and the common human coronaviruses, including types 229E, NL63, OC43, and HKU1), human metapneumovirus, influenza virus, measles, mumps, parainfluenza virus, respiratory syncytial virus, and rhinoviruses. Other viruses of special concern to travelers include Middle East respiratory syndrome (MERS) coronavirus and highly pathogenic avian influenza viruses; consider these viruses in travelers with new-onset respiratory illness, including people requiring hospitalization, when no alternative cause has been identified.

CORONAVIRUSES

Include COVID-19 in the differential diagnosis of travelers who develop evidence of upper or lower respiratory tract symptoms, anosmia, diarrhea, fever, myalgia ≤14 days after international travel, and consider referring positive specimens for genomic sequencing. Travelers can be a source of transmission of new SARS-CoV-2 variants from one geographic region to another (see Sec. 5, Part 2, Ch. 3, COVID-19, and www.cdc.gov/coronavirus/2019-ncov/index.html).

Include MERS in the differential diagnosis of travelers who develop fever and pneumonia ≤14 days after traveling from countries in or near the Arabian Peninsula. Contact with a confirmed or suspected case of MERS, or with health care facilities in a MERS transmission area, is of special concern, even in the absence of confirmed pneumonia (see Sec. 5, Part 2, Ch. 14, Middle East Respiratory Syndrome / MERS, and www.cdc.gov/coronavirus/mers/index.html).

AVIAN INFLUENZA VIRUS

Consider a diagnosis of highly pathogenic avian influenza virus (e.g., H5N1, H7N9) in patients with new onset of severe acute respiratory illness requiring hospitalization when no alternative cause has been identified. A history of recent (≤10 days) travel to a country with confirmed human or animal cases—especially if the traveler had contact with poultry or sick or dead birds—increases the likelihood of the diagnosis (see Sec. 5, Part 2, Ch. 12, Influenza, and www.cdc.gov/flu/avianflu/specific-flu-viruses.htm).

Fungi

Fungal pathogens associated with travel include *Blastomyces dermatitidis, Coccidioides* spp. (see Sec. 5, Part 4, Ch. 1, Coccidioidomycosis), *Cryptococcus gattii, Histoplasma capsulatum* (see Sec. 5, Part 4, Ch. 2, Histoplasmosis), *Paracoccidioides* spp., and *Talaromyces marneffei* (formerly *Penicillium marneffei*).

EPIDEMIOLOGIC CONSIDERATIONS

Outbreaks can occur after common-source exposures on cruise ships, in hotels, among tour groups, or during international mass gatherings (see Sec. 9, Ch. 10, Mass Gatherings). *Histoplasma capsulatum*, influenza virus, *L. pneumophila*, and SARS-CoV-2 are some of the pathogens associated with outbreaks in travelers. Groups having a greater risk for respiratory tract infection include children, older adults, and people with comorbid pulmonary conditions (e.g., asthma, chronic obstructive pulmonary disease [COPD]).

Air Quality

The air quality at many travel destinations might be poor, and exposure to carbon monoxide, nitrogen dioxide, ozone, sulfur dioxide, and particulate matter is associated with health risks, including respiratory tract inflammation, exacerbations of asthma or COPD, impaired lung function, bronchitis, and pneumonia (see Sec. 4, Ch. 3, Air Quality & Ionizing Radiation).

Air Travel

Air pressure changes during ascent and descent of aircraft can result in barotrauma and facilitate the development of sinusitis and otitis media. Direct airborne transmission of pathogens aboard commercial aircraft is unusual because recirculated air passes through a series of filters, and cabin air generally circulates within limited zones or areas of the aircraft. Despite this, COVID-19, influenza, measles, tuberculosis (TB), and other diseases have been transmitted on aircraft.

Transmission could occur via several pathways, including direct droplet spread, direct physical contact, fomites, and suspended small particles (droplet nuclei). Intermingling of large numbers of people in congregate settings (e.g., airports, cruise ships, hotels) also can facilitate transmission of respiratory pathogens.

Seasonality

The peak influenza season in the temperate Northern Hemisphere is during the winter months, typically December–February. In the temperate Southern Hemisphere, peak influenza season runs from late spring or early summer into the fall. Tropical climates have no peak season for influenza, and the risk for infection is year-round. Exposure to an infected person traveling from another hemisphere (e.g., on a cruise ship, as part of a package tour) can lead to an influenza outbreak at any time or place. The potential seasonality of COVID-19 currently is not known; transmission risk might increase during winter months, however.

Tuberculosis

Risk for TB infection among most travelers is low and correlates with the incidence of the disease in the destination country, behavior during travel, and length of stay (see Sec. 5, Part 1, Ch. 22, Tuberculosis).

CLINICAL PRESENTATION

Most respiratory infections, especially those of the upper respiratory tract, are mild. Upper respiratory tract infections often cause pharyngitis or rhinorrhea. Lower respiratory tract infections, particularly pneumonia, can be more severe. Lower respiratory tract infections are more likely than upper respiratory tract infections to cause chest pain, dyspnea, or fever. Cough is often present in either upper or lower respiratory tract infections.

People with influenza commonly have acute onset of cough, fever, headache, and myalgias. People with COVID-19 might have a similar clinical presentation, but mild disease and asymptomatic infection also are common. Consider pulmonary embolism in the differential diagnosis of travelers who present with cough, dyspnea, tachycardia, or fever and pleurisy, especially those who have recently been on long car or plane rides (see Sec. 8, Ch. 3, Deep Vein Thrombosis & Pulmonary Embolism) or who were recently infected with SARS-CoV-2.

DIAGNOSIS

Give special consideration to diagnosing patients with suspected avian influenza (see www.cdc.gov/flu/avianflu/healthprofessionals.htm), or illnesses caused by coronaviruses (e.g., COVID-19 [www.cdc.gov/coronavirus/2019-ncov/index.html], or MERS [www.cdc.gov/coronavirus/mers/interim-guidance.html]). Identifying a specific etiologic agent in immunocompetent hosts, especially in the absence of pneumonia or serious disease, is not always clinically necessary. If indicated, the following diagnostic methods can be used.

Microbiology. Gram stain and culturing of sputum can help identify a causative respiratory pathogen. Microbiologic culturing of blood, while insensitive, is also recommended as part of a diagnostic work-up.

Molecular Methods. Molecular methods are available to detect certain respiratory viruses including adenovirus, human metapneumovirus, influenza virus, parainfluenza virus, respiratory syncytial virus, SARS-CoV-2, and certain nonviral pathogens.

Rapid Diagnostic Tests. Rapid tests are available to detect some bacterial (e.g., *L. pneumophila, Streptococcus pneumoniae*, group A *Streptococcus*), viral (e.g., influenza virus, respiratory syncytial virus, SARS-CoV-2), and fungal (e.g., *Histoplasma capsulatum*) pathogens.

TREATMENT

Manage travelers with respiratory infections similarly to non-travelers, but evaluate those who are severely ill for diseases specific to their travel destinations and exposure history. Most viral respiratory infections are mild and do not require specific treatment. Treat travelers with pneumonia of uncertain etiology, as established by the presence of an infiltrate on chest radiography, with antibiotics in accordance with existing guidelines for community-acquired pneumonia. For travelers with influenza who have severe disease or who are at greater risk for complications, treat with antiviral medications. Antiviral treatment for influenza is most effective if begun ≤48 hours of symptom onset. Treat people with COVID-19 per current guidance (www.cdc.gov/coronavirus/2019-ncov/hcp/clinical-care.html).

PREVENTION

Vaccines are available to prevent a number of respiratory diseases, including COVID-19 (see www.cdc.gov/coronavirus/2019-ncov/vaccines/index.html), diphtheria, *H. influenzae* type B (in young children), influenza, measles, pertussis, *S. pneumoniae*, and varicella. Unless contraindicated, travelers should be up to date with COVID-19 and influenza vaccines and other routine immunizations, especially against *S. pneumoniae*.

Preventing respiratory illness while traveling might not be possible, but travelers can follow common-sense measures, including adhering to current recommendations regarding advisability of travel and any indicated precautions (e.g., mask wearing, physical distancing); minimizing close contact with people who are coughing and sneezing; avoiding live animal markets; frequently washing hands, either with soap and water or alcohol-based hand sanitizers containing ≥60% alcohol when soap and water are not available; and, if the traveler has a preexisting eustachian tube dysfunction, using a vasoconstricting nasal spray immediately before air travel, which might decrease the likelihood of otitis or barotrauma.

Health care workers should use appropriate infection-control measures while managing any patient with a respiratory infection (www.cdc.gov/flu/professionals/infectioncontrol).

BIBLIOGRAPHY

Brown ML, Henderson SJ, Ferguson RW, Jung P. Revisiting tuberculosis risk in Peace Corps Volunteers, 2006–13. J Travel Med. 2015;23(1):tav005.

Gautret P, Angelo KM, Asgeirsson H, Duvignaud A, van Genderen PJJ, Bottieau E, et al.; GeoSentinel Network. International mass gatherings and travel-associated illness: a GeoSentinel cross-sectional, observational study. Travel Med Infect Dis. 2019;32:101504.

German M, Olsha R, Kristjanson E, Marchand-Austin A, Peci A, Winter AL, et al. Acute respiratory infections in travelers returning from MERS-CoV-affected areas. Emerg Infect Dis. 2015;21(9):1654–6.

Hertzberg VS, Weiss H, Elon L, Si W, Norris SL; FlyHealthy Research Team. Behaviors, movements, and transmission of droplet-mediated respiratory diseases during transcontinental airline flights. Proc Natl Acad Sci. 2018;115(14):3623–7.

Jennings L, Priest PC, Psutka RA, Duncan AR, Anderson T, Mahagamasekera P, et al. Respiratory viruses in airline travellers with influenza symptoms: results of an airport screening study. J Clin Virol. 2015;67:8–13.

Matanock A, Lee G, Gierke R, Kobayashi M, Leidner A, Pilishvili T. Use of 13-valent pneumococcal conjugate vaccine and 23-valent pneumococcal polysaccharide vaccine among adults aged ≥65 years: updated recommendations of the Advisory Committee on Immunization Practices. MMWR Morb Mortal Wkly Rep. 2019;68(46):1069–75.

Salzer HJF, Stoney RJ, Angelo KM, Rolling T, Grobusch MP, Libman M, et al.; GeoSentinel Surveillance Network. Epidemiological aspects of travel-related systemic endemic mycoses: a GeoSentinel analysis, 1997–2017. J Travel Med. 2018;25(1):tay055.

Speake H, Phillips A, Chong T, Sikazwe C, Levy A, Lang J, et al. Flight-associated transmission of severe acute respiratory syndrome coronavirus 2 corroborated by whole-genome sequencing. Emerg Infect Dis. 2020;26(12):2872–80.

PERSISTENT DIARRHEA IN RETURNED TRAVELERS

Bradley Connor

Although most cases of travelers' diarrhea (TD) are acute and self-limited, a certain percentage of people afflicted will develop persistent (>14 days) gastrointestinal (GI) symptoms. Details on the management of acute TD are available in Sec. 2, Ch. 6, Travelers' Diarrhea.

PATHOGENESIS

The pathogenesis of persistent diarrhea in returned travelers generally falls into one of the following broad categories: ongoing infection or co-infection with a second organism not targeted by initial therapy; previously undiagnosed GI disease unmasked by the enteric infection; or a post-infectious phenomenon.

Ongoing Infection

Most cases of TD are the result of bacterial infection and are short-lived and self-limited. In addition to immunosuppression and sequential infection with diarrheal pathogens, ongoing infection with protozoan parasites can cause prolonged diarrheal symptoms.

11

BACTERIAL

Individual bacterial infections rarely cause persistent symptoms, but travelers infected with *Clostridioides difficile* or enteroaggregative or enteropathogenic *Escherichia coli* (see Sec. 5, Part 1, Ch. 7, Diarrheagenic *Escherichia coli*) can experience ongoing diarrhea. *C. difficile*–associated diarrhea can occur after treatment of a bacterial pathogen with a fluoroquinolone or other antibiotic, or after malaria chemoprophylaxis. The association between *C. difficile* and antimicrobial treatment is especially important to consider in patients with persistent TD that seems refractory to multiple courses of empiric antibiotic therapy. The initial work-up of persistent TD should always include a *C. difficile* stool toxin assay. Clinicians can prescribe oral vancomycin, fidaxomicin, or, less optimally, metronidazole to treat *C. difficile*.

PARASITIC

As a group, parasites are the pathogens most likely to be isolated from patients with persistent diarrhea. The probability of a traveler having a protozoal infection, relative to a bacterial one, increases with increasing duration of symptoms. Parasites might also be the cause of persistent diarrhea in patients already treated for a bacterial pathogen.

GIARDIASIS

Giardia (see Sec. 5, Part 3, Ch. 12, Giardiasis) is the most likely parasitic pathogen to cause persistent diarrhea. Suspect giardiasis particularly in patients with upper GI–predominant symptoms. Untreated, symptoms can last for months, even in immunocompetent hosts.

PCR-based diagnostics, particularly the multiplex DNA extraction PCR, are becoming the diagnostic methods of choice to identify *Giardia* and other protozoal pathogens, including *Cryptosporidium*, *Cyclospora*, and *Entamoeba histolytica*. Diagnosis also can be made by stool microscopy, antigen detection, or immunofluorescence. In the absence of diagnostics (given the high prevalence of *Giardia* as a cause for persistent TD), empiric therapy is a reasonable option in the clinical setting. Rare causes of persistent symptoms include the intestinal parasites *Cystoisospora, Dientamoeba fragilis*, and *Microsporidia*.

TROPICAL SPRUE & BRAINERD DIARRHEA

Persistent TD also has been associated with tropical sprue and Brainerd diarrhea. Tropical sprue is associated with deficiencies of vitamins absorbed in the proximal and distal small bowel and most commonly affects long-term travelers to tropical areas, as the name implies. The incidence of tropical sprue appears to have declined dramatically over the past 2 decades. Diagnosed only rarely in travelers, its cause is unknown.

Brainerd diarrhea (www.cdc.gov/ncezid/dfwed/diseases/brainerd-diarrhea/index.html) is a syndrome of acute onset of watery diarrhea lasting ≥4 weeks. Symptoms include 10–20 episodes of explosive, watery diarrhea per day, fecal incontinence, abdominal cramping, gas, and fatigue. Nausea, vomiting, and fever are rare. Although the cause is believed to be infectious, a culprit pathogen has yet to be identified, and antimicrobial therapy is ineffective as treatment. Investigation of an outbreak of Brainerd diarrhea among passengers on a cruise ship to the Galápagos Islands in 1992 identified that individuals with persistent diarrhea (range: 7 to >42 months) were more likely to have consumed contaminated water or eaten raw fruits or vegetables washed with contaminated water.

Underlying Gastrointestinal Disease

CELIAC DISEASE

In some cases, persistent symptoms relate to chronic underlying GI disease or to a susceptibility unmasked by the enteric infection. Most prominent among these is celiac disease, a systemic disease manifesting primarily with small bowel changes. In genetically susceptible people, exposure to antigens found in wheat causes villous atrophy, crypt hyperplasia, and malabsorption. Serologic tests, including tissue transglutaminase antibody testing, support the diagnosis; a small bowel biopsy showing villous atrophy confirms the diagnosis. Patients can be treated with a gluten-free diet.

COLORECTAL CANCER

Depending on the clinical setting and age group, clinicians might need to conduct a comprehensive search for other underlying causes of chronic diarrhea. Consider colorectal cancer in the differential diagnosis of patients passing occult or gross blood rectally or in patients with new-onset iron-deficiency anemia.

INFLAMMATORY BOWEL DISEASE

Idiopathic inflammatory bowel disease, including Crohn's disease, microscopic colitis, and ulcerative colitis, can occur after acute bouts of TD. One prevailing hypothesis is that in genetically susceptible people, an initiating exogenous pathogen changes the microbiota of the gut, thereby triggering inflammatory bowel disease.

Postinfectious Phenomena

In a certain percentage of patients who present with persistent GI symptoms, clinicians will not find a specific cause. After an acute diarrheal infection, patients might experience a temporary enteropathy characterized by villous atrophy, decreased absorptive surface area, and disaccharidase deficiencies, which can lead to osmotic diarrhea, particularly after consuming large amounts of fructose, lactose, sorbitol, or sucrose. Use of antimicrobial medications during the initial days of diarrhea might also lead to alterations in intestinal flora and diarrhea symptoms.

Occasionally, onset of irritable bowel syndrome (IBS) symptoms occurs after a bout of acute gastroenteritis, known as postinfectious IBS (PI-IBS). PI-IBS symptoms can occur after an episode of gastroenteritis or TD. The clinical work-up for microbial pathogens and underlying GI disease in patients with PI-IBS will be negative. Whether using antibiotics to treat acute TD increases or decreases the likelihood of PI-IBS is unknown.

EVALUATION

Traditional methods of microbial diagnosis rely on the use of microscopy. Examine stool specimens collected over 3 or more days for ova and parasites; include acid-fast staining for *Cryptosporidium*, *Cyclospora*, and *Cystoisospora*. *Giardia* antigen testing and a *C. difficile* toxin assay are appropriate elements of a work-up. In addition, a D-xylose absorption test can determine whether patients are properly absorbing nutrients. If underlying gastrointestinal disease is suspected, include serologic testing for celiac disease and consider inflammatory bowel disease during initial evaluation. Subsequently, studies to visualize both the upper and lower gastrointestinal tracts, with biopsies, might be indicated.

Diagnostic tests to determine specific microbial etiologies in cases of persistent diarrhea have advanced in the past number of years. One of the most useful tools is high-throughput multiplex DNA extraction PCR. This technology uses a single stool specimen to detect multiple bacterial, parasitic, and viral enteropathogens simultaneously. Except for *Cryptosporidium*, these assays have high sensitivity and specificity; the clinical ramifications and the economic impact of using these diagnostic molecular panels have not been determined fully, however. In some cases, molecular testing detects colonization rather than infection, making it difficult for clinicians to interpret and apply the results properly.

MANAGEMENT

Specific treatment of identified enteropathogens is usually indicated, and appropriate management of underlying gastrointestinal disease warranted (e.g., a gluten-free diet for celiac disease, medication for inflammatory bowel disease). Dietary modifications might help patients with malabsorption. Symptomatic treatment or the use of nonabsorbable antibiotics offer potential benefit if small intestinal bacterial overgrowth accompanies the symptom complex. Additionally, chronic diarrhea might cause fluid and electrolyte imbalances requiring medical management involving oral or intravenous replacement based on clinical presentation.

BIBLIOGRAPHY

Connor BA. Sequelae of traveler's diarrhea: focus on post-infectious irritable bowel syndrome. Clin Infect Dis. 2005;41(Suppl 8):S577–86.

Connor BA. Chronic diarrhea in travelers. Curr Infect Dis Rep. 2013;15(3):203–10.

Connor BA, Rogova M, Whyte O. Use of a multiplex DNA extraction PCR in the identification of pathogens in travelers' diarrhea. J Trav Med. 2018;25(1):tax087.

Duplessis CA, Gutierrez RL, Porter CK. Review: chronic and persistent diarrhea with a focus in the returning traveler. Trop Dis Travel Med Vaccines. 2017;3(9):1–17.

Hanevik K, Dizdar V, Langeland N, Hausken T. Development of functional gastrointestinal disorders after *Giardia lamblia* infection. BMC Gastroenterol. 2009;9:27.

Libman MD, Gyorkos TW, Kokoskin E, Maclean JD. Detection of pathogenic protozoa in the diagnostic laboratory: result reproducibility, specimen pooling, and competency assessment. J Clin Microbiol. 2008;76(7):2200–5.

Mintz ED, Weber JT, Guris D, Puhr N, Wells JG, Yashuk JC, et al. An outbreak of Brainerd diarrhea among travelers to the Galapagos Islands. J Infect Dis. 1998;177(4):1041–5.

Norman FF, Perez-Molina J, Perez de Ayala A, Jimenez BC, Navarro M, Lopez-Velez R. *Clostridium difficile*-associated diarrhea after antibiotic treatment for traveler's diarrhea. Clin Infect Dis. 2008;46(7):1060–3.

Porter CK, Tribble DR, Aliaga PA, Halvorson HA, Riddle MS. Infectious gastroenteritis and risk of developing inflammatory bowel disease. Gastroenterology. 2008;135(3):781–6.

Spiller R, Garsed K. Postinfectious irritable bowel syndrome. Gastroenterology. 2009;136:1979–88.

11

DERMATOLOGIC CONDITIONS

Karolyn Wanat, Scott Norton

Skin and soft tissue problems, including rashes, are among the most frequent medical concerns of returned travelers. Several large reviews of dermatologic conditions in returned travelers have shown that cutaneous larva migrans, insect bite reactions, and bacterial infections (often superimposed on insect bites) represent the most common skin problems identified during posttravel medical visits (Table 11-12).

Clinicians can use several approaches to diagnose and manage skin conditions in returned travelers. One useful approach is to consider

Table 11-12 Most common causes of skin lesions in returned travelers

DIAGNOSIS	PERCENTAGE OF ALL DERMATOLOGIC DIAGNOSES (n = 4,742)
Cutaneous larva migrans	9.8
Insect bite	8.2
Skin abscess	7.7
Superinfected insect bite	6.8
Allergic rash	5.5
Rash, unknown origin	5.5
Dog bite	4.3
Superficial fungal infection	4.0
Dengue	3.4
Leishmaniasis	3.3
Myiasis	2.7
Spotted fever group rickettsiosis	1.5
Scabies	1.5
Cellulitis	1.5
Other	32.5

Source: Modified from Lederman ER, Weld LH, Elyazar IR, von Sonnenburg F, Loutan L, Schwartz E, et al. GeoSentinel Surveillance Network. Dermatologic conditions of the ill returned traveler: an analysis from the GeoSentinel Surveillance Network. Int J Infect Dis. 2008;12(6):593–602.

whether the condition is accompanied by an elevated temperature. Few travelers' dermatoses are accompanied by fever, which could indicate a systemic infection, usually viral or bacterial, that requires prompt attention. A second consideration is the geographic and exposure elements of the travel history. A third consideration is the morphology of the lesions noted on physical examination. The most successful approach combines all 3 considerations supported by laboratory confirmation from cultures, serology, skin biopsy, or microscopy if required or indicated. Box 11-02 includes essential elements of the assessment of returned travelers presenting with skin problems.

Many dermatologic problems in returned travelers represent a flare of an existing condition, perhaps because of interruption in the usual treatment regimen while away from home. Other skin disorders might coincide with travel or appear shortly thereafter but are unrelated to travel itself.

BOX 11-02 Assessing returned travelers presenting with skin problems: essential elements

PERTINENT PAST MEDICAL HISTORY

Systemic diseases and chronic conditions, including preexisting skin conditions

Current medications and allergies

HISTORY OF THE PRESENT ILLNESS

Time of onset of lesions (during or after travel)

Associated symptoms: fever, pain, pruritus

TRAVEL HISTORY

Location and duration of travel

Exposure history: freshwater, marine water, insects, animals, plants, occupational and recreational exposures, sexual and other human contact exposures

Companion travelers with similar findings

Vaccination status

Adherence to standard travel precautions (e.g., safe food and water precautions, insect bite precautions)

Medications taken during travel (could provide adequate prophylaxis for certain conditions or might have cutaneous side effects)

PHYSICAL EXAMINATION

Shape of skin lesions (e.g., macules, nodules, papules, plaques, ulcers)

Number, pattern, and distribution of lesions

Location of lesions: exposed versus unexposed skin surfaces

FEVER & RASH

Many illnesses fall into the category of fever with a rash. Consider the following infections in the differential diagnosis of febrile travelers with rashes: cytomegalovirus, enteroviruses (e.g., coxsackievirus, echovirus), Epstein-Barr virus, hepatitis B virus, histoplasmosis, leptospirosis, measles, syphilis, and typhus. Fever and rash in returned travelers are most often, though not exclusively, due to viral infections.

Systemic Viral Infections & Illnesses

CHIKUNGUNYA

A virus transmitted by *Aedes* spp. mosquitoes, chikungunya has caused major outbreaks of illness in southeast Africa, the Americas and the Caribbean, and South Asia (see Sec. 5, Part 2, Ch. 2, Chikungunya). The rash associated with chikungunya resembles that of dengue (discussed next), but hemorrhage, shock, and death are rare with chikungunya. A major distinguishing feature of chikungunya is its associated arthritis, arthralgia, or tenosynovitis that can persist for months, particularly in older adults. As with dengue, serologic testing is available for diagnosis. After ruling out dengue, treat arthritis with nonsteroidal anti-inflammatory drugs (NSAIDs).

DENGUE

Dengue is caused by 1 of 4 strains of dengue viruses (see Sec. 5, Part 2, Ch. 4, Dengue). The disease is transmitted by *Aedes* spp. mosquitoes often found in urban areas, and its incidence continues to increase. Disease is characterized by abrupt onset of high fever, frontal headache (often accompanied by retro-orbital pain), and myalgia. A widespread but faint macular rash interrupted by islands of uninvolved pallid skin commonly becomes evident 2–4 days after illness onset. A petechial rash might be found in classic and severe dengue.

Diagnostic methods include antigen and antibody detection tests, and PCR assays. A positive IgM serology helps support the diagnosis. Treatment is supportive; avoid NSAIDs, which can increase the risk of bleeding in patients with dengue.

ACUTE HIV

Acute retroviral syndrome can present as a flulike syndrome including fever, generalized lymphadenopathy, malaise, and a generalized skin eruption. Acute HIV infection–associated skin findings are often nonspecific and present as pink to deeply red macules or papules or as a morbilliform eruption, but urticarial and pustular lesions also have been described. Oral ulcers might be present.

ZIKA

Zika is a flavivirus transmitted by *Aedes* mosquitoes. It caused major outbreaks in the Western Hemisphere beginning in 2015 (see Sec. 5, Part 2, Ch. 27, Zika). Sexual transmission has been documented for months after infection. The course of the illness is generally subclinical or mild, characterized by arthralgia, conjunctivitis, fever, lymphadenopathy, and a morbilliform ("maculopapular") rash. In pregnant people, Zika infection can cause fetal loss or fetal microcephaly and neurological damage. Zika-associated Guillain-Barré syndrome also has been reported after infection. Infection is usually diagnosed by using molecular diagnostics and serologic testing. Treatment involves supportive care.

Systemic Bacterial Infections & Illnesses

MENINGOCOCCEMIA

Invasive *Neisseria meningitidis* disease occurs worldwide and often is associated with outbreaks, especially in the meningitis belt of sub-Saharan Africa (see Sec. 5, Part 1, Ch. 13, Meningococcal Disease). Meningococcemia is characterized by acute onset of fever and petechiae that often expand into purpuric macules and patches, commonly accompanied by hypotension and multiorgan failure. Rapid diagnosis and immediate treatment can be lifesaving.

RICKETTSIOSES

AFRICAN TICK-BITE FEVER

Rickettsia africae, the bacteria responsible for African tick-bite fever (South African tick typhus), is transmitted by the bite of a hard tick (*Hyalomma* spp.). Travelers who hike and camp outdoors or who are on safari are particularly at risk for this disease, a frequent cause of fever and rash in southern Africa (see Sec. 5, Part 1, Ch. 18, Rickettsial Diseases).

Disease is characterized by fever and an eschar at the site of the tick bite. The eschar, or *tache noire*, is a mildly painful black necrotic lesion with a red rim. Several lesions might be present because people often suffer multiple tick bites. Within a few days, patients develop a fine petechial or papular rash, associated with localized lymphadenopathy. Diagnosis is usually made through clinical recognition and is confirmed by serologic testing. Treatment is doxycycline.

Other rickettsial infections (e.g., Mediterranean spotted fever, rickettsialpox, scrub typhus) might present with eschars or maculopapular, vesicular, or petechial rashes. Each has distinctive geographic or epidemiologic exposure risks.

ROCKY MOUNTAIN SPOTTED FEVER

Rocky Mountain spotted fever (RMSF) is a tickborne rickettsial disease that is more severe than the other spotted fevers. RMSF occurs in North America (the United States and Mexico) and parts of Central and South America, but it is uncommon in travelers. Nevertheless, because of its potential severity and the need for early treatment, consider RMSF when evaluating patients with fever and rash.

Most patients with RMSF develop a rash 3–5 days after illness onset. The typical rash of RMSF begins on the ankles and wrists and spreads centrally and to the palms and soles. The rash commonly starts as a blanching maculopapular eruption that becomes petechial, although in some patients it begins with petechiae. Doxycycline is the treatment of choice.

BACTERIAL SKIN INFECTIONS

Bacterial skin infections occur most frequently when the skin's surface has been interrupted, often by abrasions, bites, or minor scratches, particularly when maintaining good hygiene is difficult. Common organisms responsible are *Staphylococcus aureus* and *Streptococcus pyogenes*. Resulting infections are collectively called pyodermas (Greek for "pus skin") and can present as cellulitis and erysipelas, ecthyma (ulcers or open sores), folliculitis, furuncles (also called abscesses or boils), impetigo, and lymphangitis.

Cellulitis & Erysipelas

Cellulitis and erysipelas manifest as red, warm, edematous areas that might start at the site of a minor injury or opening in the skin, or without an obvious underlying suppurative focus. Unlike cellulitis, erysipelas tends to be raised, with a clear line of demarcation at the edge of the lesion due to involvement of superficial lymphatics, and is more likely to be associated with fever. Cellulitis, erysipelas, and lymphangitis are usually caused by β-hemolytic streptococci. *S. aureus* (including methicillin-resistant strains), and gram-negative aerobic bacteria also can cause cellulitis.

Furunculosis

People whose skin or nasal mucosa is colonized with *S. aureus* are at risk for recurrent folliculitis or furunculosis. Boils can continue to occur weeks or months after a traveler returns; if associated with *S. aureus*, treatment usually involves a decolonization regimen with nasal mupirocin and a skin wash with an antimicrobial skin cleanser. Some decolonization protocols advise similar treatment for household members and close contacts.

Many travelers who develop boils when abroad mistakenly attribute the tender lesions to spider bites. Outside a few endemic areas, however, necrotizing spider bites are extremely rare. The lesions in these cases are far more likely to be abscesses caused by methicillin-resistant *S. aureus* and should be treated accordingly.

Impetigo

Impetigo is another common bacterial skin infection, especially in children in the tropics, and is caused by *S. aureus* or *S. pyogenes*. Impetigo is a highly contagious superficial skin infection that generally appears on the arms, legs, or face as golden or "honey-colored" crusting formed from dried serum. Streptococcal impetigo is usually what causes the classic crust seen in the midface of children. Staphylococcal impetigo often appears in body folds, especially the axillae, and might present as delicate pustules.

Treatment

11

Use soap and water for local cleansing of bacterial skin infections. A topical antibiotic, preferably mupirocin, also can be used; bacitracin zinc and polymyxin sulfate (often in combination) are an alternative. Topical antibiotic ointments widely available in other countries contain neomycin (a known, common cause of acute allergic contact dermatitis) or gentamicin. Other "triple cream" type products available for purchase in low- and middle-income countries often contain ultrapotent steroids that can interfere with the healing of common infections and have their own side effects. In many low- and middle-income countries, an application of gentian violet or potassium permanganate is the treatment of choice for impetigo.

Minor skin abscesses often respond to incision and drainage without the need for antibiotics. Oral or parenteral antibiotics might be required if the skin infection is deep, expanding, extensive, painful, or associated with systemic symptoms (e.g., fever). Consider antibiotic resistance if the condition does not respond to empiric therapy. Bites and scratches from animals (both domestic and wild) can be the source of unusual gram-negative organisms and anaerobic bacteria; appropriate treatment might require care from specialists who can obtain bacterial cultures, prescribe focused antibiotic therapy, and perform surgical debridement, as needed (see Sec. 4, Ch. 7, Zoonotic Exposures: Bites, Stings, Scratches & Other Hazards).

SKIN LESION MORPHOLOGY

Linear Lesions

CUTANEOUS LARVA MIGRANS

Cutaneous larva migrans, a condition in which the skin is infested with the larval stage of cat or dog hookworm (*Ancylostoma* spp.), manifests as an extremely pruritic, serpiginous, linear lesion (see Sec. 5, Part 3, Ch. 4, Cutaneous Larva Migrans). The migrating larvae advance relatively slowly in the skin's uppermost layers. A deeper lesion that resembles urticarial patches and that progresses rapidly might be due to larva currens (running larva), caused by cutaneous migration of filariform larva of *Strongyloides stercoralis* (see Sec. 5, Part 3, Ch. 21, Strongyloidiasis).

LYMPHOCUTANEOUS OR SPOROTRICHOID SPREAD OF INFECTION

Lymphocutaneous or sporotrichoid spread of infection occurs when organisms ascend proximally along superficial cutaneous lymphatics, producing raised, cordlike, linear lesions. Alternatively, this condition can present as an ascending chain of discontinuous, sometimes ulcerated nodules (termed nodular lymphangitis) that occur after primary percutaneous inoculation of certain pathogens. Causative pathogens can be bacterial (e.g., *Francisella tularensis*; atypical *Mycobacterium* spp. [such as *M. marinum* after exposure to brackish water or rapidly growing *Mycobacteria* after pedicure footbaths]; *Nocardia* spp.), parasitic (e.g., *Leishmania* spp., particularly those responsible for causing Western Hemisphere leishmaniasis), or fungal (e.g., *Coccidioides* spp., *Sporothrix*).

PHYTOPHOTODERMATITIS & OTHER NONINFECTIOUS EXPOSURES

Phytophotodermatitis is a noninfectious condition resulting from the interaction of natural psoralens, most common in the juice of limes, and ultraviolet A radiation from the sun. The result is the equivalent of an exaggerated sunburn that creates a painful line of blisters, after which asymptomatic hyperpigmented lines appear that can take weeks or months to resolve.

Long linear lesions caused by cnidarian envenomation (e.g., stings from the tentacles of jellyfish and the Portuguese man o' war [*Physalia physalis*]), often resemble phytophotodermatitis. Another common, but self-evident, cause of an itchy, often blistering eruption, is acute contact dermatitis due to black henna. In places where temporary tattooing is practiced, paraphenylenediamine is added to red or brown henna to make a longer-lasting pigment, black henna. Travelers who receive temporary tattoos using black henna (rather than the red or brown), are at risk for developing a cutaneous reaction to paraphenylenediamine.

Macular Lesions

Macules and patches (flat lesions) are common, often nonspecific, and frequently due to drug reactions or viral exanthems. Purpura are typically macular, and any purpuric lesion associated with fever could indicate a life-threatening emergency (e.g., meningococcemia).

CORONAVIRUS DISEASE 2019

Some patients with coronavirus disease 2019 (COVID-19), particularly young children and young adults, develop a condition known as COVID toes. The condition is characterized by the sudden onset of painful, dusky red macules and patches, typically on the plantar aspect of the distal phalanges of ≥1 toes. Clinically and histologically, COVID toes resembles conditions known as chilblains (a cold weather injury) or lupus pernio (a skin finding in some patients with systemic lupus erythematosus). Although an epidemiologic link with the COVID-19 pandemic seems apparent, viral, molecular, and serologic studies have not confirmed a causal relationship. Nevertheless, young travelers who develop this medical condition warrant further evaluation for COVID-19.

LEPROSY / HANSEN'S DISEASE

Leprosy frequently presents with hypopigmented or erythematous patches that are hypoesthetic to pin prick and associated with peripheral nerve enlargement. Newly diagnosed leprosy cases occur almost exclusively in immigrants arriving from low- or middle-income countries where the disease is endemic. Diagnosis is made by skin lesion biopsies. The National Hansen's Disease Clinical Center in Baton Rouge, Louisiana, provides consultations (nhdped@hrsa.gov; 800-642-2477; www.hrsa.gov/hansens-disease/index.html).

LYME DISEASE

Lyme disease is caused by the spirochete *Borrelia burgdorferi* sensu lato (see Sec. 5, Part 1, Ch. 11, Lyme Disease). Endemic to temperate latitudes in North America, Asia, and Europe, the bacteria that causes Lyme disease is transmitted through the bite of infected hard ticks, genus *Ixodes*.

Infected travelers present with ≥1 large erythematous patch (erythema migrans). If ≥1 lesion is present, the first lesion to appear is where the tick bite occurred; subsequent lesions are due to secondary, probably hematogenous, spread of *Borrelia*, not multiple tick bites. Erythema migrans often is described as targetoid, but central clearing or red-and-white bands do not occur with every case. The lesions generally are asymptomatic. Pruritus, if present, is usually intermittent and very mild. Lesions that are severely or persistently pruritic are unlikely to be erythema migrans.

TINEA

Tinea (ringworm) is caused by a variety of superficial fungi (e.g., *Microsporum*, *Trichophyton*).

Typical lesions appear as expanding, red, raised rings, with an area of central clearing. Diagnostic methods include fungal culture, microscopy (prepare skin scraping samples using a 10% solution of potassium hydroxide [KOH]), and PCR. Treatment usually involves several weeks' application of a topical antifungal (e.g., clotrimazole, ketoconazole, miconazole, terbinafine) or a course of an oral antifungal (e.g., fluconazole, griseofulvin, terbinafine). Nystatin-based topical agents are ineffective.

For recalcitrant tinea infections associated with international travel, consider obtaining culture for species identification. Prolonged courses of higher dose oral antifungals might be needed to treat severe or recurrent infections caused by emerging resistant *Trichophyton* species.

Topical medications that combine an antifungal agent with a potent corticosteroid (e.g., betamethasone, clobetasol) are available in many countries; caution travelers against their use. Adverse events associated with steroid-containing antifungal preparations include longer-lasting infections; more extensive spread of the infection over large areas of the body; invasion of the fungal pathogen into the deeper skin layers; unusual presentation of infection (making diagnosis more challenging); and severe redness and burning.

TINEA VERSICOLOR

Caused by several species of the fungus *Malassezia* (e.g., *M. furfur* [previously *Pityrosporum ovale*], *M. globosa*), tinea versicolor is characterized by abundant, asymptomatic, round to oval skin patches. Lesions are often 1–3 cm in diameter, but dozens of lesions can coalesce to form a "map-like" appearance on the upper chest and back. Affected skin typically has a dry or dusty surface. Lesions can be skin-colored, slightly hypopigmented, or slightly hyperpigmented (*versicolor* means "changed color"), but all lesions on a person have a uniform color.

Tinea versicolor can be diagnosed in various ways. A clinical diagnosis often is based on the appearance of the lesions. Under the light of a Wood ultraviolet lamp, the lesion produces a subtle yellowish-green hue, corroborating the diagnosis. Microscopic examination using a KOH preparation can be confirmatory.

Topical azoles (e.g., clotrimazole cream, ketoconazole shampoo used as a body wash), selenium sulfide shampoo, or topical zinc pyrithione are recommended treatments. Systemic azoles (e.g., fluconazole) can be used for infections that are severe, relapsing, or recalcitrant to first-line therapies. In many countries, the most common treatment is Whitfield ointment (salicylic acid 3% and benzoic acid 6%, mixed in a vehicle such as petrolatum). Oral griseofulvin and oral terbinafine are ineffective against *Malassezia*.

Nodular & Subcutaneous Lesions

GNATHOSTOMIASIS

Gnathostomiasis is a nematode infection primarily occurring in equatorial Africa, along the Pacific coast of Ecuador and Peru, in parts of Mexico, and in Southeast Asia. Infection results from eating raw or undercooked freshwater fish, amphibians, or reptiles. Infected travelers experience transient, migratory, subcutaneous, pruritic, and painful nodules that can occur weeks or even years after exposure. Symptoms are due to migration of the nematode through the body; central nervous system involvement is possible. Eosinophilia is common, and serologic tests are available for diagnosis. Treat cutaneous gnathostomiasis with albendazole or ivermectin.

LOIASIS

Caused by *Loa loa*, a deerfly-transmitted nematode, loiasis occasionally occurs in long-term travelers living in rural equatorial Africa. Infected travelers present with transient, migratory, subcutaneous, painful, or pruritic nodules (called Calabar swellings) produced by adult nematode migration through the skin. Rarely, the worm can be observed crossing the conjunctiva or eyelid. Peripheral eosinophilia is common.

Loiasis can be diagnosed by finding microfilariae in blood collected during daytime; because microfilaremia might be indetectable, however, serologic testing is useful. Treatment is complicated, and consultation with an expert is required for nearly all cases. Two medications are required to control both the larval microfilariae and the adult filariae; the most common regimen includes use of both albendazole and diethylcarbamazine (DEC).

Due to relative contraindications for DEC use in patients with onchocerciasis, special management considerations are warranted for travelers who visited areas endemic for both loiasis and onchocerciasis. Treating loiasis with ivermectin can cause adverse neurological side effects. For additional details regarding contraindications to use of DEC and ivermectin (and a recommendation to consult a specialist in tropical diseases for management advice and support), see Sec. 5, Part 3, Ch. 9, Lymphatic Filariasis, and Sec. 5, Part 3, Ch. 17, Onchocerciasis / River Blindness).

MYIASIS

In sub-Saharan Africa, myiasis is caused by a skin infestation with the larva of the tumbu fly, also known as the mputsi fly (*Cordylobia anthropophaga* and related species). In the Western Hemisphere, larva of the botfly (*Dermatobia hominis*) cause furuncular myiasis; the botfly's range extends from central Mexico to the northern half of South America. Solitary or multiple painful nodules resembling a furuncle might be present; each lesion holds only a single larva. The center of the lesion has a small punctum through which the larva both breathes and expels waste.

More mature larvae sometimes exit on their own to pupate, or can be gently squeezed out of nodules. Extracting larva can be difficult; obstructing the breathing punctum as a first step can be helpful and is easily achieved by applying an occlusive dressing or covering (e.g., a bottle cap filled with petroleum jelly), for several hours. Removal might require minor incision, carefully performed to avoid puncturing the larval body, after which newly vacant cavity should be flushed with sterile water. Treatment for secondary infection and appropriate prophylaxis for tetanus also could be required.

TUNGIASIS

Tungiasis is a skin infestation caused by adult female sand fleas (*Tunga penetrans*). Gestating females burrow into the usually thick skin on the sole of the foot or around the toes. Most people with tungiasis have multiple lesions. Individual lesions have a strikingly uniform appearance with a round, 5 mm diameter, white, slightly elevated surface. In the center of the lesion, a minute, frequently black, opening is present, through which the embedded flea breathes, eliminates waste, and eventually extrudes eggs. Clustered lesions can appear as crusty, dirty, or draining plaques, which are typically itchy, painful, and continue to expand as the uterus of the sand flea fills with eggs.

Treatment includes extracting the burrowed fleas, empirical antibiotics for secondary bacterial infection, and appropriate prophylaxis for tetanus, if required. In many countries, extraction is performed at home using a heat-sterilized needle to pluck out the mature flea with eggs.

Papular Lesions

ARTHROPOD BITES

Arthropod bites are probably the most common cause of papular lesions. Biting arthropods include bed bugs, fleas, headlice, midges, mosquitoes, and sandflies. Itching associated with arthropod bites is due to hypersensitivity reactions to proteins and other components in arthropod saliva.

Individual bites usually appear as small (4–10 mm diameter) edematous, pink to red papules with a gentle "watch-glass" profile. The center of many bites will have a small, subtle break in the epidermis where the arthropod's mouth parts entered the surface of the skin. The pink to red color generally does not extend beyond the elevated part of the lesion, and often a subtle pale hypovascular surrounding halo is apparent.

Lesions are almost invariably quite pruritic; scratching will often excoriate or erode the skin's surface. Such bites are vulnerable to secondary bacterial infections, usually with *Staphylococcus* spp. or *Streptococcus* spp. Many types of arthropods produce bite reactions with characteristic shapes, patterns, and distributions. For example, bites from bed bugs and fleas often appear as scattered clusters of discrete red papules on unclothed surfaces of the body.

SCABIES

Scabies infestation usually manifests as a generalized or regional pruritic papular rash with erythema, abundant excoriations, and secondarily infected pustules (see Sec. 5, Part 3, Ch. 19, Scabies). Scabies generally has regional symmetry and most commonly involves the volar wrists and finger web spaces. Most boys and men with scabies will have nodular lesions on the scrotum and penis. Scabies burrows are short, delicate, linear lesions involving just the most superficial part of the epidermis; they are pathognomonic but can be difficult to detect.

OTHER PAPULAR LESIONS

Many other conditions present as widespread, extremely pruritic eruptions, often with numerous fine, slightly elevated, somewhat indistinct papules. Examples include acute allergic contact dermatitis (perhaps due to plants) and photosensitive dermatitis (often associated with photosensitizing medications, e.g., doxycycline). Onchocerciasis (specifically onchocercal dermatitis due to microfilaria migrating through the skin) can occur in expatriates living in endemic areas in sub-Saharan Africa and manifests as a generalized pruritic, papular dermatitis (see Sec. 5, Part 3, Ch. 17, Onchocerciasis / River Blindness). Swimmer's itch (cercarial dermatitis) and hookworm folliculitis are extremely itchy eruptions composed of papules on skin surfaces exposed to fresh water and fecally contaminated soils, respectively.

Ulcerative Lesions

Skin ulcers form when a destructive process damages or erodes the epidermis, the skin's superficial layer, and then enters the dermis, the skin's deeper, more leathery layer. The most frequent causes of acute (duration <1 month) cutaneous ulcers are the common pyogenic bacteria, staphylococci and streptococci. These create well-demarcated, shallow ulcers with sharp borders and are known as bacterial or common ecthyma; treatment is described earlier in this chapter.

11

ANTHRAX

Cutaneous anthrax produces a large, surprisingly painless edematous swelling. The surface develops a shallow ulcer that progresses into a necrotic black eschar. Nearly all cases of travel-associated anthrax are cutaneous and result from exposure to live cattle, goats, or sheep, or from handling unprocessed products made from animal hides or wool (see Sec. 5, Part 1, Ch. 1, Anthrax).

BURULI ULCER

Buruli ulcer is a rare infection in travelers caused by *Mycobacterium ulcerans*, a freshwater bacterium found most commonly in equatorial Africa (especially Ghana and Nigeria) and in the Australian state of Victoria. Buruli ulcers typically start as edematous nodules that arise at sites of minor skin injury. The nodules ultimately break down into expanding invasive wounds. Tropical ulcer has a similar clinical presentation but is exceptionally painful. Unlike Buruli ulcer, tropical ulcer likely represents a polymicrobial bacterial infection, including some mycobacteria.

CUTANEOUS LEISHMANIASIS

The main areas of risk for cutaneous leishmaniasis (CL) are Africa's northeastern quadrant, Latin America, south and central Asia, the Mediterranean coastal areas, and the Middle East (see Sec. 5, Part 3, Ch. 14, Cutaneous Leishmaniasis). The *Leishmania* parasite is transmitted by the bite of an infected sandfly, and CL lesions start as localized, typical insect bite reactions. Lesions then evolve slowly over several weeks into shallow ulcers with raised margins, resembling a broad, shallow, volcanic caldera; the ulcer's surface can be covered by a dried crust or a raw, fibrinous coat. In the absence of secondary bacterial infection, ulcers are generally painless.

Special techniques are necessary to confirm CL diagnosis. In travelers, pathogen speciation often is necessary to determine whether the lesion is strictly cutaneous and self-healing or will require treatment with medication (oral, topical, or intravenous) or possibly cryotherapy or heat therapy. Refer to the Centers for Disease Control and Prevention (CDC) webpage, www.cdc.gov/parasites/leishmaniasis/index.html, or call or email the CDC for recommendations on diagnosis and treatment (404-718-4745; parasites@cdc.gov).

SPIDER BITES

Necrotizing spider bites are usually caused by recluse spiders, the most common culprit being *Loxosceles reclusa*, the brown recluse, found in the south-central United States. The Mediterranean recluse spider (*Loxosceles rufescens*), native to regions around the Mediterranean Sea and the Near East, resembles the brown recluse. *L. rufescens* has become a widespread "tramp" species giving it a large, nearly worldwide distribution;

it bites only rarely and has venom of low toxicity. Many studies have shown that outside a few endemic areas, most alleged spider bites are, in fact, methicillin-resistant *S. aureus* infections and should be treated accordingly.

UNCOMMON CAUSES

A less common cause of skin ulcers is cutaneous diphtheria (*Corynebacterium diphtheriae*). On several island groups in the southwestern Pacific, *Haemophilus ducreyi* causes nonvenereal cutaneous ulcers. *Trypanosoma brucei rhodesiense*, the causative agent of African trypanosomiasis, can produce a chancre at the bite site of the transmitting tsetse fly (*Glossina* spp.). Several sexually transmitted infections (e.g., syphilis [*Treponema pallidum*], chancroid [*H. ducreyi*]), also can ulcerate the skin.

MISCELLANEOUS SKIN INFECTIONS

Bite-Associated

Wound infections after cat and dog bites are caused by a variety of microorganisms including *S. aureus*, α-, β-, and γ-hemolytic streptococci, several genera of gram-negative organisms, and several anaerobes. *Pasteurella multocida* infection classically occurs after cat bites but also can occur after dog bites. Patients lacking spleens are at particular risk for severe cellulitis and sepsis due to *Capnocytophaga canimorsus* after dog bites. Management of cat and dog bites includes consideration of rabies postexposure prophylaxis (see Sec. 5, Part 2, Ch. 18, Rabies), as well as tetanus immunization and antibiotic prophylaxis. Avoid primary closure of puncture wounds and dog bites to the hand.

Antibiotic prophylaxis after dog bites is controversial, although most experts treat patients lacking spleens prophylactically with amoxicillin-clavulanate. Consider antibiotic prophylaxis of cat bites (*P. multocida*) with amoxicillin-clavulanate or a fluoroquinolone for 3–5 days.

Monkey bite management includes wound care, tetanus immunization, rabies postexposure prophylaxis, and consideration of antimicrobial prophylaxis. Bites and scratches from Old World macaque monkeys showing no signs of illness have been associated with fatal encephalomyelitis due to B virus infection in humans (see Sec. 5, Part 2, Ch. 1, B Virus); valacyclovir is the recommended postexposure prophylaxis for high-risk macaque exposure.

Water-Associated

Skin and soft tissue infections (SSTI) can occur after exposure to fresh, brackish, or salt water, particularly if the skin's surface is compromised. Skin trauma (e.g., abrasions or lacerations sustained during swimming or wading, bites or stings from marine or aquatic creatures, puncture wounds from fishhooks) can result in waterborne infections.

The most virulent SSTIs associated with marine and estuarine exposures are due to *Vibrio vulnificus* and related non-cholera *Vibrio*. For freshwater exposures, *Aeromonas hydrophila* is the most dangerous pathogen. A variety of skin and soft tissue manifestations can occur in association with these infections, including abscess formation, cellulitis, ecthyma gangrenosum, and necrotizing fasciitis.

Pending identification of a specific organism, treat acute infections related to aquatic injury with an antibiotic that provides both gram-positive and gram-negative coverage (e.g., fluoroquinolone or third-generation cephalosporin).

MYCOBACTERIUM MARINUM

M. marinum lives in brackish water. Infection can occur on skin surfaces injured by minor abrasions or shallow puncture wounds; typical locations include knees, shins, and the dorsal surfaces of hands and feet where water-associated minor trauma occurs most commonly.

Patients often describe divergent healing patterns after minor water-associated injury—areas that were injured but not infected heal quickly, whereas areas that were injured and infected with *M. marinum* go on to develop the irregularly bordered, expanding, multinodular violaceous plaques characteristic of this infection. Treatment with antimycobacterial agents for weeks to months is required because lesions do not resolve spontaneously. Occasionally, lymphocutaneous or sporotrichoid spread of infection (see the discussion earlier in this chapter) can occur, resulting in proximal movement of lesions along superficial lymphatics.

PSEUDOMONAS AERUGINOSA

So-called "hot tub folliculitis" can occur after using inadequately disinfected swimming pools or hot tubs. Folliculitis (tender or pruritic follic-ulocentric red papules, papulopustules, or nod-ules) typically develops 8–48 hours after exposure to water contaminated with *Pseudomonas aerugi-nosa*. Usually, several dozen discrete lesions occur on skin surfaces submerged in the infectious water. Most patients have malaise, some have low-grade fever. The condition is self-limited to 2–12 days; typically, no antibiotic therapy is required.

SHEWANELLA

Shewanella, a genus of motile gram-negative bacilli found in warm marine waters worldwide, causes SSTIs that clinically and epidemiologically resemble *V. vulnificus* infections. Patients, often those with chronic liver disease, can develop sep-sis and multiple organ failure. Migrants crossing the Mediterranean with prolonged exposure of their feet and legs to contaminated seawater have developed *Shewanella* infection.

VIBRIO

Necrotizing *Vibrio vulnificus* skin infections can occur when contaminated brackish or saltwater, or the juices or drippings from contaminated raw or undercooked seafood, contact open wounds. Infections also happen from consum-ing *Vibrio*-contaminated shellfish. The illness is especially severe in people with underlying liver disease and can manifest as a dramatic celluli-tis with hemorrhagic bullae and severe sepsis. In general, infections caused by these organ-isms can be more severe in immunosuppressed people.

BIBLIOGRAPHY

Aronson N, Herwaldt B, Libman M, Pearson R, Lopez-Velez R, Weina P, et al. Diagnosis and treatment of leish-maniasis: clinical practice guidelines by the Infectious Diseases Society of America (IDSA) and the American Society of Tropical Medicine and Hygiene (ASTMH). Clin Infect Dis. 2016;63(12):e202–64.

Hochedez P, Canestri A, Lecso M, Valin N, Bricaire F, Caumes E. Skin and soft tissue infections in returning travelers. Am J Trop Med Hyg. 2009;80(3):431–4.

Jensenius M, Davis X, von Sonnenburg F, Schwartz E, Keystone JS, Leder K, et al. Multicenter GeoSentinel analysis of rickettsial diseases in international travelers, 1996–2008. Emerg Infect Dis. 2009;15(11):1791–8.

Kamimura-Nishimura K, Rudikoff D, Purswania M, Hagmann S. Dermatological conditions in international pediatric travelers: epidemiology, prevention and man-agement. Travel Med Infect Dis. 2013;11(6):350–6.

Klion AD. Filarial infections in travelers and immigrants. Curr Infect Dis Rep. 2008;10(1):50–7.

Lederman ER, Weld LH, Elyazar IR, von Sonnenburg F, Loutan L, Schwartz E, et al; GeoSentinel Surveillance Network. Dermatologic conditions of the ill returned traveler: an analysis from the GeoSentinel Surveillance Network. Int J Infect Dis. 2008;12(6):593–602.

Nordlund JJ. Cutaneous ectoparasites. Dermatol Ther. 2009;22(6):503–17.

Nurjadi D, Friedrich-Jänicke B, Schäfer J, Van Genderen PJ, Goorhuis A, Perignon A, et al. Skin and soft tissue infections in intercontinental travellers and the import of multi-resistant *Staphylococcus aureus* to Europe. Clin Microbiol Infect. 2015;21(6):567.e1–10.

Stevens MS, Geduld J, Libman M, Ward BJ, McCarthy AE, Vincelette J, et al. Dermatoses among returned Canadian travellers and immigrants: surveillance report based on CanTravNet data, 2009–2012. CMAJ Open. 2015;3(1):E119–26.

Zimmerman RF, Belanger ES, Pfeiffer CD. Skin infections in returned travelers: an update. Curr Infect Dis Rep. 2015;17(3):467.

DELUSIONAL PARASITOSIS

Susan McLellan

Delusional parasitosis (DP) is the term most often applied to a condition in which a patient presents to a health care provider with an established conviction that they are infected with an arthropod or parasite. Although not unique to travelers, many of those who present with DP have a history of travel, and travel and tropical medicine specialists often assist in evaluating these patients at the request of colleagues.

CLINICAL PRESENTATION

Primary DP is diagnosed when no underlying medical conditions typically associated with disordered thinking are present. Affected people frequently were previously successful in their professions, relationships, and other activities. In the absence of a prior history of a mental health disorder, DP is considered only after multiple visits for care. Symptoms (e.g., itching, skin sensations) are most common and lead to a preponderance of literature from the dermatologic field. Clinical manifestations also can be neurologic (e.g., "brain fog," fatigue, pain, weakness); gastrointestinal (e.g., constipation, diarrhea, sensation of movement in the gut); and auditory or visual. Morgellons syndrome is a specific variant in which sufferers see fibers emerging from the skin.

Secondary DP occurs in association with identifiable health conditions (e.g., alcoholism, bipolar disease, severe depression, drug abuse, schizophrenia, syphilis, thyroid disorders, vitamin deficiencies). In such cases, treatment of the underlying condition might resolve the fixation on parasite infestation.

Unique to DP is the conviction that the illness is due to a parasite, and the frequent auditory or visual identification of it; patients often can describe or draw the organism ("a blue and black body with 8 legs") or define activity and intent ("they buzz when they get angry"). Submitting multiple specimens collected from clothing, orifices, skin, stool, toilets, and around the house is common (the "specimen sign"). With the advent of mobile phones, we now also have the "digital specimen sign," photographs of skin lesions and purported parasites. In many cases, family members or friends are drawn into the delusion in a "folie a deux"; in a more disturbing scenario, a parent might project the delusion onto a child, resulting in potentially harmful attempts to cure the illness.

People suffering from DP can present without objective physical manifestations, or, in the classic dermatologic case, with few to extensive skin lesions attributed to the parasite. Patients might have tried multiple home therapies, including potentially toxic applications or injections (e.g., pouring permethrin in the ears to quell the buzzing of the insects, as reported by one of my patients). Patients often are prescribed empiric treatments for parasitic or arthropod infections by well-meaning practitioners. These treatments are rarely successful, but they are often reported to have provided temporary symptomatic relief—a placebo effect reinforcing the patient's erroneous belief that they are infected with a parasite.

Often, the next step is referral to a specialist, with the hope on the part of the referring provider that "they will know something I don't," "the patient will believe Dr X," or "Dr X will assume care of the patient." Eventually, depending on their presentation, description of symptoms, and the number of practitioners seen, a patient with DP will have undergone multiple examinations of specimens, biopsies of skin or other body parts, colonoscopies, imaging, and laboratory evaluations, none of which reveals a reasonable parasitic cause for their symptoms, and which are usually all "normal."

Suggestions to consider alternative diagnoses are rarely accepted; in particular, recommendations that the patient try psychiatric medications, even just for symptom relief, are frequently met with anger and rejected out of hand. Both patient and practitioner become frustrated; the patient feels they are being told "it's all in your head," and the practitioner is exhausted from the attempt to be compassionate and medically appropriate while faced with an often angry and occasionally insulting patient.

APPROACH & MANAGEMENT

Therapy for DP has relied on the use of antipsychotics. Pimozide, which selectively blocks dopamine type-2 receptors, was the drug first reported to be useful in the condition, and several series indicated a good response in most patients who accepted it. Currently, second-generation antipsychotics (SGAs) are preferred because of a lower side effect profile; no randomized clinical trials are available, however, and reported cases suggest similar efficacy.

Hence, our paradoxical "state of the art" is to treat a patient who is convinced that they do not have a mental health issue with a recognizable antipsychotic. Getting to a point where the patient will consider such medication takes nuanced communication, sympathy, and a great deal of time over multiple appointments. Referral for psychiatry consultation is notoriously unsuccessful. How best to approach the patient who presents with a fixed conviction that they have a parasite, then? Two concrete characteristics are necessary for a successful therapeutic relationship to develop: (1) the provider must be willing to take on a patient who will be complicated, emotionally challenging, needy, and time consuming; and (2) the patient must be willing and able to maintain a relationship and follow up with the provider, meaning the provider must be both geographically and financially accessible.

Ideally, the patient has a primary care provider (PCP) who can act as the long-term caregiver and assure that any other medical needs are being addressed in an integrated manner. Unfortunately, in many cases, the DP sufferer has rejected early providers and is at the stage of traveling long distances to seek out "experts" with whom they cannot feasibly establish an ongoing relationship. In such cases, one approach is for the "expert" to require that the patient identify a PCP, and to discuss the case with them with the goal of education and support, to assure a reasonable work-up for true parasites or any other underlying reversible causes, and to assist and guide them in working with the patient. Such long-distance consultation might enable rebuilding of the PCP–patient relationship with assurance that the "experts" are guiding the diagnostic and therapeutic approach.

Whichever provider accepts a patient with potential DP, a long-term relationship should be expected. Moriarty et al. have suggested a thoughtful, phased, multi-visit approach in which the health care provider takes the patient through the stages of considerate but strategic history-taking, managed expectations, appropriate diagnostic approach, and eventual introduction and maintenance of antipsychotic therapy. Low doses of medication are usually effective in improving or resolving symptoms, but maintenance should continue for months, and relapse is common. See Box 11-03 for a list of additional considerations.

Treating patients with DP can be exhausting and frustrating, and it is easy for practitioners to dismiss these patients as out of their scope of expertise and disruptive to their usual practice. If a relationship of trust can be maintained, however, pharmacologic therapy combined with ongoing behavioral support can be successful in reversing a debilitating condition. Primary care providers should be encouraged and enabled to provide these interventions; specialists with experience in DP can be invaluable as mentors, even from a distance.

BOX 11-03 Delusional parasitosis: management suggestions for health care providers

CREATE A WORKING RAPPORT

Allow the patient to tell their story but set limits on expectations for each visit.

Assure patients they are not alone in having these kinds of problems (e.g., "We have seen this before and have been able to help.").

Neither agree nor argue with patients about the delusion itself, but affirm the severity and significance of the symptoms they describe.

CONDUCT AN APPROPRIATE WORK-UP

Do not be distracted by the patient's interpretation of cause; pay attention to the history and consider alternative conditions that can cause similar symptoms.

Review records, including all medications, both prescribed and over the counter; obtain basic laboratory studies and thyroid function and sedimentation rate; consider hepatitis and HIV testing, syphilis serology, toxicology, vitamin deficiencies.

Send specimens brought in for formal analysis; allow the patient to choose the best examples.

MANAGEMENT

Reassure patients about the results of basic laboratory tests (e.g., "The labs we have done indicate that your bone marrow, kidneys, liver, thyroid, etc., are all healthy and working properly.").

As clinical reports return indicating no parasites found in specimens and no other underlying pathologies, introduce the idea of symptom control as a strategy (e.g., "We know it is safe to focus on symptoms even if we haven't found the cause.").

Don't make a distinction between mental and physical health; instead, discuss the growing understanding of the mind–body connection and how we are just learning about how neurologic signaling affects our bodily well-being.

Explain the use of an antipsychotic drug in terms of addressing the mind–body connection (e.g., "You don't have schizophrenia, but this medication has helped people who have the same kind of problem; we don't yet fully understand how or why it works.").

As much as possible, recruit the patient's family and friends to help the patient normalize what might have been a severely disrupted life.

BIBLIOGRAPHY

Freudenmann RW, Lepping P. Second-generation antipsychotics in primary and secondary delusional parasitosis: outcome and efficacy. J Clin Psychopharmacol. 2008;28(5):500–8.

Moriarty N, Alam M, Kalus A, O'Connor K. Current understanding and approach to delusional infestation. Am J Med. 2019;132(12):1401–9.

Munro A. Monosymptomatic hypochondriacal psychosis manifesting as delusions of parasitosis. Arch Dermatol. 1978;114(6):940–3.

Patel A, Jafferany M. Multidisciplinary and holistic models of care for patients with dermatologic disease and psychosocial comorbidity. JAMA Dermatol. 2020;156(6):686–94.

Pearson ML, Selby JV, Katz KA, Cantrell V, Braden CR, Parise ME, et al. Clinical, epidemiologic, histopathologic and molecular features of an unexplained dermopathy. PLoS One. 2012;7(1):e29908.

Söderfeldt Y, Groß D. Information, consent and treatment of patients with Morgellons disease: an ethical perspective. Am J Clin Dermatol. 2014;15(2):71–6.

Suh KN, Keystone JS. Delusional infestation (delusional parasitosis). In: Ryan ET, Hill DR, Solomon T, Aronson NE, Endy TP, editors. Hunter's tropical medicine and emerging infectious diseases, 10th edition. Philadelphia: Elsevier; 2020. pp. 1132–6.

... *perspectives* chapters supplement the clinical guidance in this book with additional content, context, and expert opinion. The views expressed do not necessarily represent the official position of the Centers for Disease Control and Prevention (CDC).

SEXUALLY TRANSMITTED INFECTIONS

Hilary Reno, Laura Quilter

More than 2 dozen bacterial, viral, and parasitic pathogens can cause sexually transmitted infections (STIs). STIs are among the most common infectious diseases reported worldwide. In 2018, ≈26 million new STI cases were reported in the United States; and in 2016, ≈376 million cases of chlamydia, gonorrhea, syphilis, and trichomonas were reported globally. STIs can be transmitted from person to person during sexual activity involving anal, genital, or oral mucosal contact.

EPIDEMIOLOGY

Casual sex during travel is common; a systematic review showed a 35% prevalence. In addition, some people travel for sex tourism (see Sec. 9, Ch. 12, Sex & Travel). Sex partners abroad might include commercial sex workers among whom STI prevalence is elevated. International travel was an independent risk factor for chlamydia infection in a study conducted at one sexual health clinic. Among travelers, documented risk factors for acquiring STIs or HIV include alcohol and other drug use, longer duration of travel, male gender, and increased number of new partners.

11

Before travel, counsel travelers at risk of engaging in condomless sex to have condoms available, and provide guidance regarding other risk-modifying behaviors. Providers caring for returning travelers should know where to find current information about global epidemiology and antimicrobial resistance patterns of STIs from national and international public health authorities, such as the Centers for Disease Control and Prevention (CDC) Antibiotic-Resistant Gonorrhea website (www.cdc.gov/std/gonorrhea/arg/default.htm) and World Health Organization (WHO), Gonococcal Antimicrobial Resistance (AMR) Surveillance Programme (www.who.int/data/gho/data/themes/topics/who-gonococcal-amr-surveillance-programme-who-gasp).

The epidemiology and clinical presentations of common bacterial, viral, and parasitic STIs are shown in Table 11-13, Table 11-14, and Table 11-15, respectively. Ask returning travelers about sexual activity during their trip, and include specific questions about region of travel, sexual partners, types of sexual exposure, and condom use. Assessing risk in men who have sex with men (MSM) is important because they have elevated rates of certain infections, including chlamydia, gonorrhea, lymphogranuloma venereum, and syphilis. Screen travelers seeking an evaluation for STI or with evidence of STI for other common STIs as well as HIV. For patients with HIV infection, provide information on HIV care and treatment services if they are not already receiving care.

CLINICAL PRESENTATION

Because many infections are asymptomatic, assess for chlamydia, gonorrhea, HIV, and syphilis in returning travelers who had sex outside of a monogamous relationship while traveling. Advise any traveler who develops STI symptoms (e.g., rectal, urethral, or vaginal discharge; unexplained rash or genital lesion; genital or pelvic pain) following a sexual exposure to abstain from sex and seek prompt medical evaluation.

Human papillomavirus (HPV) infection is commonly acquired ≤2 years of sexual debut and usually clears spontaneously. Although most STIs involve the genital tract, some (e.g., gonorrhea, herpes, syphilis) also cause disseminated disease. Consider STIs in returning travelers, because infection can result in serious and long-term complications including adverse birth outcomes, cancer (anal and cervical), infertility, pelvic inflammatory disease, and an increased risk for HIV acquisition and transmission.

Table 11-13 Epidemiology, clinical manifestations, diagnosis, & treatment of select bacterial STIs

STI *CAUSATIVE ORGANISM*	GEOGRAPHIC DISTRIBUTION	TYPICAL CLINICAL PRESENTATION (OFTEN ASYMPTOMATIC)	INCUBATION PERIOD	DIAGNOSIS	FIRST-LINE THERAPY
CHANCROID *Haemophilus ducreyi*	Regional (Africa, Asia, Caribbean)	Irregular, painful genital ulcer Tender, suppurative inguinal lymphadenopathy	4–7 days	Culture with specialized media	Azithromycin 1 g PO ×1 OR Ceftriaxone 250 mg IM ×1 OR Ciprofloxacin 500 mg PO BID ×3 d OR Erythromycin base 500 mg PO TID ×7 d
CHLAMYDIA *Chlamydia trachomatis*	Worldwide	Cervicitis Urethritis	7–21 days	NAAT	Doxycycline 100 mg PO BID ×7 d OR Azithromycin 1 g PO ×1
GONORRHEA *Neisseria gonorrhoeae*	Worldwide	Cervicitis Urethritis	1–14 days	NAAT	Ceftriaxone 500 mg IM ×1
GRANULOMA INGUINALE (DONOVANOSIS) *Klebsiella granulomatis*	Southern Africa Australia India Papua New Guinea	Extensive genital ulcerations with granulation and easy bleeding Tender lymphadenopathy	4–28 days	Microscopy shows Donovan bodies in macrophages	Azithromycin 1 g PO weekly ×3 weeks or until resolution OR Azithromycin 500 mg PO daily ×3 weeks or until resolution

(continued)

11

Table 11-13 Epidemiology, clinical manifestations, diagnosis, & treatment of select bacterial STIs (continued)

STI *CAUSATIVE ORGANISM*	GEOGRAPHIC DISTRIBUTION	TYPICAL CLINICAL PRESENTATION (OFTEN ASYMPTOMATIC)	INCUBATION PERIOD	DIAGNOSIS	FIRST-LINE THERAPY
LYMPHOGRANULOMA VENEREUM *Chlamydia trachomatis* serovar L1-3	Worldwide	Self-limited ulcer Tender inguinal lymphadenopathy Proctocolitis	3–30 days	NAAT, serology	Doxycycline 100 mg PO BID ×21 d
SYPHILIS *Treponema pallidum*	Worldwide	Primary syphilis Typically painless (can be painful) genital ulcer Regional lymphadenopathy Secondary syphilis Maculopapular skin rash	10–90 days	Darkfield microscopy (primary infection) Serology	Benzathine penicillin G 1°, 2°, and early latent infection: 2.4 MU IM ×1 Late latent infection or latent syphilis of unknown duration: 2.4 MU IM weekly ×3 weeks

Abbreviations: BID, twice daily; IM, intramuscularly; MU, million units; NAAT, nucleic acid amplification testing; PO, orally; STI, sexually transmitted infection; TID, 3 times daily.

Table 11-14 Epidemiology, clinical manifestations, diagnosis & treatment of select viral STIs

STI *CAUSATIVE ORGANISM*	GEOGRAPHIC DISTRIBUTION	TYPICAL CLINICAL PRESENTATION (OFTEN ASYMPTOMATIC)	INCUBATION PERIOD	DIAGNOSIS	FIRST-LINE THERAPY
HEPATITIS A Hepatitis A virus	Worldwide	Anorexia Fatigue Jaundice Malaise	28 days	Serology	Supportive care (see Sec. 5, Part 2, Ch. 7, Hepatitis A)
HEPATITIS B Hepatitis B virus	Worldwide	Anorexia Fatigue Jaundice Malaise	60–150 days	Serology	Several options available (see Sec. 5, Part 2, Ch. 8, Hepatitis B) Consult with an expert
HEPATITIS C Hepatitis C virus	Worldwide	Anorexia Fatigue Jaundice Malaise	15–50 days	Serology	Several options available (see Sec. 5, Part 2, Ch. 9, Hepatitis C) Consult with an expert
HERPES SIMPLEX Herpes simplex virus (HSV)	Worldwide	≥1 typically painful (can be painless) genital ulcers	2–7 days	Culture or PCR	Acyclovir 400 mg PO TID ×7–10 d OR Valacyclovir 1 g PO BID ×7–10 d OR Famciclovir 250 mg PO TID ×7–10 d
GENITAL WARTS Human papillomavirus (HPV)	Worldwide	Warts	14–240 days	Clinical or pathologic	Topical therapy or removal of lesions

Abbreviations: BID, twice daily; IM, intramuscularly; PCR, polymerase chain reaction; PO, orally; STI, sexually transmitted infection; TID, 3 times daily.

Monkeypox

Although not considered an STI, transmission of monkeypox virus during the 2022 multinational outbreak has been associated with close skin-to-skin contact, including that which occurs during sex. Moreover, some patients have presented with physical findings and/or symptoms that could be consistent with an STI (e.g., anogenital lesions, proctitis, dysuria). In some instances, this has resulted in misdiagnosis and delays in initiating proper medical management. In other cases, patients have been co-infected with monkeypox virus and an STI. For details on the transmission, epidemiology, and management of monkeypox during the 2022 monkeypox outbreak, see Sec. 5, Part 2, Ch. 22, Smallpox & Other

Table 11-15 Epidemiology, clinical manifestations, diagnosis & treatment of select parasitic STIs

STI *CAUSATIVE ORGANISM*	GEOGRAPHIC DISTRIBUTION	TYPICAL CLINICAL PRESENTATION (OFTEN ASYMPTOMATIC)	INCUBATION PERIOD	DIAGNOSIS	FIRST-LINE THERAPY
TRICHOMONIASIS *Trichomonas vaginalis*	Worldwide	Vaginal discharge, itching	5–28 days	NAAT	Metronidazole Females: 500 mg PO BID ×7 d Males: 2 g PO ×1 OR Tinidazole 2 g PO ×1 (both females & males)

Abbreviations: BID, twice daily; NAAT, nucleic acid amplification testing; PO, orally; STI, sexually transmitted infection

Orthopoxvirus-Associated Infections; Sec. 9, Ch. 12, Sex & Travel; and www.cdc.gov/poxvirus/monkeypox/index.html.

TREATMENT

Base STI evaluation, management, and follow-up on the most recent national and international guidelines from CDC and WHO. Because of limited availability of diagnostic testing in many countries, WHO follows a syndromic approach to STI management; in the United States, therefore, following CDC treatment guidelines is preferred. Consider drug resistance if an infection does not respond to first-line therapy. This is particularly relevant in travelers who have a persistent gonococcal infection, given the global spread of multidrug-resistant *Neisseria gonorrhoeae*.

PREVENTION

Prevention and control of STIs is based on accurate risk assessment, counseling and education, early identification of asymptomatic infection, and effective treatment of travelers; prompt evaluation and treatment of sex partners also is necessary to prevent reinfection and to disrupt STI transmission. As part of pretravel advice, include specific messages and strategies on how to avoid acquiring or transmitting STIs. Abstinence or mutual monogamy between uninfected partners is the most reliable way to avoid acquiring and transmitting STIs.

For people whose sexual behaviors place them at risk for STIs, correct and consistent use of external or internal latex condoms can reduce the risk for HIV infection and other STIs, including chlamydia, gonorrhea, and trichomoniasis. Preventing lower genital tract infections might reduce the risk for pelvic inflammatory disease in female patients. Correct and consistent use of latex condoms also reduces the risk of chancroid, genital herpes, HPV infection, and syphilis. Advise travelers to use only water-based lubricants with latex condoms, because oil-based lubricants (e.g., massage oil, mineral oil, petroleum jelly, shortening) can weaken latex. Also remind travelers that contraceptive methods that are not mechanical barriers (e.g., oral contraceptives) do not protect against HIV or other STIs, and that spermicides containing nonoxynol-9 do not prevent HIV or STIs.

Preexposure vaccination is among the most effective methods for preventing certain STIs. HPV vaccines, for example, are available and licensed for people ≤45 years of age. Both hepatitis A and hepatitis B can be transmitted sexually (see Sec. 5, Part 2, Ch. 7, Hepatitis A, and Sec. 5, Part 2, Ch. 8, Hepatitis B). The Advisory Committee on Immunization Practices (ACIP) recommends hepatitis B vaccination for all adults aged 19–59 years, and hepatitis A vaccine for MSM. Travelers at risk of acquiring HIV infection might benefit from preexposure prophylaxis (see Sec. 5, Part 2, Ch. 11, Human Immunodeficiency Virus / HIV, and www.cdc.gov/hiv/prep).

CDC website: www.cdc.gov/std

BIBLIOGRAPHY

Aung ET, Chow EP, Fairley CK, Hocking JS, Bradshaw CS, Williamson DA, et al. International travel as risk factor for Chlamydia trachomatis infections among young heterosexuals attending a sexual health clinic in Melbourne, Australia, 2007 to 2017. Euro Surveill. 2019;24(44):1900219.

Avery AK, Zenilman JM. Sexually transmitted diseases and travel: from boudoir to bordello. Microbiol Spectr. 2015;3(5):IOL5-0011-2015.

Crawford G, Lobo R, Brown G, Macri C, Smith H, Maycock B. HIV, other blood-borne viruses and sexually transmitted infections amongst expatriates and travellers to low- and middle-income countries: a systematic review. Int J Environ Res Public Health. 2016;13(12):1249.

Meites E, Kempe A, Markowitz LE. Use of a 2-dose schedule for human papillomavirus vaccination—updated recommendations of the Advisory Committee on Immunization Practices. MMWR Morb Mortal Wkly Rep. 2016;65(49):1405–8.

Newman L, Rowley J, Vander Hoorn S, Wijesooriya NS, Unemo M, Low N, et al. Global estimates of the prevalence and incidence of four curable sexually transmitted infections in 2012 based on systematic review and global reporting. PLoS One. 2015;10(12):e0143304.

Svensson P, Sundbeck M, Persson KI, Stafström M, Östergren PO, Mannheimer L, et al. A meta-analysis and systematic literature review of factors associated with sexual risk-taking during international travel. Travel Med Infect Dis. 2018;24:65–88.

Vivancos R, Abubakar I, Hunter PR. Foreign travel, casual sex, and sexually transmitted infections: systematic review and meta-analysis. Int J Infect Dis. 2010;14(10):e842–51.

Weston EJ, Wi T, Papp J. Strengthening global surveillance for antimicrobial drug-resistant *Neisseria gonorrhoeae* through the Enhanced Gonococcal Antimicrobial Surveillance Program. Emerg Infect Dis. 2017;23(13):S47–52.

Workowski KA, Bachmann L, Chan P, Johnston CM, Muzny CA, Park I, et al. Sexually transmitted infections treatment guidelines, 2021. MMWR Recomm Rep. 2021;70(RR-04):1–187.

NEWLY ARRIVED IMMIGRANTS, REFUGEES & OTHER MIGRANTS

Jennifer (Jenna) Beeler, Joanna Regan, Tarissa Mitchell, Elizabeth Barnett

Millions of travelers enter the United States every year. The majority are non-immigrants (e.g., short-term visitors, students, and temporary workers), but others are immigrants, refugees, or other migrants. Table 11-16 outlines the various immigrant and non-immigrant arrivals into the United States during fiscal year 2019. Many arriving travelers and migrants will encounter the US health care system during their stay; therefore, at some time during their careers, US health professionals likely will provide care to newly arrived foreign-born patients.

Most newly arrived travelers and migrants do not undergo an official medical examination prior to their travel to the United States, but for others, a medical examination is required by the Immigration and Nationality Act (INA). The INA mandates that all immigrants and refugees undergo a medical screening examination before travel to the United States to identify inadmissible health conditions.

The Centers for Disease Control and Prevention (CDC) develops the guidance for and monitors the quality of the screening medical examinations for people who fall under relevant categories listed in Table 11-16. CDC also provides guidance for additional pretravel public health interventions and post-arrival medical screening for US-bound refugees (described later in this chapter). In contrast, no specific guidelines cover the examination of people who do not hold an immigrant or refugee visa, or people categorized as temporary visitors or undocumented migrants.

Table 11-17 summarizes requirements and recommendations for overseas and post-arrival

Table 11-16 Immigrant & non-immigrant arrivals to the United States, fiscal year (FY) 2019

ENTRANT CATEGORY	DESCRIPTION	NUMBER OF ARRIVALS, FY 2019
IMMIGRANTS	Immigrant arrivals from foreign countries	460,000
	Lawful permanent residents[1] status–adjusters	570,000
	International adoptees	4,000
REFUGEES	For definition, see Box 11-04	30,000
NONREFUGEE MIGRANTS & OTHER TRAVELERS	Long-term visitors[2]	6 million
	Other non-immigrant entrants	180 million

[1]Also known as "Green Card holders."

[2]Includes people staying >6 months (e.g., exchange visitors, students, temporary workers).

health examinations and public health interventions for immigrants, refugees, and other migrants. For definitions of immigrants, refugees, and other migrants, and the special categories of medical professionals (i.e., panel physicians, civil surgeons) who see them before and after arrival to the United States, see Box 11-04.

THE PRETRAVEL HEALTH ASSESSMENT

Immigrants

OVERSEAS MEDICAL SCREENING EXAMINATION

A medical screening examination is mandatory for all immigrant visa applicants. CDC guidelines

Table 11-17 Health examination & intervention requirements for immigrants, refugees & other migrants

ENTRANT CATEGORY	OVERSEAS (PREDEPARTURE)			AFTER ARRIVAL
	HEALTH ASSESSMENT	VACCINATIONS	OTHER INTERVENTIONS	MEDICAL EXAMINATION
IMMIGRANTS	Required[1]	Required[2]	None[3]	None[3]
REFUGEES	Required[4]	Recommended[5]	Various (see text)[6]	Recommended (usually done)[7]
OTHER MIGRANTS	None[3]	None[3]	None[3]	None[3]

[1]See www.cdc.gov/immigrantrefugeehealth/panel-physicians.html.

[2]See www.cdc.gov/immigrantrefugeehealth/panel-physicians/vaccinations.html.

[3]No requirements or recommendations.

[4]See www.cdc.gov/immigrantrefugeehealth/guidelines/overseas-guidelines.html.

[5]See www.cdc.gov/immigrantrefugeehealth/guidelines/overseas-guidelines.html#vaccination-program.

[6]See www.cdc.gov/immigrantrefugeehealth/guidelines/refugee-guidelines.html.

[7]See www.cdc.gov/immigrantrefugeehealth/guidelines/domestic/domestic-guidelines.html.

BOX 11-04 Definitions: immigrants, refugees, other migrants & the medical professionals who see them

IMMIGRANT

A foreign-born person traveling to the United States on an official immigrant visa.

MIGRANT

Any person who moves away from their home, either temporarily or permanently, for any reason. This term is not defined under international law and can apply to a wide range of people. In this chapter, we use the term broadly to describe both immigrants and refugees, as well as other people settling in the United States, whether temporarily or permanently (e.g., undocumented immigrants and others).

REFUGEE

A refugee, according to Article 1 of the 1951 Refugee Convention, is a person who is outside their country of nationality or habitual residence; has a well-founded fear of persecution because of their race, religion, nationality, membership in a particular social group or political opinion; and is unable or unwilling to avail themselves of the protection of that country, or to return there, for fear of persecution.[1]

STATUS ADJUSTER

A person who does not arrive on an immigrant visa, but who adjusts their status to lawful permanent resident while in the United States.

TEMPORARY VISITORS

Non-immigrants in the United States for a length of time, as defined by their visa class. Temporary workers and their families, students and exchange visitors, diplomats and other foreign government officials, and people traveling for business or pleasure are all examples of temporary visitors.

CIVIL SURGEONS

US medical doctors authorized by US Citizenship and Immigration Services (USCIS) to perform official immigration medical examinations required for the adjustment of status to lawful permanent resident after arrival in the United States. Approximately 5,000 physicians have been designated as civil surgeons.

PANEL PHYSICIANS

Medical doctors practicing outside the United States, selected by the US Department of State to conduct overseas medical screening examinations for immigrants and refugees bound for the United States. More than 600 panel physicians perform these examinations worldwide.

[1]See www.unhcr.org/en-us/news/stories/2001/6/3b4c06578/frequently-asked-questions-1951-refugee-convention.html#_Toc519482140.

for this examination, referred to as Technical Instructions, are available at www.cdc.gov/immigrantrefugeehealth/exams/ti/panel/technical-instructions-panel-physicians.html. The purpose of the screening examination is to detect inadmissible health conditions, including communicable diseases of public health significance, mental health disorders associated with harmful behaviors, and substance-use or substance-induced disorders. The medical screening process includes a brief physical examination, a mental health evaluation, a review of vaccination records, testing for gonorrhea (by nucleic acid amplification), testing for syphilis (by serology), and tuberculosis (TB) screening.

Chest radiographs are required for all applicants ≥15 years of age. Applicants 2–14 years old from high TB-burden countries (i.e., countries with incidence rates ≥20 cases per 100,000 population as estimated by the World Health Organization) must have an interferon-γ release assay (IGRA); those with a positive IGRA are required to have chest radiographs. Additional acid-fast bacillus smears and sputum cultures are required for anyone whose x-ray is suspicious for TB, has signs or symptoms compatible with TB disease, or has known HIV infection. For anyone diagnosed with TB disease, CDC's Technical Instructions require *Mycobacterium tuberculosis* culture, drug-susceptibility testing, and directly observed TB therapy through the end of treatment before immigration is permitted. Pre-immigration treatment also is required for certain other inadmissible conditions, including gonorrhea, syphilis, and leprosy (Hansen's disease).

CLASSIFICATION OF MEDICAL CONDITIONS

Medical conditions of public health significance are categorized as either Class A or Class B. Class

A, or inadmissible, conditions preclude entry into the United States. An immigrant with a Class A condition might be issued a visa after the condition has been treated or after the Department of Homeland Security US Citizenship and Immigration Services (USCIS) approves a waiver of visa ineligibility. Class B conditions indicate a departure from normal well-being, and post-arrival follow-up with a health care provider is recommended.

PRE-ARRIVAL VACCINATIONS

Before immigration to the United States, immigrant visa applicants are required to receive any age-appropriate, Advisory Committee on Immunization Practices (ACIP)–recommended vaccines that are available in their country of residence. Panel physicians administer vaccines according to CDC's Vaccination Technical Instructions for Panel Physicians and Civil Surgeons (www.cdc.gov/immigrantrefugeehealth/exams/ti/panel/vaccination-panel-technical-instructions.html). These instructions are based on ACIP recommendations, with some modifications for immigrants.

HEALTH NOTIFICATIONS AT THE TIME OF ARRIVAL

CDC informs state or local health departments of all arriving immigrants who have received USCIS waivers for Class A (notifiable) conditions, as well as those who have Class B conditions for which follow-up is recommended. Panel physicians document this information in eMedical, an electronic health processing system used to record and transmit most immigrants' medical examination information. State and local health departments performing medical follow-up are asked to report their findings back to CDC, along with information about any other serious conditions of public health concern identified. This reporting helps CDC track epidemiologic patterns of disease among these populations and enables monitoring of the quality of overseas medical examinations.

Internationally Adopted Children

OVERSEAS MEDICAL SCREENING EXAMINATION

Children adopted internationally by parents residing in the United States (see Sec. 7, Ch. 5, International Adoption) are considered a subcategory of immigrants. As such, an overseas medical screening examination is mandatory, as described in the Technical Instructions.

VACCINATIONS

Parents adopting children internationally can request an immunization waiver for children <10 years of age by agreeing to begin immunizations ≤30 days of arrival in the United States; they should, however, be made aware of the potential health risks associated with delaying the immunization process, even by a month. Vaccinating children before their arrival to the United States reduces the child's risk of contracting and importing diseases of public health concern, such as measles, which was reported in unvaccinated children adopted from China in 2004, 2006, and 2013. Of note, as of October 2021, some internationally adopted children (depending on age and country of departure) are required to receive an approved coronavirus disease 2019 (COVID-19) vaccine prior to leaving for the United States.

HEALTH NOTIFICATIONS AT THE TIME OF ARRIVAL

The guidance applying to immigrants regarding health notifications at the time of arrival also applies to internationally adopted children.

US-Bound Refugees

Refugees come to the United States through the US Refugee Admissions Program (USRAP). Whereas immigrants travel to the United States individually or with their families, refugees resettle in groups, on a predetermined schedule, with a 3- to 6-month window between the required medical screening examination and departure.

OVERSEAS MEDICAL SCREENING EXAMINATION

Like immigrants, refugees resettling to the United States are required to undergo an overseas medical screening examination with a panel physician. The content and Technical Instructions for this examination are identical to those for immigrants.

PRE-ARRIVAL VACCINATIONS

Unlike immigrants, refugees bound for the United States are not statutorily required to be vaccinated, leaving them vulnerable to vaccine-preventable diseases during the migration process. In response, a voluntary global immunization program for US-bound refugees was implemented in 2012 as a public health intervention to protect the health of refugees and US health security.

Through this program, overseas panel sites offer refugees bound for the United States most ACIP-recommended vaccines (≤2 doses per vaccine) depending on age, documented immunization history or records, and vaccine availability. Pre-vaccination testing for Hepatitis B virus infection using hepatitis B surface antigen (HBsAg) is also offered where available. The vaccine schedule for US-bound refugees is based on CDC guidance and can be found at www.cdc.gov/immigrantrefugeehealth/guidelines/overseas/interventions/immunizations-schedules.html.

Resettled refugees applying for permanent residence in the United States ≥1 year after their arrival are not required to undergo a repeat medical examination; instead, they must demonstrate proof of receipt of age-appropriate, ACIP-recommended vaccinations to a US civil surgeon during the adjustment-of-status process. In some states, refugees' overseas vaccination records are transferred electronically to state immunization information systems.

OTHER OVERSEAS PUBLIC HEALTH INTERVENTIONS

The 3- to 6-month window between the predeparture medical screening examination and departure affords an opportunity to implement additional public health interventions aimed at improving the health of US-bound refugees and ensuring US health security.

PARASITIC INFECTIONS: PRESUMPTIVE TREATMENT

Many refugees resettle to the United States from places with high prevalence of region-specific parasites and other neglected tropical diseases. Depending on regional epidemiology, panel physicians offer refugees presumptive oral therapy to treat malaria (artemether/lumefantrine), intestinal roundworms (albendazole), schistosomiasis (praziquantel), and *Strongyloides stercoralis* (ivermectin) days before the refugee departs for the United States. Details on each of these diseases and their treatment can be found in Section 5, Travel-Associated Infections & Diseases.

Data from 2 large evaluations indicate that this strategy dramatically decreases the prevalence of soil-transmitted helminth infections among US-bound refugees. For further details and regional treatment recommendations, see www.cdc.gov/immigrantrefugeehealth/guidelines/overseas-guidelines.html#ipg.

FITNESS TO FLY

During the predeparture screening examination, panel physicians might identify refugees who have chronic medical conditions (e.g., cardiac disease, moderate or severe malnutrition, sickle cell disease). While these conditions do not pose a public health risk—and therefore do not make the refugee inadmissible—they can result in decompensation during air travel. CDC, in close collaboration with partners (e.g., the International Organization for Migration), has developed specific protocols to identify, manage, and stabilize refugees with various chronic medical conditions before their departure, with the goal of improving travel fitness (www.cdc.gov/immigrantrefugeehealth/panel-physicians/supplemental-guidance.html).

HEALTH NOTIFICATIONS AT THE TIME OF ARRIVAL

The guidance that applies to immigrants regarding health notifications at the time of arrival also applies to refugees bound for the United States.

NEW-ARRIVAL HEALTH ASSESSMENT

In addition to screening for diseases, consider the new-arrival health assessment as an opportunity to deliver needed health care, preventive health services (e.g., vaccines), and individual counseling. Taken together, these activities serve to establish a medical "home" where people newly arrived in the United States can receive ongoing primary care and an orientation to the US health care system.

Challenges to providing comprehensive health services to people newly arrived in the United States include a general lack of health care provider familiarity with diseases endemic to the migrant's country of origin; lack of access to trained interpreters and translators; insufficient knowledge of social and cultural beliefs and practices of immigrants and migrants; and uncertainty about which elements of the overseas pretravel assessments (screening tests, vaccinations) were completed or when. In addition, immigrants and refugees often have other resettlement priorities (e.g., attending English classes or school, locating permanent housing and work) that can take precedence over accessing health care services.

Medical Screening

Ideally, all immigrants, refugees, and other migrants should receive screening for migration-associated illnesses, communicable and non-communicable diseases, and any age-appropriate screening. Screening for infectious diseases of long latency, especially hepatitis B, HIV, and TB, is crucial for almost all groups; at each subsequent medical encounter, ensure completeness of screening.

Screening each person for diseases specific to their country of origin, migration route, and individual epidemiologic risk also is important. The Minnesota Center for Excellence in Refugee Health has developed an interactive clinical assessment tool, Clinical Assessment for Refugees (CareRef; https://careref.web.health.state.mn.us), based on CDC's Domestic Screening Guidance for Newly Arrived Refugees (www.cdc.gov/immigrantrefugeehealth/guidelines/domestic-guidelines.html). CareRef customizes screening guidance for refugees based on their age, sex, and country of origin. No standard guidelines cover other migrant groups, but the following sections provide an approach, with modified guidance based on experience with refugees and internationally adopted children.

11

Immigrants & Other Nonrefugee Migrants

Immigrants and other nonrefugee migrants enter the country in different ways, and access health care at different points and with providers who have varying levels of expertise in migrant medicine. Nonetheless, they can derive important benefits from their introduction to the US health care system and participation in a comprehensive new-arrival health assessment. Unlike refugees, who are eligible to receive Medicaid funding or Refugee Medical Assistance (described later in this chapter), immigrants and other nonrefugee migrants do not have access to funding sources to cover the costs of a standard comprehensive health assessment.

INITIAL ASSESSMENT

Initial assessment should include taking a medical and family history and reviewing all medications and treatments a person received before and during migration. Most experts agree that testing for hepatitis B, HIV, and TB should be performed for all new immigrants and other nonrefugee migrants who do not have documentation of post-arrival screening. Repeat screening for these infections if risk is ongoing.

For most people, a complete blood count with differential facilitates finding evidence of a hemoglobinopathy or diagnosing anemia or eosinophilia. Urinalysis, although no longer routinely recommended for screening of asymptomatic people, might be appropriate if the person has symptoms of renal disease or signs or symptoms of a urinary tract infection. A basic metabolic panel might be indicated, especially for people of appropriate age or with evidence of conditions such as diabetes or renal disease.

Follow age- and risk-based guidelines provided by the United States Preventive Services Task Force (USPSTF) for the general US population. Consider diagnostic testing of people who present with symptoms consistent with a particular parasite endemic to their country of origin (e.g., malaria, intestinal parasites). Consider screening for sexually transmitted or congenital infections (e.g., chlamydia, gonorrhea, hepatitis C, HIV, syphilis) beyond what is recommended for the US general population if the person's migration history places them at substantial risk. See Table 11-18 and Table 11-19 for a summary of screening tests to consider for new-arrival health assessments.

VACCINATIONS

Many people arrive to the United States without having received predeparture vaccinations. Review all immunization records, laboratory evidence of

Table 11-18 Immigrants & nonrefugee migrants to the United States: recommended new arrival infectious disease screening[1]

SCREENING TEST	AGE	POPULATION	COMMENTS
CBC with differential	All	All	Absolute eosinophilia can be evidence of parasitic infection
Hepatitis B surface antigen[2] (HBsAg)	All	Home country hepatitis B infection prevalence ≥2% People with risk factors	Consider surface antibody testing if unimmunized Consider core antibody testing If surface antibody testing is obtained before a vaccine series is complete, finish the vaccine series even if the antibody result is positive (assuming surface antigen is negative)
Hepatitis C	18–79 years	All Include people outside this age range if risk factors present	For most recent USPSTF guidelines, see Hepatitis C Virus Infection in Adolescents and Adults: Screening (www.uspreventiveservicestaskforce.org/Page/Document/RecommendationStatementFinal/hepatitis-c-screening1)
HIV	>13 years[3]	All May include others outside this age range	Test and evaluate based on standard guidelines
Malaria	All	Clinical signs or symptoms and migration route includes malaria-endemic areas	Consider malaria if symptomatic or from highly endemic area within 3 months of arrival and did not receive predeparture treatment
Parasite serology Schistosomiasis Strongyloidiasis Soil-transmitted helminths	All	Where endemic if high risk for exposure or clinical indication	Consider screening with exposure history, unexplained eosinophilia Some experts treat empirically Empiric treatment for *Strongyloides* is recommended When immigrant is about to receive steroids or become immunocompromised; If testing is unavailable; or When there is insufficient time to obtain results. CAUTION: Individuals from or who have lived in places endemic for *Loa loa*: do not treat presumptively for *Strongyloides* with ivermectin until high microfilarial load from *Loa loa* has been ruled out

(continued)

11

Table 11-18 Immigrants & nonrefugee migrants to the United States: recommended new arrival infectious disease screening (continued)

SCREENING TEST	AGE	POPULATION	COMMENTS
STI Chlamydia Gonorrhea Syphilis Others (as indicated)	15–65 years (<15 if sexually active, if concerns about congenital infection, or if concerns about sexual trauma in any age group)	All	Test choice based on standard guidelines Consider whether migration history adds increased risk
Tuberculosis screen: IGRA	≥2 years	Anyone without a prior documented positive test	Test and evaluate based on standard guidelines Rule out tuberculosis disease and offer treatment for latent tuberculosis infection to people with positive test result
Tuberculosis screen: TST	<2 years		
Urinalysis	All, if clinically indicated	Those with clinical indications	Consider if symptoms of a urinary tract infection are present

Abbreviations: CBC, complete blood count; IGRA, interferon-γ release assay; MCV, mean corpuscular volume; STI, sexually transmitted infection; TST, tuberculin skin test; USPSTF, United States Preventive Services Task Force.

[1]Recommendations outlined in this table are intended for nonrefugee migrants. For comprehensive medical screening recommendations for newly arriving refugees, consult CDC's Domestic Screening Guidance for Newly Arrived Refugees (www.cdc.gov/immigrantrefugeehealth/guidelines/domestic-guidelines.html) and CareRef (https://careref.web.health.state.mn.us/).

[2]Take into account that the prevalence of HBsAg in a country might change over time, hence older birth cohorts could have been at greater risk than younger cohorts.

[3]Consider in younger children who have signs or symptoms of disease, risk factors for transmission, or mother is missing or deceased or has illness compatible with HIV.

immunity, and history of vaccine-preventable diseases. Immunization records provided by patients can be considered valid if, at a minimum, the month and year of the vaccine are documented, and the vaccine was given at an appropriate age according to the US vaccination schedule.

Provide age-appropriate immunizations during an initial encounter with a newly arrived immigrant or migrant, and complete immunization series according to ACIP schedules during subsequent encounters (www.cdc.gov/vaccines/schedules/hcp/index.html). A vaccine series does not need to be restarted if documentation of prior doses is available.

MENTAL HEALTH SCREENING

Mental health screening includes gathering information about coping strategies and support systems, and permits appropriate and timely referral to resources if necessary.

FUTURE TRAVEL

Immigrants and other migrants are likely to travel back to their country of origin and might be at risk for travel-associated infectious diseases (see Sec. 9, Ch. 9, Visiting Friends & Relatives: VFR Travel). Ask these patients about future travel plans to allow time to plan appropriate travel vaccines, medications, and advice.

Table 11-19 Immigrants & nonrefugee migrants to the United States: recommended new arrival toxic & metabolic screening[1]

SCREENING TEST	AGE	POPULATION	COMMENTS
Blood lead level[2]	<16 years People who are pregnant or lactating Clinical indication	All	Consider if no previous lead test and additional risk factors, e.g., • Lived in highly industrialized city with potential exposure to industrial waste; • Developmental delay; or • Medical conditions consistent with lead exposure.
CBC with differential + MCV	All	All	Screen for chronic anemias
Urinalysis (basic metabolic panel)	All, if clinically indicated	Those with clinical indications	Consider if symptoms of renal disease are present

Abbreviations: CBC, complete blood count; MCV, mean corpuscular volume.

[1]Recommendations outlined in this table are intended for newly arrived nonrefugee migrants. For comprehensive medical screening recommendations for newly arriving refugees, consult CDC's Domestic Screening Guidance for Newly Arrived Refugees (www.cdc.gov/immigrantrefugeehealth/guidelines/domestic-guidelines.html) and CareRef (https://careref.web.health.state.mn.us).

[2]Lead screening recommendations are specific to immigrants and nonrefugee migrants and differ slightly from recommendations for newly arrived refugees.

Internationally Adopted Children

See Sec. 7, Ch. 5, International Adoption, for detailed guidance regarding the post-arrival health assessment of international adoptees, and preparation for the family, other household members, and close contacts. In addition, the *Red Book: Report of the Committee on Infectious Diseases*, published by the American Academy of Pediatrics (AAP), offers guidance to pediatricians and other clinicians who will serve this population after their arrival to the United States. *Red Book* is free for AAP members (http://aapredbook.aappublications.org).

Refugees

CDC, in collaboration with the US Department of Health and Human Services Administration for Children and Families' Office of Refugee Resettlement (ORR), clinical and subject matter experts outside CDC, and representatives of the Association of Refugee Health Coordinators (ARHC), has developed evidence-based guidance for domestic refugee medical screening. Comprehensive guidance outlining the screening components and recommended testing is available at www.cdc.gov/immigrantrefugeehealth/guidelines/domestic/domestic-guidelines.html. Population-specific health profiles are available for some refugee populations (Bhutanese, Burmese, Central American minors, Congolese, Iraqi, Somali, and Syrian) at www.cdc.gov/immigrantrefugeehealth/profiles/index.html.

A goal of the domestic refugee health assessment is to arrange and coordinate ongoing primary care. Many refugees have not received age-appropriate screening for chronic conditions (e.g., cancer, diabetes, heart disease; dental, hearing, or vision problems; mental health problems). These screening tests are best introduced in a culturally sensitive way and tailored to the health literacy of the individual patient. Integrating behavioral health screening and services into the domestic health assessment and subsequent primary care visits provides opportunities to screen for acute risk factors and to triage refugees in need of urgent mental health treatment.

Refugees might qualify for state Medicaid programs that cover medical screening and any needed ongoing medical care. Refugees determined ineligible for Medicaid are eligible for Refugee Medical

Assistance in many states, which provides for their medical needs for ≤8 months from their date of arrival. For more information, clinicians and refugees can contact their state health department and can access more information through ORR (www.acf.hhs.gov/programs/orr/programs/cma).

Other published resources available to clinicians include consensus documents on evidence-based screening for newly arriving refugees to Canada, provided by the Canadian Collaboration for Immigrant and Refugee Health (https://ccirhken.ca/ccirh_main).

BIBLIOGRAPHY

Liu Y, Phares CR, Posey DL, Maloney SA, Cain KP, Weinberg MS, et al. Tuberculosis among newly arrived immigrants and refugees in the United States. Ann Am Thorac Soc. 2020;17(11):1401–12.

Lowenthal P, Westenhouse J, Moore M, Posey DL, Watt JP, Flood J. Reduced importation of tuberculosis after the implementation of an enhanced pre-immigration screening protocol. Int J Tuberc Lung Dis. 2011;15(6):761–6.

Mitchell T, Lee D, Weinberg M, Phares C, James N, Amornpaisarnloet K, et al. Impact of enhanced health interventions for United States–bound refugees. Am J Trop Med Hyg. 2018;98(3):920–8.

Nyangoma EN, Olson CK, Benoit SR, Bos J, Debolt C, Kay M, et al. Measles outbreak associated with adopted children from China—Missouri, Minnesota, and Washington, July 2013. MMWR Morb Mortal Wkly Rep. 2014;63(14):301–4.

Pezzi C, Lee D, Kennedy L, Aguirre J, Titus M, Ford R, et al. Blood lead levels among resettled refugee children in select US states, 2010–2014. Pediatrics. 2019;143(5):e20182591.

Posey DL, Blackburn BG, Weinberg M, Flagg EW, Ortega L, Wilson M, et al. High prevalence and presumptive treatment of schistosomiasis and strongyloidiasis among African refugees. Clin Infect Dis. 2007;45(10):1310–5.

11

Index

For the benefit of digital users, indexed terms that span two pages (e.g., 52–53) may, on occasion, appear on only one of those pages.

Tables, figures, and boxes are indicated by *t*, *f*, and *b* following the page number

A

B

C

D

E

F

I

J

K

L

M

N

S

T

U

V

W

X

Y

Z